Vascular and Interventional Radiology THE REQUISITES

Vascular and Interventional Radiology

THE REQUISITES

JOHN A. KAUFMAN, M.D
Chief of Vascular & Interventional Radiology
Professor of Interventional Radiology
Diagnostic Radiology and Surgery
Dotter Interventional Institute
Oregon Health & Sciences University
Portland, Oregon

MICHAEL J. LEE, M.Sc., FRCPI, FRCR,
FFR (RCSI)
Professor of Radiology
Department of Radiology
Beaumont Hospital and Royal College of Surgeons
in Ireland
Dublin, Ireland

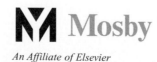

An Affiliate of Elsevier

Mosby

An Affiliate of Elsevier

The Curtis Center
Independence Square West
Philadelphia, Pennsylvania 19106

VASCULAR AND INTERVENTIONAL RADIOLOGY: THE REQUISITES

NOTICE

Radiology is an ever-changing field. Standard safety precautions must be followed, but as new research and clinical experience broaden our knowledge, changes in treatment and drug therapy may become necessary or appropriate. Readers are advised to check the most current product information provided by the manufacturer of each drug to be administered to verify the recommended dose, the method and duration of administration, and contraindications. It is the responsibility of the treating physician, relying on experience and knowledge of the patient, to determine dosages and the best treatment for each individual patient. Neither the publisher nor the authors assume any liability for any injury and/or damage to persons or property arising from this publication.

The Publisher

Library of Congress Cataloging-in-Publication Data

Kaufman, John A.
     Vascular & interventional radiology : the requisites / John A. Kaufman,
Michael J. Lee.–1st ed.
        p. ; cm.
     ISBN-13: 978-0-8151-4369-7   ISBN-10: 0-8151-4369-9
        1. Blood-vessels-Interventional radiology. 2. Interventional radiology.
     I. Title: Vascular and interventional radiology. II. Lee, Michael J. III. Title.
        [DNLM: 1. Vascular Diseases-radiography. 2. Radiography, Interventional–methods.
     WG 500 K21v 2004]
     RD598.67.K386 2004
     617.4′13059–dc22

                                                                                2003044267

ISBN-13: 978-0-8151-4369-7
ISBN-10: 0-8151-4369-9

Publishing Director, Surgery: Richard Lampert
Acquisitions Editor: Hilarie Surrena
Developmental Editor: Christy Bracken

Printed in the United States of America

Last digit is the print number: 9 8 7 6 5

For our children, Nick, Claire, and Alex. You are everything to us.

John and Cathy Kaufman

For Eileen, Aoife, Ronan, Daire and Sarah. Our Journey continues.

Michael J. Lee

Contributors

Peter Bromley, M.D., F.R.C.P.C.
Consultant Radiologist
Departments of Radiology and Surgery
Peter Lougheed Centre,
Calgary, Alberta, Canada

Jean-Louis Dietemann, M.D.
Professor of Radiology
Chief of Department
University Hospital of Strasbourg–Hautepierre
Hautepierre, France

Afshin Gangi, M.D., Ph.D.
Department of Radiology B
University Hospital
Strasbourg, France

Stéphane Guth, M.D.
Radiologie B Hospices civils CHU de Strasbourg
Clinique St Odile
Haguenau, France

William W. Mayo-Smith, M.D.
Associate Professor of Radiology
Brown University
Director of Computed Tomography
Rhode Island Hospital
Providence, RI, USA

Gary M. Nesbit, M.D.
Associate Professor
Dotter Interventional Institute
Diagnostic Radiology, Neurological Surgery, and
Neurology
Oregon Health & Science University
Portland, OR, USA

Susan Pender, F.F.R., R.C.S.I., F.R.C.R.
Consultant Radiologist
Irish National Breast Screening Programme
St Vincent's University Hospital
Dublin, Ireland

Catherine Roy, M.D.
Professor of Radiology
Department of Radiology B
University Hospital of Strasbourg
Strasbourg, France

Gregory M. Soares, M.D.
Assistant Professor
Department of Diagnostic Imaging
Brown Medical School
Rhode Island Hospital
Providence, RI, USA

Foreword

Vascular and Interventional Radiology: THE REQUI-SITES is the tenth book in a series designed to provide core material in major subspecialty areas of radiology for use by residents and fellows during their training and by practicing radiologists seeking to review or expand their knowledge.

Each book in THE REQUISITES series has offered a different set of challenges. In the case of *Vascular and Interventional Radiology: THE REQUISITES* the challenges include how to capture material in such a rapidly evolving field and how to organize and present this vast knowledge base in keeping with the philosophy of the series to emphasize essential information. Drs. Kaufman and Lee have done an outstanding job of distilling the important material and concepts of vascular and interventional radiology into a text that meets these challenges and achieves high marks for readability and accessibility. At the same time, the book is comprehensive enough to serve as an introductory text to the subject material covered and an efficient source for review prior to examinations.

Drs. Kaufman and Lee have chosen to organize their book as suggested by the title. Dr. Kaufman has taken responsibility for the chapters on vascular disease and Dr. Lee has taken the primary responsibility for the non-vascular interventional chapters. This results in an organizational structure that is both logical and at the same time allows the readers to go immediately and efficiently to the material that they are most interested in. One of the major strengths of THE REQUISITES series has been the ability of each author or team of authors to approach their subject with a fresh canvas rather than grafting new material onto an older text. Drs. Kaufman and Lee have taken advantage of this opportunity to create a book that is fresh and relevant to today's contemporary practice of vascular and interventional radiology.

One of the striking aspects of *Vascular and Interventional Radiology: THE REQUISITES* is the full recognition that this subspecialty area has become multi modality in its fundamental underpinnings. Even 10 years ago vascular imaging meant angiography and venography. Likewise the richness of the armamentarium for interventions has vastly increased for all applications. Vascular stents were just on the horizon a decade ago and now are used extensively both following angioplasty and as primary treatment. Tumor biopsy now frequently is followed by radio-frequency ablation therapy or one of several emerging alternatives.

The goal of THE REQUISITES series is to have one volume devoted to each major subspecialty area. The length and format of each volume are dictated by the material being covered, but the principal goal is to equip the reader with a text that provides the basic factual, conceptual, and interpretive material required for clinical practice. I believe residents in radiology will find *Vascular and Interventional Radiology: THE REQUISITES* to be an excellent tool for learning the subject. Drs. Kaufman and Lee have captured the most important material in a very user-friendly text.

Physicians in practice and those undertaking fellowship programs in vascular and interventional radiology will also find this book extremely useful. For seasoned practitioner and fellow alike, *Vascular and Interventional Radiology: THE REQUISITES* provides the material they need for contemporary clinical practice.

I congratulate John Kaufman and Michael Lee for their outstanding new contribution to THE REQUISITES in Radiology.

James H. Thrall, M.D.
Radiologist-in-Chief
Department of Radiology
Massachusetts General Hospital
Juan M. Taveras Professor of Radiology
Harvard Medical School
Boston, Massachusetts

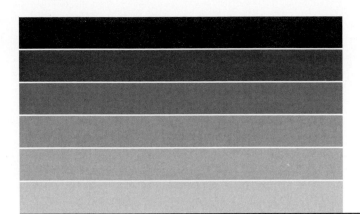

Preface

The specialty of interventional radiology has never been, and never will be, static, boring, or easily characterized. A unique combination of imaging, procedures, medicine, technology, and clinical variety, there is hardly a more exciting specialty. Image-guided, minimally invasive therapies are recognized by patients and other physicians as the way of the future, and interventional radiology is at the center.

The origins of this specialty lie in diagnostic imaging. In the era before cross-sectional imaging, the only non-operative way to evaluate many pathologic conditions was to put needles into the recesses of the body, such as blood vessels, bile ducts, renal collecting systems, subarachnoid spaces, and peritoneal cavities, and then inject contrast. In 1964, in Portland, Oregon, Charles Dotter performed the first percutaneous transluminal angioplasty (see Fig. 4-1). This shifted the whole paradigm. Radiologists who performed angiography and other special diagnostic procedures began to think of themselves as interventionalists. Not only could they diagnose the disease, but they could treat it as well.

Slowly but inevitably, procedures that once required surgeons and surgical incisions have been replaced by interventionalists using percutaneous image-guided techniques. Percutaneous catheter drainage of abdominal abscesses has all but supplanted open "I & D." More recently, transcatheter uterine artery embolization for symptomatic fibroids has become a major alternative to hysterectomy. With each technological innovation, the number and breadth of procedures increases. The impact of the percutaneously delivered intravascular metallic stent, particularly on the management of arterial occlusive and aneurysmal disease, has been enormous.

Once dismissed as fringe practitioners of dangerous and unproven arts, interventional radiologists have become indispensable to the daily functioning of the medical system. Although we will never lose our imaging roots, interventional radiologists are increasingly participants in the clinical care of many different kinds of patients. Make no mistake about it; interventional radiology is here to stay.

The impact of interventional procedures on other specialties has not gone unnoticed by those practitioners. Early in our history, cardiologists determined that cardiac catheterization should move from radiology, where it was developed, to medicine, because that was where the heart was cared for. Increasingly over the last 15 years, interventions for arterial occlusive and aneurysmal disease have been aggressively embraced by vascular surgeons, to the exclusion of many of their radiological colleagues. Lately, gynecologists have begun formulating their own credentials for performing percutaneous transcatheter uterine artery embolization for fibroids.

What does this all mean? First of all, Success! Interventional procedures are now mainstream and legitimized. Second, Excitement! There is no limit to our therapeutic horizons. Third, Change! Interventional radiologists can no longer wait for someone else to decide which procedure to order and when, but must see patients in offices or clinics, render consultations, recommend a course of action, perform the procedure, and provide follow-up. Lastly, Challenge! If only for the benefit of patients, interventional radiology must mature into the core specialty for all minimally invasive practitioners, with the basic and clinical research to support the procedures, and standards that ensure safe and effective care.

This volume of *The Requisites* is intended to whet the appetite for this exciting specialty. We have endeavored to make it accessible enough for residents, but detailed enough to be used by fellows and those seeking a current overview. The format is designed to allow quick reference for technical or diagnostic questions, but also to provide detailed but focused information. The images have been carefully selected to be representative of current practice, with the use of cross-sectional techniques whenever possible. When the book started, the authors were colleagues at the Massachusetts General Hospital, one in the Division of Vascular Radiology (Kaufman), the other in the Division of Abdominal Imaging and Intervention (Lee). Today we are international co-conspirators, so that the book reflects both North American and European practice. To sum it all up, we think interventional radiology is great, this is how we do it, and we hope you enjoy this book.

John A. Kaufman, M.D.
Michael J. Lee, M.Sc., MRCPI, FFR(RCSI), FRCR

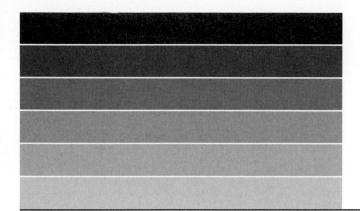

Acknowledgments

When James Thrall invited me to write this book I was simultaneously ecstatic and terrified. As a junior faculty member in his department at the Massachusetts General Hospital, the invitation was an immense honor, but I had no idea how or when I would do it. After a while (well, after a few years) Jim was probably thinking the same thing. Fortunately for me, Jim has been the most patient mentor, counselor, guide, and friend that I could have ever wished for. Without his unflagging support I could not have done this.

One of my first steps was to ask Mick Lee to collaborate on the book (read "share the pain"). Fortunately, he agreed. Mick is a superb body imager and interventionalist, great guy, and, to my chagrin, a much more efficient writer than I. Without him the book would not be. I am proud that I can link my name with his on the cover.

Accomplishments, such as a book, mirror the people in our lives. I am a radiologist because I followed the example of someone much smarter than I, my father, Sy Kaufman. During my first year of residency, I rotated on "Specials" with Alan Greenfield and John Guben. As the cliché goes, I never looked back. In July of 1991, after my fellowship with Alan, Jim Parker, and another long-time friend Mike Bettmann, I joined the Division of Vascular Radiology at MGH. Arthur Waltman welcomed me into a dream job, a professional family, and the most formative experience of my career. Over the next 9 years I learned from an outstanding group of colleagues, including Chris Athanasoulis (whose 1982 textbook *Interventional Radiology* greatly influenced this book), Chieh-Min Fan, Mark Rieumont, Kent Yucel, and Mitch Rivitz. Above all, I worked with Stuart Geller. I have never learned so much from one person, ever. I have tried to put all of it in here; I hope that I have it right.

In July 2000, I joined Fred Keller, Josef Rösch, Bryan Petersen, Rob Barton, Torre Andrews, Paul Lakin, Gary Nesbit, Stan Barnwell, and Dusan Pavcnik at the Dotter Institute in Portland, Oregon. Once again I found myself learning from, inspired by, and supported by superb interventionalists, innovators, and people. The majority of the images in this book are from the Dotter Institute and were created by these special colleagues. Phil Baker of the Portland VA Medical Center provided many outstanding MRAs.

Over the years I have been fortunate to spend time with a large number of delightful fellows and residents. They don't know it, but they are the real reason for staying in academics. They have all been incredibly generous and reliable when answering my pleas for images, especially Barry Stein in Hartford, Connecticut. One of my fellows from the Dotter Institute, Peter Bromley, not only co-authored a chapter, but created the many excellent original line drawings in this book.

Sheri Imai-Swiggart at the Dotter Institute toiled over the images in this book for 2 years. She adjusted, tweaked, and generally worked her magic on every single image (as well as about 1000 more that I didn't use ...). This project has taken so long that it has outlasted several generations of Mosby editors and production staff. Stephanie Donley, Mia Cariño, Elizabeth Corra, Hilarie Surrena, and Christy Bracken have all graciously brought this to a conclusion.

An author's family sees a different side of the process. This book was time together lost, both in person and in mind. The end product has little bearing on the real stuff of family life. Yet each and every one supported and encouraged me. Cathy, my wife, learned very quickly that this book doubled her work as a parent, which she undertook with characteristic enthusiasm. She has been my life co-author since I was 18 years old. My children, mother, and in-laws all saw "the book" as yet another work-related obsession, and adjusted accordingly. Even the dog was nice about it.

Thanks to you all.

J.A.K.

My journey in Interventional Radiology began in 1989 when I started a Fellowship in Abdominal Imaging and Interventional Radiology at Massachusetts General Hospital. Fresh from my radiology residency in Ireland, I was not sure what to expect. The teaching and professionalism of the staff at MGH soon dispelled my uncertainty. In particular, I would like to thank Peter Mueller, Nick Papanicolau, Steve Dawson, and Peter Hahn for imparting a wealth of wisdom and experience regarding all things interventional. As a fellow, one of the most satisfying achievements is to complete a technically difficult or challenging procedure without a staff supervisor taking over. I am sure it was difficult at times but thank you for not "taking over."

I believe that interventional radiologists should have a firm grasp of imaging to make correct therapeutic decisions for their patients. During my 6 years at MGH, I was fortunate to learn from some of the great imagers: Joe Ferucci, Jack Wittenberg, Joe Simeone, and Sanjay Saini to name but a few.

I would like to take this opportunity to especially thank Peter Mueller for his encouragement and support, both clinically and academically during my MGH years. Peter is a great mentor, friend, and these days an occasional antagonist during interventional radiology "Ryder cup" golf matches.

Jim Thrall, Chairman of Radiology at MGH, allowed us the freedom to develop clinical and academic skills, but also fostered leadership talents. This was accomplished with minimal fuss, but occasional gentle nudging in a certain direction.

When John Kaufman asked me to co-author this book, I was leaving MGH to take up a Chair in Radiology at the Medical School of the Royal College of Surgeons in Ireland, attached to Beaumont Hospital, Dublin. I was delighted to accept knowing that John is a great writer, interventionalist, and good friend. It has been a lengthy process but I hope you will agree worth it.

I am indebted to my colleagues at Beaumont Hospital who have allowed me the academic time to complete this project. I commissioned chapters from Susan Pender, Afshin Gangi and colleagues, and Bill Mayo-Smith and would like to thank them for their superb efforts. I would like to thank Sarah Taylor, Jill Kavanagh, and Gail O'Brien for their expert typing and organizational skills and all the staff at Mosby who have patiently reminded us over the years that this book needed to be completed. These include Elizabeth Corra and Mia Cariño in the early days and more latterly Christy Bracken and Hilarie Surrena.

Finally, and most importantly, I would like to thank my wife Eileen for taking this journey with me. Family, interventional radiology, and academic radiology are a difficult combination to balance. Writing a book, in addition to the latter, shifts the balance considerably. I could not have written this book without Eileen's support and understanding.

My father always says, "If you are going to do something, do it right." I have striven to apply this motto to the book. I hope you enjoy it.

M.J.L.

Contents

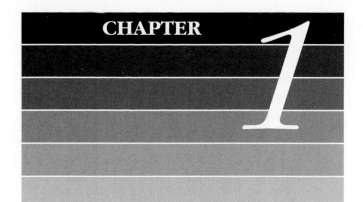

CHAPTER 1

Vascular Pathology

JOHN A. KAUFMAN, M.D.

Blood vessels are, in the simplest of terms, the plumbing of the body. Problems arise when blood flow is diminished, excessive, in the wrong direction, or when leaks occur (Table 1-1). In reality, blood vessels are complex organs within other organs, with hydrodynamic, biochemical, and cellular functions. The degree of vascular disease that can be tolerated before symptoms occur varies with the type of vessel, the nature and metabolic state of the perfused organ, and the patient. Just as vascular disease can affect an organ, disease in an organ can affect its blood vessels. Often, vascular pathology can result in loss of limb or life for a patient. The ubiquitous and serious nature of vascular disease makes this a fascinating clinical area. This chapter reviews the basic types of pathology that can occur in blood vessels. The clinical presentation, diagnosis, and therapy of disease in a particular vascular bed are addressed in specific chapters.

THE NORMAL VASCULAR WALL

The walls of arteries have three layers: the intima, media, and adventitia (Fig. 1-1). The initima forms the interface between the artery and the blood. Composed of endothelial cells, fibroblasts, and connective tissue, this is the site of much arterial pathology. The intima is a dynamic, hormonally active layer that responds to acute stress by release of substances such as prostaglandins and platelet activating factors. Chronic stress, such as turbulence, induces proliferation of the endothelial cells and fibroblasts. Any object in prolonged contact with the intima eventually becomes coated with a layer of new endothelial cells ("neo-intima"). In some circumstances, this proliferation results in local obstructive phenomena. The intima therefore has a central role in the natural history of vascular diseases and the outcome of vascular interventions.

Sandwiched between the intima and adventitia, the muscular media provides both structural support for the arterial wall as well as the ability to react acutely to sudden changes in hemodynamics. Bounded on the inside by the intima and on the outside by the adventitia, the media is made up of well-ordered layers of elastic fibers, smooth muscle cells, and connective tissue. Smooth muscle cells are orientated in both concentric and longitudinal directions. The normal media is elastic, dilating slightly with each systole and then recoiling during diastole. This is most pronounced in medium and large muscular arteries, which assists in the circulation of blood through the arterial system. In response to demands for increased blood flow the smooth muscle cells relax, resulting in enlargement of the vessel lumen (vasodilatation). Conversely, to restrict blood flow, the muscle cells contract to decrease the diameter of the lumen (vasoconstriction). With aging and certain pathologic conditions (such as atherosclerosis), the media looses this elasticity and

Table 1-1	Clinical Manifestations of Vascular Pathology[a]
Manifestation	**Example**
Obstruction to flow forward	Arterial and venous stenoses
Increased flow forward	Arteriovenous fistula, malformation
Increased flow backward	Varicose veins due to reflux through incompetent venous valves
Loss of vessel wall integrity	Aneurysm, dissection, bleeding

[a]These can occur alone or in any combination.

responsiveness as the smooth muscle cells are replaced by fibrotic tissue or become disorganized. In fact, large atherosclerotic intimal plaques can actually invade the media. The media is also the site of expression of heritable connective tissue disorders such as Marfan syndrome and Ehlers–Danlos syndrome.

The adventita is a tough filmy layer of connective tissue that forms the boundary between the artery and the surrounding structures. This layer contains collagen, fibroblasts, and some smooth muscle cells. Weaving through the interface of the adventitia and media are the small vascular channels (the vasa vasorum) that supply blood to capillaries within the adventitia and the outer third of the media. The inner part of the media and the intima receive nutrients from the blood in the vessel lumen by diffusion. The density of the vasa vasorum is highest in the thickest,

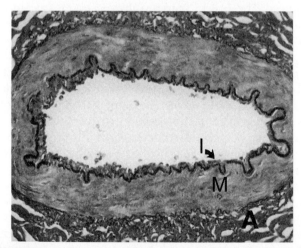

Figure 1-1   Photomicrograph of normal small muscular artery (VVG, × 650). I = single layer of intimal cells. M = media, comprised of smooth muscle cells. The wavy black line between the intima and media is the internal elastica lamina. A = adventitia. (Reproduced with permission from Johnson DE: Anatomic aspects of vascular disease. In Strandness ED, Breda AV eds: *Vascular Diseases: Surgical and Interventional Therapy*, Churchill Livingstone, New York, 1994.)

most muscular portions of the arteries, such as the ascending and transverse aorta. The adventitia also contains the adrenergic nerves (nervi vascularis) that control vasoconstriction and dilatation.

Veins also have walls with three layers, similarly termed the intima, media, and adventitia. Venous and arterial intima and adventitia are similar in composition and function. The venous intima rarely undergoes the pathologic changes seen in arteries, unless the vein is exposed to arterial pressures, high flow rates, or foreign bodies for long periods of time. Intimal hyperplasia in response to trauma, implantation of endoluminal devices, and increased flow is common. As with the arterial intima, this feature of the venous intimal cells is a major determinant of the long-term outcome of many vascular interventions.

The medial layer of veins contains far fewer smooth muscle cells than arteries, thus explaining the relatively thinner, flaccid appearance of the walls. In addition, the connective tissue component of the venous media is less pronounced than that of arteries. As result, veins contribute capacitance to the circulation. Blood flow is maintained by contraction of muscles in the surrounding structures, pressure gradients created during inspiration and expiration, and the presence of one-way bicuspid valves in the small to medium sized veins that permit flow only towards the heart. The smooth muscle cells of these small to medium veins can dilate and contract in response to stimuli, thus partially regulating flow.

ATHEROSCLEROSIS

Atherosclerosis is an arterial disease that is prevalent in industrialized nations. Veins do not develop atherosclerotic lesions unless they are exposed to arterial pressures and flow over extended periods of time. The risk factors for atherosclerosis include environmental and genetic factors (Box 1-1). There are multiple theories of causation, including intimal trauma, an autoimmune response, and infection. Whatever the underlying pathogenesis, the key point to remember is that atherosclerosis is a systemic disease, affecting arteries in all vascular beds. Patients presenting with peripheral vascular manifestations of atherosclerosis are at very high risk for ischemic coronary events (50% in 5 years).

The hallmark of an atherosclerotic lesion is the fibro-fatty plaque, which begins as microscopic lipid deposition in areas of intimal injury. Continued injury leads to a fatty streak, an accumulation of foam cells and macrophages that is the first evidence of atherosclerosis that is visible with the naked eye. As the lesion progresses, the lipid content increases and a fibrotic cap forms over the surface. The cap, composed of smooth muscle cells and collagen, isolates the highly thrombogenic contents of the plaque

Box 1-1   Risk Factors for Atherosclerosis

Genetic predisposition
Smoking
Diet
Diabetes
Chronic renal failure
Hypertension
Homocysteinuria
Advanced age
Hyperlipidemia
Obesity
Elevated lipoprotein (a)

from the blood (Fig. 1-2). If the cap is disrupted, a shower of cholesterol crystals and debris may flow downstream, producing a potentially devastating syndrome termed "cholesterol embolization." Conversely, a thrombus may form acutely on the exposed surface of the plaque. This thrombus can embolize distally, or enlarge to occlude the artery. Plaques that have little calcification and large lipid components are believed to be more prone to this complication, and have been termed "vulnerable plaque." These lesions are implicated in many acute coronary and carotid artery syndromes. There is great interest in the development of imaging techniques for identification of vulnerable plaque.

Atherosclerotic lesions can circumferentially involve the vessel wall, narrowing the arterial lumen in a concentric manner (Fig. 1-3). Plaque that predominantly affects one side of the artery wall results in an eccentric

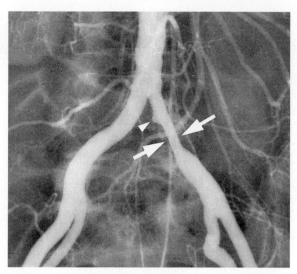

Figure 1-3   Angiographic appearance of concentric stenosis of the left common iliac artery (arrows). Irregularity (arrowhead) in the contour of the plaque may represent a small ulceration.

lesion (Fig. 1-4). Longstanding plaque can become quite bulky and calcify.

Compromise of the arterial lumen from any cause results in restriction of flow (Fig. 1-5). In general, a reduction in luminal diameter of 50% (which is equivalent to a 75% decrease in the area of the lumen) is required before a pressure drop will occur, although many other variables are important. A reduction in diameter of 75%

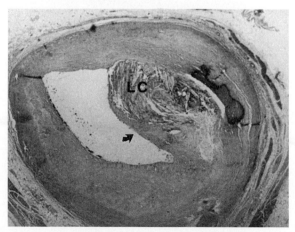

Figure 1-2   Atheromatous plaque. Eccentric atheroma, with thin fibrous cap (arrow) overlying necrotic lipid core (LC) (H&E, ×50). (Reproduced with permission from Johnson DE: Anatomic aspects of vascular disease. In Strandness ED, Breda AV eds: *Vascular Diseases: Surgical and Interventional Therapy*, Churchill Livingstone, New York, 1994.)

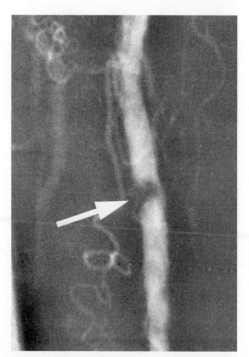

Figure 1-4   Angiographic appearance of bulky, eccentric plaque (arrow) in the superficial femoral artery.

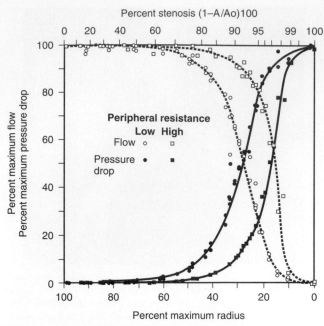

Figure 1-5   Relationship of pressure and flow to degree of stenosis. When peripheral resistance is high, the curves are shifted to the right. (Reproduced with permission from Sumner D: Essential hemodynamic principles. In Rutherford, RB ed.: *Vascular Surgery*, 5 edn, WB Saunders, Philadelphia, 2000.)

represents a >90% decrease in cross-sectional area of the lumen. However, clinical symptoms result whenever the decrease in arterial flow is sufficient to cause end-organ ischemia or dysfunction.

There is a complex relationship between arterial occlusive disease and symptoms. The mere presence of a stenosis does not mean that a patient will have symptoms. The metabolic and pathologic state of the end organ, the degree of collateralization around the stenosis, and the rapidity of onset of the reduced flow are all crucial variables. Decreased blood flow to organs or structures that are in a resting state may produce few symptoms. For example, the classic clinical presentation of chronic lower-extremity occlusive disease is ischemic muscular pain with ambulation, relieved by rest. Organs with numerous potential sources of blood supply, such as the colon, are more likely to tolerate gradual onset of occlusive disease better than organs with a solitary blood supply, such as the kidney. Gradual onset of occlusion allows existing small supplementary arteries to enlarge, forming a well-developed collateral network that may compensate for the original artery (Fig. 1-6). Acute onset of stenosis or occlusion is more likely to

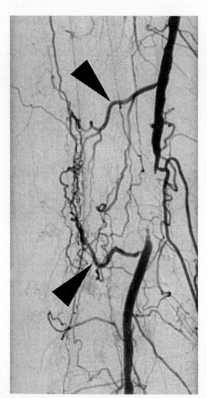

Figure 1-6   Hypertrophied collateral arteries around a short chronic occlusion of the distal superficial femoral artery (SFA). Digital subtraction angiogram (DSA) shows enlarged muscular branches (arrowheads) providing flow around the occlusion with reconstitution of the above-knee popliteal artery. Note the tapered contour of the lumen at the occlusion, which occurs just distal to a muscular branch.

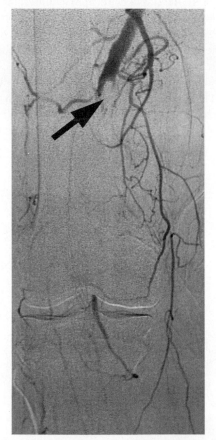

Figure 1-7   Poor collateral arterial supply around an acute occlusion due to thrombosis of a popliteal artery aneurysm. DSA showing an abrupt cutoff of flow with a filling defect (arrow) consistent with thrombus. There is a paucity of collateral vessels and lack of reconstitution of distal vessels.

produce symptoms, even at rest, if collateral vessels are poorly formed or cannot carry sufficient flow (Fig. 1-7).

INTIMAL HYPERPLASIA

Intimal hyperplasia is not a true disease or disorder, but a biologic response to injury to the vessel wall (Fig. 1-8). Whenever the intimal layer of either an artery or vein is injured, fibrin deposition and platelet aggregation occurs. Macrophages and smooth muscle cells quickly migrate into the fibrin–platelet matrix, where they proliferate. Within days of the original injury, endothelial cells appear over the surface of the matrix, extending from the adjacent intact intima and/or by direct inoculation by circulating endothelial precursor cells. This results in formation of a neo-intima over the site of injury. Over a period of approximately 12 weeks there is exuberant proliferation of smooth muscle and endothelial cells, so that some encroachment upon the vessel lumen occurs. After approximately 3 months, the entire process may slow down or stop, with thinning and stabilization of the neo-intima. For reasons that are not well understood, this process is accelerated or prolonged in some patients. The neo-intima can cause narrowing of the vessel lumen that is actually greater and more extensive than the original lesion.

Intimal hyperplasia is the bane of vascular interventions, occurring at surgical anastomoses, angioplasty sites, and after stent deployment (Table 1-2). A number of strategies have been proposed and/or are under investigation to try to reduce intimal hyperplasia, including brachytherapy (intravascular radiation), covered stents, medicated stents, gene therapy, and systemic medications. No single technique has proven successful. Currently, the best results are obtained by limiting the

Table 1-2   Causes of Intimal Hyperplasia

Cause	Examples
Injury	Surgical anastomosis, clamps, angioplasty, denudation of intima by any device
Foreign body	Stents, suture material, catheters
Abnormal flow	Arterialization of veins, turbulence

extent of intimal injury, minimizing the use of prosthetic materials, and maximizing the final diameter of the lumen.

ANEURYSMS

Aneurysms are primarily an arterial disease, although venous aneurysms do occur. Aneurysms may be either "true" or "false," depending upon whether all three layers of the vessel wall are intact (Table 1-3 and Fig. 1-9). The etiology of the aneurysm determines the type and clinical course.

True aneurysms are associated with a number of risk factors (Box 1-2). In general, focal enlargement of an artery to more than 1.5 times its normal diameter constitutes an aneurysm. The most common type of true aneurysm is degenerative. The pathogenesis of degenerative aneurysm formation is not yet fully understood, but may involve atherosclerotic, mechanical (i.e. post-stenotic dilatation), enzymatic, autoimmune, and potentially infectious mechanisms. For example, metalloproteinases are proteolytic enzymes synthesized by macrophages that have been demonstrated to be elevated in patients with abdominal aortic aneurysms. The levels drop to normal following successful repair by either surgical or endovascular techniques. Regardless of the mechanism, aneurysm formation is associated with thinning of the media, and loss of smooth muscle cells, elastic fibers, and collagen.

Degenerative aneurysms are often multifocal, occurring in large to medium-sized arteries in numerous vascular beds in a single patient. The most common arteries in which aneurysms are found are the abdominal and

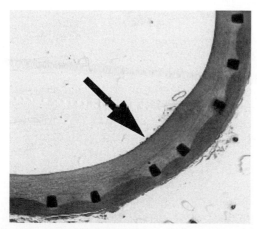

Figure 1-8   Intimal hyperplasia. Low-power micrograph showing thickened intima (arrow) lining the luminal surface of a metallic stent 6 months after placement in an external iliac artery.

Table 1-3   True versus False Aneurysms

Feature	True	False
Vessel wall	All three layers intact	Less than three layers
Etiology	Intrinsic abnormality	Trauma, rupture true aneurysm, infection
Contours	Smooth	Irregular, lobulated
Calcification	Present in intima	Absent unless chronic
Rupture	Risk increases with size	Higher risk than same size true aneurysm

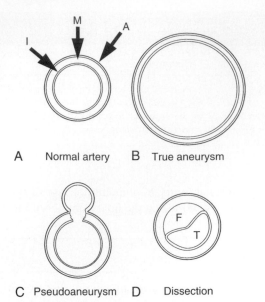

Figure 1-9 Diagram illustrating the differences between true aneurysms, false aneurysms, and dissections. **A,** The normal artery has three intact layers: I = intima, M = media, and A = adventitia. **B,** True aneurysm. All three layers of the arterial wall remain intact, although there is thinning of the media. **C,** Pseudoaneurysm. In this drawing there has been disruption of the intima and media, with formation of a saccular aneurysm contained by the adventitia. **D,** Dissection. All three layers are essentially intact, and the artery may be normal in caliber, but the intima has separated from the media, dividing the artery into two channels (T = true lumen, F = false lumen). The false lumen may be patent or thrombosed. When patent, it is frequently larger than the true lumen. (Modified with permission from Wojtowycz M: *Handbook of Interventional Radiology and Angiography*, Mosby, St Louis, 1995.)

thoracic aortas, the common iliac, internal iliac, common femoral, popliteal, subclavian, and visceral arteries. External iliac and extracranial carotid artery aneurysms are rare. Generalized enlargement without focal aneurysm formation is termed "arteriomegaly."

Box 1-2 Risk Factors for Arterial Aneurysms

Age >60 years
Hypertension
Male
Atherosclerosis
Familial
Chronic obstructive pulmonary disease (aortic aneurysms)
Heritable disorders
  Marfan syndrome
  Ehlers–Danlos syndrome
Vasculitis
Post-stenotic jet or turbulence
Repetitive trauma

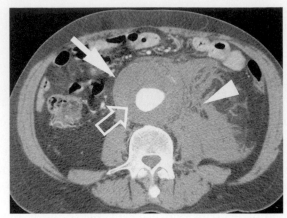

Figure 1-10 CT scan with contrast of a ruptured abdominal aortic aneurysm (AAA) (arrow). The lumen of the aneurysm is lined with mural thrombus (open arrow). There is a hematoma in the periaortic soft tissues (arrowhead).

Aneurysms of large arteries cause symptoms by rupturing (especially the aorta, common, internal iliac, and visceral arteries) (Fig. 1-10). Aneurysms of small and medium arteries (exclusive of the intracranial circulation) more often present with symptoms related to thrombosis and distal embolization (see Fig. 1-7). Symptoms related to mass effect are less common but do occur.

False aneurysms are focal enlargements of the vascular lumen due to partial or complete disruption of the arterial wall (see Fig. 1-9). The blood is contained by residual elements of the arterial wall or surrounding tissues. Also known as pseudoaneurysms (PSA), they are more prone to rupture than similar sized true aneurysms. The cause of most PSA encountered in clinical practice is iatrogenic, such as angiography (cardiac catheterizations) or percutaneous biopsies. Penetrating wounds, crush injuries, and deceleration injuries are common etiologies of PSA occurring outside of the hospital. In addition, PSA may result from contained rupture of true aneurysms or vascular infection (mycotic aneurysm).

FIBROMUSCULAR DYSPLASIA

Fibromuscular dysplasia (FMD) is a collection of fibrotic disorders of the intima, media, or adventitia of medium-sized arteries (Table 1-4). The most frequently affected arteries are the renal, extracranial internal carotid, vertebral, iliac, subclavian, and mesenteric arteries. The etiology of this nonatherosclerotic, non-inflammatory abnormality is unknown, but it tends to be found in young adult female patients. The most common subtype is medial fibroplasia, in which focal web-like stenoses alternate with small aneurysms of varying sizes ("string of natural pearls"). Fortunately, this

Table 1-4   Fibromuscular Dysplasia

Type	Incidence	Predominant Features
Medial fibroplasia	65%	Alternating webs and aneurysms
Perimedial fibroplasia	20%	Irregular, beaded stenosis
Medial hyperplasia	10%	Tubular smooth stenosis
Intimal fibroplasia	1%	Focal smooth stenosis
Periarterial fibroplasia	<1%	Tubular smooth stenosis
Medial dissection	4%	Spontaneous dissection

has a characteristic angiographic appearance (Fig. 1-11). Medial fibroplasia causes symptoms by obstructing flow (webs), distal embolization (of thrombus formed in the small aneurysms), and occlusion (spontaneous dissection). The aneurysms can grow quite large. Other forms of FMD result in tapered stenoses that are less characteristic in appearance, but unusual in that patients tend to be young and without evidence of atherosclerotic disease. Precise classification of the less common forms of FMD requires pathological specimens.

FMD is frequently a bilateral and multifocal abnormality. In the majority of cases, asymptomatic disease will remain stable throughout the patient's life. Symptomatic medial fibroplasia responds very well to balloon angioplasty. The experience with angioplasty of other forms of FMD is limited, but also favorable. Unexplained spontaneous dissection in a medium-sized artery should prompt evaluation of at least the renal arteries for FMD.

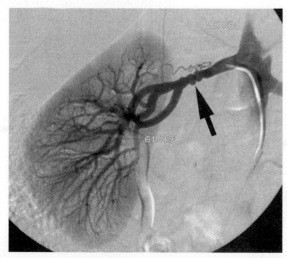

Figure 1-11   Fibromuscular dysplasia (FMD). Selective right renal artery DSA in a 48-year-old female. The irregular beaded appearance (arrow) and location of the abnormality in the distal main renal artery is typical of FMD of the medial fibroplasia type.

VASCULITIS

Vasculitides are inflammatory diseases of the vessel wall due to unknown causes. Inflammation due to infection is considered a mycotic process, and will be discussed later. Arteries are involved much more often than veins. As a rule, vasculitis is an indolent disease of patients in their third through fifth decades. There are numerous types of vasculitis, most of which are associated with constitutional symptoms such as fever, arthralgia, myalgia, rash, and malaise (Table 1-5). An elevated erythrocyte sedimentation rate (ESR) is common unless the disease has been treated or has spontaneously regressed ("burned out"). Numerous other more specific serologic markers may also be elevated, depending upon the vasculitis.

The diagnosis of vasculitis is usually well established before the patient is referred for imaging. The radiographic features of many of the different vasculitides overlap, so that a specific diagnosis may not be possible from the imaging studies. The diagnosis of vasculitis should be entertained whenever a bizarre-appearing stenosis or aneurysm occurs in an unusual location in an unusual patient.

Takayasu's arteritis is a panarteritis that involves the aorta, its major branches, and, less often, the pulmonary arteries. The cause of Takayasu arteritis is not known for certain, but it is presumed to be autoimmune. In the United States, the prevalence is roughly 0.5 persons per 100,000 person-years. There are no ethnic or racial predilections. The typical patient is a female in her second or third decade. Granulomatous changes and lymphocytic infiltration thicken the intima and media, leading to compromise of the lumen. Chronic inflammation may also result in aneurysmal changes. There are five basic patterns of distribution of lesions, with pan-aortic involvement being the most common (Fig. 1-12). It is important to note that cardiac disease is present in 40% of patients, including coronary artery stenoses, aortic and mitral valvular insufficiency, and right heart failure due to pulmonary artery stenoses. A distinctive feature of active Takayasu arteritis is wall enhancement following administration of contrast on computerized tomography (CT) or magnetic resonance imaging (MRI).

Takayasu's arteritis is also known as "pulseless disease," as stenosis or occlusion of the proximal subclavian and common carotid arteries are common (Fig. 1-13; see also Fig. 9-32). Patients may also present with renal hypertension due to abdominal aortic stenoses proximal to or involving the renal arteries. The stenotic lesions are usually long and smooth, although associated plaque may be present in longstanding aortic lesions of older patients. Aortic aneurysms, which are found in up to one-third of patients, rarely rupture. Treatment of uncomplicated Takayasu's is with steroids.

Table 1-5 Vasculitis

Syndrome	Vessels Affected	Imaging Findings
Takayasu's arteritis ("pulseless disease")	Thoracic and abdominal aorta; proximal great vessels; pulmonary arteries; coronary arteries	Thickened enhancing arterial wall on CT/MRI; long aortic stenoses; long smooth nonostial common carotid and subclavian stenoses; pulmonary artery stenosis; coronary artery stenosis; aortic aneurysm (esp. ascending)
Polyarteritis nodosa	Medium and small arteries	Microaneurysms in kidney, liver, bowel, pancreas, spleen, and extremities; stenoses and occlusion of small arteries
Giant cell arteritis	Subclavian (distal), axillary, brachial arteries; carotid artery branches; aorta	Long irregular stenoses and occlusions; rare aortic aneurysms/dissection
Buerger's disease (thromboangiitis obliterans)	Medium and small arteries of extremities; extremity veins	Occlusion of all named vessels with centripetal progression and extensive small vessel collaterals (vasa vasorum); migratory thrombophlebitis in 30%
Behçet's disease	Veins; medium and large arteries; pulmonary arteries	Venous thrombosis; peripheral and aortic aneurysms; arterial thrombosis; pulmonary artery aneurysm
Radiation	All arteries	Varies with time; early thrombosis or late stenosis, with few collaterals
Kawasaki disease (mucocutaneous lymph node syndrome)	Medium and small arteries	Coronary and medium-sized artery aneurysms
Systemic lupus erythematosus, scleroderma	Medium and small arteries, usually upper extremity	Variable-length tapered stenoses and occlusions, especially digital arteries
Rheumatoid and other HLA-B27 positive disorders	Thoracic aorta	Aortic root dilatation

CT, computerized tomography; MRI, magnetic resonance imaging.

Polyarteritis nodosa (PAN) is a systemic necrotizing vasculitis that affects primarily small and medium-sized arteries of the abdominal visceral organs, the heart, and the hands and feet. Patients are usually in their fourth or fifth decade, but may be of any age. Males are affected twice as often as females. There is a strong association between PAN and active hepatitis types B and C, as well as intravenous drug abuse, but over 50% of patients have no known cause. Patients have constitutional, dermatologic, and neurologic manifestations, as well as abdominal pain, renal insufficiency, and spontaneous intra-abdominal or retroperitoneal hemorrhage. The angiographic lesions are characteristic, with multiple small aneurysms of the renal or visceral arteries, and digital artery occlusions (Fig. 1-14). Treatment is with steroids and cyclophosphamide.

Giant cell arteritis derives its name from the presence of giant cells in the infiltrative process in all layers of the blood vessel wall. Mononuclear cells, lymphocytes, T cells, and macrophages are more commonly present. Patients with giant cell arteritis are generally much older than those affected by Takayasu's arteritis, which it can resemble. The classic patient is an elderly female with several weeks of fever, headaches, palpably tender temporal arteries, myalgias, and an extremely elevated ESR, so the disease is known also as "temporal arteritis." Acute blindness due to involvement of the ophthalmic artery is a feared complication (40% in untreated patients). Diagnosis in these patients is most often by temporal artery biopsy.

Giant cell arteritis also causes stenoses of the extremity arteries (upper more often than lower) that manifest 8–24 weeks after onset of symptoms. The arteries

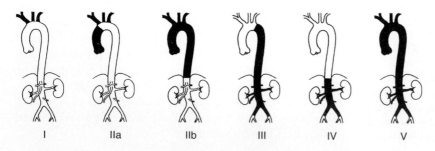

I   IIa   IIb   III   IV   V

Figure 1-12 Classification scheme of angiographic findings in Takayasu arteritis. A letter "C" is added when coronary artery involvement is present, and the letter "P" when pulmonary arteries are involved. (Reproduced with permission from Webb TH, Perler BA: Takayasu arteritis. In Ernst CB, Stanley JC eds: *Current Therapy in Vascular Surgery*, 4th edn, Mosby, St Louis, 2001.)

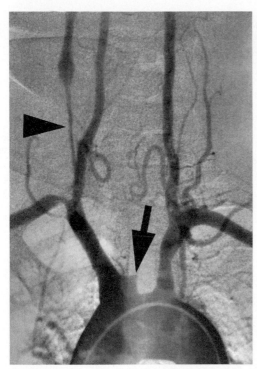

Figure 1-13   Takayasu's arteritis involving the carotid arteries in a young woman. DSA arch aortogram showing occlusion of the left CCA (arrow) at the origin, long stenosis of the right CCA (arrowhead), and stenosis of the right subclavian artery origin.

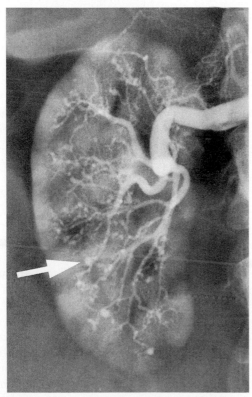

Figure 1-14   Polyarteritis nodosa (PAN). Angiogram of the right kidney shows numerous small peripheral aneurysms (arrow). These were present in the left kidney as well.

involved most often are the distal subclavian, the axillary, and the proximal brachial arteries, although a pattern very similar to Takayasu's arteritis may be seen (Fig. 1-15). These patients are more likely to be referred for angiography to evaluate upper-extremity ischemic symptoms. The appearance of multiple, long, irregular stenoses of these arteries is characteristic, although rarely other vasculitides, such as that associated with systemic lupus erythematosus (SLE), may produce similar lesions. Rarely, thoracic or abdominal aortic aneurysms may develop in patients with giant cell arteritis, and be the only presenting symptom. Rupture and dissection have been reported in these patients.

Buerger's disease is also known as "thromboangiitis obliterans" because of the inflammatory cellular debris that occludes the vessel lumen. Though the disease is a panarteritis, the vessel wall remains relatively intact, including the elastic lamellae. The distal small to medium arteries and veins of the lower and upper extremities are involved, usually with preservation of the proximal inflow vessels. Buerger's disease primarily affects male smokers younger than age 50, although females now compromise almost one-quarter of all cases. This diagnosis should be suspected in any young patient presenting with small-vessel occlusive disease in the absence of diabetes. The lower extremities are almost always involved, and the upper extremities in over one-half of patients. A migratory thrombophlebitis, usually of the superficial veins, is seen in up to 30% of patients. Fortunately, the incidence of Buerger's disease has decreased dramatically in the last 50 years, for reasons as yet unknown.

The angiographic appearance of Buerger's disease is dramatic, with occlusion of most or all named vessels below the knee or elbow (Fig. 1-16). Because the vessel wall architecture is preserved, prominent collaterals develop in the vaso vasorum of the occluded arteries. This results in a typical "corkscrew" appearance of collaterals on angiography, quite distinct from collaterals due to atherosclerotic occlusions.

Behçet's disease presents with recurrent oral and genital apthous ulcers, skin lesions, ocular inflammation, arthritis, gastrointestinal symptoms, and epididymitis. Patients are usually between the ages of 20 and 40 years. Males are affected more commonly than females, with a ratio of almost 2:1. Pathologically, Behçet's disease is an inflammatory disorder of small blood vessels, in particular venules. The clinical vascular manifestations of Behçet's disease occur in 20% of cases, with superficial venous thrombosis predominating. Aortic and pulmonary artery aneurysms, arterial occlusive disease, and central venous thrombosis occur in fewer than 5% of patients (Fig. 1-17).

Radiation arteritis is the result of injury to radiosensitive endothelial cells during external-beam radiation

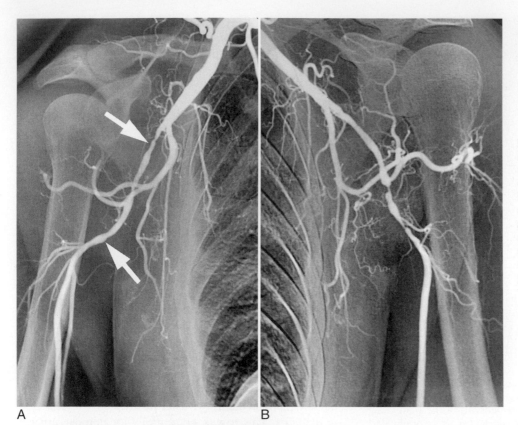

Figure 1-15   Giant cell arteritis in a middle-aged male with bilateral upper-extremity claudication and an elevated erythrocyte sedimentation rate. The aortic arch and subclavian arteries were normal. **A,** Digital angiogram showing irregular narrowing of the distal right axillary artery and proximal brachial arteries (arrows). **B,** The same findings are present on the left. The distal arteries were normal in both arms.

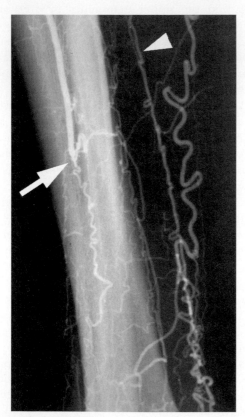

Figure 1-16   Buerger's disease. Detailed view of a lateral angiogram of the calf. The peroneal artery occludes in the mid calf (arrow). The anterior and posterior tibial arteries are occluded. There are numerous coiled collateral arteries, including one in the vasa vasorum of the occluded posterior tibial artery (arrowhead).

for malignancy. Symptoms occur when the total radiation dose exceeds 5000 rads. The clinical presentation varies with the time interval from the radiation exposure. Thrombosis is most common within 5 years of treatment. Mural fibrosis, stenosis, and occlusion with a paucity of collaterals occurs at between 5 and 10 years. Late manifestations include periarterial fibrosis and accelerated atherosclerosis, often in unusual distributions localized to the irradiated tissues (Fig. 1-18). Careful planning of radiation portals limits the incidence of this complication.

Kawasaki's disease, also known as "mucocutaneous lymph node syndrome," is a rare disease of infants and children younger than 1 year. A vasculitis affects primarily small and medium-sized arteries. The most notable presenting vascular abnormality is coronary artery aneurysm, which may thrombose or rupture. Aneurysms of other arteries occur as well. This disease has been rarely reported in patients older than 9 years of age.

Systemic lupus erythematosus (SLE) and other collagen vascular diseases are usually characterized by musculoskeletal symptoms and serologic markers. The diagnosis of these diseases is rarely made on the basis of angiographic findings alone. More commonly, patients with a known connective tissue disorder develop symptoms that suggest vascular involvement, such as digital ischemia and ulcerations in a young woman with SLE. In this case, angiography is performed

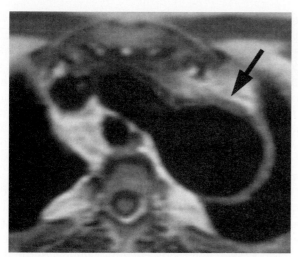

Figure 1-17 Behçet's disease. Axial T1 weighted image of the aortic arch in a young female with a focal aneurysm of the proximal descending thoracic aorta (arrow).

to exclude another, correctable problem such as digital arterial emboli. The typical angiographic findings of lupus vasculitis in the hand are focal occlusions and irregular stenoses of the palmar and digital arteries (Fig. 1-19). Similar lesions may be seen in scleroderma. Patients with

rheumatoid arthritis, ankylosing spondylitis, Reiter's syndrome, and psoriatic arthritis can develop ascending aortic dilatation with aortic valve insufficiency.

HEMANGIOMAS, VASCULAR MALFORMATIONS, AND ARTERIOVENOUS FISTULAS

Hemangiomas are congenital lesions of unknown etiology that can occur in any organ in the body (Table 1-6). Always present at birth, these lesions are never acquired. Hemangiomas are true neoplasms, but follow a benign course with spontaneous involution by age 7 years in most patients. Large lesions can be associated with platelet consumption and hemorrhagic complications, known as Kasabach–Merrit syndrome. Asymptomatic hemangiomas do not require treatment. At angiography, these lesions demonstrate normal feeding arteries, early but prolonged opacification, and normal draining veins (Fig. 1-20). In infants with large hepatic hemangiomatous lesions, transcatheter embolization may be required to decrease shunting (see Chapter 11, Fig. 11-29).

Arteriovenous malformations (AVM) are nonproliferative high-flow congenital lesions that are usually

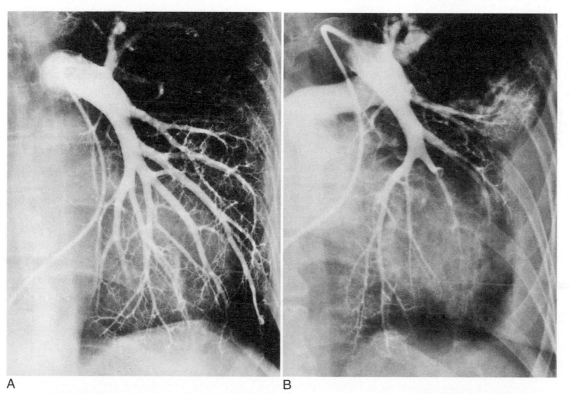

A B

Figure 1-18 Radiation arteritis. **A**, Normal pulmonary angiogram of the left lung. **B**, Left pulmonary angiogram from the same patient obtained 7 years after radiation treatment for breast carcinoma shows narrowing, branch vessel occlusions, and pleural thickening consistent with late radiation fibrosis.

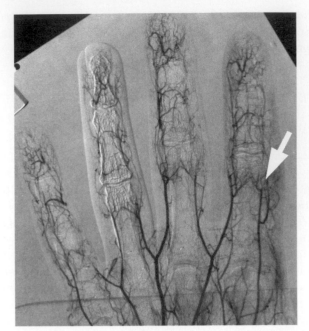

Figure 1-19 Systemic lupus erythematosis (SLE) in a teenage female with bilateral digital ulcers. Detail of a magnified, subtracted angiogram of the hand shows areas of digital artery narrowing with mulyiple occlusions (arrow). There are no intraluminal filling defects or other evidence of emboli.

single, and can occur anywhere in the body (Fig. 1-21). Approximately 60% are found in the lower limbs, 25% in the upper limbs, 12% in the pelvis and buttocks, and the remainder in other locations. These lesions are present at birth, but can remain subclinical throughout the patient's life. A characteristic feature is one or more central tangles of communicating arterioles and venules, termed the "nidus." Arteriovenous malformations grow by recruiting additional feeding arteries and draining

veins, rather than by proliferation of the component cells. Large AVMs can cause clinically symptomatic left-to-right shunts, hypertrophy of affected extremities, and bleeding (Fig. 1-22). These lesions are pulsatile, with an audible bruit, and remain distended despite elevation above the right atrium. In general, AVMs are very difficult to treat primarily with surgical resection. Careful, staged transcatheter embolization procedures using microcatheters, small particles, intravascular glue, and absolute alcohol provide excellent results in control of symptoms. Complete cure is rarely achieved.

Venous malformations are congential low-flow lesions comprised of localized dilated venous structures (Fig. 1-23). Large venous malformations can cause disfigurement, pain as a result of thrombosis or infiltration of muscle, and bleeding following minor trauma to the thin overlying skin. These lesions are soft and nonpulsatile, with no bruit, and they collapse when elevated above the right atrium. Usually single, these lesions can be associated with Klippel–Trenaunay syndrome – a complex usually affecting the lower extremities, consisting of venous malformations, varicosities, capillary malformations, hemangiomas, limb hypertrophy, and abnormal deep venous structures. Characteristically, venous malformations exhibit delayed opacification and slow flow at angiography. Direct puncture reveals a large venous space with pooling of contrast and drainage into normal veins. Lesions may have lymphatic as well as venous components. When readily accessible, these lesions respond well to direct puncture and sclerosis with absolute alcohol. These procedures are usually performed under general anesthesia for pain control in a staged fashion. Careful fluoroscopic monitoring is essential to avoid damage to normal venous structures and surrounding tissues.

Arteriovenous fistulas are almost always acquired point-to-point communications between an artery and a

Table 1-6 Features of Vascular Malformations

	Hemangioma	Arteriovenous Malformation	Venous Malformation	Arteriovenous Fistula
Etiology	Neoplasm (benign)	Congenital anomaly	Congenital anomaly	Acquired
Presentation	30% at birth, remainder within 3 months	At birth	At birth	Later in life
Cellular proliferation	First year	None	None	None
Female:male ratio	5:1	1:1	1:1	N/A
Outcome	Spontaneous involution by age 7 in 95%	Stable or grows with patient	Stable or grows with patient	Growth
Angiographic appearance	Staining, pooling of contrast; large liver hemangiomas in infants may shunt	Enlarged feeding arteries and draining veins with central nidus; rapid shunting; no parenchymal stain	Normal feeding arteries; delayed opacification of dilated venous space with slow flow	Enlarged feeding arteries and draining veins with point communication; no parenchymal stain

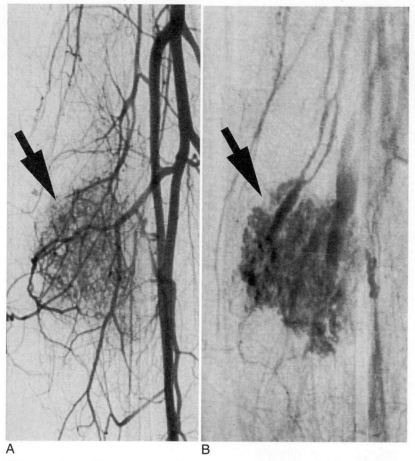

A   B

Figure 1-20   Angiographic appearance of an intramuscular hemangioma located in the calf. **A**, The tibial arteries supplying the hemangioma are normal in caliber. There is early opacification of the hemangioma (arrow), but no venous shunting. This degree of opacification is more prominent than usually seen. **B**, Late image from the same angiogram shows persistent staining of the hemangioma (arrow) and normal draining veins.

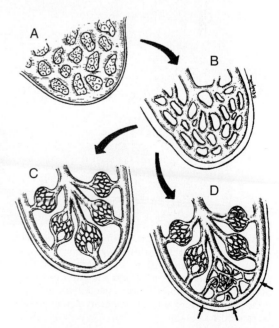

Figure 1-21   Diagram illustrating the development of arteriovenous malformations. **A**, Primitive mesenchyme with undifferentiated blood spaces. **B**, Primitive capillaries. **C**, Maturation of vascular bed with vascular stems leading to and from capillary beds. **D**, Local persistence of primitive capillary network results in an arteriovenous malformation (small arrows). (Reproduced with permission from Rosen RJ, Riles TS: Congenital vascular malformations. In Rutherford RB: *Vascular Surgery*, 5th edn, WB Saunders, Philadelphia, 2000.)

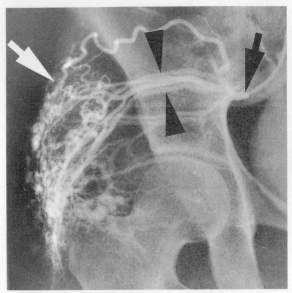

Figure 1-22 Arteriovenous malformation of the right buttock. Selective superior gluteal artery injection (black arrow) shows enlarged feeding arteries, an amorphous tangle of vessels in the soft tissues of the buttock (white arrow), and early venous enhancement (arrowheads) due to shunting.

vein (Fig. 1-24). The most common etiology in the hospital setting is iatrogenic following arterial catheterization or attempted central line placement. Small fistulas may remain asymptomatic or close spontaneously. Fistulas of all sizes can enlarge over time, resulting in recruitment of additional feeding arteries and draining veins. However, the actual communication always remains point-to-point. Lesions are pulsatile, with a palpable thrill and audible bruit, and the venous outflow remains distended when elevated above the right atrium. The clinical presentation can be similar to arteriovenous malformations, with symptomatic left-to-right shunts and pain. At arteriography, rapid shunting with hypertrophy of the feeding artery and draining veins and a single point of communication are characteristic. Occlusion of the point of communication with a stent-graft, coils (if possible), or surgical ligation is curative.

MRI (including MR angiography and venography) has proven to be an excellent imaging modality for determining the nature and extent of vascular malformations. The precise relationship to superficial and deep structures can be demonstrated, as well as the dominant vascular supply. Signal characteristics of the blood in the lesion can be used to classify the lesion, and thus plan therapy (Table 1-7).

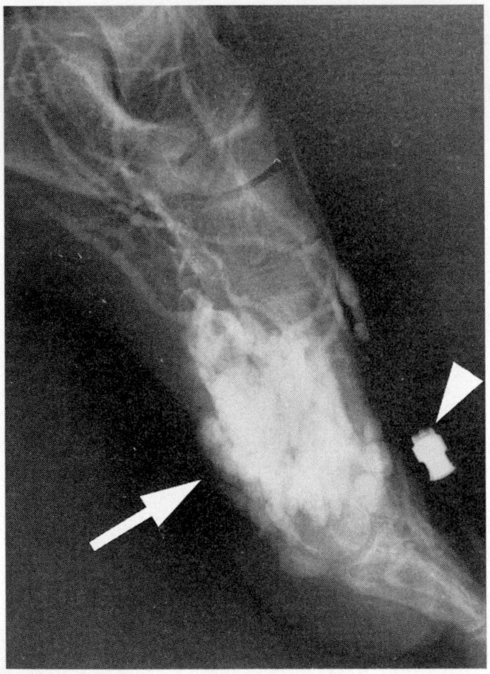

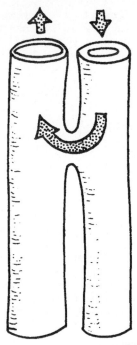

Figure 1-23 Venous malformation of the plantar aspect of the foot. Arterial injections were normal. Venography with occlusion of arterial inflow and venous outflow using a blood pressure cuff on the calf shows the extent of the venous abnormality (arrow). Contrast was injected through a catheter in a dorsal foot vein (arrowhead). Superficial venous malformations can be punctured directly.

Figure 1-24 Schematic diagram of an arteriovenous fistula. There is a direct, point-to-point communication between the artery and vein. (Reproduced with permission from Riles TS, Rosen RJ, Jacobowitz GR: Peripheral arterial fistulae. In Rutherford RB ed.: *Vascular Surgery*, 5th edn, WB Saunders, Philadelphia, 2000.)

Table 1-7	MR Characteristics of Vascular Malformations[a]
Malformation	**MR Features[b]**
Hemangioma	Dark T1; very bright T2; normal arteries and veins
Arteriovenous	Dark T1 and T2; enlarged feeding arteries and veins
Venous	Intermediate signal T1; bright T2; normal arteries and draining veins

[a]Bright signal on T1 may indicate thrombosis or hemorrhage of any of these lesions.
[b]Non-contrast scan.

NEOPLASMS

Primary vascular neoplasms are unusual, accounting for only 2 per 100,000 cases of cancer. Neoplasms arise directly from elements in the blood vessel walls, usually the smooth muscle cells. The most common primary malignant vascular neoplasms are venous leiomyosarcomas, which involve the infrarenal IVC in 60% of patients. Lipomyosarcomas, pulmonary artery sarcomas, and aortic sarcomas can also occur. Benign lesions include lipomas and leiomyomas. These lesions are discussed later in appropriate chapters.

Secondary vascular invasion by neoplasms is much more common than primary tumors of the blood vessels. Veins, in particular the IVC, are invaded more often than arteries. Tumor invasion usually indicates malignancy, and is seen in particular with renal cell carcinoma, but also with hepatoma, adrenal cell carcinoma, germ cell tumors, uterine sarcoma, and thyroid carcinoma (Fig. 1-25). Thrombus frequently forms on the intravenous portion of the tumor, and may embolize to the lungs. Depending on the vascularity of the primary tumor, angiography may demonstrate tumor vessels in the intraluminal tumor as well as the primary mass.

The angiographic appearance of a tumor varies depending on the size of the lesion, vascular supply, and vascular architecture (Figs. 1-25 and 1-26). Angiography is rarely performed to establish a diagnosis of malignancy, but occasionally to try to determine the organ of origin or extent of local invasion. An appreciation of the various appearances of malignancy on angiography remains useful (Table 1-8 and Box 1-3). As a general rule, veins are subject to compression or invasion earlier than arteries. With the exception of arterial encasement or invasion, there are few signs that can conclusively distinguish a malignant from a benign mass, although the organ of origin, the size, and the number of lesions are extremely helpful.

Neoplasms that do not arise from the vessel wall or grow into the lumen can have distinctive (but not pathognomonic) angiographic signatures. However, many tumors, especially those with little vascularity, have

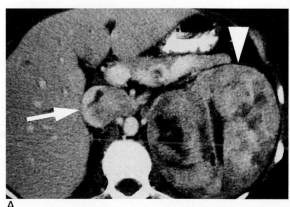
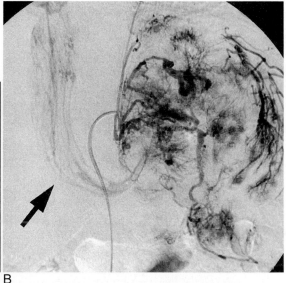

A   B

Figure 1-25   Adrenal carcinoma invading the inferior vena cava (IVC). **A**, CT scan with contrast shows a large heterogeneous mass in the retroperitoneum on the left (arrowhead). The mass is growing through the left renal vein into the IVC. The expanded appearance of the IVC (arrow) with contrast around the mass is characteristic of an intraluminal process. **B**, Digital subtraction angiogram of the left inferior phrenic artery showing a large hypervascular mass with prominent neovascularity. Tumor vessels are present in the intravenous portion of the neoplasm (arrow), which extends to the diaphragm.

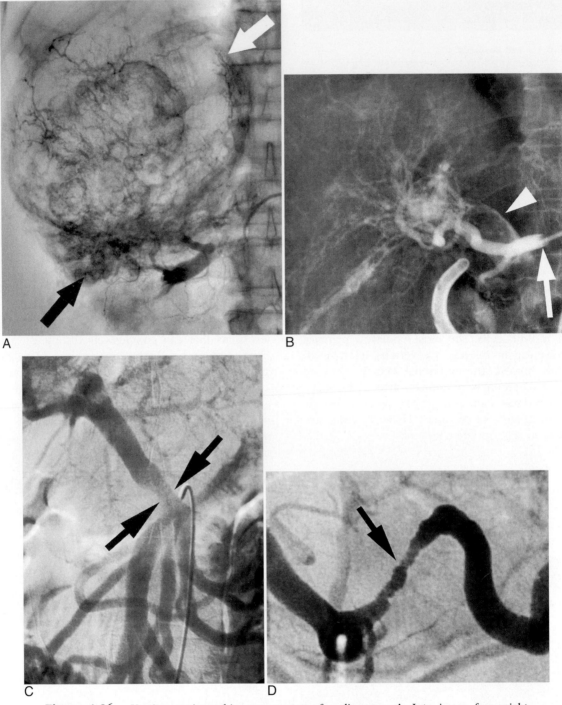

Figure 1-26   Varying angiographic appearances of malignancy. **A**, Late image from right renal angiogram in a patient with an upper-pole renal cell carcinoma showing a large mass (white arrow) with parenchymal tumor staining (black arrow). The tumor has obstructed the main renal vein, trapping contrast in the lower-pole veins. **B**, Arteriovenous shunting. Arterial phase image from a patient with a hepatoma invading the portal vein demonstrates arterial (arrow) to portal (arrowhead) shunting. **C**, Venous encasement by pancreatic carcinoma. Portal venous phase DSA image following injection of contrast into the superior mesenteric artery (SMA) showing concentric narrowing of the portal vein (arrows) consistent with tumor encasement. **D**, Arterial encasement in another patient with pancreatic carcinoma. Arterial phase celiac artery DSA demonstrates multiple irregular areas of stenosis (arrow) in the splenic artery consistent with encasement by tumor.

Table 1-8   Effects of Neoplasms on Adjacent Blood Vessels

Sign	Angiographic Appearance	Type of Neoplasm
Displacement	Vessel draped over mass	Benign or malignant
Compression	Smooth narrowing, no sharp angles	Benign or malignant
Encasement	Narrow vessel with sharp, varying angles	Malignant
Invasion	Jagged, irregular contour of lumen	Malignant
Intravascular	Vascularized mass in lumen	Malignant; rarely benign
Occlusion	Abrupt cutoff of normal vessel in mass	Benign or malignant

very nondescript angiographic appearances (Table 1-9). In addition, the appearance of a lesion on one modality, such as CT, may not be predictive of the angiographic appearance. Lastly, the sensitivity of angiography for detection of nonvascular lesions is less than with CT and MRI.

DISSECTION

Dissection is defined as disruption of the intima, entry of blood into media, with an intact adventitia so that a second, false lumen is created (see Fig. 1-9). Usually the blood cannot exit the false lumen as quickly as it enters, so that a tunnel forms in the wall of the vessel. During diastole the false lumen remains pressurized relative to the true lumen. In some circumstances, the false lumen compresses or even effaces the residual true lumen. The dissection may extend into branch vessels, tear free at the ostium, or billow over the mouth of the artery and cause an occlusion.

Dissection is almost exclusively an arterial pathology, but has been reported in veins as well. There are numerous risk factors for arterial dissection, ranging from direct trauma to inherited arterial wall abnormalities (Box 1-4). The arteries most commonly affected are the

Table 1-9   Angiographic Appearance of Selected Neoplasms

Neoplasm	Examples of Organ of Origin	Appearance
Adenocarcinoma	Bowel, pancreas, lung, breast	Hypovascular
Squamous cell carcinoma	Oropharynx, skin	Hypovascular
Leiomyosarcoma	Esophagus, bowel	Vascular
Islet cell tumor	Pancreas	Vascular
Hepatoma	Liver	Vascular
Renal cell carcinoma	Kidney	Vascular
Carcinoid metastases	Bowel	Vascular
Melanoma metastases	Skin, eye	Vascular
Benign leiomyoma	Uterus	Vascular
Angiomyolipoma	Kidney, adrenal	Vascular

aorta and medium-sized muscular arteries. When the media is normal, the dissection will usually remain localized. In the setting of an abnormal media, such as in patients with certain heritable syndromes, the dissection may extend quite far from the original tear. The symptoms of

Box 1-3   Angiographic Signs of Vascular Neoplasms

Enlarged feeding arteries[a]
Wild, random appearing arteries in mass ("neovascularity")[a]
Encasement or invasion of vessel wall
Abrupt arterial occlusion[a]
Densely staining mass[a]
Rapid shunting into veins
Intravascular extension

[a] These signs are seen with both benign and malignant neoplasms. Location of mass and clinical history are important when interpreting the angiogram.

Box 1-4   Risk Factors for Arterial Dissection

Hypertension
Atherosclerosis
Chronic obstructive pulmonary disease
Age >65 years
Chronic steroid use
Medial degeneration of any cause
Inherited disorder of the vascular wall (Marfan syndrome, Ehlers–Danlos syndrome)
Collagen vascular disease (rheumatoid arthritis, giant cell arteritis)
Fibromuscular dysplasia
Turner's syndrome
Trauma (including iatrogenic)

Table 1-10   Imaging Findings of Dissection

Modality	Findings
Angiography	Thick soft tissue density lateral to intimal calcification ("companion shadow"); contrast on both sides of intimal flap; differential flow rates in parallel lumens within same vessel; long spiral compression of true lumen; abrupt occlusion or unexplained absence of branch vessels
CT	Displacement of intimal calcification into vascular lumen; contrast on both sides of intimal flap; vascular lumen with flattened or crescentic medial contour; differential flow rates in parallel lumens within same vessel; thrombus external to intimal calcification
MR	Contrast or flow on both sides of intimal flap; vascular lumen with flattened or crescentic medial contour; differential flow rates in parallel lumens within same vessel
US	Flow on both sides of intimal flap; calcified flap in vessel lumen; expansion false lumen during diastole; vascular lumen with flattened or crescentic medial contour; differential flow rates in parallel lumens within same vessel

dissection can be variable in severity. Pain can occur, often described as "tearing," due to stretching of the artery and disruption of the media. Compression of the true lumen or involvement of critical branch vessels may result in distal organ ischemia. Rupture of the false lumen is a risk in the acute setting if blood pressure remains uncontrolled, or later if the false lumen becomes aneurysmal. Spontaneous thrombosis and obliteration of the false lumen occurs as well.

The imaging hallmark of dissection is the demonstration of blood on both sides of an intimal flap (Table 1-10 and Fig. 1-27). The true lumen is often (but by no means always) smaller and contains faster flow than the false lumen. For large vessels, such as the aorta, helical CT with contrast has exquisite sensitivity and specificity for dissection, and is usually the first cross-sectional study obtained. Angiography is used to resolve diagnostic dilemmas or prior to a catheter-based intervention. The classification system used to describe aortic dissection is discussed in Chapter 9 (see Fig. 9-22).

TRAUMA

Blood vessels are susceptible to traumatic injury by a wide variety of mechanisms (Table 1-11). High-energy injuries may result in trauma to a vessel adjacent to

but not within the area of greatest soft tissue injury. For example, high-power rifle bullets disperse destructive energy in a radius of millimeters to centimeters along their path through the soft tissues. Conversely, a knife wound creates injury only to those tissues that interact directly with the blade. However, the course of a knife blade through tissue is less predictable than that of a projectile. Consideration of the mechanism of injury is therefore important when evaluating a trauma patient for suspected vascular injury.

Traumatic vascular injuries can manifest in numerous ways (Table 1-12 and Fig. 1-28). Certain mechanisms are more likely to produce one type of injury than another, but there are no hard rules when it comes to trauma. In general, be prepared to find almost any type of injury. Common patterns of vascular injury are discussed in appropriate chapters.

A common and characteristic artifact related to power injection of contrast into normal medium and small arteries – standing waves – should not be confused with post-traumatic spasm or intimal dissection (Fig. 1-29). Usually this finding disappears on repeat injection of contrast.

VASOSPASTIC DISORDERS

Raynaud's syndrome is the most common vasospastic disorder. Primary Raynaud's is defined as reversible spasm of small arteries and arterioles (usually of the digits) in the absence of an underlying disorder. Secondary Raynaud's is vasospasm that occurs as part of a systemic disorder such as SLE (Box 1-5). A diagnosis of primary Raynaud's can only be made if symptoms are present for 2 years without an underlying explanation. The female to male ratio is 4:1, with a typical age of onset in the second and third decades. Symptoms are induced

Table 1-11   Vascular Trauma: Mechanism of Injury

Mechanism	Energy Level	Example
Penetrating	High	Bullet
	Low	Knife
Blunt	High	High speed motorcycle accident
	Low	Leg trapped between two cars
Stretch	Low	Posterior knee dislocation
Thermal	N/A	Burn
Chemical	N/A	Intraarterial injection of absolute alcohol

N/A, not applicable.

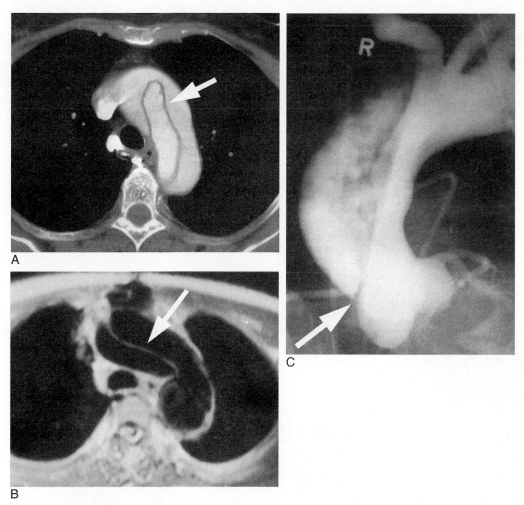

Figure 1-27   The appearance of aortic dissection is similar on different imaging modalities. **A**, CT scan with contrast through the aortic arch showing an intimal flap (arrow). Flecks of calcium can be seen in the flap, confirming its identity as intima. **B**, Axial T1 weighted MR image of the aortic arch from a different patient demonstrates an intimal flap (arrow) with a flow void on each side. The patient has undergone surgery for repair of the ascending aorta. **C**, Conventional angiogram of a patient with a dissection limited to the ascending aorta. The true lumen is compressed by the larger, less-opacified false lumen. The intimal flap (arrow) originates above the right coronary sinus.

Table 1-12   Vascular Injuries

Injury	Description
Spasm	Focal smooth narrowing; resolves spontaneously, but if severe may cause thrombosis
Wall hematoma	Focal hemorrhage into vascular wall without disruption
Intimal tear	Small intraluminal defect; usually heals with conservative management (anticoagulation); can be obstructive
Dissection	Initimal tear with creation of false lumen (frequently iatrogenic); if retrograde may heal spontaneously, but if antegrade can lead to vascular occlusion
Pseudoaneurysm	Aneurysm due to localized disruption of vascular wall (one or more layers) with blood contained by surrounding soft tissues; frequently associated with hematoma
Occlusion	Obstruction to flow caused by *in situ* thrombosis related to spasm, dissection, intimal tear, or foreign body
Transection	Circumferential disruption of vessel wall; may result in thrombosis (small vessels), pseudoaneurysm, or extravasation
AVF	Direct communication between adjacent artery and vein with left-to-right shunt

AVF, arteriovenous fistula.

by environmental factors (especially cold) in almost all patients. Patients with Raynaud's experience a predictable sequence of asymmetric digital pallor or cyanosis followed by hyperemia during episodes of vasospasm. Patients with Raynaud's disease rarely undergo angiography, but absence of intraluminal filling defects and reversible stenoses are useful diagnostic criteria in questionable cases (Fig. 1-30).

Ergotism is drug-induced vasospasm of small to medium-sized arteries caused by ergot alkaloids. These compounds are use to treat migraine, in the prophylaxis of deep vein thrombosis (DVT), and recreation

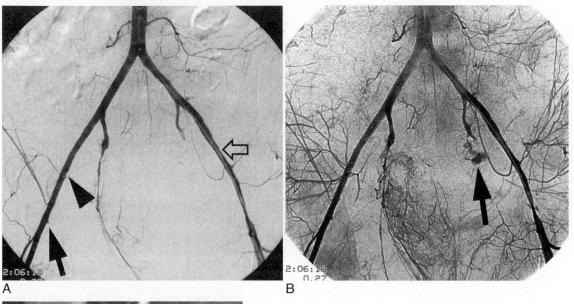

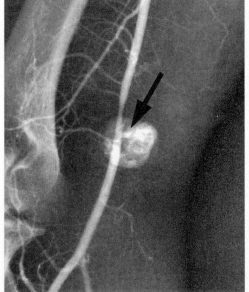

Figure 1-28   Angiographic findings in trauma. **A**, Digital subtraction angiogram of the pelvis in a pedestrian hit by a truck reveals numerous vascular injuries. There is *occlusion* of the right inferior epigastric artery (arrow) at its origin, as well as many hypogastric artery branches in the pelvis. Multiple small *intimal flaps* (arrowhead) are present in the right external iliac artery. There is *spasm* (open arrow) of the left external iliac artery. **B**, Later image from the same angiogram shows active *extravasation* (arrow) from the left hypogastric trunk. **C**, Brachial angiogram from a different patient following a stab wound to the arm shows a *pseudoaneurysm* (arrow).

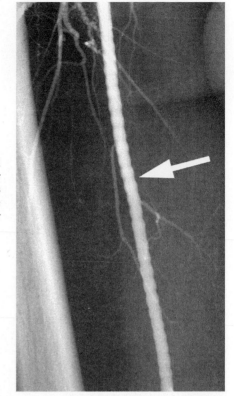

Figure 1-29   Standing waves. Detailed view of an angiogram of the superficial femoral artery shows a regular corrugated contour to the lumen (arrow). Standing waves occur in medium to small muscular arteries during contrast inject. The exact etiology is unknown, but they are harmless and usually disappear before a second injection can be performed. This appearance should be compared to spasm (Fig. 1-28) and fibromuscular dysplasia (Fig. 1-11).

Figure 1-30   Angiographic demonstration of Raynaud's syndrome. **A**, Angiogram of the hand in a patient with a long history of cold-induced blanching of the fingers and tobacco abuse. The patient was experiencing an attack during the angiogram. The arteries of the hand appear attenuated, and there is incomplete filling of the digital arteries. **B**, Following intraarterial administration of a vasodilator, there is dilatation and improved filling of the arteries, although fixed digital artery occlusions are also present.

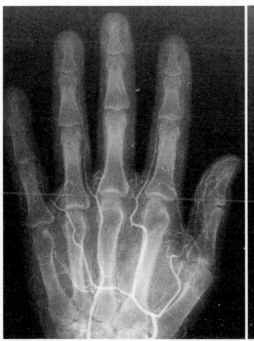

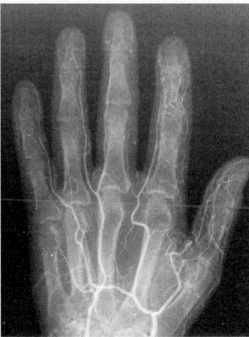

A

B

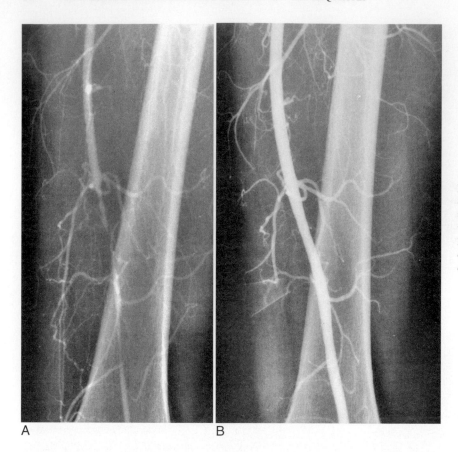

A   B

Figure 1-31   Ergotism in a patient with claudication and migraine headaches. **A,** Angiogram of the left thigh demonstrates diffuse narrowing of the superficial femoral artery (SFA) and above-knee popliteal artery. **B,** Angiogram after cessation of ergot alkaloids. The SFA and popliteal artery are entirely normal.

(lysergic acid diethylamide, or LSD). The incidence of vascular symptoms is less than one-hundredth of 1% of patients taking ergot alkaloids. Patients present with claudication and numbness, which can progress to tissue loss. Long smooth stenoses are seen at angiography, which reverse completely with cessation of ergot therapy (Fig. 1-31).

ARTERIAL EMBOLISM

The clinical presentation of an arterial embolus depends upon the size of the embolus, the organ affected, and the presence of a collateral or alternative blood supply. A small embolus to the brain can be devastating, whereas a large embolus to a hypogastric artery can be asymptomatic provided that the contralateral hypogastric artery is patent. In general, emboli lodge in vessels when there is a sudden change in caliber, such as at bifurcation points and stenoses. Emboli tend to be recurrent, multiple, and unpredictable. The most common source of macroemboli is the heart (80% of all arterial emboli), and the most common etiology is atrial fibrillation (80% of cardiogenic emboli) (Box 1-6). Other etiologies include intravascular

lesions such as exophytic aortic plaque, mural thrombus within an aortic or peripheral aneurysm, disrupted atherosclerotic plaque, and trauma (Box 1-7).

A symptomatic arterial embolus presents as an emergency when acute occlusion occurs in the absence of an established collateral blood supply. The angiographic features of emboli include abrupt occlusion with an intraluminal filling defect, lack of collateral vessels, and involvement of multiple vessels (Fig. 1-32).

Box 1-6   Cardiac Sources of Peripheral Arterial Macroemboli

Cardiac arrhythmia (especially atrial fibrillation)
Myocardial infarction (intracavitary thrombus)
Ventricular aneurysm
Prosthetic valve
Endocarditis
Cardiomyopathy
Paradoxical embolus
Intracardiac neoplasm
Rheumatic heart disease

Table 1-13   Peripheral Distribution of Symptomatic Emboli of Cardiac Origin

Location	Incidence
Common femoral artery	36%
Aortic bifurcation and common iliac arteries	22%
Popliteal artery	15%
Upper-extremity artery	14%
Visceral (renal and superior mesenteric arteries)	7%
Other	6%

Additional features that suggest emboli are occlusions in the presence of otherwise normal appearing arteries and asymmetric distribution when multiple. The anatomic distribution of emboli is determined by the source, the size of the embolus, and the flow rates. Approximately 20% emboli of cardiac origin lodge in the cerebrovascular circulation, fewer than 10% involve the visceral vessels, and the remainder lodge in the aorta and peripheral arteries (Table 1-13). When performing a diagnostic imaging study on a patient with noncardiogenic arterial embolization, it is important to evaluate the entire aorta. Recurrent embolic episodes to one limb or organ suggests an inline source close to the vascular supply of the affected anatomic region. Despite aggressive imaging with multiple modalities, a source is never found in roughly 5% of patients with arterial embolism.

Paradoxical embolism occurs when emboli of venous origin become arterial via an intracardiac (usually a patent foramen ovale) or pulmonary right–left shunt. This is believed to be an important etiology of cryptogenic embolic stroke in young patients.

Atherosclerotic microembolism (so-called "*cholesterol embolization*") represents an important subgroup of arterial embolic disorders. Platelet aggregates, cholesterol crystals, and thrombus originating from unstable or disrupted atherosclerotic plaque embolize distally and occlude small peripheral arterioles. As a result, patients may have normal pulse examination and angiographic studies despite obvious clinical findings. Patients may present with focal areas of painful discoloration (especially in the toes, known as "blue toe syndrome"), renal failure, bowel ischemia, and stroke (Fig. 1-33). Embolization is usually spontaneous, but can follow surgical or percutaneous manipulation of a diseased artery.

INFECTION

Bacterial infection of the native vessel wall can occur from several mechanisms (Table 1-14). Both arteries and veins may become infected, although venous infection

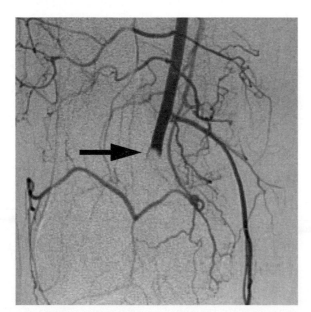

Figure 1-32   Acute arterial embolism in the above-knee popliteal artery. There is slight broadening of the contrast column and a smooth convex intraluminal filling defect (arrow) characteristic of an embolus. Notice that contrast outlines the top of the embolus. This appearance is similar to the acute *in situ* popliteal artery thrombosis shown in Fig. 1-7.

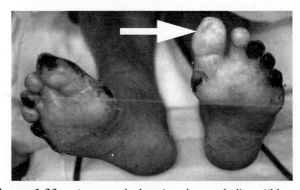

Figure 1-33   Acute and chronic atheroembolism ("blue toe syndrome") in a patient with a proximal source. Mottling consistent with acute embolism is most evident on the left great toe (arrow). The gangrenous toes are typical of chronic atheroembolism.

Table 1-14 Sources of Vascular Infection

Etiology	Examples
Hematogenous	Bacteremia following dental procedure
Embolic	Septic embolus from bacterial endocarditis
Direct inoculation	Intravenous drug abuse with nonsterile technique
Contiguous spread	Aortic infection from retroperitoneal abscess

Table 1-15 Pathogens of Isolated Mycotic Aneurysms

Pathogen	Approximate incidence
Staphylococcus aureus	30%
Salmonella species	10%
Streptococcus species	10%
Pseudomonas species	6%
Staphylococcus epidermidis	5%
Escherichia coli	3%
Klebsiella species	2%
Haemophilus influenzae	2%
Mycobacterium tuberculosis	2%
Miscellaneous	9%
Culture negative	21%

is rare. Vascular bacterial infection is a mycotic process, distinct from arteritis. Patients usually present with pain related to the infected vessel, persistent bacteremia, fever, and malaise. As the infection progresses, the vessel wall is digested, resulting in a mycotic aneurysm. This is in fact an unstable pseudoaneurysm, as the native vessel wall no longer exists, and the inflammatory process is ongoing. Mycotic aneurysms tend to be located in unusual locations, and have a wild, multilobulated appearance (Fig. 1-34). Arteries containing atherosclerotic plaque, preexisting native aneurysms, or prosthetic devices are more prone to infection by hematogenous seeding and direct inoculation than are normal vessels. The organisms that are most often responsible for mycotic aneurysms are skin, oral, and enteric flora (Table 1-15). Over 50% of mycotic aneurysms are found in the lower-extremity peripheral arteries, and one-third in the thoracic and abdominal aorta.

Syphilitic aortitis is a specific variant of vascular infection in which the treponome invades the vasa vasorum of the aorta. There are relatively more vasa vasorum in the ascending than the descending thoracic aorta,

and fewer still in the abdominal aorta. Endarteritis leads to dystrophic calcification and aneurysmal dilatation during the tertiary phase of syphilis in 10% of patients. Ascending thoracic aneurysms are most common, and abdominal aortic involvement is rare. This entity is illustrated in Chapter 9 (see Fig. 9-14).

Infection of prosthetic vascular graft material may present as fever, bacteremia, wound drainage, and pain over the graft. Thrombosis of the graft material, anastomotic pseudoaneurysm, anastomotic rupture, and aortoenteric fistula can occur. Infection of autologous vein grafts is less common, but usually is localized to the surgical anastomosis. Typical organisms include skin flora for peripheral grafts with the addition of bowel

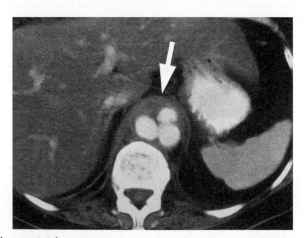

Figure 1-34 Mycotic aneurysm. CT scan with contrast at a level just proximal to the celiac artery origin in a patient with abdominal pain and *Streptococcus* species bacteremia. There is a multilobulated aneurysm with a prominent soft tissue component (arrow) typical of a mycotic aneurysm.

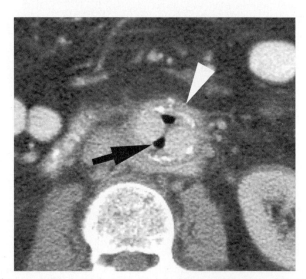

Figure 1-35 Graft infection. Axial image from a CT with contrast of a patient with fever and septicemia several years after aneurysm surgery. There is gas around the limbs of the graft (arrow) within the old aneurysm sac. There is also enhancing soft tissue density (arrowhead) around the aorta.

flora for intraabdominal grafts. At surgery, in addition to obvious signs of sepsis, lack of incorporation of the graft material into surrounding soft tissues is highly suggestive of infection. Imaging findings include perigraft soft tissue inflammatory changes, abscess formation, peri- and intragraft air, anastomotic pseudoaneurysms (frequently multiple), and intraluminal filling defects (Fig. 1-35). Imaging of the immediate postoperative patient can be confusing, but perigraft air should be absorbed within 2-3 weeks of surgery.

INHERITED DISORDERS OF THE ARTERIAL WALL

Marfan syndrome is an inherited disorder that results in vessel wall weakness due to abnormalities of type I collagen and fibrillin. The classic pathologic description is cystic medial necrosis. This autosomal dominant disease has variable penetration, with no gender difference, and is found in approximately 5 per 100,000 people. The clinical diagnosis is based upon family history and skeletal, ocular, and cardiovascular manifestations. The classic patient is tall, thin, with long arms and fingers, pectus deformities, lens subluxation, and a family history of sudden premature death due to rupture of aortic aneurysms. Cardiovascular abnormalities occur in over 95% of patients.

The most common vascular manifestation is dilatation of the ascending aorta that involves the annulus (Fig. 1-36). Aortic regurgitation and mitral valve prolapse are common. Patients with Marfan sydrome are prone to acute aortic dissection and aortic rupture.

Ehlers–Danlos syndrome is less common than Marfan's, occurring in 1 per 150,000 people. The classic patient has hyperflexible joints and elastic skin ("rubber man syndrome"). The basic defect is an abnormality in type III collagen. There are at least 12 subtypes, each with different genetic and clinical characteristics. Vascular complications, which are rare overall in this disease, are usually found in patients with type IV. However, 40% of patients with this form of Ehlers–Danlos syndrome develop vascular complications. Patients with type IV syndrome lack the typical joint and cutaneous laxity, so may be unaware of their diagnosis. Easy bruisability, and a history of spontaneous bowel perforation, splenic rupture, or pneumothorax may be present. Spontaneous dissection, aneurysm formation, and vessel rupture are the most common vascular symptoms (Fig. 1-37). Conventional angiography has an almost 70% major complication rate (dissection, rupture, major access-site bleeding) because of the abnormal arterial wall; it should be avoided when possible.

IMPINGEMENT SYNDROMES

Intermittent positional compression of a vascular structure (i.e. impingement syndrome) can be due to congenital or acquired abnormalities of form or function.

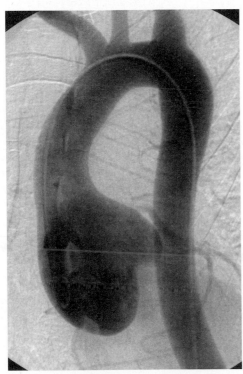

Figure 1-36   Marfan syndrome in an 18-year-old male. DSA of the thoracic aorta in the left anterior oblique projection shows dilatation of the aortic root with loss of the sinotubular ridge.

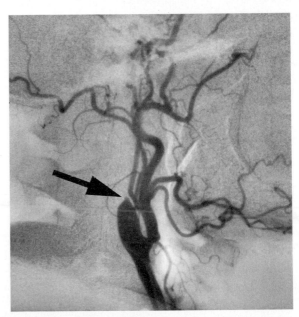

Figure 1-37   Ehlers–Danlos type IV in a 45-year-old female. This carotid angiogram shows occlusion of the internal carotid artery (arrow) due to spontaneous dissection.

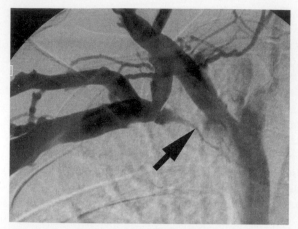

Figure 1-38 Subclavian venous stenosis in thoracic outlet syndrome. Right upper-extremity digital subtraction venogram in a 30-year-old right-handed waiter. There is severe stenosis (arrow) of the right subclavian vein at the junction with the right internal jugular vein, with enlarged collateral drainage to the external jugular vein.

These abnormalities include anomalous or hypertrophied muscles or bones, anomalous locations of vessels, and benign bony lesions such as osteochondromas. Prosthetic vascular grafts tunneled through normal muscular structures or across joints can also be subject to positional compression. Impingement syndromes are a type of repetitive trauma that result in predictable vascular lesions. In general, chronic impingement on a vein results in stenosis leading to thrombosis, whereas chronic impingement on an artery results in post-stenotic aneurysm formation with distal embolization of mural thrombus and ultimately thrombosis (Figs. 1-38 and 1-39). The two most common arterial clinical syndromes involve the subclavian artery ("thoracic outlet syndrome") and the popliteal artery ("popliteal artery entrapment;" see Fig. 15-34). The most common venous

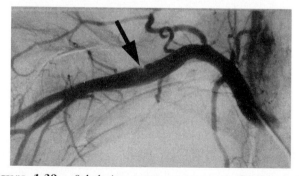

Figure 1-39 Subclavian artery aneurysm in thoracic outlet syndrome. Subtracted angiogram of the right subclavian artery demonstrates an aneurysm containing a small amount of mural thrombus (arrow). The patient had presented with recurrent embolic episodes to the right hand. The patient has a right cervical rib (not seen on this subtraction image).

Table 1-16	Difference Between Arterial and Venous Impingement Syndromes	
Feature	**Venous**	**Arterial**
Vessel abnormality	Synechia, stenosis, fibrosis	Post-stenotic aneurysm
Clinical symptoms	Limb swelling, fullness	Numbness, claudication
Complication	Thrombosis	Distal embolization, thrombosis
Treatment	Thrombolysis, decompression, anticoagulation, angioplasty/stent	± thrombolysis, decompression, surgical bypass, embolectomy

syndromes involve the subclavian vein "Paget–Schroetter" or "effort thrombosis"), and the left common iliac vein ("May–Thürner syndrome;" see Fig.16-19). These specific entities are discussed in detail in later chapters. The clinical presentation of arterial and venous impingement syndromes differ (Table 1-16). Angiographic evaluation should always include views with limbs in a position that reproduce the patient's symptoms.

ADVENTITIAL CYSTIC DISEASE

Adventitial cysitic disease is a focal arterial disorder (although affected veins have been reported) in which localized accumulations of intramural fluid compress the arterial lumen. This is a disorder of young males (male to female ratio 5:1), that is always found near a joint, usually the knee. Adventital cystic disease has also been reported in the external iliac, radial, ulnar, brachial, and common femoral arteries. This rare disorder results in fewer than 0.1% of cases of peripheral arterial occlusive disease, but should be considered in any young male presenting with claudication. The etiology is unknown, but believed to be inclusion of mucin-secreting synovial-like cells in the adventitia during fetal development. The characteristic angiographic appearance is a fixed extrinsic compression of the arterial lumen (Fig. 1-40). The only definitive treatment is surgical excision.

MONCKEBERG SCLEROSIS

Monckeberg sclerosis is medial calcification of medium and small muscular arteries in association with diabetes and renal failure. Atherosclerotic calcification is different in location and distribution, occurring in intimal plaque and involving arteries of all sizes.

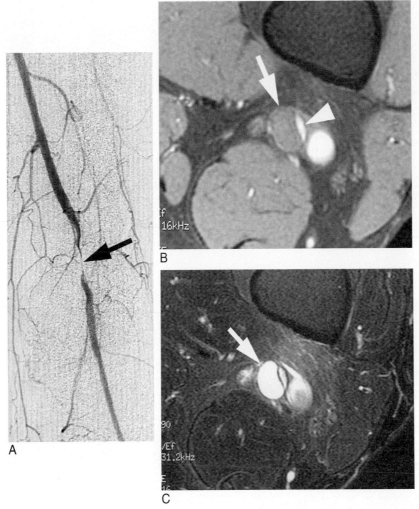

Figure 1-40   Adventitial cystic disease in a 55-year-old female with left leg claudication. **A**, Digital subtraction angiogram demonstrates focal stenosis of the popliteal artery. The lumen appears compressed by a mass rather than narrowed by intraluminal plaque. **B**, Axial T1 weighted image with gadolinium and fat suppression shows an arterial lumen (arrowhead) compressed by a mass (arrow) in the wall of the artery. The adjacent popliteal vein is normal. **C**, Axial T2 weighted image at the same level shows that the mass contains fluid (bright on T2). (Case provided by Philip Rogoff MD and Ralph Reichle MD, Mount Auburn Hospital, Cambridge, MA.)

Monckeberg sclerosis is not an obstructive process. The circumferentially calcified vessels are readily visible on plain radiographs (Fig. 1-41).

THROMBOSIS

The formation of thrombus is a normal process, essential for maintaining life (Fig. 1-42). Two pathways are recognized, intrinsic and extrinsic, which converge when factor X is activated. The intrinsic pathway is activated by contact with platelets, whereas the extrinsic pathway is activated by contact with extravascular tissues. When a vascular injury occurs, platelets become activated when the collagen in the vessel wall is exposed. Platelets adhere to the site of injury, and initiate a process of continued platelet aggregation and fibrin formation that results in a hemostatic plug.

Derangements of thrombosis result in either hypercoagulable or hemorrhagic states. Certain predisposing clinical situations for clotting disorders have been recognized. Stasis, vascular injury, and a hypercoagulable state have been associated with vascular thrombosis for over 100 years ("Virchow's triad"). A clinical example would be a patient with metastatic malignancy at bedrest who undergoes central venous line placement with subsequent subclavian vein thrombosis. A number of hypercoaguable states have been identified (Table 1-17).

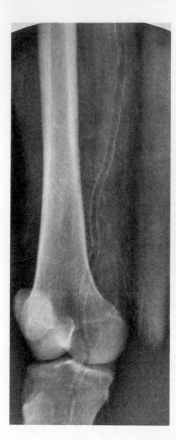

Figure 1-41 Monckeberg sclerosis. Digital image of the right thigh of a patient with diabetes and renal failure. The distal superficial femoral, popliteal, and several muscular arteries are well visualized owing to diffuse medial calcification. The patient has a normal popliteal pulse.

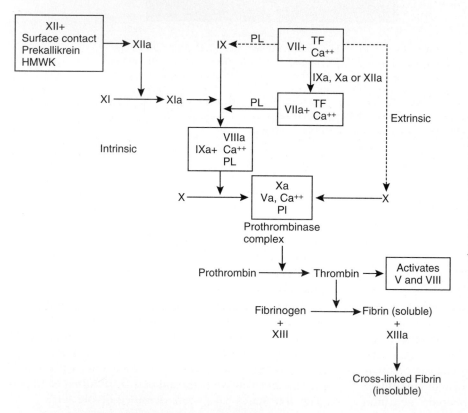

Figure 1-42 Two pathways of coagulation. The intrinsic pathway is initiated by surface contact, whereas the extrinsic pathway is triggered by release of tissue factor (TF). Phospholipid (PL) is found on activated platelets and endothelial membranes. HMWK = high-molecular-weight kininogen. (Reproduced with permission from Calaitges JG, Silver D: Principles of hemostasis. In Rutherford RB ed.: *Vascular Surgery*, 5th edn, WB Saunders, Philadelphia, 2000.)

Table 1-17   Hypercoagulable States

Condition	Mechanism	Clinical Presentation
Heparin-induced thrombocytopenia (HIT)	Type I: idiosyncratic Type II: IgG and IgM antibodies cause platelet clumping in 3-5% of patients receiving unfractionated heparin	Type I: usually subclinical; Type II: decreased platelet counts, hemorrhage, thrombosis
Antithrombin III deficiency	Failure to inhibit factors Xa, IXa, and XIa	Acute thrombosis; inherited and found in cirrhosis, nephrotic syndrome, disseminated intravascular coagulation (DIC)
Protein C and S deficiencies	Failure to inactivate factors Va, VIIIa, and tPa inhibitor	Acute thrombosis; inherited and associated with surgery, liver disease, adult respiratory distress syndrome
Resistance to activated protein C	Decreased anticoagulant function of factor V	Acute thrombosis; inherited, may be present in 50% of cases of idiopathic deep vein thrombosis
Antiphospholipid syndrome (lupus anticoagulants and anticardiolipin antibodies)	Inhibition of prostacyclin, plasminogen; protein C activation; direct platelet activation	Recurrent thrombosis, especially postoperative

Patients should be suspected of having a hypercoagulable condition when they present with venous thrombosis in unusual locations (sagittal sinus, portal venous system, deep femoral veins), recurrent DVT, and spontaneous arterial thrombosis in the absence of underlying stenosis or embolization. The diagnostic evaluation includes a search for an occult malignancy. Thrombotic complications following vascular interventions are more common in these patients.

In general, thrombus itself is not the pathology, but rather the presenting symptom. Most patients will have an identifiable underlying lesion or syndrome. Treatment of patients with acute arterial or venous thrombosis is directed towards both relief of the occlusion and diagnosis of the predisposing condition.

SUGGESTED READINGS

Abu Rahma AF, Richmond BK, Robinson PA: Etiology of peripheral arterial thromboembolism in young patients. *Am J Surg* 176:158-161, 1998.

Atalay MK, Bluemke DA: Magnetic resonance imaging of large vessel vasculitis. *Curr Opin Rheumatol* 13:41-47, 2001.

Austin OM, Redmond HP, Burke PE et al: Vascular trauma—a review. *J Am Coll Surg* 181:91-108, 1995.

Begelman SM, Olin JW: Fibromuscular dysplasia. *Curr Opin Rheumatol* 12:41-47, 2000.

Bauters C, Isner JM: The biology of restenosis. *Prog Cardiovasc Dis* 40:107-116, 1997.

Bergqvist D: Ehlers-Danlos type IV syndrome: a review from a vascular surgical point of view. *Eur J Surg* 162:163-170, 1996.

Calligaro KD, Ahmad S, Dandora R et al: Venous aneurysms: surgical indications and review of the literature. *Surgery* 117:1-6, 1995.

Caps MT: The epidemiology of vascular trauma. *Semin Vasc Surg* 11:227-231, 1998.

Coady MA, Rizzo JA, Goldstein LJ et al: Natural history, pathogenesis, and etiology of thoracic aortic aneurysms and dissections. *Cardiol Clin* 17:615-635, 1999.

Consigny PM: Pathogenesis of atherosclerosis. *Am J Roentgenol* 164:553-558, 1995.

Davies MG, Hagen PO: Pathobiology of intimal hyperplasia. *Br J Surg* 81:1254-1269, 1994.

Donnelly LF, Adams DM, Bisset GS: Vascular malformations and hemangiomas: a practical approach in a multidisciplinary clinic. *Am J Roentgenol* 174:597-608, 2000.

Epstein SE, Zhou YF, Zhu J: Infection and atherosclerosis: emerging mechanistic paradigms. *Circulation* 100:20-28, 1999.

Ernst CB, Stanley JC eds: *Current Therapy in Vascular Surgery*, 4th edn, Mosby, St Louis, 2001.

Gersony WM: Diagnosis and management of Kawasaki disease. *JAMA* 265:2699-2703, 1991.

Green RM: Vascular manifestations of the thoracic outlet syndrome. *Semin Vasc Surg* 11:67-76, 1998.

Halloran BG, Baxter BT: Pathogenesis of aneurysms. *Semin Vasc Surg* 8:85-92, 1995.

Hellmann DB: Immunopathogenesis, diagnosis, and treatment of giant cell arteritis, temporal arteritis, polymyalgia rheumatica, and Takayasu's arteritis. *Curr Opin Rheumatol* 5:25-32, 1993.

Hertzer NR: The natural history of peripheral vascular disease: implications for its management. *Circulation* 83(2 Suppl): I12-I19, 1991.

Kadir, S: *Diagnostic Angiography*, WB Saunders, Philadelphia, 1986.

Ledbetter S, Stuk JL, Kaufman JA: Helical (spiral) CT in the evaluation of emergent thoracic aortic syndromes: traumatic aortic rupture, aortic aneurysm, aortic dissection, intramural hematoma, and penetrating atherosclerotic ulcer. *Radiol Clin North Am* 37:575-589, 1999.

Mas JL: Diagnosis and management of paradoxical embolism and patent formen ovale. *Curr Opin Cardiol* 11:519-524, 1996.

Mulliken JB, Fishman SJ, Burrows PE: Vascular anomalies. *Curr Probl Surg* 37:517-584, 2000.

Orton DF, Le Veen RF, Saigh JA et al: Aortic prosthetic graft infections: radiologic manifestations and implications for management. *Radiographics* 20:977-993, 2000.

Pasic M: Mycotic aneurysm of the aorta: evolving surgical concept. *Ann Thorac Surg* 61:1053-1054, 1996.

Roseborough GS, Williams GM: Marfan and other connective tissue disorders: conservative and surgical considerations. *Semin Vasc Surg* 13:272-282, 2000.

Rutherford, RB ed.: *Vascular Surgery*, 5th edn, WB Saunders, Philadelphia, 2000.

Salvarani C, Cantini F, Boiardi L et al: Polymyalgia rheumatic and giant cell arteritis. *N Engl J Med* 347:261-271, 2002.

Strandness ED, Breda AV eds: *Vascular Diseases: Surgical and Interventional Therapy*, Churchill Livingstone, New York, 1994.

Tunaci A, Berkmen YM, Gokmen E: Thoracic involvement in Behçet's disease: pathologic, clinical, and imaging features. *Am J Roentgenol* 164:51-56, 1995.

Wigley FM, Flavahan NA: Raynaud's phenomenon. *Rheum Dis Clin North Am* 22:765-781, 1996.

Wojtowycz M: Handbook of Interventional Radiology and Angiography, Mosby, St Louis, 1995.

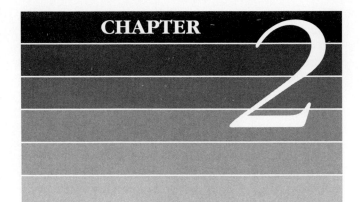

CHAPTER 2

Fundamentals of Angiography

JOHN A. KAUFMAN, M.D.

The development of modern angiography was enabled by one simple technique: the percutaneous introduction of devices into a blood vessel over a wire guide (Fig. 2-1). Described by Sven Ivan Seldinger in 1953, this elegant innovation (now known by Seldinger's name) eliminated the need for surgical exposure of a blood vessel prior to catheterization, thus allowing the transfer of angiography from the operating room to the radiology department. Virtually all vascular and many nonvascular invasive procedures are performed with Seldinger's technique.

PREPROCEDURE PATIENT EVALUATION AND MANAGEMENT

Knowledge empowers, and in interventional radiology it is the difference between unthinking completion of an assigned task and meaningful participation in the care of a patient. The interventional radiologist should not only be skilled with a catheter, but a specialist in vascular diseases. Every angiogram begins with introduction of oneself to the patient, determination of the appropriateness of the examination, and formulation of a procedural plan. Ideally, the person performing the procedure will have seen the patient previously in consultation and, in many cases, have assumed primary responsibility for management of the vascular disease. When this is not the case, the evaluation begins with a review of the requested examination: Are the diagnostic questions and the information expected from the procedure clearly understood? Are the different therapeutic options fully understood? A brief, directed history should be obtained. In particular, the symptoms or signs that precipitated the study are

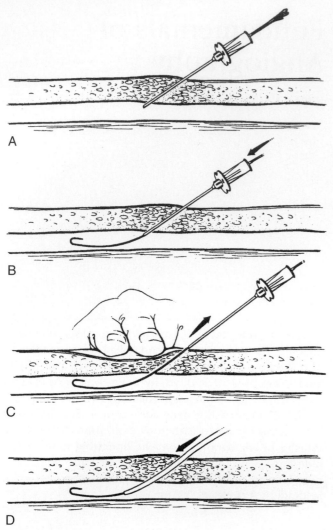

Figure 2-1 Seldinger technique. **A**, Percutaneous puncture of a blood vessel with a hollow needle. **B**, Introduction of an atraumatic guidewire through the needle into the blood vessel lumen. **C**, Needle is removed while guidewire remains in place. Compression over the puncture secures the guidewire and prevents bleeding. **D**, Angiographic catheter is advanced into vessel over the guidewire. (Reproduced with permission from Kadir S: *Diagnostic Angiography*, WB Saunders, Philadelphia, 1986.)

important, as this knowledge may impact the course of the examination and interpretation of the images. Other essential areas to cover in the history include prior surgical procedures (especially vascular); evidence of atherosclerotic disease in "index" vascular beds such as prior myocardial infarction or stroke; diabetes, with attention to medications; status of renal function; allergies; and known previous exposure to iodinated contrast agents. When available, office records or the patient's chart should be reviewed for similar information. Operative notes and reports from previous angiograms provide valuable information that may alter the entire approach to the procedure. Above all, personal review of old angiograms

or correlative imaging is essential before embarking upon an invasive procedure.

The immediate preprocedural physical examination is focused on the status of the vascular system and selection of a vascular access site. This examination should be conducted by the person who will perform the angiogram. The strength of the pulses, and the presence of an aneurysm (as suggested by a broad, prominent pulse) should be recorded using a consistent system. Cellulitis, fresh surgical incisions, a large abdominal pannus, or a scar over the vessel all impact selection of a puncture site. Pulses distal to the anticipated puncture site must be evaluated, as one of the potential complications of angiography is distal embolization. Furthermore, if an intervention is performed, this baseline information is very useful to help determine procedural endpoints. The physical examination should include both sides of the patient so that a different access site can be used during the procedure if necessary. When an upper-extremity approach is anticipated, blood pressures in both arms must be obtained.

Evidence of vascular disease such as trophic skin changes, hair loss, skin temperature, dependent rubor, the rapidity of capillary refill, ulceration, and gangrene should be noted. Classification systems for acute and chronic ischemia have been devised, which serve to decrease ambiguity when describing a patient, have prognostic implications, and allow assessment of outcomes of interventions (see Tables 15-4 and 15-10).

Whenever possible, patients should be well hydrated prior to the procedure. Outpatients should not be instructed to fast after midnight, but rather encouraged to drink clear liquids until 2 hours prior to their scheduled appointment. At the hospital an intravenous infusion of D5/0.5NS should be begun at 100 mL/h. Inpatients should stop solid food 6 hours prior to the procedure, but can be given clear liquids until 2 hours before. Inpatients should have an established intravenous infusion before arriving in the angiographic suite. Most hospitals have established guidelines for oral intake prior to invasive procedures; these must be followed, but remember that they are generally not designed for patients about to receive large doses of nephrotoxic contrast.

There are no laboratory studies that are absolutely mandatory prior to an angiogram, but since the procedure involves puncture of a blood vessel and nephrotoxic contrast, the basics are coagulation studies – international normalized ratio (INR), or prothrombin time (PT), activated prothrombin time (aPTT), and platelet count – and serum creatinine (Cr). Ideally, all patients should have normal laboratory values prior to an angiogram. When necessary, anyone can undergo an angiogram. The problems will not occur until the end of the procedure (See p. 48, "The Arterial Puncture: Common Femoral Artery").

When the PT or INR are prolonged, fresh frozen plasma given the day or night before is useless or even dangerous, as an INR drawn just after the plasma has been infused may be normal, but by the time that the procedure is performed the effect will dissipate. An abnormal aPTT is usually due to administration of heparin, which can be turned off when the patient arrives in the angiography suite. Since the half-life of heparin is roughly 60 minutes, most patients will correct sufficiently for manual compression by the end of the procedure.

In the presence of an abnormal serum Cr, the risk of renal failure after the procedure should be weighed against the benefits of the examination. When the serum Cr is ≥ 1.5 mg/dL, nonionic contrast should be used. The patient should be well hydrated before and after the examination. Prophylactic measures should be followed to maximize renal protection (see below, "Contrast Agents").

BASIC SAFETY CONSIDERATIONS

Precautions against exposure to bodily fluids should be applied to all patients, even those with no known risk factors. Masks, face shields or other protective eye-wear, sterile gloves, and impermeable gowns are the minimum. Closed flush and contrast systems minimize the risk of splatter. All materials used during the case should be disposed of in receptacles designed for biological waste.

Needles, scalpels, or any other sharp device used during a case should be carefully stored on the work surface in a red sharps container, or removed immediately after use. Recapping is not advised. The best sharps containers contain a foam block in which the point of the sharp can be imbedded. At the end of the case, it is the responsibility of the physician to dispose of the sharps in the ubiquitous hard red plastic receptacles. Puncture wounds from contaminated sharps are not only painful, but potentially life-altering events. If an accidental splash, puncture, or other exposure occurs, immediate consultation with a physician experienced in management of exposure to occupational biohazards is essential.

Radiation exposure to the patient and the staff should be kept to minimum. Use fluoroscopy only as needed. Prolonged fluoroscopy at high magnification with the x-ray tube in one position has been associated with radiation burns to the patient. Accumulative exposure to physicians can be substantial. Wrap-around lead, thyroid shields, and leaded glasses should be worn. Careful coning of the beam can reduce scatter. The operator's hands should never be visible on the fluoroscope. If a physician must remain at the bedside during filming, portable leaded shields should be positioned between the tube and the physician. Ideally, radiation badges should be worn at all times.

Some interventional radiologists report degenerative neck and back problems over time. Careful design of angiographic suites with attention to positioning of controls and monitors can reduce twisting and bending. Ultra-light protective aprons and other ergonomic innovations may also be helpful.

TOOLS

Access Needles

All angiographic procedures begin with some sort of entry needle. There is great variety in vascular access needles, but all provide a central channel for introduction of a guidewire (Fig. 2-2). Needles with a central sharp stylet that obturate the lumen have a blunted, atraumatic tip when the stylet is removed. The stylet allows the needle to puncture the vessel, but once removed theoretically reduces the risk of trauma. The stylet may be solid or hollow. In the latter case blood can be visualized on the stylet hub once the vessel lumen is entered. The stylet must be removed in order to insert the guidewire. Needles with stylets are generally used only for arterial punctures. Needles without stylets have very sharp beveled tips, a quality that is useful when attempting to puncture small or mobile vessels. As there is no stylet, the guidewire is introduced directly through the needle once the tip is fully within the vessel lumen. This style of needle is used for venous as well as arterial punctures.

The most common sizes for vascular access needles are 18- to 21-gauge in diameter, and $2\frac{1}{4}$ to 5 inches in length.

Guidewires

Guidewires are available in a profusion of thicknesses, lengths, tip configurations, stiffnesses, and materials of construction (Fig. 2-3). In general, the guidewire thickness (always referred to in hundredths of an inch; for example, 0.038 in) should match the diameter of the lumen at the tip of the catheter or device that will slide over it. Guidewires that are too big will jam inside the catheter. However, if a guidewire is much smaller than the hole at the tip of the catheter or device there will be an abrupt blunt transition between the guidewire and the catheter (Fig. 2-4).

The most commonly used type of guidewire has a central stiff core around which is tightly wrapped a smaller wire, just like a coiled spring (Fig. 2-5). The outer wire is welded to the core at the back end, but not at the tip. The purpose of the coiled wrap is to decrease the area of contact between the surface of the guidewire and the tissues. Between the inner core wire and the outer wrap is a fine safety wire that runs along the length of

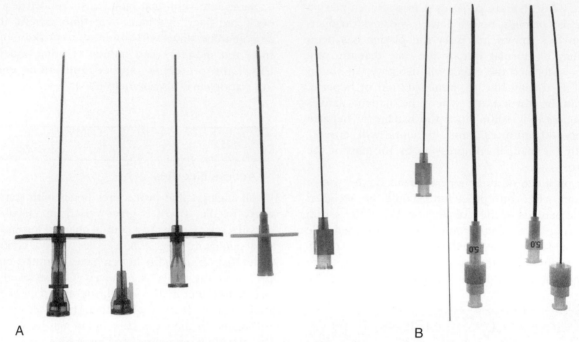

A   B

Figure 2-2 Typical access needles. **A**, *Left to right:* 18-G Seldinger needle with hollow, sharp central stylet that extends beyond the blunt tip of the needle; stylet; Seldinger needle with stylet removed; 18-G sharp hollow ("one-wall") needle; 21-G "microaccess" needle. **B**, Microaccess system. *Left to right:* 21-G needle; 0.018-inch guidewire for insertion through needle; 5-Fr dilator with central 3-Fr dilator tapered to 0.018-inch guidewire; 5-Fr dilator with 3-Fr dilator removed accepts an 0.038-inch guidewire; the 3-Fr dilator.

the guidewire and is welded to the outer wrap at both ends. The safety wire prevents the wrap from unwinding. This is the origin of the term "safety guidewire." The thickness and composition of the inner core determines the degree of guidewire stiffness (Table 2-1). Guidewires that

are very flexible are important for negotiating tortuous or diseased vessels, but stiff guidewires provide the most support for introducing catheters and devices. The ultimate variable-stiffness guidewire is one in which the core can be slid in and out of the spring wrap ("movable core guidewire") as needed. An important variation in guidewire design is the mandril wire, in which the outer wrap is limited to the soft tip of guidewire. This is a common construction for small diameter guidwires, or extra-rigid large-diameter guidewires.

The taper of the core at the leading end of the guidewire determines the softness or "floppiness" of the tip. The length and rate of transition of the taper defines the characteristics of the tip. Bentson guidewires, or movable core guidewires with the core retracted, have the softest tips. For all guidewires, the key point to

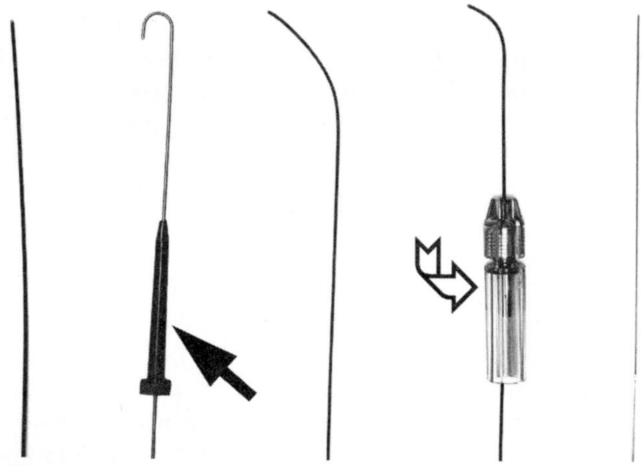

Figure 2-3 Common guidewires. *Left to right:* Straight 0.038-inch; "J"-tipped 0.038-inch with introducer device (arrow) to straighten guidewire during insertion into needle hub; angled high-torque 0.035-inch; angled hydrophilic-coated 0.038-inch nitinol wire with pinvise (curved arrow) for fine control; 0.018-inch platinum-tipped microwire.

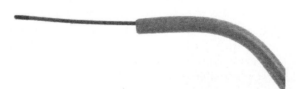

Figure 2-4 Catheter/guidewire mismatch. The catheter is tapered to 0.038 inches, but the guidewire is 0.018 inches in diameter. The tip of the catheter can "hang-up" on vessel wall, plaque, or the ostium of a branch vessel.

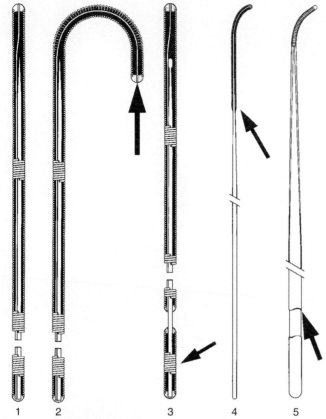

Table 2-1 Guidewire Stiffness

Guidewire	Stiffness
Movable core	0 (when core removed)
Standard 0.035-inch	++
Standard 0.038-inch	+++
Rosen	++++
Amplatz	+++++
Amplatz Super-Stiff	++++++
Lunderquist	++++++++

Figure 2-5 Basic construction of common guidewires. **1 & 2**, The straight and curved safety guidewires are basic tools. These are constructed of an outer coiled spring wrap, central stiffening mandril welded at the back end only, and a small safety wire (arrow) welded on the inside at both ends. **3**, The movable core guidewire, in which the mandril can be slid back and forth and even removed completely to change the stiffness of the wire using a handle incorporated into the back end of the guidewire (arrow). **4**, The low-profile mandril guidewire, in which the soft spring wrap is limited to one end of the guidewire (arrow). The remainder of the guidewire is a plain mandril. **5**, Mandril-guidewire coated with a hydrophilic substance (arrow) that reduces friction and increases ability to select tortuous vessels. (Drawings reproduced with permission from Cook Group Incorporated, Bloomington, IN.)

kink-resistant nitinol-based wires, and microwires are now widely available. These guidewires are the difference between routine success and failure in the most challenging cases. Hydrophilic-coated guidewires are especially useful, as they can easily get into previously inaccessible places. This type of guidewire has a central core that is coated with an outer layer of hydrophilic material (see Fig. 2-5). These guidewires should not be inserted through access needles, as the non-radiopaque coating is easily sheared off by the metal edge at the tip when withdrawn. Also, unless kept moist, hydrophilic guidewires become very sticky. When this happens it is almost impossible to advance a catheter over the guidewire, and easy to inadvertently pull the entire guidewire out of the body during an exchange.

The length of most guidewires used in angiography is 145 cm. In circumstances in which a great deal of guidewire is needed inside the body, or the devices and catheters to be placed over the guidewire are long, an "exchange length" guidewire (260–300 cm) is used. This length is not used for routine cases because the amount of guidewire outside the body is cumbersome and easily contaminated.

remember is that it is the soft end of the guidewire that goes inside the patient.

A curve in the end of the guidewire provides an additional degree of safety in diseased vessels. As the guidewire is advanced, the round presenting part bounces off plaque rather than digging into it. A curve can be added to a straight guidewire by gently drawing the floppy tip across a firm edge (such as a fingernail or closed hemostat), much like curling a ribbon. Tip-deflecting guidewires allow variation in the radius of the curve while in the patient, but these guidewires have stiff tips and should never be advanced beyond the end of the catheter (Fig. 2-6).

Specialty guidewires, such as wires coated with slippery hydrophilic substances, highly torquable guidewires,

Dilators

Vessel dilators are short tapered catheters usually made of a stiffer plastic than diagnostic angiographic catheters (Fig. 2-7). The sole purpose of a dilator is to spread the soft tissues and the wall of the blood vessel in order to make passage of a catheter or device easier. By inserting sequentially larger dilators over a guidewire, a percutaneous puncture with an 18-gauge needle can be increased to any size. Sequential dilatation is important to minimize trauma to the vessel, as small incremental steps in size (1- to 2-French) can be accomplished with much less resistance than for one giant step. The first dilator size after puncture with an 18-gauge access needle should be 5-French. Larger dilators can then be used as needed. Do not dilate a puncture site beyond 50% of the expected diameter of the artery if manual compression is anticipated; as the diameter of the hole in

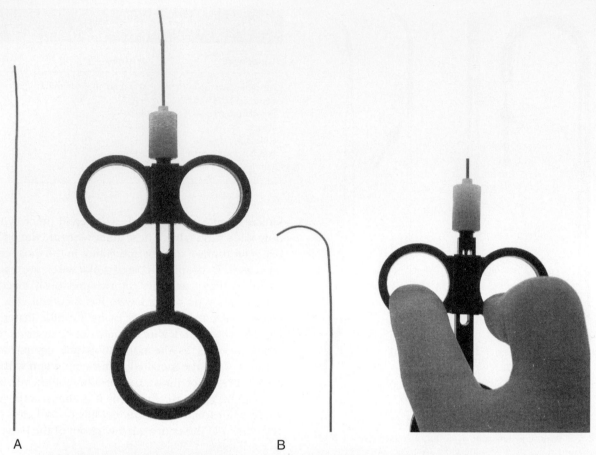

A   B

Figure 2-6   Tip deflecting guidewire. This wire has a stiff tip that is used to direct a catheter. **A,** The guidewire and the preattached handle. **B,** Deflection of the guidewire tip. The deflection is performed inside the catheter lumen. The catheter is then advanced off of the guidewire; the guidewire is never advanced beyond the tip of the catheter.

the artery approaches the diameter of the artery, the puncture becomes a partial transection.

Catheters

Angiographic catheters are made of plastic (polyurethane, polyethylene, Teflon, or Nylon). The exact catheter material, construction, coatings, inner diameter, outer diameter, length, tip shape, and hole configuration

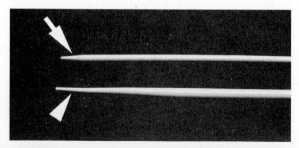

Figure 2-7   Vascular dilators. Standard-taper (arrow) and longer-taper (arrowhead) "Coons" tip. The latter is useful when more gradual dilatation is required.

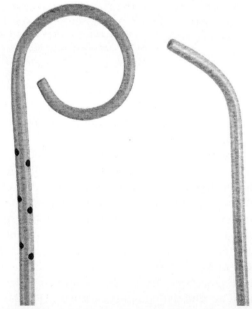

Figure 2-8   Pigtail flush catheter (left) with multiple side-holes. Selective catheter (right) with a single end-hole.

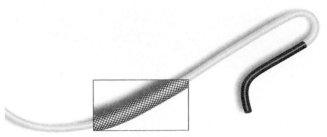

Figure 2-9 Drawing illustrating the fine wire braid in the shaft of a selective catheter. The dark color at the end of the catheter is radiopaque, facilitating visualization of the catheter. (Drawing reproduced with permission from Cook Incorporated, Bloomington, IN.)

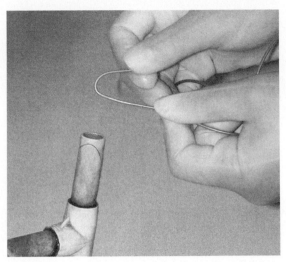

Figure 2-11 Steaming a catheter. The catheter is held in steam for 30–60 seconds, then dunked in cool sterile water to "fix" the new shape.

are determined by the intended use (Fig. 2-8). Catheters for aortography are thick-walled (to handle large-volume high-pressure injections), curled at the tip (the "pigtail", which keeps the end of the catheter away from the vessel wall) with multiple added side-holes proximal to the curl (so that the majority of the contrast exits the catheter in a cloud). Conversely, selective catheters are thinner walled with a single end-hole as injection rates are lower and directed into a small vessel. Precise control of the catheter tip is a top priority. Selective catheters usually have fine metal or plastic strands incorporated into the wall ("braid") so that the tip is responsive to gentle rotation of the shaft (Fig. 2-9).

Catheter outer size is described in French (3-French = 1 mm), while the diameter of the end-hole (and therefore the maximum size guidewire that the catheter will accommodate) is described in hundredths of an inch. The length of the catheter is in centimeters (usually between 65 and 100 cm). The shape of the tip is named for either something that the catheter looks like ("pigtail," "Cobra," "Hockey-stick"), the person who designed it (Simmons, Berenstein, Rösch), or the intended use (celiac, left gastric, internal mammary) (Fig. 2-10). There are so many different catheters that no one department

can or need stock them all. The shape of some catheters may be modified by bending into the desired configuration while heating in steam, and then rapidly dunking in cool sterile water (Fig. 2-11).

Complex catheter shapes must be reformed inside the body after insertion over a guidewire. The catheter will resume its original configuration provided that there is sufficient space within the vessel lumen and memory in the catheter material. Some catheter shapes cannot reform spontaneously, in particular the larger recurved designs such as the Simmons. There are a number of ways to reform these catheters (Figs. 2-12 to 2-16). A recurved configuration can be created from an angled selective catheter by forming a Waltman loop (Fig. 2-17).

Straight and pigtail catheters are generally used for non-selective injections. Straight catheters should be advanced

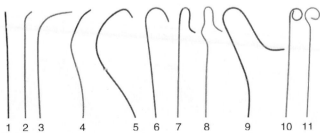

Figure 2-10 Common catheter shapes. **1**, Straight. **2**, Davis (short angled tip). **3**, Multipurpose ("hockey-stick"). **4**, Headhunter (H1). **5**, Cobra-2 (Cobra-1 has a tighter curve, Cobra-3 has a larger and longer curve). **6**, Rösch Celiac. **7**, Visceral (very similar to a Simmons 1-1). **8**, Mickaelson. **9**, Simmons-2. **10**, Pigtail. **11**, Tennis racket.

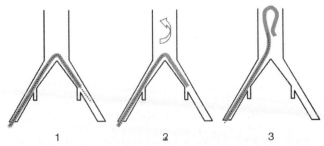

Figure 2-12 Branch technique for reforming a Simmons catheter. **1**, The catheter is advanced into the branch over a guidewire (dashed line). Aortic bifurcation is shown in this illustration. **2**, The guidewire is withdrawn proximal to the origin of the branch but still in the catheter. May also remove guidewire and reinsert stiff end to same point. Catheter is then simultaneously twisted and advanced. **3**, Reformed catheter.

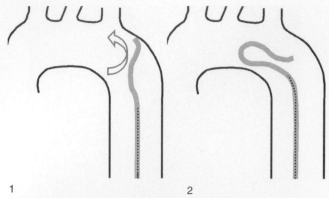

1   2

Figure 2-13   Aortic spin technique for reforming a Simmons catheter. Works best for Simmons 1-1. **1**, The catheter is simultaneously twisted and advanced in the proximal descending thoracic aorta. Note the wire is withdrawn below curved portion of catheter. **2**, Reformed catheter.

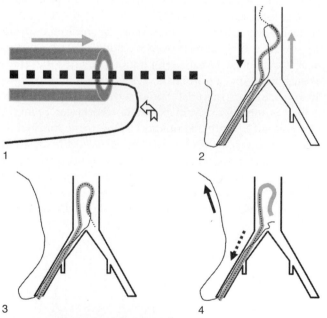

Figure 2-14   Cope string technique, which easily reforms any size Simmons. **1**, Approximately 3–4 cm of 4'0 Tevdek II (Deknatel Inc., Fall River, MA) suture material (curved arrow) has been backloaded into the catheter tip. The catheter is then advanced (arrow) on to floppy-tipped guidewire (dashed line). **2**, The catheter has been advanced over the guidewire into the aorta, with suture material exiting the groin adjacent to the catheter. Floppy portion of guidewire still exits catheter, "locking" suture material in catheter tip. Suture material is pulled gently (black arrow) as slight forward force applied to catheter (grey arrow). **3**, Simmons has been reformed. **4**, Suture removed by first retracting guidewire into catheter (dashed arrow), "unlocking" the suture material. Suture material can then gently be pulled out (black arrow).

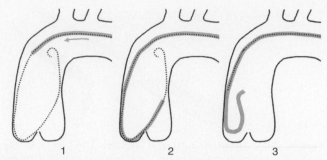

1   2   3

Figure 2-15   Ascending aorta technique for reforming a Simmons catheter. **1**, Floppy-tipped 3-J guidewire reflected off of aortic valve. The catheter is advanced over the guidewire. **2**, The catheter is advanced around a bend in the guidewire. **3**, Retraction of guidewire completes reformation.

over a guidewire; pigtail catheters can be safely advanced in normal vessels once the pigtail has reformed. Choosing a catheter shape for selection of a particular vessel is based upon anatomy (Fig. 2-18). The technique for selection varies with the type of catheter (Figs. 2-19 and 2-20). The Waltman loop is particularly useful in the pelvis for selection of branches of the internal iliac artery on the same side as the arterial puncture.

Catheters that are specially designed to fit coaxially within the lumen of a standard angiographic catheter (3-French smaller outer diameter) are termed "microcatheters" (Fig. 2-21). These soft, flexible catheters are 2- to 3-French in diameter, with 0.010- to 0.027-inch inner lumens. They are designed to reach beyond standard catheters in small or tortuous vessels. The ability to reliably select these vessels without creating spasm, dissection, or thrombosis has allowed certain subspecialties (such as neurointerventional radiology) to flourish. To use a microcatheter, a standard angiographic catheter that accepts a 0.038- or 0.035-inch guidewire is placed securely in a proximal position in the blood vessel. The microcatheter is then advanced in conjunction with a specially designed 0.010- to 0.025-inch guidewire

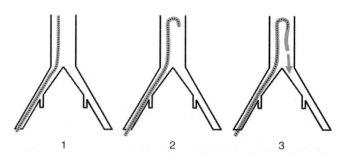

1   2   3

Figure 2-16   Deflecting wire technique (unsafe in small or diseased aortas). **1**, Deflecting wire is positioned near tip of catheter. **2**, Wire deflected, curving the catheter as well. **3**, With the guidewire fixed, the catheter is advanced (arrow) to reform Simmons.

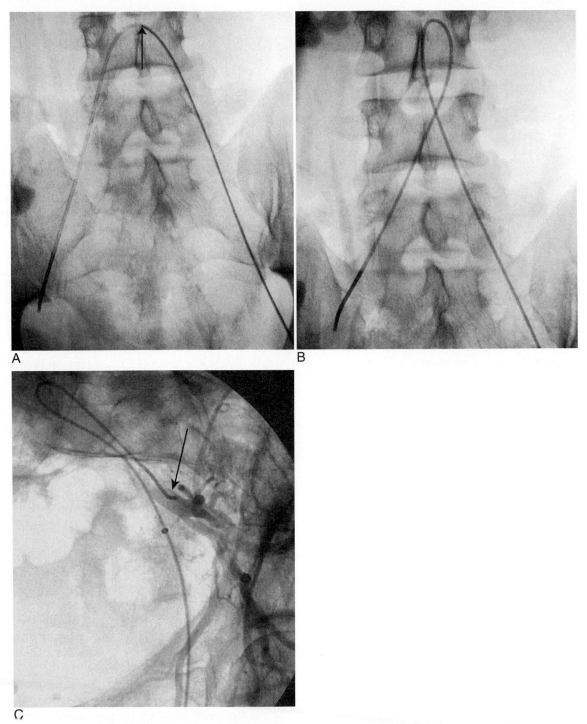

Figure 2-17   The Waltman loop, which can be formed in any major aortic branch vessel with braided selective catheters. **A,** An angled catheter positioned over the aortic bifurcation. Note the stiff end of the guidewire at catheter apex (arrow). **B,** The catheter is advanced and twisted, forming the loop. **C,** Looped catheter has been used to select the ipsilateral internal iliac artery (arrow).

through the standard catheter lumen. Once a super-selective position has been achieved with the micro-catheter, a variety of procedures can be performed such as embolization, sampling, or low-volume angiography. The high resistance to flow in the small lumen prevents

the use of microcatheters for routine angiography. Contrast and flush solutions are most easily injected through these catheters with 5-mL or smaller Luer-lock syringes.

Large guiding catheters may be used in some situations for positioning and stabilizing standard catheters.

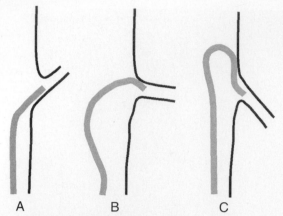

Figure 2-18   Choosing a selective catheter shape. **A**, Angled catheter when angle of axis of branch vessel from aortic axis is low. **B**, Curved catheter (such as Cobra-2 or Celiac) when angle of axis of branch vessel is between 60 and 120 degrees. **C**, Recurved catheter (such as Sos or Simmons) when angle of axis of branch vessel from aorta is great.

These nontapered catheters have extra large lumens and a simple shape that accepts standard sized catheters and devices (Fig. 2-22). There are many circumstances in which standard catheters are difficult to position selectively, such as a renal artery that arises from a tortuous or aneurysmal abdominal aorta. In this situation, a larger outer catheter that can guide the standard catheter

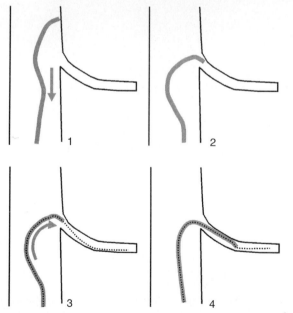

Figure 2-19   How to use a Cobra catheter. **1**, The catheter is advanced to a position proximal to the branch over the guidewire, then pulled down (arrow). **2**, The catheter tip engages the orifice of the branch. Contrast is injected gently to confirm location. **3**, Soft-tipped selective guidewire has been advanced into branch. The guidewire is held firmly and the catheter advanced (arrow). **4**, Catheter in selected position.

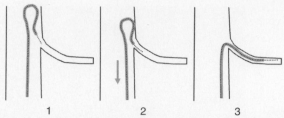

Figure 2-20   How to use a Simmons catheter. **1**, The catheter is positioned above the branch vessel with at least 1 cm of floppy straight guidewire beyond the catheter tip. **2**, The catheter is gently pulled down (arrow) until the guidewire and tip engage the orifice of the branch. **3**, Continued gentle traction results in deeper placement of catheter tip. To deselect branch, push catheter back into aorta (reverse steps 1–3). To unform the Simmons, apply continued traction after step 3.

towards the renal artery and prevent it from floundering around in the aneurysm sack is very helpful. Guiding catheters are usually shorter than standard angiographic catheters, and frequently have a radiopaque band at the tip.

Be aware that guiding catheter size in French refers to the *outer*, not the inner diameter. The inner diameter is usually described in hundredths of an inch, which must be converted to French to determine whether a standard catheter will fit (1-French = 0.012 in = 0.333 mm).

Sheaths

Most vascular interventions and many diagnostic procedures are performed through vascular access sheaths. These devices are plastic tubes of varying thickness and construction that are open at one end and are capped with a hemostatic valve at the other (Fig. 2-23). The open end is not tapered, although the edges are carefully beveled to create a smooth transition to the tapered dilator that is used to introduce the sheath over a guidewire. The valve end usually has a short, flexible, and clear side-arm that can be connected to a constant flush (to prevent thrombus from forming in the sheath) or an arterial pressure monitor. The purpose of the sheath is to simplify multiple catheter exchanges through a single puncture site. When not using a sheath, it is unwise to downsize catheters during a procedure owing to the risk of bleeding around the smaller diameter catheter. Perhaps more important, devices that are irregular in contour or even untapered can be introduced through a sheath without fear of trauma to the device or the puncture site. Long sheaths can also be used to straighten a tortuous access artery. By convention, sheaths are described by the maximum size, in French, that will fit through the sheath. Since the walls of the sheath have some thickness, this means that the actual hole in the artery is 1.5- to 2-French *larger* than the sheath "size"!

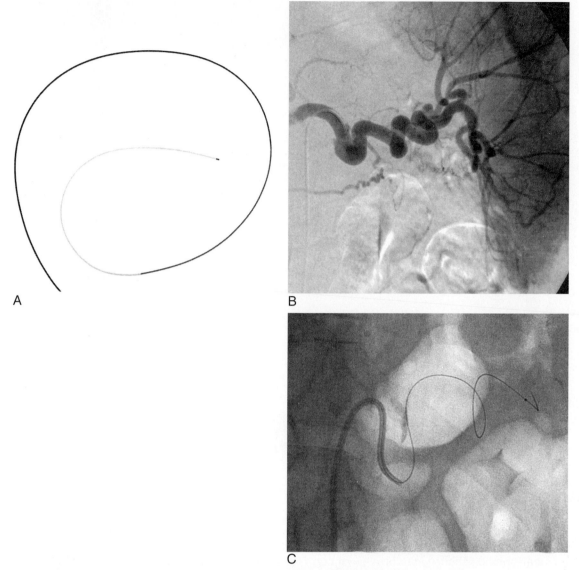

Figure 2-21   Use of a microcatheter. **A**, Typical microcatheter that tapers from 3-Fr proximally to 2.3-Fr at the tip. Note radiopaque marker at the tip. **B**, Extremely tortuous splenic artery in a patient with hypersplenism. **C**, Microcatheter has been advanced over a 0.018-inch guidewire into the distal splenic artery through a 6.5-Fr Simmons-1 catheter.

Sheaths are available in a variety of lengths, depending on the requirements of the procedure.

A useful variant is the peel-away sheath (Fig. 2-24). This device is similar in construction to a regular sheath except that the end outside of the body terminates in two plastic wings instead of a hemostatic valve. The sheath is introduced over a guidewire with a tapered plastic dilator that completely fills the lumen. Once in position, this dilator is removed. The only way to achieve hemostasis is to block the open end of the sheath with a finger, or to clamp the sheath. After inserting a device or catheter through the sheath, the plastic wings are pulled in opposite directions parallel to the skin. This "breaks" the sheath into two long strips of plastic and allows complete disengagement from the catheter without having to slide off the back end. The primary disadvantage of a peel-away sheath is that it is not hemostatic.

Contrast Agents

All of the tools described above have a single purpose, to facilitate the delivery of a contrast agent into the vascular system. The development of safe and well-tolerated contrast agents was as important to angiography as the Seldinger technique. The ideal contrast agent has excellent radiopacity, mixes well with blood, is easy to use, and does not harm the patient. Iodinated contrast agents (which are all currently based upon benzene rings with

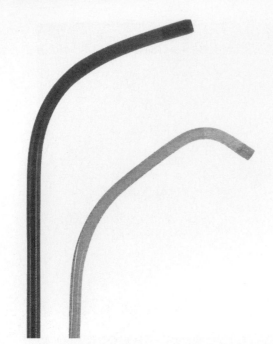

Figure 2-22 Two examples of nontapered large diameter guide catheters which can accommodate standard 5-Fr catheters. French size of guide catheters refers to the *outer* diameter.

three bound iodine atoms, termed "tri-iodinated") turn out to be as close to ideal as currently possible.

There are two major classes of tri-iodinated contrast agents: ionic and nonionic (Table 2-2). Ionic contrast agents are bound to a non-radiopaque cation, usually sodium and meglumine (N-methylglucamine), but also sometimes magnesium and calcium. This results in a highly soluble, low-viscosity, but high osmolar (two particles per iodinated ring) contrast agent. High osmolality relative to a patient's blood is believed to be a major contributing factor to adverse reactions to contrast agents. Nonionic contrast agents have no electrical charge, so cations are not necessary. This reduces the osmolality of the contrast agent (one particle per iodinated ring), which improves the safety profile, but increases viscosity. The two major classes of contrast agents are further subdivided as either monomeric (one tri-iodinated

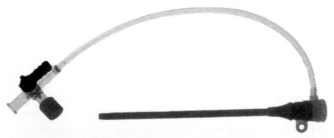

Figure 2-23 Typical hemostatic sheath. French size of sheaths refers to the *inner* diameter.

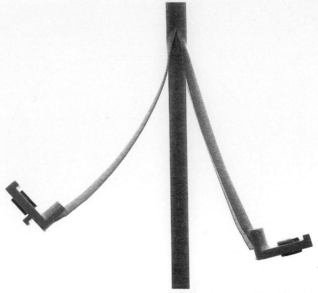

Figure 2-24 Peel-away sheath. To peel the sheath away, wings are pulled in opposite directions at 90 degrees from the catheter shaft.

benzene ring) or dimeric (two linked tri-iodinated benzene rings).

Adverse reactions to iodinated contrast agents are distressingly common, but the majority are minor, such as pain or nausea (Table 2-3). Most of the minor complications are linked to the osmolality of the contrast, so that the overall incidence is lower with nonionic contrast agents. Complications such as nausea and emesis, believed to be related to a central nervous system mechanism, are more frequent with venous than arterial injections.

The two major adverse reactions to iodinated contrast agents are anaphylaxis and renal failure. True anaphylaxis is distinguished from a vasovagal response by tachycardia and respiratory distress (Table 2-4). The incidence of life-threatening anaphylaxis due to iodinated contrast is approximately 1 per 40,000 to 170,000, with mild reactions such as urticaria and nasal stuffiness occurring more commonly (especially with ionic contrast). Contrast reactions must be treated promptly and aggressively. Keep in mind that the most common cause of death is airway obstruction (Boxes 2-1 to 2-3). The patient with a history of prior contrast allergy should receive steroid prophylaxis beginning at least 12 hours prior to the procedure (unless a true emergency exists) (Box 2-4). Patients may label many symptoms experienced during prior contrast injections as "allergy," such as nausea, vagal-nerve mediated bradycardia and hypotension, or ischemic cardiac events. Whenever the precise nature of the "allergic" reaction cannot be determined from the history, steroid prophylaxis is prudent. Nonionic contrast should be used throughout the procedure in any patient with a history of contrast allergy.

Table 2-2   Contrast Agents

Class of Contrast Agent	Contrast Agent	Commercial Names	Iodine Atoms per Molecule	Approximate Osmolality[a] (300 mg I/mL concentration)
Ionic monomer	Diatrizoate	Hypaque, Renograffin	3	1500–1700
	Iothalamate	Conray		
Nonionic monomer	Iopamidol	Isovue	3	600–700
	Iohexol	Ominpaque		
	Ioversol	Optiray		
	Ioxilan	Oxilan		
	Iopromide	Optivist		
Ionic dimer	Ioxaglate	Hexabrix	6	560
Nonionic dimer	Iodixanol	Visipaque	6	300

[a]mOsm/kg water.

Table 2-3   Contrast Reactions: Reported Rates

Reaction	Incidence Ionic Contrast	Incidence Nonionic Contrast
Nausea	4.6%	1%
Vomiting	1.8%	0.4%
Itching	3.0%	0.5%
Urticaria	3.2%	0.5%
Sneezing	1.7%	0.2%
Dyspnea	0.2%	0.04%
Hypotension	0.1%	0.01%
Sialadenitis	<0.1%	<0.1%
Death	1:40,000	1:170,000

Table 2-4   Anaphylaxis versus Vasovagal Reaction

Feature	Anaphylaxis	Vasovagal
Blood pressure	Low	Low
Pulse	Fast	Slow
Breathing	Labored, wheezes	Normal
Skin	Flushed, urticaria	Cool, clammy

Box 2-1   Treatment of Vasovagal Reactions

Lay patient down
Elevate legs
Intravenous fluid bolus (300–500 mL normal saline)
Atropine 1 mg intravenous push (note: doses less than 0.5 mg may worsen bradycardia)

Box 2-2   Treatment of Mild Contrast Reactions

Assess airway, administer 100% oxygen
Secure intravenous access
Obtain vital signs
Benadryl 50 mg intravenously
Hydrocortisone 100 mg intravenously
Observe patient for 4 hours
For mild bronchospasm:
- Albuterol 0.5 mL (2.5 mg) or metaproterenol 0.3 mL (15 mg) in 2.5 mL normal saline, inhalation nebulizer; or:
- Epinephrine (1:1000) 0.3 mL subcutaneously, repeated every 20 minutes as necessary

Box 2-3   Treatment of Severe Anaphylaxis

Call a "Code"
Secure an airway (cricothyroidotomy if necessary) and administer 100% oxygen
Secure intravenous access
Epinephrine (1:10,000) 3–5 mL intravenously or via endotracheal tube
Initiate pressor support
Methylprednisolone 125 mg or hydrocortisone 500 mg intravenously
Aggressive fluid resuscitation with normal saline or lactated Ringer's solution
Admit patient to intensive care unit

Box 2-4   Preparation of Patient with Contrast Allergy

Prednisone 50 mg (oral) on night before and morning of procedure (two doses)
Cimetidine 300 mg intravenously upon arrival in angio suite
Benedryl 50 mg intravenously on arrival in angio suite
Use nonionic contrast

Renal failure following administration of iodinated contrast agents is more common in patients with diabetes, preexisiting renal insufficiency (serum creatinine ≥1.5 mg/dL), and multiple myeloma (Box 2-5). The exact mechanism is not known, but the classic presentation is a rise in creatinine 24–48 hours following exposure to contrast, peaking at 72–96 hours. Patients are usually oliguric, but may become anuric. Management is usually expectant, as the creatinine should return to baseline in 7–14 days. However, in patients with severe preexisting renal insufficiency and diabetes, the risk of permanent dialysis may be as high as 15% despite the use of low-osmolar contrast agents and other protective measures (Table 2-5).

Contrast is administered during angiographic procedures by hand or mechanical injection. Injection by hand is useful during the initial stages of the procedure, or for low-volume and low-pressure angiograms of small vessels or through precariously situated catheters. The use of mechanical injectors is necessary for optimal contrast delivery, particularly when large volumes or high flow rates are required. In addition, there is less radiation exposure to the physician when a mechnical injector is used. Catheters are rated for both flow rates (mL/s) and maximum injection pressure in pounds per square inch (psi). This information is provided on the catheter

---

Box 2-5   Risk Factors for Contrast-induced Acute Renal Failure

Serum creatinine ≥1.5 mg/dL
Diabetes mellitus
Dehydration
Nephrotoxic medications
Age >60 years
Longstanding hypertension
Cardiovascular disease
Multiple myeloma
Hyperuricemia
High-osmolar contrast
Large volume of contrast in short period of time
Recent exposure to large contrast load

Table 2-5   Preventative Measures for Contrast-induced Acute Renal Failure

Agent	Protocol
Hydration	1 mL/kg D_5W for 12 hours prior to procedure; 0.5 mL/kg D_5W for 12 hours post procedure
Fenoldopam	*Low dose:* Begin infusion immediately before procedure at 0.05–0.1/µg/kg/min; maintain at same dose for 3–4 hours post procedure. Stop for decrease in BP systolic <100 mmHg. *High dose:* Start 2 hours prior to procedure and increase 0.1/µg/kg/min every 20 minutes to maximum 0.5/µg/kg/min or decrease in systolic blood pressure (BP) 20 mmHg (maintain systolic BP ≥100 mmHg). Infuse throughout procedure and for 4 hours post procedure. May be stopped abruptly (half-life 5 minutes).
Acetylcysteine	600 mg orally every 12 hours beginning 24 hours before the procedure, including one dose the morning of the angiogram, and one dose the night after the procedure. Total of 4 doses.
Sodium Bicarbonate	Mix 150 mEq $NaHCO_3$/1000 ml D5W. Infuse 3.5 ml/Kg for 1 hour before procedure, then 1.18 ml/Kg/hr for 6 hours post procedure. Check drug compatibilities if using one I.V. line.

---

packaging. Exceeding these limits may result in bursting the catheter (usually at the hub), or premature termination of the injection by the injector software. Careful technique is necessary when connecting a catheter to a power injector to avoid air bubbles, contamination of the catheter, or disconnection during injection (Box 2-6).

Box 2-6   Connecting a Catheter to a Power Injector

Use sterile, clear, high-pressure Luer-lock tubing between injector and catheter
If injecting through a stopcock, be sure that it is high-pressure
Turn injector tubing hub counterclockwise prior to hook-up
Allow back-bleeding from catheter and drip contrast slowly from tubing during connection
Make sure that connection is tight[a]
Withdraw contrast until blood is seen in tubing to exclude air bubbles
Advance contrast slowly to clear blood from catheter
Place sterile towel over connection in case of disconnection during injection

[a]Note that if the patient or injector is moved suddenly, the catheter can be pulled out of position.

Alternative Contrast Agents

The low but real incidence of adverse reactions to iodinated contrast agents has led to the use of alternative contrast agents in selected circumstances, particularly in patients with past histories of true anaphylactic reactions to iodinated contrast, or precarious renal function. Two alternative contrast agents have been described for patients who cannot tolerate iodinated contrast agents: carbon dioxide (CO_2) gas and gadolinium chelates.

Carbon Dioxide Gas

Experience is most extensive with CO_2, which functions as a negative contrast agent (Box 2-7). The gas briefly displaces the blood volume in the lumen of the vessel, resulting in decreased attenuation of the x-ray beam. The digital subtraction technique is therefore essential for diagnostic imaging (Fig. 2-25). The buoyant nature of CO_2 results in preferential filling of anterior structures. The CO_2 gas is highly soluble, and excreted from the lungs. The extremely low viscosity of CO_2 is advantageous for demonstration of subtle bleeding or for wedged hepatic vein portography. CO_2 can be used for abdominal aortography, selective visceral injections, lower-extremity runoffs, as well as most venous studies. For abdomen studies it is helpful to administer intravenous glucagon to decrease bowel peristalsis.

Mechanical injectors for CO_2 are not available in the United States. All injections must therefore be performed by hand (Box 2-8). Because of the invisible nature of gases, scrupulous handling of CO_2 is necessary to prevent contamination by less soluable room air. An additional key technical aspect of CO_2 angiography is to avoid explosive delivery of gas by first purging the ambient liquid in the catheter with a small volume of gas; otherwise tremendous pressure is generated as the gas is compressed behind the column of fluid.

CO_2 is contraindicated for angiography of the thoracic aorta, cerebral arteries, or upper-extremity arteries owing to potential neurological complications. Rarely, CO_2 gas can cause a "vapor lock" in a vessel, which obstructs blood flow and induces distal ischemia. An excessive volume of gas in the heart can obstruct the

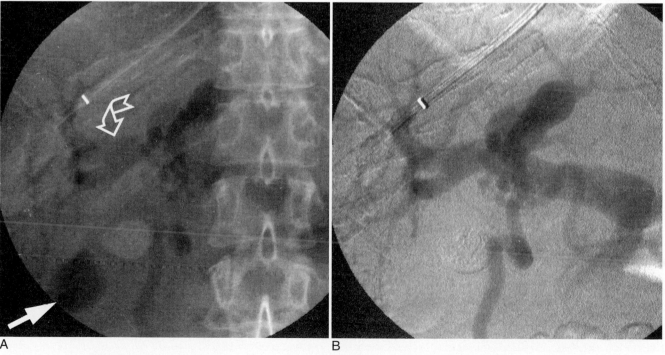

A   B

Figure 2-25 CO_2 portal venogram. **A,** Unsubtracted image from wedged hepatic venogram shows CO_2 filling portal vein (curved arrow). Density of the CO_2 is the same as gas in the bowel (straight arrow). **B,** Digital subtraction of the same frame. Visualization of the portal venous system is excellent.

Box 2-8   Simple Technique for Hand Injection CO_2 Angiography

60-mL Luer-lock syringe containing 10 mL of flush solution, equipped with stopcock

Purge all air from syringe, so that only fluid remains

Attach to purged CO_2 source

Allow 30–40 mL of uncompressed CO_2 gas to enter syringe; use stopcock to control flow

Turn stopcock to "closed" position, disconnect from CO_2 source

Keep tip of syringe pointed down

Attach to catheter while applying gentle positive pressure, ensuring "wet" connection

Purge blood from catheter with small amount of CO_2 gas

Close stopcock

Compress gas with syringe plunger

Initiate digital subtraction angiography

Open stopcock and vigorously inject compressed CO_2

---

pulmonary outflow tract, with severe cardiovascular consequences.

Gadolinium Chelates

Gadolinium chelates were developed as contrast agents for magnetic resonance imaging (MRI). The safety profile of these contrast agents is superior to that of iodinated contrast, and there appears to be lower nephrotoxicity.

There is no cross-reactivity in patients with anaphylaxis to iodinated contrast. Gadolinium has a k-edge of 50 keV, slightly higher than iodine's (33 keV). This permits visualization of gadolinium with current digital subtraction angiographic equipment (Fig. 2-26). Although the approved doses of most gadolinium-based agents are 0.1–0.3 mL/kg, volumes of 40–60 mL have been used for many years without complications and described in peer-reviewed reports. Larger volumes have also been used, but there is little published information to support this practice. Gadolinium-based contrast agents are liquids, so special injection techniques or equipment are not required. Digital subtraction angiography is necessary, as the low gadolinium concentration in the available formulations results in relatively weak opacification of deep arteries. Gadolinium-based contrast agents have been used safely in every vascular application, including carotid and coronary arteries. The main limitations of this alternative contrast are the expense, the small total volume that can be used, and the relatively low radiopacity.

INTRAPROCEDURAL CARE

Sedation

Patients undergoing invasive diagnostic and therapeutic procedures tend to be nervous, apprehensive, and ill. Frequent communication with the members of the

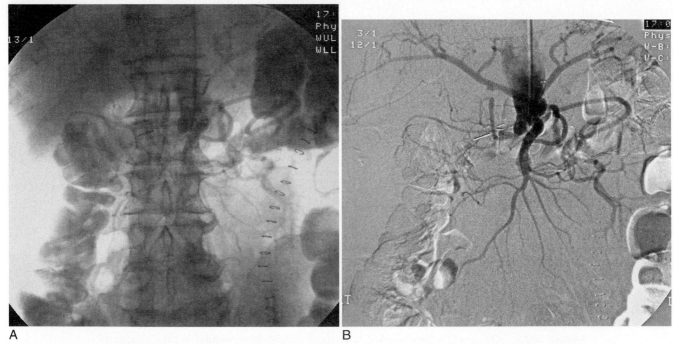

Figure 2-26   Gadolinium digital subtraction angiogram. **A,** Unsubtracted image from aortic injection in a patient with infrarenal aortic occlusion shows weak vascular opacification. **B,** Digital subtraction of the same frame. There is excellent opacification of the visceral vessels.

Table 2-6 Medications for Conscious Sedation

Medication	Type	IV Dose[a]	Duration	Antagonist
Midazolam	Benzodiazepine	0.5–1 mg[b]	30 min	Flumazenil
Diazepam	Benzodiazepine	1–3 mg[b]	6–10 h	Flumazenil
Flumazenil	Benzodiazepine *antagonist*	0.1–0.2 mg[b]	45 min	None
Fentanyl	Opioid	25–50 μg[b]	30–60 min	Naloxone
Morphine	Opioid	1–3 mg[b]	3–4 h	Naloxone
Naloxone	Opioid *antagonist*	0.1–0.2 mg[b]	45 min	None
Droperidol	Antiemetic	0.625–1.25 mg	2–4 h	None
Zofran	Antiemetic	4 mg	4–8 h	None

[a]IV, intravenous dose.
[b]Repeated as necessary until desired affect achieved.

team is greatly reassuring to the patient. Small gestures, such as alerting the patient prior to any step that may be uncomfortable, can reduce anxiety and improve cooperation. Administration of intravenous sedatives (benzodiazepines) and pain medication (opioids) is frequently necessary (Table 2-6). The goal is anxiolysis or moderate sedation, such that the patient remains responsive with spontaneous respiration and an intact gag reflex (Table 2-7). Each facility has established requirements for training of personnel providing sedation and monitoring of these patients. As a rule, blood pressure, heart rate and rhythm, respiration rate, and oxygen saturation should be monitored and recorded at regular intervals throughout the procedure. A reliable venous access is required for administration of medications and possible resuscitation. Ready access to oxygen, suction, and defibrillation equipment is necessary.

Table 2-7 Sedation/Analgesia Levels

Level	Description
Minimal sedation (anxiolysis)	Normal response to verbal commands, normal ventilation and cardiovascular function
Moderate sedation	Depressed consciousness with purposeful response to verbal commands, adequate spontaneous respiration, normal cardiovascular function
Deep sedation	Depressed consciousness, repeated or painful stimulus required for purposeful response, ability to maintain airway and ventilation may be impaired
Anesthesia	Loss of consciousness, ventilatory function often impaired, cardiovascular function may be impaired

Antibiotic Prophylaxis

Angiograms are sterile procedures. Hair at the puncture site should be shaved immediately prior to the procedure. The puncture site is scrubbed with a bactericidal liquid and sometimes painted with an antibacterial iodine solution. Patients with allergies to topical iodine can be painted with an isopropyl alcohol solution. The patient is then covered with sterile drapes so that only the puncture site is accessible. Personnel directly involved in performing the procedure should wear sterile gloves and gown, as well as a hat, mask, and splatter shield. Other personnel can wear scrub clothes, hat, and mask.

Antibiotic prophylaxis is not necessary for the majority of patients undergoing diagnostic angiography. Rare exceptions include asplenic and severely neutropenic patients. Patients with prosthetic heart valves or other indications for endocarditis prophylaxis do not require antibiotics prior to angiography. When indicated, antibiotics appropriate for skin flora should be used, such as cephazolin 1 gm, clindamycin 300 mg, or vancomycin 500 mg.

Blood Pressure Control

Anxious or uncomfortable patients may develop elevated blood pressures prior to or during the procedure. A systolic blood pressure of less than 170 mmHg is desirable to avoid cardiac ischemia in older patients and to facilitate hemostasis at the end of the procedure. In the majority of cases the blood pressure will return to normal once adequate sedation is achieved. When immediate reduction of blood pressure is indicated, or patients do not respond to sedation, pharmacologic intervention is warranted. Nitroprusside and fenoldopam mesylate (Corlapam, Abbott Laboratories, North Chicago, IL) are two intravenous medications that can be used safely in most patients (Table 2-8). When pheochromocytoma is

Table 2-8 Medications for Hypertensive Crisis

Medication	Initial Dose	Titration Schedule[a]	Duration
Nitroprusside	0.5 µg/kg/min[b]	5–10 min to desired BP	1–3 min
Fenoldopam	0.1 µg/kg/min	15 min to desired BP	5–10 min
Phentolamine	1 mg bolus[c]	5 min to desired BP	20–30 min

[a]BP, blood pressure.
[b]Avoid in patients with increased central nervous system pressures.
[c]Adrenergic crisis in patients with pheochromocytoma.

suspected as the cause of the hypertensive crisis, phentolamine, a nonselective α-adrenergic blocker should be used.

Anticoagulation

Anticoagulation during diagnostic peripheral angiography is rarely necessary in adults unless the catheter impedes flow in a diseased or small vessel. Some physicians will routinely administer heparin to patients during selective carotid angiography for occlusive disease. The typical adult dose is a 3000–5000 U intravenous bolus, followed by 1000 U each hour. The effect of the heparin can be monitored by measuring an activated clotting time (ACT), with a target of >250 seconds.

Pediatric Patients

Angiography in pediatric patients requires several modifications of standard techniques. General anesthesia is recommended for any prepubescent child, and for immature adolescents. Pediatric patients younger than 2 years should be routinely anticoagulated with heparin (100 U/kg) as catheter-induced arterial spasm and thrombosis is a risk. Microaccess needles, generous administration of perivascular lidocaine, and smaller catheter systems (4- or 5-French) should be used. Temperature control during long procedures is an important concern in infants. Nonionic contrast should always be used, with a total contrast usage not exceeding 5.0 mL/kg during short procedures in infants and toddlers. The volume of flush and test injections should be limited to 2–3 mL in small children to avoid volume overload. All children with meningomyeloceles should be assumed to be allergic to latex.

THE ARTERIAL PUNCTURE

General Considerations

The patient should be positioned on the angiographic table in such a way as to provide the easiest, most direct access to the puncture site. Patient comfort during procedures is extremely important, but the physician's ability to access the artery, manipulate the catheter, observe the puncture site, and use the table controls during the procedure are paramount. Also, be sure that all tools are nearby before beginning, so that time is not wasted during the procedure looking for something that is needed routinely. Most departments have a standardized sterile angiographic table setup that contains the basic tools necessary to begin an angiogram.

There are a few general guidelines for selecting an arterial access (Box 2-9). The area of interest should be accessible from the artery through which the catheter is introduced. The access artery must be large enough to accommodate diagnostic devices. There should be no critical or fragile organs interposed between the skin and the artery to be accessed. The puncture should be over bone whenever possible so that the vessel can be compressed against something hard at the end of the procedure. The pulse should be readily palpable to facilitate the puncture and the compression. The vessel to be punctured should be as normal as possible; bad arteries beget bad complications. Lastly, the overlying skin should be free of infection, fresh surgical incisions, or any other unpalatable features.

Common Femoral Artery

The common femoral artery (CFA) is the most frequent access site for angiography. The CFA is relatively near the surface of the skin (even in plump individuals), large enough to accommodate standard angiographic

---

Box 2-9 Prerequisites for Peripheral Arterial Access

Patent artery (not necessarily palpable)
Superficial location over bone
Healthy overlying skin
Communicates with artery of interest

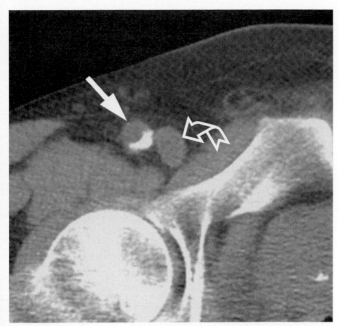

Figure 2-27   Axial CT scan without contrast at the level of the femoral head showing the relationship of the common femoral artery (CFA) (straight arrow) and common femoral vein (CFV) (curved arrow) within the femoral sheath. The femoral nerve (lateral to the CFA) is not seen on this image. Note the proximity of the CFA to the skin and the calcified posterior plaque.

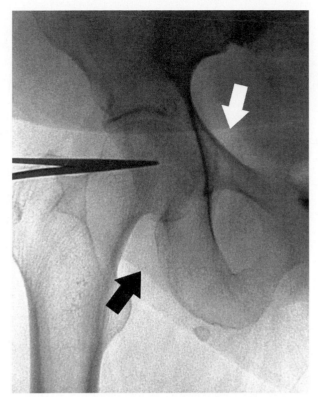

Figure 2-28   Common femoral artery (CFA) puncture in a large individual. After identifying the CFA pulse, a blunt metallic instrument is used for fluoroscopic localization of the desired site of entry into the vessel. The skin nick will be made a few centimeters distal to this point. Note the relationship of the large pannus (white arrow) and inguinal fold (black arrow) to the puncture site.

tools, and easy to compress against the underlying femoral head. Furthermore, the CFA is contained within the femoral sheath, which helps to limit peripuncture bleeding (Fig. 2-27).

The majority of CFA punctures are retrograde (against arterial blood flow) as opposed to antegrade (in the direction of arterial blood flow). Regardless of the approach, the CFA should be accessed over the middle or lower third of the femoral head to facilitate compression at the termination of the procedure. The artery is first localized by palpation. The course of the artery under the skin and the point of maximum impulse is determined. In large or elderly patients the inguinal crease cannot be relied upon to localize the common femoral artery, as it may shift downwards over the superficial femoral artery. A blunt metal instrument can then be placed on the skin at the anticipated point of access and fluoroscoped to determine its relationship to the femoral head (Fig. 2-28). The entry site in the skin should be 1–2 cm below the intended entry site into the artery (for antegrade punctures, make the skin entry the same distance above) to allow a 45-degree angle of the needle relative to the artery during puncture. The skin is anesthetized with 1–2% lidocaine injected as a superficial wheal and in the underlying deep tissues. Aspiration before injecting in the deep tissues helps to avoid intravascular lidocaine. Using the tip of a pointed (#11)

scalpel blade, a 5-mm nick is made in the skin. The skin nick and a subcutaneous tract are then dilated by gently spreading a straight surgical snap. The purpose of creating this tract is to facilitate catheter insertion during the procedure, and egress of blood in the event of bleeding afterwards.

The puncture needle is held firmly by the hub in one hand while the skin nick is straddled by the tips of the second and third fingers (either one above and one below, or one on each side) of the other hand (Fig. 2-29). The pulse should be palpable at all times during the puncture with these fingers. The needle is advanced slowly through the nick at a 45-degree angle until pulsations from the artery can be felt transmitted through the needle. The needle is then thrust forward until the underlying bone is encountered. If the needle has a stylet, this is then removed. The periosteum can be anesthetized with an additional 1 mL of lidocaine injected through the puncture needle (be sure that blood cannot be aspirated before injecting). The hub of the needle is grasped with the thumb and index finger from each hand on either side; the hub is depressed a few degrees towards the

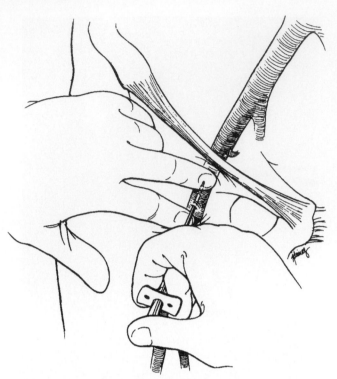

Figure 2-29   Technique for localization of the arterial pulse during puncture. (Reproduced with permission from Kadir S: *Diagnostic Angiography*, WB Saunders, Philadelphia, 1986.)

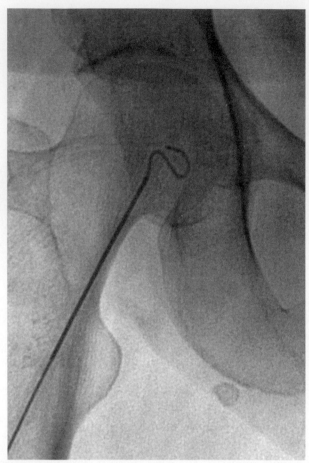

Figure 2-30   The operator felt resistance while inserting the guidewire and stopped to obtain this image. The guidewire could be extravascular, subintimal, or coiling against an obstruction. The key is to stop, look, withdraw the guidewire, and readjust the needle.

patient's thigh, and slowly withdrawn until blood spurts out of the hub. A slight "pop" is frequently felt just before this as the needle tip enters the lumen of the artery. The flow of blood should be pulsatile and vigorous. When the flow does not correlate with the quality of the pulse, the needle tip may be partially intramural ("side-walled"), under a plaque, in a vein, or in the orifice of a small branch vessel.

With one hand the needle is held steady while an atraumatic guidewire (such as a 3-J long taper or a Bentson wire) is introduced through the hub. There should be absolutely no resistance to advancement of the guidewire – stop immediately if there is any resistance (Fig. 2-30). The tip of the needle may be only partially in the artery, or directing the guidewire against the wall or under a plaque. Sometimes it is necessary to gently retract the needle to reposition the tip into the center of the vessel. When the guidewire will not advance freely, the tip should be inspected fluoroscopically while the angle of the needle is changed slightly to align with the long axis of the artery. The guidewire is then gently readvanced, with continuous fluoroscopic monitoring. When moving the needle hub slightly does not correct the problem, remove the guidewire to check for good blood return through the needle. A small injection of contrast may help sort out the problem, but only do this

if there is easy blood return. Otherwise, the injection may be into the wall of the artery and create an obstructing dissection.

Antegrade punctures can be difficult or impossible in obese patients. Sometimes a large pannus can be retracted with tape sufficiently to allow an antegrade approach. The superficial femoral artery (SFA) origin is medial and anterior to the profunda femoris artery (PFA) origin. A floppy-tipped 3-J guidewire should be used as the SFA is larger than the PFA.

Guidewires should be advanced with slow, deliberate motions. Rapid, forceful introduction of a guidewire risks dissection, kinking, or other problems. A guidewire that forms a "J" or seems to move freely is usually intravascular. A guidewire that spirals or crumples as it is advanced may have encountered an obstruction, dissected the wall of the artery, or have become extravascular (see Fig. 2-30). When this occurs, the guidewire should be pulled back until it assumes a normal shape and then gently readvanced. Sometimes it is necessary to pull out the needle completely, compress for a few minutes, check that the pulse is still good, and then repuncture.

Arterial punctures are characterized as double-walled (as described above), or single-walled. In a single-wall puncture the needle is advanced only a few millimeters after the tip touches the artery, just through the anterior wall of the vessel. This creates one hole in the artery, which is plugged with the catheter throughout the procedure, thus theoretically decreasing the chance of a bleeding complication. Single-wall punctures are more difficult than the standard double-wall technique. If the needle tip only partially enters the lumen, there will be a good blood return but the guidewire can pass into the subintimal layer as it exits the needle (Fig. 2-31).

Puncturing the nonpalpable artery (owing to an obstruction, low blood pressure, or patient obesity) can be frustrating. Puncture under ultrasound guidance is an excellent technique in this situation, eliminating all guesswork. When US is not readily available, fluoroscopic evaluation of the groin may reveal calcification in the CFA. Calcified vessels can be punctured with direct fluoroscopic guidance. Another strategy is to opacify the vessel with contrast from a catheter placed through a different access site, but this should be used only if two catheters are needed, such as prior to an intervention. Blind puncture over the medial third of the femoral head may yield success, but is least productive. If the femoral

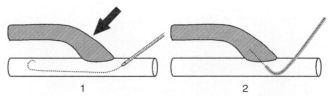

Figure 2-32   Puncture of the groin after aortofemoral bypass. **1**, The guidewire is directed into the native vessel by the access needle. Note the anterior relationship of the graft (arrow) to the native artery. **2**, A short angled catheter is used to redirect the guidewire into the graft.

vein is entered during any of these attempts, a guidewire can be inserted. This is then used as a guide to direct the needle lateral to the adjacent CFA during fluoroscopy.

Puncture of the postoperative groin requires knowledge of the type and age of the surgery, particularly if a vascular anastomosis is present. Most angiographers prefer to wait 6 weeks before puncture of a recently operated groin, as the area can be very tender, and there is a small concern about damaging the vascular suture line. In reality, the artery and graft can be punctured immediately if necessary. Antibiotics are usually not necessary when puncturing a synthetic graft. An important potential pitfall is present in the postoperative groin when the graft is anastomosed to the CFA. The graft is almost always sutured to the top of the artery, creating a wide "hood." During percutaneous puncture it can be difficult to negotiate out of the native CFA into the more anterior graft, particularly if the external iliac artery is patent (Fig. 2-32). In addition, scarring in the groin may make it difficult to introduce catheters. Overdilatation of the tract by 1 French size and a stiff guidewire may be required to introduce even a 5-French catheter.

Complications from CFA punctures are related primarily to vascular trauma and deficient hemostasis (Table 2-9). Attention to detail and a gentle touch helps to avoid most intraprocedural complications. Brute force is rarely needed and a frequent precursor to an adverse outcome in the vascular system. Dissections that occur during retrograde puncture are frequently subclinical, as antegrade blood flow tends to compress the false lumen (Fig. 2-33).

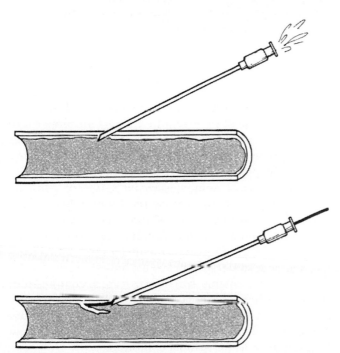

Figure 2-31   Potential mechanism of vessel wall injury during single wall puncture. *Top:* Good blood return is obtained although the needle is only partially in the lumen. *Bottom:* Guidewire passes into subintimal plane. (Reproduced with permission from Kim D, Orron DE: *Peripheral Vascular Imaging and Intervention*, Mosby, St Louis, 1992.)

Table 2-9	Complications of Common Femoral Artery Puncture	
Complication	**Acceptable Incidence**
Hematoma (requiring transfusion, surgery, or delayed discharge)	<0.5%
Occlusion	<0.2%
Pseudoaneurysm	<0.2%
Arteriovenous fistula	<0.2%

Adapted from Singh H et al. *J Vasc Interv Radiol* 13:1–6, 2002.

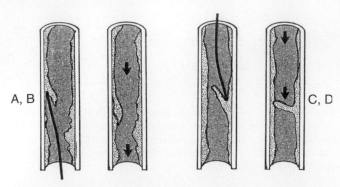

Figure 2-33 Different outcomes of retrograde and antegrade iatrogenic dissections. Arrows indicate direction of flow. **A/B**, Retrograde dissections tend to be compressed by antegrade flow. **C/D**, Antegrade dissections tend to be exacerbated and enlarged by antegrade flow. (Reproduced with permission from Kim D, Orron DE: *Peripheral Vascular Imaging and Intervention*, Mosby, St Louis, 1992.)

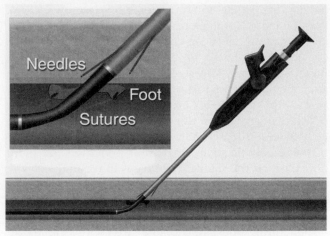

Figure 2-34 There are numerous strategies for remote closure of arterial puncture sites. Shown is a suture-based device. (Printed with permission of Abbott Laboratories Incorporated, Abbott Park, IL.)

Clinical thrombosis is unusual unless a tight stenosis is present; anticoagulation with heparin during the procedure is warranted in this situation.

The riskiest part of the procedure is actually after the catheter has been removed, when arterial bleeding may occur. Patients who received heparin during the procedure should have an ACT checked before compression. Protamine sulfate (10 mg per 1000 U heparin still active) can be given slowly to correct prolonged ACTs. Patients with an abnormal INR (>1.5) or PT (>15 seconds) can be given 2 units of FFP during the compression. Prior to removal of the catheter, the tips of the second through fourth fingers are placed so that the third finger is over the estimated *arterial* entry site (which may be above or below the skin nick). This provides proximal and distal control of the artery as well as the puncture site. The person performing the compression must know the location of the catheter entry site in the artery relative to the skin nick, and the quality of the pulse prior to the procedure. The pulse should be identified with certainty before the catheter is removed. The catheter is removed as pressure is applied. Occlusive pressure is maintained for 1–2 minutes, after which it is reduced slightly to allow some prograde blood flow (usually this results in a palpable thrill or slight pulse under the fingertips). The occlusive time should be limited to 1 minute when compressing a graft, as the likelihood of thrombosis is higher than with a native vessel. Pressure is gradually reduced over 15 minutes. Should bleeding resume, occlusive pressure is reapplied and the 15-minute clock restarted. If an obvious hematoma begins to form during compression, the pressure is either inadequate or being applied in the wrong place. Patients with heavily calcified vessels, systolic blood pressure greater than 200 mmHg, or who are systemically anticoagulated are at greater risk of bleeding and may require prolonged compressions. A sandbag should never be used to augment a compression as it is not only useless, it can also hide development of a hematoma. Patients who undergo manual compression of the puncture should remain in bed with the leg immobilized for 6 hours. The head of the bed may be elevated to 30 degrees.

There are several alternatives to manual compression of arteries. These include arterial closure devices and clamps. The advantage of closure devices is that the patient may ambulate sooner than after manual compression (Fig. 2-34). The closure strategies include remote suturing of the vessel, deposition of a hemostatic plug or procoagulant gel over the surface of the vessel, or applying a patch inside the lumen. A dense fibrotic reaction in the soft tissues may be associated with plug and patch devices. For some devices the size of the hole in the artery must be increased to introduce the closure system. All of these devices require training for proper use, and are most useful in patients at risk for bleeding after the compression, such as those on anticoagulant therapy or with low platelet count. These devices fail or require additional manual compression in 5–10% of patients. Closure devices should not be used when there is any question of contamination of the access site, such as following 24-hour lytic infusion. Infection is a reported complication, as are pseudoaneurysm formation, bleeding, and arterial occlusion. Pro-thrombotic pads can be held over the puncture site during manual compression, shortening the required bedrest. A different strategy is to substitute an external clamp for manual compression. These patients must remain at bedrest for the same length of time as for manual compression.

Axillary/High Brachial Artery

The upper-extremity approach to arterial access is an alternative to the common femoral artery in patients

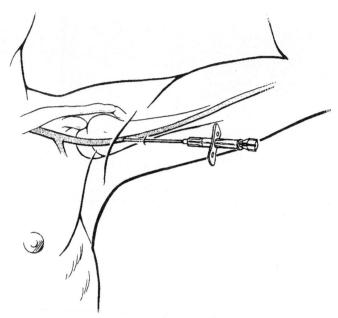

Figure 2-35   High brachial artery puncture of the left arm. The artery is entered lateral to the pectoral fold. (Reproduced with permission from Kadir S: *Diagnostic Angiography*, WB Saunders, Philadelphia, 1986.)

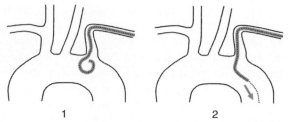

Figure 2-36   Technique to direct a pigtail catheter into the descending thoracic aorta from the left axillary approach. **1**, In the left anterior oblique (LAO) projection, the pigtail catheter is positioned at the origin of the left subclavian artery, oriented towards the descending thoracic aorta. A Cobra or other curved selective catheter can also be used. **2**, The guidewire (dashed line) is advanced, opening the pigtail, which directs the wire into the descending thoracic aorta. The catheter is then advanced over the guidewire (arrow).

with occluded femoral arteries, groin conditions that preclude safe access, when antegrade approach to visceral vessels is desirable, or cases in which an upper-extremity intervention is anticipated (Fig. 2-35). This approach is a secondary access because it introduces a small (0.5%) risk of stroke (related to the catheter crossing the origins of one or more great vessels) and peripheral upper-extremity nerve injury due to nerve compression by a hematoma in the medial brachial fascial compartment. Furthermore, the upper-extremity arteries tend to be smaller and more prone to spasm than the CFA, which limits the size of devices that can be introduced. In general, the axillary artery can accommodate up to a 7-French sheath without difficulty. Patients with uncorrected coagulopathy, uncontrolled hypertension, and morbid obesity are at higher risk for a hematoma. In addition, because the arm must be placed over and behind the patient's head for the duration of the angiogram, individuals with severe arthritis or other shoulder pathology may not be able to tolerate an upper-extremity approach. The overall incidence of complications with axillary and high brachial artery punctures is believed to be higher than with CFA puncture, primarily because of an increased incidence of neurologic, hemorrhagic, and occlusive incidents.

For procedures involving imaging of the abdominal aorta or the lower extremities, the left arm should be used if possible so that the catheter crosses only one cerebral artery (the left vertebral artery) (Fig. 2-36). When imaging the ascending thoracic aorta or selecting the cerebral vessels from an axillary approach, the right arm provides

the best access (Fig. 2-37). Prior to the procedure, the upper-extremity pulses should be palpated and the blood pressures in both arms compared. A blood pressure differential of more than 10–20 mmHg suggests the presence of stenosis in the affected extremity, and puncture should be performed in the opposite arm.

The patient is positioned on the angiographic table so that the arm is abducted 90 degrees with the elbow flexed and the hand placed under the back of the head. A pulse oximeter placed on a finger on the side of the puncture helps to monitor perfusion of the extremity during the case. The axillary artery is palpated in the axilla and as it crosses the lateral edge of the pectoralis major muscle to become the brachial artery. The preferred site of arterial puncture is actually the high brachial artery as it lies against the humerus, as this site is easier to compress than the true axillary artery. The skin overlying the artery is anesthetized, but little deep anesthesia is used to avoid an inadvertent nerve block (a confusing situation since nerve compression is a potential complication of the procedure). After making the skin nick and spreading the soft tissues, the arterial puncture is performed with the following modifications. Since the brachial and axillary arteries are more mobile than the common femoral artery, the vessel can be stabilized by placing the index and third finger side-to-side

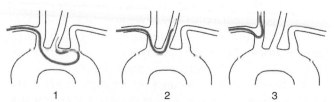

Figure 2-37   Selective catheterization of arch vessels from the right axillary approach. **1**, Simmons 1-2 catheter in the aortic arch (dashed line represents soft-tipped guidewire). **2**, Simmons 1-2 catheter in the left common carotid artery. **3**, Simmons catheter in the right common carotid artery.

over the pulse central to the puncture site (rather than one finger above and one below) so that the artery cannot slide away from the needle tip. The humerus is *superior* as well as posterior to the artery (not directly posterior like the femoral head in relation to the CFA). The needle tip is angled slightly towards the patient's head in order to hit the artery. A good initial guidewire for axillary or brachial puncture is a floppy 3-J to prevent accidental selection of the vertebral artery and other branch vessels. Many physicians routinely use ultrasound guidance and microaccess needles for brachial and axillary artery access.

Following the procedure the arm should be immobilized in a sling for 6 hours with the back of the patient's bed elevated at least 30 degrees. Patients who have had brachial or axillary artery punctures require periodic neurologic examinations during the 6-hour recovery period. Bleeding at the puncture site can result in compression of adjacent nerves. Nurses should be instructed to check grip and sensation in the hand along with vital signs and inspection of the puncture site. Weakness, parasthesias, or sensory changes in the hand following upper-extremity arterial puncture requires urgent evaluation for possible surgical decompression of the hematoma.

Translumbar Aorta

The translumbar approach to the aorta (TLA) seems like a crude and dangerous approach to angiography, but is actually a simple and safe access. The aorta is a large structure with a constant position, and the puncture is guided fluoroscopically using bony landmarks, allowing reliable access in most cases. The main disadvantages of direct aortic puncture are that selective angiography (other than the cerebral vessels) is difficult, and the patient must remain in the prone position for the examination. This access is therefore usually restricted to procedures that involve only aortic injections in patients who can lie on their stomachs for 1–2 hours.

The chief complication of translumbar aortography is retroperitoneal hematoma. Virtually all patients have a small self-contained psoas hematoma (up to $\frac{1}{2}$ unit of blood), but fewer than 1% are symptomatic. Very rarely the pleural space may be crossed, resulting in a hemopneumothorax. Visceral artery injury due to the needle has also been reported. Contraindications to TLA puncture include uncontrolled hypertension and coagulopathy, known supraceliac aortic aneurysm, a severely scoliotic spine, and dense circumferential aortic calcification.

The two types of TLA puncture are high (entry at the inferior endplate of the T12 vertebral body) and low (entry at the inferior endplate of L3) (Fig. 2-38). The high approach is most commonly used, as the low puncture is impossible in patients with infrarenal aortic occlusion (i.e., the typical TLA patient) and unwise in the presence

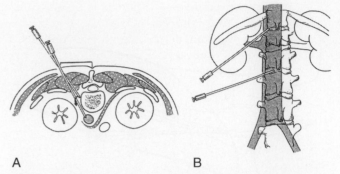

A   **B**

Figure 2-38 Translumbar puncture of the abdominal aorta. **A**, Cross-sectional diagram demonstrates anterior redirection of the needle away from the vertebral body towards the aorta. **B**, The two sites for puncture of the aorta are at the T12–L1 interspace (high) and the L2–L3 interspace (low). (Reproduced with permission from Kim D, Orron DE: *Peripheral Vascular Imaging and Intervention*, Mosby, St Louis, 1992.)

of an infrarenal abdominal aortic aneurysm. With the patient prone, the T12 vertebral body is localized as well as the iliac crest. The skin is anesthetized at a point roughly midway from the spinous process to the flank, and several centimeters below the 12th rib. If the skin nick is too medial, the needle will be blocked by a spinous process or vertebral body. An access too lateral may result in puncture of the kidney or inability to reach all the way to the aorta with the needle. Deep anesthesia can be administered with a 20-gauge spinal needle. Needles designed for TLA are usually 18-gauge, long, with preloaded coaxial Teflon dilators. The needle is advanced medially and cephalad towards the inferior endplate of T12. A skin entry site midway between the iliac crest and the 12th rib is used for a low TLA. If the vertebral body is encountered, the needle is withdrawn several centimeters, the angle changed, and the needle readvanced. Passing through the psoas muscle fascia may be uncomfortable for the patient. Deflection of aortic calcification by the needle may be visible or a transmitted aortic pulsation felt. To enter the aorta the needle is firmly advanced forward a centimeter (but not across the midline). The stylet is removed, confirming blood return (a vigorous dribble rather than pulsatile flow is usual because of the long needle) prior to introduction of a guidewire. A 0.038-inch guidewire should be used to prevent kinking in the retroperitoneal tissues during catheter exchanges. Insertion of a long 5-French sheath will allow catheter exchanges if necessary. Reversal of direction of the catheter can be accomplished by pulling a pigtail catheter or Simmons-1 catheter to the edge of the sheath to direct a floppy 3-J guidewire into the distal abdominal aorta.

The best part of a TLA is the compression: there is none. At the end of the procedure, as the patient is rolled on to their back on a stretcher, simply pull out the sheath. Patients commonly experience a mild backache due to the retroperitoneal hematoma, but otherwise should be asymptomatic. The blood pressure and vital signs should be checked frequently for several hours. Patients may ambulate after 4–6 hours of bedrest.

Unusual Arterial Access

Almost any artery in the body can be accessed percutaneously, but this is not always safe. A few unusual approaches should be kept in mind for special circumstances. The radial artery can accommodate long 4-French and smaller catheters that can be passed in a retrograde direction into the central arterial structures. The overall complication rate is low, and bedrest is not required after compression. Patients should have a normal Allen's test (compression of both arteries of the wrist followed by sequential release of the ulnar then radial arteries with inspection of the pattern of hand reperfusion) prior to catheterization as radial artery occlusion occurs in a small percentage.

The popliteal artery can be punctured in the popliteal space using ultrasound guidance. The usual indication for this access is an intervention, such as angioplasty of a superficial femoral artery origin stenosis or embolization of a distal foot lesion. Popliteal artery access is rarely necessary for diagnostic procedures. With the patient in the prone position, the popliteal artery is punctured with a microaccess needle and US guidance in a retrograde or antegrade direction as determined by the type of procedure. The popliteal vein, which lies superficial to the artery when the patient is in the prone position, should be avoided.

THE VENOUS PUNCTURE

Percutaneous puncture of deep venous structures differs from arterial access in that the veins cannot be palpated. Superficial anatomy, known anatomic relationship to palpable arterial or bony structures, or imaging with ultrasound or fluoroscopy are the major localization techniques. With the exception of femoral vein punctures, it is worthwhile to take advantage of image guidance techniques for most venous punctures.

Veins and the venous system are forgiving, as the ambient intraluminal pressure is low or even negative, and the walls of the vessels are generally soft and pliable. Large catheters and devices are readily accommodated through most percutaneous central venous punctures with satisfactory hemostasis at the end of the procedure. In comparison to arterial punctures, the primary complications associated with deep venous punctures are thrombosis, injury to adjacent arteries or organs (such as the lung), and rarely air embolism (Table 2-10).

Table 2-10	**Complications of Central Venous Punctures**
Complication	**Acceptable Incidence**
Pneumothorax[a]	<2%
Hemothorax[a]	<2%
Air embolism[a]	<2%
Hematoma	<2%
Perforation of vein	<2%
Thrombosis of puncture site (symptomatic)	<4%
Arterial injury	<1%

[a]Jugular and thoracic veins only.
Adapted from Lewis CA et al. *J Vasc Interv Radiol* 8:475–479, 1997.

Clinically important hematomas are rare, although they can occur in coagulopathic patients, especially in the presence of a central obstruction.

Common Femoral Vein

The common femoral vein (CFV) is most often accessed over the femoral head, above the junction with the deep (profunda) femoral vein and the saphenous vein (see Fig. 2-27). This segment of vein is analogous to the CFA in that it is relatively large, constant in position, and contained within the fascia of the femoral sheath. The vein lies medial and deep to the palpable arterial pulse. To access the CFV, localize the CFA, then anesthetize the skin just medial to the arterial pulse. The skin nick is usually lower than would be used for arterial puncture, as the goal is to enter the vein over the lower third of the femoral head. A sharp needle without a stylet is used, and suction is applied to the hub as the needle is advanced. Blood will be aspirated when the needle enters the vessel. Continuous localization of the arterial pulse with fingers of the other hand while advancing the needle prevents arterial puncture. If the underlying femoral head is reached without seeing a blood return, slowly withdraw the needle while maintaining suction. Remove the fingers over the femoral pulse as these may compress the adjacent vein. Vary the angle of the needle slightly with each pass if no blood return is obtained; the more lateral the trajectory, the greater the risk of arterial puncture. The femoral vein can be accessed in both the antegrade (towards the head) or retrograde (towards the foot) direction depending on the goal of the procedure. Difficult punctures can be performed with ultrasound guidance. Most femoral venous punctures for diagnostic procedures require only 5–10 minutes of compression. Interventional procedures with large sheaths in anticoagulated patients may require longer compression times. Postprocedure bedrest with the leg immobile for 3–4 hours is adequate for hemostasis.

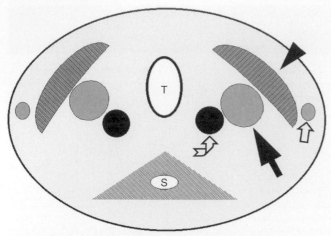

Figure 2-39 Cross-sectional vascular anatomy of the neck. Straight arrow = internal jugular vein. Curved arrow = common carotid artery. Arrowhead = sternocleidomastoid muscle. Open arrow = external jugular vein. T = trachea. S = spine.

Internal Jugular Vein

The internal jugular vein (IJV) is a valuable access for many diagnostic and interventional procedures (Fig. 2-39). The right IJV is the optimal access for insertion of dialysis catheters. The traditional approach to IJV puncture is based upon anatomic landmarks, with access from a posterior, middle, or anterior approach. Access with ultrasound guidance is the preferred method by interventional radiologists, as it is quick, safe, and reliable. Puncture of the carotid artery and pneumothorax, the major complications of blind IJV puncture, can be almost eliminated by using US guidance.

The IJ veins should be checked with US for location relative to the carotid arteries, compressibility, and change in size with respiration and cardiac cycle (indicating

central patency) prior to preparing the skin. Note the depth of the vein for future reference during the puncture. The patient should be placed in Trendelenberg or with the legs elevated on pillows to increase central venous pressure and dilate the IJ veins. Microaccess needles are ideal for US-guided IJV puncture.

The access site for an IJV puncture for diagnostic and interventional procedures is in the mid-portion of the neck, and low posterior for tunneled venous access devices. The right IJV is the easiest approach for diagnostic or interventional venous procedures involving the thorax or abdomen as it provides straight-line access to the superior vena cava (SVC). The needle is advanced under US guidance until it enters the vein or until blood can be aspirated (Fig. 2-40). Aspiration of air may indicate transgression of the pleural cavity, or (more typically) that the syringe is not attached firmly to the needle. The needle position and the status of the ipsilateral lung can be checked with fluoroscopy if there is any question. The guidewire should pass easily to the right atrium, and in many patients into the inferior vena cava (IVC). If accidental carotid puncture is suspected for any reason, either pull out everything, or insert the 3-French inner dilator from the microaccess kit over the 0.018-inch guidewire and inject a small amount of contrast.

Percutaneous access via the IJ veins has a low overall complication rate (see Table 2-10). Puncture-related thrombosis is less likely in the IJ veins than with most other venous access sites. However, a unique and potentially lethal risk of IJV (as well as subclavian vein) access is the introduction of air (air embolism) through an open catheter, dilator, or sheath (particularly the peel-way type) into the systemic circulation if the patient takes a breath at the wrong moment. A small amount of air introduced into the central venous system is harmless, but a large amount (20–30 mL) can create an obstruction in the pulmonary outflow tract. To minimize the risk of air

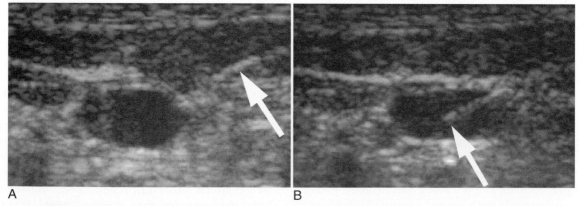

A   B

Figure 2-40 Ultrasound-guided puncture of the internal jugular vein (IJV) at the base of the neck. **A**, Axial view of the IJV showing the microaccess needle (arrow) in the sternocleidomastoid muscle. **B**, The needle tip (arrow) in the IJ vein.

embolism, the patient should be instructed to Valsalva or hum whenever a needle, catheter, or sheath is open to room air. Placing the patient in Trendelenberg also helps to decrease the risk of air embolism.

If an air embolism occurs during a procedure, first check the patient's vital signs for a drop in blood pressure or oxygen saturation (Box 2-10). The patient may complain of chest pain. A stable patient can be observed for several minutes until the air is absorbed. The air can sometimes be seen outlining the pulmonary valve with fluoroscopy. An unstable patient should be turned left side down to try to trap the air in the capacious right atrium. In severe cases, a catheter may be introduced into the right atrium in an attempt to aspirate the air.

Jugular vein punctures can be compressed with the back of the patient's bed elevated. The patient should be instructed to Valsalva during catheter removal, and occlusive pressure should be applied as the catheter is removed. Air embolism through the subcutaneous tract can occur. The duration of compression is usually only 5-10 minutes. After the procedure the patient should be at bedrest with the head of the bed upright for 1-2 hours.

Subclavian Vein

Percutaneous access to the subclavian vein has traditionally been based on superficial landmarks, similar to the IJV puncture. When this approach is used, access is achieved in 90-95% of attempts, but pneumothorax and subclavian artery puncture occur in 3-5%. With image-guided puncture, these complications are reduced to less than 1% combined, with a 100% success rate.

The safest place to access the subclavian vein is where it crosses over the anterior aspect of the first rib, lateral to the clavicle (Fig. 2-41). The vein should not be accessed under the clavicle, particularly when placing long-term central venous catheters, as this may lead to compression and fracture of the catheter ("pinch-off syndrome;" see Fig. 7-28) between the clavicle and the 1st rib. The subclavian vein is inferior and anterior to the artery over the 1st rib, and the presence of underlying bone minimizes the risk of pneumothorax during puncture. Lateral to the 1st rib the vessel becomes the axillary vein, which is best accessed over the anterior portion of the 2nd rib for the same reasons listed above.

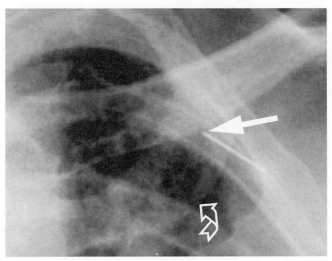

Figure 2-41   Puncture of the subclavian vein over the 1st rib. The vein was localized with contrast injection during the puncture. The tip of the needle (arrow) could be visualized over the 1st rib (curved arrow) the entire time during the puncture.

Puncture of the subclavian vein can be guided with ultrasound or fluoroscopy. The disadvantage of US is that the structures below the vein (rib and lung) may be difficult to visualize, and patency of the central veins cannot be assessed. The technique is virtually identical to that used for the IJ veins. The advantage of US guidance is that contrast is not necessary and exposure to radiation for both the operator and the patient is minimized. For fluoroscopically guided puncture, a limited upper-extremity venogram can be performed by injecting 10-20 mL of contrast material through a vein in the hand or forearm. This allows precise localization of the subclavian vein as it crosses the ribs, and confirms patency of the central venous system before beginning the procedure. Puncture can then be performed with carefully coned-down fluoroscopy over the needle tip. A micro-access needle is advanced under direct visualization until blood is aspirated or the tip hits the anterior surface of the 1st rib.

Upper-extremity Veins

When upper-extremity venous access is desired, the basilic vein should be the first target. The basilic vein is larger than the brachial veins (which are frequently multiple), and lies superficial to the nerves and brachial artery in the segment of arm immediately above the antecubital fossa (Fig. 2-42). Brachial vein puncture has the risk (albeit low) of injury to the adjacent artery or nerves. The cephalic vein can be punctured without fear of damage to surrounding structures, but this vessel is small and subject to spasm. The basilic vein is readily accessed with either ultrasound or venographic guidance.

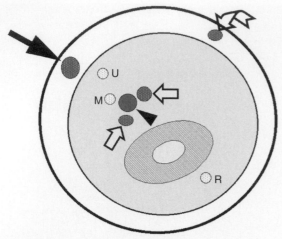

Figure 2-42   Cross-sectional anatomy of the upper arm proximal to the antecubital fossa. Straight arrow = basilic vein. Curved arrow = cephalic vein. Open arrows = brachial veins. Arrowhead = brachial artery. U = ulnar nerve. M = median nerve. R = radial nerve.

Inferior Vena Cava

Translumbar Access

Direct puncture of the IVC is used primarily for placement of long-term central venous access devices (see Fig. 7-25). Diagnostic procedures can almost always be performed from a peripheral approach. This puncture is similar in technique and materials to a low TLA (discussed above), with the difference being that the approach is from the right rather than the left.

Previous studies such as CT scans should be reviewed prior to the procedure to determine IVC anatomy, particularly in a patient with an abdominal aortic aneurysm or retroperitoneal mass. When first performing this procedure, it may be helpful to insert a small pigtail catheter into the IVC from a femoral approach to localize the cava during puncture.

The patient is placed in the left lateral decubitus position, with a small towel roll under the left flank in order to straighten the spine, or prone. A translumbar aortography needle/sheath system is inserted at a point approximately 10 cm to the right of the spinous process just above the right iliac crest. The needle is advanced at a 45-degree angle cephalad towards the top of the L3 vertebral body until the vertebral body is encountered. The needle is then withdrawn and angled more anteriorly, so that is passes just anterior to the vertebral body. The stylet is removed, and the needle withdrawn until blood can be aspirated. If a catheter has been placed previously in the inferior cava, this can be used as a target for puncture.

Entry by the needle into an arterial structure should not cause alarm unless the patient is coagulopathic; however, these patients should be observed with the same postprocedure protocol used for TLA punctures. Many patients note transient pain radiating to the right leg during the procedure. When the pain is severe the needle should be reinserted from a more lateral position to avoid the psoas muscle.

Transhepatic Access

This approach is indicated only when the thoracic veins and the infrarenal IVC are occluded. As with the translumbar puncture of the IVC, this technique is most often used for providing long-term central venous access rather than as a diagnostic procedure (see Fig. 7-25). Review of previous imaging is essential to determine hepatic anatomy and exclude dilated bile ducts, cysts, hemangiomas, or tumors along the access route. The right upper abdomen should be fluoroscoped to select a puncture site in the anterior axillary line that avoids transpleural, or at least transpulmonary, placement of the catheter. A long 21-gauge microaccess needle is advanced in a horizontal course through the liver towards the vertebral column. The needle should not be advanced beyond the mid-portion of the vertebral body. Aspiration of blood during withdrawal of the needle signifies entry into a vascular structure. Contrast should be injected to identify the vessel.

Other Venous Access

The median antecubital vein can be punctured under direct vision, but it is frequently thrombosed or already in use in hospitalized patients. The external jugular (EJ) veins are similarly easy to access, but may have an acute angle at the junction with the subclavian veins. This angle is easily negotiated with catheters and guidewires. Lastly, an enlarged collateral vein may provide access to the central circulation in patients with occlusion of the more typical access sites.

ANGIOGRAPHIC "DO'S AND DON'TS"

Never underestimate the amount of damage that can be done with a needle, guidewire, or catheter (Table 2-11). When performing an invasive vascular procedure, there

Table 2-11 Catheter-induced Complications	
Complication	**Acceptable Incidence**
Distal emboli	<0.5%
Arterial dissection/subintimal passage	<0.5%
Subintimal injection of contrast	<0.5%

Adapted from Singh H et al. *J Vasc Interv Radiol* 13:1–6, 2002.

Box 2-11   Catheter Flush Technique

Open stopcock on catheter if present

Aspirate catheter vigorously (approx 5 mL of blood) with 20 mL syringe

If no blood return, this may indicate a subintimal location; withdraw catheter while aspirating until blood appears

Attach 20 mL syringe containing 5–10 mL heparinized saline (2000 U/1000 mL) to catheter

Hold syringe tip down and tap several times to dislodge any bubbles in tip

Withdraw until a puff of blood is seen in syringe

Inject flush solution:

- For end-hole catheters, inject with mild to moderate force
- For multi-side-hole catheters, inject forcibly to ensure flush reaches catheter tip

Close stopcock if present

---

are several general guidelines that should be followed to ensure that the examination is performed safely and completely. One of the most important technical points is safe catheter flush technique (Box 2-11). This simple procedure maintains catheter patency and avoids potential embolic complications from injection of air bubbles or thrombus that can form in the catheter (Fig. 2-43).

Guidewires must be wiped with a moist nonfraying gauze or Telfa pad between exchanges or when removed from a catheter. Platelets, fibrin, and thrombus can form on guidewires. Even a thin film of material on a guidewire can make it very sticky and cause substantial

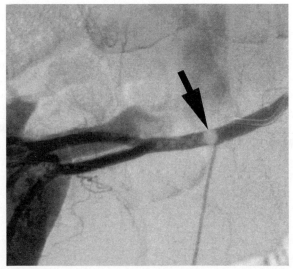

Figure 2-43   Importance of careful flush technique. Air bubbles (arrow) in an accessory renal artery during hand injection of contrast. These were easily aspirated.

resistance in a catheter. Similarly, catheters should be flushed with heparinized saline and wiped clean when first brought on to the sterile field and whenever removed from a patient. Many physicians keep guidewires and catheters in a basin of sterile heparinized saline when not in use.

During an arterial procedure it is essential to watch with fluoroscopy any time that a catheter or guidewire is moved, particularly when advancing. Very experienced operators may deviate from this when introducing a soft-tipped guidewire into a large normal vessel. New or inexperienced physicians should fluoroscope all catheter or guidewire manipulations.

Always aspirate blood before injecting anything through a catheter. Never inject when blood cannot be aspirated; the catheter tip may be subintimal, wedged in a tiny branch, or occluded. Pull the catheter back until vigorous blood return is obtained, then inject. When it remains impossible to aspirate, the catheter is most likely thrombosed. An attempt to aspirate with a 60 mL syringe may clear the thrombus. Never simply flush the catheter or ream out the thrombus with a guidewire in an artery, although this is sometimes acceptable in a vein. As a last resort the hub of the occluded catheter can be cut and a sheath advanced over the catheter as if it were a dilator. The occluded catheter can then be removed while preserving the access.

Frequently the tip of a guidewire may advance beyond the field of view of the image intensifier. This is a common situation when exchanging catheters or selecting a branch vessel. Always think about where the tip of the guidewire may be, even when it is not visible.

Diseased or delicate vessels may be easily traumatized by catheters and guidewires. In particular, patients on chronic high-dose steroids are prone to catheter-induced dissection. Straight or angled catheters should be advanced over a guidewire, whereas pigtail or recurved catheters can be safely advanced alone once they have reformed. Select diseased or delicate vessels with at least 1 cm of a soft guidewire protruding from the tip of the catheter. A soft guidewire will become very stiff if only a millimeter or two protrudes from the catheter.

Listen to the patient: if something hurts, stop and figure out why. Often, reassurance is all that is necessary, but sometimes a complication or other adverse outcome will be avoided. When something won't go, don't just push harder; try a different catheter or guidewire. When pushing a catheter at the groin, make sure the tip advances appropriately. If the tip doesn't seem to move an equal distance, stop and fluoroscope at the access site: the catheter may be coiling in the subcutaneous tissues (Fig. 2-44).

Always test inject through a catheter before a power injection after positioning or repositioning. This ensures that the catheter is in the proper position, that the tip is

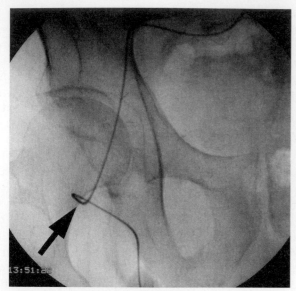

Figure 2-44 Buckling (arrow) of catheter and guidewire in the soft tissues. The patient had very tortuous arteries and a scarred groin. The operator noted that the catheter tip did not move as the catheter was pushed in.

free within the lumen rather than against the wall or subintimal, and may lead to a modification in the injection rate. Major complications can be created by large subintimal injections of contrast. Catheters should not remain connected to the power injector for more than 1-2 minutes without flushing, as thrombus will form in the tip.

Study symptomatic lesions first, particularly in the cerebral circulation. Image inflow, the lesion, and the outflow. Should an adverse event occur such as a contrast reaction or equipment failure, useful information will still have been obtained. In addition, have a low threshold for intraprocedural heparin. A groin hematoma is more acceptable than an ischemic complication.

Severely tortuous vessels are a common finding during diagnostic angiography in elderly patients. These can be difficult or impossible to negotiate safely with standard catheters and guidewires. A useful technique is to cross these vessels with a soft guidewire, followed by a hydrophilic catheter. Exchange for a stiffer guidewire through the hydrophilic catheter will enable introduction of additional catheters or devices. However, the stiff guidewire can cause distortion and "accordioning" of the artery. The vessel usually returns to normal after the stiff devices are removed (Fig. 2-45). Long sheaths that reach beyond the area of tortuosity can be extremely helpful in this situation.

Occasionally a vessel cannot be found in its usual location. A common example is failure to visualize the right hepatic artery during injection of the celiac artery. In this situation, there are several considerations, including

anomalous origin of the vessel from another location (such as the right hepatic artery from the superior mesenteric artery in the example described), occlusion by disease or other causes, congenital absence of the vessel, or surgical absence of the organ that the vessel used to supply. When the origin of a vessel cannot be selected with a catheter, but the vessel is known to be present, a severe origin stenosis may be present, or the wrong catheter shape may be employed. A moment's pause to reflect on the cause of the problem usually results in a simple solution.

Rarely, a catheter will form a true knot during extensive manipulation. This is usually the result of a combination of inattention and difficult anatomy. Knots may sometimes be undone by advancing a stiff guidewire through the catheter, forcing the catheter to unwind. Alternatively, a second catheter inserted from another access may be needed to "untie" the knot (Fig. 2-46). Small knots can be extracted through an appropriate sized sheath, but arteriotomy may be required.

IMAGING

A key element of angiography is the recording of the contrast injection (i.e., imaging). Simple observation with fluoroscopy is not sufficient (no films = no diagnosis). There are two basic modes of recording angiographic images, film-screen and digital angiography. When the latter is provided as a subtracted image, it is called "digital subtraction angiography" (DSA). Cineradiography as used in cardiac angiography has no role in noncardiac applications.

Film-screen imaging

Film-screen imaging currently provides the highest resolution, and is the traditional "gold standard" against which digital imaging is compared (Fig. 2-47). However, this modality is rapidly disappearing as all new angiographic equipment is purely digital. When film is used, the catheter is inserted and positioned using fluoroscopic guidance. A mechanical film changer is then brought into position, equipped with a magazine containing unexposed sheets of film and a receiver for exposed films. A scout film is then obtained to check patient positioning, exposure techniques, and labeling. If all is satisfactory, contrast is injected and films exposed. The films are transported to a dark room, fed through a processor, and hung on light boxes for viewing. Filming may be as rapid as 4-6 frames per second depending on the type of equipment.

There are many advantages to film-screen angiography, including a large field of view, and the ability to obtain extremely detailed magnification views by

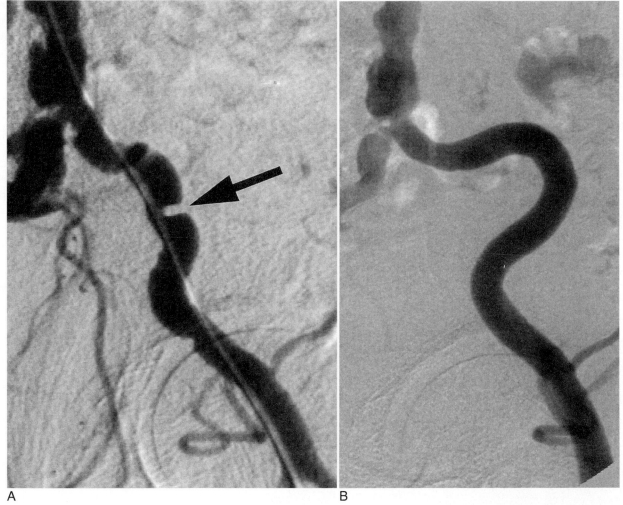

Figure 2-45   Accordion effect. **A**, Multiple eccentric, irregular stenoses (arrow) noted in the left external iliac artery during a pelvic angiogram with a stiff guidewire in place. **B**, Retrograde injection of the same vessel with the guidewire removed reveals a normal but tortuous artery. The apparent stenoses were caused when the artery was straightened and shortened by the guidewire.

manipulating distances between the patient, the tube, and the film. The limitations of film-screen angiography are poor discrimination of weakly opacified vessels, inability to film faster than 6 frames per second, the time needed to set up and process images, and the lack of replacement parts for the film changers.

Digital Subtraction Angiography

DSA is the most widely used angiographic technique. The original incarnation of DSA was a large, rapid venous injection of contrast with acquisition of digitally subtracted images timed to record arterial opacification by the bolus (IVDSA). This was an unsatisfactory application of a brilliant innovation, owing to unpredictable variations in cardiac output, poor resolution of the weakly

opacified arteries, inability to selectively inject arteries, and motion artifacts. Direct intraarterial injection of contrast, as used with film-screen angiography, rapidly supplanted IVDSA.

Digital angiography currently has lower resolution than film-screen, but provides extremely rapid acquisition of images and processing (the subtraction is performed instantaneously and displayed on a monitor), and the ability to manipulate the image appearance online to compensate for poor opacification. Most current machines utilize a 1024-pixel matrix. The interchange between fluoroscopic and angiographic modes is electronic and almost instantaneous rather than mechanical and slow. Images can be viewed in either subtracted or unsubtracted (raw) format (see Figs 2-25 and 2-26). Filming can be as rapid as 30 frames per second with some units,

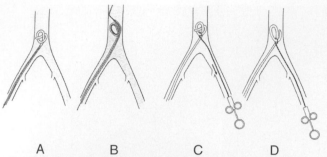

A   B   C   D

Figure 2-46   The knotted catheter. **A,** An extra-stiff hydrophilic guidewire is advanced to the knot. **B,** The knot is forced open as progressively stiffer portions of the guidewire exit the catheter. This technique is successful in the majority of instances. **C,** Alternatively, the knot can be teased open with downward traction from the opposite iliac access. A selective catheter is insinuated through the knot. Shown is a deflecting guidewire, which would be activated inside the selective catheter. **D,** The knot opens as traction is applied. (Reproduced with permission from Kim D, Orron DE: *Peripheral Vascular Imaging and Intervention*, Mosby, St Louis, 1992.)

with continuous acquisition while moving the angiographic table (bolus chase) or the tube (rotational angiography). Newer units can construct 3-dimensional models from rotational angiographic data, a useful tool during complex embolization procedures. Lower contrast concentrations can be used (30–50% less iodine than with film-screen angiography), without altering the injection rates. The exquisite sensitivity of this technique allows use of alternative negative contrast agents such as CO_2 for angiography.

The limitations of DSA, in addition to lower resolution, include subtraction artifacts from involuntary motion such as bowel peristalsis, respiration, and cardiac pulsation, and a tendency to "shoot first and ask questions later" (collect lots of images and views quickly with only superficial review of the results on a monitor during the procedure). Current residents and fellows will practice in an all-digital environment for their entire professional lives.

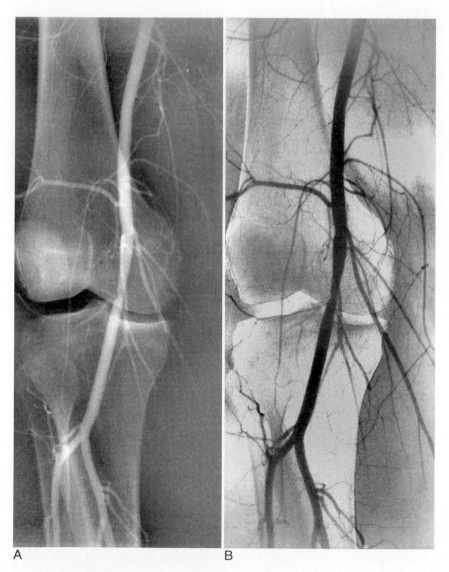

A   B

Figure 2-47   Screen-film ("cut-film") angiography. **A,** Oblique view of the popliteal artery. Detail is excellent. The bones are readily visible. **B,** Manual subtraction image of the same angiogram. The first film of the run had no visible contrast, and was used to make a mask. The mask was used to subtract the bones from the angiographic image. The patient moved slightly, so that faint outlines of bone are still visible, but smaller vessels are now easier to see.

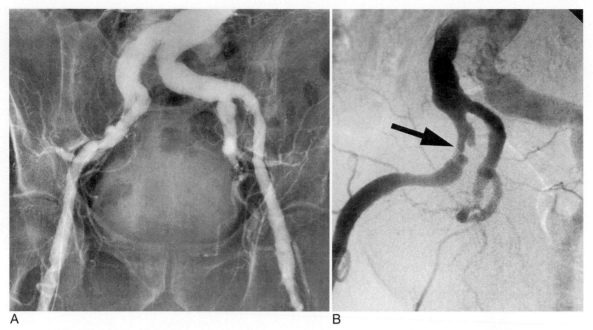

A B

Figure 2-48 Evaluation of most vascular structures requires imaging in at least two views. **A**, Screen-film pelvic angiogram in the anterior–posterior projection. There is no obvious lesion on the right, but the patient had a slightly diminished right femoral pulse. **B**, Digital subtraction view of the right external iliac artery in the right posterior oblique projection. An eccentric stenosis (arrow) is now readily visible. Note that the internal iliac artery origin is also clearly seen.

Procedural Issues

Whether using film-screen or DSA, it is necessary to determine patient positioning and filming rates for each injection. Patient positioning has been loosely standardized for most types of angiograms based on anatomy and the empiricism that two different views of the same vascular structure are necessary for evaluation of most pathologic processes ("one view = no view") (Fig. 2-48).

Similarly, contrast injection and filming rates have been developed for different studies based upon expected flow rates and pathology. Suggestions for tube angulation, patient positioning, contrast injection rates, and filming rates for specific studies can be found in later chapters. Variations in positioning, injection rates, and filming are frequently necessary to suit an individual patient, as flow may be slower or faster than anticipated, or the pathology may be visible only on delayed images. In general, film faster during the contrast injection (arterial phase), and then slow down to follow the capillary and venous phases. Large vascular spaces such as aortic aneurysms need longer injections of large volumes of contrast (not faster injection rates) to be adequately opacified; large vascular beds (such as the lower extremities) need long injections at a lower rate to ensure complete opacification, and rapidly flowing blood may require both high flow rates and large volumes (such as a thoracic aortogram in a young hyperdynamic patient).

Image intensifiers with large fields of view are desirable for most applications. Electronic magnification, careful coning of images, and application of filters enhance image quality. During prolonged procedures, pulse-mode fluoroscopy can reduce patient and operator exposure, as well as prevent tube overheating. The intensifier should always be as close to the patient as possible to minimize scatter and improve image quality.

INTRAVASCULAR ULTRASOUND

Intravascular ultrasound (IVUS) is a technology that combines features of both invasive and noninvasive imaging. Although ultrasound is generally considered noninvasive, this is true only as long as the probe is outside of the body. By placing a probe on the end of a catheter (usually 4- to 9-French in diameter), direct access to the vascular lumen can be obtained by inserting the catheter over a guidewire (Fig. 2-49). A hemostatic sheath is necessary to allow safe introduction of the IVUS probe.

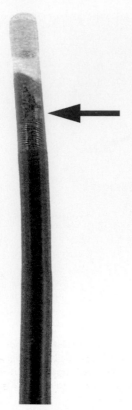

Figure 2-49 Intravascular ultrasound probe (9-Fr, 9-MHz). The transducer (arrow) is located proximal to the tip of the catheter. Smaller diameter probes that can be inserted over a guidewire are readily available.

Instead of looking from outside in, IVUS looks from inside out (Fig. 2-50). This technique is useful as an adjunct to conventional angiography to evaluate intraluminal processes such as dissections, or vessel wall abnormalities such as eccentric stenoses that are difficult to visualize on an angiogram (Fig. 2-51). Precise luminal measurements can be obtained, as well as localization of stenoses. This may be particularly useful during a complex intervention. The quality of the arterial wall can also be assessed for subtle changes of atherosclerosis, although the clinical utility of this information remains to be determined. The limitations of the technique are the expense of the additional equipment, the inability to look forward with the catheter (most designs are based on a rotating transducer that can image only in the axial plane), and the small field of view when compared to external probes.

POSTPROCEDURE CARE

The care of the patient after an angiogram is equal in importance to the procedure itself. Patients should be observed in a supervised setting for a length of time

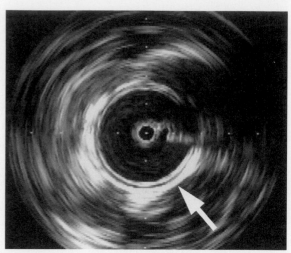

Figure 2-50 Normal intravascular ultrasound (IVUS) images of the popliteal artery. A 6-Fr probe (12.5-MHz) is visible in the center of the vessel. The echogenic intima, hypoechoic media, and echogenic adventitia are clearly visualized (arrow).

befitting the procedure and the sedation. For example, following a translumbar aortogram, a patient is kept at bedrest for 6 hours, whereas a patient may be discharged immediately following an arm venogram through a peripheral intravenous catheter performed without sedation. In general, patients should be kept at bedrest for 6 hours after puncture of an artery and 4 hours after puncture of a femoral vein with the extremity immobilized. Vary this time according to individual patient circumstances, such as increasing the duration of bedrest in patients who are anticoagulated or had a procedure with large catheters. Shorter periods of immobilization are used when closure devices or hemostatic patches have been used. The pulses at the puncture site and in the distal extremity are checked on a regular schedule, as well as the vital signs.

Patients may resume their previous diet as soon as they are awake enough to eat safely, but intravenous hydration with an appropriate solution should be continued until oral intake is satisfactory. Patients with compromised renal function should be hydrated for 12 hours following the procedure.

When discharging an outpatient after an arterial procedure, check and record the pulse and status of the puncture site, and the distal pulses. Be sure that the patient is tolerating food by mouth, and has urinated at least once. Give the patient clear instructions regarding activity for the next 24 hours, what to look for that might indicate a complication (cold extremity, painful puncture site, obvious hematoma or bleeding, or absence of urination for 24 hours), and what to do if the person suspects a complication.

When called to evaluate a patient for a suspected puncture site complication after an angiogram, be sure to

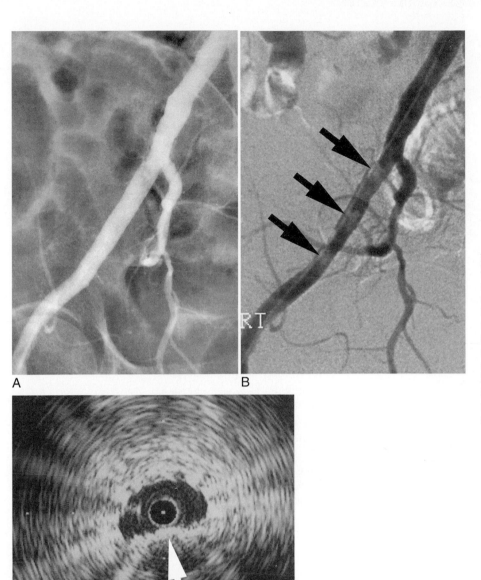

Figure 2-51 Intravascular ultrasound (IVUS) of eccentric external iliac artery stenoses. **A,** Oblique screen-film pelvic angiogram without obvious abnormality. Bulky vascular calcifications were seen on the scout films. **B,** Oblique digital subtraction angiogram of the right external iliac artery shows several areas (arrows) of decreased contrast density consistent with bulky calcified plaque. **C,** IVUS image (7-Fr, 12-MHz) of the same vessel showing one of the calcified eccentric stenoses (arrow).

bring a pair of gloves and some sterile gauze. Ischemic complications are rare, but manifest as diminished or absent pulses, rest pain, pallor, or loss of nerve function. Knowledge of the patient's preprocedural examination and the angiographic findings are important to determine whether the pulse abnormality is new. The differential diagnosis includes thrombosis of a preexisting critical stenosis, puncture site thrombosis or dissection, and distal embolization of thrombus or plaque. Rarely, a catheter may fragment and embolize distally. Management includes heparinization, emergent angiography with possible thrombolysis or stent placement, or surgical thrombectomy.

Hemorrhagic complications include overt bleeding or hematoma formation. The patient's blood pressure and pulse should be checked immediately while inspecting the puncture site. If the patient is hypotensive, a bolus of 300–500 mL of crystalloid (NS or lactated Ringer's solution) should be administered, and blood obtained for a stat complete blood count, coagulation studies, and blood bank sample. The treatment of overt bleeding or hematoma formation are identical: compression. It can be difficult to locate a pulse in the midst of a large hematoma; application of continuous firm pressure can displace the hematoma sufficiently to uncover the pulse. Knowledge of the type of puncture is essential so that pressure can be applied in the appropriate place. For example, the arterial entry site for an antegrade femoral angiogram is *distal* to the skin nick, not

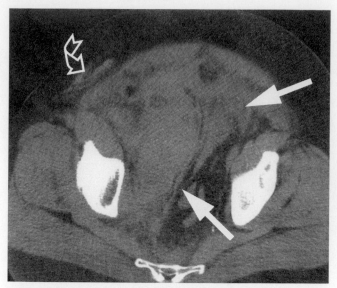

Figure 2-52   Hematomas following angiography. Noncontrast CT scan of patient who developed hypotension following a percutaneous procedure. There is a small subcutaneous hematoma (curved arrow) and a massive retroperitoneal hematoma (arrows) in the pelvis. At surgery the arterial puncture was noted to be in the external iliac artery above the inguinal ligament.

proximal. While compressing, reiterate to the patient that the extremity must be kept still. Also, check with the nurse to determine whether the patient has been following instructions. After 15 minutes, reinspect the puncture site. Be prepared to compress for an additional 15 minutes if necessary. Should bleeding persist after repeat compression, consider checking the patient's coagulation studies and platelet count if not already done. A CT scan of the abdomen and pelvis to look for a retroperitoneal hematoma should be obtained when a patient develops unexplained hypotension or a drop in hematocrit after an angiogram (Fig. 2-52). A large bleed following an angiogram is a risk factor for pseudoaneurysm formation.

Patients will experience mild to moderate discomfort at the puncture site for several days, followed by 10–14 days of slight tenderness. A small area of focal induration may develop related to resolution of subcutaneous blood. Echymosis is common, and can track into the ipsilateral thigh and perineum. Patients should be instructed to return if there is increased pain, swelling, or bleeding at the puncture site.

SUGGESTED READINGS

Baum S: *Abram's Angiography,* 4th edn. Little Brown, Boston, 1997.

Braun MA, Nemcek AA, Vogelzang RL: *Interventional Radiology Procedure Manual.* Churchill Livingstone, New York, 1997.

Johnsrude I, Jackson DC, Dunnick NR: *A Practical Approach to Angiography,* 2nd edn. Little Brown, Boston, 1987.

Kadir, S: *Diagnostic Angiography.* WB Saunders, Philadelphia, 1986.

Kandarpa K, Aruny JE: *Handbook of Interventional Radiologic Procedures,* 3rd edn. Little Brown, Boston, 2001.

Kerns SR, Hawkins IF: Carbon dioxide digital subtraction angiography: expanding applications and technical evolution. *Am J Roentgenol* 164:735–741, 1995.

Kessel D, Robertson I: *Interventional Radiology: a Survival Guide.* Churchill Livingstone, London, 2000.

Kim D, Orron DE: *Peripheral vascular imaging and intervention.* Mosby–Yearbook, St Louis, 1992.

Koenig T, Wolff D, Mettler FA et al: Skin injuries from fluoroscopically guided procedures: 1. Characteristics of radiation injury. *Am J Roentgenol* 177:3–12, 2001.

Koenig T, Mettler FA, Wagner LK: Skin injuries from fluoroscopically guided procedures: 2. Review of 73 cases and recommendations for minimizing dose delivered to patient. *Am J Roentgenol* 177:13–20, 2001.

Levitin A. Intravascular ultrasound. *Tech Vasc Interv Radiol* 4:66–74, 2001.

Lewis CA, Allen TE, Burke DR et al: Quality improvement guidelines for central venous access. *J Vasc Interv Radiol* 8:475–479, 1997.

Merten GJ, Burgess WP, Gray LV et al. Prevention of contrast-induced nephropathy with sodium bicarbonate: a randomized controlled trial. JAMA 291:2328–2334, 2004.

Mistretta CA, Crummy AB: Diagnosis of cardiovascular disease by digital subtraction angiography. *Science* 214:761–765, 1981.

Murphy TP, Benenati JF, Kaufman JA: *Patient Care in Interventional Radiology.* SCVIR, Fairfax, VA, 1999.

Seldinger SI: Catheter replacement of the needle in percutaneous arteriography. *Acta Radiologica* 39:368–376, 1953.

Singh H, Cardella JF, Cole PE et al: Quality improvement guidelines for diagnostic arteriography. *J Vasc Interv Radiol* 13:1–6, 2002.

Solomon R, Werner C, Mann D et al: Effects of saline, mannitol, and furosemide to prevent acute decreases in renal function induced by radiocontrast agents. *N Engl J Med* 331:1416–1420, 1994.

Spies JB, Bakal CR, Burke DR et al: Standards for diagnostic arteriography in adults. *J Vasc Interv Radiol* 4:385–395, 1993.

Tepel M, van der Giet M, Schwarzfeld C et al: Prevention of radiographic-contrast-agent-induced reductions in renal function by acetylcysteine. *N Engl J Med* 343:210–212, 2000.

Valji, K: *Vascular and Interventional Radiology.* WB Saunders, Philadelphia, 1999.

Wojtowycz M: *Handbook of Interventional Radiology and Angiography,* 2nd edn. Mosby–Yearbook, St Louis, 1995.

CHAPTER 3

Noninvasive Vascular Imaging

JOHN A. KAUFMAN, M.D.

The majority of patients with vascular disease are now imaged with ultrasound (US), computed tomography (CT), or magnetic resonance imaging (MRI) before (or instead of) undergoing angiography. The purpose of this chapter is to provide an understanding of the underlying principles of each of the noninvasive modalities.

ULTRASOUND

Gray-scale Ultrasound

Much of the evaluation of blood vessels with US can be accomplished with conventional gray-scale imaging. A transducer that emits high-frequency sound waves (usually 2–7 MHz) is held to the skin. A computer measures the time that it takes for the sound waves to return to the transducer, and then creates an image. Sound waves that are reflected by a tissue, such as the wall of a blood vessel, are visible as echoic structures. Sound waves that are transmitted by structures, such as the fluid-filled lumen of a blood vessel, have no echoes (anechoic).

Gray-scale US is a powerful tool for defining the morphology of blood vessels, but it has distinct limitations. Air, bone, and metal are so highly reflective that sound waves cannot penetrate to visualize underlying tissues. The two areas of the body where this is most problematic are the chest (air in the lungs) and the head (bone in the skull). Gray-scale US also provides no information about blood flow in the vessel. The presence of a vascular disease may be suspected on the basis of the gray-scale appearance of the vessel wall, such as a large echogenic plaque in an artery, but the flow is not evaluated. Fortunately, a very basic principle of US, Doppler shift, can be used to indirectly measure the velocity of flow.

Doppler Ultrasound

When a sound wave is reflected from a stationary object, the frequency of the returning wave is the same as that of the initial wave. The frequency of a wave that is reflected from an object moving towards the sound source will be higher in proportion to the speed of that object. Conversely, the frequency of a wave reflected from an object moving away from the sound source will be lower in proportion to the velocity of the object. This is why the tone of a siren drops noticeably lower as an ambulance drives by. The difference between the two frequencies is termed the "Doppler shift." This same phenomenon can be applied to flowing blood during an ultrasound examination using the sound waves emitted by the transducer.

Most diagnostic US equipment utilizes a thin beam of pulsed US (know as "pulsed-wave Doppler") because this allows precise spatial localization of the measured velocity within the tissues. Continuous-wave Doppler (such as the small hand-held units used to detect fetal heart beats) measures all flow within the emitted beam, so that overlapping structures are easily confused.

Review of the Doppler equation helps to understand the strengths and limitations of this technique. The simplified equation is as follows:

$$\text{Doppler shift}$$
$$= (F_r - F_t)$$
$$= 2 \times F_t \times V \times \cos\theta \times (1/c),$$

where F_r is the frequency of the reflected sound, F_t is the frequency of the transmitted sound, V is the velocity of flow, θ is the angle of the ultrasound beam with respect to the long axis of the vessel lumen, and c is the speed of sound in soft tissues. The velocity of flow is useful for detection of disease, so the equation can be rearranged as:

$$V\text{(cm/s)} = F_d \times (1/F_t) \times (c/2) \times (1/\cos\theta),$$

where F_d is the Doppler shift. Notice that the calculated velocity is directly proportional to the Doppler shift, but inversely proportional to $\cos\theta$ (the angle of the US beam to the direction of flow). This last fact explains why the best angles for measurement of velocity are less than 60 degrees. Below a θ of 60 degrees the value of $1/\cos\theta$ changes at a relatively leisurely rate. At a θ greater than 60 degrees the changes in the value of $1/\cos\theta$ are large with only incremental changes in θ. This leads to magnification of errors during the velocity calculation, rendering the results unreliable.

Velocity of flow is most commonly displayed as a tracing on a scale determined by the operator. By convention, flow towards the transducer is displayed above the baseline, and flow away from the transducer is displayed below. The characteristics of the tracing are determined by the type of vessel, the organ which it supplies, and the presence of disease states. Arterial flow varies with the cardiac cycle, with a rapid rise to peak velocity during systole, and gradual decrease in velocity during diastole (Fig. 3-1). A dicrotic notch representing closure of the aortic valve should be clearly visible. Blood flow to high-resistance structures, such as the leg muscles, is

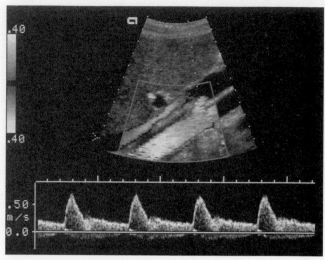

Figure 3-2   The normal Doppler waveform in a low-resistance visceral artery is biphasic: fast antegrade flow during systole with slower antegrade flow during diastole. Flow is never reversed in normal visceral arteries. A renal artery tracing is shown. (Image courtesy of Siemens Medical Solutions Inc.)

triphasic with a brief period of retrograde flow during diastole. Blood flow to low-resistance structures, such as visceral organs, remains prograde throughout diastole (Fig. 3-2). With occlusive disease the velocity of flow in the stenosis rises and the Doppler tracing thickens (termed "spectral broadening") as the range of velocities present increases (Fig. 3-3). As the stenosis progresses in severity the velocity may decrease, and the waveform dampen or disappear altogether.

Veins characteristically have a lower velocity than arteries, with a less pulsatile tracing (Fig. 3-4). The actual velocity and pulsatility will vary depending on the proximity of the vein to the heart, the health of the heart, and

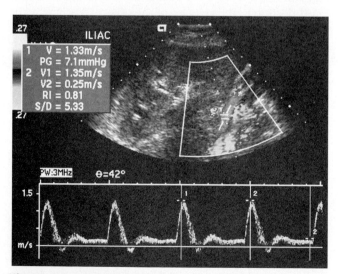

Figure 3-1   The normal Doppler waveform in high-resistance arteries is triphasic: fast antegrade flow during systole, reversed briefly at the beginning of diastole, then antegrade at a lower velocity. An external iliac artery tracing is shown.

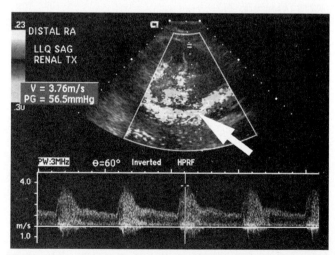

Figure 3-3   Doppler tracing from a patient with transplant renal artery stenosis shows increased velocity and broadening of the waveform in the region of greatest arterial narrowing (arrow).

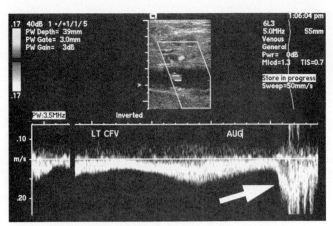

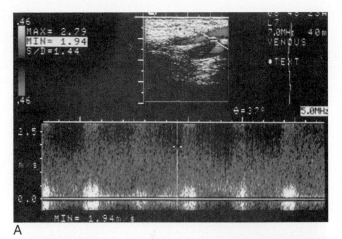

A

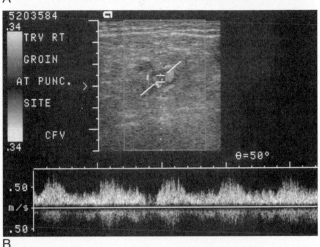

B

Figure 3-4   Doppler waveform in a normal common femoral vein shows gentle respiratory variation in flow. A sharp increase in flow (arrow) occurs with manual compression of the calf. AUG = augmentation of flow by calf compression.

Figure 3-6   Arteriovenous fistula (AVF). **A,** Doppler waveform in the fistula shows greatly accelerated velocities with extreme spectral broadening. (Image courtesy of Siemens Medical Solutions Inc.) **B,** Doppler waveform from the common femoral vein of another patient central to a post-catheterization AVF shows a pulsatile venous waveform consistent with arterialized venous flow.

the volume status of the patient. Phasic changes in velocity with respiration will also occur, with substantial increases in flow during inspiration, and dampened flow during expiration. With forced expiration (the Valsalva maneuver) flow may be completely arrested (Fig. 3-5). In general, the more distant the vein from the central circulation, the slower and more constant the flow.

Two vascular abnormalities with distinct Doppler signatures that are important to angiographers are arteriovenous fistula (AVF) and arterial pseudoaneurysm (PSA). Both lesions can occur following percutaneous vascular procedures. An AVF is a direct communication between an artery and a vein (see Fig. 1-24). The Doppler characteristics are accentuated diastolic flow (i.e., a low-resistance pattern) in the artery proximal to the AVF, a jet of extremely high-velocity flow through the point of communication, and an arterialized waveform in the vein

central to the actual fistula (Fig. 3-6). A post-catheterization PSA is a focal disruption of the arterial wall communicating with a blood-filled space that is contained by the adjacent soft tissues (see Fig. 1-9). The Doppler characteristics are a jet of high-velocity flow through the neck that may reverse during diastole ("to and-fro") with swirling flow in the pseudoaneurysm (Fig. 3-7).

Color Doppler

The Doppler shift can be assigned colors that reflect both the relative direction and velocity of the flow. All flow within a specified area of a fan beam is assigned a color, with red and blue being the most conventional. Red usually indicates flow toward the transducer, and blue represents flow away from the transducer. The color of the flow is determined by how the operator holds the transducer; one should never assume the identity of a

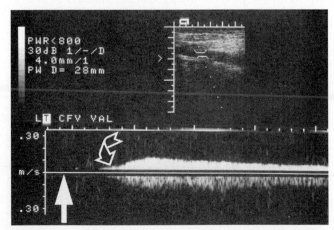

Figure 3-5   During Valsalva maneuver there is cessation of flow (straight arrow) in the common femoral vein. With relaxation flow resumes (curved arrow).

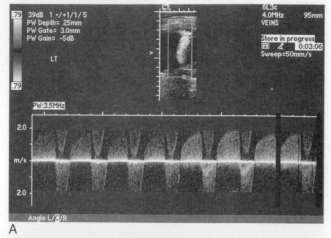

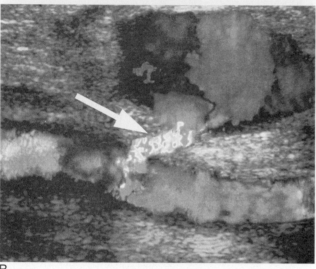

Figure 3-7   Arterial pseudoaneurysm (PSA). **A**, Doppler waveform in the neck of an iatrogenic popliteal artery PSA shows high velocity to-and-fro flow. **B**, Color flow image of an iatrogenic common femoral artery PSA shows high-velocity flow in the neck (arrow) and swirling turbulent flow in the aneurysm ("yin-yang" sign). (Images courtesy of Siemens Medical Solutions Inc.)

vessel based on the color alone. The color image is superimposed upon a gray-scale image to provide anatomic definition, and many US machines also allow simultaneous display of a pulsed-wave tracing.

With color flow Doppler, very fast flow is usually displayed as white or yellow. This helps to localize areas of stenosis or other pathologies such as an AVF or neck of a PSA by visualization of the accelerated flow. Subsequently, precise velocity measurements in the area of abnormality are obtained with pulsed-wave Doppler. The appearance of turbulent flow is exemplified by the color pattern found inside an arterial PSA, in which the color changes from red to blue as the blood swirls around in the cavity. Color imaging can be very useful when evaluating intraluminal processes, such as partially occlusive thrombus.

Power Doppler

Power Doppler is an important modification of color flow techniques. With standard color-flow imaging, the color is linked to the Doppler shift. Power Doppler uses the overall energy in the Doppler signal to assign color, without regard for the magnitude of the phase shift (velocity) or direction. Since the majority of the signal is created by moving red blood cells, this technique is more sensitive to flow than standard color imaging. Although this is useful when evaluating areas of slow flow or small structures, other movement such as transmitted pulsations or vibrations will also be more apparent on the images.

Ultrasound imaging has several limitations, some of which are related to the physics of the technique, and some to the person performing the examination. The greatest limitation is that US is reflected by bone and air–tissue interfaces. Structures surrounded by or consisting primarily of these components can be difficult or impossible to image. A second limitation is that imaging occurs in a single plane determined by the person holding the transducer. Complex nonlinear structures must be evaluated in a piecemeal fashion, with intense concentration upon the part of the examiner in order to perform a complete study. The application of 3-dimensional (3-D) image reconstruction software to US will facilitate these examinations.

Doppler imaging has several key weaknesses, including unreliable velocity calculations when the angle of insonation is above 60 degrees, as described above. Very slow flow is difficult to detect, particularly in deep vessels. This may lead to the false conclusion that a vessel is occluded, a potentially serious error when evaluating the carotid arteries. On the other hand, extremely fast flow may exceed the ability of a particular US machine to measure or display the velocity, but this is rarely an important problem in patient management.

Color-flow Doppler imaging does not display velocity as accurately as the waveform. The severity of stenosis is inferred from the visualized color changes. Selection of an inappropriate color scale may result in over- or underestimation of the degree of stenosis. Furthermore, since color-encoding is determined by the operator, the identity of a vessel cannot be assumed from the color of the flow.

TRANSESOPHAGEAL ECHOCARDIOGRAPHY

Not all ultrasound examinations are performed with hand-held external probes. Placing a probe on the end of an endoscope allows access to any hollow viscus (Fig. 3-8).

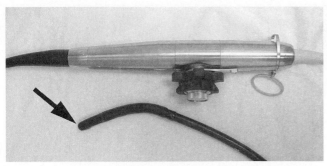

Figure 3-8 Transesophageal echo probe. The tip of the probe (arrow) is steered from the handle, allowing angulation of the transducer within the esophagus.

The esophagus is a useful access for vascular structures in the chest as it lies close to the thoracic aorta. Transesophageal echocardiography (TEE) was developed to overcome the limitations on transthoracic cardiac ultrasound imposed by the air-filled lungs. The ascending and descending thoracic aorta are easily visualized with TEE, although examination of the transverse arch is less reliable.

A more invasive examination than a transthoracic ultrasound, TEE requires intravenous sedation of the patient and administration of local anesthetic to the posterior pharynx to dull the gag reflex. Operator experience is a key element in obtaining a satisfactory examination, as manipulation of the probe requires some practice. There is a slight risk of esophageal perforation during the examination, and it should not be performed in patients with known or suspected esophageal pathology.

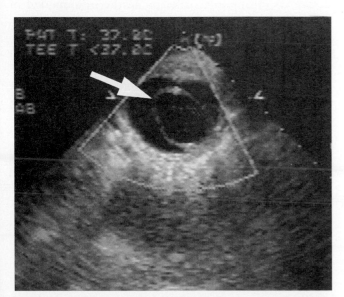

Figure 3-9 Transesophageal ultrasound of a patient with an aortic dissection. Axial image of the descending thoracic aorta shows the dissected intima (arrow) forming a central true lumen surrounded by the false lumen.

The most common applications of TEE are in the work-up of patients with acute aortic syndromes such as suspected dissection, ruptured aneurysm, and traumatic aortic transection (Fig. 3-9).

MAGNETIC RESONANCE IMAGING/MAGNETIC RESONANCE ANGIOGRAPHY

MR imaging is based upon the detection of radio-frequency signals emitted by protons within a powerful magnetic field. Protons in the tissue being imaged align their axes with the strong magnetic field in the MR scanner (longitudinal magnetization). Application of an additional radio-frequency pulse to the protons tips the spins out of alignment with the magnetic field, in a plane perpendicular to the magnetic field (transverse magnetization). The natural tendency of the protons is to realign themselves with the magnetic field (relaxation), which creates a detectable signal (echo). Images are created from the signals emitted during longitudinal (T1) or transverse (T2) relaxation of the spins. In general, images based on short echo times are T1-weighted while those based on long echo times are T2-weighted.

One of the most powerful features of MR imaging is the ability to create images in any plane, with large fields of view (Fig. 3-10). The images are acquired directly in the plane of interest, rather than recreated after the fact using processing techniques. This characteristic can be extremely useful when imaging blood vessels.

The MR signal characteristics of tissues can be complex. Normal fat, muscle, tendon, solid organs, and fluids have different signal intensities on T1- and T2-weighted images. These signal characteristics can change with the presence of pathology, bleeding, or following administration of a contrast agent. In general, fast-flowing blood is usually black, as it moves out of the image before any signal can be collected (Figs. 3-10 and 3-11). The signal characteristics of static blood (thrombus) are variable but specific with respect to the pulse sequence and the age of the thrombus (Table 3-1). After administration of contrast, blood and organs will usually become bright on most sequences. Inflammatory changes in the wall of a blood vessel will enhance. However, bone and air will always appear dark. The inability to visualize vascular calcification is an important limitation of MR imaging of vascular pathology. Nevertheless, conventional MR images are invaluable in the evaluation of most vascular diseases and should be included in most studies, with the exception of lower-extremity runoffs.

Magnetic resonance angiography (MRA) is the application of MR techniques to the imaging of flowing blood. The application was first described in 1985, and there are now numerous strategies for imaging flow in a

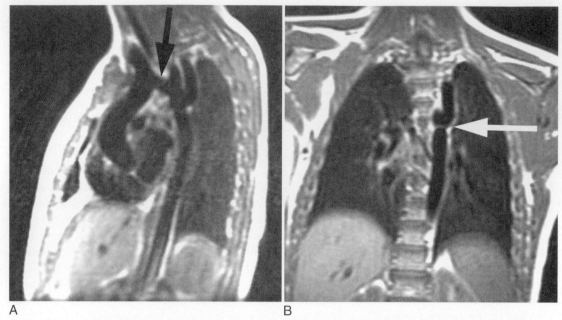

Figure 3-10   Aortic coarctation. **A**, T1-weighted oblique sagittal image of the thoracic aorta in a child with hypertension. The aortic arch is hypoplastic (arrow). Note that blood flow in the aorta is black. **B**, T1-weighted coronal image of the same patient shows a web (arrow) in the aorta. Notice the relative signal characteristics of fat, muscle, liver, lung, and the aortic lumen in these images.

magnetic field (Table 3-2). Each technique relies upon a different aspect of MR imaging to visualize blood flow. Time-of-flight (TOF) and phase-contrast (PC) sequences image flowing protons, and are susceptible to signal loss due to turbulence, slow flow, and rapid changes in velocity,

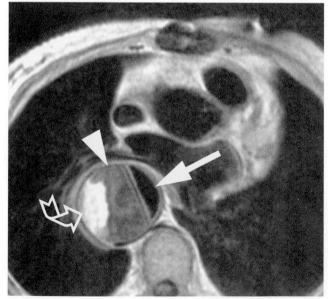

Figure 3-11   Axial T1-weighted image of chronic aortic dissection. Fast flow in the true lumen is black (straight arrow), slow flow in the false lumen is gray (arrowhead), and chronic mural thrombus in the false lumen is bright (curved arrow).

conditions which frequently exist in diseased blood vessels (Figs. 3-12 and 3-13). These techniques are used for either slice-by-slice (2-dimensional, or "2-D") or volume (3-dimensional, or "3-D") acquisitions. In general, 2-D imaging provides excellent vascular signal at the expense of image resolution, whereas 3-D imaging provides better resolution (thinner slices) but is susceptible to signal loss as volumes increase in size. Both TOF and PC imaging decreased in importance following the introduction of gadolinium-enhanced 3-D MRA by Prince in 1993.

Gadolinium-enhanced MRA images the contrast agent, with only a slight flow-related enhancement, and very little image degradation from abnormal flow patterns. The gadolinium contrast agent is injected rapidly through a peripheral vein, with image acquisition timed to occur as

Table 3-1 MR Signal Characteristics of Thrombus[a]		
Age	**T1**	**T2**
<24 hours	Intermediate	Intermediate
24–72 hours	Dark	Dark
3–7 days	Bright	Dark
7–14 days	Bright	Bright
Chronic:		
Periphery	Intermediate	Dark
Center	Intermediate	Intermediate-bright

[a] This table is a rough guide. Thrombus of varying ages may be present in the same hematoma.

Table 3-2   Magnetic Resonance Imaging Techniques

Technique	Basic Principle	Blood/Background Signal
Black-blood	No signal from rapidly flowing blood; normal signal from surrounding tissues	Dark/bright
Time-of-flight (TOF)	Signal from fresh protons in flowing blood visible against suppressed signal from background tissues; slowly moving blood may lose signal; venous/arterial selection by saturation of opposite inflow; time-consuming and limited anatomic coverage for volume imaging	Bright/dark
Phase-contrast (PC)	Measurement of phase shift of spinning proton at two time points at it moves through magnetic field; provides directional and velocity information; stationary protons have no phase shift; volume imaging time-consuming and limited anatomic coverage	Bright/dark
Gadolinium-enhanced	Signal from intravascular contrast agent (no saturation); timing critical, especially to separate arteries and veins; background signal present but minimal; quick volume imaging of large body areas	Bright/dark

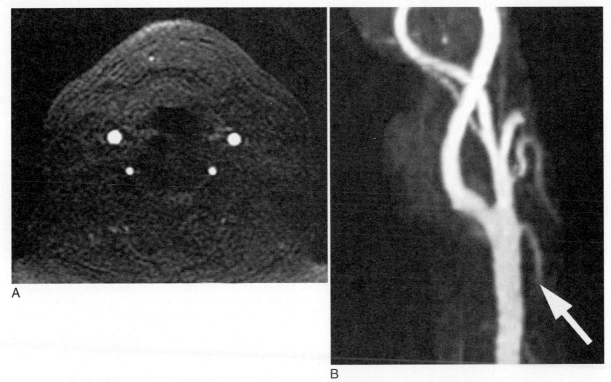

Figure 3-12   Time-of-flight (TOF) MR angiography (MRA) of the carotid arteries. TOF MRA is based upon saturation of signal from background tissues and detection of signal from "fresh" spins in blood flowing into the slice or volume. **A,** Axial 2-D TOF image of the neck. The complete study consists of many more contiguous images, collected individually and sequentially. The common carotid and vertebral arteries are visible as white structures. The signal from the background tissues is suppressed. The venous signal is eliminated by a saturation band that is positioned superior to and moves with each slice. **B,** Maximum intensity projection (MIP) of a portion of the same 2-D TOF MRA provides an angiographic view of the right carotid artery. Only the brightest pixels are displayed on the 2-D MIP image. Note the loss of signal in the superior thyroidal artery (arrow) as it reverses direction in the neck. The signal from the flow in this portion of the artery was eliminated by the saturation band used to suppress venous flow.

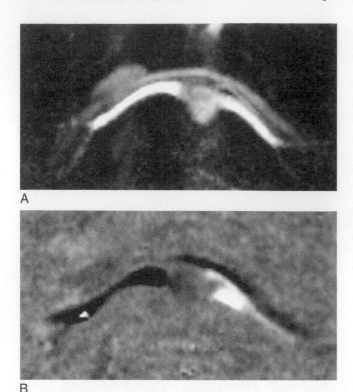

Figure 3-13 Phase-contrast (PC) MRA of the renal arteries. PC MRA is based upon measurement of phase shifts of protons moving through the magnetic field. Stationary protons have no phase shift, resulting in absence of signal from background tissues. The velocity encoding (VENC) for this study was 40 cm/s. This parameter is selected by the operator in PC MRA to purposely maximize signal from flow at a specific velocity. **A**, Axial MIP of a 3-D PC MRA of normal renal arteries. Flow in every direction is depicted as white and there is no background signal. Note the renal veins anterior to the arterial structures. A small accessory renal artery is visible on the left between the left renal artery and vein. **B**, Single slice from the same study encoded for directional flow (right to left). Flow in the left renal arteries is white, and flow in the left renal vein is black. Note that flow in the right renal artery, which is in the same direction as flow in the left renal vein, is also black. Little signal is seen in the aorta, as the predominant direction of flow is superior to inferior.

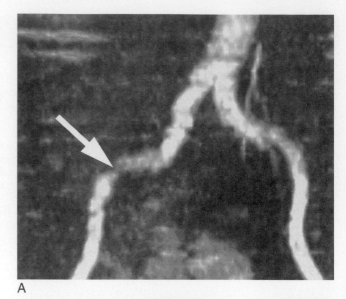

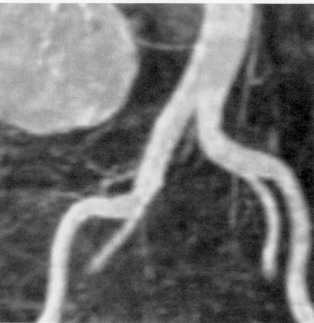

Figure 3-14 Gadolinium-enhanced 3-D MRA. **A**, Coronal MIP image of a 2-D TOF MRA of the pelvis acquired in the axial plane. There is an apparent stenosis of the right external iliac artery (EIA) (arrow). The vessels have a jagged appearance due to motion artifact. **B**, MIP image of a gadolinium-enhanced 3-D MRA of the same patient acquired in the coronal plane shows that the right EIA is normal. The signal loss in the 2-D TOF study was due to saturation of in-plane flow in the horizontal segment of the EIA. Note the smooth vessel contours in this 3-D acquisition.

the contrast enters the arterial circulation in the region of interest (Fig. 3-14). Imaging with this technique can be accomplished in a single breath-hold, encompassing large fields of view (Fig. 3-15). Although 3-D volumes are routinely used, there is no loss of signal due to saturation effects as experienced with noncontrast techniques. In fast scanners equipped with moving tables, stepping studies can be obtained that cover from the renal arteries to the ankles. Coronary and pulmonary artery MRA are a reality with gadolinium contrast and ultrafast scanners (Box 3-1).

There are fewer adverse reactions to gadolinium contrast agents than with iodinated contrast, and gadolinium appears to have little clinical nephrotoxicity.

Gadolinium-enhanced 3-D acquisitions are the most versatile and reliable technique for vascular MRA.

MR imaging techniques are subject to a number of limitations (Box 3-2). Patients with cardiac pacemakers, defibrillators, intra-ocular or intra-aural metallic foreign bodies, or claustrophobia cannot be imaged.

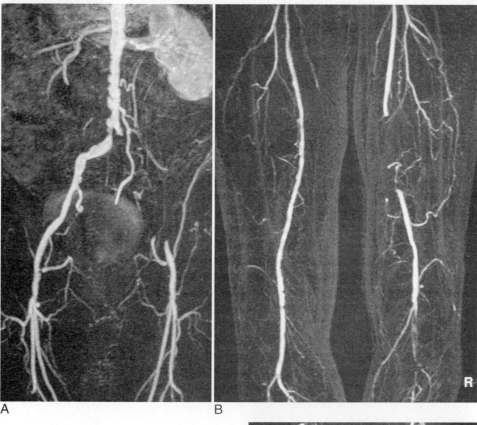

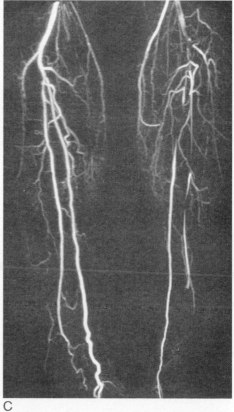

Figure 3-15   Gadolinium-enhanced 3-D MRA of the aorta and bilateral lower extremity arteries in a patient with peripheral vascular disease. The study was acquired in the coronal plane with three overlapping slabs, a moving scanning table, and a single injection of 40 mL of gadolinium. The study is displayed as MIP images. **A**, Aorta and pelvis. **B**, Superficial femoral and popliteal arteries. **C**, Tibial arteries.

Ferromagnetic objects in or adjacent to blood vessels can create susceptibility artifacts that result in signal loss (Fig. 3-16). Too much gadolinium can be a bad thing: highly concentrated gadolinium shortens T2 and results in signal loss in vessels and surrounding susceptibility artifacts (Fig. 3-17). Heavy circumferential intimal calcification in medium or small arteries may also result in susceptibility artifacts and apparent stenoses on MRA sequences. Specialized MR-compatible equipment is required for hemodynamic monitoring of unstable patients; lethal complications can occur when metallic objects are sucked into the bore while a patient is being scanned. Uncooperative or demented patients who are not be able to hold still during image acquisition can render a study useless.

CT/CT ANGIOGRAPHY

The development of helical CT scanners revitalized the vascular applications of this imaging modality. Conventional scanners imaged one slice at a time, with the table in a stationary position. Although conventional CT was recognized as an excellent modality for visualizing blood vessel morphology, imaging was too slow to be used for angiographic studies. Helical (or spiral) CT scanners image continuously as the patient is moved rapidly

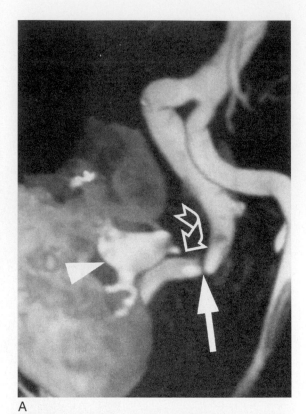

A

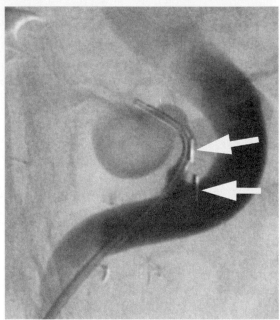

B

Figure 3-16   Signal loss due to metallic susceptibility artifact from surgical clips. **A**, Oblique MIP of a gadolinium-enhanced 3-D MRA of a renal transplant artery. There is apparent band-like stenosis of the external iliac artery (EIA) (straight arrow) and signal loss in the proximal transplant artery (curved arrow). An aneurysm of the renal artery is also present (arrow head). The femoral pulse was normal on that side. **B**, Selective digital subtraction angiogram (DSA) of the transplant renal artery shows a normal EIA, a proximal renal artery stenosis, and a distal renal artery aneurysm. Metallic clips (arrows) are adjacent to the EIA and the renal artery.

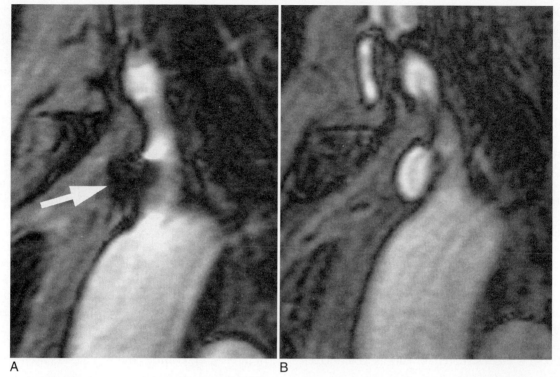

A   B

Figure 3-17   Signal loss due to concentrated gadolinium. **A,** Single slice from a gadolinium-enhanced 3-D MRA of the aortic arch obtained during injection of contrast through a left upper-extremity vein. There is a signal void in the left brachiocephalic vein (arrow) with surrounding susceptibility artifact causing an apparent bulky eccentric stenosis of the adjacent brachiocephalic artery. **B,** Single slice (same location) from the same study obtained 30 seconds after the first image. The concentration of gadolinium in the left upper-extremity veins has decreased. The brachiocephalic vein is normal and the brachiocephalic artery stenosis is less impressive.

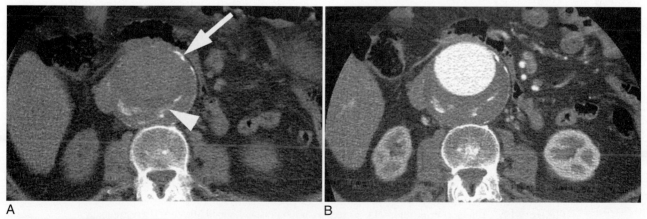

A   B

Figure 3-18   Axial CT scan of the abdominal aorta from a helical acquisition. **A,** Image without contrast of an abdominal aortic aneurysm. The wall of the aneurysm is identified by the calcification in the intimal layer (arrow). The patency of the aneurysm cannot be determined from this image, but mural thrombus containing calcium (arrowhead) is present. **B,** Contrast-enhanced image at a similar level shows the aortic lumen. The mural thrombus is now lower in density than the blood. Without the precontrast study the calcified areas in the thrombus could be misinterpreted as contrast.

through the gantry. Slip-ring technology in the CT scan gantry allows continuous rotation of the x-ray tube, without the need to stop and "rewind" between slices. Data are acquired in a volume, as with 3-D MRA, rather than as individual slices. As with conventional CT, slice thickness is determined by collimation of the x-ray beam. The scan time is dramatically reduce compared to conventional CT, so that a bolus of contrast can be tracked as it opacifies a vascular bed. Large anatomic areas can be scanned in 20–30 seconds, usually during a single breath-hold.

The initial helical scanners were equipped with a single row of detector elements. Helical scanners with multidetector row technology (MDCT) further decrease scan times, with improved image quality. Multiple interweaving helices (up to 32) can be acquired at the same time, allowing reduced scan times, reduced volumes of contrast, reduced motion and pulsatility artifacts, and improved spatial resolution. Slice thickness is determined by the thickness of the detector elements rather than beam collimation, and may be substantially less than 1 mm. Scanning of the entire vascular system from the arch to the toes in less than 30 seconds is a clinical reality. The helical data is reconstructed initially as axial images,

like conventional CT. Unstable patients can be scanned expeditiously and without special monitoring equipment.

Important information can be obtained about the vascular system without the use of intravenous contrast. All CT scans for vascular pathology should begin with a noncontrast scan. The size of the blood vessel and the degree of vascular calcification can be easily assessed on noncontrast CT (Fig. 3-18). Acute extravascular blood appears dense on noncontrast CT, so that the diagnosis of acute hemorrhage from vascular injury or rupture does not require intravenous contrast. In some situations, such as during evaluation of suspected ruptured aortic aneurysm, the CT scan can be terminated after the noncontrast images have been obtained, expediting intervention and avoiding renal exposure to iodinated contrast agents.

The basic principle of CT angiography (CTA) is a carefully timed helical acquisition during the rapid peripheral infusion of iodinated contrast. Determination of correct timing can be performed with automated techniques, test boluses, or "best guess" based upon empiric delays (Fig. 3-19). The latter method is least reliable in older patients or those with cardiac disease. The region of interest determines the parameters used for the scan.

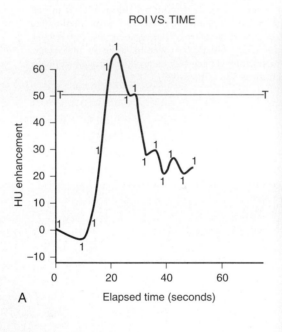

A

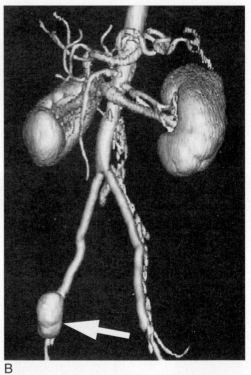

B

Figure 3-19   Timing is critical for CTA (as well as for contrast-enhanced MRA). **A,** There are many techniques for optimizing image acquisition during peak vascular opacification. Shown is a curve of opacification measured in Hounsfield units in the supraceliac aorta after injection of 10 mL of contrast. An imaging delay of 20 seconds between initial injection of contrast and scanning was used for the study based upon this curve. **B,** Oblique shaded surface display of the CTA obtained with the 20-second delay following initiation of injection of 100 mL of 60% iodine at 5 mL/s on a multidetector row CT. There is an aortobifemoral bypass graft with an anastomotic pseudoaneurysm on the right (arrow). Note the calcification in the occluded native arteries posterior to the graft.

Box 3-3 CTA Advantages

Large field of view
Vascular enhancement by contrast
Rapid scan time allows extensive longitudinal coverage
   (whole-body scan)
Limited number of variables to manipulate
Source images have valuable information
Scanners readily available
Conventional monitoring/respiratory equipment
   can be used

Box 3-4 CTA Limitations

Timing critical
Overestimates degree of stenosis, especially in
   calcified vessels
Metal and bone can obscure vascular structures
Signal-to-noise poor in large patients
Nephrotoxic contrast material
Patient motion degrades study

In general, CTA is less complicated than MRA, and faster. When protocoling studies, keep in mind that the thinner the collimation or greater the pitch, the lower the ratio of signal to noise in the image.

CTA is entirely dependent upon imaging of increased intravascular density due to a contrast agent. Information from background tissues is not suppressed, as in MRA. Three factors are important in choosing a contrast agent for CTA: injection rate, total volume, and concentration of iodine. Visualization of small vessels improves as the concentration of iodine in the blood increases. Most CTA studies utilize injection rates of 3–5 mL/s for a total volume of 70–150 mL. Contrast agents containing at least 60% iodine provide the best results in most instances.

One of the major advantages of CTA is that the source images are simply axial slices with intense vascular opacification (see Fig. 3-18). All of the information that one would normally expect regarding the vascular wall and perivascular structures on a CT scan is still present on the source images. This allows more comprehensive evaluation of the vascular structures than with MRA (Box 3-3). Although metal can create streak artifacts that degrade images, carefully windowed thin-slice CTA can be used to follow intravascular stents (Fig. 3-20).

CTA has certain important limitations (Box 3-4). Patients with contrast allergies or renal failure may not be candidates for elective studies, as well as those with contraindications to ionizing radiation (such as patients in the first trimester of pregnancy). Heavily calcified vessels are difficult to evaluate, as bulky intimal calcium can be indistinguishable from the opacified vessel lumen. Concentrated contrast can cause streak artifacts that mimic pathology or obscure detail (Fig. 3-21). Pulsatile vessels (particularly the ascending aorta) can be similarly difficult to image owing to motion artifacts. Uncooperative patients introduce motion or respiratory artifacts that seriously degrade the final images.

POST-PROCESSING

In order to view the data from MRA and CTA studies as angiograms, electronic post-processing of source digital data is necessary. This crucial step occurs after the study has been completed, and frequently after the patient has been removed from the scanner. A number of post-processing options are available, ranging from simple reformating of data into different planes (i.e., coronal

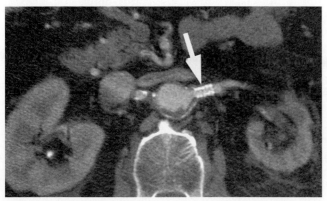

Figure 3-20   Axial source image from a CTA windowed to show a left renal artery stent (arrow).

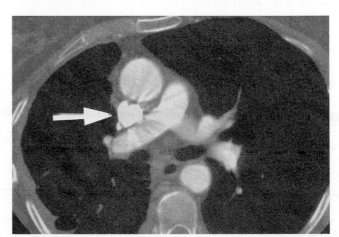

Figure 3-21   Axial CT image showing a streak artifact from dense contrast in the superior vena cava (arrow) extending into the ascending aorta and pulmonary artery.

Table 3-3 Post-processing Techniques

Technique	Basic Principle	Strengths	Weaknesses
Reformat	Allows display of all data in volume in user-defined 2-D planes, including curved	Quick; no loss of data; can display complex anatomy	Overlap of structures can be confusing, 2-D display only
Maximum-intensity projection (MIP)	Displays brightest voxels in user-defined 2-D planes; discards background information	Quick; bright vessels	Threshold for display may result in loss of critical information; 2-D display only
Shaded surface display (SSD)	Selects and displays brightest voxels as a virtual surface (i.e., empty cup) shaded to have 3-D appearance	3-D-like rendition of surface of complex structures	Model may result in loss of critical information
Volume rendering	Displays voxels as a virtual 3-dimensional volume; objects selected by setting threshold, opacity values	3-D-like rendition of selected voxel values while retaining complete data set	Threshold for model may render critical voxels transparent
Endoscopic	Displays tubular structures without intraluminal contents with 3-D appearance	Allows viewer to enter and travel through lumen of blood vessel	Intraluminal perspective only

slices from axially acquired data), to 3-dimensional renderings that permit an endoscopic viewpoint of the vascular lumen (Table 3-3 and Fig. 3-22; see also Figs 3-12 and 3-19). Excellent post-processed images can only be created from excellent original data.

The source data for MRA and CTA are composed of discrete elements termed voxels. Each voxel has only one numerical value, determined by the measured density or signal from the structures in the voxel. If a voxel contains two structures with differing values, it will be assigned a value that is an average of both. There is no way to retrospectively separate these two structures with current post-processing techniques. For this reason, small cube-shaped voxels are most desirable to maximize image detail and facilitate post-processing. If an image is constructed of large rectangular voxels, small objects may get "lost" (partial volume averaging), particularly when viewed from a perspective perpendicular to the long axis of the voxel. The regions of an image in which this becomes most apparent are curved edges or borders

of structures. However, the smaller the voxel, the greater the impact of background noise.

Post-processing is the sophisticated manipulation of voxels in order to enhance or emphasize important features of an image. With the exception of reformatting, angiographic post-processing results in loss of data as nonvascular voxels are rendered transparent or discarded. The remaining voxels are then manipulated to enhance the appearance of the final images, often by adding or further subtracting data as needed.

A few generalizations can be made regarding post-processing techniques. Most sophisticated post-processing is performed on fast independent workstations equipped with proprietary software. Datasets must be heavily edited with excision of unwanted portions of the images in order to produce satisfactory 3-D models. This requires an individual with some understanding of vascular anatomy and pathology. In addition, the source data must have excellent contrast between vascular structures and background tissues. For these reasons, all 3-D models

Figure 3-22 Image post-processing is crucial to MRA and CTA. **A**, Single axial slice from a contrast-enhanced CT showing a portion of normal renal arteries. **B**, Summation (thick slab) of several slices from the same dataset as in A shows the main renal arteries in their entirety. **C**, Sagittal midline planar linear reformation in a patient with a surgical graft for AAA. Note that all of the source data are preserved, so that perigraft thrombus (arrows) is visible. **D**, Volume rendering of the same dataset as in C, showing only the vascular structures. Note that the perigraft thrombus is no longer visible. **E**, Endoscopic view of the bifurcation of the left main renal artery from the same dataset as in Fig. 3-19.

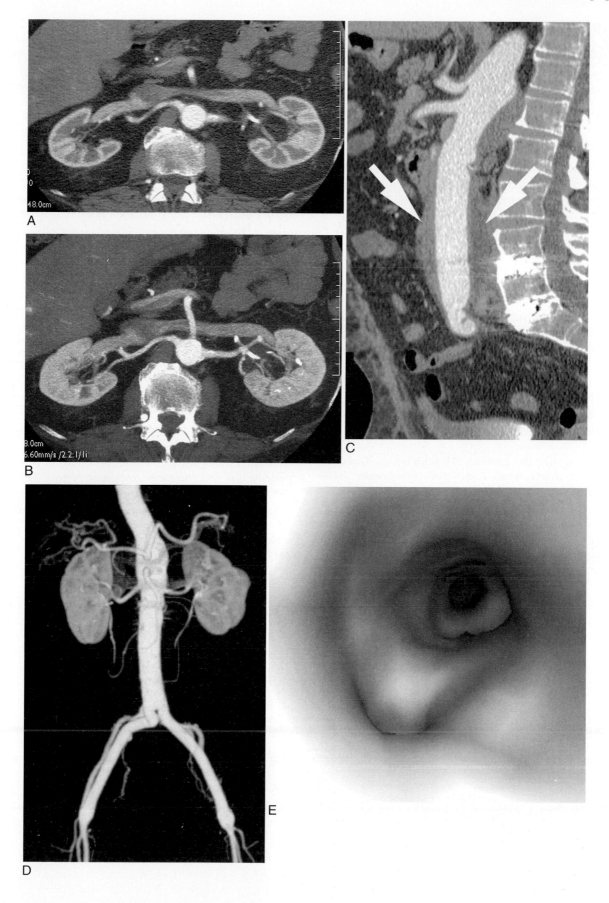

Box 3-5   Postprocessing Hints
Learn how to do it yourself Always review source data for any questionable finding Poor original data make for poor post-processed data

must be viewed with some skepticism, as important information can be omitted at several stages during creation of the final images (Box 3-5).

SUGGESTED READINGS

Fenlon HM, Yucel EK: Advances in abdominal, aortic, and peripheral contrast-enhanced MR angiography. *Magn Reson Imaging Clin N Am* 7:319-336, 1999.

Fleischmann D, Rubin GD, Bankier AA et al: Improved uniformity of aortic enhancement with customized contrast medium injection protocols at CT angiography. *Radiology* 214:363-371, 2000.

Grant EG: Sonographic contrast agents in vascular imaging. *Semin Ultrasound CT MR* 22:25-41, 2001.

Jara H, Barish MA: Black-blood MR angiography: techniques, and clinical applications. *Magn Reson Imaging Clin N Am* 7:303-317, 1999.

Kaufman JA, Hartnell GA, Trerotola SO: *Noninvasive Vascular Imaging with Ultrasound, Computed Tomography, and Magnetic Resonance.* SCVIR, Fairfax, VA, 1997.

Kuszyk BS, Fishman EK: Technical aspects of CT angiography. *Semin Ultrasound CT MR* 19:383-393, 1998.

Murphy KJ, Rubin JM: Power Doppler: it's a good thing. *Semin Ultrasound CT MR* 18:13-21, 1997.

Neimatallah MA, Chenevert TL, Carlos RC et al: Subclavian MR arteriography: reduction of susceptibility artifact with short echo time and dilute gadopentetate dimeglumine. *Radiology* 217:581-586, 2000.

Nghiem HV, Jeffrey RB: CT angiography of the visceral vasculature. *Semin Ultrasound CT MR* 19:439-446, 1998.

Prince MR: Contrast-enhanced MR angiography: theory and optimization. *Magn Reson Imaging Clin N Am* 6:257-267, 1998.

Prince MR, Yucel EK, Kaufman JA et al: Dynamic gadolinium-enhanced three-dimensional abdominal MR arteriography. *J Magn Reson Imaging* 3:877-881, 1993.

Rofsky NM: MR angiography of the aortoiliac and femoropopliteal vessels. *Magn Reson Imaging Clin N Am* 6;371-384, 1998.

Rubin GD: Techniques for performing multidetector-row computed tomographic angiography. *Tech Vasc Interv Radiol* 4:2-14, 2001.

Rubin GD, Shiau MC, Schmidt AJ et al: CT angiography: historical perspective and new state-of-the-art using multidetector-row helical CT. *J Comp Assist Tomogr* 23:S83-S90, 1999.

Scoutt LM, Zawin ML, Taylor KJ: Doppler US: II. Clinical applications. *Radiology* 174:309-319, 1990.

Stein B, Leary CJ, Ohki SK: Magnetic resonance angiography: the nuts and bolts. *Tech Vasc Interv Radiol* 4:27-44, 2001.

Strandness DE: *Duplex Scanning of Vascular Disorders*, 3rd edn. Lippincott Willams & Wilkins, Philadelphia, 2002.

Taylor KJ, Holland S: Doppler US: I. Basic principles, instrumentation, and pitfalls. *Radiology* 174:297-307, 1990.

Wedeen VJ, Meuli RA, Edelman RR et al: Projective imaging of pulsatile flow with magnetic resonance. *Science* 230:946-968, 1985.

Willens HJ, Kessler KM: Transesophageal echocardiography in the diagnosis of diseases of the thoracic aorta: II. Atherosclerotic and traumatic diseases of the aorta. *Chest* 117: 233-243, 2000.

Vascular Interventions

JOHN A. KAUFMAN, M.D.

There are four basic types of percutaneous vascular interventions: those that increase flow, decrease flow, implant devices, and remove things. The fundamentals of these interventions are the same regardless of the vessel. This chapter describes the principles of vascular interventions. The results of specific interventions are discussed in the appropriate anatomic chapters.

The history of percutaneous catheter-based vascular interventions mirrors the development of interventional radiology. Angiography was first an invasive diagnostic imaging modality. At the end of the procedure the catheter was removed and the patient went off to have surgery or medical treatment. In 1964, Charles Dotter dilated a popliteal artery stenosis using progressively larger catheters, thus performing the first percutaneous transluminal angioplasty (PTA) (Fig. 4-1). A radical new paradigm was proposed: conditions diagnosed at angiography could actually be treated by radiologists using catheters. The milestones in vascular intervention are listed in Table 4-1.

When the first image-guided intervention was performed, radiology was transformed. As the durability and acceptance of vascular interventions have grown, they have been renamed "endovascular therapy" and adopted by nonradiologic specialists. At the same time, interventional radiologists have focused on the global management of patients undergoing image-guided therapy. That is where the future of the specialty lies.

INCREASING BLOOD FLOW THROUGH VESSELS

Fundamentals

A variety of techniques have been devised to restore blood vessel patency, but all have certain elements in common (Box 4-1). This section focuses on these fundamentals, with specific interventions discussed in

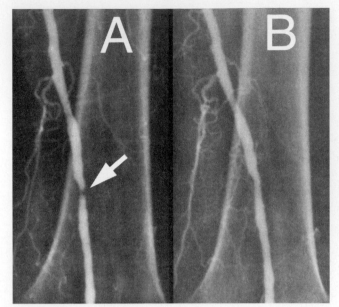

Figure 4-1   The first percutaneous angioplasty, 1964. **A**, Focal stenosis in the popliteal artery (arrow). **B**, Using progressively large coaxial catheters, the lesion was dilated. The patient's rest pain resolved and toe ulcers healed.

subsequent sections. Interventions should be performed only after a complete diagnostic evaluation in appropriately symptomatic patients. The lesion responsible for the symptoms should be identified and characterized, and both the inflow and outflow evaluated. Lesion morphology is very important in guiding intervention and predicting outcome (Fig. 4-2). For example, short concentric noncalcified atherosclerotic lesions usually respond best to simple angioplasty, whereas long, calcified occlusions may be impossible to cross or dilate. Careful review of the appearance of the lesion, sometimes in several obliquities, may be necessary.

Once the decision to intervene is made, a vascular sheath should be inserted. Medications commonly used during interventions should be prepared in advance

Table 4-1 Milestones in Vascular Intervention		
Innovation	**Year**	**Innovator**
Embolization	1960	Luessenhop
Transvascular biopsy	1962	Sakakibara
Percutaneous angioplasty	1964	Dotter
Percutaneous foreign body retrieval	1964	Thomas
Percutaneous stent	1969	Dotter
Intraarterial thrombolysis	1974	Dotter
Stent-graft	1986	Balko

Box 4-1   Basic Steps in Recanalization Procedures
Review patient history
Diagnose lesion
Administer ancillary drugs (especially heparin)
Cross lesion with selective catheter and guidewire
Confirm intraluminal position distal to lesion
Exchange for working guidewire
Perform intervention
Document result
Follow-up

(Table 4-2). The patient should be heparinized just before or immediately after crossing the lesion. The lesion is crossed with an atraumatic selective guidewire, often directed by a selective catheter (Box 4-2). Once the guidewire is across the lesion, the catheter is advanced over the guidewire, and the guidewire removed. Aspiration of blood, injection of contrast, and/or measurement of a pressure gradient across the lesion confirm that the lumen has been reached on the other side. The ability to aspirate blood is particularly important after crossing an occlusion, as the guidewire may have become and remain subintimal. In some circumstances, particularly when recanalizing long lower-extremity occlusions, a subintimal channel with re-entry distal to the lesion is purposively created with the guidewire ("subintimal angioplasty"). After confirming successful navigation across the lesion, a working guidewire is

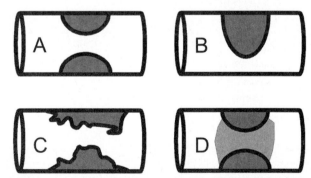

Figure 4-2   Idealized drawings of basic lesion morphologies. Any of these lesions may be soft or heavily calcified. **A**, Concentric stenosis. This is an optimal lesion for intervention, especially angioplasty alone. **B**, Eccentric stenosis. Difficult to treat with angioplasty alone as the normal wall opposing the lesion will stretch and recoil with balloon inflation. **C**, Irregular stenosis. This lesion may be more difficult to cross due to the irregularity of the surface. **D**, Occlusion. Thrombus within the lesion that, if fresh, may need to be addressed with thrombolysis or mechanical thrombectomy prior to treatment of the stenosis.

Table 4-2   Drugs Commonly Used During Revascularization Procedures

Medication	Dose	Purpose
Heparin (1000 U/mL)	3000–7000 UIA	Prevent thrombus formation
Nitroglycerin (100 μg/mL)	200–250 μg aliquots IA	Prevent/treat local spasm
Aspirin	325 mg p.o.	Prevent platelet aggregation
Glycoprotein IIb/IIIa antagonists	12–24 h infusion IV	Prevent platelet aggregation
Abciximab	0.25 mg/kg bolus, then 0.125 μg/kg/min (max 10mg/min)	
Eptifibatide	180 μg/kg bolus, then 0.5 μg/kg/min	
Tirofiban	0.4 μg/kg/min for 30 min, then 0.1 μg/kg/min	
ADP receptor antagonists		Prevent platelet aggregation
Clopidogrel	300 mg p.o. loading dose 2–3 h prior to procedure, then 75 mg daily for 1–3 months	

U, units; IA, intraarterial; IV, intravenous; ADP, adenosine diphosphate.

advanced through the catheter to provide stability for the intervention. In general, relatively stiff guidewires are used that allow devices to be advanced into position without loosing access across the lesion. Examples include the Amplatz and Rosen guidewires. Hydrophilic coated guidewires are usually not a good choice, as they easily slip out of place during catheter exchanges. Once access is secure, the intervention is performed. The outcome of the intervention is documented with angiography and/or pressure measurements. The guidewire should remain across the lesion until success has been documented. When appropriate, the status of the vessels distal to or proximal to the intervention may be re-evaluated as well. Clinical follow-up tailored to the intervention should be performed by the interventional radiologist.

Accurate device sizing (such as balloons, stents, or stent-grafts) requires consideration of several factors (Box 4-3). Oversizing of device diameters by 5–10% greater than the diameter of the normal lumen is the general rule. Very tight or calcified lesions may require progressive dilation with sequentially larger balloons. The final desired diameter of a blood vessel is determined from an adjacent normal segment of vessel, the same vessel on the other side of the body in the case of bilateral

structures, or the known average size of the vessel (i.e., "rule of thumb" technique) (Fig. 4-3). When measuring directly from images, it is helpful to calibrate to a known internal standard such as a marker catheter, but this method is not always accurate. Many digital units include measuring software. Structures are magnified by approximately 15% on screen film images. The vessel and the type of lesion also impact sizing, as veins are usually more compliant, whereas heavily calcified arteries may literally fracture when overdilated.

The length of the device should be sufficient to treat the diseased area, with minimal trauma to adjacent normal or slightly diseased vessels. When the area of disease to be treated extends up to or across a bifurcation into a smaller diameter vessel, the device should be sized or delivered in a manner that avoids trauma to the smaller or normal vessel. (See Balloon Angioplasty below.)

The optimal clinical outcome of recanalization procedures is durable improvement of the patient's symptoms.

Box 4-2   Crossing the Lesion

Be sure of lesion morphology
Choose optimal obliquity
Start slowly and gently
Use atraumatic tools
Redirect rather than push harder
Spiral or "barber pole" trajectory of guidewire
  frequently indicates subintimal location

Box 4-3   Factors to Consider when Sizing Balloons, Stents, and Stent-Grafts

Delivery System Characteristics

Catheter size
Sheath size
Flexibility of device

Lesion Characteristics

Type of vessel
Type of lesion
Initial lumen diameter
Diameter of vessel over length of lesion
Desired final diameter
Length of vessel to be treated

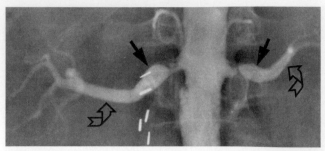

Figure 4-3   Post-stenotic dilatation (straight arrows) due to bilateral ostial renal artery stenoses. The distal renal arteries reveal the true normal diameters (curved arrows).

Since the clinical outcome cannot always be measured during a procedure, most interventionists use technical endpoints such as a residual luminal stenosis of less than 20%, or reduction of the pressure gradient across the lesion to a predetermined level. Pressure gradients across lesions are a very useful means of deciding when to perform and when to stop a procedure. Reliance upon angiographic appearance as the sole indication for intervention leads to treating the image, not the patient. Pressures are measured intravascularly, both proximal and distal to the lesion (Table 4-3). The most accurate systems obtain simultaneous pressures using two end-hole catheters, or an end-hole catheter and a sheath (Fig. 4-4). Frequently, a single catheter is pulled through the lesion with continuous recording of pressures. In many instances a catheter must be across the lesion of interest in order to obtain a distal pressure, such as in the renal artery. In this situation, it is possible that the catheter itself will accentuate the severity of the gradient by partially obstructing the lesion. Specialized pressure-sensing guidewires may be useful in these cases, but in general most interventionists feel that any *symptomatic* lesion tight enough to be partially obstructed by a 5-French catheter requires treatment. When in doubt, injection of 200–300 μg of nitroglycerine (NTG) or another

vasodilator *distal* to the lesion may induce hyperemia and unmask a gradient. Always remember that technical success and clinical success do not always coincide; pushing an intervention to an extreme in order to obtain a pretty image or perfect gradient risks harming the patient.

Procedural complications associated with opening of blood vessels are related to the patient's general status, the difficulty of the procedure, the size and type of the device, the underlying condition of the vessels, and the intensity of anticoagulation (Box 4-4). Older patients with acute illnesses, diffuse vascular disease, and concurrent major illnesses are most likely to experience a complication. Large complex devices have more complications than small simple devices.

Delayed failure (i.e., restenosis of the lesion) of a recanalization procedure occurs for different reasons at different times (Table 4-4). Most early failures are due to technical issues such as an occlusive dissection adjacent to the intervention site, elastic recoil of a fibrotic lesion,

---

Box 4-4   Complications of Recanalization Procedures

Vessel spasm
Intimal dissection
Occlusion of branch vessels
Thrombosis
Embolization:
    Atheromatous plaque
    Thrombus
    Cholesterol
Vessel rupture
Access site hemorrhage
Remote hemorrhage

Table 4-3   Acceptable Postintervention Pressure Gradients (mmHg)[a]

Anatomic Region	Parameter	At Rest	Augmented[b]
Arterial	Systolic	≤10	≤15
Venous	Mean	≤5	NA
TIPS[c]	Mean	≤12	NA

[a] Patient supine.
[b] Following injection of 200–300 μg of nitroglycerin, or 15–25 mg tolazoline distal to lesion.
[c] Transjugular intrahepatic portosystemic shunt, portal to inferior vena cava gradient.

Table 4-4   Causes of Failure of Arterial Recanalization Procedures

Etiology	0–30 days	30–60 days	3–12 months	>12 months
Occlusive dissection	×			
Elastic recoil	×			
Thrombosis	×			
Inadequate dilatation	×	×		
Missed lesion	×	×	×	
Intimal hyperplasia			×	
Progressive atherosclerosis				×
Kinked or crushed stent	×	×	×	×

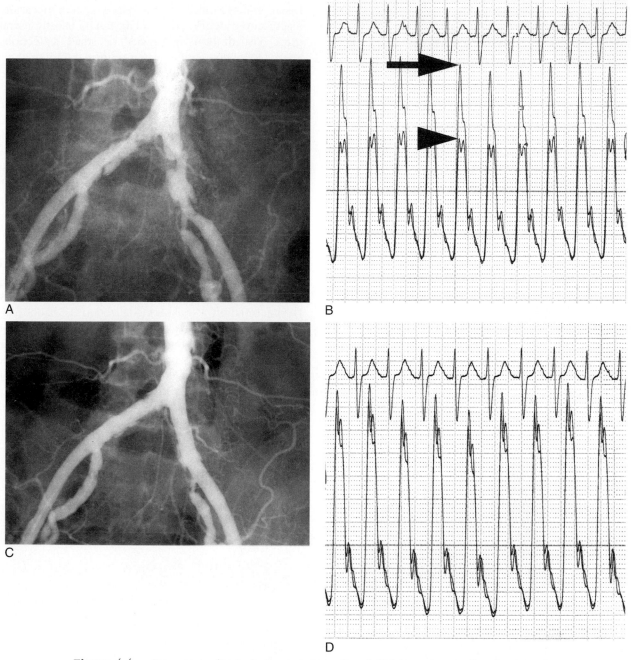

Figure 4-4   Pressure gradients during an intervention. **A**, Pelvic angiogram showing irregular bilateral common iliac artery (CIA) stenoses, right worse than left. **B**, Simultaneous pressures revealing a gradient (44 mmHg) between a catheter in the aorta (from the right common femoral artery) and a catheter in the left external iliac artery (EIA). A 30-mmHg gradient was present on the right. Arrow = aortic pressure, arrowhead = left EIA pressure. **C**, Pelvic angiogram after placement of bilateral CIA stents (balloon expandable). **D**, Final pressure measurements show superimposed aortic and left EIA pressure tracings. There was no residual gradient on the right.

or perhaps a missed lesion that continues to impair flow. After approximately 3 months, and up to 1 year from the intervention, intimal hyperplasia is the main cause of failure. The degree of intimal hyperplasia that occurs after an intervention is dependent upon the biology of the

vessel and the extent of the trauma to the endothelium (see Fig. 1-8). In general, the more extensive the area that is treated, the higher the likelihood that intimal hyperplasia will be a problem. Restenosis occurs in or adjacent to the original lesion. After 1 year, failure of a recanalization

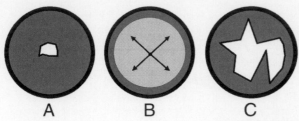

Figure 4-5 Schematic of the mechanism of angioplasty. **A,** Concentric stenosis with a small residual lumen. **B,** An appropriately sized angioplasty balloon is inflated (arrows) in the lumen. **C,** Fracturing, fissuring, and subintimal dissection of the plaque greatly increase the cross-sectional area of the lumen.

procedure is more likely to be due to progression of disease in the inflow or outflow vessels. Factors such as smoking, diet, hyperlipidemia, and homocysteinemia contribute to late failure.

Balloon Angioplasty

The primary mechanism of balloon angioplasty is controlled fracture of the obstructing plaque (Fig. 4-5). This results in formation of fissures in the plaque itself, and tearing of the edges of the plaque away from the adjacent normal intima. With proper oversizing of the balloon, the muscular media is stretched as well. Plaque is

not remodeled, redistributed, or vaporized by the balloon. Distal embolization of microscopic and, occasionally, macroscopic debris does occur, but is usually asymptomatic. Visualization of "cracks" or small dissections in lesions following angioplasty is a normal finding at angiography (Fig. 4-6). Over time these areas may remodel and the lumen resume a more normal appearance.

Andreas Gruentzig devised the first successful angioplasty balloon. The technology of balloons has become very complex, but in practical terms it can be divided into compliant and noncompliant devices (Fig. 4-7). Compliant balloons are constructed from a material such as latex that continues to expand as pressure is applied. Compliant balloons elongate and conform to the vessel walls, rather than dilate. This type of balloon is most commonly used to temporarily occlude flow.

Noncompliant balloons reach a nominal predetermined diameter during inflation, and remain close to that diameter until bursting (many of these balloons actually increase slightly in diameter as pressure increases). During inflation, a waist is visualized in the balloon at the site of maximal stenosis (Fig. 4-8). Continued inflation of the balloon ultimately obliterates the waist. For recanalization applications, noncompliant balloons are desirable, otherwise the balloon on either side of the waist will expand before the waist can be eliminated. However, some lesions cannot be dilated no matter how

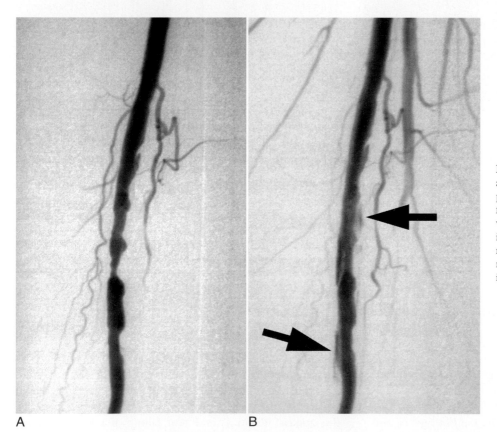

Figure 4-6 Normal angiographic appearance of an artery following angioplasty. **A,** Diseased segment of superficial femoral artery. **B,** After angioplasty with a 5-mm balloon, there is fissuring (arrows) of the plaque. This is a normal postangioplasty appearance and requires no further intervention unless it is flow-limiting.

A

B

much pressure us applied. In this situation, balloon rupture may occur, with potential trauma to the blood vessel. Burst pressures are included on the packaging of all balloons in order to avoid this situation.

The balloon material and construction determine how much pressure can be tolerated before bursting. A balloon that ruptures before the lesion is fully dilated is of little value, but a balloon that is so strong that the vessel ruptures first is potentially dangerous. Balloons are designed to split longitudinally to minimize damage to the vessel wall and facilitate removal (Fig. 4-9).

Balloon diameters range from a few millimeters to more than 3 cm, and lengths from 1 cm to greater than 10 cm. In the peripheral vessels, the sizes most commonly used are diameters of 3–12 mm and lengths of 1–4 cm (Table 4-5). When in doubt, undersize. A larger balloon can always be used if the initial result with a conservatively sized balloon is unsatisfactory, but changing to a smaller balloon will not fix a problem (such as rupture or dissection) created by a large balloon. Because of the physics of balloons (tension = pressure × radius), the larger the balloon, the lower the necessary inflation pressure.

Angioplasty balloons are mounted on angiographic catheters, usually with two lumens: one for a guidewire, and one for balloon inflation/deflation. Both the diameter of the balloon and the size of the catheter determine the overall profile of the balloon. Balloons mounted on 3- to 4-French catheters have the smallest overall profiles, and require 0.018-in or smaller guidewires. The diameters of small vessel balloons are rarely larger than 6–8 mm.

Balloon material is not radiopaque. In order to aid in positioning of the balloon, metallic rings are placed on the catheter at both ends of the balloon (Box 4-5). Dilute contrast is used to inflate the balloon to aid in visualization and facilitate rapid deflation. The balloon is centered over the lesion in order to maximize stability during inflation and force transmitted to the lesion. During inflation, the ends of the balloon inflate first, so-called "dogboning", followed by the waist (see Fig. 4-8). Soft lesions

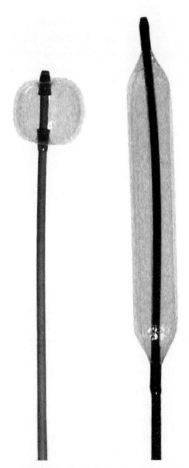

Figure 4-7   Balloon catheters. Latex occlusion balloon (*left*), 8-mm diameter angioplasty balloon on a 5-French shaft (*right*). The occlusion balloon is compliant and responds to increased pressure by enlarging. The angioplasty balloon is relatively noncompliant and reaches a fixed diameter and shape. Increased pressure may slightly increase the diameter, but primarily makes the balloon firmer. Note the short sloping "shoulders" at each end of the angioplasty balloon.

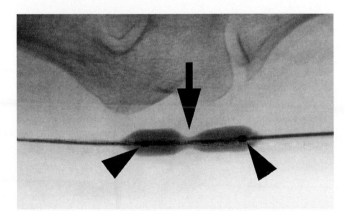

Figure 4-8   Typical appearance of a waist (arrow) in a balloon during an angioplasty (in this case dilatation of a fibrotic venous lesion). Note the radiopaque markers (arrowheads) on the balloon catheter that help in positioning the device. Disappearance of the waist is suggestive of successful angioplasty.

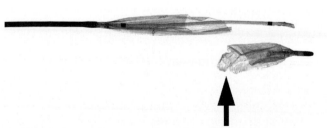

Figure 4-9   Danger of transverse rather than longitudinal balloon rupture. This balloon split circumferentially. The distal portion (arrow) was avulsed during attempted extraction because the balloon membrane mushroomed and jammed against the tip of the sheath.

Table 4-5   Typical Angioplasty Balloon Sizes

Vessel[a]	Balloon Diameter (mm)	Balloon Length (cm)
Internal carotid artery (cervical)	5-6	2-4
Subclavian artery	6-7	2-4
Abdominal aorta	10-16	2-3
Superior mesenteric/ celiac artery	6-7	1-2
Renal artery	5-6	1-2
Common iliac artery	8-10	2-4
External iliac artery	6-7	2-3
Superficial femoral artery	5-6	2-4
Popliteal artery	4-5	1-2
Tibial artery	3-4	1-4
Superior vena cava	12-18	3-4
Subclavian vein	8-16	3-4
Brachial/basilic veins	6-10	3-4
Iliac veins	10-16	3-4

[a] There is a greater range of diameters for veins owing to the distensibility of these vessels.

will dilate with relatively little pressure. Calcified or fibrotic lesions can require substantial pressure, and may never fully dilate. Inflation should be gradual, as rapid, explosive dilatation results in greater trauma to the adjacent normal vessel. In the hands of most humans a 10-mL Luer lock syringe can maximally generate 10-12 atm, which is sufficient to dilate the majority of arterial lesions. A mechanical inflation device, or a smaller syringe (5 or 3 mL) can be used to generate the higher pressures sometimes needed for fibrotic or venous lesions. Balloons are left inflated for 20-60 seconds depending upon the lesion and the vessel. The patient should be asked about discomfort during inflation. Total lack of sensation on the patient's part implies an undersized balloon (provided there is normal vascular enervation).

Box 4-5   Angioplasty Tips

Size balloon conservatively
Give heparin
Slow, steady inflation
Stabilize balloon at sheath during inflation
Maintain guidewire access across lesion until completely finished
Inflate with dilute contrast in 10-mL Luer-lock syringe
Deflate with 20-mL syringe
Counterclockwise rotation during removal from sheath

Mild pressure or pain indicates stretching of the adventitia and a properly oversized balloon. Intense, severe, or sharp pain suggests overdilatation with the associated risk of rupture. To minimize shearing trauma, balloons should not move back and forth through the lesion while inflated. Small balloons have a tendency squirt out of a lesion (similar to pinching a wet watermelon seed). This can be prevented by stabilizing the balloon shaft at the diaphragm of the sheath. Deflation of the balloon with a 20-mL syringe is quicker and more complete than with a 10-mL syringe.

When removing a balloon through a sheath, resistance may be encountered because the deflated balloon does not return to its original low profile. Continued aspiration and counterclockwise rotation as the catheter is withdrawn into the sheath rewraps the balloon around the shaft and facilitates removal.

A recent advance in balloon technology is the cutting balloon. Small longitudinal blades on the surface of the balloon create controlled shallow linear cuts during inflation rather than random intimal fractures. This enables successful angioplasty of tough, fibrotic lesions and may improve overall long-term patency.

Angioplasty of lesions that involve or are close to a bifurcation requires alteration in standard technique. In bifurcation lesions, simultaneous inflation of two balloons sized to the smaller branch vessels prevents complications such as dissection of the vessel origin (Fig. 4-10). This is known as the "kissing balloon" technique, and is used with stent deployment as well. In some cases the lesion in the branch is close to, but does not involve, the vessel origin. Since the risk of trauma to the opposing normal branch vessel origin is low but still present, a "safety wire" in the uninvolved vessel is

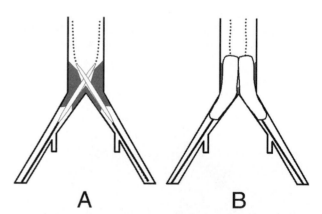

Figure 4-10   Schematic of kissing balloons. **A**, Balloon dilatation of a lesion that extends from a larger vessel (the aorta) into two smaller branches (the common iliac arteries). Each balloon is sized for the common iliac artery lesion, not the aortic lesion. **B**, The balloons are inflated simultaneously, individually dilating the common iliac arteries, and the aorta as a pair.

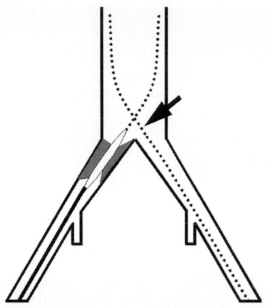

Figure 4-11   When a lesion involves the ostium of one vessel at a bifurcation, a safety wire (arrow) should be placed in the normal vessel during the intervention to preserve access should a dissection extend across the bifurcation. Alternatively, a smaller balloon can be inflated simultaneously in the normal vessel.

frequently used to preserve access should a complication occur during angioplasty (Fig. 4-11).

Specific complication rates for angioplasty of each anatomic area will be found in later chapters. One of the most potentially devastating generic complications is rupture of an intermediate to large vessel in the abdomen or chest (Fig. 4-12). Patients complain of severe pain persisting after deflation of the balloon, usually

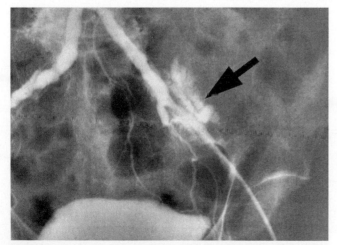

Figure 4-12   Extravasation of contrast (arrow) after angioplasty of an external iliac artery stenosis. The patient had stable vital signs but complained of persistent pain after deflation of the balloon.

Box 4-6   Arterial Rupture during Angioplasty/Stent Placement

Symptoms

Severe pain during balloon inflation, persists after balloon deflation
Hypotension
Tachycardia

Management

Maintain access across lesion with guidewire!
Check vital signs
If stable blood pressure/pulse, inject contrast and localize extravasation
If hemodynamically unstable, reinflated balloon across or proximal to lesion
Fluid resuscitation
Percutaneous stent-graft or surgical repair

(but not always) associated with hypotension and tachycardia. Immediate reinflation of the balloon across or proximal to the lesion is a life-saving maneuver (Box 4-6). Urgent surgical repair or stent-graft placement (see below) is usually required to stop the bleeding. Fortunately, the risk of vessel rupture during recanalization procedures is much less than 1%.

Cholesterol embolization is another generic complication of recanalization procedures. Although it also occurs following diagnostic procedures, interventions appear to be at higher risk. Overall, the incidence is less than 1%, but certain patients are at greater risk, such as those with extensive shaggy aortic plaque or who have had prior cholesterol embolization. The cholesterol crystals are mobilized by unroofing of soft, lipid-rich plaques during catheter and/or guidewire manipulation. Crystals continue to shower for days to weeks after the procedure. Lodging in arterioles, the crystals incite an occlusive inflammatory reaction that can lead to tissue ischemia and necrosis. Amputation, permanent renal failure, bowel ischemia, stroke, and death are all possible outcomes of cholesterol embolization (see Fig. 1-33). Other than careful technique and patient selection, there is little that can be done to prevent this complication (Box 4-7).

Stents

Stents provide an intravascular scaffold for the vessel lumen. The mechanism of action of stents is very different from angioplasty, as the plaque and vessel wall are literally pushed aside by the stent to enlarge the lumen (Figs. 4-4 and 4-13). There are many stents available, but

Box 4-7 Cholesterol Embolization

Clinical Findings

Livido reticularis
Blue toe syndrome
Bowel/renal ischemia
Transient ischemic attack/stroke (ascending and
   arch aortic source)

Laboratory Findings

Progressive renal failure
Eosinophilia (urine and serum)

few are approved for vascular use in the United States (Figs. 4-14 and 4-15). The majority of stents are approved and labeled as biliary or tracheal stents. The "off-label" use of stents in blood vessels is ubiquitous but not officially promoted by manufacturers.

Careful attention to the specific characteristics of a stent is important during procedures (Table 4-6). A self-expanding stent is desirable in a superficial location that may be subject to external compression, such as the cervical carotid artery. Conversely a balloon expandable stent is useful for precise placement in a very short segment of vessel, such as a renal artery ostium. Balloon expandable stents tend to be used in shorter or more uniform diameter lesions. Self-expanding stents are

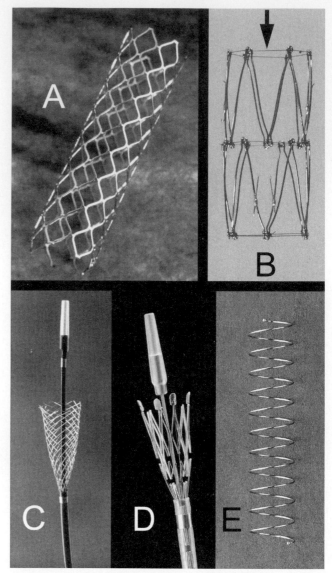

Figure 4-14   Examples of metallic stents (Reproduced courtesy of the manufacturers listed). **A**, Balloon expandable stent (© Cordis Corporation 2003). **B**, Self-expanding Gianturco–Rösch stainless steel Z-stents. Note sutures (arrow) constraining stents (Cook, Bloomington, IN). **C**, Self-expanding woven stainless steel Wallstent (Boston Scientific, Natick, MA). **D**, Self-expanding laser-cut nitinol stent (Luminexx, C.R. Bard, Covington, GA). **E**, Nitinol coil stent (with permission of *ev3* Inc., Playmouth, MN).

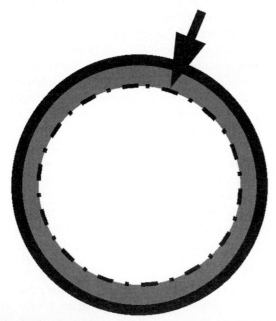

Figure 4-13   Schematic representation of a deployed stent (arrow). Compare with the postangioplasty lumen depicted in Fig. 4-5.

excellent for longer lesions that span vessels of different diameters.

The indications for stent placement are in flux, and depend on many patient-specific factors as well as the bias of the operator (Box 4-8). In practice, the tendency is to place a stent as the first intervention without trying to optimize the result of angioplasty ("primary stenting"). Although expensive (stents can cost more than $1000 each), a good result is obtained quickly and with greater certainty. Nevertheless, in many instances it is

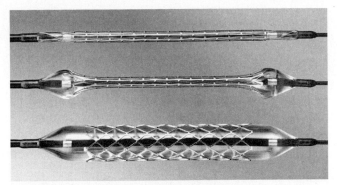

Figure 4-15   Stages of balloon-expandable stent deployment. Stent mounted on balloon (*top*); the stent expands first at the ends (*middle*); the fully deployed stent (*bottom*). Note slight decrease in overall length of the stent with full expansion. (© Cordis Corporation 2003.)

Box 4-8 Indications for Stent Placement

Arterial

Recanalization of chronic occlusion
Occlusive or flow-limiting dissection following
    angioplasty
Elastic or recurrent stenosis
Lesion suspected as source of distal emboli
Inflow lesion prior to distal surgical bypass procedure
Ostial lesion (especially renal artery)
Thoracic aortic coarctation/pulmonary artery
    stenosis (pediatric)

Venous

Recanalization of chronic occlusion
Extrinsic compression by malignancy
Elastic, fibrotic, or recurrent stenosis

Other

Bridging mouth of aneurysm prior to coil placement
Reinforce stent-graft

---

wise to attempt angioplasty first, reserving stents for failed or recurrent lesions. The long-term results of stents in most anatomic locations are better than for angioplasty alone, but not by a great amount. In certain areas, stents do not seem to offer any advantage over angioplasty, and therefore should probably be reserved to salvage failed angioplasty. Specifically, these areas are the renal artery for fibromuscular dysplasia, the infrainguinal arteries, and across joint spaces. Stents should not be placed at sites of future surgical anastomoses, as the presence of the device may complicate surgery or render it impossible. Anticoagulant and antiplatelet drugs should be used during stent placement.

Table 4-6	Stent Features
Feature	**Variables**
Metal	Stainless steel, nitinol, Elgiloy, tantalum, platinum
Construction	Laser-cut, welded, woven, wire spring, sutured
Deployment	Balloon-expanded, self-expanding, thermal memory
Precision of deployment	Stent design, deployment technique
Hoop strength	Stent design, metal
Flexibility	Stent construction, metal
Radiopacity	Type of metal, coatings, markers
Sizes	Diameter and length pre- and post-deployment
Drug eluting	Rapamycin, taxol, heparin, dexamethasone, etc.
Delivery system	French size, flexibility, guidewire requirements
Regulatory status	Approval by FDA for vascular and nonvascular use

FDA, United States Food and Drug Administration.

The techniques for stent placement vary depending upon the device, but certain broad principles can be followed. Delivery over a guidewire is essential, as almost all devices are mounted on some sort of catheter. Predilatation of the lesion with an angioplasty balloon ensures that the lesion is distensible (and thus will respond to a stent), and makes crossing the lesion with the device easier. However, in many circumstances primary stent placement reduces manipulation across the lesion and potential distal embolic complications. All stents should be just long enough to cover the lesion, with minimal extension into normal areas of the vessel. Because balloon expandable stents are mounted on the outer surface of the balloon, it may be necessary to first advance a long sheath or guiding catheter across the lesion, so that the stent can be advanced through the lesion without catching on plaque. Premounted balloon expandable stents with smooth polish edges that are firmly situated on a balloon can often be "bare-backed" through a lesion. Flexible stents mounted on small-shafted balloons can frequently negotiate tortuous vessels over a 0.018-inch or smaller guidewires.

Balloon expandable stents deploy from both ends towards the middle (see Fig. 4-15). Balloon expandable stents are sized in the same manner as angioplasty balloons, with an intentional 5–10% oversize. When mounting a stent on a balloon by hand, careful crimping is necessary to avoid dislodgment of the balloon during delivery. The stent should not be longer than the working surface of the balloon (i.e., the distance between the radiopaque marker bands on the catheter shaft inside the balloon). Each manufacturer provides information on the degree of shortening of their stent in relation to the final diameter.

Self-expanding stents are usually constrained by an outer sleeve or membrane (see Fig. 4-14). These devices usually do not require long sheaths or guiding catheters. Radiopacity of the stent is crucial to aid in correct placement and complete expansion. The nitinol-based stents can be placed with maximum precision as they have minimum shortening, but they are not reconstrainable like the Wallstent (Boston Scientific, Natick, MA). Self-expanding stents deploy from distal to proximal. The unconstrained diameter of the stent should be 10–20% larger than the normal diameter of the target vessel. Predilation of the lesion with a small balloon may be necessary to position the stent delivery catheter and allow partial expansion during deployment. The stent can then be dilated with a larger balloon to the desired final diameter. The nitinol-based self-expanding stents generally cannot be dilated beyond their rated maximal diameter. Attempts to overdilate these stents can result in device fracture or vessel injury.

Drug eluting stents can deliver agents that prevent restenosis directly to the intima. These devices are just reaching clinical implementation in the coronary arteries, but hold great promise for peripheral applications.

In general, a stent cannot do anything that a balloon cannot do first. If the lesion cannot be dilated with a balloon, then a stent will not provide any additional benefit. When the primary abnormality is chronic extrinsic compression of the lumen by an extravascular structure, placement of a stent without first relieving the compression may result in stent fracture (Fig. 4-16).

Stent placement traditionally has a higher overall complication rate than angioplasty alone owing to the larger size of the devices and more complex delivery. Most stents must be deployed through 6- or 7-French sheaths. The complication rates have decreased as experience has increased and new devices have become available. The majority of procedural complications are the same as for angioplasty. However, there are several that are

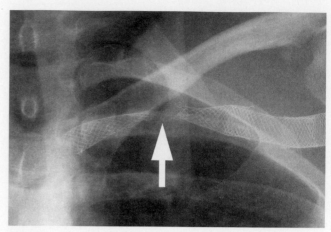

Figure 4-16   Fracture of a Wallstent (arrow) placed for venous thoracic outlet syndrome without first rib resection. Chronic compression between the clavicle and 1st rib has destroyed the metallic stent.

unique to stent placement (Table 4-7). Early thrombosis of stents is unusual unless runoff or inflow is compromised. Infection is rare but has been reported. When infection occurs pseudoaneurysm formation around the stent is common.

Stent-grafts

A stent-graft is a device constructed from a stent and a vascular conduit that is inserted using catheter techniques and image guidance. The stent serves to anchor the graft in the blood vessel lumen, and in most cases provides structural support for the graft material. The graft material provides a conduit for blood flow. The first clinically successful stent-grafts were hand-made by physicians from stents and vascular graft materials that were literally "off the shelf". There are now a wide variety of stent-grafts that are either commercially available or in clinical trials (Fig. 4-17). These devices employ a wide range of stent designs and metals, and several

Table 4-7   Complications Unique to Stent Placement

Complication	Etiology	Prevention
Stent loose on balloon during delivery	Loose crimp	Tight crimp, correct balloon size, slight positive pressure in balloon after mounting
Stent embolization after deployment	Undersized stent	Oversize stent 5–10% in diameter
Stent will not expand lesion	Nondilatable or fibrotic lesion	Test with angioplasty balloon before deploying stent; use stent with high hoop strength
Stent kinks in lesion after deployment	Angled vessel	Use flexible self-expanding stent

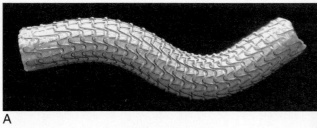

Figure 4-17   Examples of commercially available stent-grafts, fully expanded. These are delivered constrained on a catheter and expand within the vessel once released. **A**, The self-expanding ViaBahn (W.L. Gore, Flagstaff, AZ). The stent-graft is constructed from nitinol metal and expanded PTFE. This device is not approved for vascular use but is an appropriate size for medium to large vessels. **B**, The Zenith bifurcated stent-graft for abdominal aortic aneurysms (Cook Inc., Bloomington, IN). The stent-graft is constructed from stainless steel and woven polyester. Note modular components are assembled within the patient.

different types of graft materials. The stents may be located inside, outside, or in a sandwich of graft material. Nitinol, stainless steel, Elgiloy, and other metals may be used to make the stents. The graft material may be synthetic, such as woven polyester or expanded PTFE, or biologic.

The function of a stent-graft varies with the application. In occlusive disease, the stent-graft props the vessel lumen open and (theoretically) is a physical barrier to restenosis. Intimal hyperplasia at the ends of the stent-graft remains a problem. When used to treat an aneurysm, the stent-graft excludes the sac of the aneurysm from the circulation (Fig. 4-18). In the treatment of vascular injuries such as an acute arteriovenous fistula, the stent-graft seals over the hole in the wall of the vessel. In each of these cases, the basic principle is diversion of blood flow into the stent-graft. In order to function, the stent-graft must fully appose the inner walls of the vessel at the attachment sites. Otherwise, blood will leak between the stent-graft and the intimal surface. This is a fundamental difference between stent-grafts and surgical grafts, which are sewn to the vessel wall.

The indications for stent-grafts are evolving as new devices become available (Box 4-9). A widespread indication is in the treatment of arterial aneurysm disease, particularly of the abdominal aorta. There is no other endovascular therapeutic option for most large aortic aneurysms. With the exception of the transjugular intrahepatic portosystemic shunt (TIPS) procedure and some forms of acute arterial trauma, stent-grafts must compete with simpler, less costly bare metal stents in most other applications.

The technique of stent-graft delivery is determined by the design of the stent, the graft material, and the size of the delivery system. The very first clinical stent-grafts were based on balloon expandable stents. Most devices are now self-expanding, although postplacement "tacking" with a balloon is common. In addition, gentle inflation of a balloon along the length of the device may be necessary to "iron" the graft material. Each device has a its own specific delivery procedure. The size of the delivery system is determined by the amount of metal in the stent, and the thickness of the graft material.

The outcomes of stent-grafts are not clearly defined at this time. Some of the most promising applications are in treatment of aneurysms, aortic dissection, recanalization of long-segment peripheral arterial occlusions, and TIPS. In small artery occlusive disease the outcomes for

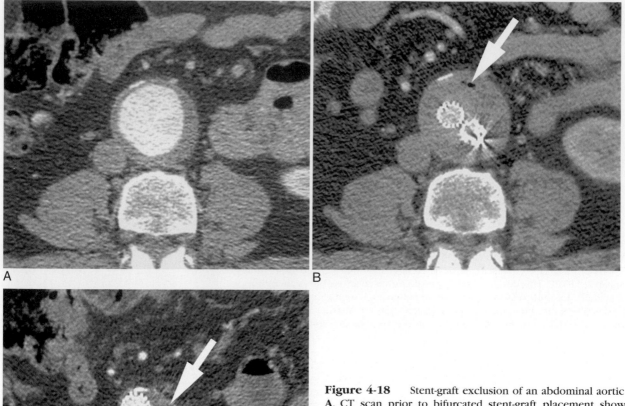

Figure 4-18   Stent-graft exclusion of an abdominal aortic aneurysm. **A**, CT scan prior to bifurcated stent-graft placement shows a patent aneurysm. **B**, CT scan at the same level 24 hours following stent-graft insertion. The lumen of the aneurysm is thrombosed. Note the air bubble (arrow) in the excluded aneurysm sac, a common early finding. **C**, CT scan 1 year later showing dramatic decrease in the diameter of the aneurysm (arrow).

Box 4-9   Indications for Stent-Grafts
Current
Aortic, iliac aneurysms/pseudoaneurysms
Transjugular intrahepatic portosystemic shunt (TIPS)
Arterial trauma
Aortic dissection
Developing
Peripheral arterial stenoses
Peripheral arterial occlusions
Dialysis access

most stent-grafts are not as good as for bare metal stents. In aneurysmal disease, late dislodgement, kinking, or shifting of the stent-graft is possible if the aneurysm shrinks.

Debulking Atheroma

Angioplasty, stents, and stent-grafts increase the size of the vessel lumen by actions that do not change the volume of preexisting disease. An alternative approach is to debulk the obstruction by removing the plaque (Fig. 4-19). This is the basic principle of surgical endarterectomy, in which the vessel is incised and the plaque cored out. Doing the same thing with a catheter is challenging, as a large plaque cannot be easily removed in one piece. A variety of devices

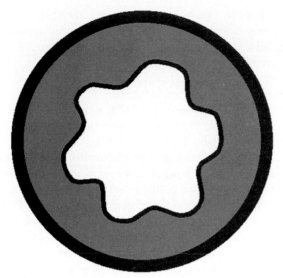

Figure 4-19   Schematic of lesion following a debulking procedure. Compare with Figs 4-5 and 4-13.

have been invented that bite, bore, or blast the plaque using augers, drills, and lasers (Fig. 4-20). Drills and lasers create a channel no larger than the diameter of the device itself, so that an additional intervention is almost always required. None has had widespread acceptance. These technologies had greater utility in the era prior to stents in the treatment of elastic lesions, postangioplasty obstructing intimal flaps, and eccentric stenoses.

Pharmacologic Thrombolysis

Thrombosis of a blood vessel rarely occurs in the absence of a lesion or systemic abnormality. Vascular thrombosis can be the result of restriction of flow, trauma, or a hypercoagulable state. Acute thrombosis is therefore a symptom of another problem, rather than an isolated pathologic process. The goals of the interventional treatment of thrombosis are to relieve the acute obstruction and unmask the underlying etiology (Fig. 4-21).

The human body has an endogenous mechanism for lysis of thrombus (Fig. 4-22). The surgical approach to thrombus management is to open the vessel and pull out the clot using balloon catheters. Interventionists employ both pharmacologic and mechanical tools for dealing with thrombus. This section will discuss the pharmacologic approach, termed thrombolysis.

The native thrombolytic system can be enhanced by the administration of drugs that ultimately activate plasminogen. Although peripheral infusion of these drugs can accomplish this to some extent, catheter-directed intrathrombus drug delivery is the core principle of the interventional radiology approach to thrombolysis.

Several thrombolytic agents are available or pending governmental approval (Table 4-8). Streptokinase was

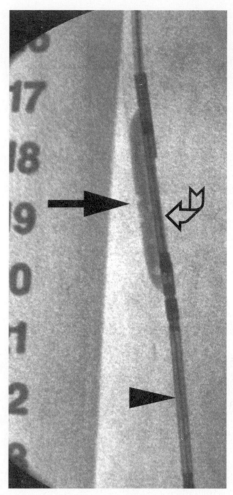

Figure 4-20   Simpson directional atherectomy device (Guidant Corporation, Indianapolis, IN). The cutting window (curved arrow) contains a motorized blade. The window is held against the plaque by a low-pressure balloon (straight arrow). Shavings are collected in the distal chamber (arrowhead) as the blade is advanced from proximal to distal across the plaque.

the first thrombolytic drug available. Streptokinase forms complexes with free plasminogen, and later plasmin, that in turn convert plasminogen to plasmin. Though inexpensive, streptokinase works slowly, which results in a high complication rate due to prolonged infusions. In addition, streptokinase is derived from streptococcal bacteria, so that allergic reactions can occur in up to 14%. Urokinase was the second thrombolytic to become available. Urokinase is a nonantigenic substance produced by human renal tissue. It is a direct plasminogen activator with little fibrin specificity, so lysis was faster and bleeding complications less common than with streptokinase. Urokinase was the dominant agent for peripheral thrombolysis for over a decade. Newer direct tissue plasminogen activators became popular in the late 1990s. These had previously been used primarily in coronary arteries. Recombinant tissue plasminogen activator (alteplase, t-PA), and a derivative (reteplase, r-PA), both have increased activity in the presence of fibrin (t-PA greater than r-PA). The duration of lytic therapy is shorter than with urokinase, but bleeding complications may be higher. Many other agents have been studied, but few have reached clinical practice. The doses of each agent vary based upon the vascular bed, the volume of thrombus, and the method of delivery.

All thrombolytic agents ultimately result in dissolution and fragmentation of thrombus. The fresher the thrombus, the faster and more complete the thrombolysis. Chronic organized thrombus that has become fibrotic and endothelialized is less likely to be successfully thrombolysed. Inability to cross the thrombus with a guidewire is a rough predictor of unsuccessful thrombolysis. Mechanical disruption of the thrombus seems to accelerate thrombolysis by exposure of a larger surface area to the thrombolytic agent, leading to improved delivery of the agent and activation of local plasminogen.

Thrombolytic agents do not prevent formation of new thrombus or platelet aggregation. Systemic heparinization (lower doses with t-PA and r-PA) and platelet inhibition are frequently used during lysis procedures.

The indications for catheter-directed thrombolysis in most vascular beds are acute or subacute thrombosis resulting in clinical symptoms that require urgent resolution (Box 4-10). There are a few notable exceptions. Thrombosed dialysis grafts cause no immediate symptoms, but require treatment. Occasionally a brief course of thrombolysis prior to angioplasty or stenting is employed when fresh thrombus is suspected in a chronic lesion.

Success of a thrombolytic procedure can be defined as technical, hemodynamic, or clinical. Technical success is restoration of prograde blood flow with less than 5% residual thrombus. Hemodynamic success is the return of the patient to the preocclusive vascular status. Clinical success is the relief of acute symptoms with return to baseline functional level. In peripheral arterial thrombolysis,

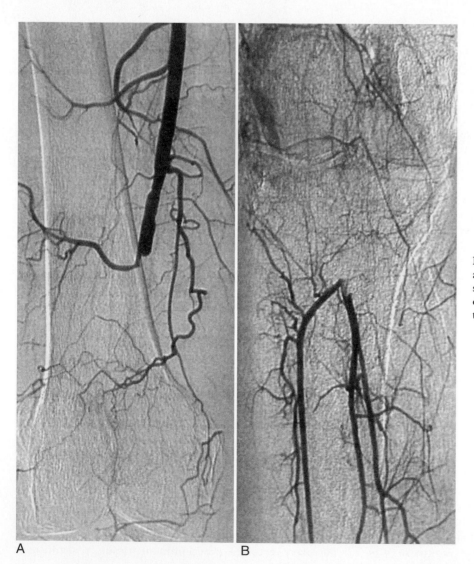

A   B

Figure 4-21   Thrombolysis of popliteal artery thrombosis. **A,** Popliteal artery occlusion in a patient with sudden increase in calf claudication. **B,** There is reconstitution of the tibial arteries.   (*Continued*)

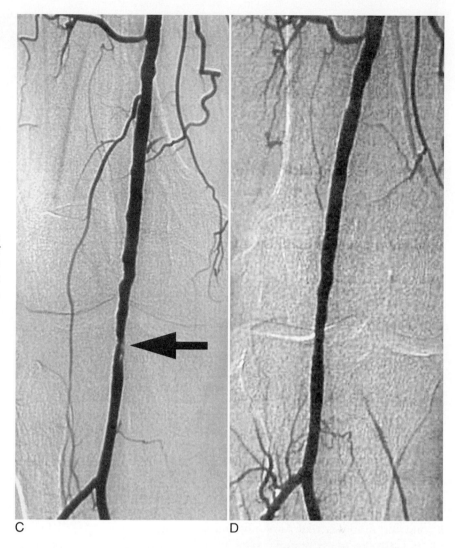

C   D

Figure 4-21   cont'd C, Following over-night thrombolysis, there is complete clearing of thrombus which reveals a focal stenosis (arrow). **D,** The lesion was dilated with a 5-mm balloon. (Case courtesy of Thomas Burdick, M.D., Seattle, Washington.)

amputation rates at 1 year are also an important measure of success.

The established contraindications to thrombolysis are generally related to bleeding in undesirable locations or the complications of revascularization of already dead tissue (Box 4-11). Thrombolytic drugs cannot distinguish between "good" thrombus, such as at an arterial puncture site, and the "bad" thrombus in a stenosis. In addition, pre-existing lesions (such as vascular brain metastases) that have a tendency to bleed spontaneously will be more likely to do just that during thrombolysis. Limbs or organs that are irreversibly ischemic should not undergo

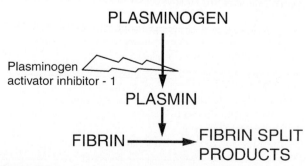

**Figure 4-22   ** The final steps in the lytic pathway.

PLASMINOGEN

Plasminogen
activator inhibitor - 1

PLASMIN

FIBRIN ⟶ FIBRIN SPLIT
PRODUCTS

Box 4-10 Indications for Thrombolysis

Arterial occlusions with viable extremity/organ[a]
Thrombotic occlusion of dialysis graft[a]
Conversion of thrombotic occlusion to stenosis prior to angioplasty/stent
Acute thrombotic stroke (anterior circulation <6 hours, posterior circulation 12–24 hours)
Extensive deep venous thrombosis[a]
Massive pulmonary embolism[a]
Central venous access catheter malfunction

[a]<14 days old, but exceptions may be made in specific cases.

Table 4-8 Thrombolytic Agents

Agent	Trade Name	Description	Half-life	Mechanism of Action
Streptokinase (SK)	Streptase	Derived from group-C β-hemolytic streptococci	20 min	Indirect; streptokinase–plasminogen and plasmin complexes activate plasminogen; no fibrin specificity
Urokinase (UK)	Abbokinase	Derived from fetal kidney cells	14 min	Direct; no fibrin specificity
Recombinant urokinase(r-UK)	r-UK	Recombinant double-chain analogue of UK	7 min	Direct: no fibrin specificity
Recombinant pro-urokinase (pro-UK), or single-chain UK-type plasminogen activator (scu-PA)	Saruplase	Recombinant single-chain precursor of UK	7 min	Direct; fibrin-specific
Alteplase (rt-PA)	Activase	Recombinant tissue plasminogen activator, (527 unit amino acid chain)	5 min	Direct; moderate fibrin specificity
Reteplase (r-PA)	Retevase	Recombinant mutein of tissue plasminogen activator (355-unit amino acid chain)	15 min	Direct; low fibrin specificity
TNK-tissue plasminogen activator (TNK-t-PA)	Tenecteplase	Modified recombinant mutein of tissue plasminogen activator	20 min	Direct; high fibrin specificity; only agent resistant to inactivation by plasminogen activator inhibitor-1

thrombolysis, as reperfusion of dead tissue may lead to severe metabolic disturbances (termed "reperfusion syndrome") (see Box 15-10). Furthermore, vessels opened during thrombolysis that have no runoff will not stay open. Lastly, an uncooperative patient cannot undergo this procedure.

The two basic techniques for thrombolysis are drip infusion and pulse-spray. The essential feature of a drip infusion is to span the entire length of the thrombus with a catheter (Box 4-12). The catheter(s) should be

Box 4-11 Contraindications to Thrombolysis

Irreversible limb/organ ischemia
Active hemorrhage
Recent major surgery
Recent intraocular surgery/bleeding
Craniotomy within 2 months
Brain tumor (primary or metastatic)
Completed stroke within 6 months
History of spontaneous intracranial hemorrhage
Uncooperative or demented patient

Box 4-12 Catheter-directed Thrombolysis

Position catheter system across entire length of thrombus
• 5-Fr multiple side-holes catheter with coaxial 3-Fr catheter
• One side-hole should be just proximal to top of thrombus
Infuse equal doses of thrombolytic agent through each catheter
Dosage (these are empirical total hourly doses)[a]
• Urokinase: 100,000 U/h
• rt-PA: 0.5–1.0 mg/h
• r-PA: 0.5–1.0 U/h
Infuse with high-pressure mechanical pumps
Concurrent heparin/platelet inhibitor therapy (lower doses with tissue plasminogen activators)
Secure catheter at insertion site
Frequent monitoring of access site for bleeding
Strict bedrest with access limb immobilized
Frequent monitoring of limb for changes in vascular examination
Foley bladder catheter
Minimize blood draws, no arterial punctures

[a]Risk of bleeding complication increases as dose increases.

positioned so that the top of the thrombus is bathed by the thrombolytic agent, otherwise the distal thrombus will lyse leaving an obstructing proximal plug (Fig. 4-23). Dosage is controversial, with passionate advocates for all regimens, but in general complications are fewer and results satisfactory using modest doses. Drip infusions usually require 8–24 hours depending on the drug (shorter with tissue plasminogen activators, longer with urokinase), so patients must be monitored in a controlled setting. In most hospitals this will be an intensive care unit. When concurrent anticoagulation is used, lower doses of heparin should be used with t-PA and r-PA than with urokinase, and the PTT should be followed during treatment. Daily hematocrit and serum creatinine should also be obtained. Fibrinogen levels and fibrin split products have little correlation with outcomes.

Pulse-spray thrombolysis (also known as pharmaco-mechanical thrombolysis) uses a catheter with multiple side-holes or slits positioned across the thrombus (Box 4-13). Small aliquots of concentrated thrombolytic drug are forcibly injected through the catheter at short

Box 4-13   Pulse Spray Pharmacomechanical Thrombolysis
Position catheter across thrombus Urokinase: 250,000 U in 9 mL sterile water plus 5000 U heparin (1 mL) • Inject 0.2–0.3 mL every 30 seconds t-PA: 2 mg in 10 mL (+/− heparin; may precipitate) • Inject 0.2 mL (0.04 mg) every 30 seconds r-PA: 2 U in 10 mL (+/− heparin) • Inject 0.2 mL (0.04 mg) every 30 seconds Concurrent heparin/platelet inhibitor therapy (lower doses with tissue plasminogen activators) Immobilize catheters at insertion site Frequent monitoring of access site for bleeding Frequent monitoring of limb for changes in vascular examination

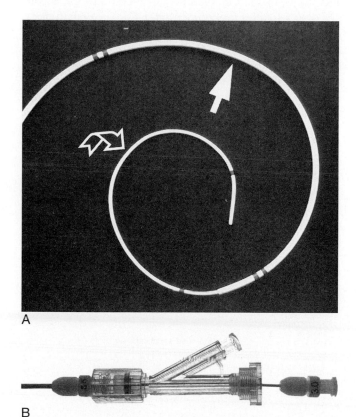

A

B

Figure 4-23   Example of coaxial catheter infusion system for thrombolysis infusion. **A**, The outer 5.5-Fr catheter (straight arrow) has multiple side-holes between the paired radiopaque marker bands. The 3-Fr inner coaxial catheter (curved arrow) with multiple side-holes between the single marker bands. **B**, Close-up of the Y-adaptor that allows simultaneous infusion through both catheters.

intervals (Fig. 4-24). The numerous jets of fluid disrupt the thrombus as well as deliver the drug, resulting in a shorter lysis time, frequently 1–2 hours. The patient remains in the angiography suite for the duration of the procedure. A mechanical injector is available.

Thrombolysis with urokinase, t-PA, or r-PA has an 80–90% technical success rate for recent occlusions in most applications. Success rates decrease with the age of the occlusion and vary among different vascular beds and types of lesions. Clinical success in peripheral arterial occlusions, defined as limb salvage, is approximately 70% at 1 year. The results with streptokinase were less favorable, and required longer infusions.

The majority of complications of thrombolytic procedures are hemorrhagic involving the access site (Table 4-9). Careful technique during arterial puncture, the use of vascular sheaths, immobilization of the limb on the side of access, and gentle anticoagulation will minimize this problem. Central nervous system bleeding occurs in 0.5–2.0% of cases, with apparent higher risk with r-UK, t-PA, and r-PA. The risk of central nervous system bleeding seems to persist for at least 12–24 hours following termination of therapy. Distal embolization of fragments of thrombus occurs in up to 20% of peripheral arterial thrombolysis procedures as flow is restored. Patients complain of sudden acute worsening of ischemic symptoms just when things seemed to be getting better. Known as the "darkness before the dawn," this situation will resolve in almost all cases within an hour or two with continued therapy as the embolized thrombus lyses. Persistence of symptoms requires return to the angiography suite or surgical thrombectomy.

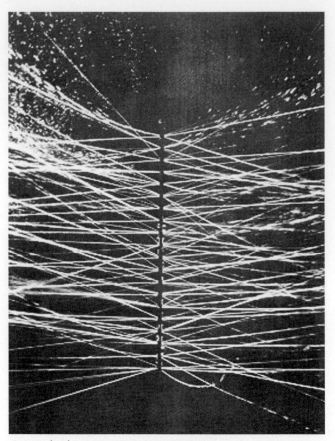

Figure 4-24   Photograph of multiple fluid jets exiting from a pulse-spray catheter (Courtesy of Angiodynamics Inc., Queensbury, NY).

Percutaneous Mechanical Thrombectomy

An alternative to a pharmacologic approach to thrombolysis are mechanical devices that can pulverize and/or remove thrombus. A number of devices have been designed that utilize impellers, fluid jets, brushes, baskets, lasers, and ultrasound to break thrombus into fragments small enough to be aspirated through a catheter or released into the circulation (Fig. 4-25). The goal of all of these devices is rapid restoration of blood flow by rapid reduction of the volume of thrombus.

Mechanical thrombectomy devices vary in sheath requirements and their ability to be advanced over a guidewire. These devices are most widely applied for declotting surgical dialysis access. Most are not approved for use in native arteries or veins, although they are frequently used in these areas. Fresh thrombus responds best, particularly within surgical grafts. A common problem is an inability to satisfactorily clear thrombus in large-diameter vessels such as the inferior vena cava. However, when used appropriately, excellent results can be obtained. One area in which these devices may be particularly useful is in the treatment of massive pulmonary embolism, when fragmentation of the embolus frequently results in major improvement in pulmonary arterial flow.

A very simple mechanical approach to removal of fresh thrombus that uses readily available equipment is suction thrombectomy. For this procedure, a sheath should always be used at the access site. A nontapered catheter large enough to accommodate the thrombus and still fit inside the vessel is advanced into the thrombus over a smaller tapered catheter. The inner catheter is removed, and an empty 60-mL syringe is attached to the nontapered catheter. A vigorous, continuous suction is then applied to the catheter as it as advanced into, and then withdrawn through, the thrombus. Suction is applied without interruption until the catheter is removed completely from the sheath, otherwise thrombus may dislodge from the catheter and embolize (Fig. 4-26). This quick technique is particularly useful for management of acute intraprocedural thrombus in medium to small-diameter vessels, or removal of embolized atheromatous debris.

The complications of mechanical thrombectomy are somewhat device-dependent, and include embolization, hemolysis, and volume overload. Unusual problems such as device fracture can result from improper or prolonged use.

Table 4-9   Complication Rates with Peripheral Arterial Thrombolysis[a]

Complication	Streptokinase	Urokinase	t-PA and Derivatives
Access-site bleeding			
Minor[b]	20–40%	20–40%	20–40%
Major[c]	10–20%	5%	5–15%
Intracranial bleed	0.5%	0.5%	0.5–3%
Distal embolization	15%	15%	15%
Failed procedure	30–40%	5–10%	5–10%

[a] These complication rates are generalizations based upon highly inhomogeneous (and sometimes suspect) data and vary greatly with the dose of lytic agent, age of occlusion, length of therapy, and concurrent anticoagulation.
[b] In reality almost all patients develop a small access-site hematoma.
[c] Requires transfusion or operative therapy.

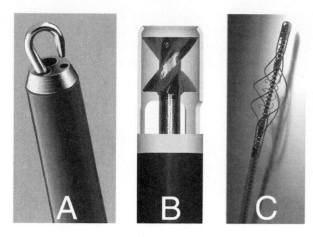

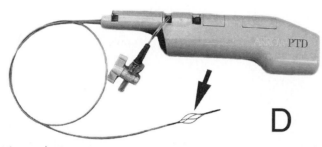

Figure 4-25 Mechanical thrombectomy devices. **A**, Oasis catheter (Courtesy of Boston Scientific Corp., Natick, MA). Saline injected through the curved metal tube at the tip enters opposing channel, creating a Bernoulli effect that disrupts and removes thrombus. **B**, Helix Clot Buster thrombectomy device (with permission of *ev3* Inc., Plymouth, MN). The impeller within the housing creates a vortex that fragments thrombus. **C**, Solera device (Courtesy of Bacchus Vascular, Santa Clara, CA). The outer basket is stationary, the rotating middle coil disrupts the thrombus, and the rotating innermost spiral catheter extracts the thrombus (Archemedes' screw). **D**, Arrow–Trerotola PTD Device (Arrow International, Reading, PA). Battery-powered motor-driven rotating basket (arrow) very effectively pulverizes thrombus (Image courtesy of Scott Trerotola, MD, Philadelphia, PA).

In general, these are very safe devices when used properly.

Vasodilating Drugs

Vascular spasm can restrict blood flow to the point of occlusion in the absence of an underlying structural lesion. Spasm can be caused by external trauma to the vessel, guidewire manipulation in the vessel lumen, shock, or the use of vasoconstrictor drugs. Vasoactive drugs can be used intra-arterially to reverse or reduce vasospasm (Table 4-10). When induced by a guidewire or catheter, removal of the offending device frequently allows the spasm to resolve (Fig. 4-27). The most useful drug for acute intraprocedural spasm is nitroglycerin, which can be given every 5–10 minutes until the spasm improves or the blood pressure drops. Tolazoline, a potent alpha blocker, also has a relatively short half-life. When more prolonged therapy is required, an infusion of papaverine may be used. In cases of severe procedure-related spasm that does not resolve quickly, heparin should be given to prevent thrombosis.

DECREASING BLOOD FLOW THROUGH VESSELS

Fundamentals

Partial or complete occlusion of blood flow using catheter-based techniques is desirable for many conditions, including holes in blood vessels, tumors (both benign and malignant), abnormal communications between blood vessels, and abnormal blood vessels. Although the pathologies are varied, the basics of the procedures are the same. The essential considerations are the underlying lesion, the clinical problem that needs to be addressed, the feasibility of a percutaneous approach to the lesion, the ability to accomplish what is required by the clinical

Table 4-10	Vasodilating Agents		
Drug	**Dose**	**Half-life**	**Mechanism of Action**
Nitroglycerin	100- to 250-µg bolus IA (100 µg/mL)	4–6 min	Direct vasodilator (metabolized to nitric oxide)
Tolazoline	25- to 50-mg bolus IA (in 10 cc NS slowly)	3–12 h (varies with urine output)	Alpha blocker
Papaverine	30–60 mg/h infusion IA (1 mg/mL NS)	30–120 mins	Direct smooth muscle relaxant (inhibits cyclic nucleotide phosphodiesterase)
Nifedipine	10 mg p.o.	2–5 h	Calcium-channel blocker
Verapamil	2.5 mg bolus IV	2–5 h	Calcium-channel blocker

IA, intraarterial; IV, intravenous; p.o. = oral (alternatively pill can be punctured and contents administered sublingually).

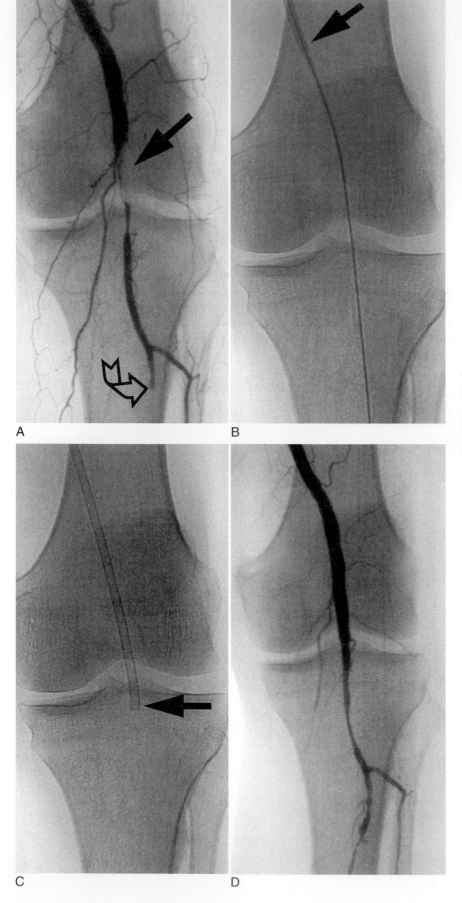

A

B

C

D

Figure 4-26 Aspiration thrombectomy. **A,** Embolus in the popliteal artery (straight arrow) and tibioperoneal trunk (curved arrow). **B,** After crossing the occlusions with a guidewire, an 8-Fr nontapered guiding catheter (arrow) is advanced over a 5-Fr catheter beyond the embolus. **C,** The guidewire and inner catheter are removed. Suction is applied to the guiding catheter (arrow) with a 60-mL syringe as it is withdrawn through the occlusion. **D,** Postaspiration run shows patent vessels, although there is now some spasm in the distal popliteal artery.

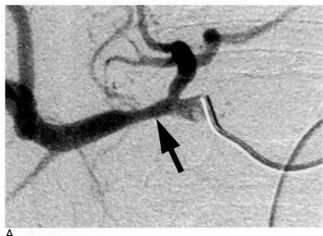

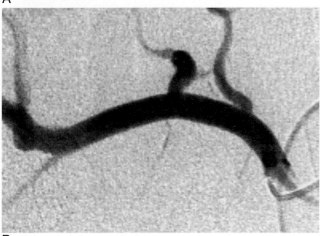

Figure 4-27 Catheter-induced vasospasm. **A**, Proper hepatic angiogram through a 5-Fr catheter shows focal, smooth, concentric narrowing (arrow) consistent with spasm. **B**, After withdrawing the catheter slightly and injecting 200 µg of nitroglycerin into the artery, the spasm has resolved.

situation, and the management plans for the patient after the procedure.

The lesions most amenable to treatment with percutaneous vascular occlusion techniques are those that involve or are supplied by blood vessels. Avascular lesions usually cannot be treated effectively through an intravascular route.

A clear understanding of the clinical problem is essential to the procedure (Table 4-11). The rapidity with which the occlusion must be achieved, the occlusive technique, and the tolerance for complications can be very different depending on the goals of the procedure. For example, both life-threatening postpartum hemorrhage and symptomatic uterine fibroids can be treated with transcatheter embolization of the uterus, but the approach to each procedure is very different.

In order to perform the procedure, it is necessary to gain access to the lesion, and to be able to deliver a device or drug that will be effective. Access can be accomplished

Table 4-11	Planning an Occlusion Procedure
Category	**Considerations**
Goal of procedure	Decrease flow; complete occlusion; deliver drug; kill organ
Level of occlusion	Proximal; distal; capillary
Precision of delivery	Exact; flow-directed; regional
Delivery system	Microcatheters; diagnostic catheters; direct puncture
Vascular anatomy	Approach; major blood supply; accessory/collateral vessels
Adjacent structures	Risks of nontarget organ embolization

through a blood vessel, or by direct puncture. Very tortuous vessels can be successfully negotiated with specialized microcatheters (see Fig. 2-21). However, an effective occlusive agent may be impossible to deliver through such a small catheter. Careful review of available imaging studies and performance of a complete diagnostic angiogram (when the clinical situation allows) assist in formulation of a successful strategy. A crucial step in this process is consideration of potential collateral or accessory blood supply to a lesion, as failure to identify these vessels may result in a failed procedure (Fig. 4-28).

Knowing the next step in management of the patient following embolization has great bearing on the specifics of the occlusion procedure. When additional therapy will be based on the results of the embolization, the procedure should be tailored to enhance the results of the second procedure. For example, embolizing an organ that will be subsequently removed surgically is approached differently from an organ that must remain in the patient and be functional.

A variety of tools and techniques can be used to slow down flow or occlude blood vessels (Table 4-12). Matching the tools and techniques to the clinical situation is frequently a matter of judgment, experience, and device availability.

Embolization

There are a large number of embolic agents, with varying physical properties, methods of delivery, and permanence (Table 4-13). Selection of an embolic agent depends on the clinical factors and the technical aspects of the procedure. There are a few basic rules for embolization procedures that, when followed, lead to a successful procedure with minimal complications (Box 4-14).

Proximal vessel occlusion is useful when a single vessel supplies the target area, a quick result is necessary, or preservation of distal collateral vessels is desirable. Large agents such as coils or detachable balloons are ideal for

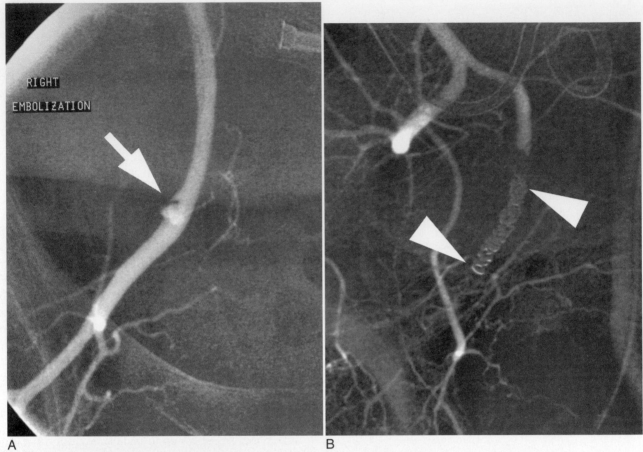

Figure 4-28   Embolization of an inferior gluteal artery to treat a pseudoaneurysm following transgluteal abscess drainage. Coils were used in this case. **A**, Digital angiogram showing the pseudoaneurysm (arrow) of the inferior gluteal artery. **B**, Coils have been densely packed on both sides of pseudoaneurysm (arrowheads). This was done to block antegrade perfusion from the hypogastric artery, and retrograde perfusion from collaterals to the distal inferior gluteal artery from the superior gluteal and profunda femoris arteries. Simply embolizing the inferior gluteal artery proximal to the pseudoaneurysm would have been inadequate treatment.

Table 4-12	Techniques and Tools for Vascular Occlusion

Technique	Sample Tools
Intraluminal obstruction	Steel coils; thrombin injection
Delivery of chemotherapeutic agent	Ethiodol
Vasoconstriction	Pitressin drip
Sclerosis of lumen	Absolute ethanol
Sealing hole in vessel wall:	
Intraluminal approach	Stent-graft
Extraluminal	US-guided compression; thrombin injection into pseudoaneurysm

this situation. Distal occlusion has a higher chance of tissue infarction. Liquid agents penetrate more deeply than solid agents. Detachable coils and balloons are the most precise embolic agents, as they can be repositioned or removed if placement is unsatisfactory. Lastly, secure placement of large embolic agents in natural areas of narrowing prevents distal migration.

Coils

Embolization coils are available in a variety of sizes, lengths and shapes (Fig. 4-29). Coils are lengths of coil-spring wire (usually stainless steel or platinum) that may be preformed into any number of shapes. Wire diameters range from 0.010 to 0.052 inches. Tufts of polyester fibers may be attached to the coil to promote platelet aggregation and thrombosis. Coils occlude vessels by physically obstructing the vessel. Packaging for coils usually is labeled with the diameter of the wire, the length of the coil wire, and the diameter when re-formed.

Table 4-13   Embolic Agents

Agent	Properties	Durability	Vessel Size	Delivery
Coils (stainless steel, platinum wire)	Solid; obstructs flow	Permanent	Large, medium, small	Push or inject through catheter; some detachable
Balloons	Solid; filled with liquid after positioning; obstructs flow	Permanent, but may deflate	Large, medium	Detachable from catheter
Ivalon (polyvinyl alcohol)	Solid; obstructs flow	Permanent	Small	Injected
Acrylic spheres	Solid; obstructs flow	Permanent	Small	Injected
Gelfoam (gelatin sponge)	Solid; obstructs flow	4–6 weeks	Medium to small	Injected; pushed
Autologous clot	Solid; obstructs flow	4–7 days	Medium	Injected
Glues and Polymers	Liquid/solid; varying agents; obstructs flow	Permanent	Determined by vessel lumen	Injected
Ethiodol (iodized oil)	Liquid; obstructs flow	Permanent	Small to capillary	Injected
Thrombin	Liquid; induces thrombosis	Permanent	Large to capillary	Injected
Sotradecol	Liquid; sclerosant	Permanent	Medium to capillary	Injected
Ethanol (95% ETOH)	Liquid; sclerosant	Permanent	Large to capillary	Injected

Careful attention to the labeling is necessary to avoid inserting inappropriately sized devices (Fig. 4-30). Coils are supplied straightened in a metal or plastic tube. This tube must be placed firmly into the hub of the catheter, and the coil pushed into the catheter with the back end of a guidewire or other straight wire (Box 4-15). The diameter of the coil wire should always match the inner diameter of the delivery catheter, otherwise the coil may begin to re-form and jam in the catheter. The coil is then pushed through the catheter with a floppy-tipped guidewire or coil pusher that matches the inner diameter of the catheter. Gentle but firm forward pressure on the catheter may be necessary during the final stages of coil delivery to prevent "bucking" of the catheter or improper placement. Alternatively, when catheter position is secure, coils may be injected using 1-mL Luer lock syringes.

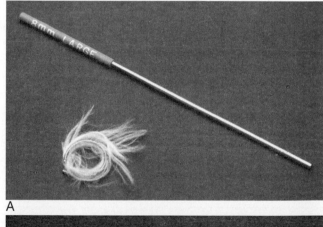

A

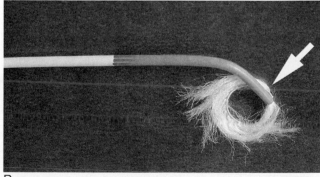

B

Box 4-14   Embolization Rules

Have a plan
Be sure of the pathology and anatomy
Maintain stable, secure catheter position
Embolize antegrade (with flow) when possible
Use coaxial microcatheters for small vessels
If image quality is poor, don't embolize
Embolize to a predetermined endpoint
Avoid "just one more for good luck"; it's frequently one too many
Document results: always check for collateral reconstitution distal to occlusion
Consider prophylactic antibiotics (primarily solid organ embolization)

Figure 4-29   Embolization coils. **A**, Coils are supplied pre-loaded in tubes. Shown is a standard Gianturco stainless steel coil with polyester fibers (Cook, Bloomington, IN). **B**, Delivery of a coil through a catheter (arrow). The coil can be pushed with a soft guidewire, or injected.

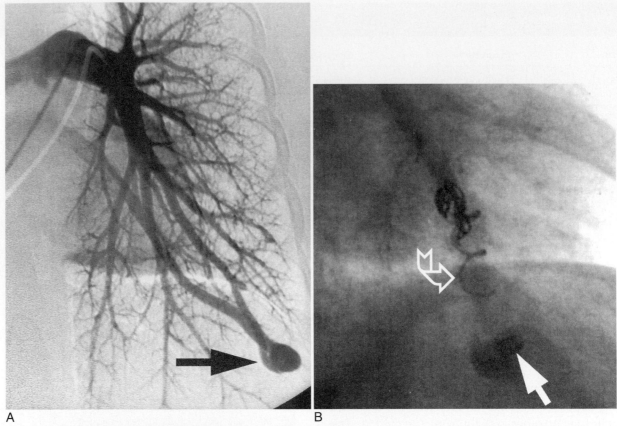

A   B

Figure 4-30   Improper coil selection. **A**, Pulmonary arteriovenous malformation (arrow). **B**, One coil was too small and embolized into the malformation (straight arrow). This could have been a disaster. Another coil was too big, and could not adequately re-form in the feeding pulmonary artery (curved arrow).

Detachable coils are available that remain connected to the pusher wire until an electric current is applied or other technique is used to release the coil. These are particularly useful in neuroembolization procedures when precise placement is critical. Another specialty

coil is the "liquid coil," an extremely limp length of nonfibered platinum coil that, when injected through a microcatheter, piles up in the target vessel like soft-serve ice-cream.

Detachable Balloons

Detachable balloons were originally developed for neuroembolization procedures (Fig. 4-31). These are silicone or latex balloons with one-way valves that admit a small catheter but seal when the catheter is removed. Balloons are available in a variety of maximum sizes; lower inflation volumes result in smaller diameter balloons. Detachable balloons are first tested on the angiography table for leaks, and all air is evacuated. The deflated balloon is advanced into position on the end of a small delivery catheter, usually through a guiding catheter. The balloon is then inflated with an isotonic mixture of saline and contrast, and the placement confirmed. The balloon is released by gentle traction on the delivery catheter. Over time, silicone balloons may "deflate" if the fluid mixture in the balloon is hypotonic. Conversely, a balloon filled with a hypertonic solution may continue to enlarge and ultimately rupture.

Box 4-15   Coil Tips

Read labels carefully: be sure of coil dimensions before it goes into the patient

Final diameter of coil should be slightly larger than target vessel

Match diameter of coil wire to catheter lumen; smaller coils will jam in catheter

Push coils with guidewire/pusher that matches catheter lumen, otherwise pusher will jam along side coil in catheter

Platinum coils are softer and easier to see than steel coils

Avoid sharp angles or redundancy in delivery catheter

Flush gently after each coil is placed and contrast injections

Coils can be injected with 1-mL Luer-Lock syringes

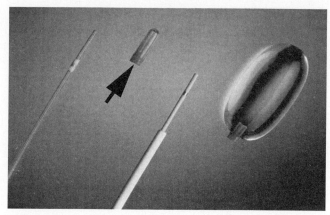

Figure 4-31   Detachable balloons. Detachable balloons with delivery catheters before inflation (arrow on valve) and after.

Box 4-16   Ivalon Tips

Mix particles in clean small bowl with 2:1 mixture of contrast and 5% albumin (irregular particles only)

Inject using 1-mL or 3-mL Luer lock syringes

Use 700 µm or smaller particles through microcatheters

Flush catheter with 1- to 3-mL table flush after each syringe of Ivalon

Blocked catheters can be cleared by flushing with 1-mL Luer lock syringe

Inject Ivalon using fluoroscopic guidance ("road mapping" if available)

Embolize until stasis or visible reflux along catheter

Polyvinyl Alcohol Particles (Ivalon)

Ivalon is an inert, permanent particulate embolic agent that is injected through a catheter (Fig. 4-32). Once released from the catheter, the particles are carried to the site of embolization by the arterial flow (Box 4-16). Correct sizing of the Ivalon is critical to prevent blockage of the delivery catheter and to achieve the desired embolization. Ivalon is supplied dry in vials as irregular or spherically shaped particles in sizes from 50 to 1200 µm in diameter. Each vial usually contains particles that are within a 150- to 200-µm range. The particles are not visible radiographically, so they are usually suspended in contrast prior to injection. Adding albumin to

the suspension helps prevent clumping of irregular particles. The particles are delivered by gently injecting with 1- to 3-mL syringes using a pulsing motion during fluoroscopy. Embolic endpoints are determined by the quality of flow in the vessel. As the embolization approaches completion, flow becomes slower. Forceful injection of particles or contrast during the procedure may result in reflux out of the target vessel into another vessel.

Acrylic Spheres

Acrylic spheres are a permanent, flow-directed, solid embolic agent that are perfectly round and slightly deformable (Fig. 4-33). The spheres can compress by approximately 20% in diameter, a feature that requires consideration when selecting a size. The spheres range in diameter from 200 to 1200 µm, and are available suspended in an aqueous solution. Because the spheres are

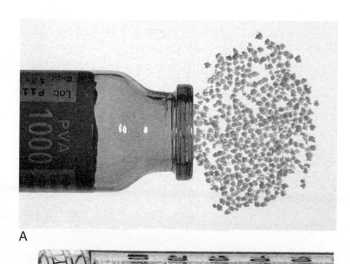

Figure 4-32   Polyvinyl alcohol particles. **A**, These particles are very large (up to 1000 µm in diameter). **B**, Particles suspended in a 1-mL syringe: a 2:1 mixture of contrast and 5% albumin.

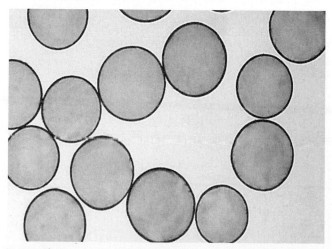

Figure 4-33   Embospheres (Courtesy of BioSphere Medical, Rockland, MA). Note the uniform shape.

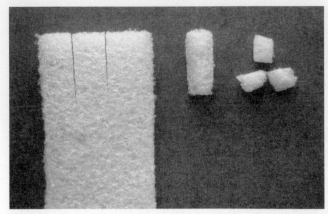

Figure 4-34   Gelfoam brick cut into "torpedo" and small cubes.

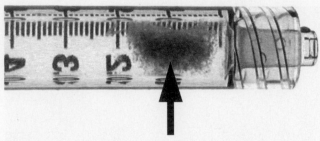

Figure 4-35   Gelfoam "torpedo" (arrow) suspended in a 1-mL Luer lock syringe.

not radiopaque, they should be mixed with contrast before injection. Clumping is less of a problem with the spheres owing to their smooth contour. However, over-compression of the spheres by forcing them through too small a catheter can result in cracking of the spheres and allows biodegradation over time.

Gelfoam

Gelfoam (gelatin sponge) is one of the oldest and most versatile of all flow-directed embolic agents. This substance is compressible and absorbed over a period of 4–6 weeks. Gelfoam is supplied in small sterile bricks or a fine (approximately 50-μm) powder (Fig. 4-34). The brick can be cut to the size needed to occlude the vessel of interest, compressed to fit through a catheter, and then injected into the vessel where it will expand to a larger size than when dry (Box 4-17). Gelfoam pieces can be suspended in contrast prior to injection to aid in fluoroscopic visualization (Fig. 4-35). Gelfoam can also be soaked in thrombin or a sclerosing agent prior to injection. As with all particulates, over-forceful injection

can result in reflux of the Gelfoam into a nontarget vessel. Gelfoam pieces are very useful any time that temporary occlusion is desired. In addition, Gelfoam torpedoes can be used in combination with coil emboliza-tion; after initial placement of a few coils, Gelfoam pieces are injected which lodge in the coils and complete the occlusion, after which coils can be placed to finalize the embolization (the "Gelfoam sandwich").

Gelfoam powder frequently results in permanent occlusion owing to the small size of the particles. The level of occlusion is so distal that tissue necrosis can occur.

Autologous Clot

Rarely used except when very temporary (hours to days) occlusion is desired, autologous clot was actually one of the first solid embolic agents. Pieces of thrombus formed in a bowl from the patient's blood are injected in a similar fashion as for Gelfoam.

Glues and Polymers

Liquid embolic materials that can be injected through a small catheter and then solidify to occlude a larger space

---

Box 4-17   Gelfoam Tips

Cut dry brick with scalpel or scissors
Place piece(s) in syringe
Soak in syringe with contrast
Long "torpedoes" can be delivered individually with 1-mL syringes
Multiple small cubes can be injected with 3- to 5-mL syringe
Smaller pieces are necessary for microcatheters
Flush catheter with 1-mL syringe after each Gelfoam syringe
Gelfoam stuck in syringe can be cleared with 1-mL syringe

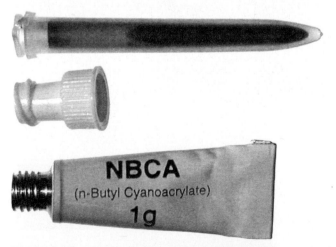

Figure 4-36   Tube of N-butyl cyanoacrylate and a vial of tantalum powder. The powder is sometimes mixed in the glue to enhance radiopacity.

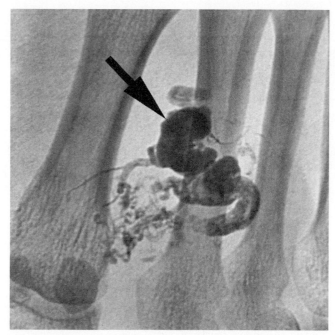

Figure 4-37   Glue cast (arrow) in an arteriovenous malformation of the foot.

are very useful flow-directed agents (Fig. 4-36). These agents flow into complex vascular structures and then solidify (Fig. 4-37). This is of particular value in treatment of arteriovenous malformations, in which a central nidus with multiple feeding arteries and draining veins can be effectively treated. Cyanoacrylate glues and derivatives "set" upon contact with ionic solutions such as blood or saline. The time required for the glue to set can be adjusted by mixing with varying amounts of iodized oil (Box 4-18).

Box 4-18   Glue Tips

Use a coaxial microcatheter system
Angiogram through microcatheter at 1 frame/s to estimate rate of flow in lesion
Mix oil and glue in a ratio to obtain an appropriate "set" time
Add tantalum powder as necessary to increase radiopacity
Flush catheter with 5% dextrose solution before introducing glue
Inject glue with 1- to 3-mL syringe
Once glue begins to set, inject until no forward flow
Immediately retract microcatheter to avoid glue "tail" on catheter
Aspirate microcatheter while removing from patient
Use new microcatheter for each glue injection

In addition, the oil opacifies the otherwise radiolucent glue. Meticulous technique is required to prevent solidification in the catheter; the catheter must be flushed with a glucose solution prior to injection of glue. Once injected, the catheter must be withdrawn to avoid cementing the catheter in place.

Numerous new polymerization agents are becoming available that are easier to use than glues. Ethelyene vinyl alcohol copolymer (EVOH) is a biocompatible agent that is dissolved in dimethyl sulfoxide (DMSO). Upon contact with an aqueous solution it precipitates into a spongy mass. The EVOH mass is not adhesive to the catheter, although specialized delivery systems that are compatible with the DMSO solvent are necessary.

Ethiodol

An inert iodinated oil, ethiodol, obstructs small vessels owing to its high viscosity relative to blood. Supplied in 10-mL vials, it is frequently used as a vehicle for chemotherapy in embolization of hepatic tumors. Hepatomas have a specific affinity for iodinated oil (Fig. 4-38). Delivery is by gentle injection. Because it is iodinated, Ethiodol is readily visible during injection, which facilitates a controlled delivery. Ethiodol should not be used in high-flow tumors with large arteriovenous shunts.

Thrombin

Topical thrombin is a potent agent that induces rapid thrombosis when injected intravascularly (Fig. 4-39). Approved only for topical use, it is used intravascularly to treat aneurysms or induce thrombosis during stubborn embolization cases. Thrombin powder is reconstituted in saline and injected slowly in aliquots of 500–1000 units. When contrast is not added to make the solution radiopaque, extreme care must be taken to prevent reflux into the systemic circulation. Following injection of thrombin, the catheter should be flushed gently to evacuate any residual thrombin. Lesions with rapid washout, such as high-flow arteriovenous malformations or fistulas, should not be treated with thrombin. Entire limbs or vascular beds may occlude if too much thrombin refluxes or washes out into nontarget vessels. Thrombosis is initiated instantly upon injection, but may take several minutes to complete. Gentle injections of contrast can help determine the progress of the thrombosis without refluxing residual thrombin or fresh thrombus out of the target artery.

Sotradecol

Sotradecol is a 1–3% solution of sodium tetradecyl sulfate. This is a mild sclerosing agent that induces thrombosis, inflammation, and eventually obliteration of the vascular lumen. Commonly used to obliterate superficial lower-extremity venous varicosities, this agent can also be used in arteries. Supplied as a liquid, it is injected

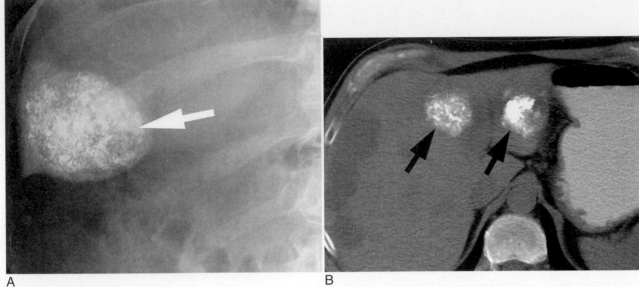

Figure 4-38   Oil-based chemoembolization of hepatoma. **A**, Dense staining and oil uptake in a right lobe hepatoma (arrow) following chemoembolization. **B**, Noncontrast CT scan from another patient with multifocal hepatoma following chemoembolization shows oil uptake in several tumors (arrows).

slowly into the target vessel in 1- to 2-mL aliquots. The maximum dose is 10 mL. This agent should not be used in high-flow situations, or when reflux into nontarget vessels is likely. In some situations, a balloon occlusion catheter can be used to occlude inflow and prevent reflux. Because it is a relatively mild sclerosant, damage of adjacent tissue is uncommon when small doses are used.

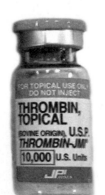
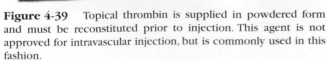

Figure 4-39   Topical thrombin is supplied in powdered form and must be reconstituted prior to injection. This agent is not approved for intravascular injection, but is commonly used in this fashion.

Absolute Ethanol

Dehydrated alcohol (95% ethanol) is a powerful sclerosing agent that produces intravascular thrombosis, vessel wall sclerosis, and death of perfused tissue. Absolute ethanol does not simply cause occlusion of flow, but ablates tissue as well. This quality is an advantage when trying to treat certain types of vascular malformations or tumors. Supplied in vials, it is injected slowly in small volumes sufficient to fill the vessel or vascular bed to be obliterated. Large volumes can result in systemic ethanol toxicity. The pain associated with ethanol embolization can be so severe that many patients require general

Box 4-19   Ethanol Tips

Use only 95% ethanol
Do not dilute ethanol
General anesthesia for superficial vascular lesions
Use 3- to 5-mL syringes
Use balloon occlusion catheter in arteries; test with contrast to confirm position and occlusion
Inject slowly
Inject volume of alcohol sufficient to fill target vessel
Wait 5–10 minutes
Aspirate residual alcohol *before* deflating occlusion balloon
Confirm occlusion with gentle injection of contrast

anesthesia for treatment of superficial vascular malformations. Control of flow is essential when using alcohol, as rapid washout causes dilution and limits contact with the vessel wall (Box 4-19). For this reason, balloon occlusion catheters are frequently employed so that the alcohol can dwell in the target vessel for several minutes. Balloon occlusion catheters also prevent reflux into nontarget organs. The specific gravity of ethanol is lower than that of blood, so anterior structures are particularly at risk when reflux occurs.

Chemoembolization

The treatment of certain tumors (particularly primary and metastatic hepatic lesion) with intravascular delivery of chemotherapeutic agents can be performed alone or in conjunction with other therapies such as radiofrequency ablation or surgical excision. A wide variety of chemotherapeutic regimens are used, with great variation from one institution to another. In general, vascular tumors respond best to chemoembolization. The chemotherapy is usually mixed with an embolic agent that slows flow and allows the active drugs to remain in the organ of interest for a prolonged period of time. Particles such as Ivalon or Gelfoam powder, or iodized oil, are used most often (see Fig. 4-38). The goal of chemoembolization is to deliver the chemotherapy, not occlude the vessel, as multiple treatments are frequently required. Patients require antibiotic and antiemetic prophylaxis. The results of chemoembolization are promising when applied to appropriate lesions.

Vasoconstricting Drugs

Blood flow can be diminished without obstructing an artery by inducing vasoconstriction. This is a particularly useful strategy when the goal is to temporarily decrease the pressure or volume of blood reaching a specific area. A common example would be gastrointestinal bleeding from sigmoid colon diverticulosis, in which preservation of flow is desired to prevent bowel infarction, but decreased flow is necessary to allow the natural hemostatic mechanism to work. Vasconstricting agents have little value in the venous system.

The most commonly used agent is vasopressin (Box 4-20). This drug causes smooth muscle contraction in the peripheral arteries, and water retention by the kidneys. The indication for intraarterial use is intestinal bleeding. Because of the potential for systemic vasoconstriction, patients with symptomatic coronary artery disease should not be treated with vasopressin. The initial dose is 0.2 u/min, with a maximum dose for all patients of 0.4 u/min. Patients frequently have abdominal cramping with initiation of therapy, and may evacuate bloody colonic contents. This should not be confused with either intestinal ischemia or recurrent bleeding.

Box 4-20   Vasopressin (Pitressin)

Localize bleeding source with arteriography
Place catheter in proximal superior or inferior mesenteric artery
Infusion dosage:
- Infuse 0.2 units/min for 30 minutes, then reassess with angiography
- If still bleeding, increase to 0.3 or 0.4 units/min for 30 minutes
- Repeat angiogram; if still bleeding, pursue different therapy
When bleeding controlled, secure catheter
Infuse at successful dose for 12–24 hours
Monitor serum sodium, serial hematocrit
For rebleeding during therapy, check:
- Patient is still getting the drug
- Catheter is not dislodged (inject contrast at bedside with portable abdominal film)
- Increase to maximum dose (0.4 units/min)
Taper to normal saline over 12 hours
Leave catheter in place for 6 hours after Pitressin stopped before removal

Epinephrine can be used for arterial injection to cause transient vasoconstriction, but should not be used for infusions. There are currently few applications for this drug, but at one time it was felt to be useful in the angiographic diagnosis of tumors. On occasion it is still used to decrease renal arterial flow to allow satisfactory renal venography. For this application a mixture of 2 µg/mL is prepared by diluting 1 mL of 1:1000 epinephrine in 500 mL of 5% dextrose or saline. Injection of 10-12 µg in the renal artery immediately prior to the retrograde renal venogram decreases flow sufficiently to allow a filling of the intrarenal venules. Smaller doses (5–6 µg) are used in diagnosis of renal and hepatic tumors.

Treatment of Arterial Access Pseudoaneurysms

Pseudoaneurysms at the site of an arterial puncture occur in less than 5% of cases. Large catheter size, anticoagulation, calcified arteries, hypertension, puncture of the superficial femoral rather than the common femoral artery, and obesity are contributing factors. On physical examination, patients have a pulsatile hematoma at the puncture site, frequently with a bruit. A discrete pulsatile mass may or may not be present. Color-flow ultrasound allows rapid diagnosis (see Fig. 3-7). Many pseudoaneurysms will resolve spontaneously, particularly when small in size and in the absence of anticoagulation.

However, rupture and infection can occur. The conventional treatment of pseudoaneurysms is surgical repair.

There are two image-guided therapies for pseudoaneurysms. Ultrasound-guided compression of the neck of the pseudoaneurysm is successful in approximately 80% of attempts. This procedure requires careful identification of the neck of the pseudoaneurysm, and the ability to compress this neck without obliterating the lumen of the underlying normal vessel. This can be a very uncomfortable procedure for the patient, particularly those with fresh pseudoaneurysms and large hematomas. Compression for 20–30 minutes may be required. Complications with this procedure are rare, but distal embolization or thrombosis can occur. The rate of recurrence of the pseudoaneurysm is less than 5%.

As an alternative to compression therapy, direct percutaneous injection of the pseudoaneurysm with thrombin using ultrasound guidance results in rapid thrombosis of the pseudoaneurysm. A discrete neck should be identified by ultrasound, and the presence of an arteriovenous fistula excluded. Meticulous sterile technique is essential for the entire procedure, including the skin preparation. A small needle (21-gauge) is advanced into the center of the pseudoaneurysm using ultrasound. The thrombin is prepared in a concentration of 1000 U/mL. Small aliquots of thrombin (500–1000 U) are injected gently through the needle using a 1-mL syringe. Thrombosis of the pseudoaneurysm is usually instantaneous, but a small additional injection may be required. Reflux of thrombin into the systemic circulation can result in arterial thrombosis distal to the pseudoaneurysm. Careful positioning of the needle away from the pseudoaneurysm neck and gentle injection of small volumes of thrombin help avoid this complication. Recurrence of the pseudoaneurysm occurs in fewer than 5% of cases.

PUTTING THINGS INTO BLOOD VESSELS

The insertion of intravascular devices for purposes other than increasing or decreasing blood flow has become an important part of vascular and interventional radiology. The two devices most commonly inserted are central venous access catheters and vena cava filters. These subjects are covered in detail in Chapters 7 and 13.

TAKING THINGS OUT OF BLOOD VESSELS

Intravascular Foreign-body Retrieval

Basic Principles

This is a fun procedure. However, certain criteria must be satisfied for a successful retrieval (Box 4-21). The most

---

Box 4-21 Intravascular Foreign Body Retrieval

Is it necessary to remove foreign body (what is risk of just leaving it)?
Is it really intravascular?
Is it accessible from a peripheral access?
Can it be moved (i.e., is not sewn, stapled, glued, or otherwise permanently attached to blood vessel)?
Can it be moved without endangering patient?
Size of object allows removal from a peripheral location?

---

important consideration is whether or not the object needs to be retrieved. This is often a judgment based upon individual opinion, rather than scientific fact, but should always be considered. The most common "lost" objects are central venous catheter fragments. Fortunately, these are among the easiest objects to retrieve as they are flexible, narrow, have well-defined ends, and are usually lodged in a capacious low-pressure vessel. Retrieval of objects from the arterial system differs from the venous system in that the clinical presentation may be ischemia, prompting a more urgent procedure. This is logical, in that objects lost in veins tend to move centrally, whereas objects lost in arteries move peripherally. Almost every object conceivable has been retrieved from the vascular system, including embolization coils, pacemaker wires, stents, stent-grafts, vena cava filters, and fragments of angiographic catheters.

Devices used for retrieval are listed in Table 4-14. The most ubiquitous and simple device is the snare (Figs. 4-40 and 4-41, Box 4-22). Other devices include wire baskets that can engage an object in a similar manner, special forceps that actually grasp an object, multistranded "mops" that can be used to entangle a coil, and large nontapered catheters than can be used to aspirate a small object.

Table 4-14 Retrieval Devices

Device	Mechanism
Snare	Encircles
Basket	Encircles
Forceps	Pincer
Aspiration catheter	Suction
Balloon	Dislodgement

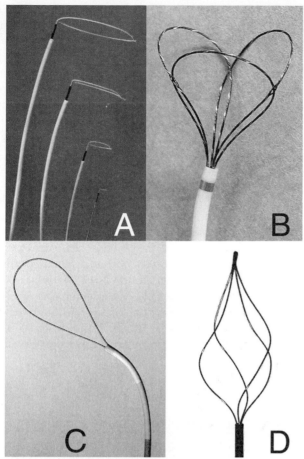

Figure 4-40 Different retrieval devices. **A**, Amplatz gooseneck snares (with permission of *ev3* Inc., Plymouth, MN). **B**, EnSnare (MD Tech, Atlanta, GA). **C**, Snare formed by looping a guidewire through a catheter. **D**, Basket

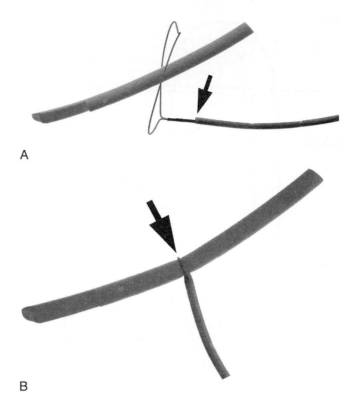

Figure 4-41 How a snare works. **A**, Snare is looped around one end of the catheter fragment. Note that this snare forms at a right-angle to the guiding catheter (arrow). **B**, The snare is locked down on the fragment (arrow) by advancing the guiding catheter to close the loop.

Special Retrieval Techniques

When a catheter fragment is positioned so that neither end is free, retrieval is still possible with a snare if one end can be dislodged. Pigtail or recurved catheters can be used to hook the central portion of the fragment. Applying traction can pull an end of the fragment free. A deflecting guidewire advanced to the end of the catheter (but not beyond) may be needed to provide extra stiffness when the fragment cannot be easily repositioned. Another strategy is to use a recurved catheter to pass a guidewire over the fragment. The guidewire can then be snared from below, forming a closed loop that can dislodge even the most stubborn objects (Fig. 4-42).

Rarely, an object will get away from the operator during a procedure but still be on the guidewire. Though embarrassing, this is actually the ideal situation for snare retrieval. A typical example would be a stent that becomes dislodged from an angioplasty balloon, but remains on the guidewire in the vessel (Fig. 4-43). The loop of a snare can be placed over the back end of the guidewire, and advanced to the stent using the guidewire as a monorail. The loop is then carefully advanced over the stent without pushing it off of the guidewire. Once engaged, the loop is closed over the stent and guidewire, and retrieved through a large-caliber sheath or guide catheter.

Box 4-22   Using a Snare
Select loop diameter equal to or slightly larger than lumen in which object is located
Insert sheath large enough to accommodate snare and object
Engage object with snare (selective catheter very useful to direct snare)
Advance catheter over snare to close loop and lock object
Apply firm, continuous traction on snare wire from now on ("death grip")
Using continuous fluoroscopic monitoring, withdraw snare and object
Release death grip only when object and snare are outside of body

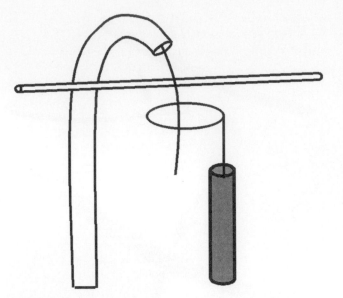

Figure 4-42 When the ends of an object are not free, a snare can be formed around the object. A wire is passed over the object and snared. The snare and the wire are brought out through the same sheath, forming a loop around the object. A guiding catheter can be advanced over both ends of the wire to the object, completing the snare.

Great care should be taken to keep the stent on the guidewire at all times, as retrieval of a free-floating stent can be extremely difficult.

In some circumstances it may possible to engage a large object, but not remove it percutaneously. In this situation the object can move to peripheral location, where a simple cut-down can be performed. This is usually preferable to a major operation.

Transvascular Biopsy

Indications

Transvascular biopsy of masses or organs is a valuable technique when conventional percutaneous biopsy has a high risk of hemorrhagic complication, or the only access is through a blood vessel. The basic premise of transvascular biopsy is that any potential bleeding from the biopsy site will be into a blood vessel. The most common indication is suspected liver parenchymal disease in patients with coagulopathy or ascites, although renal biopsy is becoming more common (Table 4-15). Focal liver and renal masses are, in general, more successfully

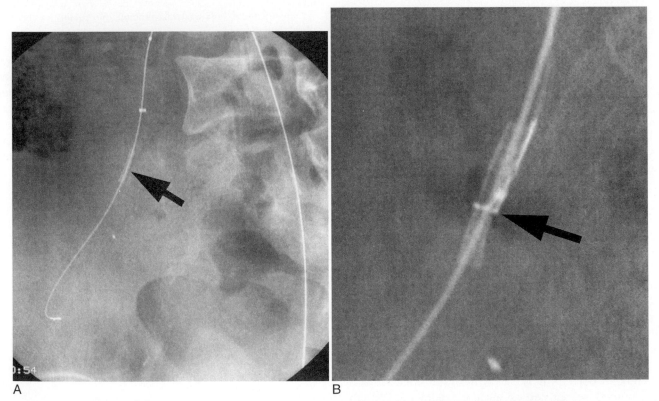

A   B

Figure 4-43 Snaring a stent that is free on a guidewire. **A,** A stent (arrow) has become dislodged from the balloon during an intervention on a transplant renal artery. The stent remains on the guidewire. **B,** A snare (arrow) has been passed over the guidewire and used to capture the stent.

Table 4-15	Indications for Transvascular Biopsy
Organ	**Indications**
Liver	Coagulopathy; ascites; failed percutaneous attempt
Renal	Coagulopathy; failed percutaneous attempt
Intravascular masses	Only available access route

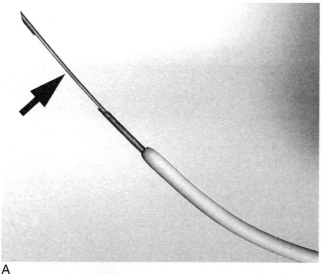

A

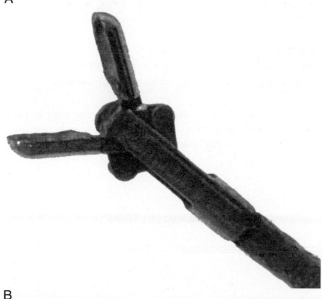

B

Figure 4-44 Intravascular biopsy devices. **A,** Close-up of cutting needle (arrow) used for transjugular liver biopsy. The needle extends beyond the curved 7-Fr guiding catheter. **B,** Close-up of clam-shell biopsy forceps in the open position. The actual catheter diameter is 4-Fr.

biopsied in a conventional manner using a cross-sectional imaging modality such as CT, US, or MRI. Some vascular tumors present as entirely intraluminal masses, particularly venous and arterial leiomyosarcomas. These lesions are ideal for transvascular biopsy.

Principles

The access route is determined by the organ or vessel that is involved. For liver and kidney biopsies a transvenous route from a jugular access is preferred, as the hepatic and renal veins are easy to catheterize from this approach and hemostasis at the venapuncture site is readily achieved with compression. The appropriate lab slips and solutions should be determined in advance for each type of specimen.

Dedicated transvascular biopsy kits are available that utilize automated cutting needles to obtain a core of tissue (e.g., Quick Core 18-gauge needle from Cook Inc.) (Fig. 4-44). These are primarily designed for liver or renal biopsy through a 7-French sheath and a curved inner metal cannula. A modified needle with a shorter intraparenchymal excursion is available for renal biopsies. Other biopsy tools include biting clam-shell forceps, similar to devices used during endoscopy. Guiding catheters are helpful to position these devices adjacent to the mass. Occasionally, an atherectomy device can be used to obtain shavings from an intravascular mass.

Complications

The overall complication rate of transvascular liver and renal biopsy is less than 6%, with the majority being hemorrhagic. This tends to occur when the liver or renal capsule is inadvertently transgressed during the biopsy. Deaths have been reported. Patients should be observed for several hours after a biopsy in a monitored setting. When hemorrhage is suspected, a noncontrast CT scan should be obtained.

SUGGESTED READINGS

Athanasoulis CA, Pfister RC, Greene RE et al. eds: *Interventional Radiology,* WB Saunders, Philadelphia, 1982.

Balko A, Piasecki GJ, Shah DM et al: Transfemoral placement of intraluminal polyurethane prosthesis for abdominal aortic aneurysm. *J Surg Res* 40:305 309, 1986.

Banares R, Alonso S, Catalina MV et al: Randomized controlled trial of aspiration needle versus automated biopsy device for transjugular liver biopsy. *J Vasc Interv Radiol* 12:583-587, 2001.

Becker, GJ: Vascular stents. In Baum S, Pentecost MJ eds: *Abram's Angiography: Interventional Radiology,* Little, Brown, Boston, 1997, 85-118.

Block PC, Myler RK, Stertzer S et al: Morphology after transluminal angioplasty in human beings. *N Engl J Med* 305:382-385, 1981.

Bolia A: Percutaneous intentional extraluminal (subintimal) recanalization of crural arteries. *Eur J Radiol* 28:199–204, 1998.

Cluzel P, Martinez F, Bellin MF et al: Transjugular versus percutaneous renal biopsy for the diagnosis of parenchymal disease: comparison of sampling effectiveness and complications. *Radiology* 215:689–693, 2000.

Dotter CT: Transluminally-placed coilspring endarterial tube grafts: long-term patency in canine popliteal artery. *Invest Radiol* 4:329–332, 1969.

Dotter CT, Judkins MP: Transluminal treatment of arteriosclerotic obstruction: description of a new technic and a preliminary report of its application. *Circulation* 30:654, 1964.

Dotter CT, Rösch J, Seaman AJ: Selective clot lysis with low dose streptokinase. *Radiology* 111:31, 1974.

Drooz AT, Lewis CA, Allen TE et al: Quality improvement guidelines for percutaneous transcatheter embolization. *J Vasc Interv Radiol* 8:889–895, 1997.

Fattori R, Piva T: Drug-eluting stents in vascular intervention. *Lancet* 361:247–249, 2003.

Kandarpa K, Becker GJ, Hunink MG et al: Transcatheter interventions for the treatment of peripheral atherosclerotic lesions: I. *J Vasc Interv Radiol* 12:683–695, 2001.

Kandarpa K, Becker GJ, Ferguson RDG et al: Transcatheter interventions for the treatment of peripheral atherosclerotic lesions: II. *J Vasc Interv Radiol* 12:807–812, 2001.

Kasirajan K, Haskal ZJ, Ouriel K: The use of mechanical thrombectomy devices in the management of acute peripheral arterial occlusive disease. *J Vasc Interv Radiol* 12:405–411, 2001.

Katzen BT, Kaplan JO, Dake MD: Developing an interventional radiology practice in a community hospital: the interventional radiologist as an equal partner in patient care. *Radiology* 170 (3 Pt 2):955–958, 1989.

Katzen BT: Endovascular stent grafts: the beginning of the future, or the beginning of the end? *J Vasc Interv Radiol* 7: 469–476, 1996.

Kinney TB, Rose SC: Intraarterial pressure measurements during angiographic evaluation of peripheral vascular disease: techniques, interpretation, applications, and limitations. *Am J Roentgenol* 166:277–284, 1996.

Luessenhop AJ, Spence WT: Artificial embolization of cerebral arteries. *JAMA* 172:1153, 1960.

Ouriel K, Gray B, Clair DG et al: Complications associated with the use of urokinase and recombinant tissue plasminogen activator for catheter-directed peripheral arterial and venous thrombolysis. *J Vasc Interv Radiol* 11:295–298, 2000.

Patel N, Sacks D, Patel RG et al: SCVIR reporting standards for the treatment of acute acute limb ischemia with the use of transluminal removal of arterial thrombus. *J Vasc Interv Radiol* 12:559–570, 2001.

Pentecost MJ, Criqui MH, Dorros G et al: Guidelines for peripheral percutaneous transluminal angioplasty of the abdominal aorta and lower extremity vessels: a statement for health professionals from a special writing group of the Councils on Cardiovascular Radiology, Arteriosclerosis, Cardio-Thoracic and Vascular Surgery, Clinical Cardiology, and Epidemiology and Prevention, the American Heart Association. *Circulation* 89:511–531, 1994.

Perler BA, Becker GJ eds: *Vascular Intervention: a Clinical Approach*, Thieme Medical Publishers, New York, 1998.

Pollack JS, White RA: Mechanical embolic agents. In Baum S, Pentecost MJ eds: *Abram's Angiography: Interventional Radiology*, Little, Brown, Boston, 1997, 55–79.

Ryan JM, Dumbleton SA, Smith TP: Technical innovation: using a cutting balloon to treat resistant high-grade dialysis graft stenosis. *Am J Roentgenol* 180:1072–1074, 2003.

Sacks D, Marinelli DL, Martin LG et al: Reporting standards for clinical evaluation of new peripheral arterial revascularization devices. Technology Assessment Committee. *J Vasc Interv Radiol* 8:137–149, 1997.

Sakakibara S, Kono S: Emdomyocardial biopsy. *Jpn Heart J* 3:537, 1962.

Sousa JE, Costa MA, Sousa AG et al: Two-year angiographic and intravascular ultrasound follow-up after implantation of sirolimus-eluting stents in human coronary arteries. *Circulation* 107:381–383, 2003.

Thomas J, Sinclair-Smith B, Bloomfield D et al: Nonsurgical retrieval of a broken segment of steel spring guide from the right atrium and inferior vena cava. *Circulation* 30:106, 1964.

Watson HR, Bergqvist D: Antithrombotic agents after peripheral transluminal angioplasty: a review of the studies, methods and evidence for their use. *Eur J Vasc Endovasc Surg* 19: 445–450, 2000.

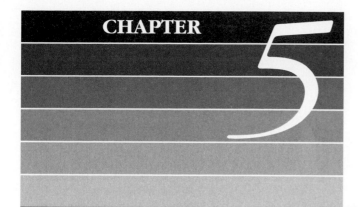

CHAPTER 5

Carotid and Vertebral Arteries

JOHN A. KAUFMAN, M.D.

GARY M. NESBIT, M.D.

The organ at risk from carotid and vertebral artery disease is the brain. Central nervous system ischemia can be severely debilitating and even lethal. Vascular imaging has a central role in diagnosis of all aspects of cerebrovascular disease. Catheter-based interventions have a rapidly expanding role in the therapy of occlusive disease and acute stroke.

ANATOMY

The right common carotid artery (CCA) arises from the brachiocephalic artery, while the left CCA usually takes its origin directly from the aortic arch (Fig. 5-1). The common carotid arteries ascend through the mediastinum and lie posterior and medial to the internal jugular veins in the neck (see Fig. 2-39). Typical internal diameters of the CCA are 6-8 mm. The CCA bifurcates into the external carotid artery (ECA) and internal carotid artery (ICA) in the upper neck, typically at the upper edge of the thyroid cartilage (between the 3rd and 5th cervical vertebrae). The ICA arises posterolateral to the ECA in approximately 90% of individuals; a medial origin is present in the remaining 10%. The ICA and ECA are normally the only branches of the CCA; small cervical branches directly from the CCA are extremely rare (Fig. 5-2).

The external carotid artery (ECA) supplies the structures of the neck, face, and scalp (Fig. 5-3). The ECA branches that supply the midline structures of the face frequently anastomose with each other. Many memorable mnemonics have been devised for the branches of the ECA. Unfortunately, none is suitable for publication here.

The ICA is usually a branchless vessel until it reaches the base of the skull (Fig. 5-4). The internal diameter of this vessel ranges from 4 to 6 mm. Rarely, persistent embryonic branches to the basilar artery from the cervical ICA may be encountered at the C1–C2 (persistent hypoglossal artery) and C2–C3 (proatlantal intersegmental artery) levels. At the skull base the internal carotid artery enters the serpentine carotid canal within the petrous bone, traveling medial and anterior towards the cavernous sinus. Small branches can communicate from this portion of the ICA with the internal maxillary artery. The ICA exits the petrous canal into the cavernous sinus. An anomalous branch from the cavernous ICA to the basilar artery, the persistent trigeminal artery, is found in 0.5% of patients (Fig. 5-5). Typically, the opthalmic artery is the first major branch of the distal ICA, arising just above the cavernous sinus. The posterior communicating and anterior choroidal arteries arise from the ICA within the subarachnoid space just prior to the bifurcation into anterior and middle cerebral arteries.

The vertebral arteries arise from the proximal subclavian arteries in almost 95% of patients, traveling in a posterior and medial direction towards the skull (Fig. 5-6). In 5% of patients the left vertebral artery arises directly from the aortic arch. The diameter of the cervical vertebral artery is 3–5 mm. The left vertebral artery is equal to or larger than the right in 75% of individuals. Unlike the CCA and ICA, the cervical portion of the vertebral artery has many small unnamed muscular branches. The vertebral arteries lie within a series of bony rings formed

119

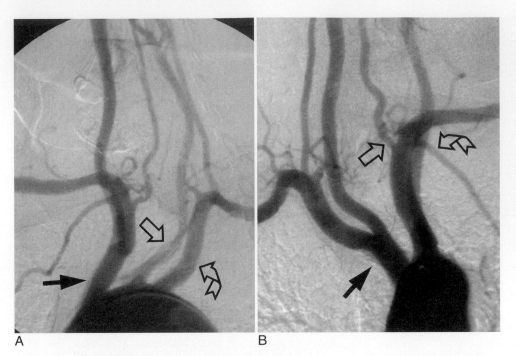

A   B

Figure 5-1 Normal great vessel origin anatomy. **A**, Digital subtraction (DSA) arch aortogram in the left anterior oblique (LAO) projection. The brachiocephalic (solid arrow), left common carotid (open arrow), and left subclavian artery origins (curved arrow) are visualized in this obliquity. The bifurcation of the brachiocephalic artery into the right subclavian and common carotid artery origins is obscured in this projection. **B**, DSA arch in the right anterior oblique (RAO) projection allows evaluation of the bifurcation of the brachiocephalic artery (solid arrow) into the right subclavian and common carotid arteries. The left vertebral (open arrow) and internal mammary (curved arrows) artery origins are seen best in this projection.

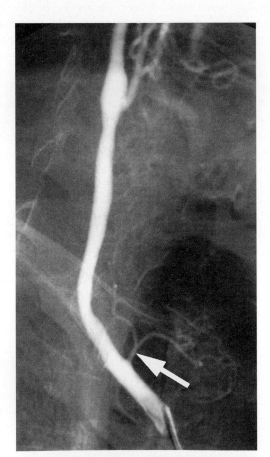

Figure 5-2 Branches from the common carotid artery (CCA) are very rare. An artery to the isthmus of the thyroid (arrow) arises from the right CCA in this patient.

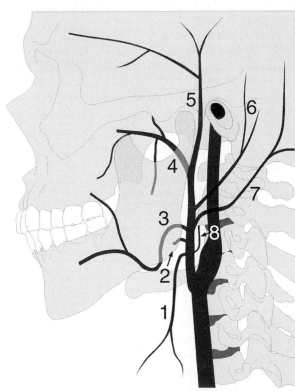

Figure 5-3 Line drawing of the external carotid artery (ECA) branches. **1**, Superior thyroidal artery. **2**, Lingual artery. **3**, Facial artery. **4**, Internal maxillary artery. **5**, Superficial temporal artery. **6**, Posterior auricular artery. **7**, Occipital artery. **8**, Ascending pharyngeal artery.

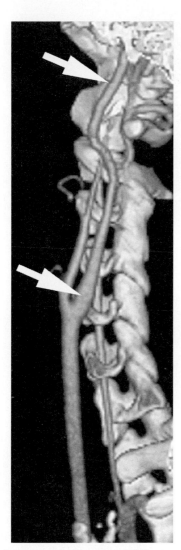

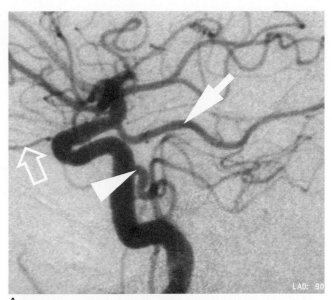

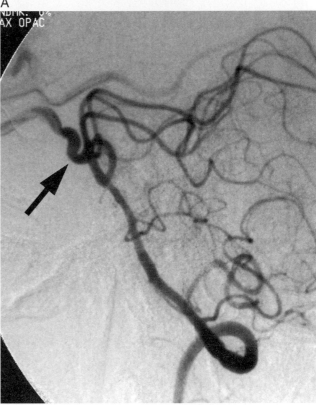

Figure 5-4 Internal carotid artery (ICA) anatomy shown on volume rendering of CT angiogram. The cervical ICA (arrows) is a branchless vessel.

by the C6 to C1 transverse processes, before looping posteriorly into the spinal canal between the skull base and C1. The paired vertebral arteries enter the skull through the foramen magnum, giving off the posterior inferior cerebellar arteries before joining to form the basilar artery. The basilar artery, which runs along the posterior surface of the clivus, terminates by branching into the posterior cerebral arteries. Numerous small branches to the pons, as well as the paired anterior inferior and superior cerebellar arteries, arise from the basilar artery before it bifurcates.

The majority of anatomic variations of the CCA, ICA, and vertebral arteries occur at vessel origins (Table 5-1). These anomalies are related to the development of the thoracic arch (see Chapter 9).

Figure 5-5 Anomalous branches of the ICA. **A**, Lateral view of the cavernous ICA. Two anomalous branches are present, a posterior cerebral artery (arrow) (termed a fetal origin, found in 30% of patients, bilateral in 8%), and a trigeminal artery (arrowhead). The ophthalmic artery (open arrow) is a normal branch of the cavernous ICA. **B**, Lateral view of vertebral artery injection in the same patient confirms the identity of the trigeminal artery (arrow).

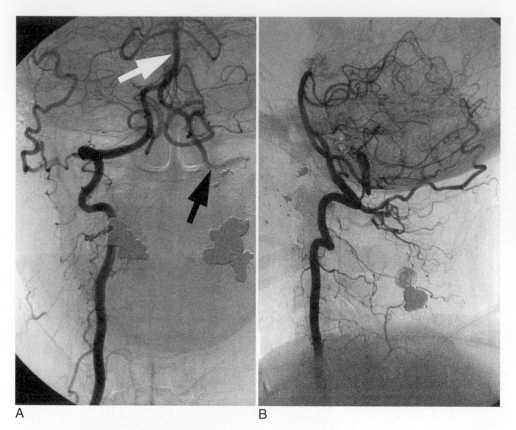

A   B

Figure 5-6 Vertebral artery anatomy. **A**, Anteroposterior view of right vertebral artery injection in a patient with traumatic occlusion of the left vertebral artery (black arrow). The vertebral arteries join to form the basilar artery (white arrow). **B**, Lateral view from the same injection.

KEY COLLATERAL PATHWAYS

There are two levels of cerebrovascular collaterals; extra- and intracranial. The ECA is an important source of collateral blood supply to both the ipsilateral and contralateral ICA. In the setting of a proximal ICA occlusion, retrograde flow in the opthalmic artery can reconstitute

Table 5-1 Anatomic Variants of the Carotid and Vertebral Arteries

Variant	Incidence
Left common carotid artery from brachiocephalic artery ("bovine arch")	22%
Left vertebral artery directly from aortic arch	5%
Combined left common carotid and left subclavian artery origin	1%
Aberrant right subclavian artery (last branch from aortic arch)	1%
Persistent trigeminal artery	0.5%
Persistent hypoglossal artery	0.03%
Congenital absence of the internal carotid artery	0.01%

the intracranial portion of the distal ICA, thus supplying the brain (Fig. 5-7). With occlusion of a CCA, collateral flow from the opposite ECA and the ipsilateral vertebral artery can reconstitute the cervical ICA (Fig. 5-8). Rarely, the superficial temporal and middle meningeal arteries can provide collateral supply through the skull to leptomeningeal arteries on the surface of the brain.

In the neck the vertebral artery is an additional potential source of collateral blood supply to the carotid arteries. Muscular branches of the vertebral artery communicate with the occipital branch of the ECA, which can then reconstitute the ICA. Conversely, the ECA can provide collateral blood supply to the distal cervical vertebral artery through the same pathway. The distal cervical vertebral artery can be reconstituted by muscular arteries of the neck such as the ascending cervical artery.

Within the skull the anterior (carotid) and posterior (vertebral) circulations communicate through a vascular ring, the Circle of Willis, that is located at the base of the brain (Fig. 5-9). This network potentially allows perfusion of the entire brain via any one of four vessels that supply the head. Similarly, the Circle of Willis serves as a potential collateral pathway to the upper extremities. The Circle of Willis is incomplete or contains hypoplastic elements in more than 50% of individuals. One or both posterior communicating arteries are absent in up to a third

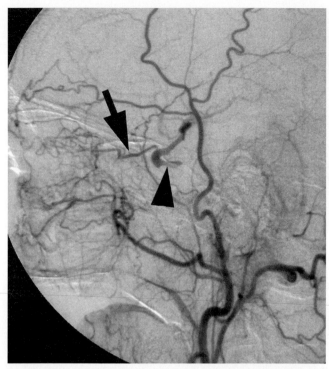

Figure 5-7   Lateral view (anterior is to left of image) showing reconstitution of the cavernous portion of the ICA (arrowhead) from retrograde flow in the opthalmic artery (arrow) in a patient with occlusion of the cervical ICA.

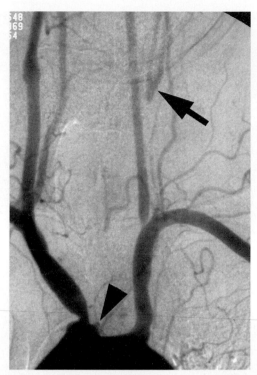

Figure 5-8   Reconstitution of the cervical ICA from retrograde flow in ECA branches. LAO arch aortogram in a patient with left CCA origin occlusion (arrowhead) and innominate artery stenosis. The left CCA bifurcation (arrow) appears to be "floating" in the neck.

of patients. A hypoplastic or absent A1 segment of the anterior cerebral artery is found in approximately 15%. The posterior cerebral artery arises directly from the ICA in up to 20%. These variants can occur in isolation or in conjunction with other circle anomalies.

IMAGING

The most widely used imaging tool for the extracranial cerebral circulation is ultrasound (US) with pulsed Doppler and Duplex color-flow. Gray-scale imaging with a 5- to 7.5-MHz linear array transducer is sufficient in most patients to identify the CCA, ICA, and ECA, and areas of plaque. Gray scale imaging alone does not perform well in the determination of the degree of stenosis, as hypoechoic "soft" plaque may be indistinguishable from the residual lumen, and calcification in the anterior wall of the vessel can reflect the US beam so that the lumen cannot be visualized. Sometimes it can be difficult to distinguish the ICA from the ECA. Doppler interrogation of flow improves identification of the vessels and quantification of stenoses. The normal CCA, ICA, and ECA have distinctive Doppler waveforms (Fig. 5-10). The CCA, ICA, and vertebral artery have low-resistance waveforms, whereas the ECA has a high-resistance waveform.

Color flow is helpful in localizing vessels and selecting the best place to measure velocities in a stenosis.

The intracranial arteries cannot be directly visualized with current ultrasound units owing to the reflective properties of the skull. Transcranial Doppler (TCD) uses low-frequency (2-MHz) pulse-wave Doppler to evaluate the intracranial arteries. The low frequency sound waves

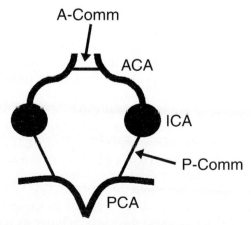

Figure 5-9   Diagram of the circle of Willis. A-Comm = anterior communicating artery. ACA = A1 segment of the anterior cerebral artery. ICA = internal carotid artery. P-Comm = posterior communicating artery. PCA = posterior cerebral artery.

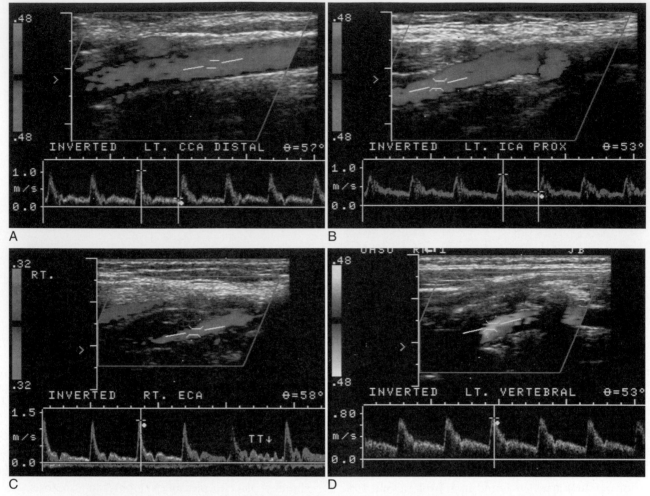

Figure 5-10   Normal Doppler waveforms and flow velocities in the cervical carotid and vertebral arteries. **A**, CCA. The waveform is low-resistance. **B**, ICA. The waveform is noticeably more low-resistance than the CCA. **C**, ECA. Note the high-resistance waveform. TT = tapping over temporal artery, used to confirm the identity of the artery being imaged. **D**, Vertebral artery. The waveform is low-resistance.

can penetrate the thinner portions of the skull. The arteries of the Circle of Willis can be evaluated through the temporal bone, the ophthalmic artery through the orbit, and the vertebral artery through the foramen magnum. Direction of flow and alterations in flow velocity and waveforms can be used to infer the presence of occlusive disease.

A number of potential pitfalls exist with carotid US. The quality of the study is very dependent upon a skilled and knowledgeable sonographer. The great vessel origins cannot be reliably imaged. A complete study may not be possible in a patient with a high carotid artery bifurcation situated behind the ramus of the mandible. Lastly, the cervical vertebral arteries are difficult to image in their entirety with US owing to the surrounding bony vertebra, although direction of flow can be readily determined.

The cervical vessels are excellent subjects for magnetic resonance angiography (MRA). Two-dimensional time-of-flight (2-D TOF) MRA with a superior saturation band is commonly used to image the cervical arteries (see Fig. 3-12). The superior saturation band eliminates jugular venous flow, but will also mask reversed flow in a vertebral artery. Reversal of flow in the vertebral arteries can be elegantly demonstrated with an 2-D phase-contrast acquisition to detect flow in the superior to inferior direction (Fig. 5-11). Calcification of lesions does not impair the ability of MRA to image the carotid arteries, but the degree of stenosis is routinely overestimated. The great vessel origins cannot be adequately evaluated with 2-D TOF, and flow in kinked or tortuous carotid arteries loses signal due to saturation. Lastly, very slow flow distal to a severe stenosis may become completely saturated and produce no signal, so that the vessel appears occluded.

Dynamic gadolinium-enhanced 3-D sequences overcome many of the limitations of 2-D TOF carotid MRA.

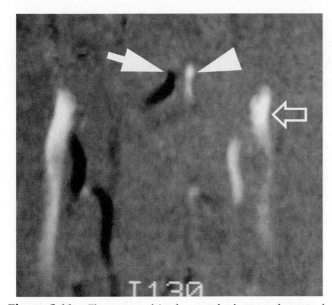

Figure 5-11   Flow reversal in the vertebral artery due to subclavian artery origin stenosis. Coronal 2-D phase-contrast (PC) of the neck. Flow in the superior–inferior direction is white. There is prograde flow in the right vertebral artery (arrow), and retrograde flow in the left vertebral artery (arrowhead). Note that the direction of flow in the left vertebral artery is the same as in the neck veins (open arrow).

Rapid acquisitions during breath holding are necessary to avoid enhancement of the adjacent jugular veins. However, stenosis, tortuosity, and slow flow do not impair gadolinium-enhanced 3-D carotid MRA. The absence of signal loss from turbulence allows more accurate grading of stenoses. A larger field of view may be utilized than with 2-D TOF MRA, so that diagnostic images can be obtained from origin of the great vessels to the carotid siphon (Fig. 5-12). Dedicated, separate sequences should be used to image the Circle of Willis and the intracranial circulation. When coupled with anatomic and perfusion/diffusion brain imaging, MR with MRA have the potential to provide complete cerebrovascular evaluation.

Limitations of all forms of carotid MRA include signal loss due to metal (such as stents or adjacent surgical clips), motion artifacts (such as swallowing or talking during the study), and spatial image resolution.

CT angiography (CTA) has also been used successfully to image the cervical carotid arteries (see Fig. 5-4). Rapid bolus injection of iodinated contrast with a short delay is necessary to avoid venous enhancement. Thin collimation allows accurate evaluation of stenoses. Slow flow in a vessel distal to a pinpoint lesion can be detected

Figure 5-12   Three-dimensional gadolinium-enhanced MRA of the carotid arteries. **A**, Anterior maximum intensity projection (MIP) shows from the great vessel origins to the Circle of Willis. The left CCA arises from the innominate artery (arrow). **B**, Oblique MIP from the same study showing normal CCA bifurcations (arrows).

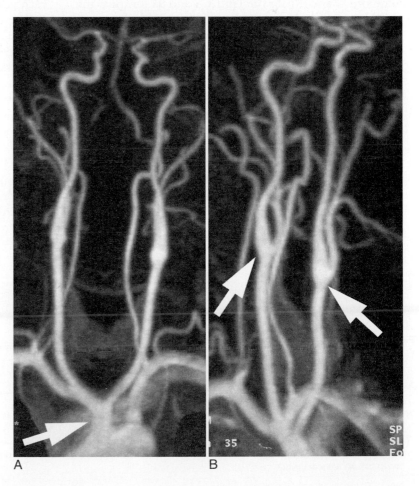

A   B

with CTA. The degree of calcification is readily apparent. Although acquisition times are short and multidetector row CT scanners are readily available, this modality has been utilized less than US or MRA.

Catheter angiography of the extracranial carotid and vertebral arteries is the standard against which other imaging modalities have been validated. Though infrequently used for routine preoperative planning, this modality remains important for resolving diagnostic dilemmas and as a prelude to interventions. The study should begin with a flush aortic injection through a 5- or 6-French pigtail catheter positioned so that the sideholes are in the transverse portion of the aortic arch. Filming should be rapid (4–6 frames per second) in the LAO projection (the exact degree depends on the patient anatomy, but is usually about 45 degrees). This obliquity opens up the arch to show the origins of the brachiocephalic, left common carotid, and left subclavian vessels to best advantage. If there is a question about the right common carotid or subclavian artery origin, a second injection in the RAO projection should be obtained (see Fig. 5-1). The common carotid arteries can be selected with 5-French catheters, usually with an H-1, Davis, or Berenstein-type shape (Table 5-2). When the great vessels arise from the arch at a steep angle, a Simmons shape (S1 for the left CCA and S2 for the right CCA) may be necessary. A short segment (1–2 cm) of soft guidewire should protrude from the tip of the catheter during selection of the vessel to minimize the risk of trauma. Selection of the ICA and ECA can be accomplished with the same catheters and a hydrophilic-coated guidewire. Filming in an anterior oblique view may be necessary to profile ICA and ECA origins.

Vertebral arteries can be visualized from subclavian artery injections, or selected with the same catheter shapes as used for CCA. Filming of selective injections should be in at least two planes (AP and lateral) (see Fig. 5-6).

In the unusual situation of performing selective carotid angiography from the upper extremity approach, use the *right* arm for access and a Simmons catheter (see Fig. 2-37).

Selection of the right CCA is difficult from a left axillary artery approach.

Extreme care is necessary when manipulating or flushing any catheter in the aortic arch or cerebral vessels, as small thrombi or air bubbles create huge problems in this vascular bed. Double flush all catheters in these locations every 90 seconds. Many angiographers administer a bolus of 3000–5000 U of heparin during diagnostic studies after obtaining vascular access. The risk of permanent stroke during cerebral angiography is less than 1%. Reversible ischemic events occur in as many as 3% of patients.

ATHEROSCLEROTIC OCCLUSIVE DISEASE

Approximately 550,000 strokes occur each year in the United States, with a 30-day mortality of 17%. An ischemic etiology is responsible for almost 85% of strokes, of which the majority are believed to be the result of cerebrovascular occlusive disease. Approximately 15% of strokes are hemorrhagic in nature, due to hypertensive vasculopathy, ruptured cerebral aneurysms or arteriovenous malformations, and hematologic disorders. The estimated total cost of the care of patients with stroke approaches $30 billion each year.

The most common pathology in the extracranial carotid and vertebral arteries is occlusive atherosclerotic disease. Over 90% of carotid artery stenoses are localized to the bifurcation of the CCA or the proximal ICA. Origin stenoses of the common carotid artery are present in fewer than 5% of patients with concurrent disease at the CCA bifurcation (see Fig. 5-8). Similarly, stenosis resulting in a greater than 50% reduction in luminal diameter of the intracranial portion of the ICA are found in 5% of patients with ICA bifurcation disease. Stenoses of the cervical vertebral arteries are found in approximately one-third of patients with ICA stenosis, but are rarely symptomatic.

The definition of carotid stenosis is, unfortunately, not uniform among physicians. The most widely accepted

---

Table 5-2 Injection Rates for Carotid and Vertebral Angiography

Location	Injection Rate	Total Volume	Projections	Filming Rate	Duration
Arch	20–25 mL	30–50 mL	LAO, RAO	4–6 s	10 sc
CCA	7–9 mL	11–12 mL	AP, Lat, AO	2–4 s	15 s
ECA	3–5 mL	5–7 mL	AP, Lat	2–4 s	15 s
ICA	6–7 mL	8–9 mL	AP, Lat, AO	2–4 s	20 s
Vertebral	3–5 mL	5–7 mL	AP, Lat	2–4 s	15 s

CCA, common carotid artery; ECA, external carotid artery; ICA, internal carotid artery; LAO, left anterior oblique; RAO, right anterior oblique; AP, anterior–posterior; Lat, lateral; AO, anterior oblique.

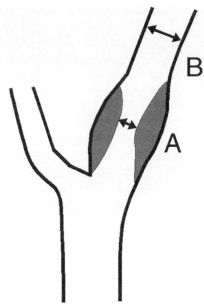

Figure 5-13   Technique to measure ICA stenosis. The diameter of the lumen in the most narrow portion is divided by the diameter of the most normal appearing adjacent cervical ICA. The degree of stenosis is $(\frac{B-A}{B}) \times 100$.

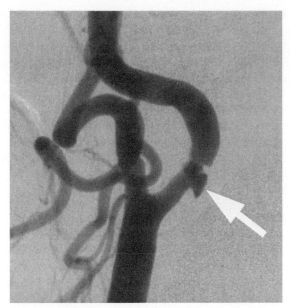

Figure 5-14   DSA in the anterior oblique projection showing a stenotic proximal ICA with an ulcer (arrow). The clinical importance of this angiographic appearance is not certain, but would be suspicious as a source of emboli in a patient with recurrent transient ischemic attacks.

technique for determination of carotid stenosis on MRA, CTA, and catheter angiography is to determine the ratio of the diameter of the lumen at the point of maximal stenosis to the diameter of the lumen in the closest normal segment of cervical internal carotid artery (Fig. 5-13). The estimated or true maximal diameter of the ICA bulb or CCA should not be used. As an alternative, a metallic pellet or other object with a known diameter placed on the neck provides calibration for measurements of luminal diameter from conventional angiograms.

Carotid stenosis is associated with ipsilateral stroke when the vessel lumen is reduced by 50% or more in diameter (Box 5-1). The mechanism of stroke due to carotid disease is believed to be embolic, either from thrombus or platelet aggregates that form within a lesion, or debris released when an unstable plaque ruptures

into the vessel lumen. Irregularities of the plaque surface that look like pits are termed ulcers, and may have a higher propensity for causing stroke (Fig. 5-14). Acute carotid occlusion can result in ipsilateral stroke when the intracranial collateral circulation is insufficient or thrombus embolizes from the ICA, but in many cases is a clinically silent event.

Patients with carotid stenosis may present with symptoms of transient cerebral or retinal ischemia, presumably due to small emboli that spontaneously lyse or fragment. These events occur in up to one-third of patients prior to a permanent stroke. Termed a transient ischemic attack (TIA), these result in a neurologic or visual abnormality that reverses completely within minutes, but may last up to 24 hours. The risk of a stroke increases 10-fold in patients with TIAs.

Two important prospective studies of carotid artery stenosis were completed in the 1990s and profoundly influenced the management of this disease. The North American Symptomatic Carotid Endarterectomy Trial was a randomized comparison of optimal medical therapy and combined surgical endarterectomy and medical therapy in patients with carotid stenosis and documented neurologic symptoms within 120 days of enrollment in the study. For patients with stenoses 70–99%, the cumulative risks of any ipsilateral stroke at 2 years were 26% in the medical and 9% in the surgical patients. For a major or fatal ipsilateral stroke, the corresponding risks were 13.1% versus 2.5%. Similar benefit of surgery was not found in symptomatic patients with stenoses that

Box 5-1   Risk Factors for Stroke

Smoking
Hypertension
Diabetes
Elevated cholesterol
Male sex
Advanced age
African-American or Asian
Family history

were less than 70%. This study was followed by the Asymptomatic Carotid Atherosclerosis Study (ACAS). In ACAS, 1662 asymptomatic men and women with stenoses 60% or greater of the ICA were randomized to either surgical or medical therapy. The aggregate risk of stroke at 5 years was 5.1% for the surgical group and 11% for medical therapy. This study established 60% diameter reduction of the ICA as the threshold for intervention in patients with asymptomatic stenoses.

TIAs due to vertebral and basilar artery occlusive disease have a different clinical presentation from those due to ICA stenosis. Because the neurologic territory at risk involves the brainstem, cerebellum, and posterior cerebral lobes, the complex of symptoms are referred to as vertebrobasilar syndrome (Box 5-2). Occlusive lesions of the subclavian artery origin (resulting in a retrograde flow in the vertebral artery) can produce identical symptoms.

When carotid occlusive disease is suspected, the first imaging examination for the majority patients is grayscale and Doppler ultrasound (Fig. 5-15). Velocity measurements proximal, within, and distal to the area of stenosis allows accurate determination of the degree of stenosis (Table 5-3). The flow through an area of stenosis is at first accelerated, and remains so until the lumen becomes severely narrowed. Flow then decreases, and may be barely detectable by ultrasound. Doppler waveforms distal to the stenosis broaden with a loss in amplitude and ultimately pulsatility. Estimation of flow velocities can quantify the degree of luminal narrowing, although several different schemes exist for interpreting these velocities. The generally accepted sensitivity and specificity of US for clinically significant carotid stenosis are each 95%.

The presence of severe disease or occlusion in one ICA may result in US overestimation of the degree of stenosis in the other ICA owing to normal compensatory increased flow. A pinpoint residual ICA lumen with very slow distal flow may be indistinguishable from a total occlusion by ultrasound. This distinction is important as the management is different, as described below.

MRA has a sensitivity of >90% and a specificity of >90% for the detection of hemodynamically significant

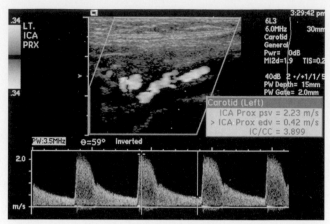

Figure 5-15 Ultrasound of carotid stenosis. Spectral broadening and elevated velocities in a patient with left ICA stenosis.

(greater than 50% reduction in luminal diameter) carotid stenosis (Fig. 5-16). However, as a rule, the degree of stenosis is overestimated by MRA, particularly on 2-D TOF sequences. Precise determination of the degree of stenosis requires high-resolution gadolinium-enhanced 3-D sequences. The vertebral arteries are reliably imaged with MRA techniques, although signal loss as the vessels enter the spinal canal is common in 2-D TOF images, and the origins can be seen with confidence only with gadolinium enhanced 3-D sequences.

The sensitivity and specificity of CTA for detection of carotid stenoses are also reported to be >90% each (Fig. 5-17). The vertebral arteries can be evaluated for patency, but direction of flow cannot be determined. Heavily calcified plaque and vascular tortuosity can make image interpretation difficult.

Selective common carotid angiography remains widely accepted as a reliable technique for evaluation of ICA stenosis. However, owing to the cost and small risk of stroke, routine use of angiography is uncommon. The current indications for catheter angiography include

Box 5-2	Clinical Features of Vertebrobasilar Insufficiency

Bilateral motor/sensory deficits
Ataxia
Diplopia
Dysarthria
Dysmetria
Bilateral homonymous hemianopsia

Table 5-3	US Evaluation of Internal Carotid Artery Stenosis		
Lesion Severity	**PSV (cm/s)**	**EDV (cm/s)**	**VICA/VCCA**
≥50%	150	60	2.5
≥60%	175	70	2.75
≥70%	225	90	3.75
≥80%	300	100	5

PSV, peak systolic velocity in lesion; EDV, end diastolic velocity in lesion; VICA/VCCA, ratio of ICA PSV to the PSV of the middle/distal CCA.

Modified from Grant EG, Duerinckx AJ: Noninvasive diagnosis of carotid stenosis: technique, normal anatomy, and new observations in light of the NASCET study. *RSNA Categorical Course in Vascular Imaging* 211–221, 1998.

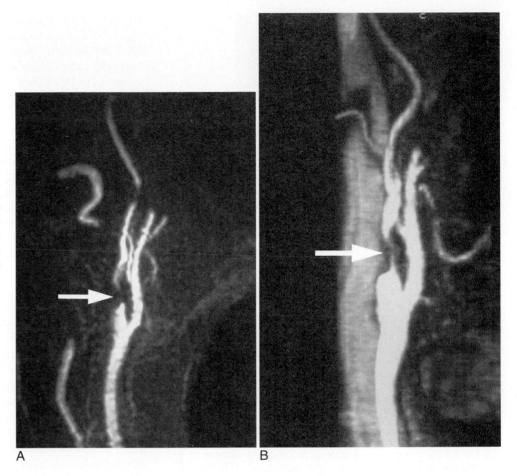

Figure 5-16 MRA of ICA stenosis. **A**, Oblique MIP of a 2-D TOF MRA showing the signal void indicative of a stenosis (arrow). **B**, Oblique MIP of a 3-D gadolinium-enhanced MRA showing the irregular stenosis (arrow). There is no signal loss.

A

B

discordant results of noninvasive imaging modalities, technically inadequate noninvasive studies, suspected concurrent great vessel origin or intracranial ICA occlusive disease, acute or delayed operative failures, and differentiation of severe stenosis from occlusion of the ICA. Delayed filming in the lateral plane should be obtained in order to detect a "string sign" whenever a critical stenosis, rather than occlusion, is suspected (Fig. 5-18).

There is great debate over the timing and type of intervention for ICA stenosis. The entire debate is framed by the morbidity and mortality of the intervention versus the risk of medical management. The intervention that is used as a benchmark is surgical carotid endarterectomy, which has a reported operative stroke rate of 2–3%, mortality of <1%, and a symptomatic restenosis rate of 1–2% (Fig. 5-19).

Catheter-based carotid interventions are emerging as alternatives to conventional surgery. The enabling technology is the metal stent; angioplasty alone has limited success in this vascular territory. Although there is much less experience with carotid stents than endarterectomy, the procedure has been embraced with enthusiasm. The essential steps involve meticulous technique (one small air bubble can ruin everything), accurate localization of

the stenotic area, aggressive procedural anticoagulation and administration of antiplatelet drugs, initial dilatation of the lesion with an undersized balloon with short inflation times, and deployment of a self-expanding stent with postdilatation to the presumed native vessel diameter (Fig. 5-20). In order to minimize manipulation of the lesions, guiding catheters (6- or 7-French) are positioned in the CCA, and small balloon and stent systems that require 0.018- or 0.014-inch guidewires are used. Typical angioplasty balloon diameters are 4–6 mm for the internal carotid artery. Stent placement across the origin of the ECA is frequently necessary to adequately treat ICA-origin stenoses and is well tolerated. Stretching of the carotid bulb can trigger a reflex bradycardia or asystole, so atropine 1 mg may be given intravenously prior to balloon inflation, and a transvenous or transcutaneous pacemaker should be close at hand. The goal of the procedure is to increase flow across the lesion, not make it equal or better than new. This is a vascular bed in which the old adage "the enemy of good is better" applies.

The use of distal "neuroprotective" devices during the procedure such as an occlusion balloon or an endovascular "net" may prove important in reducing

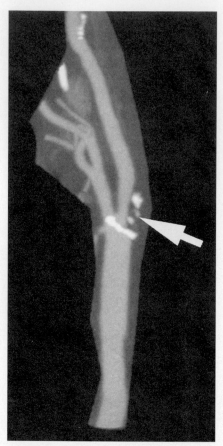

Figure 5-17   Sagittal reformat of a CTA showing calcified ICA origin stenosis (arrow). (Courtesy Larry Tanenbaum M.D., Edison Imaging, NJ.)

procedural morbidity. The obvious concern during this procedure is distal embolization of plaque fragments or thrombus. In skilled hands and selected patients the procedural success rate is over 95% and the permanent stroke rate is reported to be under 2%, equal or less than that of open surgery, although the restenosis rate has yet to be defined. Careful patient selection is crucial. Specifically, the procedure should be avoided in patients with poor access (i.e., tortuous or diseased iliac arteries or thoracic aorta), coiled or redundant carotid arteries, heavily calcified lesions, and multiple or tandem lesions especially those involving the carotid siphon.

FIBROMUSCULAR DYSPLASIA (FMD)

The internal carotid artery is the second most common site of fibromuscular dysplasia (FMD), with the renal arteries being the first. Overall, FMD of the ICA is found in just under 1% of patients undergoing carotid arteriography. There are a number of forms of FMD (see Table 1-4), but 65% of cases are of the medial fibroplasia

type which has a distinctive "string of pearls" appearance (Fig. 5-21). FMD is localized to the cervical portion of the ICA in 90% of cases, above the bifurcation. This process can also involve the vertebral artery (10–40%). Lesions are bilateral in up to two-thirds of patients. Approximately 20% of patients with carotid FMD also have intracranial aneurysms.

The presence of FMD in the carotid or vertebral circulation is frequently an asymptomatic incidental finding on imaging studies. However, patients can present with transient ischemic attacks (TIAs), presumably due to embolization of small thrombi that form in the "pearls." Other sources of emboli, such as a routine atherosclerotic ICA stenosis, should be excluded before attributing these symptoms to FMD. Spontaneous ICA or vertebral artery dissection can be due to underlying FMD, although establishing the diagnosis after the dissection has occurred is difficult unless FMD can be found in the other nondissected ICA or vertebral artery.

The most sensitive imaging modality for detecting FMD is conventional angiography. Subtle FMD can be difficult or impossible to visualize with MRA and CTA because image resolution is too low. A flow disturbance or area of stenosis may be detected by ultrasound, but the full extent of the FMD in the cervical ICA cannot be determined with this modality.

Intervention in carotid FMD is warranted in symptomatic patients (such as TIA without another source), or when a critical stenosis is present. Surgical resection of the abnormal segment may be possible if the FMD is low enough and limited in extent. However, medial fibroplasia is ideally suited for angioplasty (and stents when necessary), as distal lesions can be treated. Results in small series of patients undergoing ICA angioplasty for FMD have been excellent and durable.

VASCULITIS

Vasculitides involving the carotid and vertebral arteries are rare in North America, but much more common in portions of Asia and South America. Long, smooth stenoses are characteristic, although irregular lesions or a "sausage link" appearance may be present. Concurrent atherosclerosis can be seen in older patients or with radiation vasculitis.

The best known vasculitis that affects the carotid arteries is Takayasu's arteritis. This giant-cell arteritis can involve the CCA, great vessel origins, subclavian arteries, thoracic and abdominal aorta, coronary arteries, visceral arteries, and pulmonary arteries (Figs 5-22 and 9-32). Patients present with signs of a systemic illness such as fever and malaise, but many have vascular occlusion as their only symptom. The typical patient is a young woman (20–40 years), although the disease has been reported in males, children, and septuagenarians as well.

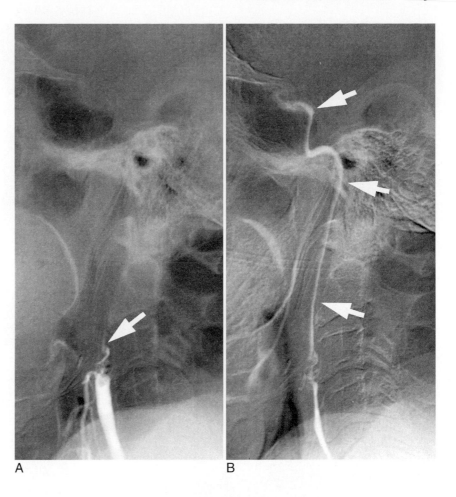

Figure 5-18   String sign. **A**, Early lateral film from selective CCA injection shows filling of a few ECA branches and what appears to be an ICA occlusion (arrow). **B**, Later image from the same injection shows layering of contrast and slow prograde flow in a patent ICA (arrows) beyond a severe origin stenosis. Delayed filming is necessary to detect a string sign.

A   B

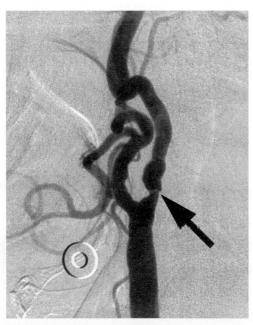

Figure 5-19   Lateral DSA showing focal restenosis (arrow) after carotid endartectomy. The metal washer has been placed on the patient's neck as a reference for measurements.

Angiographically, long smooth stenoses of the common carotid and subclavian arteries are characteristic. A thickened, enhancing arterial wall can be seen with US, CT, and MR. Angioplasty of Takayasu's arteritis during the inactive or "burned out" phase has been successful.

Radiation vasculitis occurs months to years following external beam therapy. The typical appearance is diffuse stenosis that can look very much like atherosclerosis with intimal calcification and focal irregularity. The distribution of the lesions is the key to the diagnosis, as they are localized to the radiation portal and involve many vessels. Patients may present with acute stroke or chronic ischemic symptoms. Intervention is difficult as the vessels do not respond well to angioplasty, and the surgical field is challenging owing to the location of the lesions and scarring.

SPONTANEOUS CAROTID AND VERTEBRAL DISSECTION

Spontaneous (i.e., in the absence of trauma) dissection of the CCA, ICA, or vertebral arteries is a rare but

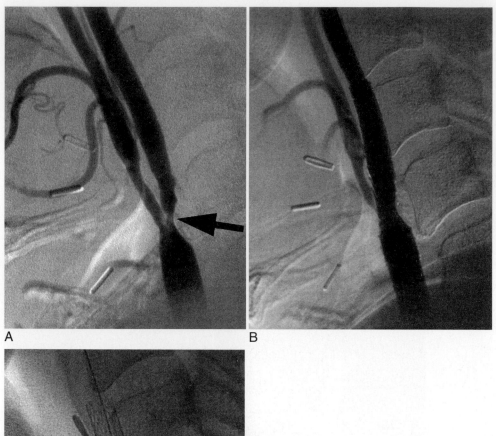

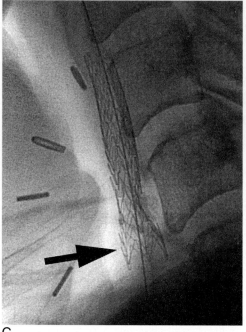

Figure 5-20 Carotid stenosis treated with metallic stent in a patient with previous neck surgery. **A,** Lateral DSA showing stenosis of the CCA bifurcation extending into the ICA (arrow) and ECA. **B,** Lateral DSA after placement of a self-expanding stent. The ICA is widely patent, but the ECA does not fill as well as before. **C,** Unsubtracted lateral image showing that the stent extends from the distal CCA (arrow) into the ICA. This placement is intentional in order to treat the full length of the stenosis. Note that the guidewire remains in place across the stent until the very end of the procedure.

potentially devastating event. The incidence is unknown, and the etiology may be multifactorial (Box 5-3 and Fig. 1-37). Patients tend to be in their fourth or fifth decade, but dissection can occur in any age group. The presenting symptoms can be misleading and result in delay in diagnosis. Ipsilateral headache is characteristic, but incomplete Horner's syndrome, cranial nerve dysfunction (VII, IX, X, and XII), and focal cerebral ischemic events can also occur (Box 5-4). The neurologic findings may be delayed by hours, days, and even months.

Box 5-3   Etiologies of Carotid Dissection

Trauma
Hypertension
Marfan syndrome
Ehlers–Danlos syndrome
Fibromuscular dysplasia

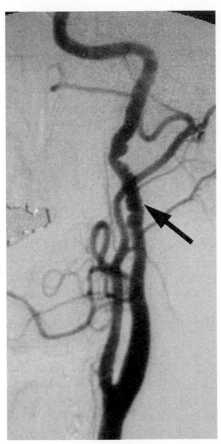

Figure 5-21 Fibromuscular dysplasia of the ICA. Lateral DSA of the left ICA showing a beaded appearance (arrow) of the distal cervical ICA typical of medial fibroplasia.

CT, MRI, and US are particularly useful for diagnosis of carotid and vertebral dissection. The intimal flap or a compressed true lumen may be visualized (Fig. 5-23). Slow flow or a thrombosed false lumen may appear bright on both T1- and T2-weighted MRI, depending upon velocity of flow or the age of the thrombus. Compression or even long tapered occlusion of the lumen are characteristic on angiography. Dissection of

Box 5-4   Symptoms of Carotid Dissection

Unilateral headache
Neck pain
Loss of superficial temporal artery pulse (with common carotid artery involvement)
Horner syndrome (ptosis, miosis, and unilateral anhidrosis)
Aphasia
Unilateral facial weakness
Transient ischemic attack
Hemiparesis

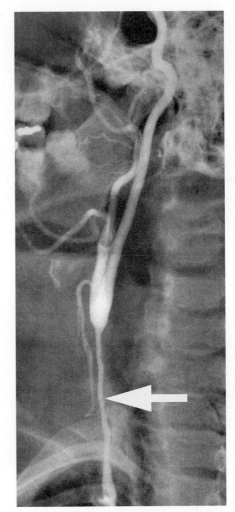

Figure 5-22 Takayasu's arteritis involving the carotid arteries in a young woman. Selective right CCA angiogram showing the long, smooth stenosis (arrow) that spares the bifurcation, ICA, and ECA (see Fig. 1-13).

the ICA may extend into the cavernous portion of the artery.

The majority of patients can be successfully managed with long-term anticoagulation. Stent placement in the true lumen may be necessary to restore cerebral perfusion. Identification and, if possible, modification of underlying risk factors is crucial. However, in the majority of patients, no etiology can be found.

TRAUMA

Traumatic lesions to the extracranial cervical vessels can be caused by any mechanism, but are most commonly related to penetrating, blunt, hyperextension, and blast injuries. Common associations include cervical fractures and dislocations, and airway and esophageal trauma. Injury can occur to both the arteries and the veins,

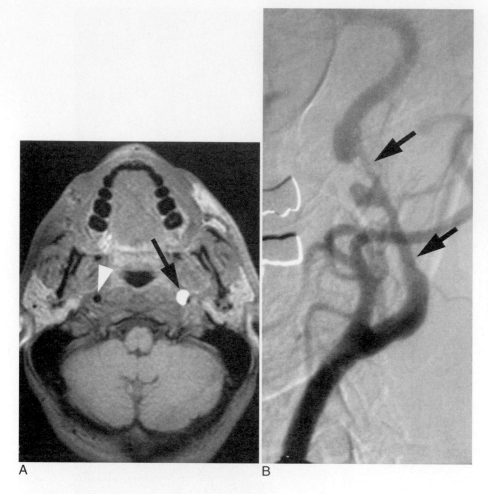

Figure 5-23 Spontaneous carotid dissection. **A**, Axial T1-weighted MR image showing the true lumen of the left ICA lumen compressed by a false lumen that has bright signal (arrow) consistent with thrombus or slow flow. The right ICA (arrowhead) is normal. **B**, DSA in the same patient showing the compressed true lumen of the left ICA (arrows). The false lumen does not fill.

A   B

particularly the internal jugular vein. Clinical presentation varies with the type and mechanism of trauma, and severity of other injuries. The full spectrum of vascular injuries may be present, ranging from spasm to transection with active extravasation (Fig. 5-24).

Penetrating neck injuries result in vascular injury in up to 25% of patients, and have an overall mortality rate of approximately 5%. The neck is divided into three vascular zones (Table 5-4). Zone 3 and 1 injuries are extremely difficult to approach surgically (the mandible obstructs access to zone 3, and thoracotomy is required for zone 1). Vascular injuries in zone 1 have a 12% mortality rate. Stable patients with suspected vascular injury in these zones usually undergo angiography or CT scans. Injuries to zone 2 are not only more common (60–70%), but are readily accessible for physical examination and surgery. Stable patients may undergo exploratory surgery, angiography, US examination, or serial physical examinations, depending on the local standard of care.

The majority of major vascular injuries in the neck due to penetrating wounds involve the carotid arteries, although the vertebral arteries are injured in up to 4% of patients (Fig. 5-25). Branches of the external carotid artery

may be involved as well as the major veins. Angiography for trauma of the cervical vessels should therefore always include delayed images that visualize the veins.

Blunt injury to the neck from a direct blow, the shoulder strap of seat belts, and strangulation result in arterial injury in fewer than 1% of cases. Intimal dissection and occlusion are more common with blunt injury than with penetrating wounds. The most common location is the cervical ICA, extending into the skull base. Vertebral artery dissection may be found in as many as 20% of patients (Fig. 5-26). Up to two-thirds of patients develop symptoms within the first 24 hours, but only 10% have focal

Table 5-4	Vascular Zones in Penetrating Neck Trauma
Zone	**Definition**
1	Below cricoid cartilage to clavicles
2	Cricoid cartilage to mandibular angle
3	Above angle of mandible to skull base

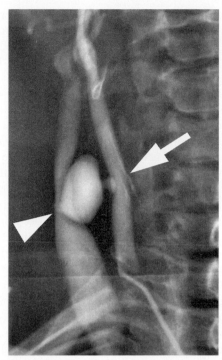

Figure 5-24   Angiogram showing CCA (arrow) to internal jugular vein (arrowhead) fistula with an associated pseudoaneurysm following a stab wound to the neck. (Attempted central line placement at the bedside.)

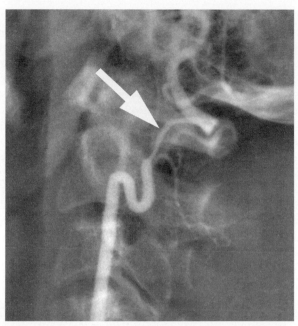

Figure 5-26   Lateral angiogram of a patient with neck pain following a boxing match. There is segmental narrowing of the vertebral artery (arrow) characteristic of dissection.

Figure 5-25   Vertebral artery pseudoaneurysm due to penetrating injury. **A**, CT scan of the neck showing a wood splinter through the neural foramina (arrow). There is a large hematoma in the neck that displaces the airway. **B**, Selective vertebral angiogram after removal of the splinter shows a small pseudoaneurysm (arrow). This was treated by balloon occlusion of the vertebral artery proximal and distal to the lesion after ensuring that the left vertebral artery was normal.

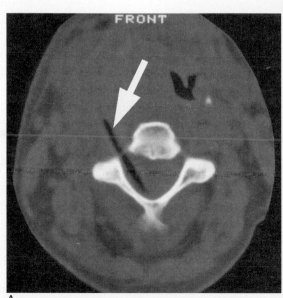

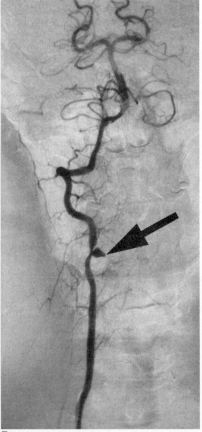

A

B

neurologic findings on initial presentation. Symptoms may develop weeks to months following injury. The etiology of the delayed symptoms is believed to be emboli originating from the dissection, rather than compromise of ICA flow. A high level of suspicion is necessary to diagnose these lesions. US, MRI/MRA, CT, and angiography are all used for evaluation of suspected carotid injury in blunt trauma.

Intervention in carotid and vertebral injury is determined by the type of injury, symptoms, accessibility of the vessel, and the overall status of the patient. Spasm, intimal tears, and nonocclusive dissection may be managed with anticoagulation alone. Stent placement (bare metal or covered) may be feasible in zone 1 and 3 dissections and pseudoaneurysms. Embolization of surgically inaccessible transected vessels can be performed with coils, detachable balloons, or other devices. These procedures are usually tolerated well in patients with intact intracranial collateral pathways.

EPISTAXIS

Nose-bleeds are common and usually due to a source in the anterior portion of the nose. These bleeds usually stop spontaneously, or can be readily visualized and treated with local measures. Posterior epistaxis occurs in a more inaccessible region and is much more difficult to control. In addition, bleeding in this location is more typical of older patients with multiple medical problems.

Uncommon etiologies include tumors, penetrating trauma, and carotid artery laceration in the siphon due to fractures of the skull base. Up to 25% of patients with Osler–Weber–Rendu disease have frequent bleeding from nasopharyngeal telangiectases.

The initial management of severe posterior epistaxis is resuscitation (including blood products), correction of coagulopathies, intravenous vasoconstrictors, and application of direct pressure to the area with nasal packing. The latter is extremely uncomfortable and fails in roughly 25% of cases. The arterial supply to the posterior nasal cavity is primarily from the internal maxillary artery. Surgical ligation or clipping of the internal maxillary artery has a 10–30% failure rate. Endoscopic cautery has a similar rate of success and rebleeding. Selective catheterization of the internal maxillary artery and embolization with particles (such as Ivalon) and Gelfoam successfully controls bleeding in 75–95% of cases. Adjunctive coil embolization can also be considered in patients with intractable non-recurrent epistaxis, but not in those with expected recurrence such as patients with Osler-Weber Rendu. Bilateral embolization should be performed to prevent reconstitution of the distal internal maxillary branches from the opposite side (Fig. 5-27). Collateral supply to the posterior nasopharynx from sources such as the facial artery should be evaluated when internal maxillary artery embolization is insufficient. Epistaxis due to rupture of the ICA in the siphon is managed with proximal and distal balloon occlusion.

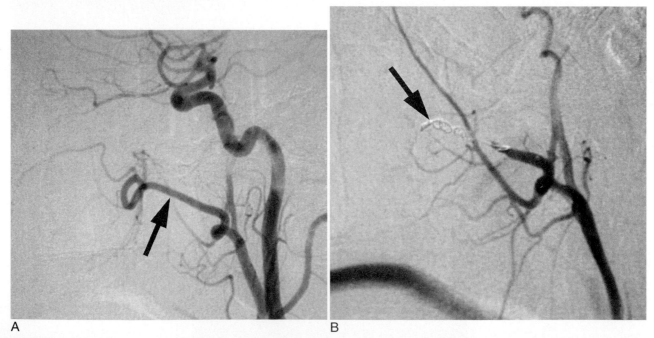

A   B

Figure 5-27   Embolization of the internal maxillary artery in a patient with epistaxis unresponsive to conservative treatment. **A**, Lateral DSA with injection into the CCA. The internal maxillary artery (arrow) is well visualized, but no extravasation is present. **B**, Selective ECA injection following embolization with Ivalon particles and microcoils (arrow). The contralateral internal maxillary artery was subsequently embolized with Ivalon particles until flow was sluggish (not shown).

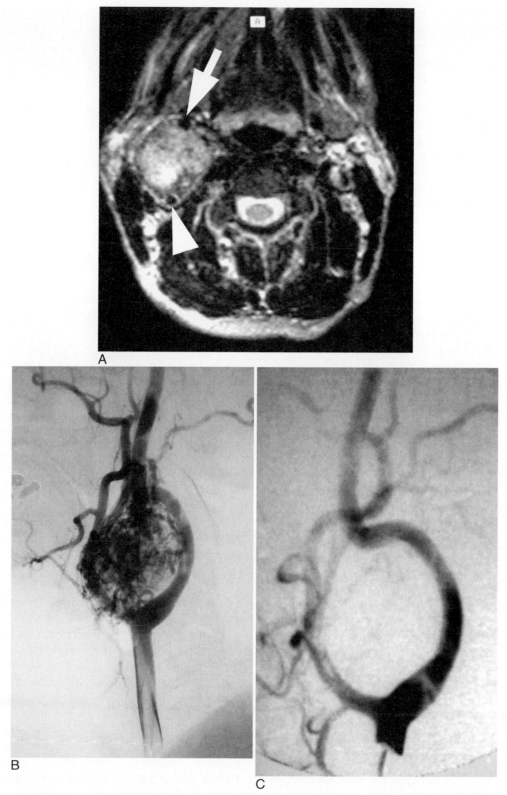

Figure 5-28 Carotid body tumor. **A,** T2-weighted MR image showing the tumor splaying the ICA (arrowhead) and ECA (arrow). **B,** Lateral CCA DSA showing a hypervascular mass splaying the ICA and ECA. **C,** Following embolization, the mass is devascularized. The patient then underwent uncomplicated surgical resection.

CAROTID BODY TUMORS

The carotid body comprises neural tissue located in the adventitia of the posterior medial CCA bifurcation. The carotid body is a chemoreceptor that is responsive to hypoxia, hypercapnia, and acidosis, producing an increased respiratory and heart rate, tidal volume, blood pressure, and circulating catecholamines.

Tumors of the carotid body are rare; 5% are bilateral (unless familial, in which bilateral lesions are found in one-third), about 5% are endocrinologically active, and up to 50% are malignant (although metastases are present in fewer than 5%). The typical presentation is a painless neck mass at the angle of the mandible. Carotid body tumors are highly vascular, receiving arterial blood supply from the ECA in the majority of cases. Splaying of the CCA bifurcation by a vascular mass is a characteristic finding on imaging studies (Fig. 5-28). Large lesions can encase the ICA and ECA.

The treatment of carotid body tumors is surgical excision because of the progressive growth and malignant potential of these masses. Preoperative embolization reduces blood loss. Selective catheterization of supplying arterial branches and embolization with small-diameter particles is performed shortly prior to surgery.

HEAD AND NECK MALIGNANCY

Primary tumors of the carotid arteries are exceedingly rare, but secondary involvement by head and neck tumors is a well-known phenomenon. Arterial encasement and invasion of the CCA, ICA, or ECA occurs in at least 5% of patients with squamous cell carcinomas. Rarely, stent placement is required to relieve symptomatic CCA or ICA compression by an unresectable tumor. Massive arterial bleeding may occur due to direct tumor invasion, infection, tumor necrosis, iatrogenic injury, or radiation necrosis. Endovascular treatment of bleeding with embolization (including carotid artery occlusion) or stent-graft may be temporarily life-saving (Fig. 5-29).

CATHETER-DIRECTED THROMBOLYTIC THERAPY FOR STROKE

Restoration of blood flow to ischemic brain tissue within 6 hours of onset of ischemia can limit permanent damage or even restore normal function in the majority of patients. Thrombolysis in the setting of acute anterior circulation (ICA territory) stroke makes sense even though most strokes in this area are due to emboli, as the embolus itself may be thrombotic in origin, or secondary thrombosis may widen the area of ischemia.

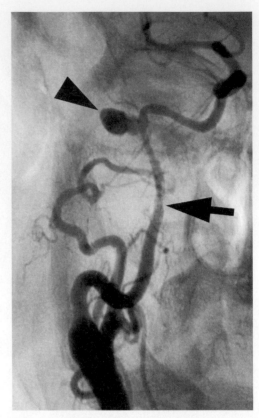

Figure 5-29   Massive intermittent posterior pharyngeal bleeding in a patient with inoperable squamous cell carcinoma who has been treated with radiation. Unsubtracted DSA in the anterior projection showing a diffusely narrowing cervical ICA (arrow) and a pseudoaneurysm (arrowhead). This was treated with balloon occlusion of the ICA proximal and distal to the lesion. Prior to balloon occlusion, an injection in the left CCA was performed while compressing the right CCA to confirm that the right anterior and middle cerebral arteries would fill from the left ICA. The patient tolerated the balloon occlusion without complication.

Posterior circulation (vertebral artery distribution) is more likely to be caused by local thrombosis due to an underlying stenosis, in which case thrombolysis is also potentially beneficial. Intravenous infusion of rt-PA in large randomized trials yielded improved outcomes compared to placebo in 30–40% of patients who were treated within 3 hours of onset of neurologic symptoms. Patients with uncontrolled hypertension, CT evidence of intracranial bleeding, or a completed stroke were excluded. Intracerebral hemorrhage was seen in 6% of patients. Catheter-directed thrombolysis with recombinant pro-urokinase (UK) was compared to heparin alone in the randomized Prolyse in Acute Cerebral Thromboembolism (PROACT II) study using similar entry criteria. Although the rate of intracranial hemorrhage was 10% in patients who underwent thrombolysis, significantly more had improved clinical outcomes compared to controls (40% versus 25%).

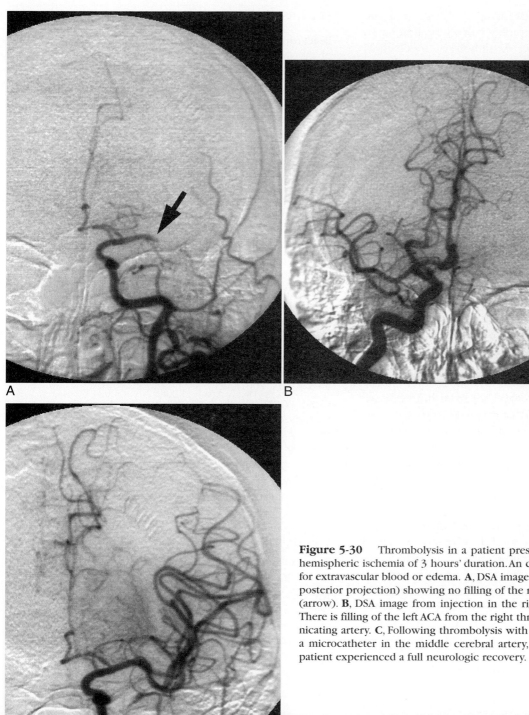

Figure 5-30   Thrombolysis in a patient presenting with acute onset of left hemispheric ischemia of 3 hours' duration. An emergent head CT was negative for extravascular blood or edema. **A**, DSA image from left ICA injection (anteroposterior projection) showing no filling of the middle cerebral artery branches (arrow). **B**, DSA image from injection in the right ICA shows normal vessels. There is filling of the left ACA from the right through a patent anterior communicating artery. **C**, Following thrombolysis with urokinase (700,000 U) through a microcatheter in the middle cerebral artery, the vessel in now patent. The patient experienced a full neurologic recovery.

Catheter-directed thrombolytic therapy in acute stroke is a promising but rapidly evolving technique. In addition to pharmacologic thrombolysis, mechanical thombectomy devices may also be beneficial. Patients considered for thrombolytic therapy should have onset of symptoms within 6 hours, be conscious, with no clinical or CT evidence of acute intracranial hemorrhage, mass lesion, or arteriovenous malformation. In addition, blood pressure should be <180 mmHg systolic and 100 mmHg diastolic, and there should be no evidence of an acute lacunar stroke or prior stroke within 6 weeks.

Thrombolysis is performed after a quick angiographic survey of the intracranial circulation to determine the status of the collateral supply and the extent of the obstruction (Fig. 5-30). The majority of emboli to the anterior circulation lodge in the middle cerebral artery (MCA). The risk of procedural bleeding increases with the duration of occlusion of the lenticulostriate arteries arising from the horizontal portion of the MCA (M1 segment). All glucose-containing fluids are banned from the procedure. The patient should be heparinized with a low systemic dose, such as a 2000-U bolus. Using a guiding catheter in the ICA, a coaxial superselective catheter is advanced into the thrombus. The dosage of thrombolytic agent is currently in flux, but most infusions are limited to 2 hours (Table 5-5). Combined intravenous and intraarterial administration of low doses of thrombolytic agents has been advocated.

Restoration of prograde flow is a hopeful angiographic sign, particularly in the lenticulostriate arteries. Repositioning of the microcatheter may be necessary during the procedure to thrombolyse small distal emboli that result from dissolution of the original obstruction. Thrombolysis should be stopped and heparin reversed immediately if an intracranial bleed is suspected. Following successful thrombolysis of an ICA territory thrombosis, heparin is stopped within 4 hours and the patient is usually managed with aspirin alone. The patient is carefully followed for clinical or imaging signs of stroke or bleed. In the posterior circulation, thrombolysis frequently reveals an underlying stenosis which may require angioplasty if flow remains marginal.

Table 5-5	Suggested Thrombolytic Dosages for Catheter-directed Stroke Therapy[a]	
Agent	**Dosage**	**Total Dose**
Urokinase	250,000 to 500,000 U/h	1,000,000 to 2,000,000 U
Pro-urokinase	4.5 mg/h	9 mg
rt-PA	2.5 mg/h	5 mg

[a] These dosages are in flux and should be used as a rough guide.

SUGGESTED READINGS

Begelman SM, Olin JW: Nonatherosclerotic arterial disease of the extracranial cerebrovasculature. *Semin Vasc Surg* 13: 153–164, 2000.

Executive Committee for the Asymptomatic Carotid Atherosclerosis (ACAS) Study: Endarterectomy for asymptomatic carotid artery stenosis. *JAMA* 273:1421–1428, 1995.

Foo TK, Ho VB, Choyke PL: Contrast-enhanced carotid MR angiography: imaging principles and physics. *Neuroimag Clin N Am* 9:263–284, 1999.

Frerichs K, Baker J, Norbash A: Intra-arterial stroke thrombolysis and carotid stenting: methods for the treatment of ischemic cerebrovascular disease. *Semin Roentgenol* 37:255–265, 2002.

Furie DM, Tien RD: Fibromuscular dysplasia of arteries of the head and neck: imaging findings. *Am J Roentgenol* 162: 1205–1209, 1995.

Furlan A, Higashida R, Wechsler L et al: Intra-arterial pro-urokinase for acute ischemic stroke. The PROACT II study: a randomized controlled trial. Prolyse in Acute Cerebral Thromboembolism. *JAMA* 282:2003–2011, 1999.

Goddard AJ, Mendelow AD, Birchall D: Computed tomography angiography in the investigation of carotid stenosis. *Clin Radiol* 56:523–534, 2001.

Grant EG, Duerinckx, AJ: Noninvasive diagnosis of carotid stenosis: technique, normal anatomy, and new observations in light of the NASCET study. *RSNA Categorical Course in Vascular Imaging* 211–221, 1998.

Hu WY, Ter Brugge KG: The role of angiography in the evaluation of vascular and neoplastic disease in the external carotid artery circulation. *Neuroimag Clin N Am* 6:625–644, 1996.

Kellogg JX, Nesbit GM, Clark WM et al: The role of angioplasty in the treatment of cerebrovascular disease. *Neurosurgery* 1998; 43:549–555.

Kendall JL, Anglin D, Demetriades D: Penetrating neck trauma. *Emerg Med Clin N Am* 16:85–105, 1998.

Kremer C, Mosso M, Georgiadis D et al: Carotid dissection with permanent and transient occlusion or severe stenosis: long-term outcome. *Neurology* 60:271–275, 2003.

North American Symptomatic Carotid Endarterectomy Trial (NASCET) Collaborators: Beneficial effect of carotid endarterectomy in symptomatic patients with high-grade carotid stenosis. *N Engl J Med* 325:445–453, 1991.

Moreau S, De Rugy MG, Babin E et al: Supraselective embolization in intractable epistaxis: review of 45 cases. *Laryngoscope* 108:887–888, 1998.

Morrissey DD, Andersen PE, Nesbit GM et al: Endovascular management of hemorrhage in patients with head and neck cancer. *Arch Otolaryngol Head Neck Surg* 123:15–19, 1997.

Muhm M, Polterauer P, Gstottner W et al: Diagnostic and therapeutic approaches to carotid body tumors: review of 24 patients. *Arch Surg* 132:279–284, 1997.

Mulloy JP, Flick PA, Gold RE: Blunt carotid injury: a review. *Radiology* 207:571–585, 1998.

Osborn AE: *Diagnostic Cerebral Angiography*, 2nd edn, Lippincott Williams & Wilkins, Philadelphia, 1999.

Phan T, Huston J, Bernstein MA et al: Contrast-enhanced magnetic resonance angiography of the cervical vessels: experience with 422 patients. *Stroke* 32:2282-2286, 2001.

Polak JF: Carotid ultrasound. *Radiol Clin N Am* 39:569-589, 2001.

Rao AB, Koeller KK, Adair CF, Armed Forces Institute of Pathology: Paragangliomas of the head and neck: radiologic-pathologic correlation. *Radiographics* 19:1605-1632, 1999.

Rothwell PM, Pendlebury ST, Wardlaw J et al: Critical appraisal of the design and reporting of studies of imaging and measurement of carotid stenosis. *Stroke* 31:1444-1450, 2000.

Schievink WI: Spontaneous dissection of the carotid and vertebral arteries. *N Engl J Med* 344:898-906, 2001.

Valavanis A, Christoforidis G: Applications of interventional neuroradiology in the head and neck. *Semin Roentgenol* 35: 72-83, 2000.

Wasserman BA: Clinical carotid atherosclerosis. *Neuroimag Clin N Am* 12:403-419, 2002.

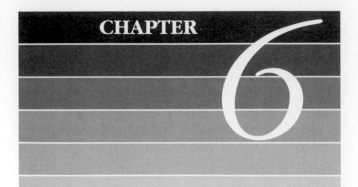

CHAPTER 6

Upper-extremity Arteries

JOHN A. KAUFMAN, M.D.

Arterial disease is diagnosed less commonly in the upper extremity than in the lower extremity, and much less often than venous diseases of the upper extremity. Unusual pathologies such as vasculitis, entrapment syndromes, and trauma make up a higher proportion of cases of symptomatic arterial disease in the upper extremities than in the lower extremity. This variety keeps upper-extremity arterial diagnosis and intervention very interesting.

NORMAL AND VARIANT ANATOMY

The arterial blood supply of the upper extremities originates with the subclavian arteries. The right subclavian artery arises from the brachiocephalic artery, whereas the left subclavian artery is a branch directly from the aorta (see Fig. 5-1). The subclavian arteries are defined as the segment of vessel between the aortic arch or brachiocephalic artery bifurcation and the lateral border of the 1st rib. The subclavian artery exits the thoracic cavity between the anterior and middle scalene muscles, and then passes between the clavicle and 1st rib (Fig. 6-1). The typical diameter of the subclavian artery is 8–10 mm. The subclavian arteries provide blood to the upper chest, the arms, and the central nervous system (through the vertebral artery).

The internal mammary arteries are constant vessels that arise from the anterior inferior aspect of the subclavian arteries just opposite or slightly distal to the vertebral arteries. These vessels course anteriorly and medially along the inner surface of the chest wall. The internal mammary arteries are important potential sources of collateral blood supply in cases of thoracic or abdominal aortic obstruction (via the anterior anastomoses with the intercostal arteries in the former, and the inferior epigastric arteries in the latter). The internal mammary arteries can provide collateral supply to bronchial arteries as well.

The other named branches of the subclavian arteries are highly variable in origin, but relatively constant in presence. The thyrocervical trunk frequently arises just distal to the internal mammary arteries from the superior surface of the subclavian artery. This vessel is subject to enormous variability, but is often the origin of the inferior thyroidal, superficial cervical, and suprascapular arteries. Only slightly more than 50% of individuals have this classic anatomy. Independent origins of one or more of these vessels from the subclavian artery are common. The next major branch of the subclavian artery is the costocervical trunk, which gives rise to the ascending cervical, supreme intercostals, and occasionally the anterior spinal arteries (Fig. 6-2). The supreme intercostal artery contributes to the blood supply of the 1st through 3rd ribs. This anatomy is found in approximately 80% of individuals, with the most common variants being independent origins of the two branches.

The axillary artery begins at the lateral margin of the 1st rib, extending to the lateral margin of the teres minor muscle where it becomes the brachial artery. Thus, a portion of the axillary artery is located quite medial to the axilla. The branches of the axillary artery are highly variable in origin. These are the superior thoracic artery (to the anterior portions of the first through third

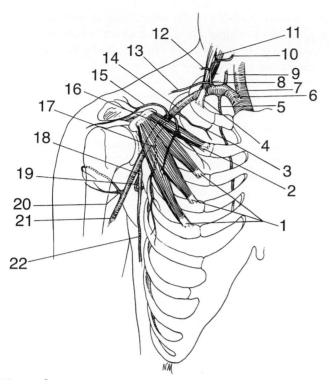

Figure 6-1 Line drawing of subclavian and axillary artery anatomy. The clavicle is not shown. **1**, Pectoralis minor muscle. **2**, Pectoral branch of the thoracoacromial artery. **3**, Superior thoracic artery. **4**, Anterior scalene muscle. **5**, Internal mammary artery. **6**, Subclavian artery. **7**, Right common carotid artery. **8**, Thyrocervical trunk. **9**, Vertebral artery. **10**, Inferior thyroid artery. **11**, Ascending cervical artery. **12**, Superficial cervical artery. **13**, Suprascapular artery. **14**, Axillary artery. **15**, Acromial branch of the thoracoacromial artery. **16**, Thoracoacromial artery. **17**, Lateral thoracic artery. **18**, Subscapular artery. **19**, Circumflex scapular artery. **20**, Circumflex humeral artery. **21**, Brachial artery. **22**, Thoracodorsal artery. (Reproduced with permission from Kadir S: *Atlas of Normal and Variant Anatomy*, WB Saunders, Philadelphia, 1991.)

intercostal spaces); the lateral thoracic artery (to the lateral chest, with a prominent mammary branch in women); the thoracoacromial artery (with branches to the clavicle, the acromion, and deltoid); the subscapular artery, which gives rise to the thoracodorsal artery (supplying the musculature along the lateral margin of the scapula); and the scapular circumflex artery (supplying the muscles of the back deep to the scapula). The last branch of the axillary artery is the circumflex humeral artery, which supplies the humeral head and the surrounding soft tissues. All of the axillary and subclavian artery branches (exclusive of the vertebral artery) have potential anastomoses with each other that become evident in the presence of occlusive disease or vascular tumors. Of great importance are the close proximity of the radial, ulnar, and median nerves to the axillary artery. Contained in a sheath of connective tissue along with the artery, these neural structures are at risk for compression by hematoma after axillary artery punctures.

Lateral to the teres major muscle the axillary artery becomes the brachial artery which continues to the forearm (Fig. 6-3). Variants of the brachial artery itself are uncommon, but include a small accessory branch to the radial artery (persistent superficial brachial artery, 1–2%) and duplication (0.1%). The profunda brachialis artery is usually the first major branch of this vessel, traveling with the ulnar artery in a posterolateral course around the humerus. This vessel supplies the muscular structures of

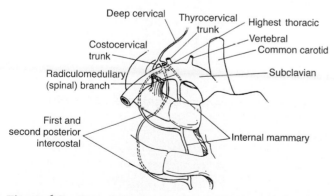

Figure 6-2 Line drawing of costocervical trunk anatomy. (Reproduced with permission from Kadir S: *Atlas of Normal and Variant Anatomy*, WB Saunders, Philadelphia, 1991.)

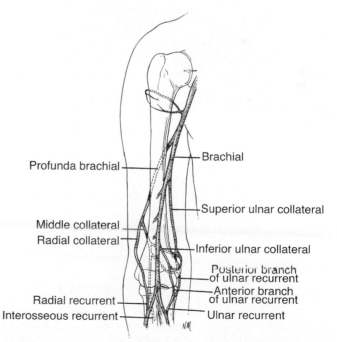

Figure 6-3 Line drawing of normal brachial artery anatomy. (Reproduced with permission from Kadir S: *Atlas of Normal and Variant Anatomy*, WB Saunders, Philadelphia, 1991.)

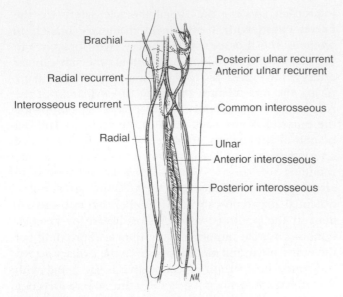

Figure 6-4 Line drawing of normal forearm arterial anatomy. (Reproduced with permission from Kadir S: *Atlas of Normal and Variant Anatomy*, WB Saunders, Philadelphia, 1991.)

the posterior aspect of the upper arm, as well as providing collateral supply around the elbow. There are many unnamed muscular branches of this artery, but those that anastomose to muscular branches distal to the elbow joint are termed collateral vessels. These variable vessels are named after the forearm vessel to which they collateralize (e.g., ulnar collateral artery).

The terminal branches of the brachial artery are the radial, ulnar, and interosseous arteries (Fig. 6-4). Anomalous high origins of the radial or ulnar artery from the brachial or axillary arteries are present in 15% and 3% of patients, respectively. These variants are potential sources of confusion during upper-extremity angiography if the catheter is unknowingly placed distal to an anomalously high origin (Fig. 6-5). The forearm arteries supply the adjacent muscles, while the radial and ulnar arteries continue into the hand. The interosseous artery frequently divides into an anterior and posterior branch. In most cases the radial and ulnar arteries both supply the hand, although one vessel may dominate. In fewer than 2% of individuals the interosseous artery may continue into the hand as the median artery (Fig. 6-6).

The classical arterial anatomy of the hand includes two complete palmar arcades, each of which receives

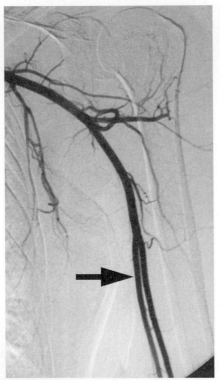

Figure 6-5 Proximal origin of the radial artery. Digital subtraction angiogram (DSA) of the left upper arm with injection in the subclavian artery showing a large branch (arrow) arising from the proximal brachial artery and continuing towards the hand. This proved to be the radial artery on distal images.

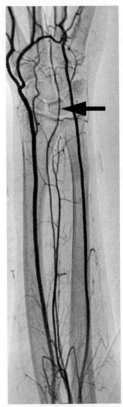

Figure 6-6 Median artery. DSA of the forearm with the hand in the anatomic position. The interosseous artery continues across the wrist as the median artery (arrow).

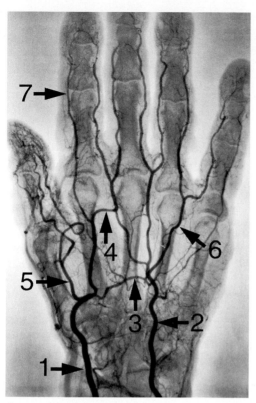

Figure 6-7   Subtracted angiogram of the hand in a 54-year-old male smoker. There are distal occlusions of the proper palmar digital arteries, and the palmar metacarpal arteries are not visualized. **1**, Radial artery. **2**, Ulnar artery. **3**, Deep palmar arch. **4**, Superficial palmar arch. **5**, Princeps pollicis artery. **6**, Common palmar digital artery. **7**, Proper palmar digital artery.

contributions from both the radial and ulnar arteries (Fig. 6-7). The more proximal arcade is the deep palmar arch, primarily supplied by the radial artery. The more distal arcade is the superficial palmar arch, supplied primarily by the ulnar artery. Variations upon this anatomy are so numerous and common that both "classical"

Table 6-1 Variant Arterial Anatomy of the Hand	
Variant	**Approximate Incidence**
Incomplete superficial arch	55%
Ulnar artery supplies entire incomplete superficial arch	13%
Superficial arch from median and ulnar arteries	4%
Superficial arch from radial, median, and ulnar arteries	1%
Independent radial, median, and ulnar arteries (no arch)	1%
Incomplete deep arch	5%

arcades described above are present in fewer than 50% of patients (Table 6-1). Rather than try to memorize all of these variants, just remember that they are the rule, rather than the exception.

The blood supply to the fingers is derived from the paired palmar metacarpal and common palmar digital arteries that originate from the deep and superficial palmar arches, respectively. These arteries join at the interdigital webspace to form the paired proper palmar digital arteries of the fingers. The radial artery is usually the dominant blood supply to the thumb and the second digit, while the ulnar artery supplies the fourth and fifth digits. The third digit may be supplied by either artery. The dominant blood supply to the fingers varies with the arch anatomy.

KEY COLLATERAL PATHWAYS

The potential collateral blood supply in the presence of subclavian artery origin stenosis or occlusion are numerous, including all of the branches of the subclavian and axillary artery. One pattern, subclavian steal, describes retrograde flow in the ipsilateral vertebral artery (Figs 6-8 and 5-11). Subclavian steal is associated with arm pain or central neurologic symptoms in a third of patients. Symptoms may be exacerbated with use of the arm (Box 6-1). Bilateral subclavian steal is uncommon.

Steal physiology can affect other vessels in the upper extremity. Proximal occlusion of the brachiocephalic artery origin can result in retrograde flow down the right common carotid artery as well as the right vertebral artery. Reversal of flow can occur in smaller subclavian artery branches such as the thyrocervical trunk and the internal mammary artery. In patients with cardiac bypass surgery based upon an internal mammary artery, proximal subclavian stenosis can cause a steal phenomenon involving the internal mammary artery that results in angina (Fig. 6-9).

Axillary artery occlusion is usually well compensated by the rich potential collateral pathways around the

Box 6-1   Symptoms of Subclavian Steal
Vertebrobasilar insufficiency
Dizziness
Drop attack
Ataxia
Vertigo
Syncope
Exercise-induced upper-extremity ischemia
Hemispheric transient ischemic attack

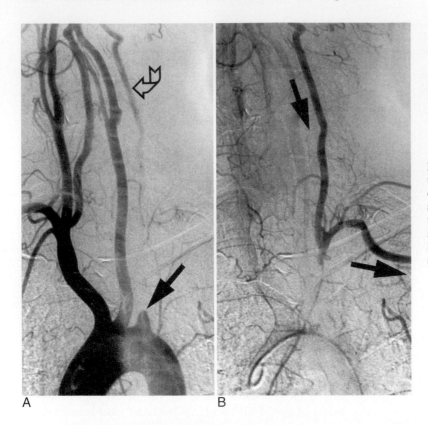

A   B

Figure 6-8   Subclavian steal. **A**, DSA of the arch in the left anterior oblique (LAO) projection. There is occlusion of the left subclavian artery origin (straight arrow). Faint retrograde opacification of the left vertebral artery is present (curved arrow). **B**, Later image from the same injection showing retrograde flow in the left vertebral artery reconstituting the left subclavian artery. Arrows indicate direction of blood flow.

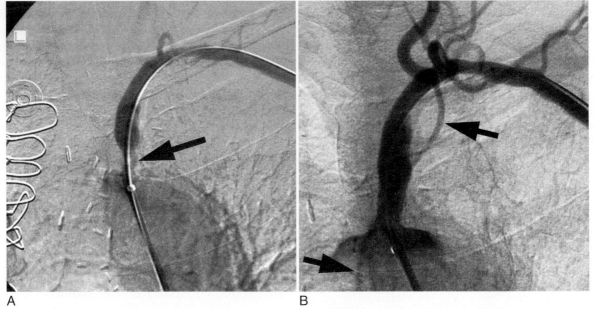

A   B

Figure 6-9   Symptomatic left internal mammary artery (LIMA) steal in a patient who developed recurrent angina several years following coronary artery revascularization with the LIMA. A coronary angiogram showed retrograde flow in a patent LIMA away from the heart. **A**, Selective left subclavian artery DSA shows absent filling of both the LIMA and the vertebral artery. The origin of the subclavian artery is stenotic (arrow). **B**, Following stent placement in the subclavian artery origin there is antegrade flow in the LIMA (arrows) as well as the vertebral artery. The patient's angina resolved.

scapula and humerus. Frequently, the subscapular artery assumes a dominant role in reconstituting the distal axillary artery. In addition, the intercostal arteries can provide collateral blood supply to the upper extremity through anastomoses with the vessels of the chest wall such as the lateral thoracic artery. Occlusion of the distal brachial artery results in collateral supply from the profunda brachialis artery high in the arm and around the elbow through the radial and ulnar collateral arteries to radial and ulnar recurrent arteries.

Occlusion of either the radial or ulnar artery is well tolerated by the fingers provided that one or both arches are intact. When the deep and superficial arches are incomplete or absent, acute occlusion of a forearm artery may result in severe digital ischemia. Over time, collateral supply can develop from the opposite forearm vessel or the interosseous artery.

IMAGING

Ultrasound (US) examination of the upper-extremity arteries distal to the clavicle is relatively straightforward. Standard Duplex color-flow ultrasound techniques can be used for the peripheral vessels (a high-resistance Doppler waveform is normal). A complete examination is time-consuming, especially in the forearm and hand where there are many vessels. Nevertheless, the superficial location of these vessels facilitates visualization with US. Medial to the clavicle the vessels dive deep into the mediastinum, beyond the reach of surface probes. To fully evaluate the subclavian artery origins and brachiocephalic artery, a transesophageal probe is needed. However, even with this technique the origins of the arteries may not be completely visualized.

CT angiography (CTA) of the upper-extremity vessels is an excellent modality for evaluation of the axillosubclavian arteries, especially within the mediastinum. CTA requires the patient to breath-hold, with a short delay after injection of contrast. As a general rule, a noncontrast scan should be obtained prior to contrast injection. Thick collimation, such as 7–10 mm, is appropriate for the noncontrast scan. Thinner effective collimation, such as 1–3 mm, should be used for the contrast scan. The area of coverage should include the proximal neck to the hand for complete upper-extremity studies. A very important technical consideration is the route of administration of contrast. Contrast injected into an upper-extremity vein remains extremely dense on CT before it reaches the central circulation. This causes streak artifacts that degrade image quality, particularly across the great vessel origins. The arm opposite to the side of interest should therefore be used for contrast administration. The vessels can be evaluated using simple postprocessing techniques such as reformatting (Fig. 6-10).

The upper-extremity arteries are well suited for evaluation with MR angiographic techniques. Gadolinium-enhanced 3-dimensional (3-D) acquisitions provide excellent images of the arch and proximal portions of the upper-extremity arteries (Fig. 6-11). Acquisitions oriented in the coronal plane can include both the arch and the upper-extremity vessels to the shoulder. An important pitfall is signal loss due to susceptibility artifact from adjacent veins caused by undiluted gadolinium injected in an upper-extremity vein (see Fig. 3-17). As with CTA of the upper extremities, contrast should be injected into the extremity opposite to the side of clinical interest. Imaging of the arteries of the arm and hand can be accomplished with either contrast-enhanced 3-D or non-contrast 2-dimensional time-of-flight (2-D TOF) acquisitions. Small coils can be used to maximize image detail (Fig. 6-12).

Angiographic studies of the upper-extremity arteries are preceded by a bilateral pulse examination, and bilateral

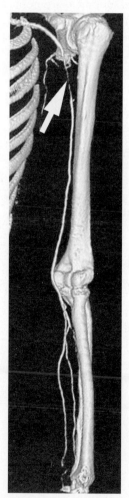

Figure 6-10   Volume rendering of a CT angiogram (CTA) of the left upper extremity of a woman with a diagnosis of giant-cell arteritis. There is narrowing of the proximal brachial artery (arrow).

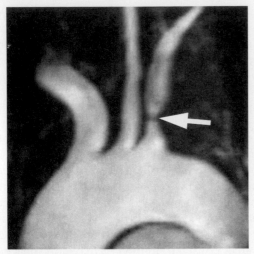

Figure 6-11 Gadolinium-enhanced 3-D MRA viewed in the LAO projection showing a focal proximal left subclavian artery stenosis (arrow). (Courtesy of Barry Stein M.D., Hartford Hospital, Hartford, CT.)

brachial blood pressure measurements (even if it is a unilateral problem). The axillary, brachial, radial, and ulnar pulses should be documented. A subclavian artery aneurysm may be palpable as a pulsatile mass in the supraclavicular fossa, although a tortuous but normal-caliber artery may feel similar.

The complete angiographic study of the upper extremity involves visualization from the aortic arch to the tips of the fingers. Anything less risks missing pathology. Exceptions to this rule should be made only after careful analysis of the clinical scenario and the patient. For each injection it is essential to ensure that there is satisfactory overlap of coverage with the preceding injection so that the extremity is imaged in its entirety.

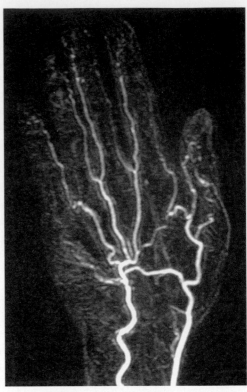

Figure 6-12 MIP image of a normal 3-D gadolinium-enhanced MRA of the hand. The image spatial resolution is not sufficient for evaluation of the digital arteries.

An arch aortogram in the left anterior oblique (LAO) projection will profile the origins of the great vessels (see Fig. 6-8). To open the brachiocephalic artery bifurcation, filming in the right anterior oblique (RAO) projection is necessary (see Fig. 5-1). The pigtail catheter should be positioned in the ascending aorta just proximal to the

Table 6-2	Upper-extremity Angiography			
Vessel	**Catheter**	**Position**	**Projection**[a]	**Injection**[b]
Great vessel origins	Pigtail	Ascending aorta	LAO	20/30
Right subclavian origin	Pigtail	Ascending aorta	RAO	20/30
	H-1, Davis[c]	Brachiocephalic	RAO	5-8/12-16
Subclavian	H-1, Davis	Proximal subclavian	AP	6-8/12-16
	Simmons-1 or -2			
Axillary	H-1, Davis	Distal subclavian	AP	5-8/10-16
Brachial	H-1, Davis	Distal subclavian	AP	5-8/10-16
Forearm	H-1, Davis	Mid-brachial	AP, hand in anatomic position	5-8/10-16
Hand	H-1, Davis	Mid-brachial	AP, hand in anatomic position[d]	5-6/20-30

[a] Projection = filming obliquity.

[b] Injection = rate per second/total volume.

[c] H-1 = Headhunter 1; Davis = Davis A1.

[d] Flow augmentation with: warming of hand with heat lamp or by holding hot pack during examination; inject vasodilator (priscoline, 25 mg in 10-mL table flush) immediately before contrast; reactive hyperemia (2-3 minutes).

LAO, left anterior oblique; RAO, right anterior oblique, AP, anteroposterior projection.

brachiocephalic artery origin. Specific injection and exposure rates are provided in Table 6-2. When upper-extremity arterial embolus is suspected clinically, the catheter should be positioned just above the aortic valve so that the entire ascending aorta can be inspected. To select the subclavian arteries, the pigtail catheter is exchanged for a 5-French 100-cm length catheter with a gentle angle at the tip, such as Davis or H-1 (see Fig. 2-10). Arteries that arise from the arch at an acute angle can be selected with a Simmons-2 (right subclavian) or Simmons-1 (left subclavian). With the tube angled to show the arch in an LAO projection, the catheter is positioned in the aorta proximal to the great vessel origins. The catheter is then turned so that the tip points towards the head and slowly withdrawn until it pops up into a great vessel origin. Leading with 1 cm of soft guidewire (such as a Bentson) minimizes the risk of vessel trauma. In older patients there is frequently enough calcification at the ostia of the great vessels to provide a fluoroscopic landmark. A gentle test of contrast (*no air bubbles!*) can be used to identify the vessel. The subclavian artery can be selected using almost any atraumatic guidewire, but the two most commonly used are a 3-J long taper or an angled hydrophilic guidewire. If the guidewire passes into the neck towards the head, it may be in a vertebral artery or, on the right, in the common carotid artery. When selecting the right subclavian artery, remember that the origin is usually *posterior* to the right common carotid artery (see Fig. 5-1).

The subclavian and axillary arteries can usually be included on one image with the catheter tip positioned just beyond the origin of the vertebral artery. Nonionic contrast should be used to minimize patient discomfort during the examination. An angled hydrophilic guidewire is very useful to advance the catheter. The brachial artery should be imaged with the catheter in the proximal axillary artery in order to avoid causing spasm or missing a high origin of an ulnar or radial artery. Once these anomalies have been excluded, the catheter can be positioned in the mid-portion of the brachial artery for angiography of the forearm or hand. The hand should be in anatomic position (palm up and hand flat on the table) for forearm angiography (see Fig. 6-6). Otherwise it can be extremely difficult to identify vessels in the forearm or hand. Selective angiography of the forearm arteries requires the use of small atraumatic catheters as these vessels are very subject to spasm when manipulated.

The hand can be maintained in anatomic position (palm up) or placed completely flat with the fingers spread slightly for the hand angiogram (see Fig. 6-7). Since the digital arteries are small and numerous, magnification views and vasodilation are frequently necessary to obtain the best images. Vasodilation of the arteries of the hand can be induced by wrapping the hand in warm towels or having the patient hold a warm pack during the initial parts of the examination. Another effective method is reactive hyperemia with a blood pressure cuff on the upper arm. Intraarterial injection of a vasodilating agent (such as tolazoline 25 mg) through the catheter just before injection of contrast can also be used, but it seems to be less effective than the other techniques described. There are few radiographic images more distinctive and beautiful than high-quality magnification arteriograms of the human hand.

VASOSPASTIC DISORDERS

Raynaud's syndrome is the most common cause of symptomatic upper-extremity ischemia (see Box 1-5). More common in cold climates, the classic presentation is onset of a white digit or digits in response to cold exposure, followed by transition to blue, then red. The duration of the attack may be up to 1 hour, but patients with Raynaud syndrome usually have a normal baseline physical examination. Though rarely performed, angiography demonstrates reversible vasospasm (induced by cold and ameliorated by heat or vasodilators) (see Fig. 1-30). Patients with associated connective tissue disorders, atherosclerosis, and history of repetitive trauma may have underlying fixed small vessel arterial obstruction.

CHRONIC OCCLUSIVE DISEASE

Symptomatic chronic ischemia of the upper extremities can be divided into small (hand) or large (wrist to arch) vessel etiologies (Boxes 6-2 and 6-3). Atherosclerotic occlusive disease of the upper extremities represents approximately 5% of all cases of clinically evident limb ischemia. The muscle mass of the upper body is smaller than in the lower limbs, and is used less vigorously (perhaps if we walked on all fours symptomatic upper-extremity arterial disease would be more common). In addition, the collateral pathways are numerous and well developed at

---

Box 6-2 Upper-extremity Occlusive Disease: Small Vessel

Raynaud syndrome/disease
Atherosclerosis
Connective tissue disease
Vibration injury
Buerger's disease
Hypercoagulable syndrome
Frostbite
Chronic renal failure
Diabetes

Box 6-3 Chronic Upper-extremity Occlusive Disease: Large Vessel

Atherosclerosis
Trauma
Recurrent embolization
Thoracic outlet syndrome
Vasculitis
    Giant-cell arteritis
    Takayasu's arteritis
    Radiation arteritis
    Buerger's disease
Fibromuscular dysplasia

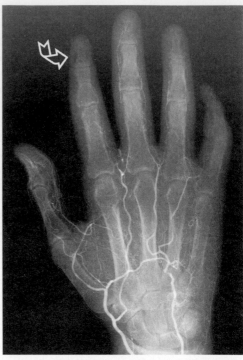

Figure 6-13 Severe atherosclerotic occlusive disease of the arteries of the hand and digits in a patient with chronic renal failure, tobacco abuse, and ulceration of the tip of the second finger (arrow).

multiple levels. The most frequent etiology of chronic large vessel upper-extremity occlusive disease is atherosclerosis. The risk factors for atherosclerotic disease of the upper-extremity arteries are the same as everywhere else in the body. Patients are usually older, with other manifestations of atherosclerosis. True arm claudication, rest pain, or tissue loss are rare. When rest pain and ulceration occurs, it is usually in the fingers.

On physical examination, diminished pulses or a lower blood pressure in an arm may indicate the presence of proximal occlusive disease. The Allen test (compression of both the radial and ulnar artery to prevent blood flow to the hand followed by sequential release of the arteries and inspection of pattern of reperfusion) is a simple measure that gauges the relative contribution of the radial and ulnar arteries to the hand.

Atherosclerotic occlusive disease can occur anywhere in the upper-extremity arteries, but is most often manifested clinically when it is located at the subclavian artery origins (see Figs 6-8 and 6-9). The left subclavian artery is affected more often than the brachiocephalic artery or the right subclavian artery. Obstruction at the ostia of the left subclavian artery is the result of aortic plaque, a characteristic that has an impact on the types and outcomes of interventions. Ostial stenosis of the right subclavian artery may also involve the right common carotid artery origin. Subclavian artery occlusive disease proximal to the vertebral artery frequently results in subclavian steal physiology (see Key Collateral Pathways above, and Fig. 6-8).

Atherosclerotic digital arterial occlusive disease is more prevalent than it is symptomatic. Abnormal digital arteries are often found in smokers, patients with renal failure, diabetics, and individuals who perform heavy manual work (Fig. 6-13). Symptoms may be precipitated be creation of a proximal surgical dialysis access which effectively "steals" arterial blood from the hand, or after placement of a radial arterial catheter in an intensive care unit in a patient with an occluded ulnar artery.

The subclavian artery origins are difficult to visualize with ultrasound, but abnormal pulsatility and flow velocities can infer a proximal lesion. The vertebral arteries are easily interrogated, as are the extremity arteries distal to the clavicle. Detailed evaluation of the small vessels of the hand is possible but tedious.

CTA and contrast-enhanced MRA are excellent modalities for evaluation of the occlusive disease of the subclavian artery origins (see Fig. 6-11). MRA seems better suited than CTA for evaluation distal to the axillary artery. Retrograde flow in the vertebral artery due to a proximal subclavian stenosis will be indistinguishable from antegrade flow on CTA and contrast-enhanced MRA. Noncontrast 2-D TOF or phase contrast (PC) images of the vertebral artery can provide accurate information about directional flow. Neither CTA nor MRA are currently suitable for routine vascular imaging of the hand owing to limited resolution and the small size of the vessels.

Conventional angiography remains the definitive imaging modality for evaluation of symptomatic chronic upper-extremity ischemia. Injections in the aortic arch should always precede selective angiography. Magnification angiography is usually necessary to adequately evaluate the hand vessels.

Direct surgical access to subclavian artery origin stenoses through a thoracotomy is needed for transaortic

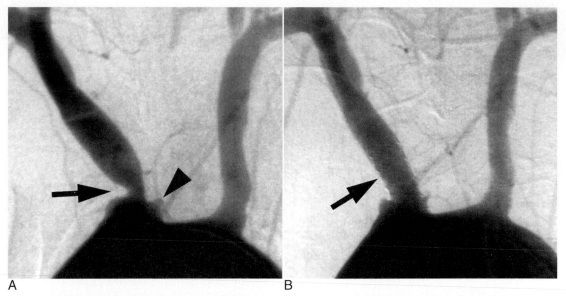

Figure 6-14   Innominate artery stenosis treated with stent placement in a 47-year-old male smoker. **A**, DSA of the arch in the LAO projection shows a focal stenosis of the innominate artery origin (arrow) and occlusion of the left common carotid artery origin (arrowhead). **B**, DSA in the same projection following placement of a balloon expandable stent (arrow) dilated to 9 mm in the innominate artery.

endarterectomy or bypass with a graft from the ascending aorta. However, bypass from a more accessible inflow source, such as the ipsilateral common carotid artery, is usually performed unless the arch disease involves multiple great vessel origins. Inflow for bypass can also be from the contralateral common carotid or axillary arteries. In extreme situations, a common femoral to axillary artery bypass can be constructed. Thoracic sympathectomy may delay or prevent amputation in patients with intractable digital ischemia due to fixed occlusive disease.

The most frequent percutaneous intervention in chronic upper-extremity arterial occlusive disease is angioplasty and/or stent placement in the subclavian and innominate artery origins (Figs 6-9 and 6-14). This procedure can be performed from either a femoral or brachial artery access. The relationship of the stenosis to the origin of cerebral branches and the status of the other cerebral arteries are key considerations when planning the procedure. Occlusion of a vertebral artery origin by a dissection flap during subclavian artery angioplasty, though rare, could result in a stroke in a patient with poor intracranial collateral circulation. Common balloon sizes range from 6 to 10 mm in diameter in the subclavian and innominate arteries. Balloon expandable stent placement is frequently necessary when the lesion involves the ostium of the artery. Careful stent positioning is required when the stenosis involves the right subclavian artery origin, in order to avoid compression of the orifice of the right common carotid artery. Self-expanding stents can be used in more peripheral locations. However,

stents should be avoided in the segment of the subclavian artery between the clavicle and the 1st rib, as they can be crushed by the bony structures. The technical success rate of subclavian and innominate artery angioplasty and stent placement is greater than 90%, with a complication rate (stroke and distal embolization) of less than 1%. There is relatively little information on the long-term patency of these procedures, but reported results are excellent.

ACUTE UPPER-EXTREMITY ISCHEMIA

Acute upper-extremity ischemia usually presents with digital and hand symptoms. Mild ischemia may result in simply a cold hand with delayed capillary refill, whereas severe ischemia produces a cadaveric extremity. The pulse examination is dependent upon the level of occlusion; severe digital ischemia with normal pulses at the wrist is not uncommon. Always examine both upper extremities. When a patient presents with digital ischemia, the location of the pathology may be suggested by the distribution of affected fingers.

The patient history is helpful in suggesting a cause of the ischemia and directing subsequent imaging. The most common cause of acute upper-extremity ischemia is an embolus of cardiac origin (Boxes 6-4 and 6-5). Current or recurrent atrial arrhythmia is suggestive of a cardiac source in a patient presenting with acute arm ischemia. Recurrent emboli limited to one arm indicate a

---

Box 6-4 Causes of Acute Upper-extremity Ischemia

Embolus
Trauma
Brachial, radial artery catheterization
Hypercoagulable syndrome
Aortic dissection
"Steal" after creation of dialysis graft/fistula
Vasospasm
Compartment syndrome

Table 6-3 Location of Upper-extremity Emboli

Location	Incidence
Brachial artery	60%
Axillary artery	23%
Subclavian artery	12%
Forearm and digital arteries	5%

---

source localized to that extremity, such as an aneurysm or a stenosis (see Thoracic Outlet Syndrome below). Other etiologies include trauma, aortic dissection, thrombosis of an existing lesion, and *in situ* thrombosis due to a hypercoagulable syndrome. Acute ischemia localized to the digits is more common in smokers, diabetics, and patients with chronic renal failure or malignancy.

Patients on hemodialysis can develop acute hand ischemia following surgical creation of a proximal dialysis access. These patients frequently have preexisting occlusive disease of the forearm and digital arteries. When an arteriovenous communication is created from the radial or brachial artery, reversal of flow in the palmar arches with "stealing" of blood from the digits can occur.

Physical examination and history alone may be enough to allow a management decision such as urgent surgical exploration of the brachial artery (Table 6-3). The most expeditious imaging of acute upper-extremity ischemia is with angiography, as everything between the aortic valve and the finger tips can be visualized (Fig. 6-15). Noninvasive imaging modalities do not yet provide sufficient anatomic coverage and resolution of detail.

Box 6-5 Sources of Upper-extremity Emboli

Heart
   Left ventricle
   Left atrium
   Aortic valve
Upper-extremity artery aneurysm (subclavian, axillary, ulnar)
Atherosclerotic plaque
Ascending aortic aneurysm
Subclavian and axillary artery fibromuscular dysplasia
Iatrogenic
   Dialysis access declotting
   Cardiac surgery
Paradoxical

Magnification views of the fingers may be essential to distinguish between embolic occlusion (intraluminal filing defects) and other causes. The subclavian artery should be carefully inspected for the presence of a subtle aneurysm or an ulcerated plaque. The finding of small emboli in proximal branch vessels supports the diagnosis of embolus. Though rare, aneurysms can occur at any point beyond the subclavian artery. The findings of a focal aneurysm or occlusion of the ulnar artery in the base of the hand is suggestive of hypothenar hammer syndrome (see Trauma below). When hand ischemia occurs in the presence of a dialysis graft or fistula, injections with temporary occlusion of the venous outflow (usually by manual compression) are necessary to assess the hand arteries (see Fig. 7-30).

Patients with critically ischemic extremities should undergo surgical thromboembolectomy. The latter can be very difficult when the small vessels of the hand are involved. Proximal surgical thromboembolectomy has been combined with local, distal intraoperative thrombolysis in these cases.

Intervention in acute upper-extremity ischemia is less commonly performed than in the lower extremities, perhaps because the problem is less prevalent and the usual etiology is a brachial embolus of cardiac origin. The extremity must be viable in order to consider percutaneous intervention. Thrombolysis may be helpful when extensive thrombus is present, particularly in the small vessels of the hand. Catheter-directed thrombolysis can be performed from either the femoral artery or an antegrade brachial artery approach, depending upon the location and extent of the thrombus (Fig. 6-16). Thrombolysis of proximal subclavian artery thrombus risks vertebral artery embolization and stroke. When the hand and digital arteries are involved, a microcatheter may be required to deliver the thrombolytic agent into the radial or ulnar artery. Excellent results are frequently obtained with the catheter positioned in the distal brachial artery to perfuse the entire forearm and hand. When a femoral artery approach is used, anticoagulation with heparin is important to prevent pericatheter thrombus formation in the subclavian artery and subsequent embolization up the vertebral artery. There is limited

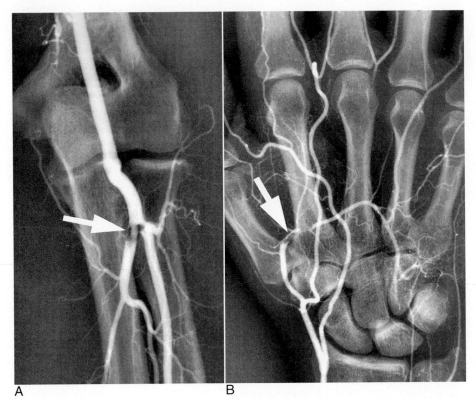

A   B

Figure 6-15   Patient with atrial fibrillation who presented with acute hand ischemia. The pulse examination was normal to the antecubital fossa, where the brachial pulse seemed more prominent than usual ("water hammer" pulse). Distal pulses were absent. **A,** Brachial artery angiogram showing an embolus (arrow) lodged at the bifurcation of the brachial artery. There is diminished filling of the ulnar artery. **B,** Detailed view of the angiogram of the hand showing a fragment of embolus in the deep arch (arrow). The ulnar artery and superficial arch are not opacified.

published experience with upper-extremity thrombolysis, but the results are promising with few complications in properly selected patients. Mechanical thrombectomy devices may have a role in this anatomic bed.

When the source of distal embolization is a focal atherosclerotic lesion in the subclavian or axillary artery, this may be treated with dilation and stent placement (Fig. 6-17). Acute hand ischemia following placement of a surgical dialysis access can be managed by reversal of the access. Occasionally, coil occlusion of the radial artery distal to the arterial anastomosis of a Brescia–Cimino fistula is required to prevent steal from the fingers through the palmar arches.

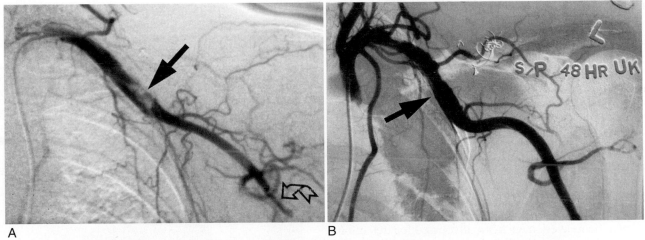

A   B

Figure 6-16   Acute left upper-extremity ischemia in a patient with a chronic nonunion of a displaced clavicular fracture and multiple failed attempts at operative reduction. **A,** Selective DSA of the left subclavian artery showing thrombus in the axillary artery (straight arrow) and proximal brachial artery (curved arrow). The distal arteries reconstituted and were patent. **B,** Subtracted angiogram following a 48-h urokinase infusion into the axillary and brachial arteries from a femoral approach showing a subclavian and proximal axillary artery aneurysm (arrow). The aneurysm is most likely due to chronic impingement related to the clavicle fracture. The brachial artery is now patent.

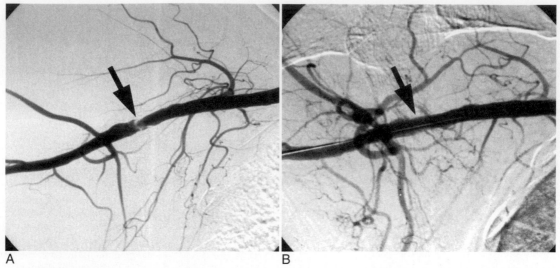

Figure 6-17   Ulcerated plaque in the axillary artery causing acute and chronic digital artery atheroembolization in a 58-year-old female vasculopath presenting with finger gangrene, ulcerations, and superimposed acute digital ischemia. The brachial pulse was diminished. **A**, Irregular, web-like stenosis of the axillary artery (arrow). The arterial inflow was normal. **B**, The stenosis was treated with primary stent placement (arrow) using a self-expanding nitinol stent (8 mm × 20 mm), followed by angioplasty to 7 mm. A self-expanding stent was used because of the peripheral location of the lesion. The patient had immediate relief of her hand pain with improved perfusion. She was subsequently managed with chronic anticoagulation with healing of her digital ulcerations.

THORACIC OUTLET SYNDROME

Symptomatic extrinsic compression of the neurovascular structures of the upper extremity as they exit the bony thorax is termed "thoracic outlet syndrome." Neurologic symptoms are by far the most common manifestation, accounting for 90% of cases. Neurogenic thoracic outlet syndrome is most often found in women (female/male ratio 4:1) between the ages of 20 and 50. Symptomatic arterial thoracic outlet syndrome is unusual, comprising roughly 1% of cases. The usual patient with arterial thoracic outlet syndrome is a young, athletic male. Patients may present with hand numbness, tingling, or coolness with activities that require arm abduction, and diminished extremity pulses. Acute embolic events to the forearm and hand occur in up to 40% of patients, and may be the initial presenting symptom. Combined neurologic and vascular symptoms may be present.

The physical examination is usually unremarkable, but a pulsatile mass may be present in the supraclavicular fossa with diminished distal pulses (Fig. 6-18). Several evocative maneuvers have been advocated for detection of arterial thoracic outlet syndrome, such as Adson's (caudal traction on the arm, the head turned towards the arm, and inspiration) and 90-degree abduction and external rotation. However, compression of the subclavian artery resulting in diminished distal pulses is very common (at least 50%) in normal patients.

There are three locations in which thoracic outlet syndrome can occur: in the scalene triangle; the costoclavicular space; and the subpectoral space. The most common site of arterial compression is the scalene triangle, followed by the costoclavicular space. Compression of arterial structures in the subpectoral space is extremely rare. Arterial compression may be due to hypertrophy of normal structures, or anomalous muscular, ligamentous, or bony structures. Repetitive crushing of the artery with arm motion results in development of a focal narrowing

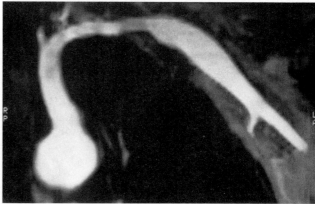

Figure 6-18   Coronal reformat of a 3-D gadolinium-enhanced MRA showing an aneurysm of the distal subclavian and axillary arteries in a female who presented with a cervical rib and pulsatile supraclavicular mass. The distal pulses were normal. The aneurysm and rib were resected without additional imaging.

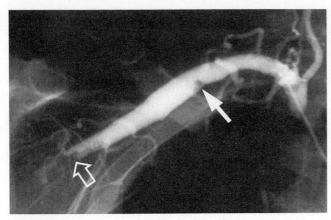

Figure 6-19 Chronic right-hand ischemia in a 45-year-old right-handed painter treated initially for carpal tunnel syndrome. The patient had a right cervical rib. Right subclavian artery angiogram shows mural thrombus (arrow) in a subclavian–axillary artery aneurysm, and embolic occlusion of the brachial artery (open arrow). This constellation of findings is diagnostic of arterial thoracic outlet syndrome.

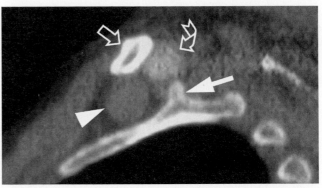

Figure 6-20 Right-handed male tennis player with a pulsatile mass in the supraclavicular fossa. Sagittal reformation of a CTA shows an exostosis arising from the 1st rib (arrow), the subclavian artery aneurysm (curved arrow), the subclavian vein (arrowhead), and the clavicle (open arrow). The aneurysm was caused by chronic compression of the artery against the clavicle by the exostosis.

and post-stenotic dilatation. Thrombus may form in these dilated or aneurysmal segments, with subsequent distal embolization (Figs 6-19 and 1-39).

Imaging of thoracic outlet syndrome must include both the inside and the outside of the arteries. The structures around the subclavian artery are imaged in order to determine the cause of the compression. The arterial lumen is imaged in order to confirm the compression and diagnose a complication of the syndrome such as distal embolization. Imaging should begin with a simple chest radiograph, which may reveal a cervical rib or other bony anomaly. Cross-sectional imaging of the upper thorax with CT/CTA or MR/MRA is useful for evaluating both the artery and the surrounding soft tissues (see Fig. 6-18). Careful postprocessing of the CTA or MRA may be needed to identify the cause of the aneurysm (Fig. 6-20). The goals of angiography in these patients are to evaluate the subclavian artery for stenosis, aneurysmal change, and the presence of thrombus, and to detect distal emboli. A complete angiographic examination from the aortic arch to the hand is necessary. The subclavian aneurysms can be quite subtle, so comparison with the opposite side is very useful. Injections with the arm in neutral position, and one with the arm in a position that elicits symptoms, have been considered essential in the past. As noted above, evocative maneuvers can induce arterial compression in half of normal patients (Fig. 6-21). In positive cases both subclavian arteries should be studied.

Definitive therapy requires surgical decompression of the thoracic outlet, resection of the aneurysm, and placement of a bypass graft. Patients that present with distal emboli may first undergo thrombolysis. Exclusion

of the aneurysm can also be accomplished with a stent-graft, but prior decompression of the extrinsic structures is necessary.

ANEURYSMS

Upper-extremity artery aneurysms are unusual, representing fewer than 2% of all peripheral aneurysms. There are numerous etiologies of upper-extremity aneurysms, several of which are discussed in other sections of this chapter (Box 6-6). Degenerative aneurysms are uncommon, but usually involve the proximal or intrathoracic portion of the subclavian artery. These aneurysms are associated with atherosclerosis and aortic, contralateral subclavian, or visceral artery aneurysms in up to 50% of patients. Elderly males are most often affected. Aneurysms of the extrathoracic subclavian and proximal axillary artery are typically due to thoracic outlet syndrome, and more distal aneurysms are often traumatic in origin. A detailed history and careful imaging are essential to determine the nature of the aneurysm.

Central (intrathoracic) aneurysms can present with pain, compression of adjacent structures such as veins and nerves (including hoarseness when the right recurrent laryngeal nerve is involved), distal thromboembolism, and rupture. Extrathoracic subclavian and more distal aneurysms present with distal embolization and thrombosis.

Aberrant right subclavian arteries (arising as the last branch of the arch) occur in 1% of individuals. The origin of this artery is frequently patulous, termed a diverticulum of Kommerell. Aneurysmal dilatation (diameter larger than 2 cm) is common. In 80% of patients the aberrant subclavian artery lies posterior to the esophagus, in 15%

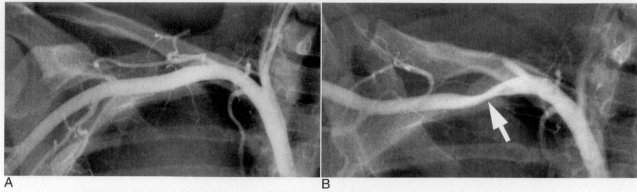

Figure 6-21 Evocative maneuvers in a patient with suspected arterial thoracic outlet syndrome. **A,** The subclavian artery appears normal in neutral position. **B,** With the arm abducted 90 degrees, there is compression of the subclavian artery (arrow). Care in interpretation of this result in the absence of a subclavian artery aneurysm is necessary as this same finding can be induced in asymptomatic individuals.

between the esophagus and trachea, and anterior to both in 5%. Aneurysms of this artery can compress and obstruct the esophagus resulting in difficulty swallowing (dysphagia lusoria). These aneurysms appear to be at high risk of rupture, and are usually surgically resected when diagnosed (Fig. 6-22). Though extremely rare, the same pathology can be found in an aberrant left subclavian artery in patients with right-sided aortic arches.

Imaging with US, CTA, and MRA is frequently sufficient to detect an upper-extremity aneurysm and differentiate it from a tortuous but otherwise normal artery. CTA and MRA can often provide definitive evaluation of aneurysms of the intrathoracic subclavian artery. Etiologies of intrathoracic subclavian aneurysms other than degeneration should be carefully excluded, particularly trauma and chronic dissection. Angiography may not be necessary

unless the relationship of the aneurysm to cerebral artery origins or the aorta cannot be determined.

Therapy of upper-extremity aneurysms is determined by the etiology, size, and location. The majority of aneurysms are treated surgically with excision and bypass, although stent-grafts may have a role in the future.

VASCULITIS

The arteries of the upper extremity can be affected by any of the arteritides (Box 6-7). The typical patient is younger than would be expected for atherosclerotic disease, and usually has constitutional symptoms such as arthralgias, myaglias, or skin rashes. Patients may present with intermittent or fixed ischemic symptoms, ranging from diminished upper-extremity pulses to digital ulceration. A frequent association is Raynaud syndrome.

Imaging of vasculitides that have a more central distribution, such as Takayasu's, can be initiated with cross-sectional techniques such as CT or MR. Wall thickening that enhances with contrast, central stenoses, and central aneurysms suggest a vasculitis. When there is digital involvement, angiography is necessary to differentiate between embolic, atherosclerotic, and inflammatory diseases.

The location of the vascular abnormality is somewhat helpful in classifying the vasculitis, although rules in this situation are destined to be broken. Proximal stenoses and occlusions (brachiocephalic and subclavian arteries) strongly suggests Takayasu's disease (see Fig. 1-13). Subclavian, axillary, and proximal brachial artery occlusions suggest giant-cell arteritis (see Figs 6-10 and 1-15). These occlusions are usually well collateralized, with preservation of the distal runoff to the forearm and hand. The patient history is equally important in determining

---

Box 6-6 Etiologies of Upper-extremity Aneurysms

True

Thoracic outlet syndrome
Chronic dissection (originating in aorta)
Degenerative
Marfan syndrome
Vasculitis

False

Trauma
Infection
Ehlers–Danlos syndrome
Behçet's disease

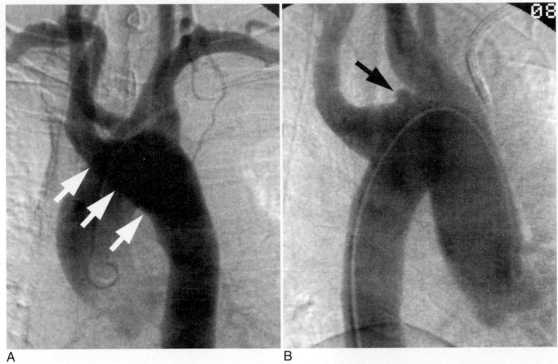

A   B

Figure 6-22   Ruptured aneurysm of aberrant right subclavian artery in a 49-year-old hypertensive female presenting with acute chest pain and transient hypotension. **A**, DSA of the aorta in the anterior–posterior projection shows the origin of the aberrant right subclavian artery (arrows) projected posterior to the arch. **B**, DSA of the aorta in the RAO projection showing the aneurysmal origin of the aberrant right subclavian artery and a contained rupture (arrow). (Case courtesy of Drs. John Thomas, San Antonio, and Charles Trinh, Houston, TX.)

Box 6-7   Vasculitides Affecting the Upper Extremities

Digital

Systemic lupus erythematosus
Scleroderma
Rheumatoid
Buerger's disease
Polyarteritis nodosa

Forearm

Buerger's disease

Axillary artery

Giant cell
Systemic lupus erythematosus (rare)

Subclavian artery

Takayasu's arteritis
Behçet's disease

---

the etiology of the lesion. For example, radiation treatments that included the extremity in the therapy portal may result in radiation vasculitis.

Buerger's disease (thrombangiitis obliterans) affects the upper extremities in over two-thirds of patients with this disorder. Occlusion of named arteries and hypertrophy of small perineural vessels and vasa vasorum are characteristic (Fig. 6-23). In addition to tobacco abuse, frequent use of marijuana also appears to be a risk factor.

The angiographic appearance of systemic lupus erythematosus (SLE), scleroderma, rheumatoid arthritis, and many other connective tissue disorders is similar (see Fig. 1-19). In general there are multiple occlusions of the medium to small arteries of hand, particularly in the digits, with poor collateralization. The occlusions are usually tapered, although there may be intimal irregularity and abrupt changes in caliber of the patent vessels. The absence of intraluminal filling defects is a key diagnostic feature. The arteries of the upper arm and forearm are usually spared, although axillary occlusion has been reported in SLE. The presence of multiple small aneurysms is typical of polyarteritis nodosa (PAN), but atypical with other vasculitides.

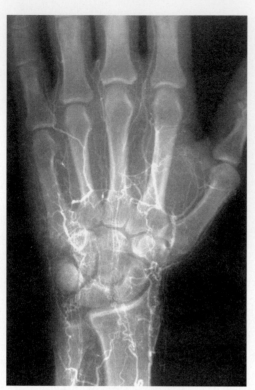

Figure 6-23   Upper-extremity Buerger's disease in a 33-year-old male heavy smoker (not just tobacco). Angiogram of the hand shows widespread arterial occlusions with numerous corkscrew collaterals.

TRAUMA

The upper limb is involved in approximately 40% of all cases of penetrating trauma to the extremities. The likelihood that there is an arterial injury that requires intervention is 40–50% when hard clinical findings are present (Box 6-8). Angiography is the optimal imaging modality, as it can be both diagnostic and therapeutic. The diagnostic angiographic examination in trauma patients is focused on the injured limb segment. The full range of vascular injuries may be found, including spasm, intimal tear, pseudoaneurysm, extravasation, occlusion, and arteriovenous fistula (Fig. 6-24). Branch vessel pseudoaneurysms and arteriovenous fistulas can be easily treated by transcatheter embolization. Similar injuries to the subclavian and axillary arteries can be effectively stabilized with stent-grafts.

In the absence of hard clinical signs a major vascular injury is unlikely, and patients are managed conservatively with observation and clinical follow-up. Vascular ultrasound has been used to confirm absence of vascular injury when clinical suspicion is low, but is probably unnecessary. Shotgun wounds are an exception, as the

---

Box 6-8   Clinical Signs of Vascular Injury

Hard

Active arterial hemorrhage
Thrill or bruit
Expanding hematoma
Extremity ischemia
Pulse deficit

Soft

Adjacent fracture
Adjacent nerve injury
Stable hematoma
Delayed or decreased capillary refill
History of hypotension or bleeding
Extensive soft tissue injury

---

large area of soft tissue trauma and the multiple pellets makes physical examination difficult and less reliable. These patients undergo angiography despite the absence of hard clinical signs. Penetrating injury to the chest in the vicinity of the intrathoracic portions of subclavian artery is also considered differently, as physical examination of these vessels is impossible, and surgical repair requires a thoracotomy. Angiography is warranted if vascular injury is suspected, even in the absence of objective evidence of vascular injury.

Stretch as a mechanism of injury is somewhat unique to the upper extremities, particularly the axillosubclavian arteries (Fig. 6-25). This occurs when there is sudden

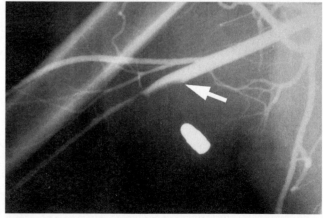

Figure 6-24   Angiogram showing intimal irregularity and narrowing (arrow) of the brachial artery in a patient with diminished distal pulses following a gunshot wound in the vicinity of the brachial artery. These findings are consistent with intimal tear, spasm, and superimposed formation of thrombus. This injury requires surgical repair.

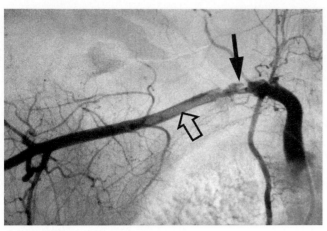

Figure 6-25   Subtracted angiogram showing intimal irregularity (arrow) and intraluminal thrombosis (open arrow) of the subclavian and axillary arteries in a patient who had diminished right upper-extremity pulses and a brachial plexus injury after falling from a tree. The patient tried to grab a branch half way down.

extreme traction on the arm, such as when trying to stop a fall from a tree by grabbing a branch, or dislocation. The artery is stretched along its long axis, resulting in intimal tears and disruption of the media. Small branch arteries may be sheared away. Secondary thrombosis with distal embolization may complicate the injury. Concomitant neurologic injury occurs in over 40% owing to avulsion of the brachial plexus nerve roots. The combination of neurologic and vascular injury can be devastating, with poor long-term functional results. Chronic forceful stretching, such as in baseball pitchers, may result in localized arterial dissection or thrombosis.

Iatrogenic injuries to the upper-extremity arteries occur most often during central venous access procedures or placement of an arterial line for hemodynamic monitoring. When central lines are placed using blind bedside techniques, the incidence of inadvertent arterial puncture may be as high as 2%. The arteries most commonly injured are the subclavian and carotid, although other branch vessels such as the internal mammary artery and thyrocervical trunk can be involved. In the majority of instances the arterial puncture is of no consequence. Arterial dissection can result from attempts to cannulate the artery with a guidewire or large central venous access device. Pseudoaneurysms and arteriovenous fistulas are more likely to occur in patients with coagulation disorders. Sudden widening of the mediastinum or hemo-pneumothorax after placement of a central line should suggest an unrecognized arterial injury. Further evaluation may be attempted with US (if the suspected location of the injury is peripheral), or contrast-enhanced CT. Angiography is both definitive and possibly therapeutic. Keep in mind that during bedside attempts to place central venous catheters nobody *really* knows how deep or far the needle went.

The brachial artery can be injured by blunt trauma to the inside of the upper arm such as might occur with chronic improper use of crutches. Aneurysmal degeneration of the artery leads to thrombus formation with local occlusion or distal embolization. Stretch injury, thrombosis, and transection can occur in association with dislocations and fractures. Extravasation from disrupted branch arteries can be managed with embolization in the majority of instances (Fig. 6-26).

Chronic trauma to the base of the hand, such as occurs when the "butt" of the hand is used as a hammer, can result in intimal injury and aneurysm formation in the ulnar artery as it cross the base of the metacarpals (Fig. 6-27). An underlying intrinsic abnormality of the ulnar artery, such as fibromuscular dysplasia, has been proposed as a contributing factor. Symptoms occur when the aneurysms or intimal irregularities become a source of digital emboli, characteristically to the third through fifth fingers. This complex is termed "hypothenar hammer syndrome." Angiography remains the best imaging modality for this entity, although US may be used to determine the size of the aneurysm. Digital artery emboli with an ulnar artery aneurysm or focal ulnar occlusion at the hypothenar eminence are diagnostic findings.

Self-administered drugs injected directly into an upper-extremity artery can result in pseudoaneurysms, arteriovenous fistulas, dissections, and thrombosis. Acute hand and digital ischemia may complicate the local arterial injury. Mycotic pseudoaneurysms are prevalent in this patient population.

FIBROMUSCULAR DYSPLASIA

Fibromuscular dysplasia (FMD) may affect any medium-sized artery in the body. As a group, the subclavian, axillary, and brachial arteries are the fifth most common location for this process (Fig. 6-28). Ulnar and radial artery involvement has also been reported. Patients may be asymptomatic, or present with distal embolization. The diagnosis is usually not suspected prior to imaging, but angiography is required for confirmation. Both upper extremities should be studied, as FMD is frequently bilateral. Angioplasty of symptomatic lesions is safe and effective.

PRIMARY HYPERPARATHYROIDISM

Hyperparathyroidism can be divided into three forms. Primary hyperparathyroidism is due to independent secretion of parathyroid hormone (PTH) by an adenoma in the gland (Box 6-9). Secondary hyperparathyroidism is

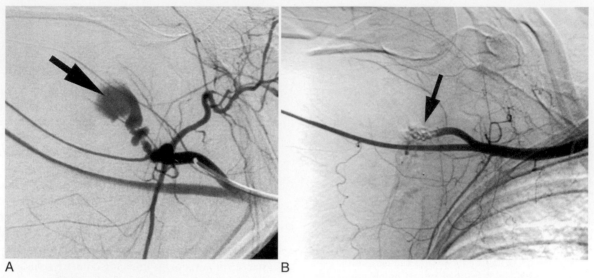

A   B

Figure 6-26   Alcoholic female who stumbled over her cat, resulting in a right humeral fracture. Patient presented to the emergency room 6 hours after the fall when she noted swelling of her upper arm and hand weakness. Distal pulses were diminished. **A**, Selective DSA of the subscapular artery showing extravasation (arrow) of contrast directly from the subscapular artery. The distal arterial runoff was intact. **B**, Completion DSA after successful coil embolization (arrow) of the subscapular artery. The patient required surgical evacuation of the hematoma to relieve nerve compression.

due to stimulation of PTH by hypocalcemia. The tertiary form is due to autonomous hypersecretion of PTH due to chronic hypocalcemia or chronic renal failure. Vascular imaging and intervention has a role in the diagnosis and treatment of primary hyperparathyroidism.

There are normally four parathyroid glands, each residing posterior to the poles of the thyroid. Ectopic parathyroid glands can occur in the neck and mediastinum. The blood supply to normally situated glands is from the inferior and superior thyroidal arteries. Rarely, a small branch may arise directly from the aortic arch (thyroid ima).

Imaging of patients with suspected primary hyperparathyroidism is usually with neck US, CT, MRI, and

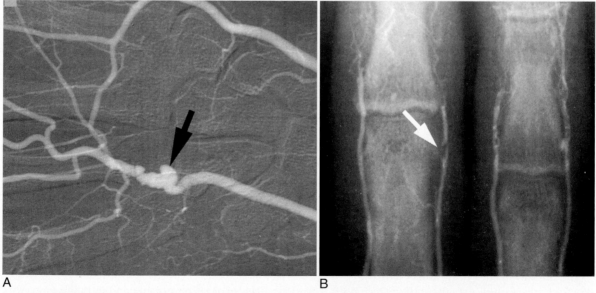

A   B

Figure 6-27   Hand angiogram in a 37-year-old male mechanic presenting with recurrent episodes of digital ischemia. **A**, There is irregularity and enlargement of the ulnar artery (arrow) in the region of the hamate bone. **B**, Magnified view of one of the digital arteries showing an intraluminal filling defect characteristic of an embolus (arrow) and multiple distal occlusions.

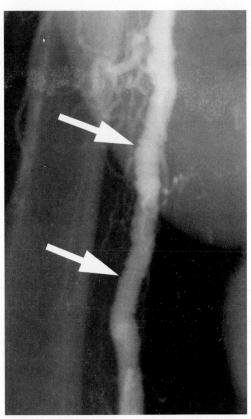

Figure 6-28   Angiogram of the right brachial artery showing the characteristic beaded appearance of medial fibroplasia (arrows).

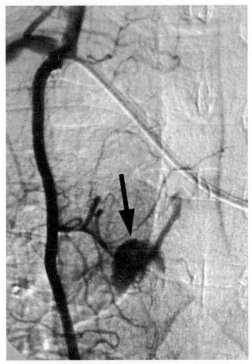

Figure 6-29   Selective DSA of the right internal mammary artery in a patient with persistent hyperparathyroidism after neck exploration. There is a densely staining, well-circumscribed right paratracheal mass (arrow). This proved to be an adenoma in an ectopic parathyroid gland.

technetium-99^m sestamibi scans. Angiography or venous sampling is not indicated in patients when first diagnosed with primary hyperparathyroidism. Neck exploration, inspection of all four parathyroid glands, and resection of the abnormal gland is curative in 90–95%. Those that continue to manifest primary hyperparathyroidism should undergo angiography followed by venous sampling (discussed in Chapter 7).

Selective injection of the thyrocervical trunk, the internal mammary arteries, and external carotid or superior thyroidal arteries should be performed (Fig. 6-29). Parathyroid adenomas appear as densely staining masses on angiography. Angiographic localization is successful in 60-70%. An aortic arch injection in the LAO projection is necessary to identify a thyroid ima artery.

Wedged injection of hypertonic contrast or absolute alcohol into a parathyroid adenoma results in cure in 60-70% of patients, but most reoccur within 5 years. This can be a valuable therapy in those rare patients who have failed repeated surgical exploration.

Box 6-9   Primary Hyperparathyroidism

Incidence 4–6 per 100,000
Female:male ratio 3:2
Fifth and sixth decades
Single adenomas in 80%
Multiple adenomas in 15%
Ectopic adenomas 1%
Parathyroid carcinoma 1%
Usually sporadic, but associated with multiple
  endocrine neoplasia syndromes

SUGGESTED READINGS

Angle JF, Matsumoto AH, McGraw JK et al: Percutaneous angioplasty and stenting of left subclavian artery stenosis in patients with left internal mammary-coronary bypass grafts: clinical experience and long-term follow-up. *Vasc Endovasc Surg* 37: 89–97, 2003.

Aqel MB, Olin JW: Thromboangiitis obliterans (Buerger's disease). *Vasc Med* 2:61–66, 1997.

Davidian M, Kee ST, Kato N et al: Aneurysm of an aberrant right subclavian artery: treatment with PTFE-covered stentgraft. *J Vasc Surg* 28:335–339, 1998.

Disdier P, Granel B, Serratrice J et al: Cannabis arteritis revisited: ten new case reports. *Angiology* 52:1–5, 2001.

Doherty GM, Doppman JL, Miller DL et al: Results of a multidisciplinary strategy for management of mediastinal parathyroid adenoma as a cause of persistent primary hyperparathyroidism. *Ann Surg* 215:101–106, 1992.

Dorman RL, Kaufman JA, La Muraglia GM: Digital emboli from brachial artery fibromuscular dysplasia. *Cardiovasc Intervent Radiol* 17:95–98, 1994.

Durham JR, Yao JS, Pearce WH et al: Arterial injuries in the thoracic outlet syndrome. *J Vasc Surg* 21:57–69, 1995.

Edwards JM, Porter JM: Upper extremity arterial disease: etiologic considerations and differential diagnosis. *Semin Vasc Surg* 11:60–66, 1998.

Ferris BL, Taylor LM, Oyama K et al: Hypothenar hammer syndrome: proposed etiology. *J Vasc Surg* 31:104–113, 2000.

Gaines PA, Swarbrick MJ, Lopez AJ et al: The endovascular management of blue finger syndrome. *Eur J Vasc Endovasc Surg* 17:106–110, 1999.

Hallisey MJ, Rees JH, Meranze SG et al: Use of angioplasty in the prevention and treatment of coronary–subclavian steal syndrome. *J Vasc Interv Radiol* 6:125–129, 1995.

Hood DB, Kuehne J, Yellin AE et al: Vascular complications of thoracic outlet syndrome. *Am Surg* 63:913–917, 1997.

Jaeger HJ, Mathias KD, Kempkes U: Bilateral subclavian steal syndrome: treatment with percutaneous transluminal angioplasty and stent placement. *Cardiovasc Interv Radiol* 17: 328–332, 1994.

Johnson SP, Durham JD, Subber SW et al: Acute arterial occlusions of the small vessels of the hand and forearm: treatment with regional urokinase therapy. *J Vasc Interv Radiol* 10:869–876, 1999.

Joseph S, Mandalam KR, Rao VR et al: Percutaneous transluminal angioplasty of the subclavian artery in nonspecific aortoarteritis: results of long-term follow-up. *J Vasc Interv Radiol* 5:573–580, 1994.

Kadir S: Arteriography of the upper extremities. In Kadir S: *Diagnostic Angiography*, WB Saunders, Philadelphia, 1986.

Katras T, Baltazar U, Rush DS et al: Subclavian arterial injury associated with blunt trauma. *Vasc Surg* 35:43–50, 2001.

Kieffer E, Bahnini A, Koskas F: Aberrant subclavian artery: surgical treatment in thirty-three adult patients. *J Vasc Surg* 19: 100–109, 1994.

Krinsky G, Rofsky NM: MR angiography of the aortic arch vessels and upper extremities. *Magn Reson Imaging Clin N Am* 6: 269–292, 1998.

Landry GJ, Edwards JM, McLafferty RB et al: Long-term outcome of Raynaud's syndrome in a prospectively analyzed patient cohort. *J Vasc Surg* 23:76–85, 1996.

Nehler MR, Taylor LM, Moneta GM et al: Upper extremity ischemia from subclavian artery aneurysm caused by bony abnormalities of the thoracic outlet. *Arch Surg* 132:527–532, 1997.

Nomura M, Kida S, Yamashima T et al: Percutaneous transluminal angioplasty and stent placement for subclavian and brachiocephalic artery stenosis in aortitis syndrome. *Cardiovasc Interv Radiol* 22:427–432, 1999.

Owens LV, Tinsley EA, Criado E et al: Extrathoracic reconstruction of arterial occlusive disease involving the supraaortic trunks. *J Vasc Surg* 22:217–221, 1995.

Pillai L, Luchette FA, Romano KS et al: Upper-extremity arterial injury. *Am Surg* 63:224–227, 1997.

Roddy SP, Darling RC, Chang BB et al: Brachial artery reconstruction for occlusive disease: a 12-year experience. *J Vasc Surg* 33:802–805, 2001.

Rose SC: Noninvasive vascular laboratory for evaluation of peripheral arterial occlusive disease: III. Clinical applications: nonatherosclerotic lower extremity arterial conditions and upper extremity arterial disease. *J Vasc Interv Radiol* 12:11–18, 2001.

Rose SC, Kadir S: Arterial anatomy of the upper extremities. In Kadir S ed: *Atlas of Normal and Variant Anatomy*, WB Saunders, Philadelphia, 1991.

Sueoka BL: Percutaneous transluminal stent placement to treat subclavian steal syndrome. *J Vasc Interv Radiol* 7:351–356, 1996.

Ulfacker R: Arteries of the upper extremities. In Ulfacker R: *Atlas of Vascular Anatomy: an Angiographic Approach*, Williams & Wilkins, Baltimore, 1997.

Yao JS: Upper extremity ischemia in athletes. *Semin Vasc Surg* 11:96–105, 1998.

CHAPTER 7

Upper-extremity, Neck, and Central Thoracic Veins

JOHN A. KAUFMAN, M.D.

The veins of the neck, arms, and chest are visited frequently by interventional radiologists. Placement of long-term central venous access catheters is a common yet essential procedure. The upper-extremity veins are of critical importance for dialysis patients, whether they are managed with venous catheters or surgically created access. Upper-extremity and central venous occlusion are recognized as clinically important entities, and effective strategies for recanalization now exist. Procedures involving the veins of the upper body comprise a large portion of many interventional practices.

ANATOMY

Veins of the Neck

The internal jugular veins (IJV) are the largest veins of the head and neck. These valveless veins begin at the sigmoid fossa of the skull and anastomose with the subclavian veins at the base of the neck, behind the proximal head of the clavicle. There is frequently a valve in the IJV at this junction. Within the middle and lower neck the IJV lies within the carotid sheath anterior and slightly lateral to the carotid artery and beneath the sternocleidomastoid muscle (see Fig. 2-39). The right IJV is commonly larger than the other IJV, or "dominant." Important tributaries of the IJVs include the inferior petrosal sinuses (venous blood from the pituitary) at the jugular foramen, and the superior and middle thyroidal veins in the neck (Fig. 7-1). The inferior thyroidal vein is usually a single structure that drains vertically into the left brachiocephalic vein.

The external jugular veins (EJVs) are much smaller in size than their internal counterparts (see Fig. 7-1). The EJVs drain soft tissue structures of the face and scalp. Superficial in location, these veins are frequently visible as they pass over the upper sternocleidomastoid muscle and travel in an oblique course towards the supraclavicular fossa. The EJVs enter the subclavian veins just lateral to the IJVs. Additional drainage of the head and neck is provided by the vertebral veins, which also drain into the subclavian veins.

Key Collateral Pathways

The major draining veins of the neck are the IJVs. There are numerous potential collateral drainage pathways via the external jugular, vertebral, and muscular veins of the neck. In general, obstruction of the internal

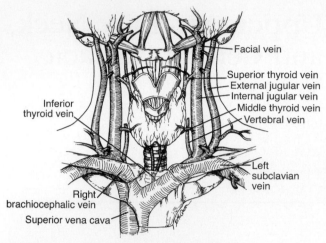

Figure 7-1 Drawing of the venous anatomy of the neck. (Reproduced with permission from Lundell C, Kadir S: Superior vena cava and thoracic veins. In Kadir S ed: *Atlas of Normal and Angiographic Anatomy,* WB Saunders, Philadelphia, 1991.)

jugular veins is well tolerated provided that the central thoracic veins are intact.

Veins of the Upper Extremities

The veins of the upper extremities are divided into superficial and deep systems. From the hand to the shoulder, the superficial veins are the major drainage pathway. At the shoulder the deep veins become the primary drainage route. This is different from the anatomy of the lower extremities, where the deep veins are dominant throughout.

The superficial veins of the forearm are the cephalic along the anterior radial edge, the basilic along the posterior ulnar edge, and the median along the anterior aspect in the midline (Fig. 7-2). At the antecubital fossa just below the elbow joint the cephalic vein sends a branch, the median cubital vein, obliquely across to join

the basilic vein, which swings anteriorly in the upper third of the forearm to meet this branch. The median vein of the forearm drains into the median cubital vein.

In the upper arm the cephalic vein lies in the groove between the biceps and brachialis muscles. At the shoulder the cephalic vein passes between the pectoralis and deltoid muscles, then dives over the medial edge of the pectoralis minor muscle to join the deeper axillary vein. There are no critical arterial or neural structures near the cephalic vein. The basilic vein ascends along the medial border of the biceps muscle, superficial to the brachial fascia, accompanied by only a few small superficial nerves. The brachial artery, veins, and associated major nerves lurk below the brachial fascia. At the junction of the distal and middle thirds of the upper arm the basilic vein pierces the brachial fascia to join the deep (brachial) veins. The basilic vein becomes confluent with the brachial veins at the lower border of the teres major muscle to form the axillary vein. The basilic vein is easily identified in the upper arm as the largest single, most superficial medial draining vein.

The deep veins of the arm are small paired structures that parallel their associated namesake arteries (Fig. 7-3). Predictably, the deep veins of the forearm are the ulnar, interosseous, and radial veins. These drain into the paired brachial veins at the level of the antecubital fossa. In the upper arm, the brachial veins are closely related to the brachial artery and the median and radial nerves. At the lateral border of the teres major muscle the brachial veins fuse with the basilic vein to form the axillary vein. Up until this point, the deep veins are smaller in size

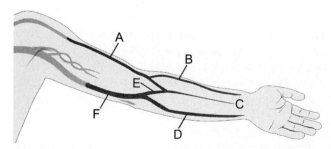

Figure 7-2 Drawing of the superficial veins of the arm. **A,** Cephalic vein in upper arm. **B,** Cephalic vein in forearm. **C,** Median vein of forearm. **D,** Basilic vein in forearm. **E,** Median cubital vein. **F,** Basilic vein in upper arm.

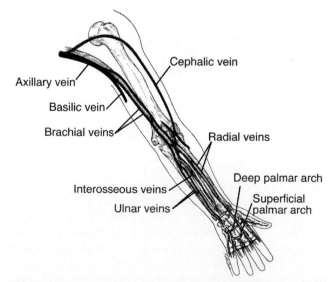

Figure 7-3 Drawing of the deep upper-extremity veins. (Reproduced with permission from Lundell C, Kadir S: Upper extremity veins. In Kadir S ed: *Atlas of Normal and Angiographic Anatomy,* WB Saunders, Philadelphia, 1991.)

than the superficial veins. However, from the axillary vein centrally the deep veins assume dominance. The axillary vein lies slightly inferior and anterior to the axillary artery. At the lateral edge of the 1st rib the axillary vein changes its name and becomes the subclavian vein. This vein passes between the 1st rib and the clavicle to combine with the internal jugular vein at the thoracic inlet to form the brachiocephalic veins. Of all the upper-extremity veins, only the subclavian vein is consistently valveless.

Key Collateral Pathways

The venous drainage of the upper extremities is rich with potential collateral pathways. Because of the multiplicity of veins in the arm, occlusion of a basilic or brachial vein is usually well tolerated. Occlusion of an axillary or subclavian vein results in collateral flow through muscular and superficial veins about the shoulder, scapula, and chest wall. Dilated subcutaneous veins over the upper chest and shoulder are frequently visible in patients with occluded subclavian veins. Potential decompressive pathways include the ipsilateral internal jugular vein, the ipsilateral intercostal veins, and the contralateral jugular or subclavian veins (Fig. 7-4).

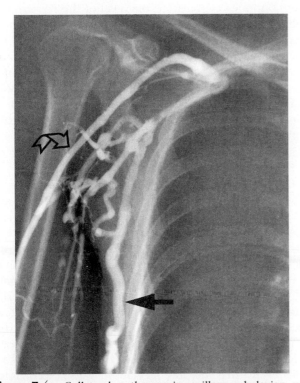

Figure 7-4   Collateral pathways in axillary–subclavian vein occlusion. Right upper-extremity venogram in a patient with long-standing subclavian vein occlusion shows drainage via a large chest wall collateral (arrow). Note the course of the cephalic vein (curved arrow).

Central Thoracic Veins

Blood from the upper extremities and the head returns to the heart through the brachiocephalic (or innominate) veins and the superior vena cava (SVC) (Fig. 7-5). The right brachiocephalic vein is a short (2- to 3-cm) structure that has a vertical trajectory into the SVC. The left brachiocephalic vein, fully 2–3 times longer than the right, crosses from the left side of the mediastinum anterior to the great vessels to join the right brachiocephalic vein. This defines the origin of the superior vena cava. Important tributaries of the brachiocephalic vein include the internal mammary, vertebral, pericardiophrenic, and the first intercostal veins. On the left, the inferior thyroidal vein drains into the superior aspect of the brachiocephalic vein at the midpoint.

The left brachiocephalic vein crosses the midline to join the right in more than 99% of normal individuals. In less than 1% of patients without congenital heart disease, the left brachiocephalic vein does not anastomose with the right but drains into the coronary sinus through a second, left-sided SVC (Fig. 7-6). This anomaly is observed in 4–5% of patients with congenital heart disease.

The SVC is generally 6–8 cm in length, and up to 2 cm in diameter. The main tributaries of the SVC are the brachiocephalic veins and the azygos vein. The SVC generally enters the pericardium below the orifice of the azygos vein. In more than 99% of individuals this vessel is single, right-sided, and drains into the right atrium.

The azygos and hemiazygos veins are posterior mediastinal structures that originate at the L1–L2 level (Fig. 7-7). The azygos vein ascends anterior to the thoracic spine to the right of the midline, while the hemiazygos vein lies slightly to the left of the midline anterior to the spine. Both veins receive blood from ascending lumbar, intercostal,

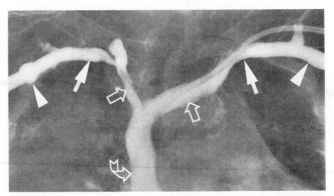

Figure 7-5   Central venogram obtained by simultaneous injection of both upper extremities. The patient has bilateral indwelling subclavian vein catheters. Arrowhead = axillary vein; solid arrow = subclavian vein; open arrow = brachiocephalic vein; curved arrow = SVC.

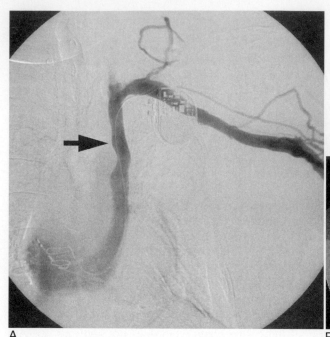

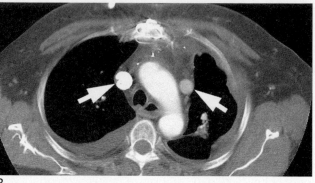

Figure 7-6 Persistent left superior vena cava (SVC). **A,** Digital subtraction venogram from the left arm showing the left SVC (arrow) draining directly into the right atrium. There is no communication with the right SVC. **B,** Axial CT scan in same patient after contrast injection in the right arm shows both SVCs (arrows). The right SVC is densely opacified relative to the left.

A   B

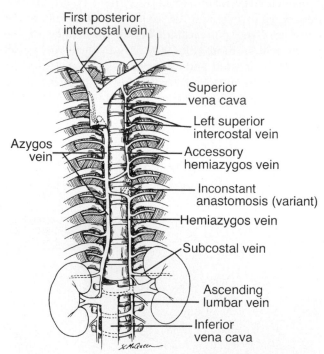

Figure 7-7 Drawing of the azygos veins. (Reproduced with permission from Lundell C, Kadir S: Superior vena cava and thoracic veins. In Kadir S ed: *Atlas of Normal and Angiographic Anatomy*, WB Saunders, Philadelphia, 1991.)

subcostal, esophageal, and bronchial veins. The hemiazygos vein crosses anterior to the spine at the level of the T8 vertebral body to join the azygos vein. The azygos vein continues cephalad to the level of the T4 vertebral body, where it passes anteriorly over the right hilum to empty into the SVC. The accessory hemiazygos vein is a small, left-sided tributary of either the azygos or hemiazygos vein that drains the upper (through T8) intercostal veins. This vein will sometimes empty anteriorly and superiorly into the left brachiocephalic vein, in which case it can be visualized along the lateral border of the proximal descending thoracic aorta.

Key Collateral Pathways

Occlusion of a brachiocephalic vein results in obstruction of flow from both the ipsilateral arm and neck. Facial swelling on the side of the occlusion is rare as long as the contralateral internal jugular vein is patent. The venous blood from the arm may drain across the back, chest, and neck via deep and superficial collaterals to the opposite jugular, subclavian, and brachiocephalic veins. The superficial chest wall veins such as internal mammary and intercostal veins may also serve as collateral drainage pathways. These veins drain into the azygos vein on the right and hemiazygos vein on the left, or may continue down the abdominal wall to the inferior epigastric veins. Pericardial and phrenic veins may also be recruited as collateral drainage pathways.

The level of occlusion of the SVC determines which collateral pathway will be dominant. When occlusion is above the azygos vein, the collateral drainage involves

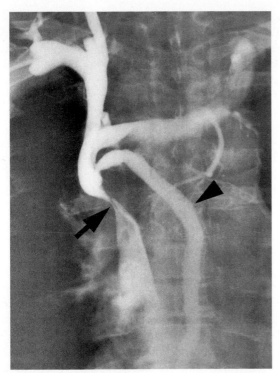

Figure 7-8   Collateral pathways in SVC obstruction. Venogram showing severe stenosis of the central SVC (arrow) with collateral drainage via the azygos vein (arrowhead).

the azygos vein, flow reverses in this vein with drainage into the inferior vena cava (IVC) (Fig. 7-8). Chest wall and pericardial collaterals may also develop. Occlusion of the SVC above and below the azygos veins results in azygos and hemiazygos drainage into the IVC, as well as extensive chest wall and pericardial collateral veins.

IMAGING

The superficial veins of the neck and upper-extremity can be readily imaged with ultrasound (US). When evaluating a patient for upper-extremity central venous thrombosis, the neck as well as the upper-extremity veins should be studied, as the jugular veins are frequently involved. Gray-scale imaging with compression, and Doppler with color flow, can provide information about venous patency and direction of flow (Fig. 7-9). The central veins such as the brachiocephalic veins and SVC cannot be directly imaged satisfactorily with external US transducers owing to the surrounding bone and lung. The patency of the central vessels can be inferred by studying subclavian vein and IJV Doppler waveforms at rest and in response to respiration and Valsalva. However, the impact of central stenoses on flow in the more peripheral veins has not been carefully worked out, and may be masked by a well-developed collateral network. If, for some reason, US examination of the intrathoracic veins is strongly desired, then a transesophageal study is required.

Contrast-enhanced computed tomography (CT) is an excellent modality for evaluation of the jugular, proximal subclavian, brachiocephalic, and central veins. The veins

primarily the chest wall and intercostal veins, emptying into the azygos system. The direction of flow within the azygos veins remains towards the SVC. Some drainage through the pericardial and abdominal wall veins may be present as well. When the occlusion is localized below

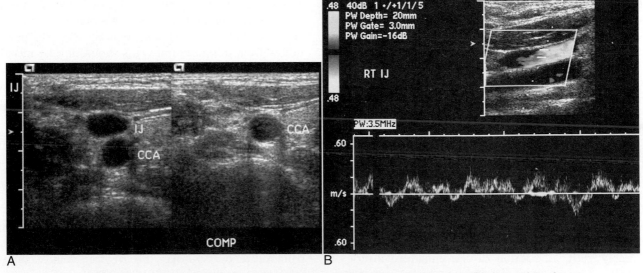

Figure 7-9   US of jugular veins. **A,** Gray-scale image showing normal, compressible internal jugular vein (IJ). CCA = common carotid artery. Comp = compression. **B,** Normal IJV Doppler waveform.

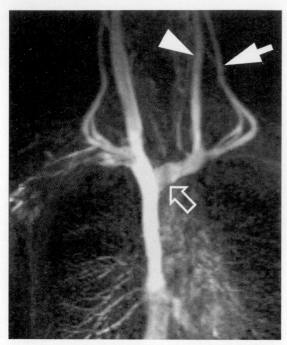

Figure 7-10 Gadolinium-enhanced 3-D MR venogram of normal neck and central veins. The deep and superficial neck veins (closed arrow on left IJV, arrowhead on left EJV) are well visualized. An impression (open arrow) from the brachiocephalic artery can be seen on the left brachiocephalic vein. The heart and subclavian veins are not included in this restricted maximum-intensity projection (MIP). (Courtesy of Barry Stein M.D., Hartford Hospital, CT.)

from the forearm to the axilla are difficult to image with CT. The advantages of this modality are the ability to map out collateral pathways, such as superficial chest wall veins in SVC obstruction, as well as revealing extrinsic causes of venous obstruction. Injection of contrast into the upper extremity of the side of interest is advised, as this will provide the best opacification of the unobstructed and collateral veins. When bilateral obstruction is suspected, bilateral contrast injections may be necessary. A delayed scan after the initial contrast injection may be necessary to obtain maximum opacification of veins not filled from the arm injection. However, the density of venous contrast in these scans can be poor. Careful postprocessing is very useful when tracing collateral pathways and determining the etiology of extrinsic compression.

MR venography (MRV) is also an excellent cross-sectional modality for evaluating the upper-extremity, neck, and central veins (Fig. 7-10). Suppression of signal from background structures results in images that are easy to view, in comparison to CT in which bone and other tissues can obscure the veins. The most robust techniques involve gadolinium-enhanced acquisitions, preferably with subtraction of the enhanced arteries. The side of injection of contrast is not an issue with this technique, with the exception that concentrated

gadolinium may result in signal loss due to dominance of T2 shortening effects (see Fig. 3-17). This is easily solved by sequential acquisitions over several minutes, during which time the gadolinium becomes diluted. Conventional 2-dimensional time-of-flight techniques (2-D TOF) have also been used with great success, although multiple acquisitions with careful orientation of the slices and saturation bands is necessary to image all of the veins (e.g., axial slices with inferior saturation for the jugular veins and SVC, but sagittal slices with medial saturation slabs for the brachiocephalic and subclavian veins). The highly motivated MR imager can study the veins of the arms, but this usually requires the patient to lie in the scanner with arms extended (US imaging of these veins is much simpler). Although MRV is excellent for visualizing the veins, the surrounding structures are not well seen. Conventional anatomic T1-weighted images are necessary to see the adjacent soft tissues, except bone. When a bony cause for venous obstruction is suspected, CT is a better choice of imaging modality.

Arm venography is a simple, quick procedure for evaluation of the upper-extremity and central veins. The internal jugular veins are not routinely studied with this technique. For arm venography, an 18- to 20-gauge IV should be started in a vein in the hand or forearm. When using an existing IV, test it first to make sure that it is patent and in a vein. Injection of antecubital vein or upper-arm cephalic vein may fail to opacify the basilic, brachial, and proximal axillary veins. Two or three 20-mL syringes of dilute contrast (20–30% iodine) are injected by hand. A tourniquet in the axilla enhances filling of deep and superficial veins. The hand should be in anatomic position (palm up) with the arm positioned slightly abducted. In large patients, compression by the chest wall can cause pseudostenoses of the veins in the medial aspect of the upper arm (Fig. 7-11). Both spot films and digital subtraction images are satisfactory for the arm veins. Digital subtraction is usually required to adequately visualize the brachiocephalic veins and SVC. Unopacified inflow from other central veins should not be mistaken for thrombus or other filling defects. Bilateral injections can be performed to evaluate central processes (see Fig. 7-5). One of the major advantages of conventional arm venography is that there is an option to proceed directly to an intervention if an amenable abnormality is found.

UPPER-EXTREMITY VENOUS THROMBOSIS

Acute thrombosis of a single peripheral upper-extremity vein rarely results in arm swelling, but patients may have pain and tenderness over the involved vein. A common etiology is intravenous injection of medication or illicit drugs. The treatment is oral anti-inflammatory agents

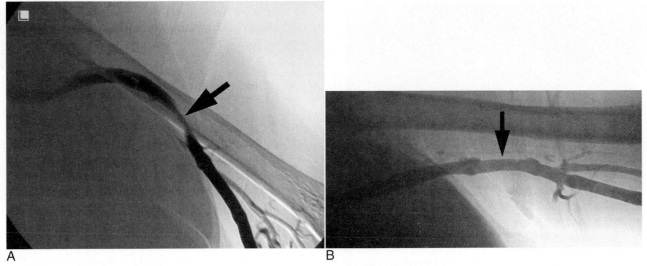

Figure 7-11   Basilic vein pseudolesion due to compression by chest wall soft tissues in an obese patient. **A,** Digital image of left upper-extremity venogram with the arm at the patient's side. There appears to be a stenosis (arrow) of the basilic vein. Note the copious soft tissues of the chest. **B,** Digital image of the same patient with the arm abducted. The area of stenosis is now normal (arrow).

and local measures such as heat packs. Thrombosis of central veins such as the axillary, subclavian, or brachiocephalic veins may result in arm swelling and cyanosis, especially when the limb is dependent. Patients frequently report noticing a tight ring or wristwatch as the first symptom. Acute thrombosis may also be locally painful, possibly due to the expansion of the vein by thrombus or firm edema of the extremity. When the jugular vein is involved patients may complain of neck stiffness or tenderness, or swelling of the face on the affected side. Phlegmasia (alba or cerulea dolens) is extremely rare in the upper extremity. Pulmonary embolization from the upper extremity is thought to occur in 15–30% of cases.

Chronic occlusion of the peripheral upper-extremity veins produces a hard, cord-like vein, but is usually otherwise symptomatically innocuous. Chronic central thrombosis is suggested by the presence of well-developed superficial chest wall collateral veins. Patients may complain of arm swelling, particularly with use of the limb, but many are asymptomatic.

Central venous catheterization is the most common underlying etiology of upper-extremity and jugular thrombosis (Box 7-1). Approximately 40–60% of all patients with chronic indwelling subclavian venous catheters develop some thrombus around the catheter, although fewer than 5% are symptomatic (Fig. 7-12). There are many factors that influence the incidence of this complication in specific patient populations, such as catheter size, location, and the presence of an underlying hypercoagulable state. Prophylaxis with 1 mg of coumadin a day has been shown to dramatically decrease

this complication. Venous stenosis and subsequent thrombosis may also present at a time remote from the venous catheterization. The incidence of occlusive thrombosis around transvenous pacemaker wires is approximately 10% (Fig. 7-13).

Several imaging findings of acute venous thrombosis are common to most imaging modalities, although each has additional specific findings (Boxes 7-2 and 7-3). Patients should be initially evaluated with US, although the ability of this modality to image the central veins is limited. CT or MR allows diagnosis and determination of the extent of central venous obstruction. In addition, an underlying etiology may be found in the perivascular tissues. Venography is not usually necessary unless the diagnosis

---

Box 7-1   Risk Factors for Upper-extremity and Central Venous Thrombosis

Central venous catheter
Pacemaker
Hypercoagulable syndromes
Malignancy
Extrinsic compression
  Lymph node
  Tumor
  Musculoskeletal
Tumor invasion (Pancoast)
Injection of sclerosing medications
Trauma

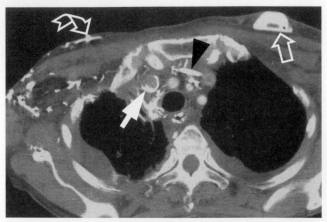

Figure 7-12   Axial CT with scan injection through the right arm showing thrombus in the right brachiocephalic vein (straight arrow) and extensive chest wall collaterals (curved arrow). The patient has a left chest port (open arrow) with a catheter (arrowhead) visible in the unopacified left brachiocephalic vein.

is uncertain, or an intervention is contemplated. Chronic venous thrombosis has a different appearance from acute, but both can coexist (Box 7-4).

The treatment of upper-extremity central venous thrombosis depends upon the chronicity, underlying cause, and the clinical scenario. Acute thrombosis associated with a central line may be managed with simple local measures such as arm elevation, or full anticoagulation. Most other patients are managed with anticoagulation, when possible. Evaluation for a prothrombotic state

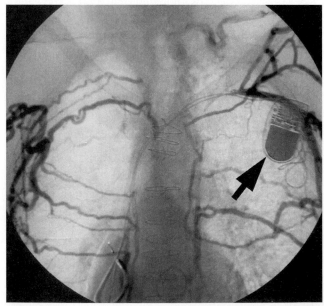

Figure 7-13   Digital venogram showing central venous occlusions in a patient with a left-sided pacemaker (arrow) and previous right subclavian catheters.

Box 7-2   Imaging Features of Acute Venous Thrombosis Common to All Modalities

Intraluminal filling defect
Absent flow
Expansion of vein
Increased flow through collateral veins

is important when the etiology is cryptic. Very symptomatic patients should be evaluated for potential thrombolysis, although this is pursued less often when an indwelling catheter is the culprit.

Thrombolysis of acute upper-extremity venous thrombosis is useful to relieve symptoms and potentially unmask the underlying etiology. US- or venographically guided puncture of the ipsilateral basilic vein (when patent) with a microaccess needle allows a direct approach to subclavian thrombosis. Femoral or jugular vein access may be used as well. The area of thrombosis should be crossed with a selective guidewire, followed by a multi-side-holed infusion catheter. Pharmacologic thrombolysis with concurrent anticoagulation has excellent outcomes with low complication rates. The results of mechanical thrombectomy devices are less predictable in

Box 7-3   Imaging Features of Acute Venous Thrombosis with US, CT, MR, and Venography

Ultrasound

Noncompressible vessel
Hypoechoic to slightly echogenic lumen
Absent Doppler signal in lumen

Computed Tomography

Increased density in lumen on noncontrast scan
Lack of opacification of lumen on contrast scan
Wall enhancement on delayed images

Magnetic Resonance

Increased signal in lumen (varies with age and pulse
    sequence; see Table 3-1)
Absent signal in lumen on flow sequences
Wall enhancement on delayed contrast images

Venography

Intraluminal filling defect
Abrupt concave cutoff of contrast column
Poorly developed collateral drainage

Box 7-4 Imaging Findings of Chronic Venous Thrombus

Occluded, string-like vessel
Linear intraluminal webs
Mural irregularity and thickening
Stenoses
Hyperechoic intraluminal filling defects (US finding)
Dilated, well-developed collateral drainage

large-diameter veins, and certain devices may traumatize the venous intima. When a venous stenosis is unmasked by this process, angioplasty should be considered if thoracic outlet syndrome has been excluded as a potential etiology (see below). Most patients require long-term anticoagulation following successful thrombolysis.

In rare cases, patients with acute upper-extremity thrombosis may have documented symptomatic pulmonary embolism and a contraindication to anticoagulation. Placement of a superior vena cava filter may be necessary (Fig. 7-14).

Asymptomatic patients with chronic occlusions do not require treatment unless the vein is needed as a conduit for another procedure. Symptomatic patients with chronic occlusions may benefit from angioplasty and stent placement. However, the restenosis rate approaches 45% at 1 year for stents.

THORACIC OUTLET SYNDROME

Venous thoracic outlet syndrome usually first presents with acute thrombosis (Box 7-5). Also known as Paget Schroetter or effort thrombosis syndromes, this diagnosis should be suspected in any young, healthy

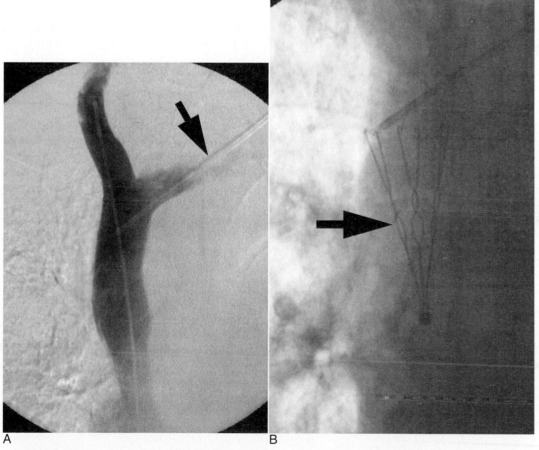

A   B

Figure 7-14   Filter in the SVC in a patient with massive upper-extremity thrombosis, pulmonary embolism, and contraindication to anticoagulation. **A,** Venogram showing the right and left brachiocephalic veins and the SVC. A triple-lumen catheter (arrow) is present in the left brachiocephalic vein. **B,** A 12-Fr Greenfield vena cava filter (Boston Scientific, Natick, MA) (arrow) has been placed with the feet just below the confluence of the brachiocephalic veins and the apex oriented towards the right atrium.

(especially athletic) patient presenting with unexplained acute subclavian vein thrombosis. Fewer than 5% of all cases of acute upper-extremity venous thrombosis are due to thoracic outlet syndrome. Extrinsic compression of the subclavian or axillary vein by a cervical rib, bony exostosis, anomalous ligament or muscle, or hypertrophied scalene muscles (exercise can be dangerous) results in intimal hyperplasia and gradual stenosis (see Fig. 1-38). Collaterals develop that compensate for the obstruction and prevent symptoms, although many patients give a history of arm swelling and heaviness when questioned. Thrombosis isolated to the residual lumen is usually accompanied by only minimal symptoms. However, when thrombus propagates retrograde into the collateral veins acute obstruction of venous outflow results. Patients frequently report onset of symptoms after vigorous upper-body activity, such as painting a ceiling. Pulmonary embolus from upper-extremity thrombosis due to thoracic outlet syndrome is unusual, as the underlying pathology is a fixed venous obstruction. The long-term natural history is not well known, but estimates of chronic disability due to swelling and discomfort range from 10 to 60%.

In patients with acute symptoms and suspected thoracic outlet syndrome, the chest radiograph should be reviewed for anomalous cervical ribs. The presence of thrombus can be confirmed with US or venography. MRI or CT of the thoracic outlet is helpful to evaluate for anomalous muscles or ligaments. When thoracic outlet syndrome is suspected in the absence of acute symptoms, the same imaging studies can be obtained. Venography should performed with the arm positioned to reproduce the patient's symptoms. Specific maneuvers include Adson's, in which the shoulder is depressed with the arm at the side and the patient's head turned toward the shoulder. When thoracic outlet syndrome is found or suspected, bilateral subclavian venograms should be obtained. However, be wary, as subclavian vein compression with extreme abduction of the arm can be induced in half the asymptomatic population (Fig. 7-15).

Thoracic outlet syndrome is initially managed with heparinization and catheter-directed thrombolysis, usually from an ipsilateral upper-extremity approach (Fig. 7-16). This quickly reduces arm swelling, and allows delineation of the underlying venous lesion. The cause of the extrinsic compression must also be determined, as the second step in treatment is decompression of the thoracic outlet. Repeat venography is performed after surgical decompression, with angioplasty of residual stenoses. Stents may be necessary when stenoses are recurrent and

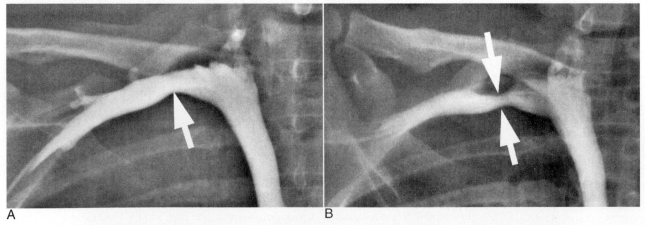

Figure 7-15   Compression of the subclavian vein in a normal individual. **A,** Venogram with the arm in neutral position shows minimal inferior indentation (arrow) of the subclavian vein. Note the absence of collateral veins. **B,** Venogram with the arm abducted shows partial compression of the subclavian vein (arrows). Again note the absence of collateral veins.

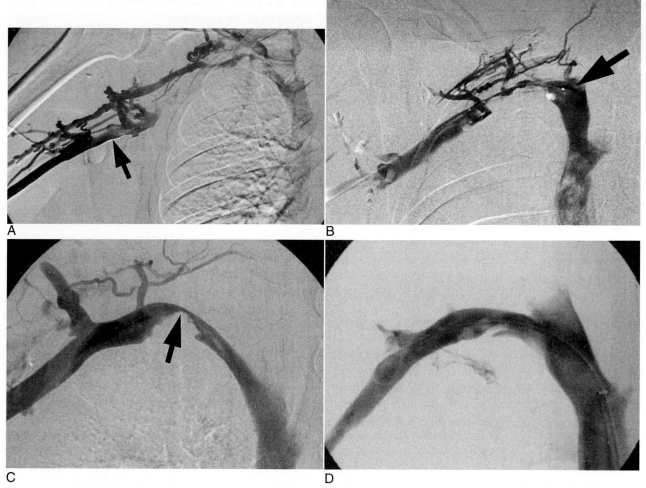

Figure 7-16 Upper-extremity venous thrombosis in a young athlete. **A,** Right upper-extremity venogram in a healthy young male with acute arm swelling. There is obstruction at the level of the axillary vein (note the intraluminal filling defect characteristic of thrombus (arrow) and the drainage through collateral veins). **B,** Venogram after 4 hours of thrombolysis shows multi-side-hole catheter positioned across the thrombus with the tip (arrow) in the right brachiocephalic vein. **C,** After 24 hours of catheter-directed thrombolysis, a focal, bulky stenosis (arrow) is present at the junction of the subclavian and internal jugular vein. **D,** Venogram following 1st rib resection with subsequent angioplasty (12-mm diameter balloon) shows minimal residual stenosis.

severely symptomatic, but the poor long-term patency and the young age of most of these patients should discourage routine use. Stents should not be placed without surgical decompression of the thoracic outlet, or the stent may be crushed or fractured (see Fig. 4-16).

SUPERIOR VENA CAVA SYNDROME

Abrupt occlusion of the SVC results in a characteristic syndrome of facial and upper-extremity edema, superficial venous distension, and cyanosis. These patients are usually extremely uncomfortable, especially when lying flat. Acute SVC syndrome is considered a medical emergency.

Chronic occlusion or stenosis may be asymptomatic or cause moderate facial edema or pressure that improves when the patient is upright. The level of obstruction is important, as occlusion below the azygos vein may be well tolerated if the azygos drainage is robust (see Fig. 7-8). Obstruction of the SVC may be due to intrinsic or extrinsic causes (Box 7-6). The most common etiology (>80%) is compression by thoracic malignancy, usually originating in the lung. Patients with SVC syndrome caused by malignancy have less than 50% survival at 6 months.

Although SVC syndrome is a clinical diagnosis, imaging is necessary for confirmation and planning of therapy. The most expeditious imaging modality is contrast-enhanced CT, as this allows evaluation of venous patency and the surrounding tissues (see Fig. 7-12). Injection of contrast into the upper extremity with filling of abdominal wall collateral veins is indicative of central stenosis or occlusion (Fig. 7-17). Opacification of the more central veins may be delayed, so a repeat scan may be necessary to avoid overestimating the extent of occlusion. The lower neck should be included in the area scanned so that jugular vein patency can be assessed. Gadolinium-enhanced MR venography is also very useful in the evaluation of suspected SVC syndrome. Upper-extremity venography with simultaneous injection of contrast into both arms defines the status of the veins, but does not provide information about the adjacent structures (see Fig. 7-13).

Symptomatic chronic SVC stenosis should be managed by angioplasty first, with stents reserved for recurrent or recalcitrant lesions (Fig. 7-18). Identification of the underlying etiology is essential to provide proper treatment. Thrombosis of a chronic lesion is usually amenable to thrombolysis. Indwelling long-term central venous access catheters are frequently present, and can be repositioned into a jugular or subclavian vein during placement of an SVC stent. Stents can be placed over pacemaker wires when necessary. Balloon and stent diameters range from 8 mm to 16 mm, but must be tailored to the patient and the underlying pathology. Re-establishment of inline drainage from one jugular vein to the right atrium is usually sufficient to relieve head and neck symptoms acutely. Extension of stents into the right atrium may induce arrhythmia and should be avoided.

Recanalization of an occluded SVC is frequently successfull when combined IJV and femoral venous approaches are used. Access through the right IJV is preferred as this provides a short, straight path to the right atrium. A second catheter placed in the residual patent SVC below the obstruction from a femoral approach can be used to guide recanalization. Care must be taken not to perforate the SVC below the azygos vein, as this portion is frequently intrapericardial and may result in hemopericardium with tamponade. Stent placement is almost always required in these patients. Surgical bypass of the SVC can be performed, with reported 60–70% patency rates at 1 year.

Acute SVC syndrome is not treated surgically. External radiation can rapidly shrink some mediastinal tumors that cause SVC obstruction by compression. Interventional radiology has much to offer patients with acute SVC syndrome, particularly when there is a large thrombus burden or an intrinsic lesion within the SVC. Thrombolysis restores patency and reveals the underlying lesion, but is frequently not possible in patients with advanced malignancy complicated by brain or pericardial metastases. Stent placement is almost always necessary in these patients, and can be performed in the presence of thrombus. Flexible, self-expanding stents are ideal for extensive reconstructions. After crossing the thrombosed SVC, the self-expanding stent can be deployed and then post-dilated. This minimizes the risk of massive pulmonary embolization. The relief of symptoms can be so dramatic that the patient feels improved by the end of the case. The goal is palliation, not perfection.

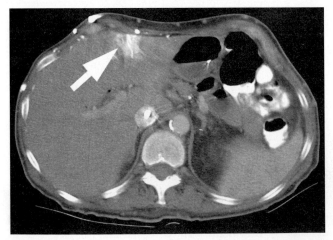

Figure 7-17   Characteristic enhancement of segment IV (arrow) of the liver by chest and mediastinal collateral veins in a patient with SVC syndrome following injection of contrast in an upper-extremity vein. Note the numerous collateral veins in the abdominal wall.

CENTRAL VENOUS ACCESS

One of the most common vascular interventional procedures currently performed is placement of long-term

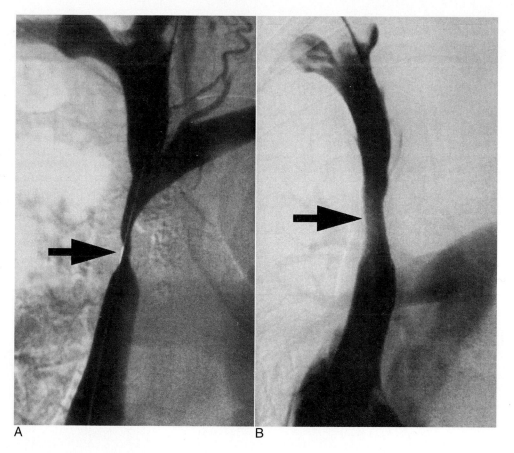

Figure 7-18   SVC syndrome due to mediastinal fibrosis in a patient with histoplasmosis exposure. **A**, Contrast venogram performed by injection from the right internal jugular vein showing severe SVC stenosis (arrow) and reflux into the left brachiocephalic vein. **B**, Contrast venogram following stent placement (arrow) dilated to 10 mm, at which point the patient complained of chest pain. Note absence of reflux into other mediastinal veins.

A   B

central venous access devices. A large variety of venous access devices are available (Fig. 7-19 and Table 7-1). There are several basic configurations of catheter tips, including open and valved (Fig. 7-20). Valves can also be incorporated into the hub of the catheter. Valved catheters are useful for patients with heparin allergies, as the flush solution can be sterile saline. However, valves prevent high flow rates, so dialysis and plasmapheresis catheters are open-ended. Suggestions for specific flush solutions for various devices are listed in Table 7-2.

Image-guided placement of long-term venous access devices is safe, cost-effective, and efficacious. Selection of an appropriate device requires familiarity with the access device, an understanding of the patient's access needs, and knowledge of the patient's venous anatomy. Many patients will have specific requests regarding location of devices that should be taken into consideration.

Table 7-1   Types of Central Venous Access Devices

Device	Duration	Uses
Non-tunneled central catheter	7–14 days	Resuscitation; acute dialysis; stem cell harvest
Non-tunneled PICC	1–12 weeks	Antibiotics; TPN
Tunneled catheter	>1 month	Chemotherapy; TPN; dialysis; plasmapheresis
Implantable port	>3 months	Chemotherapy; dialysis (specialized devices)

PICC, peripherally inserted central catheter; TPN, total parenteral nutrition.

Table 7-2   Flush Solutions for Long-term Central Venous Access Devices

Catheter	Solution
PICC	Heparin 100 U/mL; can use saline if valved
Hickman	Heparin 100 U/mL; can use saline if valved
Port (non-dialysis)	Heparin 100 U/mL; can use saline if valved
Port (dialysis)	Per manufacturer
Pheresis	Heparin 1000 U/mL
Dialysis	Heparin 5000 U/mL

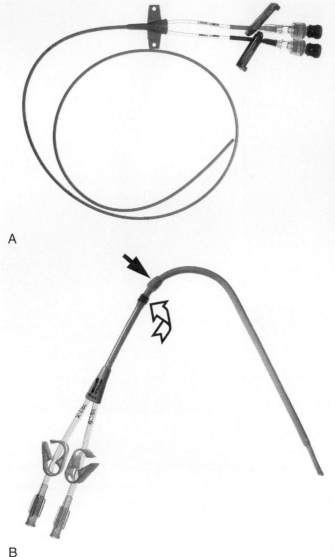

A

B

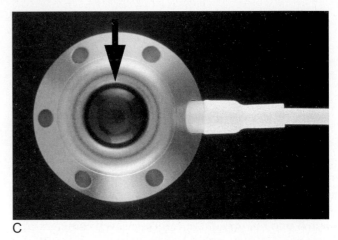

C

Figure 7-19   Typical long-term central venous access devices. **A,** Peripherally inserted central catheter (PICC), double-lumen. Catheter may be silicone or polyurethane, 3- to 6-Fr, single- or double-lumen, valved or nonvalved. There is no cuff for tissue ingrowth. **B,** Tunneled catheter (in this case for dialysis). Tunneled catheters may be silicone or polyurethane, up to 16-Fr or larger, have up to three lumens, and be valved or nonvalved. Tunneled catheters are characterized by the presence of a cuff for tissue ingrowth (straight arrow) that stabilizes the catheter after 3–4 weeks. The catheter shown here also has a silver-impregnated cuff (curved arrow) to reduce tunnel infections. **C,** Port for subcutaneous implantation. A silicone membrane (arrow) for access with a noncoring needle is characteristic. Ports may be metal or plastic, single- or double-lumen, with a range of sizes suitable for arm or chest placement. Catheters are silicone or polyurethane, 5- to 12-Fr in diameter.

Basic Principles of Device Implantation

There are a few guidelines to follow during insertion that are applicable to all venous access devices. The right internal jugular vein is the preferred access for most devices because it is large, close to the skin, and provides a short straight route to the superior vena cava. This vein should be used whenever possible for dialysis catheters to avoid compromise of subclavian veins and the left brachiocephalic vein, which are important for the success of upper-arm surgical dialysis access (shunts and fistulas) (Table 7-3). Techniques for puncture of internal jugular, subclavian, and upper-extremity veins are described in Chapter 2. The one potential procedural complication

that can result in immediate death to the patient is massive air embolism through large peel-away sheaths during catheter insertion. Specific measures to avoid and manage this complication are described in Chapter 2 (Venous Access, Internal Jugular Vein, and Box 2-10). In addition, tunneled catheters should be flushed, clamped, and capped prior to insertion into the patient to prevent inadvertent aspiration of air through an open catheter.

The tip of a long-term central venous access device should lie in the high right atrium (Fig. 7-21). Catheter tips that end in the SVC or brachiocephalic vein have a higher incidence of catheter malfunction due to formation of fibrin sheaths, as well as catheter-related central venous stenosis and thrombosis (Fig. 7-22). The etiology of

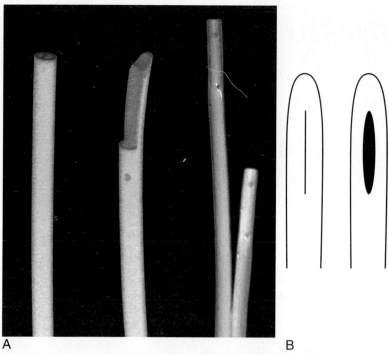

A   B

Figure 7-20   Catheter tips. **A** (from left to right), Nontapered dual-lumen; staggered-tip dual-lumen; split catheter. **B,** Schematic of mechanism of action of a Groshong valve-tipped catheter. The end of the catheter is sealed, and flow is through a slit in the side near the tip. *Left:* Resting closed state. *Right:* With aspiration or injection the slit opens to allow flow.

stenotic complications are not known with certainty, but are probably related to irritation of the endothelium by the catheter tip and the injected medications. Catheter tips in the high right atrium are rarely in contact with endothelium. During positioning of the catheter in a supine patient, it is important to note that chest wall tissues may drop and the mediastinum lengthen when the patient stands or sits upright. Catheters will

Table 7-3   Preferred Veins (in Order) for Long-term Central Access

Device	Vein
PICC line[a]	Basilic, cephalic[b], brachial[c] veins
Dialysis	RIJ, REJ, LIJ, LEJ; avoid LSCV, RSCV
Non-dialysis tunneled	RIJ, LIJ, RSCV, LSCV
Implantable ports	RIJ, LIJ, RSCV, LSCV

[a]Should not be placed in arm in patients with renal failure. Use neck veins.
[b]More subject to spasm, angle in shoulder can be difficult to negotiate.
[c]Close to brachial artery, radial and median nerves.

RIJ, right internal jugular vein; REJ, right external jugular vein; LIJ, left internal jugular vein; LEJ, left external jugular vein; LSCV, left subclavian vein; RSCV, right subclavian vein.

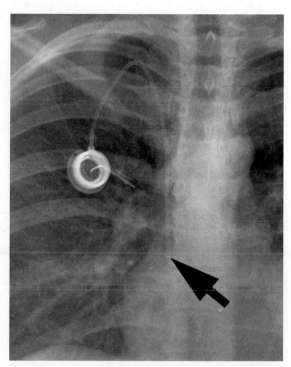

Figure 7-21   Chest radiograph after insertion of a single-lumen chest port through the right IJV. The catheter tip is in the high right atrium (arrow).

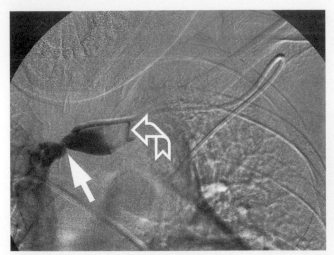

Figure 7-22   Consequences of catheter malpositioning. The tip of this chest port has withdrawn into the left brachiocephalic vein. A stenosis (straight arrow) has developed central to the catheter tip. A fibrin sheath has formed around the catheter tip, so that blood could not be aspirated. Contrast injected through the catheter tracks underneath the fibrin sheath, entering the vessel lumen through gaps in the fibrin (curved arrow).

withdraw a few centimeters when this happens (Fig. 7-23). To compensate for this natural pull-back the catheter tip should be placed a few centimeters deeper into the atrium than the intended final location, especially in patients with loose chest wall tissues. Most conventional catheters can be trimmed to length by the operator after determining the amount of catheter needed to reach a desired central location. Special-use catheters, such as for dialysis, have staggered tip configurations that should not be altered.

When placing tunneled catheters or ports, infected or irradiated skin should be avoided. An appropriate thickness of skin and subcutaneous tissue over the device is 5–10 mm. Otherwise, erosion may occur, particularly in oncology patients who may lose substantial amounts of weight during their illness. Conversely, ports should not be placed too deep under the subcutaneous tissues, as they become difficult to access. In women, it is always wise to avoid placing the port in breast tissue as access is uncomfortable and inconvenient, and scarring will be created that will confuse the mammographers.

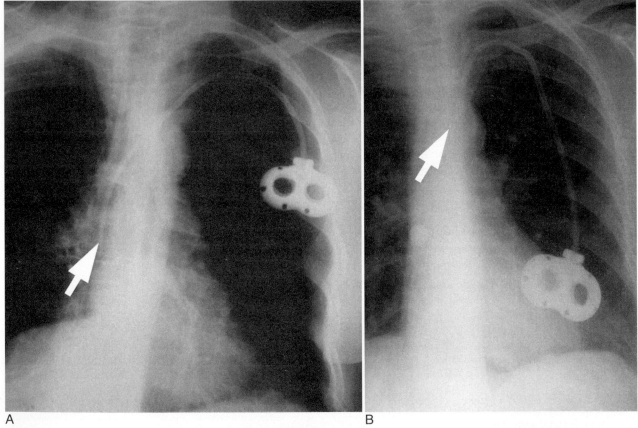

A   B

Figure 7-23   Positional change in catheter tip location in patient with abundant, loose chest wall tissues. **A,** Chest radiograph in supine position shows catheter tip (arrow) in a central location. **B,** Same patient in upright position during full inspiration a few minutes later. The port is located lower on the chest wall, and the catheter tip has withdrawn to a less central position (arrow).

Box 7-7 PICC-line Placement

Peripheral intravenous catheter on side of access
Surgical arm prep
Basilic or cephalic vein preferred
Arm venogram to confirm venous anatomy/patency
 Alternatively, ultrasound arm veins
Access vein with micropuncture needle
Advance wire to SVC
Determine appropriate intravascular length of catheter
 Tip should be in high right atrium
Insert peel-away sheath
Advance catheter through sheath
Suture to skin with Nylon sutures

Box 7-9 Port Placement

Confirm patency of access site
Surgical prep skin
+/− Prophylactic antibiotics
Surgical scrub operator hands
Image-guided access
 Micro-access needle
Insert catheter through peel-away sheath
 Valsalva, Trendelenburg position to prevent air
 embolism
Position catheter tip in high right atrium
Create pocket
Tunnel catheter into pocket
Trim catheter, assemble port, flush
Secure in port in pocket
 3'0 slowly absorbable suture
Close skin in layers
 3'0 absorbable suture deep layer
 5'0 Nylon interrupted mattress or 4'0 absorbable
 suture subcuticular skin
Access port, confirm correct function, flush

The use of prophylactic antibiotics during device insertion varies from one institution to another. One dose of an antibiotic that provides coverage for *Staphylococci aureus*, such as cefazolin or vancomycin, can be given immediately prior to the procedure. Tunneled or implanted devices should not be placed into patients with ongoing sepsis, or who have been febrile within the previous 48 hours.

Each type of device has certain unique aspects of the insertion procedure (Boxes 7-7 to 7-9). Generally, it is best not to tunnel or create pockets until venous access has been obtained. Tunneling devices are used to pull catheters through subcutaneous tunnels without damaging the catheter tips. The majority of implantation

procedures can be performed with local anesthetic and light conscious sedation.

Patients with occlusion of conventional access sites represent a particular challenge. Image-guided placement of central venous access devices may be life-saving in these patients (Box 7-10). The first option to consider is recanalization of an already occluded vein (Fig. 7-24). This preserves future alternative access sites, without risking a new occlusion. Standard recanalization techniques should be used to allow passage of a catheter to a central position. Stent placement is not necessary unless the occlusion was symptomatic. When recanalization is not possible, several alternative access techniques have been described, including translumbar to the IVC,

Box 7-8 Placement of Tunneled Catheters

Confirm patency of access vein
Surgical prep skin
+/− Prophylactic antibiotics
Surgical scrub operator hands
Image-guided access
 Micro-puncture needle
Determine appropriate intravascular length with
 guidewire
 Tip should be in high right atrium
Tunnel catheter to puncture site
 Tunnel on chest wall should have gentle curve to
 access site
Insert catheter through peel-away sheath
 Valsalva, Trendelenburg position to prevent air
 embolism during catheter insertion
Close venous access site with 4'0 Nylon suture
Secure catheter to skin

Box 7-10 Alternative Access Routes for Long-term Central Venous Access

Recanalization of occluded central vein
Translumbar IVC
Collateral vein
Femoral vein
Direct right brachiocephalic vein
Transhepatic IVC

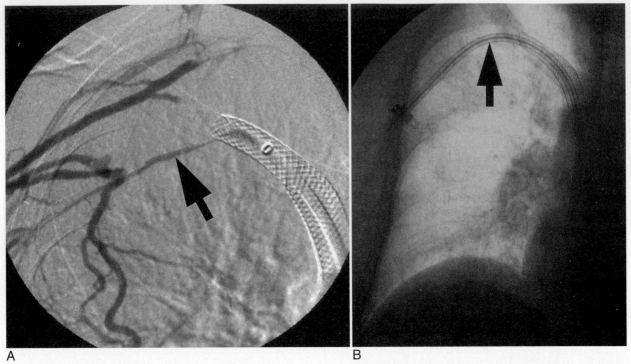

A   B

Figure 7-24   Recanalization of the right subclavian vein in a chronic dialysis patient with occlusion of both IJVs and the left brachiocephalic vein. **A,** Digital subtraction venogram showing a severely stenotic right subclavian vein (arrow) and stent. The vein was dilated with a 6-mm angioplasty balloon from a femoral vein access, and then punctured lateral to the stent with a micropuncture needle. **B,** Final radiograph showing a 16-Fr dialysis catheter (arrow) inserted through the subclavian vein and stent.

transhepatic to the IVC, common femoral vein, direct suprasternal puncture of the right brachiocephalic vein, and through collaterals (Fig. 7-25). These puncture techniques are described in Chapter 2. The greatest experience has been accumulated with translumbar IVC catheters, with a lower than 5% rate of caval thrombosis. Although once discouraged, femoral venous access is becoming more widely accepted. In all cases the tip of the catheter should be positioned in the right atrium to maximize the functional life of the device. In extreme cases, direct surgical placement into the right atrium is possible.

Complications of Venous Access Devices

Procedural complications of central venous catheter placement are related primarily to the venous access, such as injury to adjacent structures (lung or artery), and air embolism (Table 7-4). Meticulous technique, image-guided venous puncture, and image-guided catheter insertion will minimize complications. Infection, catheter malfunction, and venous thrombosis comprise the majority of post-placement complications. Careful device selection, placement, and education of the staff using the device can minimize late complications.

Catheter malfunction, defined as suboptimal infusion or aspiration of blood, is the most common problem encountered after catheter placement. This is usually due to fibrin deposition in or around the tip of the catheter, but may also be caused by venous thrombosis, catheter

Table 7-4	Complications of Central Venous Catheters

Complication	Incidence
Insertion procedure	
Pneumothorax	<2%
Air embolism	<2%
Arterial puncture	1%
Failure to insert catheter	<1%
Catheter malposition	<1%
Indwelling catheter	
Catheter malfunction	10–20%[a]
Symptomatic venous thrombosis	5–15%[b]
Infection	5–10%
Catheter fracture	<1%

[a] Most catheter malfunctions are transitory.
[b] Varies by access site, catheter size, and patient factors. Highest for large subclavian catheters in patients with cancer.
Adapted from Lewis CA et al. J Vasc Interv Radiol 8:475-479, 1997.

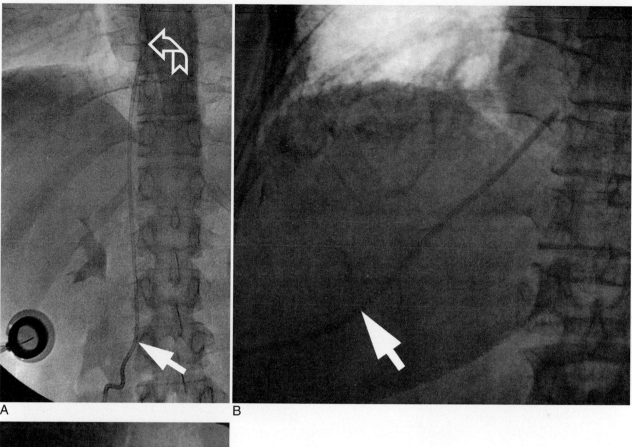

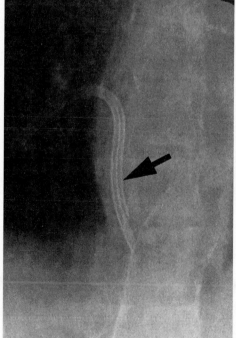

Figure 7-25   Alternative access sites for long-term central venous catheter placement. **A,** Translumbar placement of a port through the inferior vena cava (IVC) in a patient with SVC occlusion. The catheter enters the IVC at the level of the L3 vertebral body (straight arrow). The tip is in the RA (curved arrow). **B,** Transhepatic placement of a tunneled catheter (arrow) through the middle hepatic vein. The patient had occlusion of the infrarenal IVC as well as the SVC. **C,** Direct right atrial catheter (arrow) inserted surgically in a patient with thrombosis of all central veins.

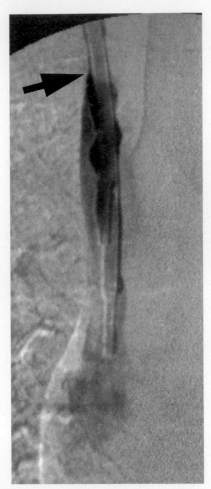

Figure 7-26 Typical appearance of fibrin sheath on a split-tip dialysis catheter. Injection through the proximal lumen shows contrast collecting around the catheter and tracking retrograde (arrow) before it enters the vessel lumen.

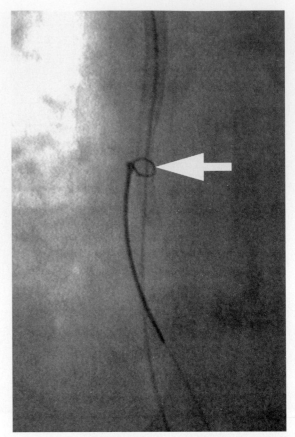

Figure 7-27 A snare can be used to pull a fibrin sheath off a catheter. A guidewire through the catheter was used to guide the snare over the catheter. The snare was tightened to the point where it would slide down the catheter with moderate force, stripping off the fibrin. In this image, the snare (arrow) is almost at the tip of the catheter.

malpositioning, catheter kinking, or catheter fracture (Fig. 7-26). Any patient that complains of pain during injection through a catheter should be evaluated promptly with a chest radiograph followed by injection of contrast through the catheter. In the majority of patients, catheter malfunction can be managed with a simple algorithm involving administration of thrombolytic agents, mechanical stripping of the fibrin from the catheter, or catheter replacement (Fig. 7-27 and Box 7-11). When the cause is central venous thrombosis, thrombolysis through the catheter followed by anticoagulation may restore function. Catheters that have migrated into unsatisfactory locations can be repositioned with percutaneous techniques, but frequently return to the poor position. Revision or replacement of the catheter is usually necessary. Tunneled catheters that have no outward signs of infection can usually be replaced over a guidewire through the original tunnel. There are no proven preventative measures for catheter malfunction, but new strategies such as

low-molecular-weight heparin, weekly catheter flushes with a thrombolytic agent, or catheters coated with sheath-inhibiting drugs may reduce this problem.

Thrombosis of the access vein may be asymptomatic, but can cause pain at the insertion site, and limb swelling if an arm vein has been used. Catheter-related central venous thrombosis can be a source of pulmonary emboli. In most cases the catheter is still fully functional unless the thrombus extends to centrally to the catheter tip. Whenever possible, the catheter should be left in place while the thrombosis is treated with anticoagulation, unless the patient no longer requires venous access.

Catheter fracture is extremely rare owing to the durability of silicone and polyurethane. When fracture occurs it is frequently due to unusual stress upon the catheter. "Pinch-off" syndrome, in which a catheter is compressed between bony or ligamentous structures, predisposes to catheter fracture (Fig. 7-28). This occurs most often with blind subclavian vein puncture when the catheter enters

---

Box 7-11   Management of the Malfunctioning Catheter

Check catheter position on chest radiograph
Fill catheter with small dose thrombolytic agent (e.g., tPA 1-2 mg, urokinase 5000 U)
Check catheter function after 30-60 minutes
If no change, repeat dose of thrombolytic agent
Check catheter function after 30-60 minutes
If no change, obtain contrast study of catheter:
- For extensive fibrin sheath, infuse thrombolytic agent for 4-8 hours (e.g., t-PA 1 mg/h, urokinase 50,000 U/h). Should this fail, consider stripping with snare, or catheter exchange over a guidewire. Balloon may be used to disrupt sheath
- For central venous thrombosis, infuse thrombolytic agent through catheter for 8-12 hours
- For catheter malpositioning, reposition catheter tip or replace. Tip must be in high right atrium at end of procedure

---

the vein under the clavicle from an inferior approach. The extravascular portion of the catheter is subject to compression and shearing between the 1st rib and the clavicle.

Infection of a venous access device may range from purulence at the tunnel or port pocket to fever with no other obvious cause. The latter scenario is the most difficult to manage, as the catheter is often presumed to be the culprit without proof. This can lead to repeated catheter removals and insertions. Culturing the catheter tip may provide an answer, but usually the patient is already on antibiotics. Removal is rarely an emergency procedure unless the patient is neutropenic or septic. Whenever feasible, the patient should be afebrile for 48 hours with negative blood cultures after removal of a presumed infected device before reinsertion.

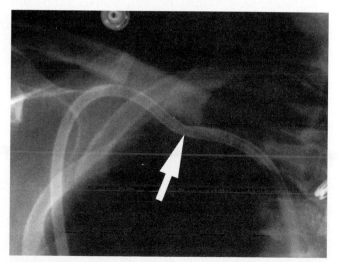

Figure 7-28   Pinch-off syndrome. Compression (arrow) of a 16-Fr catheter between the clavicle and the 1st rib. Ultimately this will lead to catheter fracture with central embolization of the distal fragment. The catheter was removed and replaced through the right IJV.

Device Removal

Removal of venous access devices is part of the responsibility of insertion. Catheters containing concentrated heparin, such as dialysis catheters, should be aspirated before manipulation to avoid inadvertent injection of a large bolus of heparin. Patients with central venous catheters should be placed flat in the supine position for the removal procedure. Non-tunneled catheters can be removed by compressing over the skin entry site and gently pulling the catheter. Tunneled catheters that have been in place for less than 2 weeks can removed in a similar fashion. Cuffed tunneled catheters that have been in place for more than 2 weeks have usually become incorporated into the soft tissues unless the tunnel is infected. The cuff should be identified and the area around it infiltrated with local anesthetic. When the cuff is close to the skin exit site a blunt instrument can be used to free the cuff. Occasionally a small incision directly over the cuff is necessary. Overaggressive traction can cause catheter fracture in the tunnel. Immediate pressure should be applied over the tunnel when this occurs to prevent air embolism or excessive blood loss. After catheter removal, pressure should be held over the exit site for 5 minutes. The skin exit site can be closed with a steri-strip or simply covered with a small sterile dressing. The device should be inspected to ensure that it has been removed in one piece.

To remove a noninfected port, the area around the device is extensively infiltrated with local anesthetic. Incision through the scar from the insertion may be desirable cosmetically, but usually makes the dissection more difficult. Incision directly over the upper edge of the pocket provides ready access to the port. Once the pocket has been entered, fibrotic bands that have formed through suture holes on the port are broken, freeing the device. Careful control of the catheter is necessary at all times to prevent accidental detachment during removal. The pocket should be closed in layers unless infection is suspected. Infected pockets should be packed with sterile gauze with daily changes, allowing healing by secondary intention.

PERMANENT DIALYSIS ACCESS

Over 250,000 patients are on permanent hemodialysis in the United States. Goals for optimized care of these patients have been formulated by the National Kidney Foundation (NKF) and disseminated as the Dialysis Outcomes Quality Initiative (DOQI guidelines). This is a living public document that can be accessed electronically through the NKF website. A major goal of the document is improvement of the outcomes of dialysis access.

Venous catheters do not provide reliable long-term access owing to infection and malfunction rates. Permanent access for dialysis is usually accomplished by surgical creation of an arteriovenous fistula or interposition of a short bridge of synthetic vascular graft material between an artery and vein in a superficial location (Box 7-12 and Fig. 7-29). The anastomoses are usually end-to-side for both fistulas and bridge grafts to preserve the continuity of the native vessels. Grafts are typically polytetrafluorethylene (PTFE) material, 6 mm in diameter and 6–12 cm in length in the forearm.

Fistulas have a superior longevity in comparison to bridge grafts (85% vs 50% patency at 2 years), but require several months for the veins to enlarge sufficiently to accommodate the large needles and flow rates used during dialysis. As many as 30% of fistulas fail to mature or

Box 7-12   Surgical Dialysis Access

Arteriovenous Fistula
Radial artery to cephalic vein at wrist
Brachial artery to antecubital, cephalic, or transposed
    basilic vein in forearm

Bridge Grafts
Forearm:
    Radial to antecubital, basilic, or brachial vein
        straight/curved
    Brachial artery to antecubital, basilic, or brachial vein
        loop
Upper arm:
    Brachial artery to brachial or axillary vein
        straight/curved
    Axillary artery to axillary vein loop
Leg:
    Femoral artery to saphenous or femoral vein loop
Chest:
    Axillary artery to contralateral axillary vein
    (necklace)

thrombose acutely. Conventional and MR venography can be useful to evaluate the upper-extremity veins prior to creation of the fistula. Once established, fistulas can maintain patency despite flow rates as low as 80 mL/min. Late failures occur most often due to venous outflow stenosis or, less often, anastomotic stenoses. Bridge grafts can be accessed sooner after creation than fistulas, but are more prone to development of stenoses at the venous anastomosis and in the outflow veins. Stenosis at the arterial anastomosis occurs in fewer than 4% of patients. Bridge grafts require flow rates >450 mL/min to prevent thrombosis. A healthy surgical dialysis access has a strong pulse throughout its course with a palpable thrill at the arterial anastomosis. The pressure within the graft just distal to the arterial anastomosis usually falls to one-half the systemic arterial pressure.

Venous stenoses in the dialysis access patients are usually fibrotic, hyperplastic, and elastic lesions. The increased flow and pressure in the veins that results from arterial shunting is believed to contribute to formation of these lesions. Central stenoses are typically the sequelae of prior central venous catheterization (see Figs. 7-5 and 7-22).

The most common acute complications of surgical creation of dialysis access are thrombosis or inadequate flow rates. The cause is usually an unrecognized venous outflow obstruction, but may also be arterial inflow disease or a technical error. Surgical thrombectomy and revision is the appropriate treatment, although venography may be useful to delineate venous anatomy. During the life of the dialysis access, thrombosis and inadequate flow rates account for over 85% of all complications. The remainder includes infection (higher with PTFE grafts than AVFs), pseudoaneurysm formation, and steal syndrome. The latter occurs in up to 5% of patients, usually in diabetics, most commonly with dialysis grafts, and twice as often with upper- rather than lower-arm grafts (Fig. 7-30). Symptoms may occur immediately or months later, and vary from a cool extremity to digital ischemia. Correction of inflow arterial stenoses, ligation of the access, bypass of the arterial anastomosis, or occlusion of the artery distal to the access may be necessary.

Both fistulas and bridge grafts are accessed for dialysis by inserting a large-bore needle in the vein or graft close to the arterial anastomosis and the other in a more central location in a dilated vein (fistulas), or close to the venous anastomosis of the graft. Blood is aspirated from the first (termed "arterial") needle and returned through the second (termed "venous") needle. Inability to aspirate blood at a satisfactory flow rate indicates an inflow problem such as stenosis at the arterial anastomosis or, less often, a stenosis in the native artery proximal to the access. Low pressures in both the arterial and venous needles have the same implication. When excessive pressure is required to return blood through the venous needle, or clearance of metabolites is very slow, a venous

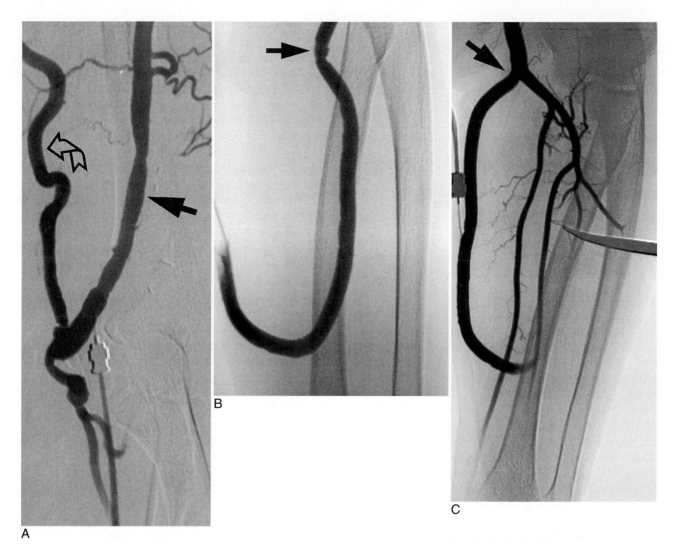

Figure 7-29   Permanent surgical dialysis access. **A,** Arm fistula: brachial artery to cephalic vein. The venous outflow was compressed with a clamp during contrast injection, allowing visualization of the vein (straight arrow) and inflow artery (curved arrow). **B,** Forearm bridge graft. Injection of contrast without occlusion of venous outflow shows the venous anastomosis (arrow). **C,** Contrast injection in the same graft with compression of the outflow with a clamp shows the arterial anastomosis (arrow) and a portion of the arterial inflow.

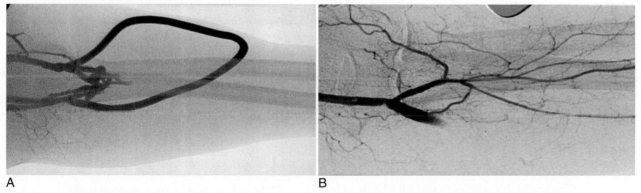

Figure 7-30   Patient with hand ischemia developing several months after placement of a bridge graft. Symptoms are worse during dialysis. **A,** Angiogram showing a patent bridge graft, but no visible distal runoff. **B,** Angiogram with compression of the venous outflow shows opacification of forearm arteries.

Table 7-5 Surgical Dialysis Access Parameters

Parameter	Value
Maximum flow rate bridge graft	800 mL/min
Maximum flow rate forearm fistula	300 mL/min
Maximum flow rate upper arm fistula	1000 mL/min
Indicators of venous outflow stenosis (grafts):	
Intraaccess flow measurements	<600 mL/min or decreased by 25%
Venous pressure[a] at flow rate of 200 mL/min	>125 mmHg
Ratio of venous to systemic arterial pressure[b]	>0.4

[a] Pressure measured in dialysis needle returning blood to patient during dialysis.
[b] Baseline venous pressure in dialysis access compared to ipsilateral upper arm cuff pressure.

outflow lesion may be present (Table 7-5). Complete absence of a pulse in a surgical dialysis access usually indicates thrombosis. Screening of dialysis access to detect correctable lesions before thrombosis by physical examination and careful analysis of flow parameters during dialysis allows early intervention, but may not ultimately prolong the life of the access.

Imaging of a patent dialysis access is indicated when flow rates are unsatisfactory, physical examination suggests decreased flow (for example, loss of a palpable thrill), or the patient develops upper-extremity swelling or hand ischemia (Table 7-6). Duplex color-flow US can be used to evaluate the access and upper-extremity veins for stenosis, but it is limited in ability to image the central veins. Imaging with MRA and MRV is used in some centers, as these combined techniques can visualize both the arterial and venous structures.

Conventional venography allows both diagnosis and intervention during the same procedure (see Fig. 7-29). The approach used most widely is to insert a short 18-gauge peripheral intravenous catheter that can accommodate a 0.035-inch guidewire directly into the access with local anesthesia after a standard sterile skin preparation. Aspiration of blood confirms an appropriate location. The needle is generally oriented towards the venous anastomosis (or outflow in the case of a fistula) unless an arterial inflow lesion is suspected. Nonionic contrast is injected by hand (using an extension tubing so the radiologist can stand behind a lead shield) and filmed with DSA technique. Images from the access to the right atrium should be obtained with careful overlap of each field of view. The arterial anastomosis is visualized by injection while obstructing the venous outflow. This allows contrast to reflux into the artery. The hand or arm should be rotated to improve visualization of the anastomosis. Patients do not need immediate dialysis following venography unless volume status is tenuous.

Angioplasty and Stents

The diagnostic examination can be converted to an intervention by exchanging the 18-gauge catheter for a 5- or 6-French sheath over a 0.035-inch guidewire. When the lesion is located in a direction opposite to that of the initial 18-gauge catheter, a second puncture in an appropriate direction is made. The patient should be anticoagulated with 3000–5000 units of heparin. Stenosis of the venous anastomosis of a bridge graft is usually dilated with a 6 or 7-mm diameter balloon (Fig. 7-31). Lesions in outflow veins can be dilated with larger or smaller balloons as appropriate. The use of high-pressure balloons

Table 7-6 Venography of Surgical Dialysis Access

Indication	Technique	Imaging Goals
Access planning	Venogram from dorsum of hand	Document patency of upper-extremity veins from forearm to right atrium
Malfunctioning but patent dialysis access	Venogram from access; include view of arterial anastomosis	Localize and correct stenotic lesions in inflow and outflow from arterial anastomosis to right atrium
Thrombosed dialysis access	5-Fr catheter from access into patent outflow veins; injection in access after declotting	Prior to declotting, document absence of thrombus in outflow veins; following declotting, identify and correct stenotic lesions in access or at anastomoses
Upper-extremity swelling with patent dialysis access	Venogram from access	Localize and correct obstruction of outflow from upper-extremity veins to right atrium
Upper-extremity ischemia with patent dialysis access	5-Fr catheter retrograde from access to aortic arch, or from femoral arterial access	Aortic arch injection to show subclavian artery origin, selective injection upper extremity arteries, and injection with obstruction of venous outflow to visualize arteries distal to access

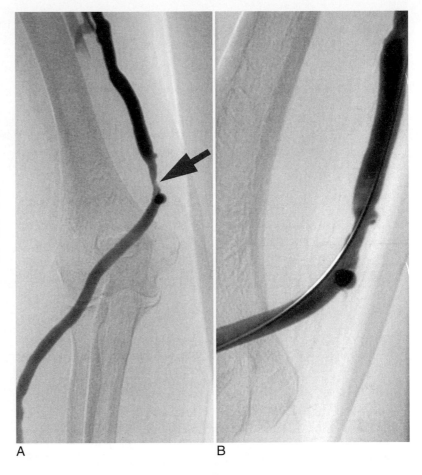

Figure 7-31   Angioplasty of a venous anastomotic stenosis. **A,** Digital angiogram showing stenosis (arrow) at the anastomosis with the basilic vein. **B,** Postangioplasty venogram showing improved caliber of the lumen. The thrill returned in the graft, and the patient resumed successful dialysis. In dialysis angioplasty, good is often good enough.

A   B

(15-20 atmospheres or more), or a cutting balloon, may be necessary to successfully dilate these fibrotic lesions. Multiple, slow, and prolonged (5 minutes or more) inflations may be required to prevent recoil. Patients may experience considerable pain during angioplasty. Inflow lesions in the forearm arteries can be angioplastied with 0.018-inch based systems. Lesions in the venous anastomosis or outflow veins that do not respond to angioplasty can be treated with a cutting balloon, metallic stent, short stent-graft, or surgical revision (when accessible). Central venous stenoses or occlusions should be angioplastied first, with stents reserved for recurrences or inadequate acute results (Fig. 7-32). In most instances self-expanding rather than balloon-expandable stents are used. Arterial inflow lesions that cannot be dilated are usually managed with surgical revision. The endpoints of these procedures are restoration of a palpable thrill and pulse in the access, improved intra-graft flow rates, or a venous to brachial artery pressure ratio less than 0.4.

Removal of the sheaths can be safely performed while the patient is still anticoagulated. Gentle compression or a cerclage suture can be used to obtain hemostasis (Fig. 7-33). When a suture is placed, the patient should be instructed to return for removal before the next dialysis session.

Satisfactory dialysis can be achieved after intervention in 90-95% of patients. Stenoses at the bridge-graft venous anastomoses recur within 6 months after angioplasty in at least 50% of patients. The results of angioplasty and stents in lesions within the outflow veins are slightly better, approaching 60% primary patency at 6 months (Table 7-7).

The acute complications of angioplasty and stent placement in dialysis access include thrombosis, dissection, and rupture (Fig. 7-34). Acute thrombosis responds well to pharmacologic or mechanical thrombectomy

Table 7-7   Outcomes of Venous Angioplasty/Stents in Dialysis Access

Outcome	Percent
Technical success angioplasty	90
Technical success stents	95
Primary patency venous angioplasty at 6 months	65
Primary patency venous angioplasty at 12 months	30
Primary patency stents at 12 months	50

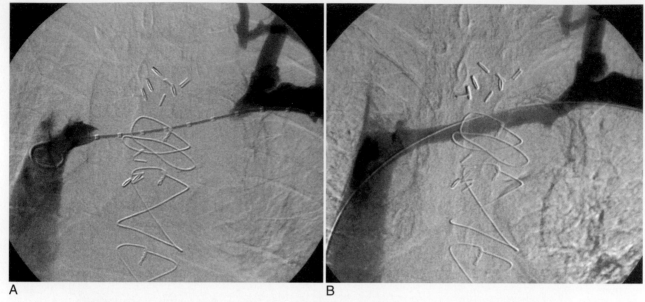

Figure 7-32   Patient with a left forearm dialysis fistula and high venous pressures at dialysis. The fistula and veins in the arm were normal, but the brachiocephalic vein was occluded. **A,** Central image showing a measuring catheter in place to determine the length of the occlusion. This aids in selection of a stent. **B,** Digital subtraction venogram after placement of a self-expanding stent due to unsatisfactory result with angioplasty alone.

(see next section). Dissection of a vessel can be managed by prolonged balloon inflation to tack down the flap (with aggressive anticoagulation to prevent thrombosis of the entire access). When this fails, stent placement is usually curative. Rupture of a vessel in the arm can sometimes be treated successfully with 10–15 minutes of manual compression or prolonged balloon inflation across the site of rupture. The vein remains patent, while extravasation ceases. When this technique fails, placement of a bare metal stent across the defect in the vessel wall can stop extravasation, possibly by eliminating any outflow obstruction. Stent-grafts can also be used, particularly for central ruptures.

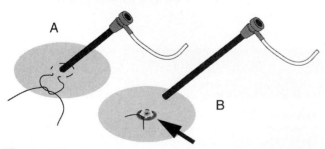

Figure 7-33   Cerclage or "purse-string" suture for removal of sheaths following dialysis intervention. **A,** A monofilament Nylon suture has been placed in the skin around the sheath and a half-hitch thrown. **B,** As the sheath is removed the purse-string is tightened (arrow) to obtain hemostasis.

Management of the Thrombosed Dialysis Access

Acute thrombosis of a mature dialysis access requires urgent, but not emergent intervention. Patients in need of immediate dialysis can be managed with placement of a short-term non-tunneled dialysis catheter. The two basic approaches for declotting a dialysis access are surgical cutdown with extraction of the thrombus with a small balloon catheter, and percutaneous methods. The latter can be accomplished with pharmacological thrombolysis, mechanical thrombolysis, or a combination of both techniques. In all cases, identification of an underlying lesion that predisposed to thrombosis is of paramount importance. Regardless of the technique used to restore patency, thrombosis is associated with a 50–70% rate of irreversible failure of the access within one year.

There are a number of general principles common to all percutaneous declotting techniques (both pharmacologic and mechanical) (Box 7-13). First, bridge grafts are easier to declot than fistulas because the anatomy is straightforward and the thrombus is usually limited to the graft, between the arterial and venous anastomoses. The anatomy of dialysis fistulas is less predictable, and the presence of multiple side-branches may complicate the declotting procedure. Second, grafts and fistulas almost always thrombose due to a stenotic lesion; the goal of the declotting procedure is to find and treat this lesion. Third, there is always a hard plug of white thrombus (platelets and fibrin)

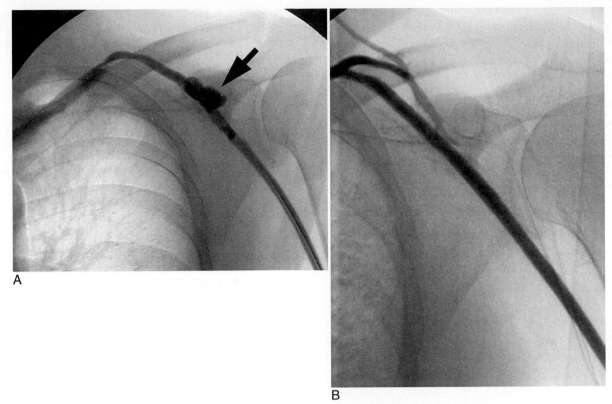

Figure 7-34   Vein rupture during angioplasty of stenotic venous outflow in a dialysis patient. **A,** Venogram after angioplasty shows vein rupture and a pseudoaneurysm (arrow). Reversal of heparin, prolonged balloon inflations across the rupture, and manual compression failed and the patient developed an expanding hematoma. **B,** Venogram after placement of a stent-graft across the rupture site. Flow in the graft remains excellent 6 months after placement of the stent-graft.

Box 7-13   Common Principles of Dialysis Declot Procedures

Do not perform procedure in patients with
- Known central right-to-left shunts
- Limited pulmonary reserve
- Severe pulmonary hypertension or right heart failure
- Dialysis access infection
- Emergent need for immediate dialysis

Determine type of access from history or records

Localize all anastomoses

Examine access for pulse, thrill, aneurysm, and evidence of infection

Use sterile technique

Anticoagulate patient with 3000–5000 units heparin during procedure

Use low-pressure injections in clotted access

Avoid CO_2 gas as contrast agent

Document patency of central veins before restoring flow

Identify and correct stenotic lesions after declotting

Keep your hands out of the x-ray beam

Use careful radiation protection measures

---

at the arterial anastomosis, whereas thrombus in the access and at the venous end is soft and red (full of red blood cells). Fourth, when puncturing a clotted dialysis access dark blood or no blood may be aspirated. A small, very low-pressure injection of contrast can be used to document correct position of the needle. A large or forceful injection should be avoided, as this may cause reflux of thrombus into the arterial circulation and an ischemic hand. Fifth, the venous system central to the dialysis access must be patent before embarking on a declotting procedure. This can be easily determined by advancing a short 5-French catheter centrally from the clotted access while injecting contrast until patent veins are found. Lastly, declotting procedures should not be performed in patients with suspected graft infection, severely limited cardiac reserve (as small asymptomatic pulmonary emboli are common during the procedure), or known central right-to-left shunts (due to the risk of paradoxical embolism).

Pharmacologic Thrombolysis

There are many techniques described for pharmacologic thrombolysis of dialysis access, but the two most popular are "pulse-spray" and "lyse-and-wait". (See Box 4-13.) These two techniques are preferred because they are the quickest. The pulse spray technique, described by Bookstein, is a pharmaco-mechanical process in which a specially design 5-French multiple-sidehole catheter is inserted into the thrombosed portion of the dialysis access through a 5- or 6-French sheath and small aliquots of a thrombolytic agent are forcefully injected using a 1-mL Luer-lock syringe (see Fig. 4-24). The jets of fluid exiting the side-holes act to fragment the thrombus, while the thrombolytic agent induces fibrinolysis. Two catheters are used, each inserted pointing towards the opposite anastomosis (Fig. 7-35). This allows lytic agent to be deposited along the entire length of the access. The catheters cross at the midpoint of the access, and the tips can be positioned beyond the entry site of the opposing catheter. Injection of small amounts of contrast during

the process is used to assess progress. Once satisfactory lysis has been achieved (the definition of this varies, but generally indicates substantial reduction of the volume of thrombus), the venous anastomosis is angioplastied, usually with a balloon sized to the bridge graft (typically 6-mm diameter). This relieves any potential outflow obstruction. The arterial anastomosis is cleared by pulling the plug into the access with a 4- to 5-mm Fogarty balloon. This is accomplished by advancing the deflated balloon through the arterial anastomosis, over a guidewire, and then withdrawing the gently inflated balloon into the access. Any arterial inflow obstruction can then be angioplastied.

The "lyse-and-wait" technique, described by Cynamon, varies from the pulse-spray in that the thrombolytic agent is introduce into the thrombus approximately 15–30 minutes before the procedure is initiated (Box 7-14). A thrombolytic agent is mixed to a total volume of 7–10 mL. An 18- to 22-gauge intravenous catheter is inserted into the access as close to the arterial anastomosis as possible pointing towards the venous outflow. The arterial anastomosis and venous anastomosis of bridge grafts should be compressed while the thrombolytic agent is slowly injected. This prevents reflux of thrombus into the arterial supply as well as trapping the lytic agent in the dialysis access. The catheter is then capped for 15–30 minutes (longer with urokinase, shorter with t-PA, r-PA, or other newer thrombolytic drugs). A small amount of contrast is then injected to determine the extent of thrombolysis. Typically, the

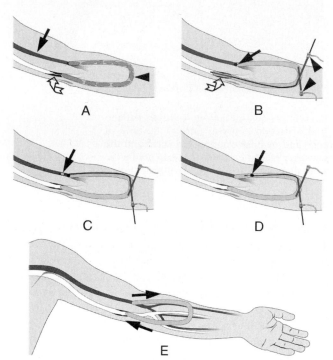

Figure 7-35 Basic elements of restoring flow in a thrombosed bridge graft. **A,** Thrombosis of a synthetic dialysis graft from the brachial artery to basilic vein. (Arrow = brachial artery, curved arrow = basilic vein with intimal hyperplasia at anastomosis, arrowhead = thrombosed graft). **B,** Sheaths have been placed (arrowheads) to allow access to both the arterial and venous anastomoses; a diagnostic venogram was performed through a 5-Fr catheter advanced beyond the venous anastomosis to confirm patent outflow veins, and the thrombus in the graft was then thrombolysed. At this point, a 6-mm × 2-cm angioplasty balloon is used to dilate the region of the venous anastomosis (curved arrow), opening the outflow. Note the platelet plug (straight arrow) obstructing flow through the arterial anastomosis. **C,** A Fogarty-type balloon (arrow) is advanced past the platelet plug and gently inflated in the brachial artery. **D,** As the balloon is withdrawn into the graft, the plug (arrow) is pulled with it, restoring inflow. **E,** The graft is now patent. Arrows show the direction of flow.

Box 7-14   "Lyse and Wait" Technique for Dialysis Access Declot

Insert 18- to 22-gauge intravenous catheter into access in direction of venous outflow
Compress arterial and venous anastomosis (bridge graft)
Compress arterial anastomosis and distal extent of palpable thrombosed vein (fistula)
Inject thrombolytic agent slowly:
• Urokinase 250,000 U plus 5000 units heparin (total volume 6 mL)
• t-PA 5 mg (total volume 5 mL)
• r-PA 5 U plus 5000 units heparin (total volume 6 mL)
Wait for:
• 30–60 minutes urokinase
• 15–30 minutes t-PA, r-PA
Exchange intravenous catheter for 5- to 6-French sheath
Angioplasty venous outflow stenosis
Insert 5- to 6-French sheath in direction towards arterial anastomosis
Dislodge arterial plug

thrombolysis within the bridge graft or fistula is complete with the exception of the arterial plug and venous anastomosis. The intravenous catheter is then exchanged over a guidewire for a 5- or 6-French sheath for intervention on the venous outflow. A second sheath is inserted in the direction of the arterial anastomosis for dislodgement of the arterial plug.

Pharmacologic thrombolysis techniques are successful in restoring patency of bridge grafts in over 90% of patients. Intervention is almost universally required, usually for an outflow lesion. Rethrombosis occurs within 6 months in over 50% of bridge grafts and 30% of fistulas.

Percutaneous Mechanical Thrombectomy

There are a number of mechanical thrombectomy devices available (see Fig. 4-25 and Table 7-8). Each is based upon a different mechanical principle, with the common goal of fragmenting the thrombus into pieces small enough that they can be either released into the systemic circulation or removed through the device. The purpose of these devices is to rapidly declot the graft without the need for a thrombolytic agent. The arterial and venous anastomoses are still managed with balloons, in the same way as during pharmacologic thrombolysis. Patients should be adequately heparinized during the procedure to prevent rethrombosis before outflow and inflow are restored.

Mechanical thrombectomy devices are inserted into the thrombosed graft following the same principles as thrombolysis catheters. The status of the central venous outflow is documented at the beginning of the procedure prior to initiating thrombectomy. The sheath requirements for each device should be carefully checked to ensure compatibility. Some devices can be utilized over a guidewire, whereas others do not have this capability. Not all devices are approved for use in native vessels, so the anatomy of the graft should be well understood before inserting the device. The duration of activation of the device must be carefully monitored, as the mechanical elements may fracture with prolonged use, or cause clinically significant hemolysis. Overall procedural times are shorter with mechanical rather than pharmacologic thrombolysis. The success rates and

Table 7-9 Procedural Complications of Percutaneous Declotting Procedures

Complication	Incidence
Immediate thrombosis	5%
Vein rupture (usually peripheral)	2%
Arterial embolization	2%
Pseudoaneurysm (immediate and delayed)	1%
Infection	<1%

Adapted from Aruny JE et al. J Vasc Interv Radiol 10:419-498, 1999.

outcomes of mechanical thrombectomy in bridge grafts are similar to pharmacologic thrombolysis.

Complications of Dialysis Access Declotting

Complications of thrombolysis and mechanical declotting procedures are similar (Table 7-9). Arterial embolization due to reflux of thrombus can be successfully managed with percutaneous methods, such as withdrawing the embolus into the dialysis access with a Fogarty balloon or thrombolysis, but surgical embolectomy may be necessary (Fig. 7-36). Lethal complications are rare, but can occur, usually due to pulmonary embolization in patients with limited pulmonary arterial reserve.

PRIMARY HYPERPARATHYROIDISM

The clinical features of hyperparathyroidism are discussed in Chapter 6 (see Box 6-9). Venous sampling is indicated in patients with persistent primary hyperparathyroidism following neck exploration. Venous sampling is usually performed following unsuccessful localization by angiography.

The technique of venous sampling ideally involves selection of the superior, middle, and inferior thyroid, thymic, and vertebral veins, as well as a peripheral vein. However, many of the thyroidal veins may have been ligated during surgery, and the anatomy is highly variable. Samples from multiple levels in the brachiocephalic vein, IJV, and SVC are generally easier to obtain and allow lateralization of the adenoma. An angled 5-French catheter with an added side-hole at the tip, such as a Davis, can be used with an angled 0.038-inch hydrophilic guidewire to select these veins. Crossing the valve at the junction of the IJV and subclavian vein can be difficult. Having the patient inhale, turn the head, or shrug can open the valve. Test injection of contrast confirms the identity of the vein before sampling. Careful labeling and

Table 7-8 Mechanical Thrombectomy Device Principles

Principle	Examples
Fragmentation	Rotating baskets; brushes; vortex
Venturi effect	Saline jets directed into catheters
Aspiration	Reciprocating clot spoon

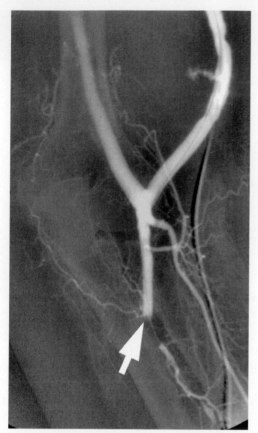

Figure 7-36 Brachial artery embolus (arrow) during declotting of a dialysis graft. The embolus was successfully treated with catheter-directed thrombolysis.

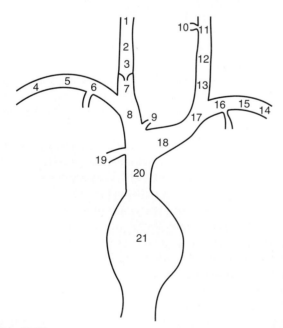

Figure 7-37 Diagram of the venous samples obtained in a patient with failed surgical localization of a parathyroid adenoma. Precise labeling and recording of sampling locations is critical.

recording of each sample is critical (Fig. 7-37). Samples are analyzed for parathyroid hormone (PTH).

Venous sampling is successful in lateralizing an adenoma in approximately 80% of cases. A ratio of at least 2:1 compared to a peripheral vein sample is considered diagnostic.

SUGGESTED READINGS

Allon M, Bailey R, Ballard R et al: A multidisciplinary approach to hemodialysis access: prospective evaluation. *Kidney Int* 53:473–479, 1998.

Aruny JE, Lewis CA, Cardella JF et al. Quality improvement guidelines for percutaneous management of the thrombosed or dysfunctional dialysis access. *J Vasc Interv Radiol* 10: 491-498, 1999.

Bern MM, Lokich JJ, Wallach SR et al: Very low doses of warfarin can prevent thrombosis in central venous catheters: a randomized prospective trial. *Ann Intern Med* 112: 423–428, 1990.

Borsa JJ, Patel NH: The venous system: normal developmental anatomy and congenital anomalies. *Semin Interv Radiol* 18: 69–82, 2001.

Burkhart HM, Cikrit DF: Arteriovenous fistulae for hemodialysis. *Semin Vasc Surg* 10:162–165, 1997.

Clark TW, Hirsch DA, Jindal KJ et al: Outcome and prognostic factors of restenosis after percutaneous treatment of native hemodialysis fistulas. *J Vasc Interv Radiol* 13:51-59, 2002.

Cynamon J, Lakritz P, Wahl S et al: Hemodialysis graft declotting: description of the "lyse and wait" technique. *J Vasc Interv Radiol* 8:925-929, 1997.

Falk A, Mitty H, Guller J et al: Thrombolysis of clotted hemodialysis grafts with tissue-type plasminogen activator. *J Vasc Interv Radiol* 12:305–311, 2001.

Ferral H, Bjarnason H, Wholey M et al: Recanalization of occluded veins to provide access for central catheter placement. *J Vasc Interv Radiol* 7:681–685, 1996.

Gray RJ, Sacks D, Martin LG et al: Reporting standards for percutaneous interventions in dialysis access. Technology Assessment Committee. *J Vasc Interv Radiol* 10:1405-1415, 1999.

Hingorani A, Ascher E, Hanson J et al: Upper-extremity versus lower extremity deep venous thrombosis. *Am J Surg* 174: 214-217, 1997.

Kaufman JA, Kazanjian SA, Rivitz SM et al: Long-term central venous catheterization in patients with limited access. *Am J Roentgenol* 167:1327-1333, 1996.

Kearns AE, Thompson GB: Medical and surgical management of hyperparathyroidism. *Mayo Clin Proc* 77:87-91, 2002.

Kidney DD, Nguyen DT, Deutsch LS: Radiologic evaluation and management of malfunctioning long-term central vein catheters. *Am J Roentgenol* 171:1251-1257, 1998.

Kinney TB, Valji K, Rose SC et al: Pulmonary embolism from pulse-spray pharmacomechanical thrombolysis of clotted hemodialysis grafts: urokinase versus heparinized saline. *J Vasc Interv Radiol* 11:1143-1152, 2000.

Kreienberg PB, Chang BB, Darling RC et al: Long-term results in patients treated with thrombolysis, thoracic inlet decompression, and subclavian vein stenting for Paget–Schroetter syndrome. *J Vasc Surg* 33: S100–S105, 2001.

Kroencke TJ, Taupitz M, Arnold R et al: Three-dimensional gadolinium-enhanced magnetic resonance venography in suspected thrombo-occlusive disease of the central chest veins. *Chest* 120:1570–1576, 2001.

Laissy JP, Fernandez P, Karila-Cohen P et al: Upper limb vein anatomy before hemodialysis fistula creation: cross-sectional anatomy using MR venography. *Eur Radiol* 13:256–261, 2003.

Lau TN, Kinney TB: Direct US-guided puncture of the innominate veins for central venous access. *J Vasc Interv Radiol* 12: 641–645, 2001.

Lawler LP, Fishman EK: Multi-detector row CT of thoracic disease with emphasis on 3D volume rendering and CT angiography. *Radiographics* 21:1257–1273, 2001.

Lewis CA, Allen TE, Burke DR et al: Quality improvement guidelines for central venous access. The Standards of Practice Committee of the Society of Cardiovascular & Interventional Radiology. *J Vasc Interv Radiol* 8:475–479, 1997.

Lundell C, Kadir S: Upper-extremity veins. In Kadir S ed: *Atlas of Normal and Angiographic Anatomy*, WB Saunders, Philadelphia, 1991.

Lundell C, Kadir S: Superior vena cava and thoracic veins. In Kadir S ed: *Atlas of Normal and Angiographic Anatomy*, WB Saunders, Philadelphia, 1991.

McGee DC, Gould MK: Preventing complications of central venous catheterization. *N Engl J Med* 348:1123–1133, 2003.

Miller DL, O'Grady NP: Guidelines for the prevention of intravascular catheter-related infections: recommendations relevant to interventional radiology. *J Vasc Interv Radiol* 14(2 Pt 1):133–136, 2003.

Murphy GJ, White SA, Nicholson ML: Vascular access for haemodialysis. *Br J Surg* 87:1300–1315, 2000.

Murray BM, Rajczak S, Ali B; Herman A, Mepani B: Assessment of access blood flow after preemptive angioplasty. *Am J Kidney Dis* 37:1029–1038, 2001.

Namyslowski J, Patel NH: Central venous access: a new task for interventional radiologists. *Cardiovasc Interv Radiol* 22: 355–368, 1999.

Nicholson AA, Ettles DF, Arnold A et al: Treatment of malignant superior vena cava obstruction: metal stents or radiation therapy. *J Vasc Interv Radiol* 8:781–788, 1997.

Ray CE, Shenoy SS, McCarthy PL et al: Weekly prophylactic urokinase instillation in tunneled central venous access devices. *J Vasc Interv Radiol* 10:1330–1334, 1999.

Rutherford RB: Primary subclavian-axillary vein thrombosis: the relative roles of thrombolysis, percutaneous angioplasty, stents, and surgery. *Semin Vasc Surg* 11:91–95, 1998.

Schindler N, Vogelzang RL: Superior vena cava syndrome: experience with endovascular stents and surgical therapy. *Surg Clin N Am* 79:683–694, 1999.

Sharafuddin MJ, Hicks ME: Current status of percutaneous mechanical thrombectomy: I. General principles. *J Vasc Interv Radiol* 8:911–921, 1997.

Sharafuddin MJ, Hicks ME: Current status of percutaneous mechanical thrombectomy: II. Devices and mechanisms of action. *J Vasc Interv Radiol* 9:15–31, 1998.

Sharafuddin MJ, Hicks ME: Current status of percutaneous mechanical thrombectomy: III. Present and future applications. *J Vasc Interv Radiol* 9:209–224, 1998.

Shinde TS, Lee VS, Rofsky NM et al: Three-dimensional gadolinium-enhanced MR venographic evaluation of patency of central veins in the thorax: initial experience. *Radiology* 213:555–560, 1999.

Silberzweig JE, Sacks D, Khorsandi AS et al: Reporting standards for central venous access. *J Vasc Interv Radiol* 11:391–400, 2000.

Sugg SL, Fraker DL, Alexander R et al: Prospective evaluation of selective venous sampling for parathyroid hormone concentration in patients undergoing reoperations for primary hyperparathyroidism. *Surgery* 114:1004–1009, 1993.

Trerotola SO: Hemodialysis catheter placement and management. *Radiology* 215:651–658, 2000.

Valji K, Bookstein JJ, Roberts AC et al: Pulse-spray pharmacomechanical thrombolysis of thrombosed hemodialysis access grafts: long-term experience and comparison of original and current techniques. *Am J Roentgenol* 164:1495–1500, 1995.

Vesely TM, Hovsepian DM, Pilgram TK et al: Upper-extremity central venous obstruction in hemodialysis patients: treatment with wallstents. *Radiology* 204:343–348, 1997.

Vesely TM: Central venous catheter tip position: a continuing controversy. *J Vasc Interv Radiol* 14:527–534, 2003.

Pulmonary Circulation

JOHN A. KAUFMAN, M.D.

The lungs are unique in that they receive output from both ventricles – the entire volume of the right heart and also a small fraction of blood from the left heart via the bronchial arteries. The lungs are the site of oxygenation of venous blood. In addition, the lungs are the venous waste processing plant of the body, routinely trapping and disposing of small bits of venous "trash." The clinical evidence for this is compelling, in that otherwise healthy individuals with intrapulmonary arteriovenous shunts are at high risk for embolic stroke and brain abscess due to paradoxical bland and infectious emboli. Pulmonary arterial imaging and intervention therefore frequently has a clinical impact that extends far beyond the lungs.

ANATOMY

The pulmonary vascular circuit comprises the pulmonary arteries, the alveolar capillary network, and the pulmonary veins. Systemic venous blood exits the heart from the right ventricle through the main pulmonary artery, an anterior intrapericardial structure. After a distance of approximately 3-5 cm, the main pulmonary artery bifurcates into right and left main pulmonary arteries. The right main pulmonary artery crosses to the right hilum posterior to the ascending aorta and superior vena cava (SVC) and anterior to the carina and the esophagus (Fig. 8-1). Within the right hemithorax the artery branches first into upper and lower trunks, and then into segmental vessels that roughly follow the bronchial segments. Beyond this point pulmonary artery anatomy becomes extremely variable. Common variants of the right pulmonary artery include an accessory branch to the posterior segment of the upper lobe from the lower trunk, and two arteries to the middle lobe.

After the bifurcation of the main pulmonary artery, the left main pulmonary artery continues superiorly and posteriorly towards the left hilum for a short distance (see Fig. 8-1). The left pulmonary artery lies anterior to the descending thoracic aorta, in close approximation to the undersurface of the arch. At the hilum, the vessel gives off multiple individual or paired segmental branches to the upper lobe. A single common trunk is seen in fewer than 20% of individuals. The lingula is usually supplied from the descending portion of the left pulmonary artery before it divides into the lower lobe vessels. As with the right pulmonary artery, the division of vessels approximates the segmental bronchial anatomy of the left lung, but is highly variable.

The pulmonary arteries are elastic vessels that contain only small amounts of smooth muscle cells down to the level of fifth-order branches. Conversely, the pulmonary arterioles are very muscular. Because of the elastic nature of the pulmonary arteries and the extensive capillary network, the capacity of this vascular bed is enormous. Normal main pulmonary artery pressures are in the range of 22/8 mmHg, with a mean of 13 mmHg.

The diameter of the individual pulmonary capillaries averages 8-9 μm. The capillary bed is vast (almost 90 square meters), which permits efficient and rapid gas

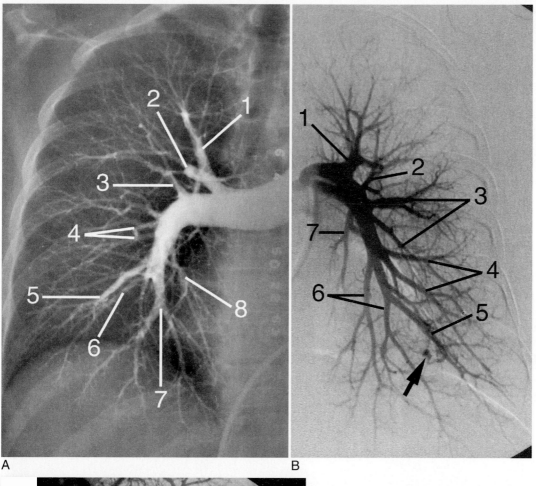

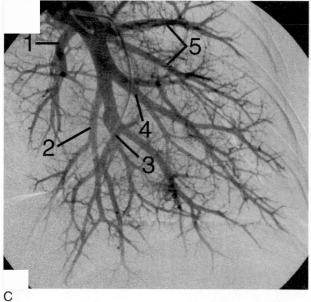

Figure 8-1   Pulmonary artery anatomy as seen on bilateral selective pulmonary angiograms. **A**, Right pulmonary angiogram using cut-film technique: **1**, Apical posterior branch right upper lobe (RUL). **2**, Anterior branch RUL. **3**, Superior branch right lower lobe (RLL). **4**, Middle lobe branches. **5**, Lateral basal branch RLL. **6**, Anterior basal branch RLL. **7**, Posterior basal branch RLL. **8**, Medial basal branch RLL. **B**, Left pulmonary artery using digital subtraction technique: **1**, Apical posterior branch left upper lobe (LUL). **2**, Anterior branch LUL. **3**, Lingular branches. **4**, Anteromedial branch left lower lobe (LLL). **5**, Lateral branch LLL. **6**, Posterior branch LLL. **7**, Superior branch LLL. Arrow = small pulmonary arteriovenous fistula. **C**, Left posterior oblique magnification selective left pulmonary angiogram. The basal vessels are displayed to best advantage in this view. **1**, Superior branch LLL. **2**, Posterior branch LLL. **3**, Lateral branch LLL. **4**, Anteromedial branch LLL. **5**, Lingular branches.

exchange at the alveolar level. This bed also performs another important function – filtration of solid material from the venous blood before it reaches the left side of the heart and the systemic arteries. The small size but immense number of capillaries allows filtration of large quantities of particulate material without compromising gas exchange or blood flow. Active intrinsic thrombolytic and phagocytic systems in the lung rapidly dispose of normal physiologic debris.

Oxygenated blood is returned to the left atrium by the pulmonary veins (Fig. 8-2). Typically, one upper and two lower veins are formed from the segmental veins in each lung. The right pulmonary veins lie inferior to the pulmonary artery and posterior to the SVC. The right middle lobe usually drains into the upper vein, but may empty directly into the left atrium. On the left, the pulmonary veins also lie inferior to the pulmonary artery, and anterior to the descending thoracic aorta. The lingular veins drain with the upper lobe segments. Anomalous venous drainage to the superior vena cava, systemic thoracic veins, or coronary sinus may be found in association with congenital heart disease, pulmonary sequestration, or as an isolated occurrence (Fig. 8-3).

At any point in time, 30% of pulmonary blood is in the arteries, 20% is in the capillaries, and 50% is in the veins. In the supine position the blood volume is relatively evenly distributed between the upper and lower lobes. When upright, the lower lobes are preferentially perfused.

The bronchial arteries, branches of the thoracic aorta, provide blood supply to the airways. Bronchial arteries are normally small vessels that are highly variable in number, but the most common pattern (45%) is two on the left and one on the right (Fig. 8-4). The right bronchial artery arises from a common intercostal trunk in over 70% of individuals, but only 5% of left bronchial arteries have a common origin with an intercostal artery. One quarter of individuals will have single bronchial arteries bilaterally, whereas 30% will have four or more. Right and left bronchial arteries have a common origin in about 40% of individuals (Fig. 8-5). Bronchial arteries usually are located on the anterolateral surface of the thoracic aorta just below the ligamentum arteriosum at the level of the T3–T4 vertebral bodies. Variant sites of origin include the inner surface of the aortic arch (15%), internal mammary, brachiocephalic, inferior thyroidal, and subclavian arteries. Bronchial arteries (especially those on the right) have

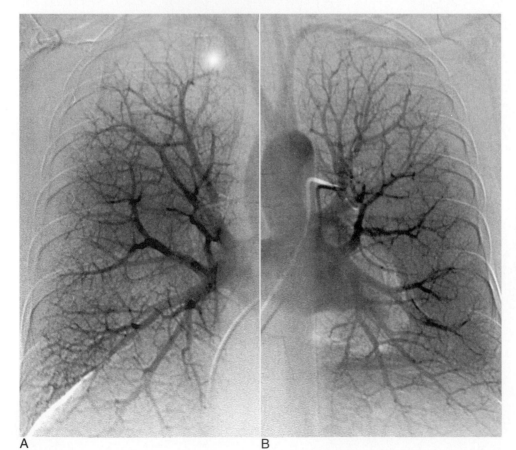

A   B

Figure 8-2 Pulmonary veins seen on the late phase of selective digital subtraction pulmonary angiograms. Note the opacification of the thoracic aorta on both studies. **A**, Right pulmonary veins. **B**, Left pulmonary veins.

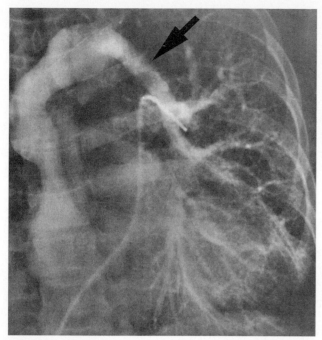

Figure 8-3   Partial anomalous venous return of the left lung demonstrated on late image from cut-film selective left pulmonary angiogram. The pulmonary vein (arrow) draining the left upper lobe and lingula empties directly into the left brachiocephalic vein and then returns to the heart. A pigtail catheter can be seen in the left main pulmonary artery.

communication with the anterior spinal artery in 10% of patients. Anastomoses may also be present with the coronary arteries. The venous drainage of the bronchi is through both the systemic veins of the thorax and the pulmonary veins.

KEY COLLATERAL PATHWAYS

Pulmonary arteries are considered end arteries, in that few normal intrapulmonary anastomoses exist. Proximal occlusion of a pulmonary artery segment usually results in distal infarction of the subtended lung parenchyma. Congenital proximal pulmonary artery obstruction is relieved by flow through a patent ductus arteriosum, as well as the bronchial arteries and other mediastinal arteries. In adults with longstanding acquired pulmonary artery occlusions, reconstitution of peripheral pulmonary arteries by small distal intrapulmonary collaterals can occur. The bronchial arteries provide collateral supply to the lung parenchyma, and can contribute to the pulmonary arterial flow as well (Fig. 8-6). In addition to bronchial arteries, almost every artery that supplies the thorax (including the diaphragm) can provide collateral supply to the lungs. When systemic arteries provide substantial collateral flow to the pulmonary arteries, a measurable left-to-right shunt may develop.

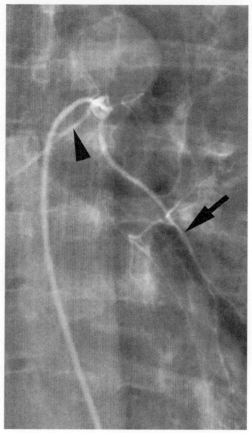

Figure 8-4   Selective left bronchial artery injection showing a normal-caliber vessel (arrow). In this patient, a right bronchial artery branch (arrowhead) arises with the left.

Bronchial arteries and the lung parenchyma have multiple potential sources of collateral supply (Box 8-1). These usually develop in response to increased arterial flow to the lung tissues in patients with chronic pulmonary infections, granulomatous diseases, and tumors,

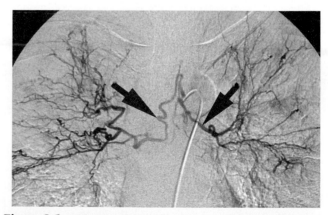

Figure 8-5   Digital subtraction angiogram (DSA) showing conjoint origin of hypertrophied right and left bronchial arteries (arrows) in a patient with cystic fibrosis (compare to Fig. 8-4).

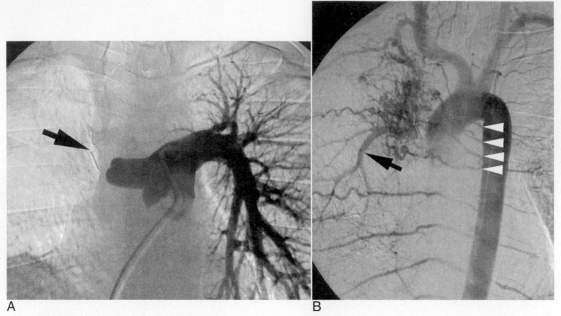

A   B

Figure 8-6   Systemic to pulmonary artery collateralization due to iatrogenic pulmonary artery occlusion following right upper lobectomy for chronic inflammation. **A**, Main pulmonary angiogram showing occlusion of the right pulmonary artery. Note the surgical clip in the right hilum (arrow). **B**, Aortogram showing numerous bronchial and intercostal arteries (arrowheads) supplying hypervascular lung tissue and reconstituting the pulmonary artery (arrow).

as well as in congenital pulmonary or acquired pulmonary artery obstruction (Fig. 8-7). Knowledge of these collateral pathways becomes important during interventions for bronchial artery bleeding. Successful occlusion of the bronchial arteries may fail to control bleeding in patients with well-developed collaterals.

IMAGING

Pulmonary Circulation

The optimum imaging modality for the pulmonary vasculature depends on the clinical question, the vessels

---

Box 8-1   Sources of Potential Collateral Supply to Bronchial Arteries

Intercostal arteries
Branches of the subclavian artery
   Thyrocervical trunk
   Internal mammary artery
   Lateral thoracic artery
   Long thoracic artery
Phrenic arteries
Coronary arteries

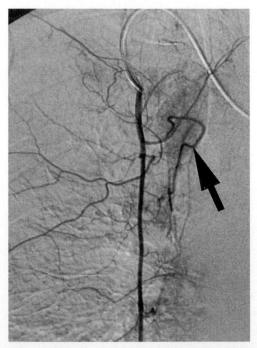

Figure 8-7   Collateral supply to the bronchial circulation in a patient with cystic fibrosis (see Fig. 8-5). Selective right internal mammary artery DSA showing an enlarged branch (arrow) to the lung parenchyma.

of interest, available technology, and available technique. There is no consensus on the optimum modality, although each has major advantages and some disadvantages.

Helical CT of the pulmonary arteries provides fast, accurate, and comprehensive imaging. A noncontrast scan should be obtained first, followed by a breath-hold thin-section (1–3 mm) contrast-enhanced scan. The scan delay should be short (5–10 seconds) so that opacification of pulmonary arteries is optimized (Fig. 8-8). When possible, injection of contrast through a peripheral vein in the right upper extremity minimizes artifact from dense contrast in the brachiocephalic vein. Power injection of 80–120 mL of contrast at 3–5 mL/s is crucial to obtain satisfactory images. Streak artifact from contrast in the SVC can interfere with evaluation of the main right pulmonary artery (see Fig. 3-21). The proximal pulmonary arteries can be reliably depicted with single-detector CTA, although subsegmental arteries can be difficult to interpret unless a multidetector (four or more) scanner is used. Delayed scans can be useful when evaluating pulmonary veins and vascular masses.

Careful postprocessing on an independent workstation facilitates inspection of the pulmonary vasculature. One of the great advantages of CT is the vast amount of additional information about the lung parenchyma, mediastinal structures, and thoracic arteries that can be acquired by simply viewing the same data at different window levels. Patients with suspected pulmonary arterial pathology often have alternate thoracic disease processes that explain or contribute to their symptoms.

Pulmonary arterial MRA requires contrast enhancement with gadolinium in order to obtain satisfactory images (Fig. 8-9). The surrounding aerated lung and cardiac motion limits conventional spin-echo images to evaluation of the central pulmonary arteries. The intrinsic black-blood nature of these images is useful for depiction of central vascular tumors or thrombi. Acquisition times for conventional time-of-flight (TOF) angiographic techniques are too long, and signal loss from in-plane flow is problematic. The most promising techniques are breath-hold fast 3-dimensional (3-D) gradient echo sequences with bolus injection of gadolinium. Ultra-fast scanners

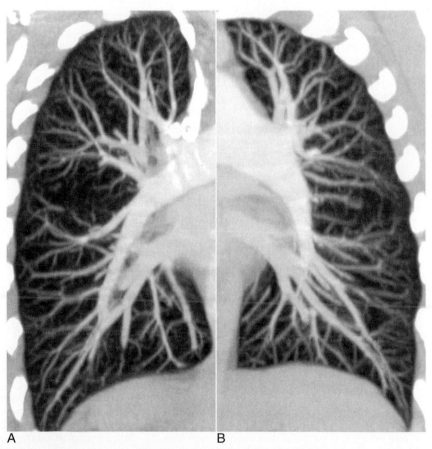

A   B

Figure 8-8   Pulmonary CT angiogram (16 detector row) displayed as thick coronal maximum-intensity projections (MIPs) showing the level of detail that can be obtained. These views exclude some of the pulmonary artery branches, and include pulmonary veins. **A**, Right pulmonary artery. **B**, Left pulmonary artery.

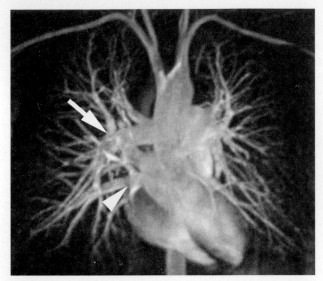

Figure 8-9   Pulmonary artery MR angiogram using gadolinium-enhanced 3-D acquisition displayed as a coronal MIP projection. The pulmonary artery (arrow) and veins (arrowhead) are visualized, as well as the thoracic aorta. (Courtesy of Barry Stein M.D., Hartford Hospital, CT.)

MRA is the poor discrimination of small peripheral vessels with current technology.

Catheter angiography remains the most accurate modality for imaging the peripheral pulmonary arterial circulation. Selective pulmonary arteriography with a pigtail catheter and low-osmolar contrast agents is more invasive than either CT or MR, but safe and definitive in experienced hands.

Pulmonary angiography can be performed from either the femoral (most commonly) or jugular venous approach. Nonselective injection of contrast into the vena cava, right atrium, or main pulmonary artery usually does not provide satisfactory visualization of the peripheral pulmonary vessels and requires very large volumes of contrast. Selective pulmonary angiography is safer and provides the best images. Large pigtail catheters (7- or 8-French) that can tolerate high flow rates without whipping in the artery or unwinding are used. The catheter is advanced to the right atrium, and then through the heart selectively into a right or left pulmonary artery. Several techniques can be used to catheterize the pulmonary arteries, including a deflecting wire to direct a standard pigtail catheter through the valves, or manipulation of a preshaped catheter (Figs 8-10 and 8-11). Ventricular arrhythmias as the catheter is manipulated through the right ventricle are common, but almost always self-limited. As soon as the catheter is positioned in the pulmonary artery, a pressure measurement should be obtained. Careful and frequent flushing of the catheter is important to prevent thrombus formation in the lumen, which, if injected into the lung during

can image the contrast bolus at each step in the pulmonary circuit. Very powerful and fast gradients are required in order to obtain the extremely short echo times used for time-resolved pulmonary MRA. Conventional scanners can produce excellent images using 20- to 30-second duration gadolinium-enhanced 3-D gradient echo sequences. A limitation of pulmonary

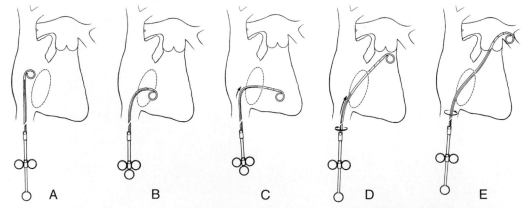

Figure 8-10   Deflecting wire technique for selective catheterization of the pulmonary arteries. Note that the wire *never* exits the catheter. **A,** The deflecting wire is positioned in the catheter just below the pigtail. **B,** The wire is deflected, directing the catheter towards the tricuspid valve. **C,** The catheter is advanced off the wire into the right ventricle. **D,** The deflection is released, and the wire advanced into the catheter without deflection for stiffening. The catheter is advanced through the pulmonary valve while being rotated counterclockwise. **E,** The deflecting wire can be used to direct the catheter from the left to the right pulmonary artery by deflecting and rotating the catheter in a clockwise direction. (Adapted with permission from Kadir S: Pulmonary angiography. In Kadir S ed: *Diagnostic Angiography*, WB Saunders, Philadelphia, 1986.)

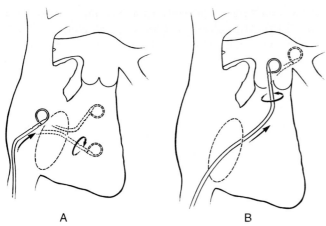

Figure 8-11   Grollman catheter technique. **A,** A pigtail catheter with a secondary curve is advanced across the tricuspid valve. **B,** Using a rotary motion the catheter is advanced through the pulmonary valve. (Adapted with permission from Kadir S: Pulmonary angiography. In Kadir S ed: *Diagnostic Angiography,* WB Saunders, Philadelphia, 1986.)

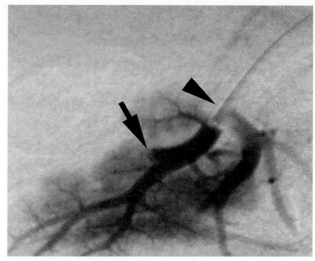

Figure 8-12   Balloon occlusion catheter (arrowhead) in the right lateral basal segmental artery demonstrating a small embolus (arrow).

the study, mimics small emboli peripheral from a peripheral source. Normal contrast injection rates are 25–30 mL/s for 2 seconds (see Fig. 8-1). In patients with uncompensated pulmonary hypertension, the rate and volume of contrast should be reduced to avoid acute right heart failure. There is no generally agreed guideline for contrast reduction, but if the end-diastolic pressure in the right ventricle is greater than 20 mmHg, then the study should be terminated. Equally important for setting contrast injection parameters is observation of a small test dose (8–10 mL) of contrast injected by hand. Brisk flow, even in the setting of extremely elevated pressures, indicates adequate right ventricular function and the ability to tolerate high injection rates. In the setting of a normal or elevated heart rate, slow flow and delayed washout of test contrast in the pulmonary arteries is ominous, suggesting an impaired right ventricle. Contrast volumes should be reduced appropriately in this situation.

The choice of imaging projection depends on the clinical question, but usually an anteroposterior (AP) view of the entire lung and a posterior oblique magnification view of the lung base with the catheter advanced beyond the upper lobe branches is sufficient for pulmonary embolism studies (see Fig. 8-1). When basilar lung segments are atelectatic, the anterior oblique view may provide the best view of the lower-lobe pulmonary arteries. Rapid filming (at least four frames per second) is necessary. Imaging should be continued into the venous phase to evaluate the pulmonary veins (see Figs 8-2 and 8-3). Low-osmolar contrast reduces coughing during filming and is safer in patients with elevated pulmonary artery pressures. In rare instances, a balloon occlusion catheter may be necessary to isolate a pulmonary artery segment to image a peripheral or high-flow abnormality (Fig. 8-12).

There is a lot of lore about the proper way to remove a pigtail catheter from the pulmonary artery. The theoretical concern is that the catheter will become entangled in valve elements, and either tear them or become trapped. The most conservative approach is to open the pigtail with a soft-tipped guidewire in the pulmonary artery before removing it. Gentle withdrawal of the closed pigtail while observing under fluoroscopy seems to work well. The pigtail frequently opens while exiting through the tricuspid valve, with no sequelae. Do not spin the pigtail, especially if it seems to get stuck, as this may entangle it. Either push it back into the heart, or insert a soft straight guidewire to open the pig should this happen.

Overall complication rates of pulmonary angiography are less than 3%, with the majority related to access site issues or contrast-induced nephropathy. The mortality rate is under 1%, and usually occurs in critically ill patients with acute right heart strain, pulmonary hypertension, or elevated cardiac troponins due to the thromboembolic event (Box 8-2). Since pulmonary angiography requires right-heart catheterization, there is a small risk

---

Box 8-2 Risk Factors for Pulmonary Angiography

Complete left bundle branch block
Severe uncompensated right heart failure
Severe pulmonary hypertension
Acute myocardial infarction
Pulmonary edema
History of anaphylaxis to iodinated contrast

of temporary paralysis of the right bundle of His and complete heart block during catheter manipulation in patients with preexisting complete left bundle block. These patients can be safely studied following placement of a temporary transvenous pacing electrode or external pacemaker pads.

Right ventricular overload is avoided by reduction of contrast rate and volume in patients with elevated pulmonary artery pressures. Once induced, acute right ventricular failure is difficult to reverse. Extreme care is necessary with all catheter flushes and injections in patients with pulmonary arteriovenous malformations as these patients are at risk of stroke from introduced catheter thrombi and air bubbles.

Bronchial Arteries

Bronchial artery angiography is usually performed as part of an embolization procedure for hemoptysis. Fortunately, the normally small bronchial arteries are typically hypertrophied in these patients. Nonionic contrast should be used. A digital subtraction aortogram in the AP projection with a pigtail catheter positioned in the transverse arch and injection of full-strength contrast at 20–30 mL/s for 2 seconds will allow rapid identification of the enlarged and tortuous bronchial arteries (see Fig. 8-6). The arteries can then be selected with 5-French catheters using a variety of shapes, such as Cobra 2, Simmons 1, and Shepard's Crook. Gentle hand injection of small volumes of contrast (3–10 mL) will usually be sufficient unless massive collaterals have developed. Branches to intercostal arteries, the esophagus, and the spinal cord may be seen (see Figs 8-4 and 8-5). When more selective catheterization is required, a 3-French microcatheter can be advanced into the bronchial artery. In patients with chronic pulmonary inflammatory processes, multiple selective injections of sources of potential collaterals, such as the internal mammary and other subclavian artery branches, may be necessary to map out the entire bronchial arterial supply (see Fig. 8-7).

The most feared complication of bronchial arteriography is paraplegia due to transverse myelitis. The exact mechanism is unknown, but it is exceedingly rare (much less than 1%) with current catheters and contrast agents. However, all patients must be advised of this potential complication prior to bronchial angiography.

ACUTE PULMONARY EMBOLISM

Acute thrombotic pulmonary embolism (PE) occurs when thrombus that has formed in the systemic veins breaks free and is carried by the venous return to the heart and, ultimately, the lungs. *In situ* formation of thrombus in the pulmonary arteries is rare, and usually related to a surgical procedure or proximal obstruction (Fig. 8-13). Thrombus in the lung is almost always embolic in origin. The actual incidence of PE is not known, but is suspected to be more than 600,000 cases per year in the United States. Untreated, it is thought that the mortality rate of acute PE is 30%. However, despite a high level of clinical concern, acute PE is probably underdiagnosed.

The clinical effects, and therefore the presenting symptoms, of acute obstruction of the pulmonary arteries are dependent upon the following factors: degree and level of obstruction; baseline conditions of the pulmonary vasculature and lung parenchyma; and the status of the heart. Healthy patients with normal lungs and hearts can tolerate massive pulmonary emboli, whereas elderly patients with end-stage pulmonary diseases may succumb to relatively small emboli. In general, large emboli lodge in the central pulmonary arteries and present with cardiopulmonary collapse, elevated right heart pressures, and hypoxia with evidence of poor oxygen exchange (the so-called "death embolus") (Fig. 8-14). Small emboli lodge in peripheral pulmonary arteries and cause infarcts, which result in pleuritic chest pain and tachypnea, but stable hemodynamic parameters and normal oxygenation (Fig. 8-15). Subsegmental emboli tend to be multiple, bilateral, and in the lower lobes. One confusing scenario is the patient who presents with a

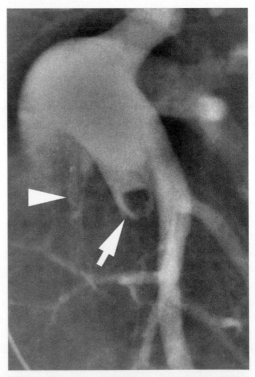

Figure 8-13 Selective pulmonary angiogram demonstrating thrombus (arrow) in a pulmonary artery stump following lower lobectomy. (Arrowhead on surgical staples in lung.)

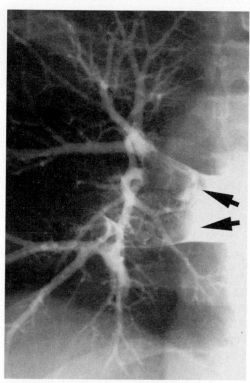

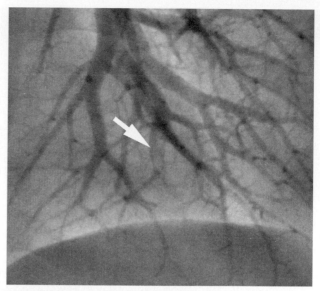

Figure 8-15   Subsegmental pulmonary embolus (arrow) shown on magnification view of the left base. The patient presented with pleuritic chest pain.

Figure 8-14   Massive saddle embolus (arrows) occluding the right upper and lower pulmonary arteries. The patient presented with sudden, transient hypotension.

large central embolus, is anticoagulated, and then approximately 3–7 days latter develops pleuritic chest pain. The explanation is frequently not recurrent PE, but peripheral embolization of small fragments of the large embolus as it undergoes lysis.

A source of acute PE is found in only 30% of patients, with lower-extremity deep vein thrombosis (DVT) being the most common (Box 8-3). Conversely, 50% of patients with DVT have abnormal ventilation/perfusion (V/Q) scans that are consistent with PE, despite the lack of pulmonary symptoms.

Suspicion of acute PE is the most common indication for imaging the pulmonary vasculature. The diagnostic algorithm is in flux owing to the increasing acceptance of cross-sectional imaging (namely helical CT angiography) in the diagnosis of PE. Historically, the plain radiograph is useful only to identify alternate explanations for the patient's pulmonary symptoms, and as a correlate for other studies. Peripheral wedge-shaped infiltrates can be seen in pulmonary infarcts, but emboli by themselves are not visible.

The V/Q scan is commonly used in the evaluation of patients with suspected PE. Unlike other imaging tests, the V/Q scan compares pulmonary perfusion with pulmonary ventilation. Ventilation of nonperfused areas of lung that are normal on chest radiograph allows a presumptive

diagnosis of pulmonary artery obstruction. Conversely, perfusion of areas of nonventilated lung are not explained by PE. This test is most useful in cooperative patients with normal chest radiographs. Uncooperative patients with obvious chest radiograph abnormalities are poor candidates for V/Q scans as perfusion abnormalities may result from pneumonia, atelectasis, and other nonembolic causes. This modality was validated in a landmark multicenter trial (Prospective Investigation of Pulmonary Embolism Diagnosis; PIOPED) that comprised 933 patients.

Readers are referred to another volume in this book series, *Nuclear Medicine: the Requisites,* for a complete description of V/Q scan interpretation (Box 8-4). In summary, the results of V/Q scans are expressed in terms of probability of pulmonary embolism. Patients with the most convincing V/Q scans ("high probability") and clinical histories for acute PE had only a 4% chance of

---

Box 8-3   Sources of Acute Pulmonary Emboli

Lower-extremity deep venous thrombosis
Pelvic vein thrombosis
Gonadal vein thrombosis (postpartum)
Renal vein thrombosis
Upper-extremity central vein thrombosis
Vascular invasion by malignancy (renal cell carcinoma, adrenal carcinoma, hepatoma)

Box 8-4 Modified PIOPED Criteria

Normal

No perfusion defects

Low Probability: <20%

Any perfusion defect with a substantially larger
radiographic abnormality

Matched ventilation and perfusion defects with a
normal chest radiograph

Nonsegmental perfusion defects (for example:
cardiomegaly, aortic aneurysm, hilar mass, mediastinal
mass, elevated diaphragm, small pleural effusion with
blunting of costophrenic angle)

Small subsegmental perfusion defects

Medium Probability: 20–80%

One moderate mismatched segmental defect with a
normal radiograph

One large and one moderate mismatched segmental
defect with a normal radiograph

Difficult to categorize as high- or low-probability

Not meeting the stated criteria for high- or
low-probability

High Probability: >80%

Two or more large mismatched segmental defects
without a radiographic abnormality (or the
perfusion defect is substantially larger than the
radiographic abnormality)

Any combination of mismatched defects equivalent to
the above (two moderate defects = one large defect)

Table 8-1 Mismatched Vascular Defects (Large or Moderate-sized Segmental Perfusion Defects) and Positive Predictive Value (PPV) for Pulmonary Embolism

Defects	Prior Cardiopulmonary Disease PPV (%)	No Prior Disease PPV (%)
0	33	41
1	68	80
2	77	89
3	80	91
4	84	89
5	89	92
6	93	94
7	92	96
≥8	91	95

Modified from Gottschalk A: New criteria for ventilation-perfusion lung scan
interpretation: a basis for optimal interaction with helical CT angiography.
Radiographics 20:1206–1210, 2000.

an alternate diagnosis in the original PIOPED study.
Conversely, PE will be found at angiography in 4–8% of
patients with low-probability or near-normal *V/Q* scans
but a high clinical suspicion for PE. However, a definitive
diagnosis or exclusion of PE based upon *V/Q* scanning
alone is possible in fewer than 50% of patients. For this
reason, a number of strategies have been proposed
to enhance the diagnosis of PE using *V/Q* scans.
Interpretation of scans based upon the number of vascular defects with consideration of preexisting cardiopulmonary disease, and combination with the results
of lower-extremity venous ultrasound (US) or pulmonary
CTA, have been proposed (Table 8-1).

All vascular imaging modalities (CTA, MRA, and conventional angiography) base the diagnosis of PE on the
same criteria: visualization of an intraluminal filling
defect. An intraluminal filling defect is defined as an
unopacified object in the vessel lumen surrounded by
contrast-enhanced blood. This finding is not exclusive to
PE, but must be interpreted in the context of the patient's

history, as postoperative changes and pulmonary artery
tumors may also produce intraluminal filling defects.
Acute emboli fill the lumen of the artery, have smooth
contours, and are most common at bifurcation points in
the pulmonary artery (see Figs 8-14 and 8-15). Subacute
or partially lysed emboli appear contracted, with slightly
irregular contours (Fig. 8-16). All other "signs" of PE are
secondary and possibly explained by nonembolic etiologies (Box 8-5). When undertaking imaging for PE, plan to
make a definitive diagnosis; the answer should be either
"positive" or "negative."

Helical CTA is the imaging modality used most often
for patients with suspected acute PE. Emboli appear as
nonenhancing intraluminal filling defects (Fig. 8-17).

Box 8-5 Imaging Criteria for Diagnosis of PE

Absolute

Intraluminal filling defect

Secondary

Abrupt cutoff of pulmonary artery

Abrupt-transition artery diameter without branch

Unexplained absence of pulmonary artery branch(es)

Oligemia of lung parenchyma

Slow flow in pulmonary artery segment

Absent venous drainage of lung segment

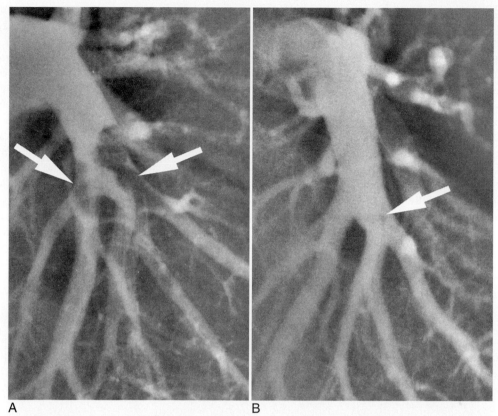

Figure 8-16   Subacute pulmonary embolus with resolution on anticoagulant therapy. **A**, Selective left lower-lobe pulmonary angiogram obtained several days after symptoms of pulmonary embolism developed. Multiple nonocclusive, irregular filling defects (arrows) consistent with subacute emboli. **B**, Repeat angiogram 6 weeks later (patient was treated with anticoagulation) shows substantial resolution of emboli with only minimal residual intraluminal abnormality (arrow).

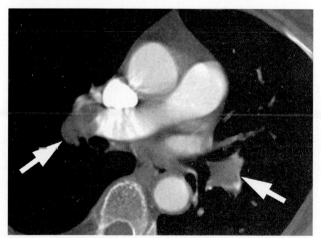

Figure 8-17   CT angiogram of acute pulmonary embolism in an elderly woman with progressive shortness of breath. There are large bilateral proximal filling defects consistent with extensive pulmonary emboli (arrows).

Areas of decreased perfusion on lung windows are suggestive of pulmonary artery obstruction, but cannot be used to diagnose PE in the absence of an intraluminal filling defect. False positive diagnoses can result from volume averaging of extrapulmonary structures, particularly peribronchial lymph nodes. Atelectasis, tumors, and infiltrates can make interpretation of studies difficult. The sensitivity and specificity of CTA for acute PE are approximately 95% for central emboli (presuming an interpretable study). As emboli become more peripheral, sensitivity and specificity decrease. CTA has limited utility when searching for small peripheral emboli. A major advantage of CTA is the vast amount of information that is acquired about the other intrathoracic structures, which sometimes leads to the alternate and correct diagnosis.

Gadolinium-enhanced MRA has performed well in the diagnosis of proximal and central PE, but clinical application remains limited. Emboli are seen as intraluminal filling defects. Sensitivity and specificity for central emboli approach 95% each. The ability of this modality to diagnose small peripheral PE is unknown, but probably similar to that of CTA. Fast gadolinium-enhanced 3-D gradient echo acquisitions can be acquired in a single breath-hold with most current equipment. As more MR scanners become available, use of MRA for diagnosis of acute PE may increase.

Pulmonary angiography remains an important modality for diagnosis of acute PE. When performed properly, it is a safe examination, even in very ill patients. As with both CTA and MRA, the definitive diagnosis of PE is made by finding an intraluminal filling defect in the pulmonary artery (see Fig. 8-14). The most common location for emboli to lodge is at bifurcation points, so these areas should be inspected carefully. Overlap of pulmonary arteries may obscure or mimic PE, so a second view in a different projection is frequently obtained. When

peripheral emboli are suspected, magnification views (sometimes in multiple obliquities) may be necessary (see Fig. 8-15). A filling defect due to an embolus is constant on several images. Inflow of unopacified blood can mimic an embolus on a single image, but is easily identified on serial images by its changing morphology (Fig. 8-18). Secondary signs of PE are helpful but do not substitute for a filling defect. Injection of a sufficient volume of contrast with rapid filming are the keys to obtaining diagnostic pulmonary angiograms. However, contrast volumes and rates have to be adjusted based on pulmonary artery pressures and qualitative assessment of flow.

The lung of interest should be studied first, based on either clinical symptoms or other imaging tests. The right lung may be studied first when there is no obvious

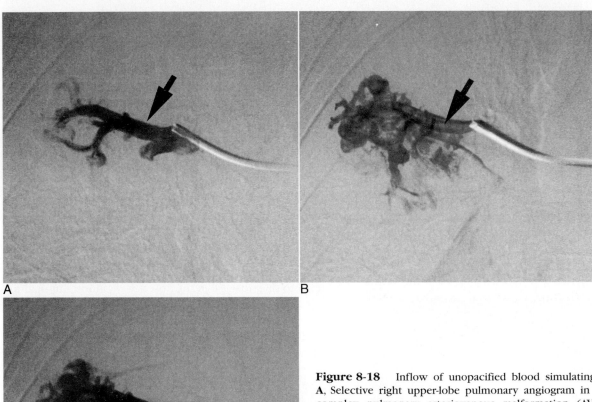

Figure 8-18 Inflow of unopacified blood simulating a filling defect. **A**, Selective right upper-lobe pulmonary angiogram in a patient with a complex pulmonary arteriovenous malformation (AVM). The feeding artery (arrow) is completely opacified with contrast. **B**, The next frame shows unopacified blood in the center of the feeding artery (arrow), surrounded by slower moving contrast-enhanced blood along the walls of the vessel, causing the appearance of a filling defect. Note the numerous communicating branches with the AVM. **C**, A few frames later (during diastole) the feeding artery is again completely opacified. A single draining vein is now visible (arrow).

choice, as it is harder to catheterize than the left. When the diagnosis is made on the first run, obtain at least one view of the opposite lung unless contraindicated by the patient's condition. A small number of patients will be suspected of having recurrent PE during initiation of therapy, and baseline studies will be helpful during interpretation of repeat studies. Cardiac and respiratory motion can seriously degrade digital subtraction acquisitions.

The treatment of acute PE has two objectives: (1) permit or enhance lysis of the embolus by the intrinsic thrombolytic pathways of the lung, and (2) prevent additional emboli from occurring. Both objectives are usually successfully accomplished with anticoagulation, which prevents formation of additional thrombus. Patients may be treated with unfractionated heparin followed by warfarin for 6 months, or low-molecular-weight heparin compounds. The duration of anticoagulation should be at least 6 months, and possibly for life in some patients. Symptomatic repeat PE occurs in almost 5% of patients during the initial phase of anticoagulation, half of which are fatal. The ability of normal lung to lyse thrombus is remarkable (see Fig. 8-16).

Rarely, acute relief of obstruction is required to save a patient's life. Indications for aggressive treatment of PE include evidence of acute right heart failure, severely elevated pulmonary artery pressures, hypoxia, and hypotension. Thrombolytic agents can be administered either through a peripheral vein or through a catheter directly into the pulmonary arteries (Table 8-2). A small decrease in arterial obstruction can result in major clinical improvement. Thrombolysis has a 25% risk of bleeding complications in some reports, and is contraindicated in patients with recent major surgery, hemorrhagic stroke, or contraindications to anticoagulation. Mechanical fragmentation of large emboli can be achieved using devices intended for declotting dialysis grafts or a rotating pigtail catheter. A guiding catheter is necessary with most devices for stabilization and direction of the device. Emergency surgical pulmonary thromboembolectomy should be considered when intervention must be immediate.

Table 8-2	**Thrombolytic Dosing for Pulmonary Emboli**	
Drug	**Systemic Dose**	**Catheter-directed**
rt-PA	100 mg over 2 h	1-2 mg/h over 12-24 h
r-PA	Unknown	1 U/h for 12-24 h
UK	4400 IU/kg over 10 min, then 4400/kg/h for 12-24 h	100,000-200,000 IU/h over 12-24 h

IU, International Units.

When anticoagulation is not feasible, or an additional PE would be life-threatening, interruption of the inferior vena cava (IVC) with a filter may be indicated (see Chapter 13).

CHRONIC PULMONARY EMBOLISM

Although the lungs are capable of absorbing relatively large acute embolic loads, repeat embolization over a long period leads to permanent pulmonary artery damage. Failure of lysis results in occlusion of pulmonary artery branches. Partial recanalization of emboli results in luminal compromise by web-like stenoses, linear strands of organized intraluminal thrombus, and mural thrombus. As the available pulmonary artery vascular bed decreases, pulmonary artery pressure increases, the main pulmonary arteries and right ventricle become enlarged, and gas exchange is compromised. Ultimately, right heart failure ensues.

The diagnosis of chronic PE is frequently arrived at during evaluation for other more common disorders such as pulmonary fibrosis. Patients with chronic PE frequently have no history of prior documented PE or DVT. Fewer than 1% of patients diagnosed with acute PE develop chronic PE. Symptoms include dyspnea on exertion, pulmonary artery hypertension, right heart failure, as well as nondescript complaints such as fatigue and failure to thrive. Acute PE can coexist with chronic PE.

The approach to imaging patients with suspected chronic PE is somewhat different from acute PE. Patients are usually stable, although sometimes very ill. Accurate determination of the extent of pulmonary artery involvement is crucial for planning therapy. Emergent imaging is rarely necessary.

As with acute PE, the plain radiograph is rarely useful in the diagnosis of chronic PE other than to possibly provide alternative diagnoses. Enlarged central pulmonary arteries, absence or "pruned" appearance of peripheral pulmonary artery branches, and wedge-shaped peripheral infarcts have all been reported in chronic PE.

The findings at V/Q scan for chronic PE are the same as in acute PE (Table 8-3). Nevertheless, the study is useful in that a normal examination excludes chronic PE as an explanation for dyspnea, pulmonary artery hypertension, and right heart failure. In order to develop these symptoms, a large quantity of the pulmonary vasculature must be obstructed.

Helical CTA is an excellent modality for evaluation of suspected chronic PE. The typical findings include mural thrombus in the pulmonary arteries, stenoses, central pulmonary artery enlargement, as well as parenchymal abnormalities such as a mosaic pattern and peripheral nodules (Fig. 8-19). MRA provides similar information

Table 8-3 Findings in Chronic Pulmonary Embolism

Finding	V/Q	CTA	MRA	Angio
Perfusion/ventilation mismatch	+[a]	N/A	N/A	N/A
Mural thrombus	N/A	+	+	−
Enlarged central PA	N/A	+	+	+
PA stenoses/webs	N/A	+	+	+
Proximal PA occlusions	N/A	+	+	+
Peripheral PA occlusions	N/A	−	−	+
PA hypertension	N/A	−	−	+[b]

[a] Also found in acute pulmonary embolism.
[b] Direct measurement.
PA, pulmonary artery; N/A, not applicable.

about the vasculature, but is not as useful for the pulmonary parenchyma.

The angiographic findings of chronic PE are listed in Table 8-3. Angiography allows direct determination of right heart and pulmonary artery pressures. Subtle intimal irregularities stenoses, occlusions, and a "pruned" or branchless appearance of the pulmonary artery are all typical of chronic PE (see Fig. 8-19). Remnants of recanalized emboli can be seen as linear filling defects, termed "synechia." An important limitation of angiography is the inability to characterize the extent of mural thrombus in the pulmonary artery. However, angiography provides an overall assessment of the extent of chronic embolism.

An important aspect of the treatment of chronic PE is based on preventing further emboli from occurring. Long-term anticoagulation prevents development of new peripheral sources of thrombus that may embolize. Many of these patients are candidates for IVC filters, as even small emboli may be life-threatening. Surgical removal of the chronic thrombus (pulmonary thrombo-endarterectomy) results in substantial improvement.

PULMONARY ARTERY STENOSIS

There are multiple causes of pulmonary artery stenoses in adults (Table 8-4). In children, pulmonary artery stenosis may be associated with congenital heart defects such as Tetralogy of Fallot.

The etiology of pulmonary stenosis may be suggested by the appearance (Table 8-5). Stenoses which are focal, smooth, and with obtuse angles imply extrinsic compression by masses (Fig. 8-20). Diffuse smooth stenoses are more likely to be due to congenital abnormalities of the pulmonary artery or vasculitis (Fig. 8-21; see also Fig. 1-18). Stenoses that are irregular with acute angles or obvious webs imply an intrinsic lesion such as chronic PE (see Fig. 8-19). Other important factors are the

Table 8-4 Causes of Pulmonary Artery Stenoses

Etiology	Central	Peripheral
Chronic PE	+	+
Vasculitis		
Takayasu's	+	+
Radiation	+	+
Chronic inflammation	+	+
Tumor	+	+
Congenital rubella	+	−
Adenopathy	+	−
Fibrosing mediastinitis	+	−
Aortic aneurysm	+	−

Table 8-5 Pulmonary Artery Stenosis

Etiology	Extrinsic	Intrinsic
Chronic PE	−	+
Vasculitis		
Takayasu's	−	+
Radiation	−	+
Congenital rubella	−	+
Post lung transplant	−	+
Williams syndrome	−	+
Chronic inflammation	+	−
Tumor	+	−
Adenopathy	+	−
Fibrosing mediastinitis	+	−
Aortic aneurysm	+	−

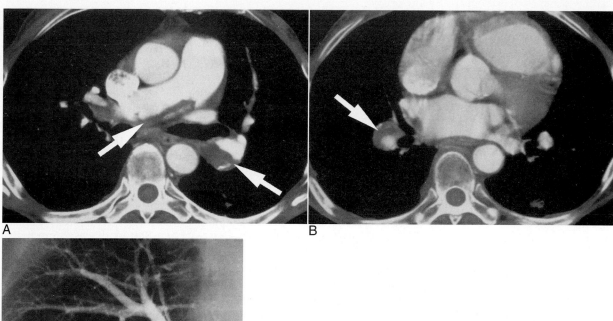

Figure 8-19 Chronic pulmonary embolism (PE). **A**, Contrast-enhanced CT in a patient with chronic PE showing mural thrombus (arrows) lining the left and right pulmonary arteries. **B**, Lower image from the same CT showing recanalized embolus (arrow) in the right lower lobe. (Compare with the acute PE in Fig. 8-17.) (Courtesy of David Levin M.D. and Thomas Kinney M.D., UCSD Department of Radiology, San Diego, CA.) **C**, Selective right pulmonary angiogram from a different patient with chronic PE showing webs (arrow), partially recanalized occlusions (arrowhead), and diminished parenchymal vascularity.

patient's age, associated conditions, and past history. Plain radiographs may reveal calcified lymph nodes, pulmonary fibrosis, or masses. Conventional CT and MRI of the chest are extremely useful for evaluation of the mediastinal and hilar structures, as well as the lung parenchyma. CTA and MRA accurately depict central pulmonary artery stenosis. Pulmonary angiography is necessary to diagnose peripheral stenoses, as cross-sectional imaging lacks the required resolution.

Therapy is determined by the severity of the symptoms and the underlying etiology of the lesion. Stenoses due to chronic PE may be amenable to thromboendarterectomy. Focal proximal lesions may respond to placement of a balloon-expandable stent.

PULMONARY ARTERIOVENOUS FISTULAS AND MALFORMATIONS

Congenital pulmonary artery arteriovenous fistulas (AVF) and malformations (AVM) are abnormal direct communications between a pulmonary artery and pulmonary vein (Fig. 8-22; see also Figs 8-18 and 4-30). Blood is shunted directly from the right heart to the left, without benefiting from two major functions of the pulmonary capillary bed: oxygenation and filtration. Patients with pulmonary arteriovenous lesions may present with symptoms of hypoxia due to shunting, high-output cardiac failure, or, more seriously, paradoxical embolization. Dyspnea

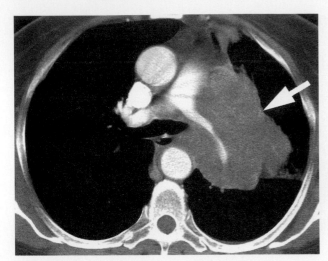

Figure 8-20 Contrast-enhanced CT of a patient with a large lung carcinoma (arrow) encasing and compressing the right pulmonary artery.

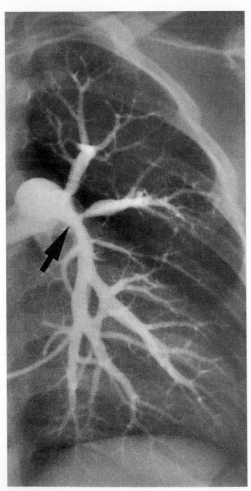

Figure 8-21 Selective left pulmonary artery angiogram in a child with congenital rubella infection showing pulmonary artery stenoses (arrow).

and hypoxia due to shunting that are worse with standing is typical in patients with large lower-lobe lesions (platypnea and orthodeoxia, respectively). The presence of an intrapulmonary shunt allows otherwise innocuous venous debris to pass directly into the systemic arterial circulation. Transient ischemic attacks, strokes, brain abscesses, and peripheral arterial emboli may occur. The risk of paradoxical embolus increases with the number of malformations and the size of the feeding arteries. A rare complication is acute hemorrhage, either intrapulmonary or intrapleural, particularly in pregnant women.

Pulmonary AVFs and AVMs occur sporadically (15%) or as part of an autosomal dominant disorder (85%) known as either hereditary hemorrhagic telangectasia (HHT) or Osler–Weber–Rendu disease. Rarely, patients with cirrhosis can develop multiple symptomatic fistulas at the lung base (hepatopulmonary syndrome). Patients with HHT have AVFs or AVMs in multiple organs, including bowel, upper respiratory tract, central nervous system, liver, and skin. Presenting symptoms of lesions in these areas include bleeding and peripheral shunting. The overall incidence of HHT is between 2 and 5 per 100,000, with pulmonary involvement in one-quarter of affected patients. Pulmonary lesions are multiple in 35–58% of patients, bilateral in 40%, and predominantly in the lower lobes. Simple AVFs (supply from one artery) occur in 80%, and AVMs (complex supply from multiple arteries) in 20%. A new diagnosis of HHT should prompt two actions – a search for pulmonary AVFs in the patient, and a search for HHT in the patient's relatives.

Calculation of intrapulmonary shunting is a useful parameter in the diagnosis and postintervention follow-up. The normal shunt is <5%, and more than 95% of patients with pulmonary AVFs will have a shunt >5% while breathing 100% oxygen. Pulmonary AVFs appear on chest radiographs as smooth, round or lobulated mass lesions, and are frequently initially thought to represent solid tumors. The presence of large vessels extending from the mass to the hilum is highly suggestive of an AVF. A normal chest radiograph does not exclude the presence of pulmonary AVF.

The sensitivity and specificity of thin-section CT for clinically relevant pulmonary AVFs is so high that a negative examination excludes the diagnosis (Fig. 8-23). Tiny AVFs that have a low risk for paradoxical shunting may be missed. Thin-section noncontrast scans, as well as CTA, allow accurate planning for therapy. Contrast-enhanced 3-D MRA has also been used for evaluation of these patients. With both CT and MRA, great care must be observed during insertion of the peripheral intravenous catheter and injection of contrast to avoid introduction of air bubbles.

Pulmonary angiography for pulmonary AVF is performed to confirm the diagnosis prior to embolotherapy. Angiographic technique must be fastidious. Intravenous

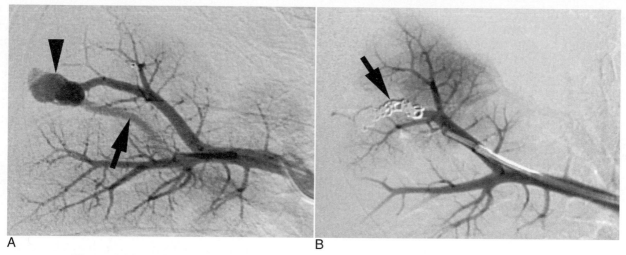

Figure 8-22   Pulmonary arteriovenous fistula in a patient with hereditary hemorraghic telangiectasia syndrome (HHT). **A,** Selective right upper-lobe pulmonary artery DSA showing an arteriovenous fistula (arrowhead) with a single enlarged feeding artery and early filling of a draining pulmonary vein (arrow). Multiple lesions were also present on the left. **B,** Angiogram after successful coil occlusion (arrow) of the feeding artery.

lines should be free of air bubbles and have particulate filters. Heparinization with a bolus of 3000–5000 units after introduction of the catheter provides a measure of security against thrombus formation in or around the catheter. All catheter and guidewire manipulations should be conducted in a manner as to prevent air from entering the catheter. Frequent catheter flushing with bubble-free flush solution is a critical point of technique.

Patients with pulmonary AVFs are generally young and nervous about their diagnosis, factors that result in a hyperdynamic state. Pulmonary angiography in this population may require higher flow rates (30–35 mL/s for 2 seconds) than the typical older patient with thromboembolic disease. Complete angiography with multiple views of both lungs should be obtained to identify all pulmonary AVFs. Small AVFs may be missed at CT, and detection at angiography is important when planning long-term follow-up. AVFs are identifiable by one or more large feeding arteries and a large draining vein that opacifies before the remainder of the pulmonary veins. The actual arteriovenous communication is frequently saccular or aneurysmal in appearance.

The therapy of the majority of simple and complex pulmonary AVFs is embolization. AVFs with feeding pulmonary arteries that are 3 mm or greater in diameter should be occluded. Long guiding catheters are used to stabilize the system in the pulmonary artery (see Fig. 8-22). After selection of a feeding branch, hand injection of contrast in multiple views may be necessary to define the anatomy. The guiding catheter is then advanced as close to the actual shunt as possible. Occlusion of the feeding artery can be accomplished with coils or detachable balloons. Coils are easy to obtain, and therefore used most often. The occluding coils should have a diameter at least 20% larger than the vessel to be embolized to avoid becoming a paradoxical embolus (see Fig. 4-30). The first coil should be relatively large, and placed close to the shunt in the feeding artery. Additional coils more

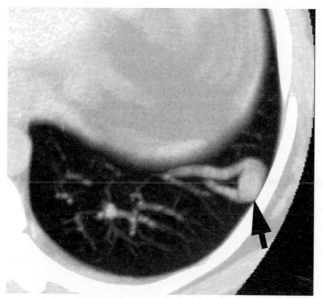

Figure 8-23   Noncontrast enhanced CT scan of a simple lower lobe pulmonary arteriovenous fistula. Several axial images were stacked to show the fistula (arrow) with feeding artery and draining vein.

closely sized to the artery are then deposited until there is no longer filling of the AVF.

Recurrence after embolization is unusual (<5%). Slow progressive enlargement of small AVFs over time mandates follow-up for life for patients with multiple lesions. Complications of embolization are rare, but include systemic embolization of the coil or balloon (<1%), and air embolus to the right coronary artery (<5%). Many patients have transient pleural pain and fever following embolization.

PULMONARY SEQUESTRATION

Pulmonary sequestration is a focus of lung that either has no connection to the bronchi or pulmonary arteries, or derives its major blood supply from an aberrant systemic artery (Fig. 8-24). This artery typically originates from the distal descending thoracic or the upper abdominal aorta. Sequestrations are either contained within the pleura of the normal lung (intralobar), or have their own separate pleura (extralobar). Intralobar sequestrations drain to the pulmonary veins, are usually found in adults, and are more common than extralobar sequestration. Extralobar sequestration is found in children, is less common than the intralobar variety, and drains to the systemic veins. Both types of sequestration occur more commonly at the left lung base.

Sequestration appears as a mass lesion on chest radio-graphs. Large anomalous vessels may be seen arising from the distal thoracic aorta on contrast-enhanced CT. The main role of angiography in patients with suspected sequestration is to conclusively demonstrate the arterial supply to the abnormal lung tissue. In addition to pulmonary angiography, aortography and selective injection of the aberrant arterial supply should be performed.

PULMONARY ARTERY TUMORS

Primary malignant pulmonary artery tumors are rare, accounting for fewer than 1% of thoracic tumors. These are usually sarcomatous lesions, such as leiomyosarcoma (Box 8-6). The tumors commonly occur in a central location, but can be multifocal. Pulmonary artery invasion by adjacent tumor can also occur with bronchogenic carcinoma, germ-cell tumors, and other mediastinal malignancies. The prognosis of primary and secondary pulmonary artery tumors is poor.

Patients may be asymptomatic when the mass is nonobstructive or slowly enlarging. These lesions may be identified incidentally during evaluation of suspected thoracic malignancy or pulmonary embolism. Large central masses may obstruct the main pulmonary artery, resulting in hypoxia, syncope, and right heart failure.

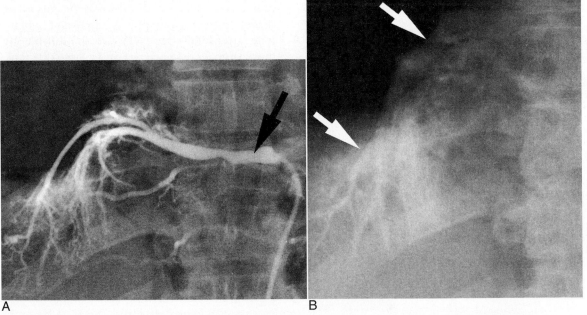

A　　　　　　　　　　　　　　　　　　　　　　B

Figure 8-24　Angiographic findings of intralobar pulmonary sequestration. **A,** Selective injection of an anomalous large artery (arrow) arising from the distal thoracic aorta opacifies a portion of right lower lobe lung parenchyma. **B,** Later image from the same injection shows filling of pulmonary veins (arrows).

Box 8-6   Primary Pulmonary Artery Tumors

Leiomyosarcoma
Spindle cell sarcoma
Malignant fibrous hystiocytoma
Fibrosarcoma
Fibromyxosarcoma
Rhabdomyosarcoma
Chondrosarcoma

The CT and MR findings of a primary pulmonary artery tumor are an enhancing intraluminal mass that may partially or completely obstruct the lumen (Fig. 8-25). This is a critical distinguishing feature between a mass and a large embolus, which will not enhance. Secondary involvement of the pulmonary arteries by a primary mediastinal or lung tumor is usually easily determined on the basis of cross-sectional imaging findings. Angiography demonstrates intraluminal filling defects, frequently with a lobulated contour. Intravascular biopsy can be performed to obtain a tissue diagnosis. Therapy, when possible, is

surgical resection. Stent placement to relieve obstructive symptoms can be beneficial as palliative therapy.

PULMONARY ARTERY ANEURYSMS AND PSEUDOANEURYSMS

There are numerous etiologies of pulmonary artery aneurysms and pseudoaneurysms (PSA) (Box 8-7). As a rule, these are rare lesions. The clinical presentation and course vary with the etiology. Aneurysms are often identified incidentally during evaluation of unrelated pulmonary diseases (Fig. 8-26). However, hemoptysis is a common acute presenting symptom, particularly with PSAs. When the etiology is tuberculosis, the PSAs are termed "Rasmussen's aneurysms."

The most commonly encountered pulmonary artery PSAs are iatrogenic, usually related to flow-directed balloon-tipped catheters placed for hemodynamic monitoring in acutely ill patients (Fig. 8-27). Although the balloons are made from compliant materials, inflation in a small pulmonary artery branch can lead to rupture of the vessel and a PSA. Alternatively, the catheter itself may perforate the wall of the artery. The estimated incidence is as high as 1 in 1600 insertions. Acute hemoptysis is the

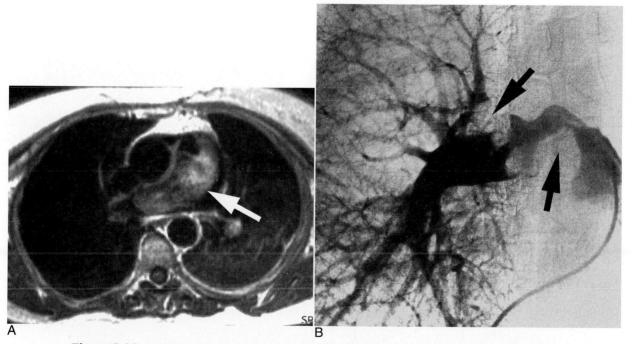

A   B

Figure 8-25   Pulmonary artery sarcoma (malignant fibrous hystiocytoma). **A**, Axial T1-weighted MR image after administration of gadolinium shows an enhancing mass in the main pulmonary artery (arrow) extending into the right pulmonary artery. The left pulmonary artery was completely occluded by the mass. **B**, Selective right pulmonary angiogram shows a bulky filling defects (arrows) and attenuation of the central contrast density consistent with a tumor. Note that although contrast refluxed to the main pulmonary artery, there was no filling of the left pulmonary artery.

Box 8-7   Pulmonary Artery Aneurysms

True

Chronic pulmonary hypertension
Pulmonic valve stenosis
Behçet's disease
Takayasu's arteritis
Congenital
Hugh Stoven syndrome
Marfan syndrome

False

Infection
   Endocarditis
   Septic emboli
   Necrotizing pneumonia
   Tuberculosis
Trauma
   Penetrating
   Deceleration
   Swan–Ganz

typical presentation, occurring at the presumed time of arterial injury. Hemoptysis may be massive, life-threatening, and recurrent. Pulmonary artery hypertension, anticoagulation, and concurrent cardiopulmonary bypass contribute to the severity of the presentation. Untreated, the mortality approaches 20% from pulmonary bleeding, but is higher overall owing to underlying illness.

Chest radiographic findings of pulmonary PSA vary over time. Initially, a focal area of consolidation consistent with pulmonary hemorrhage may be seen. Over time, resolution of the hemorrhage may reveal a new lung mass. Retrospective review of serial radiographs may identify a Swan–Ganz catheter in a peripheral location that correlates with the new mass.

Pulmonary CTA can show a focal enhancing lesion surrounded by pulmonary parenchymal hemorrhage and bronchial blood. However, when this diagnosis is highly likely, proceeding directly to pulmonary angiography may be warranted as this provides an opportunity for definitive treatment. Frequently these patients are quite ill with multiple medical problems, so the number of stops in the radiology department should be kept to a minimum. Pulmonary angiography should be performed in the usual fashion.

Pulmonary artery PSAs can be safely embolized in a manner similar to AVFs. Unlike with AVFs, the risk of paradoxical embolization is nonexistent, but the fragile PSAs are more prone to rupture during manipulation. Once the PSA is identified and localized, the pigtail catheter is exchanged for a guiding catheter. A selective catheter should then be used to deposit coils in the artery that feeds the PSA. Since the pulmonary arteries are essentially end-arteries, there is no concern for retrograde perfusion of the PSA. In some cases, coils can be gently packed into the PSA to promote thrombosis.

Experience with coil embolization is limited. Occlusion of the PSA is achieved in the majority of cases,

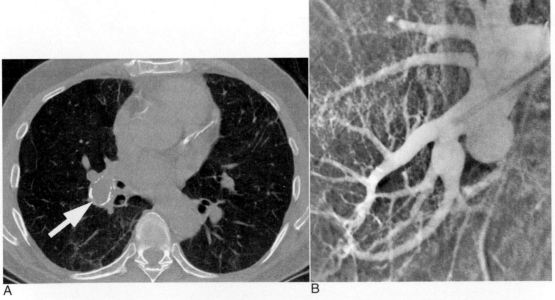

Figure 8-26   Pulmonary artery aneurysms in an adult with a history of tricuspid valvular bacterial endocarditis as a child. **A**, Axial CT scan without contrast windowed to show a calcified right pulmonary artery aneurysm (arrow). **B**, Selective right pulmonary angiogram shows multiple aneurysms.

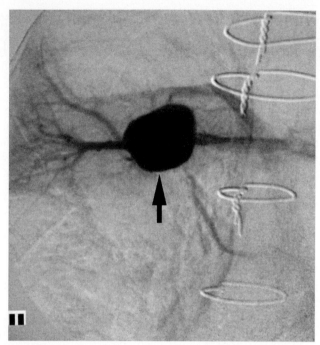

Figure 8-27 Pulmonary artery pseudoaneurysm due to a Swan–Ganz catheter placed in the operating room during coronary artery surgery. The patient developed intermittent massive hemoptysis in the postoperative period. Selective injection of the right upper-lobe pulmonary artery shows a large pseudoaneurysm (arrow). This was successfully embolized with coils.

with cessation of bleeding. Mortality remains high in reported series owing to concurrent severe medical and surgical illnesses. Surgical therapy is an alternative but has a higher mortality rate.

BRONCHIAL ARTERY BLEEDING

Hypertrophy of the bronchial arteries usually occurs as a result of chronic inflammatory processes in the lung (Box 8-8). Bronchial and parenchymal inflammatory processes derive their blood supply from the bronchial arteries rather than the pulmonary arteries (see Fig. 8-5). Chronic inflammation and hyperemia leads to enlargement of bronchial arteries and recruitment of collaterals from other systemic thoracic arteries (see Fig. 8-7 and Box 8-1). Pulmonary artery occlusion can also lead to bronchial and collateral artery enlargement due to systemic to pulmonary shunting (see Fig. 8-6).

Patients with enlarged bronchial arteries present with bleeding from the mucosa overlying the hypertrophied vessels. The triggering event for bleeding is frequently infection with mucosal inflammation and erosion. In patients with systemic to pulmonary shunting, the enlarged arteries can erode into the airway. Patients typically can sense and localize the onset of bleeding.

Box 8-8 Conditions Leading to Bronchial Artery Hypertrophy

Cystic fibrosis
Chronic infection
    Fungal
    Tuberculosis
    Pneumonia
    Abscess
Chronic granulomatous disease
    Sarcoidosis
    Wegener's granulomatosis
Bronchiectasis
Congenital pulmonary stenosis/atresia with
    systemic–pulmonary collaterals
Acquired pulmonary artery stenosis/occlusion
Tumor (rare)

Endobronchial blood is very irritating to the airway, leading to coughing and production of large clots intermixed with sputum. Patients should lie with the source lung dependent during acute bleeding.

The definition of massive hemoptysis differs from that employed in most other types of arterial bleeding. Airway compromise and aspiration of blood are of greater risk to the patient than exsanguination. Hemoptysis of more than 300 mL of blood in 24 hours is therefore considered massive. Intervention should not be delayed until the patient has a measurable drop in hematocrit or hypotension.

Patients with suspected bronchial artery bleeding require immediate evaluation. A chest radiograph followed by emergency bronchoscopy should be obtained when patients have massive hemoptysis for the first time. Selective intubation or a bifurcated double-barrel endotracheal tube may be necessary to protect the non-bleeding lung. Correction of any underlying coagulopathy is essential. Careful exclusion of an alternative diagnosis is important before proceeding to angiography and embolization (Box 8-9).

Angiography is for both diagnosis and therapy (by embolization) of bronchial artery bleeding. CTA and MRA have no role in acutely bleeding patients. Airway protection is a major concern during angiography, as patients must lie on their back and be sedated. In addition to the usual risks of angiography and embolization, patients should be counseled on the risk (albeit low) of paralysis from inadvertent embolization of a spinal artery. Knowledge of the suspected side of bleeding (based on bronchoscopy or the patient's history) is useful to direct the study. The angiographic technique is described above.

Hypertophied bronchial arteries characteristically have a wild random appearance that extends to the

Box 8-9 Differential Diagnosis of Hemoptysis

Pulmonary

Bronchial artery (e.g., chronic inflammatory processes)
Pulmonary infarct
Pulmonary artery PSA
Pulmonary artery AVM
Malignancy
Mitral stenosis
Autoimmune (e.g., Goodpasture syndrome, Wegener's
  granulomatosis)
Pneumonia
Aortopulmonary fistula

Oropharyngeal

Inflammatory
Trauma (intubation)
Malignancy
Aspirated from nasal airway (e.g., epistaxis)

Gastrointestinal

Aspirated from upper GI tract

abnormal area of lung parenchyma as well as the hilum. These abnormal vessels are frequently so large that they are readily visible from the aortogram. A parenchymal blush, shunting to the pulmonary arteries, and pulmonary veins may be seen, but extravasation is rare. Selective injection of the subclavian artery, thyrocervical trunk, internal mammary artery, anterior chest wall arteries (such as the long thoracic artery), intercostals arteries, and phrenic arteries may be necessary in patients with extensive pulmonary pathology, prior embolizations, or prior surgery. Bronchial, intercostal, and thyrocervical angiograms must be carefully inspected for branches to the anterior spinal artery. A normal diameter artery with absent parenchymal staining or venous shunting essentially excludes a systemic arterial etiology of bleeding (see Fig. 8-4). When an arterial source cannot be identified, pulmonary angiography should be considered in patients with cavitary lung lesions or a history of recent Swan–Ganz catheterization.

The goal of embolization of bronchial arteries (or hypertrophied collateral arteries) in patients with hemoptysis is to decrease blood supply without infarcting tissue (Fig. 8-28). Owing to the chronic nature of the underlying pathology, embolization alone is rarely

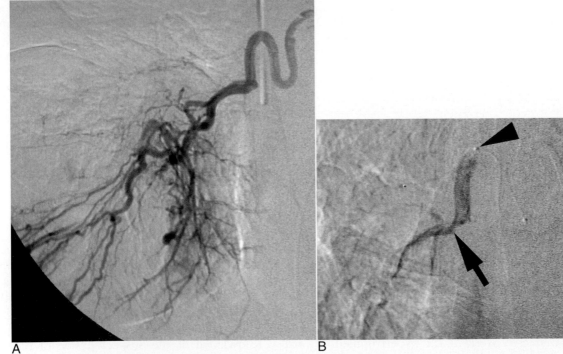

A   B

Figure 8-28   Embolization of a right lower lobe bronchial artery in a patient with cystic fibrosis. **A,** DSA prior to embolization shows an enlarged artery with dense parenchymal stain. **B,** Selective injection following embolization through a microcatheter (arrowhead) with Ivalon particles (300–500 µm) shows stasis of flow (arrow).

definitive. Particulate agents between 300 and 700 μm should be delivered through a selective catheter (frequently a microcatheter) that is securely placed in the artery. When embolization of a bronchial artery that gives rise to a spinal artery is necessary, the catheter should be advanced beyond the critical branch, and the large size particles should be used. The particles are injected carefully to avoid reflux into the aorta or critical side-branches. The endpoint of embolization is stasis of flow in the target vessel. Alcohol, ethiodol, and fine powders are contraindicated. Coils should not be used in the ostium of the artery, as repeat embolization may be necessary. In certain vessels (such as the internal mammary artery), placement of a coil or Gelfoam plug *distal* to the origin of the collateral branches to the bronchial arteries redirects the flow of embolic agent and prevents nontarget embolization of abdominal or chest-wall soft tissues.

Technical and clinical success in embolization for hemoptysis is dependent upon the ability to selectively catheterize the bronchial blood supply. The first procedure usually has the best results, with greater than 90% technical and clinical success. Each subsequent procedure becomes more difficult as smaller and smaller collateral branches are recruited. More intensive selective catheterization is required for repeat embolizations. The long-term success varies with the underlying etiology, but rebleeding is frequent in patients with ongoing chronic inflammatory processes. Ultimately, pulmonary resection may be required, but it can have a high mortality owing to dense vascular pleural adhesions.

SUGGESTED READINGS

American College of Emergency Physicians Clinical Policies Committee: Clinical policy - critical issues in the evaluation and management of adult patients presenting with suspected pulmonary embolism. *Ann Emerg Med* 41:257-270, 2003.

Arcasoy SM, Kreit JW: Thrombolytic therapy of pulmonary embolism: a comprehensive review of current evidence. *Chest* 115:1695-1707, 1999.

Bartter T, Irwin RS, Nash G: Aneurysms of the pulmonary arteries. *Chest* 94:1065-1075, 1988.

Brinson GM, Noone PG, Mauro MA et al. Bronchial artery embolization for the treatment of hemoptysis in patients with cystic fibrosis. *Am J Respir Crit Care Med* 157:1951-1958, 1998.

Cox JE, Chiles C, Aquino SL, Savage P, Oaks T: Pulmonary artery sarcomas: a review of clinical and radiologic features. *J Comput Assist Tomogr* 21:750-755, 1997.

De Gregorio MA, Gimeno MJ, Mainar A et al. Mechanical and enzymatic thrombolysis for massive pulmonary embolism. *J Vasc Interv Radiol* 13:163-169, 2002.

Do KH, Goo JM, Im JG et al: Systemic arterial supply to the lungs in adults: spiral CT findings. *Radiographics* 21:387-402, 2001.

Fedullo PF, Auger WR, Kerr KM, Rubin LJ: Chronic thromboembolic pulmonary hypertension. *N Engl J Med* 345:1465-1472, 2001.

Felker RE, Tonkin IL: Imaging of pulmonary sequestration. *Am J Roentgenol* 154:241-249, 1990.

Goldhaber SZ: The current role of thrombolytic therapy for pulmonary embolism. *Semin Vasc Surg* 13:217-220, 2000.

Goodman LR, Lipchik RJ, Kuzo RS et al: Subsequent pulmonary embolism: risk after a negative helical CT pulmonary angiogram - prospective comparison with scintigraphy. *Radiology* 215:535-542, 2000.

Gottschalk, A: New criteria for ventilation–perfusion lung scan interpretation: a basis for optimal interaction with helical CT angiography. *Radiographics* 20:1206-1210, 2000.

Gottschalk A, Sostman HD, Coleman RE et al: Ventilation/perfusion scintigraphy in the PIOPED study: II. Evaluation of scintigraphic criteria and interpretations. *J Nucl Med* 34:1119-1126, 1993.

Henk CB, Grampp S, Linnau KF et al: Suspected pulmonary embolism: enhancement of pulmonary arteries at deep-inspiration CT angiography: influence of patent foramen ovale and atrial–septal defect. *Radiology* 226:749-755, 2003.

Hudson ER, Smith TP, McDermott VG et al: Pulmonary angiography performed with iopamidol: complications in 1434 patients. *Radiology* 198:61-65, 1996.

Johnson MS: Current strategies for the diagnosis of pulmonary embolus. *J Vasc Interv Radiol* 13:13-23, 2002.

Kadir S: Pulmonary angiography. In Kadir S ed: *Diagnostic Angiography*, WB Saunders, Philadelphia, 1986, 584-616.

Loud PA, Katz DS, Bruce DA, Klippenstein DL, Grossman ZD: Deep venous thrombosis with suspected pulmonary embolism: detection with combined CT venography and pulmonary angiography. *Radiology* 219:498-502, 2001.

Nicod P, Peterson K, Levine M et al: Pulmonary angiography in severe chronic pulmonary hypertension. *Ann Intern Med* 107:565-568, 1987.

The PIOPED Investigators: Value of the ventilation/perfusion scan in acute pulmonary embolism: results of the prospective investigation of pulmonary embolism diagnosis (PIOPED). *JAMA* 263:2753-2759, 1990.

Roberts AC: Bronchial artery embolization therapy. *J Thorac Imaging* 5:60-72, 1990.

Ray CE, Kaufman JA, Geller S et al: Embolization of pulmonary catheter-induced pulmonary artery pseudoaneurysms. *Chest* 110:1370-1373, 1996.

Remy-Jardin M, Remy J: Spiral CT angiography of the pulmonary circulation. *Radiology* 212:615-636, 1999.

Rosado-de-Christenson ML, Frazier AA, Stocker JT, Templeton PA: From the archives of the AFIP. Extralobar sequestration: radiologic-pathologic correlation. *Radiographics* 13:425-441, 1993.

Tunaci M, Ozkorkmaz B, Tunaci A et al: CT findings of pulmonary artery aneurysms during treatment for Behçet's disease. *Am J Roentgenol* 172:729-733, 1999.

Uflacker R: Interventional therapy for pulmonary embolism. *J Vasc Interv Radiol* 12:147–164, 2001.

White RI, Pollak JS, Wirth JA: Pulmonary arteriovenous malformations: diagnosis and transcatheter embolotherapy. *J Vasc Interv Radiol* 7:787–804, 1996.

Woodard PK, Yusen RD: Diagnosis of pulmonary embolism with spiral computed tomography and magnetic resonance angiography. *Curr Opin Cardiol* 14:442–447, 1999.

Zuckerman DA, Sterling KM, Oser RF: Safety of pulmonary angiography in the 1990s. *J Vasc Interv Radiol* 7:199–205, 1996.

Thoracic Aorta

JOHN A. KAUFMAN, M.D.

Thoracic aortic diseases can be some of the most challenging vascular problems to manage. The organs that are supplied directly by this segment of aorta (heart, brain, and spine) are intolerant of ischemia for more than a few minutes. Flow disturbances in the aorta impact the entire body. Surgical access requires a thoracotomy and possibly cardiopulmonary bypass. Imaging and percutaneous intervention in the thoracic aorta is one of the most exciting areas of interventional radiology.

NORMAL ANATOMY

The thoracic aorta begins at the heart, at the level of the aortic valves. The thoracic aorta becomes the abdominal aorta at the diaphragm, just proximal to the celiac artery origin, usually at the T12 vertebral body. The thoracic aorta is divided into ascending, transverse, and descending portions (Fig. 9-1). The ascending aorta extends from the aortic valve to the origin of the first great vessel (usually the innominate artery). The transverse aorta is also termed the "arch," the aortic segment that contains the origins of the great vessels. The descending thoracic aorta begins just distal to the left subclavian artery, ending at the diaphragm.

The normal area of the aortic valve is 2.5–3.5 cm². There are usually three valve leaflets, named for the coronary artery that originates in the coronary sinuses (sinuses of Valsalva) above each leaflet; the right, left, and noncoronary. The coronary sinuses have a characteristic slight bulge in contour (see Fig. 9-1). Immediately above the coronary sinuses the ascending aorta is typically 2.5–3.5 cm in diameter. The transverse and descending thoracic aorta are frequently slightly narrower than the ascending aorta, with diameters rarely greater than 2.5 cm in normal individuals.

The major noncoronary branches of the thoracic aorta are (in order) the innominate (also known as the brachiocephalic) artery, the left common carotid artery, and the left subclavian artery. The innominate artery bifurcates into the right common carotid and right subclavian arteries. Rarely (<1%) a small artery to the isthmus of the thyroid (the thyroid ima) may arise from the aortic arch. When present, this vessel arises more commonly from the innominate artery (3%) or right common carotid artery (1%) (see Fig. 5-2).

The proximal descending thoracic aorta frequently has a slight bulge in contour along the inner anterior surface just distal to the left subclavian artery, termed a "ductus bump" (see Fig. 9-1). This is named after the ductus arteriosus, the structure that connects the fetal pulmonary circulation to the aorta at this site. Rarely, a small portion of the ductus remains patent, resulting in an outpouching of the aorta at this point, termed a "ductus diverticulum" (Fig. 9-2). This structure invariably has a broad mouth and totally smooth walls, important features to consider when evaluating patients for aortic trauma.

The descending thoracic aorta gives origin to a number of small, but clinically important arteries. These vessels supply the bronchi, esophagus, intercostal muscles, and the spinal cord. The bronchial arteries are discussed in Chapter 8. The intercostal arteries arise from the posterolateral aspect of the thoracic aorta from the level of the T3 vertebral body to T12 (see Fig. 9-1). The arteries to

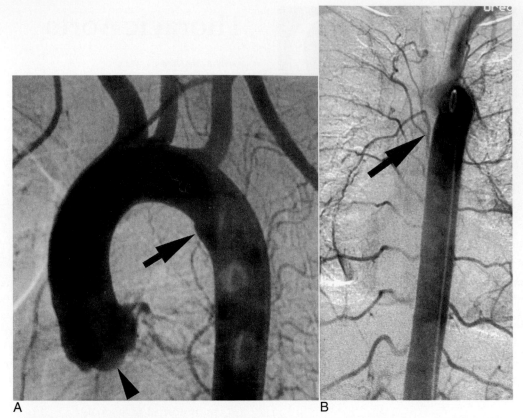

Figure 9-1   Normal thoracic aorta. **A**, Digital subtraction angiogram (DSA) of the aorta in the left anterior oblique (LAO) projection with the catheter positioned just above the aortic valve (arrowhead). The ascending aorta, transverse arch, great-vessel origins, and proximal descending aorta are well visualized in this projection. The subtle bulge in proximal descending thoracic aorta is a "ductus bump" (arrow). Note the smooth contours. (The oval lucencies projected over the distal aorta are subtraction artifacts from the spine.) **B**, DSA aortogram in the anteroposterior (AP) projection with the catheter positioned just distal to the left subclavian artery. The paired intercostal arteries are well visualized, with the arteries to the upper ribs arising from common trunks (arrow).

the first through the third intercostal spaces usually arise from a pair of common trunks on each side of the aorta, termed the supreme intercostals arteries. From T4 to T12 each intercostal space has its own pair of arteries. These vessels have multiple anastomoses, including the internal mammary arteries anteriorly and the chest wall arteries laterally. Less constant are anastomoses to the anterior spinal and bronchial arteries.

The arterial supply to the thoracic portion of the spinal cord is derived from the upper and lower thoracic aorta. The anterior spinal artery at the T4–T5 level is variably supplied from intercostal and bronchial arteries. The anterior spinal artery at the level of the T6–T12 vertebral bodies, the Artery of Adamkiewicz, originates from the intercostal arteries (usually the left) in 75% of individuals at these levels (Fig. 9-3). Spinal arteries have a characteristic appearance with a hairpin turn and a midline course.

There are many important variants of thoracic aortic arch anatomy, usually involving branching patterns of the great vessels and location of the descending thoracic aorta in relation to the spine. Familiarity with these variants is crucial to avoid diagnostic errors and therapeutic misadventures. A brief review of the embryology of the thoracic aorta makes understanding the variations very easy. The thoracic aorta is derived from the embryonic primitive ventral and dorsal aortae that are connected by six paired branchial arches (Fig. 9-4). Between the sixth and eighth weeks of life, selected arches appear and regress, resulting in a single aorta with three major noncoronary branches. The first arch forms the maxillary and external carotid arteries. The second arch forms the stapedial arteries. The third arch forms the carotid arteries, while the fourth arch forms the aortic arch and the proximal subclavian arteries. The fifth arch is present in only 50% of fetuses and regresses completely. The sixth

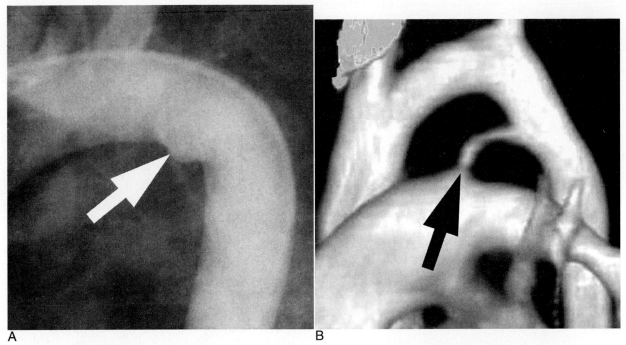

A   B

Figure 9-2   The ductus region of the thoracic aorta. **A**, In comparison to Fig. 9-1A, a more defined, focal bulge is termed a "ductus diverticulum" (arrow). Again note the smooth contours and lack of acute angles. **B**, Patent ductus arteriosus (arrow) seen on volume rendering of a CT angiogram (CTA).

arch forms the pulmonary arteries. All of the anomalies of aortic branching can be traced to variations in the pattern of branchial arch regression.

The most common variant (20%) of aortic arch anatomy is the left common carotid artery arising from the brachiocephalic artery ("bovine arch") (Table 9-1). Other frequent variants include direct origin of the left vertebral artery from the arch between the left common carotid and left subclavian arteries, and aberrant origin of the right subclavian distal to the left subclavian artery (Fig. 9-5). Aberrant right subclavian arteries lie posterior to the esophagus in 80% of patients, between the esophagus and trachea in 15%, and anterior to both in 5%. This vessel is more prone to aneurysm formation than right subclavian arteries that arise in a normal location (see Fig. 6-22). Similarly, in patients with a right-sided aortic arch, the left subclavian artery may arise aberrantly from the descending thoracic aorta.

The arch and descending thoracic aorta lie to the right of the spine in fewer than 1% of individuals (Fig. 9-6). This anomaly is the result of regression of left-sided rather than right-sided branchial arches. There are great-vessel origin variants (most commonly an aberrant left subclavian artery) in most adults with right-sided arches. Over 90% of individuals with normal branching pattern of the right arch ("mirror image") have severe congenital cardiac defects.

Bilateral ("duplicated") aortic arches are a rare variant that results from failure of regression of branchial arches on both sides (Fig. 9-7). The arches may be equal or disproportionate in size, with variable great-vessel branching patterns. The arch segments arise from a single ascending aorta, pass lateral to both sides of the trachea and esophagus, and join posteriorly to form the descending thoracic aorta. Duplicated arches account for over 40% of all cases of thoracic vascular rings. Found most often in infancy or childhood, symptoms include recurrent pneumonia, stridor, apnea, choking, and dysphagia due to compression of the encircled trachea and esophagus. Other etiologies of vascular rings include right aortic arch with a left ligamentum arteriosum (25%), right aortic arch with anomalous innominate artery (17%), and pulmonary artery sling (5%).

Additional arch variants include the cervical arch, in which the aortic arch is derived from the third rather than the fourth branchial arch (Fig. 9-8). These arches are recognizable by their unusually high location in the chest, frequently appearing to occupy the apex of the hemithorax. Additionally, cervical arches tend to be somewhat ectatic and elongated, with associated anomalous great vessel origins.

Coarctation of the thoracic aorta is a congenital fibrous narrowing of the distal arch or, most often, the proximal descending thoracic aorta distal to the left

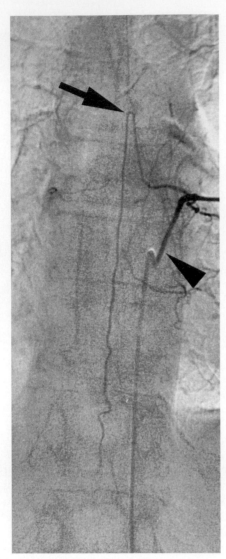

Figure 9-3   Artery of Adamkiewicz (arrow) seen on selective DSA of the left T9 intercostal artery (arrowhead). Note the classic hairpin turn in the spinal artery.

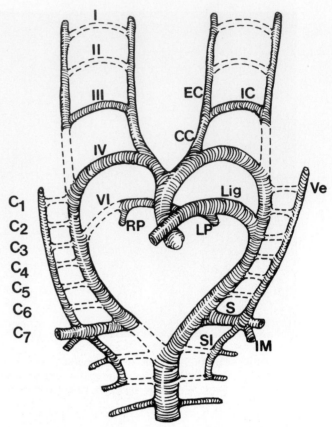

Figure 9-4   Diagram illustrating the development of the thoracic aorta, great vessels, and pulmonary arteries. I, II, III, IV, VI = paired branchial arches between the ventral and dorsal aorta. C1–C7 = cervical intersegmental arteries. CC = common carotid artery. EC = external carotid artery. IC = internal carotid artery. IM = internal mammary artery. Lig = ligamentum arteriosus. LP = left pulmonary artery. RP = right pulmonary artery. S = subclavian artery. SI = superior intercostal artery. Ve = vertebral artery. (Reproduced with permission from Kadir S: *Atlas of Normal and Variant Anatomy*, WB Saunders, Philadelphia, 1991.)

subclavian artery (Fig. 9-9; see also Fig. 3-10). The narrowing can be variable in severity, but with hemodynamic significance manifests as upper-extremity hypertension with decreased lower-extremity pressures in young patients. Aortic dissection is a recognized complication. Hypertrophy of collateral arteries (discussed below) is a hallmark of a severe stenosis. Untreated, this condition leads to left ventricular hypertrophy with eventual dysfunction (Box 9-1). In older hypertensive adults the descending thoracic aorta may become elongated and tortuous, simulating a congenital coarctation. The lack of a significant pressure gradient (>20 mmHg) distinguishes this entity as a pseudo-coarctation.

KEY COLLATERAL PATHWAYS

Obstructive lesions of the thoracic aorta are uncommon, but when they are present the collateral supply is determined by the location of the lesion. In the unusual situation of coarctation of the aorta between the left common carotid and left subclavian artery origins, there is low or reversed flow in the left subclavian artery. The descending thoracic aorta also receives collateral supply from right subclavian artery branches through communication with mediastinal and intercostal arteries. The lower extremities receive additional collateral supply via communication between the right internal mammary artery and the inferior epigastric artery in the anterior abdominal wall. The right subclavian artery and its

Table 9-1   Aortic Arch Variants

Variant	Incidence
Common origin innominate and left common carotid arteries	20%
Left vertebral arising from aorta	5%
of which:	
Between left common carotid and left subclavian artery,	4%
Distal to left subclavian artery,	<1%
Common origin carotid arteries	1%
Aberrant right subclavian artery (left arch)	1%
Right aortic arch	<0.1%
of which:	
Mirror image,	65%
Aberrant left subclavian/other variation great vessel origin	35%
Duplicated arch	<0.1%
Cervical arch (right more common than left)	<0.1%
Coarctation	<0.1%

branches can become quite enlarged in patients with longstanding distal arch coarctation.

The more common location for coarctation is the proximal descending thoracic aorta just beyond the left subclavian artery. This results in hypertrophy of both subclavian arteries and their muscular branches (see Fig. 9-9). There is reversal of flow in intercostal arteries distal to the obstruction (usually beginning with the intercostal artery pair at T4), which are supplied from the internal mammary and other chest wall muscular arteries. In this situation, both internal mammary arteries supply the lower extremities via the epigastric arteries.

IMAGING

Chest radiographs provide a large amount of information about thoracic aortic anatomy and pathology. This is probably the only vascular bed in which plain radiographs have an important role in imaging. Views should be obtained in both the anteroposterior (AP) and lateral projections, in full inspiration (Fig. 9-10). The location of the arch impression on the trachea is an important clue to the relationship of the arch to the spine (the side of the impression indicates the side of the arch). The diameter of the aorta, presence of calcification, width of the mediastinum, deviation of mediastinal structures, and presence of pleural effusion should be evaluated. The bony structures should also be carefully inspected for evidence of prior surgery (such as sternal wires or rib resections), or enlarged collateral arteries (such as scalloping of the inferior margins of the lower ribs due

to hypertrophied intercostals arteries in coarctation). As is always the case with imaging studies, comparison with old studies is crucial.

Helical CT with CT angiography (CTA) is an excellent modality for evaluation of the thoracic aorta. Multidetector array and other high-speed scanning techniques have further improved image quality (Fig. 9-11). A high-quality CT is frequently sufficient for definitive diagnosis and planning of an intervention. Prior to injection of contrast, a noncontrast acquisition should almost always be obtained. This allows assessment for wall calcification, intramural hematoma, and other high-density lesions that may be obscured by the presence of contrast (see Aortic Dissection below). The slice thickness for the noncontrast scan can be 7–10 mm in order to reduce time and radiation exposure. The contrast-enhanced scan should be performed with rapid injection of contrast (3–5 mL/s for total volume of 80–120 mL) through a peripheral intravenous (IV) line, the arms raised over the patient's head, and with an appropriate scan delay. When evaluating a patient for great-vessel origin pathology, contrast should be injected through an IV in the right hand to avoid artifact from dense contrast in the left brachiocephalic vein. Slice thickness of 1.5–3 mm can be achieved with fast scanners, allowing extremely detailed images (see Fig. 9-2). Careful inspection of other thoracic structures frequently yields important additional findings. Postprocessing is essential when evaluating tortuous or aneurysmal aortas.

MR of the thoracic aorta provides excellent anatomic (MRI) and vascular (MRA) images (see Figs. 9-7, and 9-12). Fast pulse sequences, cardiac gating, and breathhold techniques optimize image quality. Anatomic images are acquired in orthogonal planes (axial, sagittal, and coronal), and in an oblique orientation through the arch. These images are essential for determining true aortic size, evaluating for pleural effusion, mediastinal hematoma, and other pathology. MRA is usually performed with a 3-dimensional (3-D) fast-gradient echo acquisition and injection of gadolinium through a peripheral vein. The acquisition plane varies with the type of pathology and area of interest in the aorta, but generally a coronal slab is adequate. Slice thickness should be as thin as feasible in order to maximize resolution but without comprom-ising anatomic coverage. As with CT, contrast should be injected from the right upper extremity when possible. An appropriate scan delay is used, but serial acquisition of scans immediately following initiation of contrast injection allows dynamic imaging. The absence of calcium on MR images is an advantage compared to CT, but artifact from metal remains a major limitation. In addition, certain patients, such as those with pacemakers, cannot undergo MR scans. Postprocessing is necessary to create angiographic views.

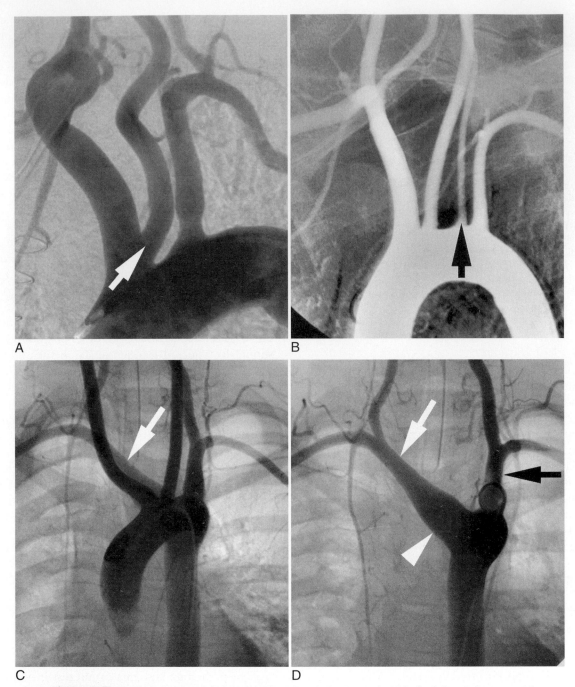

Figure 9-5   Variant anatomy of great-vessel origins. **A**, Bovine arch, with the left common carotid artery (arrow) arising from the brachiocephalic artery rather than the aortic arch. **B**, Origin of the left vertebral artery (arrow) directly from the aortic arch. **C**, Aberrant right subclavian artery (arrow) arising distal to the left subclavian artery. **D**, The same patient with the catheter positioned in the descending thoracic aorta. The right subclavian artery (white arrow) has a patulous origin (arrowhead) termed a "diverticulum of Kommerell." The left subclavian artery (black arrow) is normal.

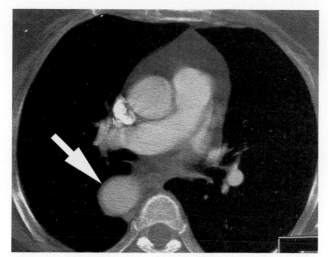

Figure 9-6   Axial CT scan showing the descending thoracic aorta (arrow) to the right of the spine in a patient with a right-sided arch.

Angiography is usually performed from a femoral approach, although the axillary artery can also be used. When selecting an axillary artery approach, the right should be chosen in patients with dissection or if injections will be limited to the ascending aorta or arch. When catheter placement in the descending thoracic aorta is certain, the left axillary artery approach is preferable (see Fig. 2-36). Injection rates for contrast vary from 20 to 35 mL/s for 2 seconds, so a reasonably sized pigtail catheter (6- to 7-French) is necessary. In young trauma patients with high cardiac outputs, an 8-French catheter and injection rates of 40–45 mL/sec for 2 seconds may be required. The first view that should be obtained when evaluating the thoracic aorta is the left anterior oblique projection with the catheter approximately 2 cm above the aortic valve (see Fig. 9-1). This view opens the aortic arch and places the great-vessel origins in profile. By carefully positioning the pigtail above the aortic valve, the risk of inadvertent injection into a coronary ostium or the left ventricle if the catheter jumps forward and unwinds can be minimized. Right anterior oblique and anteroposterior projections are also obtained (see Fig. 9-5). Occasionally, a true lateral view is necessary to evaluate pathology arising directly anterior from the aorta. The field of view should encompass from the proximal great vessels to the diaphragm for initial injections. The catheter should be positioned at the level of the pathology whenever additional views are necessary.

Breath-holding is necessary for catheter aortography. Digital subtraction acquisitions (DSA) with rapid filming (4–6 frames/s) are desirable, especially in young, hyperdynamic patients. For patients with slow flow or suspected dissection, extended filming for as long as 30 seconds may be necessary. Full-strength contrast (at least 30% iodine) should be used unless patient factors require diluted contrast. In patients with large aneurysms and sluggish flow, slower filming with an elongated contrast injection (increased total volume over a longer period of time) improves opacification, but these are frequently

Ultrasound of the thoracic aorta can be performed with external (transthoracic) and internal (transesophageal) probes. Transthoracic US requires no patient preparation and, usually, no sedation. The ability to evaluate the distal arch and the descending thoracic aorta is limited owing to the distance from the anterior chest wall and surrounding lung. Insertion of transesophageal echocardiography (TEE) probes requires some patient preparation and sedation, but the ability to visualize the deeper aortic structures is greatly improved over transthoracic probes (see Figs. 3-8 and 3-9). Both studies are highly operator-dependent for acquisition of diagnostic images, and require 30–45 minutes to complete.

Catheter angiography retains an important but limited role in the diagnosis of thoracic aortic diseases (Table 9-2). The noninvasive modalities described above have supplanted catheter angiography in most patients.

Table 9-2   Thoracic Aortography

Projection	Catheter position[a]	Injection (mL/s)[b]	Filming (Frames/s)	Application
LAO	Ascending	30–40	4–8	Trauma; aneurysm; dissection
RAO	Ascending	30–40	4–8	Trauma; aneurysm; dissection
LAO	Arch	20–30	4–8	Great-vessel origins
AP, lateral	Distal arch	20–30	4–8	Trauma; dissection; aneurysm; localization of bronchial arteries

[a]Pigtail catheter 6- to 8-Fr for injection in the ascending aorta; 5-Fr can be used when injection is limited to arch or descending aorta.
[b]For 2 seconds.
  LAO, left anterior oblique; RAO, right anterior oblique; AP, anterior projection.

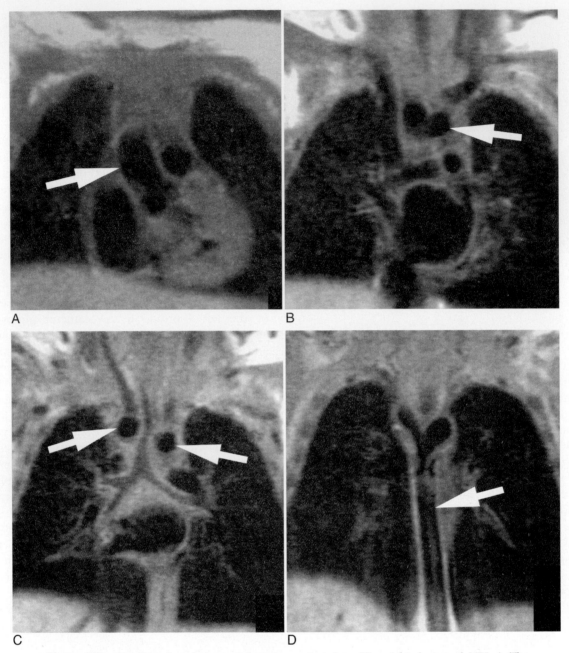

Figure 9-7   Duplicated arch in an infant demonstrated on T1-weighted coronal MRI. **A,** The ascending aorta (arrow) is normal. **B,** The ascending aorta bifurcates (arrow) into two arches. **C,** The arches (arrows) pass on either side of and compress the trachea. Note the right common carotid artery visible arising from the right arch. **D,** The arches join posteriorly into a single descending thoracic aorta (arrow).

the least satisfactory studies. Mask and pixel shifting are usually necessary even in cooperative patients who remain motionless during the injection, as cardiac motion introduces noticeable artifacts. Screen-film angiography can be performed when available, but most angiographers prefer DSA images, as the juxtaposition of lung and mediastinum makes the screen-film technique

challenging. The patient's arms should be raised over the head for biplane and true lateral filming unless contraindicated by clinical circumstances (e.g., trauma). Careful and frequent double flushing of the catheter is essential to avoid catheter-related embolic complications. Carbon dioxide gas is contraindicated as a contrast agent in the thoracic aorta.

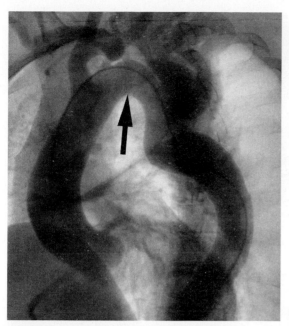

Figure 9-8   Cervical arch demonstrated on thoracic aortic angiogram in the LAO projection showing the elongated aorta (arrow) extending into the left lung apex.

Box 9-1   Thoracic Aortic Coarctation

Associated with bicuspid aortic valve in 80%
Congenital cardiac anomalies in 50%
    Patent ductus arteriosus
    Ventricular septal defects
    Mitral valve abnormalities
Life expectancy (untreated) is 35 years
Complications
    Hypertension (upper body)
    Left ventricular failure
    Aortic dissection
    Bacterial endocarditis
    Mycotic aneurysm
    Intracranial berry aneurysms
    Intracranial hemorrhage

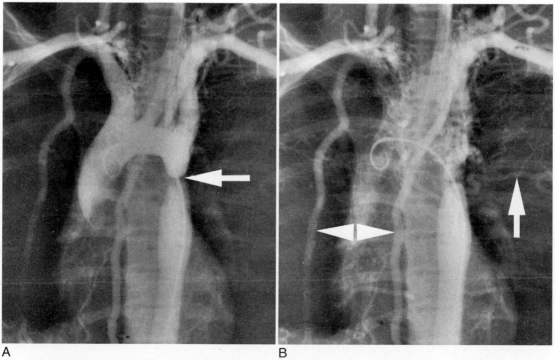

A   B

Figure 9-9   Descending thoracic aortic coarctation. **A**, Conventional angiogram in a patient with a coarctation (arrow). **B**, Later image from the same angiogram showing the extensive collateralization that occurs. (Arrow = enlarged intercostal artery reconstituting the distal thoracic aorta; arrowheads = enlarged internal mammary arteries providing collateral supply to the lower extremities).

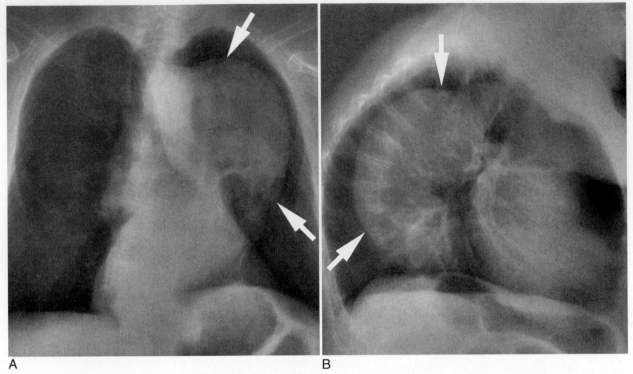

Figure 9-10 Chest radiograph in an elderly patient presenting with recurrent pneumonia. **A,** Anteroposterior view showing a large mass in the left chest (arrows) that displaces the trachea to the right and obscures the aortic arch. **B,** Lateral view of the same patient showing that the mass (arrows) is a large aneurysm of the descending thoracic aorta.

ANEURYSMS

Thoracic aortic aneurysms are less common than those of the abdominal aorta, but the range of etiologies is broader (Box 9-2). The majority of thoracic aneurysms (80%) are degenerative in etiology, occurring in older patients. Systemic atherosclerosis, hypertension, chronic obstructive pulmonary disease, and a history of aneurysms in other locations are frequent associations. Younger patients typically have nondegenerative aneurysms, such as those caused by vasculitis and connective tissue diseases, and post-traumatic false aneurysms. Thoracic aortic aneurysms are usually asymptomatic and discovered on chest imaging performed for other reasons (see Fig. 9-10). Large aneurysms may become clinically evident due to compression of adjacent structures, such as the central airways, pulmonary arteries, and superior vena cava (Box 9-3 and Fig. 9-13). Paralysis of a vocal cord can result from stretching of the recurrent laryngeal nerve by a large aneurysm. Rapid expansion or rupture of an aneurysm causes chest pain and hypotension. The differential diagnosis in these patients includes

acute myocardial infarction, pulmonary embolism, and aortic dissection.

Thoracic aortic aneurysms are described by their location: ascending aorta, arch, or descending aorta. Aneurysm location has a major impact upon management, as both the surgical and endovascular approach to repair is determined by the relationship of the aneurysm to the aortic valve, the great-vessel origins (in particular the left subclavian artery), and the abdominal visceral arteries. Aneurysms distal to the left subclavian artery may be treated with endovascular techniques or surgically through a left thoracotomy with a clamp placed distal to the great-vessel origins. Ascending aortic or arch aneurysm repair requires median sternotomy and, frequently, cardiac bypass.

Cross-sectional imaging of thoracic aortic aneurysms with CT or MR frequently provides satisfactory information for following progression of the aneurysm or planning intervention. When angiographic sequences are employed, both imaging modalities can allow precise delineation of extent of involvement, status of the great vessels, and associated thoracic pathology. It is actually much easier to image thoracic aortic aneurysms with

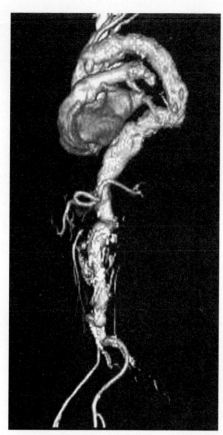

Figure 9-11   Oblique volume rendering of aortic CT angiogram (CTA) in an elderly patient with extensive atherosclerosis. This scan was obtained in less than 20 seconds on a multidetector row scanner.

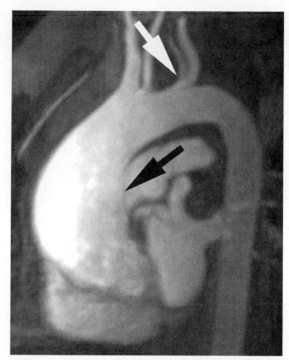

Figure 9-12   Oblique sagittal maximum-intensity projection (MIP) of a gadolinium-enhanced 3-D MRA showing a dilated ascending aorta (black arrow) in a patient with a bicuspid aortic valve. Note the left vertebral artery (white arrow) arising anomalously from the origin of the left subclavian artery. (Image courtesy of Barry Stein M.D., Hartford Hospital, Hartford, CT.)

cross-sectional techniques than with conventional angiography. Careful postprocessing of images yields excellent diagnostic information. The large capacity of the aorta, slow flow, tortuosity of the anatomy, and cardiac motion conspire to make conventional angiography difficult.

Ascending Aortic Aneurysms

The etiology of ascending aortic aneurysms determines, in the majority of cases, the appearance on imaging studies. The age of the patient is also helpful in predicting the etiology, with collagen vascular and inflammatory diseases most often found in younger patients. The most common underlying pathology in older patients is atherosclerosis. In these patients, the aortic valve is usually normal in diameter, with fusiform dilation of the aneurysm beginning distal to the sinotubular ridge (see Fig. 9-12). Severe aortic valvular stenosis may lead to post-stenotic dilatation of the ascending aorta. Although there are no universally accepted size criteria for surgical repair, aneurysms greater than 6 cm in diameter warrant consideration.

Dilation of the aortic valve and effacement of the sinotubular ridge is characteristic of Marfan syndrome, but may be seen with other connective disorders as well (see Fig. 1-36). Other features of Marfan syndrome include autosomal dominant inheritance (but spontaneous mutation accounts for 15–30% of cases), asthenic body habitus, arachnodactyly, pectus deformities, subluxation of the lens, and increased risk of aortic rupture or dissection. Isolated ectasia of the aortic root can occur without other manifestations of Marfan syndrome. Less commonly, other heritable and connective tissue diseases can also cause dilation of the aortic root and sinotubular ectasia, such as osteogenesis imperfecta, Ehlers–Danlos syndrome, and rheumatoid arthritis.

Fusiform ascending aortic aneurysms may be seen rarely in patients with Takayasu's arteritis. Aortic wall thickening on cross-sectional imaging is characteristic. Syphilitic aortitis occurs in 10% of patients with untreated tertiary syphilis and was, at one time, the most common cause of thoracic aortic aneurysm (Fig. 9-14). The characteristic features of syphilitic aneurysms are sparing of the sinotubular junction (although aortic

Box 9-2   Thoracic Aortic Aneurysms

Ascending

Degenerative (associated with atherosclerosis)
Syphilis
Marfan syndrome
Arteritis
    Giant-cell
    Takayasu's
    Rheumatoid
    Ankylosing spondylitis
Post-coronary bypass

Arch

Degenerative (associated with atherosclerosis)
Syphilis
Infection
Arteritis
    Giant-cell
    Takayasu's
    Behçet's disease

Descending

Degenerative (associated with atherosclerosis)
Arteritis
    Giant-cell
    Takayasu's
    Behçet's disease
Post-traumatic
Post-coarctation
Ductus diverticulum
Infection

Box 9-3   Complications of Thoracic Aortic Aneurysms

Rupture
Distal embolization
Compression of adjacent structures
    Trachea
    Esophagus
    Pulmonary artery or vein
    Superior vena cava
    Recurrent laryngeal nerve
Fistula
    Trachea or bronchus
    Superior vena cava
    Esophagus
Infection
Erosion of adjacent vertebrae

Aneurysms of the Transverse Arch

Fusiform aneurysms of the transverse aortic arch are almost always degenerative in nature, and contiguous with either an ascending or descending aortic aneurysm. Common features on cross-sectional imaging are intimal calcification with bulky plaque or mural thrombus, tortuosity and elongation of the arch, and deviation of

regurgitation and aneurysms of the Sinus of Valsalva can occur), saccular aneurysms in 75% with fine linear calcification and shaggy "tree-bark" intima upon which is superimposed atherosclerotic disease. The finding of extensive calcification of the ascending aorta on a chest radiograph strongly suggests syphilitic aortitis. Half of the aneurysms are located in the ascending aorta, one-third in the arch, one-fifth in the descending thoracic aorta, and rarely in the abdominal aorta.

Aneurysms of the Sinus of Valsalva may be due to acute infections and chronic infection, vasculitis such as Kawasaki's, and following valvular surgery. Large focal saccular aneurysms of the ascending aorta at the implantation sites of coronary artery grafts may represent anastomotic pseudoaneurysms.

The treatment of ascending aortic aneurysms remains surgical replacement. The status of the aortic valve, coronary arteries, and great vessels influences the extent of the repair.

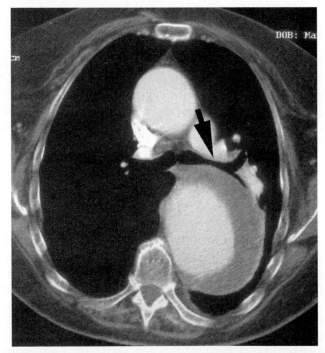

Figure 9-13   Axial CT scan showing compression of the left main bronchus (arrow) by a large descending thoracic aortic aneurysm (same patient as Fig. 9-10).

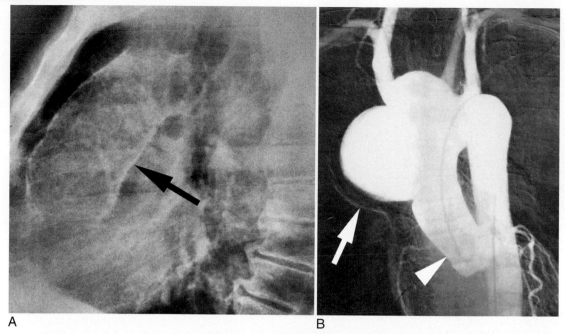

A   B

Figure 9-14   Syphilitic aortic aneurysms. **A**, Lateral chest radiograph shows dilatation and dense calcification of the ascending thoracic aorta (arrow). **B**, Angiogram in the anteroposterior projection from another patient showing a lobulated aneurysm (arrow) of the ascending aorta and arch with preservation of the aortic valve and sinuses of Valsalva (arrowhead) and the descending thoracic aorta.

mediastinal structures such as the trachea or esophagus. The most critical feature with respect to operative repair is the relationship of the aneurysm to the great-vessel origins.

Saccular aneurysms of the transverse arch are also most commonly degenerative in origin, but several additional etiologies should be considered. A focal aneurysm in an otherwise normal-diameter but atherosclerotic aortic arch may be a contained rupture due to a penetrating ulcer. An "aortic blister" may result from deep excavation of an aortic plaque, with formation of a localized aneurysm without rupture. Mycotic aneurysms are usually associated with an irregular contour and perianeurysmal inflammatory changes. As noted above, one-third of syphilitic aneurysms occur in the arch, and are most commonly saccular in appearance.

Aneurysms involving the transverse arch currently are managed with surgical repair and reimplantation of the great vessels.

Aneurysms of the Descending Thoracic Aorta

Most aneurysms of the descending thoracic aorta in older patients (>60 years) are degenerative in origin. These may be localized or diffuse, but are usually fusiform in contour, have calcified intima, contain mural thrombus, and have some associated aortic tortuosity (Fig. 9-15). This tortuosity is most notable at the diaphragmatic hiatus,

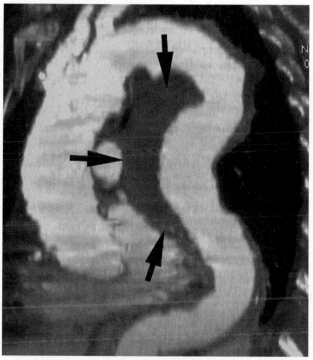

Figure 9-15   Descending thoracic aortic aneurysm in an elderly female with chest pain and a history of two prior surgical repairs of suprarenal abdominal aortic aneurysms. Oblique sagittal MIP of CTA (single detector) showing a tortuous aorta, diffuse atherosclerosis, and an aneurysm of the proximal descending aorta containing mural thrombus (arrows). The aneurysm begins several centimeters distal to the left subclavian artery. Note the horizontal segment of distal aorta typical in aneurysm disease.

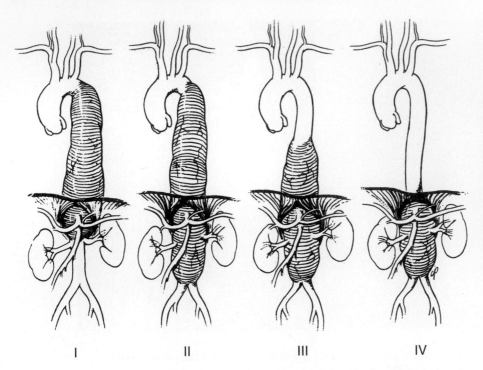

I   II   III   IV

Figure 9-16 The Crawford classification of thoracoabdominal aneurysms. I: Descending thoracic aorta to surparenal aorta. II: Proximal descending thoracic aorta to infrarenal aorta. III. Mid-descending thoracic aorta to infrarenal aorta. IV. Supravisceral aorta to infrarenal aorta. (Reproduced with permission from Cambria RP: Management of thoracoabdominal aortic aneurysms. In Gewertz BL, Schwartz LB eds: *Surgery of the Aorta and Its Branches*, WB Saunders, Philadelphia, 2000.)

where the descending thoracic aorta may actually make a 90-degree turn, run parallel to the diaphragm for a short distance, and then make another 90-degree turn to pass through the hiatus. Aortic diameters measured from axial images in areas of tortuosity are easily overestimated if the long diameter of an in-plane segment of vessel is measured. As a rule, always take the shorter diameter of noncircular segment of vessel as the true diameter.

As with ascending thoracic aortic aneurysms, exact size criteria for intervention have not been formulated, but aneurysms <5 cm in diameter are usually observed. Focal proximal aneurysms are simpler to repair with endovascular than surgical techniques. When the aortic dilatation extends below the diaphragm, the aneurysm is termed thoracoabdominal. The Crawford classification designates the types of thoracoabdominal aneurysms, with type IV analogous to an abdominal aortic aneurysm with supraceliac extension (Fig. 9-16). These are generally more complex to treat in that the abdominal visceral arteries are included in the aneurysm.

Fusiform descending thoracic aortic aneurysms may be found in patients with Takayasu's arteritis, other vasculitides, and Marfan syndrome. These patients are generally young, without evidence of coexistent atherosclerotic disease.

Saccular aneurysms of the descending thoracic aorta are usually not simple atherosclerotic lesions. When localized to the proximal descending thoracic aorta,

chronic aortic transection should be a strong consideration in a young patient, particularly if the aneurysm is heavily calcified with normal adjacent aorta (Fig. 9-17). Aneurysms that arise from the underside of the proximal descending aorta and burrow into the middle mediastinum towards the pulmonary artery may be aneurysms of the ductus remnant, termed a ductus aneurysm (Fig. 9-18). Focal pseudoaneurysms in otherwise normal-caliber but atherosclerotic aortas may occur due to penetrating ulcers (Fig. 9-19). An important differential in this situation is a mycotic aneurysm, which is usually multilobulated, and has a predilection for the distal aorta at the diaphragm, but may occur at any level (Fig. 9-20; see also Fig. 1-34). Vasculitis, such as Behçet's, may also result in focal saccular descending thoracic aortic aneurysms (see Fig. 1-17).

When imaging any thoracic aortic aneurysm, it is essential to know whether the patient has symptoms of pain, acute onset of hoarseness, hemoptysis, or dysphagia. These symptoms suggest an active process, such as rapid expansion or rupture. For example, a new left pleural effusion in the setting of an intact descending thoracic aortic aneurysm and acute onset of back pain suggests impending rupture. Stranding of the soft tissues in the mediastinum, or extravascular blood in the presence of a degenerative aneurysm, suggest rapid expansion or contained rupture, respectively. Mycotic aneurysms are by definition contained ruptures, and may have a prominent inflammatory response in the

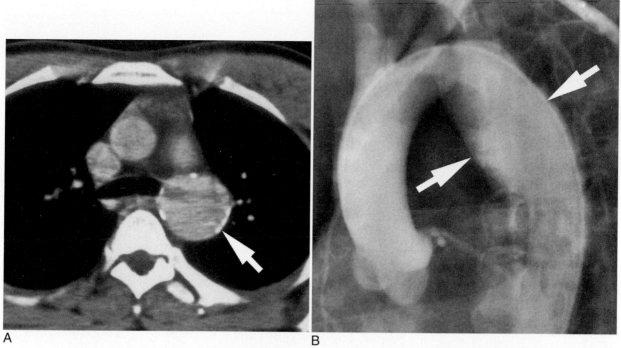

Figure 9-17   Pseudoaneurysm due to chronic untreated aortic transection in a 25-year-old male 7 years following a high-speed motor vehicle accident. A calcified proximal descending thoracic aneurysm was noted on a chest radiograph obtained to rule out pneumonia. **A,** Axial image from a chest CT shows an aneurysm with a calcified wall consistent with an old pseudoaneurysm (arrow). The remainder of the aorta was normal. **B,** Angiogram in the LAO projection showing the focal proximal descending thoracic aneurysm (arrows). The patient underwent uneventful surgical repair.

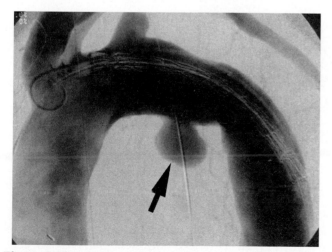

Figure 9-18   Focal saccular aneurysm (arrow) in the region of the ductus in a 75-year-old man. The true size of the aneurysm was much larger, but contained mural thrombus not visualized on this DSA aortogram. This was treated with a stent-graft (visible prior to deployment in aorta).

surrounding soft tissues. In acute situations, helical CT is an excellent imaging modality for assessing the thoracic aorta.

The relationship of the aneurysm to the left subclavian artery and the abdominal visceral arteries greatly impacts the approach and complexity of treatment. Involvement of these major aortic branches in the aneurysm increases the difficulty and morbidity of intervention. In general, operative repair of descending thoracic aortic aneurysms has a mortality of 5–10%. Paraplegia due to spinal cord ischemia occurs in 5–10% of patients, depending on such factors as the location of the aneurysm, extent of repair, number of patent intercostals arteries, and age of the patient. Other major morbidities include renal failure, stroke, and respiratory failure.

Endovascular repair of descending thoracic aortic aneurysms is a promising alternative to open surgical repair (see Fig. 9-19). Patients with aneurysms that have 1.5–2 cm of normal aorta distal to the left subclavian or left common carotid artery and proximal to the celiac artery are potential candidates for stent-grafts (Box 9-4). When the distance between the left subclavian artery

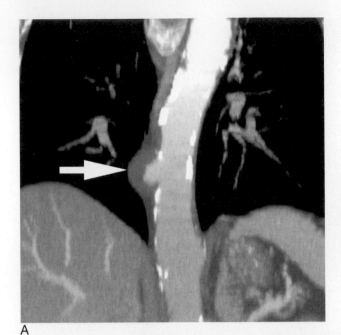

Figure 9-19   Focal descending thoracic pseudoaneurysm (symptomatic with back pain) in an 83-year-old woman probably due to a penetrating aortic ulcer. It was treated with a stent-graft. **A**, Coronal reformat from a CTA (single detector) showing the focal pseudoaneurysm (arrow), in essence a contained rupture of the distal descending thoracic aorta. **B**, DSA aortogram obtained immediately prior to deployment of a stent-graft (arrowhead) shows the pseudoaneurysm (arrow). **C**, DSA after deployment of the stent graft showing exclusion of the pseudoaneurysm.

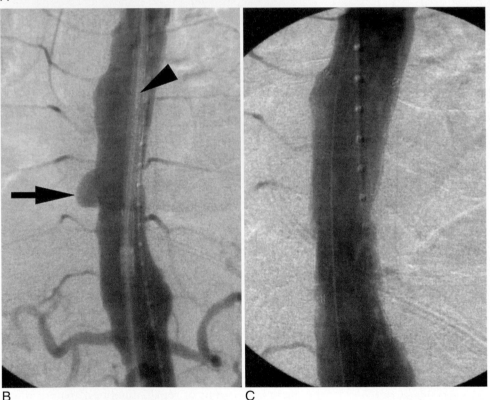

and the aneurysm is shorter than 1.5 cm, the endograft can be placed across the left subclavian artery origin provided that the left vertebral artery is dispensable. Most patients tolerate left subclavian artery occlusion without incident. Alternatively, surgical transposition of the left subclavian artery to the left common carotid artery can create a suitable proximal attachment site. Though the majority of patients treated with stent-grafts have degenerative aneurysms, acute and chronic dissections and transections have also been successfully treated.

Delivery systems for thoracic stent-grafts tend to be large, so assessment of the iliac arteries and abdominal

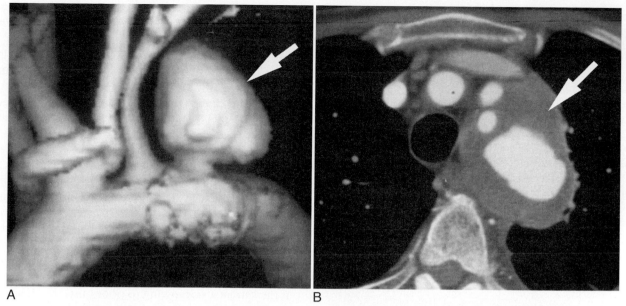

A   B

Figure 9-20   Saccular mycotic aneurysm of the proximal descending thoracic aorta in an octogenarian. **A**, Shaded surface display of a CTA showing the aneurysm (arrow). **B**, Axial source image shows a large amount of thrombus (arrow) that engulfs the adjacent left subclavian and left common carotid arteries.

aorta is necessary when evaluating a patient for one of these procedures. Surgical placement of a temporary graft to the common iliac artery or distal aorta may be required to deliver the endograft in patients with small or diseased pelvic arteries.

Approximately 90% of aneurysms undergo thrombosis after placement of a stent-graft, with an overall major procedural complication rate less than 10%. Paraplegia occurs in fewer than 3% of patients, usually when there has been prior or concomitant abdominal aortic aneurysm repair. With the development of branched stent-grafts, and stent-grafts with aortic valves, this technology will become applicable to arch and ascending aortic aneurysms.

Box 9-4   Stent-graft Repair of Thoracic Aortic Aneurysm

Proximal landing zone:
- 1.5–2 cm normal aorta distal to left subclavian artery or left common carotid

Left subclavian artery cannot be sacrificed:
- Consider subclavian–carotid artery bypass

Distal landing zone:
- 1.5–2 cm normal aorta above celiac artery

Acceptable landing zone diameters:
- Varies with device

Angulation of proximal or distal aorta:
- Preferably less than 90 degrees

Prior abdominal aortic aneurysm repair:
- Increased risk of paraplegia with thoracic aortic stent-graft

Patency and caliber of pelvic arteries:
- Large delivery systems may require direct access to common iliac artery or abdominal aorta

---

AORTIC DISSECTION

Aortic dissection is the separation of the intima from the adventitia by blood within the medial layer of the artery (see Fig. 1-9). The lumen lined by intima is the "true" lumen, while blood in the media forms the "false" lumen. In most instances, extensive aortic dissection can occur only if the media is abnormal, such as in patients with longstanding atherosclerosis, Marfan syndrome, or other connective tissue disorders (Box 9-5). The presumed etiology is a defect in the intima that allows blood to enter the media. This defect may be a linear tear, or a penetrating ulcer in an aortic atherosclerotic plaque. Pressurized blood then dissects antegrade, retrograde, or in both directions. As the intima is pulled away from the media, small tears ("fenestrations") occur at the origins of branch vessels. In these instances the blood supply to the branch vessel may be entirely from the false lumen. Alternatively, the dissection may extend into the branch vessel, causing compromised flow. A variant of dissection is spontaneous intramural hematoma, which is defined as

Box 9-5 Conditions Associated with Aortic Dissection

Hypertension
Atherosclerosis
Inherited disorder
  Marfan syndrome
  Ehlers–Danlos syndrome
  Osteogenesis imperfecta
  Turner syndrome
  Polycystic kidney disease
Autoimmune
  Giant-cell arteritis
  Relapsing polychronditis
  Systemic lupus erythematosus
Pregnancy (etiology of 50% of dissections in women
  <40 years)
Congenital vascular anomalies
  Coarctation
  Bicuspid/unicuspid aortic valve
Iatrogenic
  Aortic catheterization
  Aortic surgery
  Intraaortic balloon pump
Cocaine abuse

blood in the wall of the aorta with no definable entry tear (Fig. 9-21). Usually, with detailed evaluation, an inciting lesion can be found.

Aortic dissection is classified according to the location of the entry tear and the extent of the false lumen (Fig. 9-22). Classification systems for aortic dissection are based on the clinical outcomes. Dissection involving the ascending aorta is usually repaired surgically on an emergent basis owing to involvement of the aortic valve and coronary ostia (50% of patients), and the high risk of rupture into the pericardium or pleural cavity. Dissection isolated to the descending thoracic aorta is usually managed medically with aggressive blood pressure control unless critical organ ischemia is present. With time, the false lumen may thrombose if there is no outflow (Table 9-3).

The critical physiology of dissection is that the false lumen tends to remain at near systolic pressure throughout the cardiac cycle, owing to poor outflow. This results in progressive enlargement of the false lumen and compression of the true lumen during diastole (Fig. 9-23). When a critical branch vessel is supplied from a compressed true lumen, organ ischemia can result.

Patients with acute aortic dissection present with sudden onset of severe anterior or posterior chest pain,

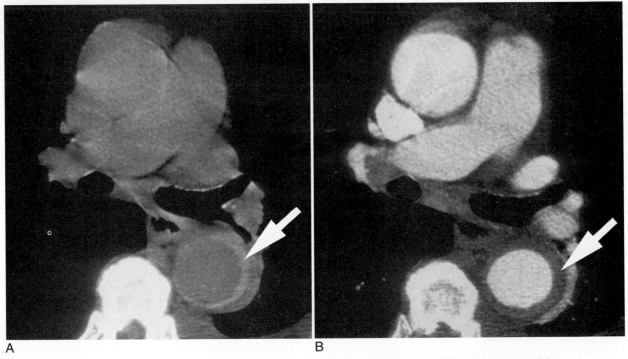

A   B

Figure 9-21   Intramural hematoma. **A**, Noncontrast axial CT image shows high density (arrow) in the wall of the descending thoracic aorta representing an intramural hematoma. **B**, Contrast-enhanced axial CT image at the same level. No intimal flap is visible. Relative to the contrast-enhanced blood, the wall of the aorta now appears thickened by low density (arrow). This underscores the importance of always obtaining an initial noncontrast scan before giving contrast when evaluating a patient for acute aortic pathology.

Table 9-3   Aortic Dissection[a]

	Incidence
Origin in and isolated to ascending aorta	15%
Origin in ascending aorta with extension to descending aorta	35%
Origin in descending aorta	50%
Mortality (*untreated*) at 2 weeks:	
Origin in ascending aorta	80%
Origin in descending aorta	40%
Five-year survival, treated	50%

[a] The male to female ratio is 2:1.

often described as "tearing." Unfortunately, these same symptoms may be found in patients with ruptured thoracic aortic aneurysms, acute myocardial infarction, pulmonary embolism, and other thoracic emergencies. The pain may wax and wane, and be associated with evidence of branch vessel occlusion such as stroke, abdominal pain, or limb ischemia. Rarely, organ or limb ischemia may be the only presenting symptom. The majority of patients with dissection are in their sixth through eighth decades, with underlying atherosclerosis and hypertension. Aortic dissection in a young individual without coarctation is suspicious for an inherited abnormality of the arterial wall or a connective tissue disorder.

Helical CT without and with contrast is an excellent modality for imaging of patients with acute aortic dissection (see Fig. 1-27). The value of the noncontrast scan is the conspicuity of acute intramural blood, which may be less obvious after administration of contrast (see Fig. 9-21). Other acute aortic pathologies, such as ruptured aneurysm, are easily distinguished from dissection on CT. A normal aortic CT in a patient with suspected dissection effectively excludes the diagnosis, provided that the quality of the study is satisfactory. In the region of the aortic root, artifacts due to motion, metal, and dense venous contrast can make interpretation difficult (see Figs. 9-11 and 3-21). Nevertheless, the overall sensitivity and specificity exceeds 95% for contrast-enhanced helical CT. MR with angiographic sequences has similar sensitivity and specificity, but can be difficult to obtain in acute, hemodynamically unstable patients. In addition, slowly flowing blood in the false lumen may produce a signal that can be confused with thrombus on spin-echo images. MRI is an excellent modality for long-term follow-up of dissections because of the ability to acquire images in multiple planes and avoid nephrotoxic contrast agents (see Fig. 3-11). TEE is also an excellent imaging technique for dissection, but requires sedation and is not as readily available as CT (see Fig. 3-9). TEE has

Figure 9-22 Classification of aortic dissection. Arrows indicate site of entry tear. (Reproduced with permission from Gertler JP, Tsukurov O: The spectrum of thoracoabdominal aortic disease. In Gewertz BL, Schwartz LB eds: *Surgery of the Aorta and Its Branches*, WB Saunders, Philadelphia, 2000.)

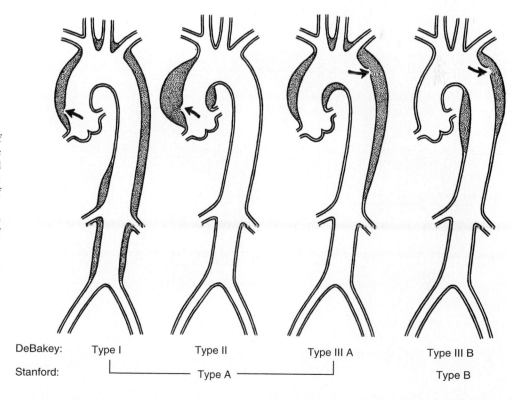

DeBakey: Type I   Type II   Type III A   Type III B

Stanford: └──────── Type A ────────┘   Type B

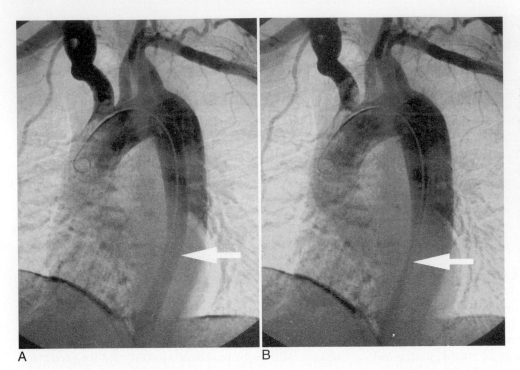

Figure 9-23 True and false lumen physiology of acute aortic dissection. **A,** DSA aortogram in the LAO projection of a patient with a dissection of the descending thoracic aorta extending into the left subclavian artery. The false lumen fills slowly owing to lack of a distal communication with the true lumen. During systole the true lumen (arrow) is partially distended and almost equal in size to the false lumen. **B,** During diastole the true lumen (arrow) is almost obliterated by the pressured false lumen.

an only 80% sensitivity and specificity for diagnosis of dissection.

Conventional angiography can be safely performed in patients with acute dissection, but is rarely necessary unless an intervention is planned. The common femoral artery approach usually allows access to the true lumen, as dissections rarely extend into the external iliac arteries.

However, if the true lumen cannot be entered from below, right axillary artery puncture frequently provides access to the true lumen in the ascending aorta. Opacification of both the true and false lumen, especially in the ascending aorta, is important to determine involvement of critical aortic branches and the aortic valve by the dissection (Figs. 9-23 and 9-24).

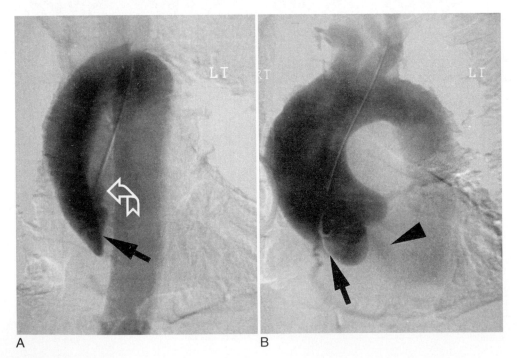

Figure 9-24 Catheter positioning in angiography of aortic dissection. **A,** DSA angiogram performed from the left axillary approach with injection into the false lumen. The catheter has inadvertently been inserted through an intimal tear (curved arrow) into the false lumen (arrow). Note that the aortic valves, coronary arteries, and great vessels are not visualized. **B,** After repositioning the catheter in the true lumen, the dissection flap is visible (arrow) as well as both the true and false lumens. There is slight aortic valve regurgitation (arrowhead). This is the desired catheter position.

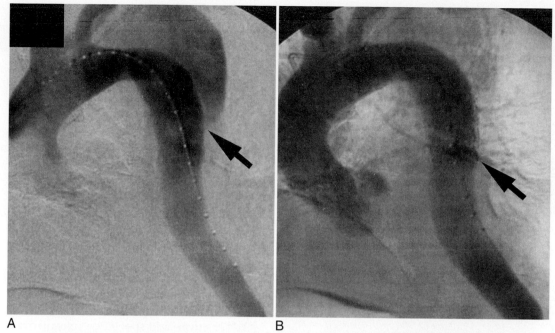

A   B

Figure 9-25   Stent-graft treatment of aortic dissection. The goal of therapy is to seal the entry tear, allowing depressurization and thrombosis of the false lumen with improved perfusion of the true lumen. **A**, DSA aortogram of a patient with a Stanford type B dissection (arrow). **B**, After placement of a stent-graft (arrow) over the entry tear in the true lumen of the descending thoracic aorta, the false lumen no longer fills. (Images courtesy of Michael Dake M.D., Stanford University Medical Center, Stanford, CA.)

The traditional therapy for type A dissection is emergent surgical replacement of the ascending aorta, with or without valve replacement. This stabilizes the process in the ascending aorta, but distally the false lumen may remain patent. Type B dissections usually do not require surgery in the acute phase unless the patient cannot be managed with blood pressure control alone. When aneurysmal change of the false lumen occurs, repair may be necessary to avoid rupture. Intramural hematoma without free flow in the false lumen is managed as if it were a classic dissection.

Several percutaneous options for management of acute and chronic dissection are available. Placement of a stent-graft over the entry tear has been shown to lead to depressurization of the false lumen and restoration of normal flow dynamics in the true lumen (Fig. 9-25). Initial results with this technique have been promising. Critical organ ischemia due to extension of the dissection into a branch vessel may be relieved by placement of stents in the true lumen. Percutaneous fenestration of the aortic flap (intentional creation of a large distal exit tear) can decompress the false lumen and relieve obstruction of the true lumen. Fenestration is accomplished by crossing the intimal flap with an intravascular needle using fluoroscopy or intravascular ultrasound to guide the thrust. Large angioplasty balloons are

then inflated across the flap to create an exit tear (see Fig 10-33).

TRAUMA

Aortic injury may result from rapid deceleration, crush injuries, penetrating wounds, or instrumentation during surgical or angiographic procedures. In general, suspected aortic injury requires rapid evaluation, and, if found, emergent treatment.

The majority of thoracic aortic injuries are due to blunt trauma. When a rapidly moving person suddenly comes to a halt, structures inside the body keep moving. This leads to injury of these organs, as they have very short vascular tethers. In the thoracic aorta, this manifests as either partial or complete tear through the layers of the aortic wall. This is termed *traumatic transection*. Patients with free rupture of the aorta die within seconds of exsanguination. When the rupture is contained by aortic or periaortic tissues, the patient may survive long enough to enter the emergency medical care system. These patients usually have multiple injuries, including to the head, spine, and abdomen.

Transections of the ascending aorta are rarely encountered in the hospital setting as these lesions are almost

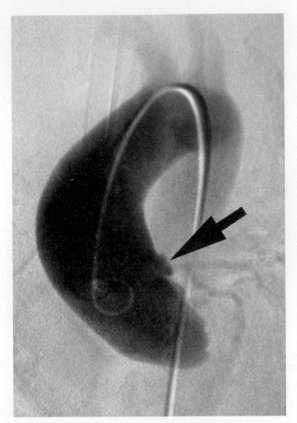

Figure 9-26   Ascending aortic laceration in an older trauma patient with a mediastinal hematoma on chest CT. DSA aortogram performed in the anterior projection shows a small tear (arrow) in the ascending aorta. The patient underwent successful surgical repair.

Table 9-4   Aortic Injury due to Blunt Trauma Seen at Imaging

Location	Incidence
Proximal descending thoracic aorta	90%
Great-vessel origin (innominate artery most common)	7%
Mid or distal descending thoracic aorta	2%
Ascending thoracic aorta	<1%

aortic transection (Box 9-6). Diagnosis requires confirmatory imaging, most often with contrast-enhanced helical CT (see Fig. 9-27). Mediastinal blood should raise the suspicion of aortic injury, but may be due to bony trauma or disruption of venous structures. A normal-appearing aorta on a good-quality helical scan with satisfactory vascular enhancement reliably excludes aortic injury, with >98% sensitivity and specificity. Irregularity of the aortic lumen or an obvious pseudoaneurysm on CT are consistent with transection. In many cases, postprocessing of the helical CT provides sufficient information to plan surgical repair, such as identification of additional aortic injuries and arch anomalies. Conventional aortography should be obtained in any patient with an equivocal CT. In general, it is far wiser to perform an angiogram rather than try to be definitive on the basis of a marginal CT scan. Intravascular ultrasound can be used to identify subtle aortic wall injuries and small intimal flaps.

At aortography, a transection appears as an irregular collection of contrast beyond the normal aortic lumen (see Figs. 9-27, 9-28 and 9-29). The tear may be partial or circumferential, and more than one vascular injury may be present. Along the underside of the aorta just distal to the left subclavian artery there is frequently a slight bulge in the region of the ductus, the "ductus bump." These always have smooth walls, with a very gently contour, and no acute angles or irregularity (see Fig. 9-1). Rarely, a small true saccular out-pouching or even an

uniformly lethal (Fig. 9-26). The lack of surrounding connective tissue results in rapid exsanguination, or bleeding into the pericardial space and acute tamponade. Patients who survive aortic injury usually have tears in the descending thoracic aorta, just distal to the origin of the left subclavian artery (Table 9-4 and Fig. 9-27). The mechanism of injury in this area may be due to either traction of the relatively mobile arch against the fixed descending thoracic aorta, or compression and shearing of the aorta between the head of the clavicle and the spine. In either case, survival beyond the initial injury occurs only when a pseudoaneurysm forms that is contained by adventitial or periadventitial mediastinal tissues. The resulting pseudoaneurysm is very unstable, with an extremely high risk of rupture. Untreated, mortality from aneurysm rupture exceeds 90% within a month.

Aortic transection in a trauma patient can be reliably excluded if the chest radiograph is pristinely normal. However, in reality, supine chest radiographs in patients with massive trauma are rarely normal. Numerous chest radiograph findings have been evaluated that suggest

Box 9-6   Chest Radiograph Findings Suggestive of Thoracic Aortic Injury

Widened mediastinum
Obscured aortic contour
Deviation of esophagus and trachea to right
Depression of left main bronchus
Apical cap
Left-sided pleural effusion

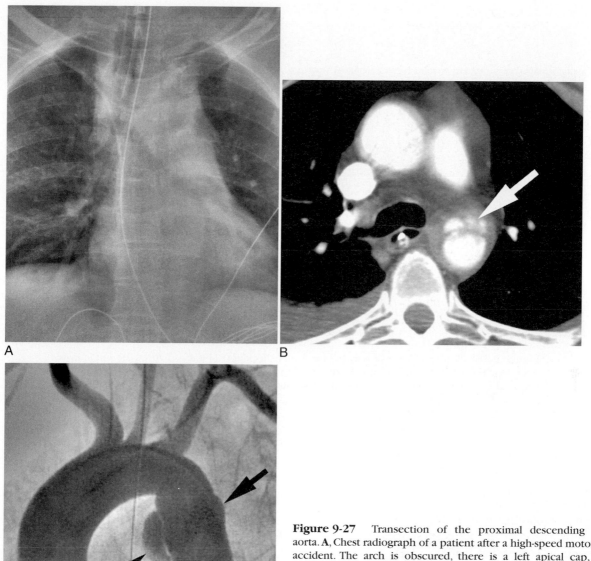

Figure 9-27   Transection of the proximal descending thoracic aorta. **A**, Chest radiograph of a patient after a high-speed motor vehicle accident. The arch is obscured, there is a left apical cap, the left mainstem bronchus is depressed, and the mediastinal tubes are displaced to the right. **B**, Axial CT image of the same patient shows mediastinal hematoma and irregularity of the aortic lumen (arrow). **C**, DSA aortogram in the LAO projection showing circumferential transection of the proximal descending thoracic with a large pseudoaneurysm (arrows).

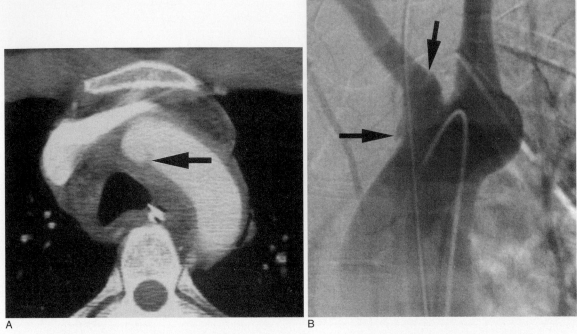

A   B

Figure 9-28   Traumatic transection (motor vehicle accident) of the origin of the innominate artery. **A**, Axial CT image showing mediastinal blood and irregularity of the origin of the innominate artery (arrow). **B**, DSA aortogram in the RAO projection clearly shows the pseudoaneurysm (arrows) at the base of the innominate artery.

aneurysm is found at this location, termed a "ductus diverticulum" (see Fig. 9-2). These are broad-mouthed, with smooth walls, and no sharp angles. Differentiation from a transection can be difficult when there is a large surrounding mediastinal hematoma, but the presence of any sharp or irregular contour represents a transection until proven otherwise (Fig. 9-30).

The conventional therapy of aortic transection is surgery with placement of a short tube graft. This surgery has a 5–10% risk of spinal cord ischemia, but otherwise has excellent long-term results. Rarely, patients with undiagnosed aortic transection survive to present years later with focal calcified descending thoracic aortic aneurysm (see Fig. 9-17). However, this does not occur with enough reliability to offer observation as a reasonable therapeutic alternative. Stent-grafts can be used to exclude the traumatic aortic pseudoaneurysm. When appropriate devices become available this may become the preferred initial management in the multi-trauma patient, followed later by elective surgical repair.

Penetrating aortic and great vessel injury is thought to be present in up to 5% of gunshot and 2% of knife wounds to the chest. Patients present with cardiac arrest, hypotension, hemothorax, hemomediastinum, or pseudoaneurysm. In the stable patient, definitive diagnosis, usually with angiography, should be accomplished quickly (Fig. 9-31). Endovascular repair with stent-grafts may be possible for injuries of the proximal great vessels or

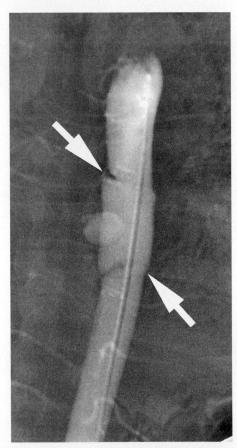

Figure 9-29   Transection of the mid-descending thoracic aorta (arrows) in a victim of a motor vehicle accident. The patient also had spinal injuries.

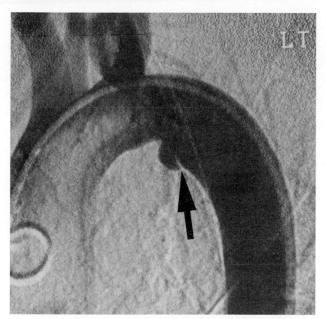

Figure 9-30 Focal aortic transection, surgically proven. This lesion can be differentiated from a ductus diverticulum (see Fig. 9-2) by the presence of sharp contour (arrow).

descending thoracic aorta. The majority of patients require immediate thoracotomy, but even so mortality rates remain above 80%.

VASCULITIS

Occlusive disease of the thoracic aorta due to atherosclerosis is virtually nonexistent. Whenever a patient presents with stenoses in the descending thoracic aorta that are not due to coarctation, vasculitis is the most likely etiology (Table 9-5). Patients usually have additional signs of vasculitis, such as constitutional and joint symptoms, abnormal rheumatologic profiles, and angiographic findings in other arteries consistent with vasculitis.

Long, smooth stenoses of varying severity are typical of arteritis. On cross-sectional imaging, a thickened aortic wall that enhances with contrast indicates an active process (Fig. 9-32). A thick, calcified wall with little or no enhancement after contrast administration suggests a burned out or treated vasculitis. These findings can be

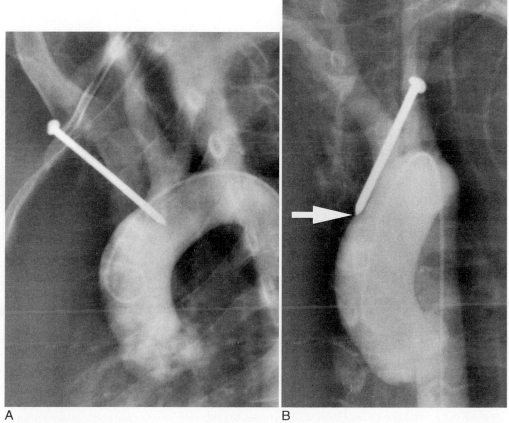

A   B

Figure 9-31 Aortography to evaluate penetrating injury of the thoracic aorta in a patient involved in a work-related incident. **A,** In the LAO projection a nail appears to pierce the ascending thoracic aorta. **B,** In the RAO projection the tip of the nail can be seen alongside the aorta (arrow). Would you pull it out? (Case courtesy of Frederick Keller M.D., Dotter Interventional Institute, Portland, OR.)

Table 9-5	Thoracic Aortic Vasculitis
Condition	**Aortic Manifestation**
Takayasu's arteritis	Long segment stenoses, also involving proximal great vessels; rarely, focal aneurysms, dissection
Giant-cell arteritis	Aneurysm; dissection; rupture
Rheumatoid arthritis	Aortic insufficiency; ascending aortic aneurysm
Ankylosing spondylitis	Aortic insufficiency; sinotubular ectasia
Relapsing polychondritis	Aneurysm; dissection
Behçet's disease	Focal aneurysms
Polymyalgia rheumatica	Aneurysm; dissection

made at both contrast-enhanced helical CT and MRI. The lack of signal from calcium makes MRI easier to read, but calcification can be important for a correct differential diagnosis and assessment of the activity of the disease. At angiography, these lesions have an appearance and location atypical for atherosclerotic disease, and may be associated with other unusual lesions such as great-vessel stenoses, aortic aneurysms, pulmonary artery aneurysms or stenoses, or abnormalities of the abdominal aorta. When performing conventional angiography as part of a vasculitis work-up, images from the aortic valve to the femoral arteries should be acquired, with selective injection of any suspicious-appearing visceral or other branch vessel (see Fig. 1-13).

The therapy for thoracic aortic vasculitis is first medical with anti-inflammatory agents, and only secondarily surgical with bypass procedures. Angioplasty and stent placement have been successful when attempted, but there is insufficient follow-up to determine the outcome of percutaneous intervention.

SUGGESTED READINGS

Atalay MK, Bluemke DA: Magnetic resonance imaging of large vessel vasculitis. *Curr Opin Rheumatol* 13:41–47, 2001.

Chen MY, Regan JD, D'Amore MJ et al: Role of angiography in the detection of aortic branch vessel injury after blunt thoracic trauma. *J Trauma* 51:1166–1171, 2001.

Cid MC, Font C, Coll-Vinent B, Grau JM: Large vessel vasculitides. *Curr Opin Rheumatol* 10:18–28, 1998.

Coady MA, Rizzo JA, Goldstein LJ, Elefteriades JA: Natural history, pathogenesis, and etiology of thoracic aortic aneurysms and dissections. *Cardiol Clin* 17:615–635, 1999.

Dake MD, Miller DC, Semba CP et al: Transluminal placement of endovascular stent-grafts for the treatment of descending thoracic aortic aneurysms. *N Engl J Med* 331:1729–1734, 1994.

Dake MD, Kato N, Mitchell RS et al: Endovascular stent-graft placement for the treatment of acute aortic dissection. *N Engl J Med* 340:1546–1552, 1999.

Demetriades D: Penetrating injuries to the thoracic great vessels. *J Card Surg* 12(2 Suppl.): 173–179, 1997.

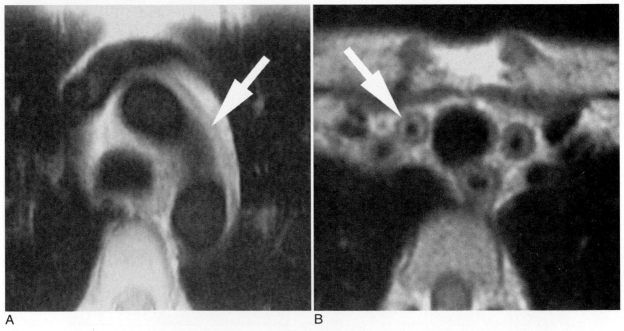

A   B

Figure 9-32   Takayasu's arteritis. **A**, Axial T1-weighted MRI at the level of the aortic arch shows a thickened, aortic wall (arrow) with intermediate signal intensity. **B**, Axial T1-weighted image through the proximal great vessels shows similar findings (arrow on left common carotid artery). (Image courtesy of David Bluemke M.D., Johns Hopkins University Hospital, Baltimore, MD.)

Fuster V, Andrews P: Medical treatment of the aorta: I. *Cardiol Clin* 17:697–715, 1999.

Ganaha F, Miller DC, Sugimoto K et al: Prognosis of aortic intramural hematoma with and without penetrating atherosclerotic ulcer: a clinical and radiological analysis. *Circulation* 106: 342–348, 2002.

Gavant ML: Helical CT grading of traumatic aortic injuries: impact on clinical guidelines for medical and surgical management. *Radiol Clin N Am* 37:553–574, 1999.

Kadir S: Regional anatomy of the thoracic aorta. In Kadir S ed: *Atlas of Normal and Variant Anatomy*, WB Saunders, Philadelphia, 1991.

Kelley MJ, Bettmann MA, Boxt LM et al: Blunt chest trauma: suspected aortic injury. American College of Radiology. ACR Appropriateness Criteria. *Radiology* 215(Suppl.):35-39, 2000.

Krinsky G: Gadolinium-enhanced three-dimensional magnetic resonance angiography of the thoracic aorta and arch vessels: a review. *Invest Radiol* 33:587–605, 1998.

Ledbetter S, Stuk JL, Kaufman JA: Helical (spiral) CT in the evaluation of emergent thoracic aortic syndromes. *Radiol Clin N Am* 37:575–589, 1999.

Mirvis SE, Shanmuganathan K: MR imaging of thoracic trauma. *Magn Reson Imaging Clin N Am* 8:91–104, 2000.

Moes CA, Freedom RM: Rare types of aortic arch anomalies. *Pediatr Cardiol* 14:93–101, 1993.

Orford VP, Atkinson NR, Thomson K et al: Blunt traumatic aortic transection: the endovascular experience. *Ann Thorac Surg* 75:106–111, 2003.

Prendergast BD, Boon NA, Buckenham T: Aortic dissection: advances in imaging and endoluminal repair. *Cardiovasc Interv Radiol* 25:85–97, 2002.

Sakai T, Dake MD, Semba CP et al: Descending thoracic aortic aneurysm: thoracic CT findings after endovascular stent-graft placement. *Radiology* 212:169–174, 1999.

Savage CO, Harper L, Cockwell P, Adu D, Howie AJ: ABC of arterial and vascular disease: vasculitis. *Br Med J* 320:1325–1328, 2000.

Shkrum MJ, McClafferty KJ, Green RN, Nowak ES, Young JG: Mechanisms of aortic injury in fatalities occurring in motor vehicle collisions. *J Forensic Sci* 44:44–56, 1999.

Svensson LG: Natural history of aneurysms of the descending and thoracoabdominal aorta. *J Card Surg* 12(2 Suppl.): 279–284, 1997.

Tunaci A, Berkmen YM, Gokmen E: Thoracic involvement in Behçet's disease: pathologic, clinical, and imaging features. *Am J Roentgenol* 164:51–56, 1995.

Wall MJ, Hirshberg A, Le Maire SA, Holcomb J, Mattox K: Thoracic aortic and thoracic vascular injuries. *Surg Clin N Am* 81:1375–1393, 2001.

Williams DM, Lee DY, Hamilton BH et al: The dissected aorta: percutaneous treatment of ischemic complications – principles and results. *J Vasc Interv Radiol* 8:605–625, 1997.

Williams DM, Lee DY, Hamilton BH et al: The dissected aorta: III. Anatomy and radiologic diagnosis of branch-vessel compromise. *Radiology* 203:37–44, 1997.

Zabal C, Attie F, Rosas M, Buendia-Hernandez A, Garcia-Montes JA: The adult patient with native coarctation of the aorta: balloon angioplasty or primary stenting? *Heart* 89:77–83, 2003.

CHAPTER 10

Abdominal Aorta and Iliac Arteries

JOHN A. KAUFMAN, M.D.

The abdominal aorta and pelvic arteries supply blood to all of the structures below the diaphragm. The pathologic processes that involve these vessels are varied and have major morbidity. This chapter covers aortic–iliac arterial diseases, including the male and female reproductive organs. The renal and mesenteric arteries are discussed in separate chapters.

NORMAL AND VARIANT ANATOMY

Abdominal Aorta

The abdominal aorta begins at the level of the diaphragmatic crura and terminates in a bifurcation into the common iliac arteries. This bifurcation is usually in the region of the L4–L5 disk interspace. The major blood supply to the abdominal viscera is derived from the aorta (Fig. 10-1). The aorta is constant in location and presence, although there is extensive variability of the anatomy of the branch vessels. The average diameter of the abdominal aorta is 1.5–2.0 cm at the diaphragm and 1.5 cm

below the renal arteries. The anterior branches of the abdominal aorta are the celiac, superior mesenteric (SMA), gonadal, phrenic, and inferior mesenteric arteries (IMA). The lateral branches are the renal and middle adrenal arteries (Table 10-1). The posterior branches are the lumbar arteries (one pair for each lumbar vertebra) and the middle sacral artery (arising at the aortic bifurcation). Clinically, the abdominal aorta is frequently divided into supra (above) and infra (below) renal artery segments. The impetus for this division is the higher incidence of atherosclerotic and aneurysmal disease in the infrarenal abdominal aorta, and the increased complexity of interventions that involve the suprarenal portion.

The anatomy of the testicular and ovarian arteries is similar in the abdomen, but divergent in the pelvis. In 70% of individuals the gonadal arteries arise from the anterior surface of the abdominal aorta just below the renal arteries (see Fig. 10-1). The most common variant location for gonadal artery origins is the renal arteries (20%), followed by the adrenal, lumbar, or even iliac arteries. The gonadal arteries pass to the pelvis along the anterior surface of the psoas muscles, adjacent to the gonadal veins and ureters, and anterior to the iliac vessels.

In the pelvis, the testicular arteries have a lateral course, entering the spermatic cord to continue into the scrotum. These arteries are the sole blood supply to the testes. The ovarian arteries have a more medial path, through the suspensory ligament of the ovary. The ovarian artery provides branches to the ovary and Fallopian tubes. The artery then continues medially to the uterus, where it anastomoses with the uterine artery in the broad ligament.

The lumbar arteries are paired vessels that arise from the posterior wall of the abdominal aorta at the levels of the lumbar vertebrae. The origins of the paired lumbar arteries may be separate, or conjoint. These vessels anastomose with the intercostal and other chest wall arteries superiorly, the epigastric arteries anteriorly, and the

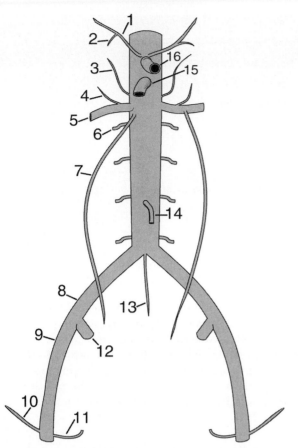

Figure 10-1   Drawing of the abdominal aorta and iliac arteries. **1**, Superior phrenic artery. **2**, Superior adrenal artery. **3**, Middle adrenal artery. **4**, Inferior adrenal artery. **5**, Renal artery. **6**, Lumbar artery. **7**, Gonadal artery. **8**, Common iliac artery. **9**, External iliac artery. **10**, Deep iliac circumflex artery. **11**, Inferior epigastric artery. **12**, Internal iliac (hypogastric) artery. **13**, Median sacral artery. **14**, Inferior mesenteric artery. **15**, Superior mesenteric artery. **16**, Celiac artery.

Table 10-1 Major Branches of the Abdominal Aorta	
Artery	**Approximate Level of Origin**
Celiac	T12–L1
Superior mesenteric	L1–L2
Renal	L2
Inferior mesenteric	L3–L4
Common iliac	L4–L5

angiographically from the superior hemorrhoidal branch of the IMA by its posterior location and lack of a terminal bifurcation.

Iliac Arteries and their Branches

The aorta bifurcates at the level of L4 or L5 interspace into the right and left common iliac arteries (Figs. 10-1 and 10-2). The common iliac arteries are symmetric structures that usually have no major side-branches. In the adult, the average common iliac artery is 8–10 mm in diameter, and 3–6 cm in length. The course of the artery is caudal, lateral, and slightly posterior into the pelvis. The right common iliac artery lies anterior and across the left common iliac vein. A small branch arising from a common iliac artery and taking a superior course into the abdomen will most likely be an accessory lower-pole renal artery. Occasionally, a middle sacral artery may arise from a common iliac artery.

The common iliac arteries terminate when they bifurcate into the internal and external iliac arteries. The internal iliac (also known as the "hypogastric") artery originates posterior and medial from the common iliac artery. This vessel is 1–4 cm in length, and bifurcates into an anterior and posterior division (see Fig. 10-2). The divisional arteries then give rise to the major visceral and muscular arteries of the pelvis (Box 10-1). There is great variation in the branching patterns of the pelvic arteries. When these variants are encountered, identification of vessels should be based on what they supply rather than the location from which they arise.

The branches of the posterior division are the iliolumbar, superior gluteal, and lateral sacral arteries. The iliolumbar artery is usually the first branch, although it may arise from the proximal internal iliac or, rarely, the common iliac artery. The iliolumbar artery courses superiorly along the sacroiliac joint. There is usually an anastomosis between this artery and the lowest lumbar artery. The superior gluteal artery is the largest component of the posterior division. This artery exits the bony pelvis through the greater sciatic foramen, superior to the piriformis muscle, to supply the muscles of the

internal iliac arteries inferiorly. These anastomoses can form the basis of collateral supply to the lower extremities in cases of distal aortic occlusive disease. The lumbar arteries supply the musculature of the abdominal wall, as well as the branches to the vertebral bodies and the contents of the spinal canal. This latter fact is of paramount concern whenever embolization of a lumbar artery for a nonneurologic indication is contemplated. In a small percentage of patients, the lower anterior spinal artery (artery of Adamkiewicz) will arise from an L1 or L2 lumbar artery.

The median sacral artery arises from the posterior wall of the aorta just proximal to the aortic bifurcation or as a common trunk with the L5 lumbar arteries (see Fig. 10-1). Occasionally, the median sacral artery will arise from a common iliac artery. This artery maintains a midline course in the pelvis, providing branches to the sacrum and coccyx. The median sacral artery is distinguished

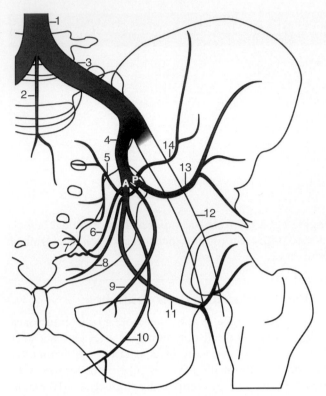

Figure 10-2 Drawing of conventional internal iliac artery anatomy. There is extensive variability of the anatomy of this vessel. **1**, Aorta. **2**, Median sacral artery. **3**, Common iliac artery. **4**, Internal iliac artery (A = anterior division; P = posterior division). **5**, Lateral sacral artery. **6**, Uterine artery. **7**, Middle rectal (hemorrhoidal) artery. **8**, Vesical artery. **9**, Obturator artery. **10**, Internal pudendal artery. **11**, Inferior gluteal artery. **12**, External iliac artery. **13**, Superior gluteal artery. **14**, Iliolumbar artery. (Drawing provided by R.T. Andrews, M.D., Seattle, WA.)

posterior pelvis. The lateral sacral arteries are named for their origins relative to the sacrum, rather than their course in the pelvis. These arteries are small in caliber and frequently multiple. They travel medially towards the sacrum, with anastomoses to the median sacral artery and the opposite lateral sacral vessels.

The anterior division of the hypogastric artery supplies the visceral and muscular contents of the pelvic cavity. The visceral branches are the internal pudendal, vesicle, middle rectal, and in females, the uterine and vaginal arteries (Figs. 10-2, 10-3 and 10-4). Discrete superior and inferior vesicle arteries are usually present. In females, the inferior vesicle artery becomes one of the vaginal arteries. The middle rectal artery, frequently a branch of the inferior vesicle artery, anastomoses with the IMA through the superior hemorrhoidal artery. The uterine artery courses medially in the broad ligament superior to the ureter. At the uterus the artery assumes a characteristic corkscrew configuration as it travels parallel to the uterine body. The uterus is a very vascular organ that stains or enhances intensely, particularly in

menstruating women. The uterine arteries anastomose with both the ovarian artery and the vaginal arteries. The internal pudendal artery supplies the external genitalia. Accessory pudendal branches may arise from other anterior division arteries. The internal pudendal artery exits the floor of the pelvis between the piriformis and coccygeus muscles, after which it travels anteriorly along

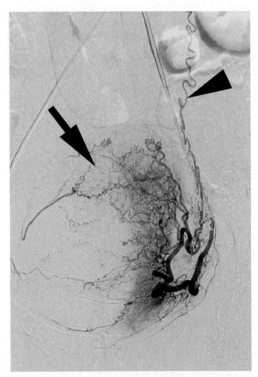

Figure 10-3 Selective injection of the left uterine artery in a patient with fibroids shows the hypervascular benign tumor (arrow) and reflux into the left ovarian artery (arrowhead). (Image courtesy of Hal Folander M.D., St Luke's Hospital & Health Network, Bethlehem, PA.)

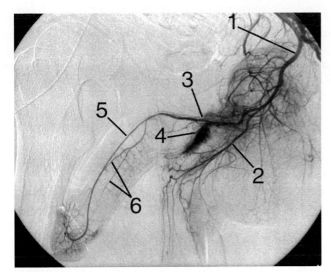

Figure 10-4 Normal internal pudendal arteriogram in a male. The arterial anatomy is usually symmetric. **1**, Internal pudendal artery. **2**, Perineal artery. **3**, Common penile artery. **4**, Normal cavernosal blush. **5**, Dorsal penile artery. **6**, Deep penile artery (in this individual both arise from the left).

frequently provide branches to the bladder. The obturator artery arises from the anterior division in 50% of individuals. This vessel exits the pelvis through the obturator canal, where it has a characteristic bifurcation. In approximately 15% of people the artery may take its origin from the inferior gluteal or the internal pudendal arteries. The obturator artery arises from the superior gluteal artery (a branch of the posterior division) in 20%, and from the common femoral or inferior epigastric arteries in 20% of individuals. The inferior gluteal artery is a branch of the anterior division in 75% and of the posterior division in 25% of individuals. The artery exits the pelvis between the piriformis and the coccygeus muscles, in the lower portion of the sciatic notch. The inferior gluteal artery accompanies the sciatic and posterior femoral cutaneous nerves, terminating in branches to the buttocks and posterior thigh.

The external iliac arteries provide blood supply to the lower extremities. The typical diameter of the external iliac artery is 5–7 mm. The artery angles anteriorly and laterally from the common iliac artery bifurcation, passing under the inguinal ligament to form the common femoral artery. The only branches of the external iliac artery are usually the circumflex iliac arteries (deep and superficial) arising laterally, and the inferior epigastric artery medially (see Fig. 10-1). These branches demarcate the transition from the external iliac to common femoral arteries.

the lateral border of the pelvis. The inferior rectal artery arises as a branch of the internal pudendal in this region. In males, the internal pudendal artery bifurcates into the perineal artery to the scrotum, and a common penile artery. The common penile bifurcates into deep penile (in the center of the corpus collosum) and dorsal penile (along the dorsal surface of the corpus cavernosum) arteries as it travels beneath the pubic symphysis. In females, the internal pudendal artery has a similar branching pattern that supplies the labia and the clitoris.

The obturator and inferior gluteal arteries are the primary musculoskeletal branches of the anterior division of the internal iliac artery (see Fig. 10-2). Both vessels

KEY COLLATERAL PATHWAYS

A large number of potential collateral arterial pathways are present in the abdomen and pelvis (Table 10-2). The pathway that becomes dominant in a particular patient depends upon the level and length of the

Table 10-2 Collateral Pathways in Aortoiliac Arterial Occlusion

Source	Example
Thoracic aorta	1. Superior to inferior epigastric to common femoral arteries
	2. Intercostal to lumbar arteries to aorta
Mesenteric arteries	Inferior mesenteric to hemorrhoidal to internal iliac to external iliac arteries (see Chapter 11)
Lumbar arteries	1. Lumbar to iliolumbar to internal iliac to external iliac arteries
	2. Lumbar to iliac-circumflex to common femoral arteries
Median sacral artery	Median sacral to lateral sacral to internal iliac to external iliac artery
Internal iliac artery	To opposite side of pelvis: internal iliac to lateral sacral and anterior division arteries across midline to same arteries on contralateral side
	To common femoral artery on same side of pelvis:
	1. Internal iliac to posterior division branches to iliac circumflex to ipsilateral common femoral artery
	2. Internal iliac to both anterior and posterior divisions to profunda femoris branches to common femoral artery

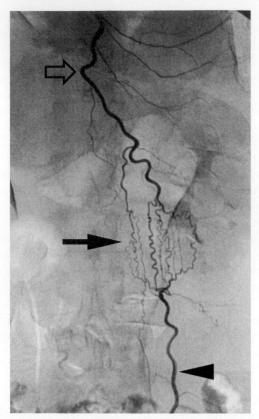

Figure 10-5   Internal mammary artery (open arrow) angiogram centered over the abdomen in a patient with aortoiliac occlusion showing collateralization (arrow) to the inferior epigastric artery (arrowhead), providing blood supply to the left lower extremity. This is known as "nature's axillofemoral bypass."

obstruction, and whether one or both sides of the pelvis are affected (Fig. 10-5). Multiple collateral pathways frequently coexist in the same patient.

The collateral supply to the uterus in the presence of uterine artery occlusion is from the gonadal and vaginal arteries. In general, central pelvic structures may be supplied by branches from either side of the pelvis, the distal aorta, the IMA, the gonadal arteries, or even branches of the profunda femoral artery. Structures lateral to and including the iliac bones may be supplied by multiple branches of the internal iliac artery, lumbar arteries, or branches of the distal external iliac artery or the common femoral artery. Conversely, the ovaries can receive collateral supply from the uterine arteries.

IMAGING

Ultrasound (US) of the abdominal aorta is an excellent modality for screening for abdominal aortic aneurysms (AAA), but performs poorly as a means of detecting occlusive disease. In many patients the aorta is a deep structure, surrounded by air-filled bowel, making

US imaging technically difficult. Tortuosity of the aorta and mural calcification can also limit US imaging. These same restrictions apply to US imaging of the common and internal iliac arteries. With the addition of intravenous US contrast agents, this modality may become more useful in the evaluation of aortoiliac arterial occlusive disease.

Perhaps the single most useful cross-sectional imaging modality for the abdominal aorta is helical CT. Aortic vascular studies should begin with a noncontrast scan to assess calcification and detect fresh hemorrhage. Contrast-enhanced CT scans should be performed with a power injector (3–5 mL/s contrast for a total volume of 80–120 mL) on a high-speed scanner using thin (1–3 mm) effective collimation. The scanning delay for contrast injection can be determined with a test bolus or automated triggering software. The field of view should be reduced to emphasize the central vascular structures. Images obtained in this manner can be postprocessed into elegant CT angiograms (Fig. 10-6; see also Fig. 11-1).

CTA has excellent sensitivity and specificity (each >99%) for detection of abdominal and iliac artery aneurysms. Aortic occlusive disease is readily evaluated with CTA, but this modality is less successful with iliac occlusive disease. The iliac arteries, particularly tortuous and small external iliac arteries, can be difficult to evaluate with confidence with CTA.

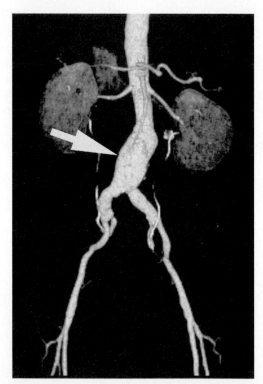

Figure 10-6   Volume rendering of CT angiogram (16-detector row) of the aorta and iliac arteries in a patient with an infrarenal abdominal aortic aneurysm (AAA) (arrow).

Magnetic resonance (MR) imaging of the abdominal aorta is relatively straightforward and accurate. With the exceptions of an inability to demonstrate calcium and artifact from metal, there are few limitations of this modality. The aortic wall can be evaluated from T1-weighted images in three orthogonal planes, but the best vascular imaging is obtained with gadolinium-enhanced 3-dimensional (3-D) MR angiography (MRA) (Fig. 10-7). The volume of gadolinium ranges from 20 to 40 mL, injected at 2–3 mL/s, 15–20 seconds before the scan is obtained (or with a delay determined from a test dose). For aortoiliac disease, the images are obtained as a coronal slab. The gadolinium-enhanced 3-D volume can then be postprocessed into angiographic images. Imaging of the major pelvic arteries is slightly superior with gadolinium-enhanced MRA compared to CTA, but the lack of visualization of calcium can be a limitation. Although there is no nephrotoxicity with MRA, metal clips, orthopedic and spinal hardware, and certain stents can create artifacts.

Conventional angiography of the abdominal aorta is usually performed with a 5- or 6-French pigtail or other flush catheter. The tip of the catheter is positioned at or just above the origin of the celiac artery (usually the T12–L1 interspace) (Table 10-3). If the renal artery origins are obscured, repositioning the catheter at the level of the renal arteries and filming with 10- to 15-degree left

Table 10-3 Abdominal Aortography

Parameter	Recommendations
Catheter	5- or 6-Fr pigtail or equivalent
Catheter position	T12–L1
Contrast	30% Iodine or greater
Injection rate	20–25 mL/s for 2 seconds
Views	Anteroposterior and lateral
Filming rate	4–6 frames/s
Additional views	10–15 degrees left anterior oblique with catheter at renal origins

anterior oblique angulation will display the vessels to best advantage (Fig. 10-8). In patients with contraindications to iodinated contrast, CO_2 or gadolinium can be used, although CO_2 may become trapped in large aneurysm sacs. When evaluating a patient with an AAA prior to an endograft, a graduated measuring catheter should be used and the distance from the renal arteries to the internal iliac arteries should be included in the field of view.

Flush pelvic angiography can be performed with the same catheter positioned 2–3 cm proximal to the aortic bifurcation to ensure that all of the side-holes are in the aorta (Table 10-4). The area included in the field of view should extend from the distal aorta to just below the common femoral artery bifurcation. Oblique views are crucial owing to the natural tortuosity of the pelvic arteries and to visualize the internal iliac artery origins. The posterior oblique projection usually displays the internal iliac artery origin to best advantage (Fig. 10-9; see also Fig. 2-48).

Angiography of the internal iliac artery or its branches requires a selective end-hole catheter. Usually both internal iliac arteries can be selected from a single femoral artery access. The contralateral internal iliac artery is selected in an antegrade fashion with a Cobra 2 or other angled catheter by crossing the aortic bifurcation, usually in

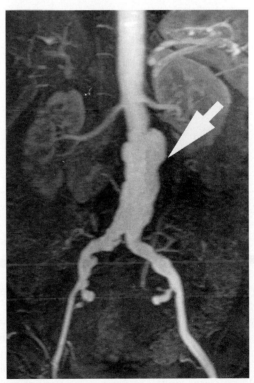

Figure 10-7 Coronal maximum-intensity projection (MIP) of gadolinium-enhanced 3-D MRA showing an infrarenal AAA (arrow).

Table 10-4 Pelvic Angiography

Parameter	Recommendations
Catheter	5- or 6-Fr pigtail or equivalent
Catheter position	2–3 cm proximal to aortic bifurcation
Contrast	30% Iodine or greater
Injection rate	7–15 mL/s for 2–4 seconds
Views	Anterior-posterior, 30–45 degrees oblique (bilateral)
Filming rate	2–6 frames/s

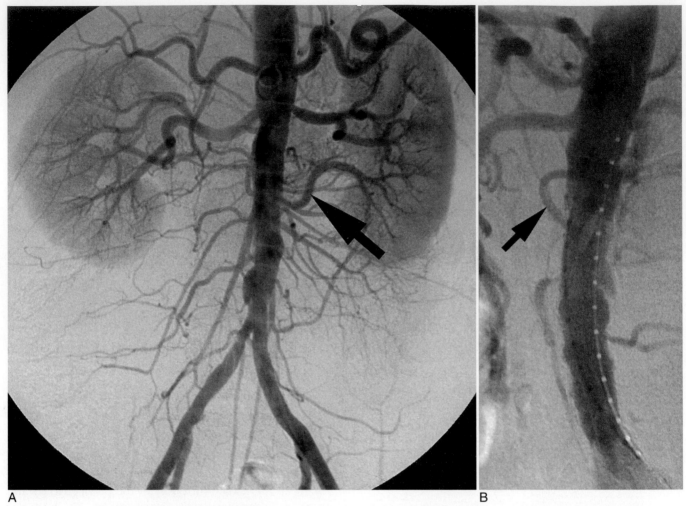

A   B

Figure 10-8 DSA aortography in a patient with diffuse aortic atherosclerosis. **A**, Anteroposterior angiogram obtained with a pigtail catheter placed just proximal to the level of the renal arteries. Incidentally, there is an accessory lower pole renal artery on the left (arrow). **B**, Lateral view in the same patient. Note the course of the accessory renal artery (arrow).

conjunction with an angled steerable hydrophilic guidewire. The ipsilateral internal iliac artery can be selected from the same femoral artery access with a pull-down technique using a Waltman loop or a Simmons-shaped catheter, or sometimes by antegrade cannulation with an angled catheter (see Fig. 2-17). The posterior oblique projection is most useful to visualize the origin of the internal iliac artery (see Fig. 10-9). However, the opposite (i.e., anterior) oblique view opens up the anterior and posterior divisions. In young patients, especially women, the internal iliac branches are prone to spasm, so gentle manipulation and generous utilization of intraarterial nitroglycerin (150- to 200-µg aliquots) may be necessary. Injection rates for these vessels vary, but are usually 3–5 mL/s for 2–3 seconds.

ANEURYSMS

There are numerous etiologies of aortic and iliac aneurysms (Box 10-2). Degenerative aneurysms are the most commonly encountered type in clinical practice, occurring in older patients with generalized atherosclerotic disease (Table 10-5; see also Fig. 3-18). The size of the aneurysm determines timing of elective therapy, and the extent of involvement of the aorta and pelvic arteries determines the approach. Aneurysms involving the descending thoracic as well as the abdominal aorta are difficult to treat with endovascular techniques, and require more extensive surgical exposure. In general, degenerative aortoiliac aneurysms are asymptomatic

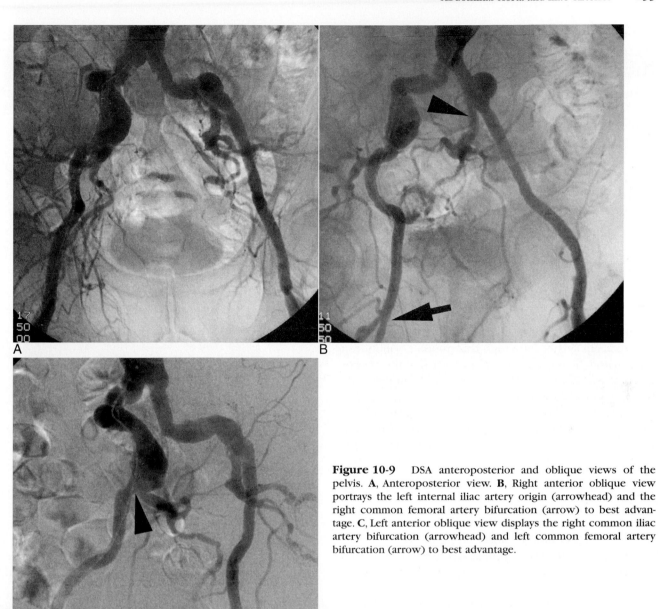

Figure 10-9   DSA anteroposterior and oblique views of the pelvis. **A**, Anteroposterior view. **B**, Right anterior oblique view portrays the left internal iliac artery origin (arrowhead) and the right common femoral artery bifurcation (arrow) to best advantage. **C**, Left anterior oblique view displays the right common iliac artery bifurcation (arrowhead) and left common femoral artery bifurcation (arrow) to best advantage.

until they rupture, so that preemptive treatment is desirable.

The etiology of degenerative aortoiliac aneurysms is multifactorial and incompletely understood. The different potential mechanisms are detailed in Chapter 1, but include familial, enzymatic, and possibly infectious causes. Atherosclerotic changes including calcification of the intima are prominent features of these aneurysms. An AAA is defined as a fusiform or saccular enlargement of the aorta that is 1.5 times greater in diameter than a normal aorta, or more than 3.0 cm in diameter. Aneurysms are frequently lined with mural thrombus, although the volume and distribution is variable (see Fig. 3-18).

The most feared complication of AAA is rupture, which occurs without warning often in a patient unaware of the presence of the aneurysm. The risk of rupture is proportional to aneurysm diameter, but is felt to be negligible below a diameter of 5.0 cm. Elective repair of aneurysms is usually performed when the diameter exceeds 5.0 cm, although this number continues to be debated. In addition to rupture, other complications are rare but include distal embolization of mural thrombus, thrombosis, and infection.

Aortic aneurysms that occur in young patients, in unusual locations, or under unusual circumstances are usually not degenerative in etiology. Underlying connective tissue disorders, trauma, vasculitis, and infection are more common in these patients. Often these are actually pseudoaneurysms, which are at greater risk of rupture than similar sized degenerative aneurysms.

Degenerative aneurysms of the iliac arteries usually involve the common and internal iliac arteries. Aneurysms of the external iliac artery are rare. Isolated degenerative common iliac artery aneurysms are also unusual, with more than 99% found in association with AAA (Fig. 10-10). The male to female ratio for isolated iliac artery aneurysms is 3–4:1, and 50% are bilateral. In general, common iliac aneurysms warrant repair when they reach a diameter of 3.0 cm. Isolated internal iliac artery aneurysms are even less common than isolated common iliac aneurysms (Fig. 10-11).

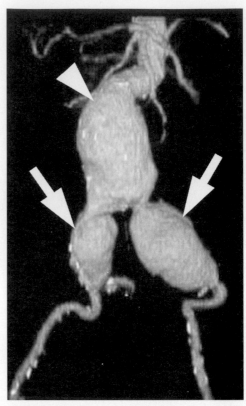

Figure 10-10   Volume rendering of a CTA showing an abdominal aortic aneurysm (arrowhead) and bilateral common iliac artery aneurysms (arrows).

Inflammatory aneurysms comprise 5% of all AAA. These are not infected aneurysms. The characteristic appearance is an enhancing mantle of tissue circumferentially or partially surrounding the infrarenal aorta (Fig. 10-12). This distinguishes an inflammatory aneurysm from a localized rupture, in which the periaortic tissue

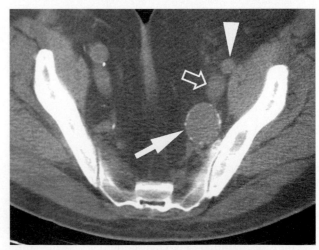

Figure 10-11   Axial CT scan of the pelvis without contrast showing an isolated 3-cm diameter left internal iliac artery aneurysm (solid arrow). The external iliac artery (arrowhead) is normal. (Open arrow = external iliac vein.)

Table 10-5   Abdominal Aortic Aneurysm

Factor	Reported values
Male:female	4:1
Prevalence	5–9% males aged 65
Average rate of growth	0.2–0.4 cm/yr
Risk of rupture at 5 cm diameter	5%/yr
Risk of rupture at 7 cm diameter	20%/yr

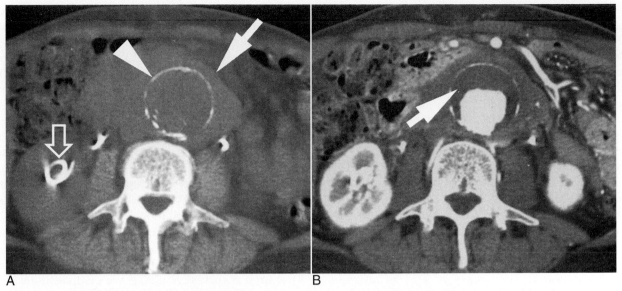

Figure 10-12   Inflammatory abdominal aortic aneurysm in a 53-year-old male. **A,** Axial CT scan without contrast shows a thick rind (solid arrow) around the aortic aneurysm (arrowhead). The patient has bilateral ureteral stents (open arrow) due to obstruction by the inflammatory mass. **B,** Axial CT scan with contrast at the same level. The inflammatory rind enhances slightly in comparison with the mural thrombus in the aneurysm (arrow).

will not enhance. The etiology is unknown, occurring in slightly younger patients than bland degenerative AAA. The presenting symptoms may be abdominal pain and aortic tenderness, similar to a contained aortic rupture. The inflammatory mantle involves the duodenum in 90%, the IVC and left renal vein in 50%, and ureters in 25%.

Imaging of aortoiliac aneurysms has several objectives: detection of aneurysms, monitoring size, preintervention planning, and postintervention follow-up. Preprocedural planning requires evaluation of specific anatomic features of the aneurysm (Box 10-3). Ultrasound is an excellent and inexpensive modality for detection and monitoring of AAA, with somewhat less success in the iliac arteries (especially internal iliac). However, US cannot provide sufficient information for planning intervention, or follow-up of interventions. Both CT with CTA and MRI with MRA can provide most of the information needed to plan interventions, as well as detection and monitoring of AAA (see Figs. 10-6 and 10-7). Postprocessing of good-quality studies is necessary to obtain the pertinent information to determine suitability for and plan an endograft procedure. However, aneurysm size is best measured from raw or reformatted images, as volume and surface renderings may show only the opacified lumen (see Fig. 3-22C,D). MR imaging is limited by an inability to show calcification, so a noncontrast CT scan is frequently also obtained when planning an endovascular repair using MR.

Conventional angiography is not necessary in the majority of patients undergoing repair of AAA. Aneurysm

---

Box 10-3   Preintervention Evaluation of Abdominal Aortic Aneurysms

Maximum diameter of aneurysm
Diameter and quality of normal infrarenal aorta
Quality and anatomy of renal and visceral arteries
Relationship of aneurysm to renal arteries:
- Infrarenal: >1 cm length normal aorta below renal arteries (>1.5 cm required for most endografts)
- Juxtarenal: Aneurysm begins within 1 cm of renal arteries
- Suprarenal: Aneurysm extends above renal arteries
Diameter and length of normal aorta distal to aneurysm (if present)
Relationship of aneurysm to aortic bifurcation
Distance from lowest renal artery to aortic bifurcation
Associated common and internal iliac artery aneurysms:
    Diameter and length of common iliac arteries
    Diameter of external iliac artery
Presence of occlusive disease in iliac and common femoral arteries
    Calcification, tortuosity
Venous anatomy
    Inferior vena cava, left renal vein
Renal anatomy
    Horseshoe, pelvic kidney

size is not accurately depicted, as mural thrombus can reduce the diameter of the patent lumen so that the true vessel diameter is not appreciated. Conventional angiography remains important in evaluation of patients with complex AAA, such as juxtarenal or suprarenal aneurysms, unusual renal artery anatomy such as horseshoe kidney, suspected visceral artery occlusive disease, and iliac occlusive disease. Conventional angiography may be obtained prior to endovascular repair in addition to CT to measure distances, determine the patency of renal and visceral arteries, or assess the access arteries. A graduated measuring catheter should used for these studies. Intravascular ultrasound (IVUS) can also be used to measure the internal diameters of vessels and distances.

Aneurysm rupture can be either free, contained, or into an adjacent venous structure (Figs. 10-13 and 10-14; see also Fig. 1-10). Most free ruptures are associated with large retroperitoneal hematomas as well as intraperitoneal blood. Early or small ruptures may be subtle, with the only evidence being stranding in the periaortic fat. In comparison, chronic contained ruptures are usually focal saccular contour abnormalities associated with localized disruption of intimal calcification and little or no surrounding soft tissue reaction. These localized chronic ruptures may contain thrombus. Patients with rupture into an adjacent vein (left renal vein, IVC, or common iliac vein) may present with hematuria, flank pain, or high-output cardiac failure. When acute AAA rupture is suspected in a hemodynamically stable patient, CT scan is the imaging modality of choice. This should be performed first without contrast, followed by contrast, unless rupture is diagnosed on the noncontrast images.

Treatment of infrarenal AAA is by surgery or placement of a stent-graft. Surgical repair involves an abdominal or retroperitoneal incision, placement of a proximal clamp on the aorta (preferably infrarenal), placement of a distal clamp, incision of the aneurysm with evacuation of mural thrombus, suture ligation of patent lumbar arteries and the IMA, suturing of a synthetic graft that extends from the proximal clamp to either the distal aorta, common iliac or femoral arteries, and then closure of the incisions (Fig. 10-15; see also Figs. 3-22C,D). Repair of suprarenal AAA is more difficult and morbid as a supraceliac clamp is required and the major visceral branches must be reimplanted. The mortality rate is 3–6% for elective surgery, and 25–50% for emergent repair of a ruptured aneurysm. Acute severe complications include bowel ischemia (2%), limb ischemia (0.5%), and cardiopulmonary disorders (15%). Repair of inflammatory aneurysms is more difficult owing to the periaortic rind.

Late complications of surgical repair are infrequent (Box 10-4). The two that are most dreaded are graft infection and aortoenteric fistula. Graft infection may present as sepsis, a draining wound, graft thrombosis, abscess formation, or an anastomotic aneurysm (see Fig. 1-35). Aortoenteric fistula usually occurs at the proximal anastomosis and presents as upper gastrointestinal bleeding (usually duodenal) of catastrophic proportions.

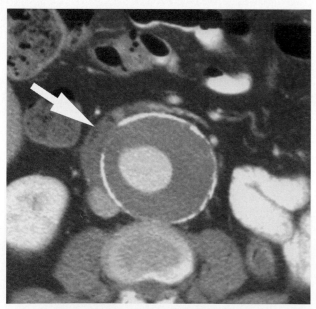

Figure 10-13   Subtle rupture (surgically proven) of the abdominal aorta in an elderly man with an episode of acute back pain. There is focal increased density of the periaortic soft tissues (arrow) adjacent to an interruption in the intimal calcification. Compare with Fig. 1-10.

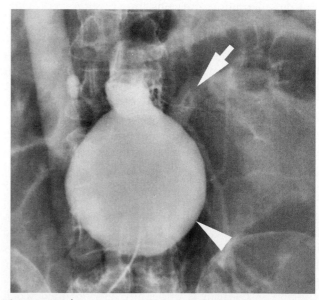

Figure 10-14   Rupture of a large abdominal aortic aneurysm (arrowhead) into a retro-aortic left renal vein (arrow). The patient presented with acute onset of left flank pain, hematuria, and high-output cardiac failure.

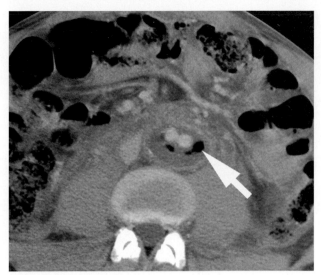

Figure 10-15   Axial CT scan with contrast obtained 48 hours after surgery for aortic aneurysm. Perigraft gas (arrow) is present around the graft within the aneurysm sac, but is a normal finding up to 3 weeks after surgery. Compare with Fig. 1-35. It is essential to know the date of surgery when interpreting postoperative scans.

By definition, graft material involved in aortoenteric fistulas is infected, but massive bleeding dominates the clinical scenario. Graft–enteric fistulas can occur anywhere along the graft, and present with chronic bleeding and infection (Box 10-5).

Endovascular repair of infrarenal AAA with stent-grafts is an alternative to surgical repair (Box 10-6). Aortic stent-grafts are available in three basic configurations (Fig. 10-16). Patients must meet anatomic criteria involving the proximal and distal attachment sites, angulation and tortuosity of the aorta and pelvis, and the presence of calcification and occlusive disease in the access arteries. The specific requirements vary for each manufacturer. The devices are modular in construction; i.e the endograft is assembled in the patient. The materials used in construction of endografts are biocompatible metals such as nitinol, stainless steel, and Elgiloy, and proven vascular graft materials. Endografts function by depressurizing the aneurysm sac. Two critical differences from surgery are the absence of sutured anastomoses to blood vessels, and the potential for continued patency of branch vessels arising from the sac such as lumbar

---

Box 10-5   Aortoenteric Fistula

Clinical presentation includes massive hematemesis, lower gastrointestinal tract bleeding, sepsis, abdominal pain

Usually at anastomotic suture lines (<1% aortic repairs), but can occur with native aneurysm

Duodenum most common site, but can occur at any point where bowel and graft are in contact

On CT, no definable fat plan between graft and bowel, +/− perigraft gas

Angiography may be negative, small "nipple" at anastomosis, or aneurysm; extravasation rare

At upper endoscopy, graft may be visible in base of duodenal erosion

---

Box 10-6   Indications and Contraindications for Endografts in Abdominal Aortic Aneurysm

Indications

AAA ≥5.0-cm diameter
Rapidly expanding (>5 mm/yr) smaller AAA
Contained-rupture AAA
Inflammatory AAA
High risk for complication with open repair

Contraindications

No suitable proximal/distal attachment site
Severe iliac occlusive disease
Mycotic aneurysm
Marfan syndrome
Ehlers Danlos syndrome
Unstable ruptured aneurysm
Associated visceral occlusive disease
Indispensable IMA
Life-threatening contrast allergy
Long life expectancy
Poor compliance with follow-up

AAA, abdominal aortic aneurysm; IMA, inferior mesenteric artery.

Box 10-4   Complications of Surgical Aortic Aneurysm Repair

Bowel ischemia (usually acute, inferior mesenteric artery distribution)
Graft thrombosis
Aneurysm formation above or below graft
Anastomotic pseudoaneurysm (frequently at more than one anastomosis)
Aortoenteric fistula
Graft infection
Graft degeneration

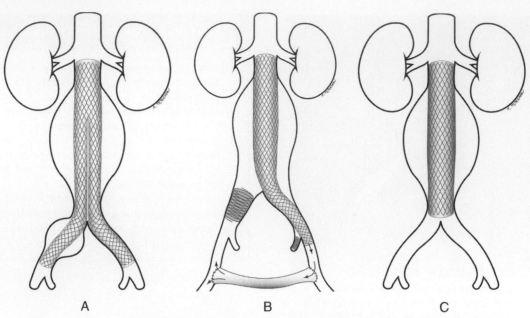

A   B   C

Figure 10-16 Endograft configurations. **A**, Bifurcated extending into either the common or external iliac arteries. This is the most common type of endograft. **B**, Aorto-unilateral iliac (AUNI) graft with surgical femoral–femoral bypass. This type is used when the patient's anatomy is not suited to a bifurcated graft. **C**, Tube graft. This is rarely used owing to the lack of adequate distal landing zones in the aorta below the aneurysm. (Reproduced with permission from Kaufman JA, Geller SC, Brewster DC et al: Endovascular repair of abdominal aortic aneurysms: current status and future directions. *Am J Roentgenol* 175:289–302, 2000.)

arteries and the IMA. Most patients treated with current devices receive bifurcated endografts. In general, only one-half to two-thirds of patients with AAA amenable to surgery can be managed with current endografts. Up to a third of these patients require preimplantation embolization of an internal iliac or accessory renal artery, or other percutaneous intervention in order to become anatomically suitable for an endograft (Fig. 10-17). As many as 30% of patients who undergo internal iliac artery embolization develop transient buttock claudication.

The exact technique of endograft placement varies with each device, but certain commonalities exist. Most important is careful preprocedural planning, especially device selection, as none is retrievable. For most manufacturers, the diameters of the device at the attachment sites should be at least 10–15% greater than the artery (measured adventitia to adventitia). Excellent intraprocedural imaging is mandatory. Precise localization of critical branch vessels such as the renal and internal iliac arteries prevents inadvertent occlusion by graft overlay. In general, an aortogram is obtained centered on the renal arteries, followed by deployment of the proximal portion of the device (Fig. 10-18). Once this has been accomplished, the distal portion is deployed after localization of the internal iliac arteries. Most modular

bifurcated devices require catheterization of at least one limb stump, usually from the opposite common femoral artery, to complete construction of the endograft. The device delivery systems range in size from 12- to 21-French. Large-diameter introduction systems require surgical exposure of the common femoral arteries.

Placement of endografts is successful in more than 95% of attempts, provided patients are carefully selected. In approximately 15–30% of patients additional endovascular procedures are necessary to improve the technical and clinical success of the procedure (Box 10-7). The major complication rate is less than 5%, with most complications related to the vascular access. Patients usually are discharged home by the third postprocedure day.

Continued opacification of the aneurysm sac by contrast following endograft placement (termed "endoleak") is found on CT scans in 30–40% of patients acutely, and 20–40% during follow-up (Table 10-6 and Fig. 10-19). This finding correlates with near-systemic or systemic arterial pressures in the aneurysm sac. The etiology of the majority of early and late sac perfusion is type II, although types I and III can occur at any time. Type IV perfusion generally resolves spontaneously within 48 hours of endograft placement. Many endoleaks can be treated with percutaneous methods, such as insertion of endograft extensions for type I leaks, embolization of

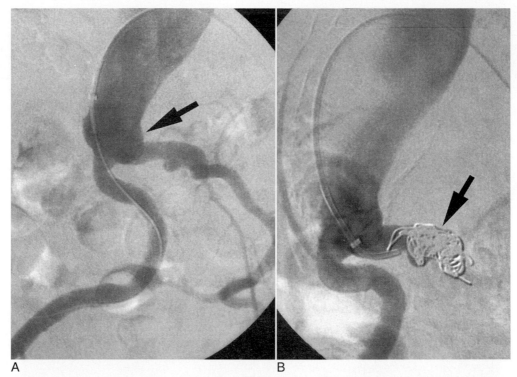

Figure 10-17   Embolization of the internal iliac artery prior to stent-graft placement. **A,** Right posterior oblique DSA showing a common iliac artery aneurysm that involves the origin of the right internal iliac artery (arrow). The landing zone of the stent-graft on this side will be the external iliac artery. **B,** Postembolization DSA showing proximal, compact placement of the coils (arrow) in the internal iliac artery. Notice that the approach was over the bifurcation in this patient. Often an ipsilateral approach is easier.

branch vessels or the sac for type II leaks, and insertion of endograft "patches" for type III leaks (Fig. 10-20).

The most important outcome of endografts is freedom from AAA rupture. Delayed rupture is reported in fewer than 0.1% of patients. Most patients have stabilization or decrease in the volume of the aneurysm sac (see Fig. 4-18). However, continued sac growth is seen in at least 5% of patients. Shrinkage of the perianeurysmal fibrosis after

endograft placement has been reported in patients with inflammatory aneurysms.

Plain films as well as CT scans (or some other reproducible imaging technique) are essential parts of the follow-up of these patients. Patients must be studied at regular intervals for the remainder of their lives after endograft placement. As the AAA sac decreases in volume, the endograft may become distorted, with limb

---

Box 10-7   Adjunct Procedures Prior or During Endovascular Repair of Aneurysms

Branch vessel embolization (internal iliac, accessory renal, or inferior mesenteric artery)

Angioplasty of iliac artery stenosis during device delivery

Stent reinforcement of endograft limb

Stent for access artery dissection

Stent-graft extension or surgical bypass for access artery rupture

Surgical placement of conduit graft to common iliac artery or aorta

---

Table 10-6   Endoleak Classification

Type	Definition
I	Attachment: lack of seal between endograft and wall of artery
II	Branch-to-branch: retrograde flow in IMA, lumbar, gonadal, or median sacral artery
III	Device integrity: hole in graft material, separation of modular elements
IV	Porous graft material: "bleed-through" due to interstices in fabric of graft material
V	Endo-tension: No visible contrast or flow in aneurysm sac, but continued expansion
Early	Within 30 days of procedure
Late	After 30 days

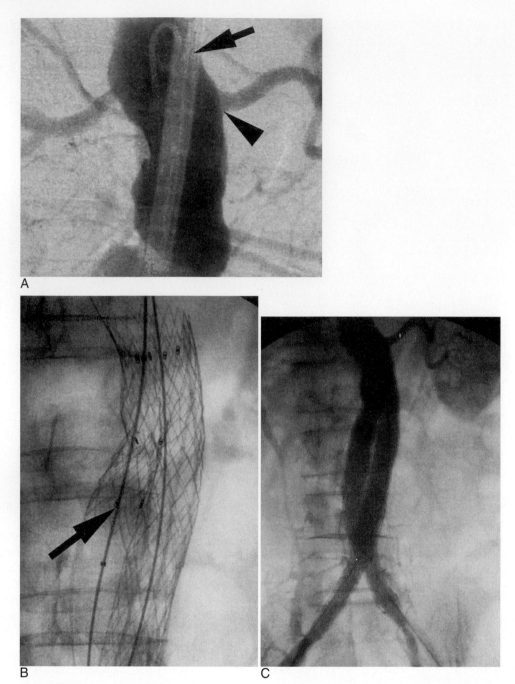

Figure 10-18   Basic elements of deployment of a modular bifurcated endograft. **A**, Magnified DSA with craniocaudad angulation centered over the renal arteries. The top of the endograft (arrow) can now be repositioned below the lowest renal artery (arrowhead) prior to deployment. **B**, Catheterization of the contralateral stump (arrow) with a guidewire after deployment of the main body of the endograft. This was accomplished in a retrograde manner. **C**, Final DSA aortogram showing exclusion of the aneurysm and excellent endograft position.

kinking, separation, and even disengagement from attachment sites. The incidence of complications is increasing as longer follow-up is accumulated. The future role of endografts for AAA remains to be determined as these late outcomes become known.

Isolated degenerative common iliac artery aneurysms can be managed with stent-grafts, often percutaneously.

The same principles apply as for AAA endografts: adequate proximal and distal attachment sites, and the ability to deliver the device through the external iliac artery. Embolization of the proximal internal iliac artery is frequently required to avoid a type II endoleak. Internal iliac artery aneurysms can be effectively managed by embolization of all outflow branches, followed by embolization of the proximal internal iliac artery or overlay by a stent-graft extending from the common to external iliac arteries.

OCCLUSIVE DISEASE

The most common cause of aortoiliac occlusive disease is atherosclerosis (Box 10-8). Isolated aortic lesions are unusual, occurring in 5% of patients with symptoms of chronic lower-extremity arterial insufficiency. These manifest as calcified bulky intraaortic plaque ("Coral reef" plaque) usually in the visceral artery segment, or focal infrarenal stenoses (Figs. 10-21 and 10-22). Combined aortic and iliac artery occlusive disease is the most common pattern, with associated infrainguinal occlusive disease in 65% (Fig. 10-23). When the occlusive disease is limited to the aortoiliac segment, the male to female ratio is 1:1. This ratio

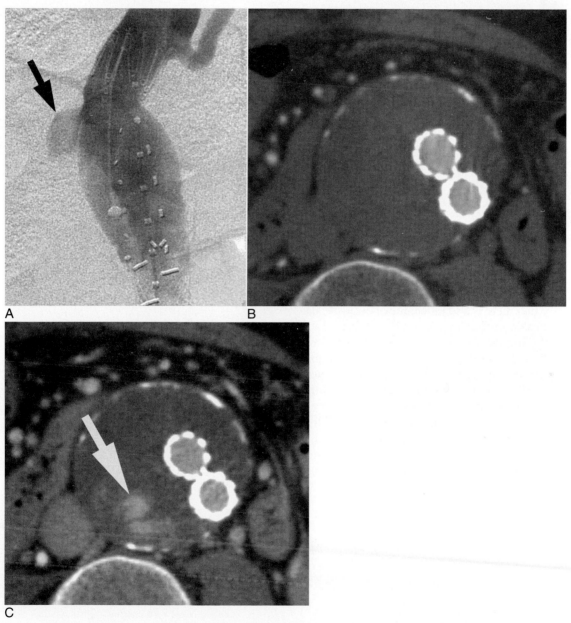

Figure 10-19   Sac perfusion after endograft placement ("endoleaks"). **A,** Type I perfusion. Intraprocedural DSA showing a jet of contrast (arrow) entering the aneurysm sac around the proximal attachment. This was eliminated by gentle inflation of a large angioplasty balloon across the proximal attachment site. **B,** CT scan 12 months after endograft placement during the arterial phase. No contrast is seen in the sac (see C and D). **C,** Image at the same level from the delayed phase (90 seconds after contrast injection) now shows contrast in the sac consistent with an endoleak (arrow). This illustrates the importance of the delayed scan when evaluating endografts.

(Continued)

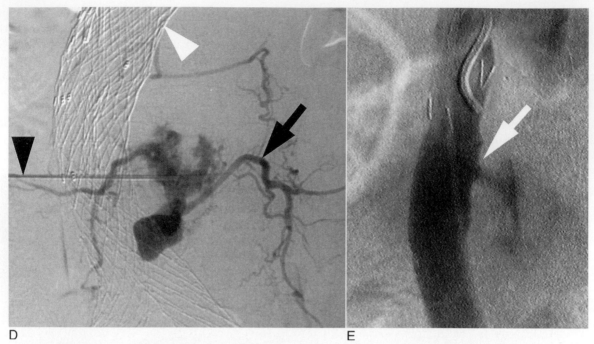

D   E

Figure 10-19   cont'd D, Type II perfusion. DSA after direct sac puncture in the same patient as B and C showing filling of an intra-aneurysmal space with communication with the lumbar arteries (arrow). The access needle (black arrowhead) passes behind the graft (white arrowhead). The pressure in the sac was near systemic. **E,** Type III perfusion. Selective injection in the limb of a bifurcated modular endograft showing a hole (arrow) in the fabric (proven surgically).

becomes 6:1 when there is also infrainguinal occlusive disease. With occlusion of the distal aorta there is retrograde propagation of thrombus to the level of the next proximal patent aortic branch vessel. When this vessel is a lumbar or inferior mesenteric artery, the lumen of the aorta tapers to the origin of that vessel. Retrograde thrombosis to the renal arteries results in an occlusion just at or immediately below the renal artery orifices (Figs. 10-24 and 10-25).

Patients with aortoiliac occlusive disease usually present with leg claudication or ischemia. Symptoms can be unilateral or bilateral depending on the level of

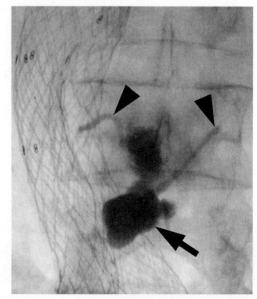

Figure 10-20   Digital image of the same patient as in Figs. 10-19B,C following embolization of the sac with N-butyl cyanoacrylate. Glue has filled the space in the sac (arrow) and occluded the proximal lumbar arteries (arrowheads).

**Box 10-8   Etiologies of Aortoiliac
Occlusive Disease**

Atherosclerosis
Hypoplastic aorta syndrome
Vasculitis
Radiation arteritis
Dissection
Neurofibromatosis
Fibromuscular dysplasia

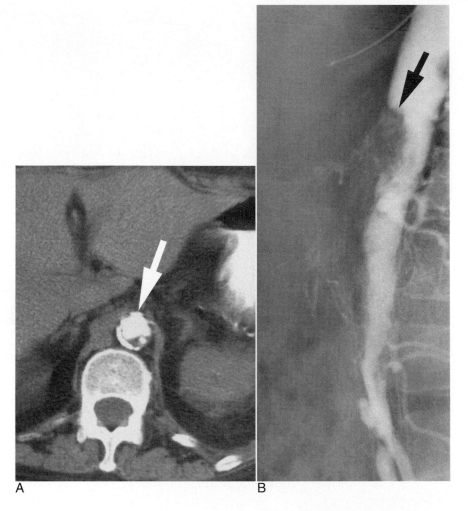

Figure 10-21 Bulky aortic plaque ("coral reef") in a patient with chronic postprandial abdominal pain. **A,** Axial noncontrast CT scan at the level of the celiac artery origin showing heavily calcified intraluminal plaque (arrow). The dense calcium in the aorta could have easily been overlooked if the noncontrast scan had not been obtained prior to contrast. **B,** Lateral aortogram showing the bulky plaque (arrow) obstructing the celiac and superior mesenteric artery origins.

A   B

obstruction and collateral pathways. Patients may complain of upper-thigh claudication and proximal leg weakness with severe pelvic occlusive disease. Bilateral buttock claudication, impotence, and diminished femoral pulses in men is termed "Leriche syndrome," usually indicating severe disease of the distal aorta and common iliac arteries. This constellation of symptoms is present in up to one-third of men with severe aortoiliac occlusive disease, but is frequently not discussed. Aortic and iliac plaque can also be a source of distal atheroemboli ("blue-toe syndrome"). An iliac source should be suspected when there are recurrent episodes involving one foot; an aortic source is suggested when both feet are involved.

Noninvasive studies of patients with isolated aortoiliac occlusive disease reveal diminished femoral pulses, decreased ankle–brachial indices, and reduced segmental pressures or pulse volume recordings (PVR) in the thigh, with normalized distal wave-forms (see Chapter 15). However, PVRs cannot precisely localize the level of proximal disease, as common femoral artery occlusion will produce the same distal waveform and pressure abnormalities as a more proximal lesion. Imaging of aortoiliac occlusive disease with US is less accurate than other modalities owing to iliac artery tortuously, the depth of the vessels in the pelvis, and calcification. Contrast-enhanced MRA detects aortoiliac disease with greater than 95% sensitivity and specificity (see Figs. 10-24 and 3-15). A coronal gadolinium-enhanced 3-D acquisition centered on the aortic bifurcation will usually cover from the renal arteries to the femoral artery bifurcation. The presence of intravascular metal stents (particularly those made from stainless steel) can create artifact that obscures the vessel lumen, so that MRA may not be useful in these patients. CTA has similar sensitivity and specificity, and also tends to overestimate the degree of stenosis. Unlike MRA, intravascular stents do not degrade CTA, but heavy calcification can obscure the lumen of a small-diameter vessel. Greater image postprocessing is required with CTA than MRA to eliminate bone and surrounding soft tissues. MRA and CTA

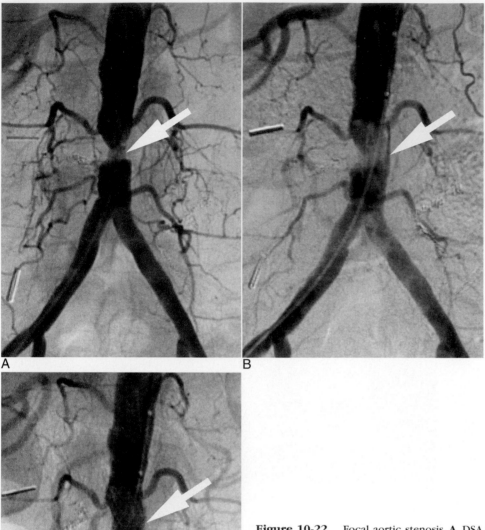

Figure 10-22 Focal aortic stenosis. **A**, DSA of the distal abdominal aorta showing a focal atherosclerotic stenosis (arrow). There was a 50-mmHg gradient across the stenosis. **B**, Following angioplasty with a 12-mm diameter balloon there is persistent stenosis (arrow) with only slight reduction in the gradient. **C**, DSA after placement of a balloon expandable stent (arrow). The gradient was obliterated.

can be used to both diagnose occlusive disease and plan for an intervention.

Conventional angiography should be obtained when intervention is required, or a diagnostic dilemma exists that cannot be resolved with noninvasive techniques. Angiography provides accurate morphologic as well as physiologic information. Care is required in interpretation of DSA images, as artifacts can be caused by motion, dense bone, and bowel gas. Bowel gas artifact in the abdomen can be minimized by intravenous injection of glucagon 1 mg prior to aortography. Oblique views are essential when evaluating the iliac arteries (see Figs. 10-9 and 2-48). Pressure measurements (preferably simultaneous with pharmacologic induction of distal

Type I   Type II   Type III

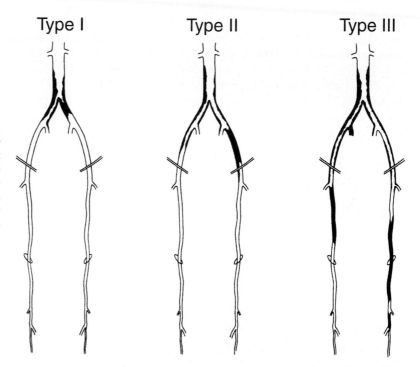

Figure 10-23   Patterns of aortoiliac occlusive disease. *Type 1:* Distal aorta and common iliac arteries. *Type 2:* Aorta and generalized pelvic arterial disease with intact distal runoff. *Type 3:* Multilevel disease including the aorta, pelvis, and distal runoff. This pattern carries the worst prognosis. (Reproduced with permission from Brewster DC: Direct reconstruction for aortoiliac occlusive disease. In Rutherford RB ed: *Vascular Surgery*, 5th edn, WB Saunders, Philadelphia, 2000.)

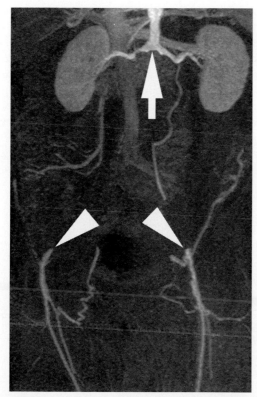

Figure 10-24   Chronic proximal aortic occlusion. Coronal MIP of gadolinium-enhanced MRA showing occlusion of the abdominal aorta just below the renal arteries (arrow) and reconstitution of the distal runoff at the level of the common femoral arteries (arrowheads).

hyperemia) obtained across lesions allows definitive determinations of severity and need for intervention (see Fig. 4-4). When desired, IVUS can be used to further evaluate a lesion (see Fig. 2-51).

The indications for intervention in patients with aortoiliac occlusive disease are disabling claudication, threatened limb loss, or a hemodynamically obstructive lesion prior to a distal revascularization procedure. Recommendations for the type of intervention based upon lesion morphology and distribution have been

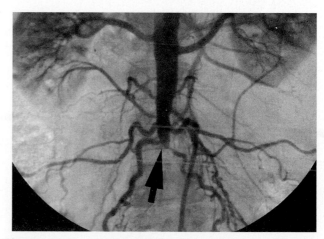

Figure 10-25   Chronic distal aortic occlusion. DSA of the aorta showing distal occlusion (arrow). Note the enlarged lumbar arteries.

developed (Box 10-9). The surgical options include aortofemoral bypass, axillofemoral bypass, femoral–femoral bypass, and aortic endarterectomy (Figs. 10-26 and 10-27). An end-to-side proximal anastomosis is employed when residual flow in the native aorta is to be preserved. The femoral anastomoses are also usually end-to-side, with the graft material anterior to the native artery (see Fig. 2-32). The best long-term surgical results are for aortofemoral bypass or aortic endarterectomy (70% primary 10-year patency), although the latter is rarely performed in most centers. Axillofemoral and femoral–femoral bypasses (both considered "extraanatomic" as the grafts do not follow the natural course of the arteries that they replace) have lower patency

rates owing to factors which include external compression and length of the graft. Complications are similar to those listed in Boxes 10-4 and 10-5 (see Fig. 3-19).

Angioplasty of aortic stenosis can be performed with a single low-profile low-pressure large-diameter balloon (10–16 mm) from one arterial access, or two smaller balloons (8- to 10-mm diameter) with kissing technique from bilateral access (see Fig. 10-22). Kissing technique is commonly used for aortic lesions that also involve the common iliac artery origins (see Fig. 4-10). The long-term results of angioplasty of focal aortic stenoses are excellent, but these are rare lesions. Stent placement is indicated for eccentric lesions, recanalization of complete occlusions, or lesions that are believed to be a source of atheroemboli (see Fig. 10-22). Stent-grafts may be used to exclude symptomatic ulcerated plaque, but otherwise currently have little role for aortic occlusive disease.

Isolated, concentric, and focal iliac stenoses that are at least 1 cm from the aorta or iliac artery bifurcation respond well to angioplasty alone, with a 4-year patency of almost 80%. In general, stents should be required only in approximately 50% of cases when strict hemodynamic criteria are followed (Box 10-10). However, it is very hard to suppress the "oculostenting reflex," so most iliac lesions are now treated primarily with stents (see Fig. 4-4). Typical balloon diameters for the common iliac artery are 8–10 mm. When a lesion involves the proximal common iliac artery or the origin, a second access from the opposite side is useful (see Fig. 4-11). This allows control injections for precise positioning of the stent, simultaneous pressure measurements, and inflation of an undersized balloon in the normal common iliac artery orifice during stent deployment to prevent distal embolization of plaque. Bilateral stent placement is often required to protect a relatively normal contralateral common iliac artery when treating origin disease. Treatment of disease involving both common iliac artery origins involves reconstruction of

---

Box 10-9   TransAtlantic Inter-Society Consensus (TASC) Recommendations for Iliac Interventions

Lesion Type A

Endovascular is treatment of choice
1. Single stenosis <3 cm of CIA or EIA (unilateral/bilateral)

Lesion Type B

Endovascular frequently used but insufficient scientific evidence
2. Single stenosis 3–10 cm in length, not involving CFA
3. Total of two stenoses <5 cm in CIA/EIA, not involving CFA
4. Unilateral CIA occlusion

Lesion Type C

Surgical treatment used more often but insufficient scientific evidence
5. Bilateral stenosis 5–10 cm in length of CIA/EIA, not involving CFA
6. Unilateral EIA occlusion, not involving CFA
7. Unilateral EIA stenosis, extending into CFA
8. Bilateral CIA occlusion

Lesion Type D

Surgery is treatment of choice
9. Diffuse unilateral stenoses of CIA, EIA, and CFA; usually >10 cm in length
10. Unilateral occlusion of both CIA and EIA
11. Bilateral EIA occlusions
12. Diffuse aortic and iliac disease
13. Iliac stenosis in patient that requires aortic or iliac surgery for aneurysm, etc.

CIA, common iliac artery; EIA, external iliac artery; CFA, common femoral artery.

Box 10-10   Indications for Stent Placement in the Aorta and Iliac Arteries

Failed angioplasty (residual pressure gradient >10 mmHg at rest, 15 mmHg with distal vasodilatation, or residual stenosis ≥30%)
Common iliac artery origin lesion
Recurrent stenosis
Anastomotic stenosis
Occlusive dissection flap
Recanalization of total occlusion
Ulcerated plaque
Planned distal revascularization procedure

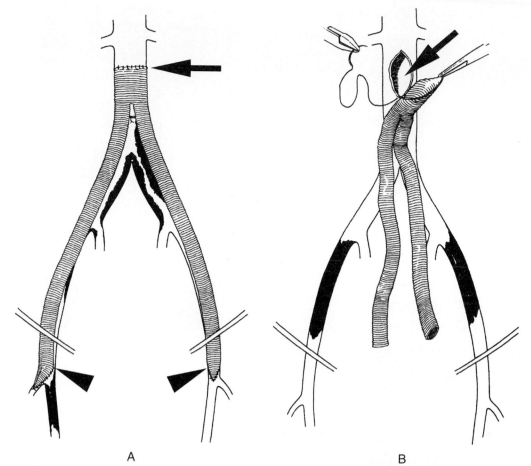

A   B

Figure 10-26   Surgical options for aortoiliac occlusive disease. The distal anastomosis is typically to the common femoral artery or lower when bypass is performed for occlusive disease. **A**, Aortobifemoral graft with end-to-end proximal (arrow) and end-to-side distal anastomoses (arrowheads). **B**, Aortobifemoral graft with an end-to-side proximal anastomosis (arrow) that preserves flow to the distal lumbar and pelvic arteries. (Reproduced with permission from Brewster DC: Direct reconstruction for aortoiliac occlusive disease. In Rutherford RB ed: *Vascular Surgery*, 5th edn, WB Saunders, Philadelphia, PA, 2000.)

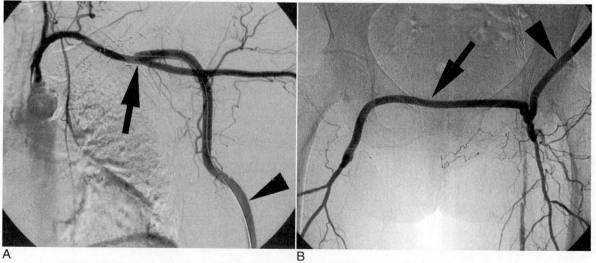

A   B

Figure 10-27   Axillobifemoral graft. **A**, DSA of the proximal left upper-extremity arteries showing the proximal anastomosis (arrow) of an axillobifemoral bypass (arrowhead). **B**, DSA of the pelvis showing the axillofemoral bypass graft (arrowhead) with a cross femoral bypass (arrow) to the right profunda femoris artery.

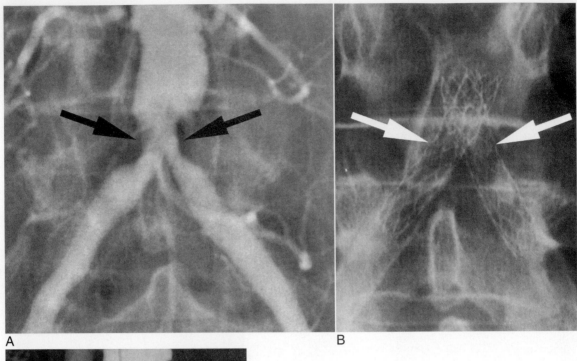

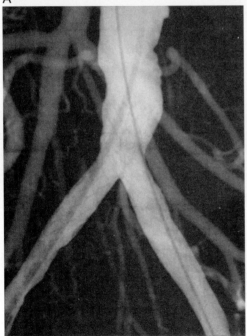

Figure 10-28 Kissing common iliac artery stents. **A**, Angiogram showing stenosis of the distal aorta (arrows) and both proximal common iliac artery origins. **B**, Digital image showing kissing iliac stents (arrows) extending into the distal aorta. **C**, Angiogram following bilateral stent placement.

the aortic bifurcation with bilateral stents that extend equally into the distal abdominal aorta (Fig. 10-28).

Common iliac artery occlusions can be crossed from either a retrograde or antegrade approach. Generally, a retrograde approach is easier as the path from the access to the lesion is short and straight (Fig. 10-29). An angled catheter and a straight or angled hydrophilic guidewire can be used to probe the lesion for a "soft spot." Working over the bifurcation requires a sturdy recurved catheter

that allows probing of the occlusion (Fig. 10-30). Failure to cross the lesion occurs in about 5% of cases. Aggressive recanalization utilizing the back end of a guidewire or even a long needle from a transjugular trans-hepatic portal access kit (see Fig. 14-19) can be used for stubborn lesions, although there is increased risk of vessel perforation. When fresh thrombus is present or suspected, a short course of thrombolysis will reduce the risk of distal embolization during stent placement. Stent placement in

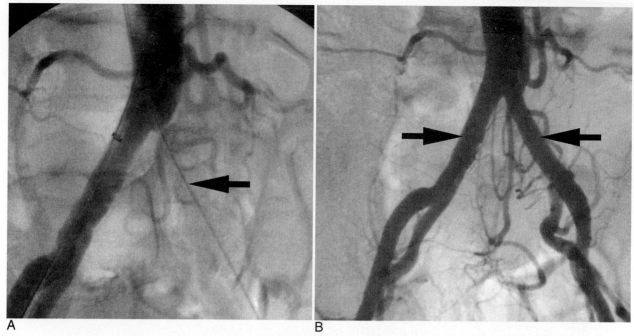

A   B

Figure 10-29   Occluded left common iliac artery recanalized in a retrograde fashion. **A**, Angiogram obtained after occlusion has been crossed (arrow) in a retrograde fashion from the left common femoral artery with hydrophilic guidewire and an angled catheter. The proximal occlusion is flush with the origin of the common iliac artery; compare with the occlusion in Fig. 10-30. **B**, Angiogram after bilateral common iliac artery stent placement (arrows). The right stent was necessary because the left stent extended into the distal aorta.

occlusions have improved patency rates over angioplasty alone, equal to that of stented stenoses (Table 10-7).

Internal iliac artery origin lesions can be treated through a sheath placed across the aortic bifurcation from the opposite groin. This provides an antegrade approach to the internal iliac artery, as well as proximal contrast injections during the procedure. Angioplasty or stent placement can be performed, but stents should be positioned carefully to avoid extension into the common iliac artery.

External iliac artery angioplasty and stent placement is technically similar to the treatment of common iliac artery lesions. The external iliac artery is more prone to rupture than the common iliac artery, so balloon sizing should be less aggressive (see Fig. 4-12). Extension of stents over the internal iliac artery origin usually does not jeopardize the patency of that vessel. However, placement of stents in the common femoral artery has generally been avoided owing to the relative ease of open endarterectomy of this vessel, and concerns about future percutaneous access and flexion across the hip joint.

The role of stent-grafts in iliac artery occlusive disease is currently under investigation. Intimal hyperplasia at the ends of the stent-graft remains a serious problem. The indications include ulcerated plaque, angioplasty-induced iliac artery rupture, and perhaps recanalization of long occlusions. Drug-eluting stents offer great promise for improved long-term patency.

Major complications of aortoiliac angioplasty and stent placement include distal dissection, embolization, thrombosis, and rupture. These occur in fewer than 5% of patients, but are more frequent when recanalizing occlusions. These complications can be minimized by careful balloon selection, heparinization during the intervention, and remembering the dictum that "the enemy of good is better."

Table 10-7   Results of Aortoiliac Angioplasty and Stents (generalized)

Iliac artery lesion	Procedure	Initial Success	4-year Primary Patency
Stenosis	Angioplasty	95%	65%
Stenosis	Stent	95%	77%
Occlusion	Angioplasty	85%	54%
Occlusion	Stent	85%	61%

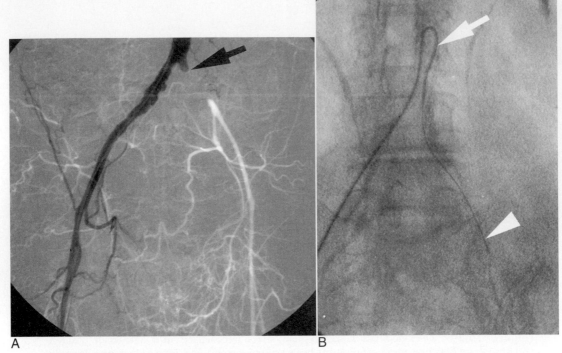

Figure 10-30   Crossing a common iliac artery occlusion using antegrade technique. **A**, DSA angiogram masked to demonstrate left common iliac occlusion (arrow) with late reconstitution of the left external iliac artery via retrograde flow in the internal iliac artery. **B**, The occlusion has been crossed by pulling a Simmons 1 catheter (arrow) into the "nipple" of the occlusion and advancing a hydrophilic guidewire (arrowhead) through the occlusion.

DISSECTION

Isolated spontaneous dissection of the abdominal aorta and iliac arteries is extremely rare (Box 10-11). A dissection in this vascular territory is usually an extension of a spontaneous thoracic aortic dissection, or iatrogenic following a surgical or angiographic procedure. Rarely, abdominal or limb symptoms due to acute branch vessel occlusion are the first presentation of a dissection originating in the thoracic aorta. Patients may have vague abdominal or low back pain, or full-blown visceral or limb ischemia. Symptoms due to branch vessel involvement occur in almost one-third of patients with aortic dissection. Ischemic symptoms are characteristically severe owing to the acuity of onset, but may wax and wane as the true lumen perfusion changes. Rupture of the false lumen of a dissected aorta in the abdomen is much less common than in the thorax.

Iatrogenic retrograde dissections created during angiographic procedures are frequently innocuous, as the false lumen tends to collapse rather than expand (see Fig. 2-33). However, occlusive antegrade dissection may occur following angioplasty or stent placement, particularly in the external iliac arteries.

Imaging of aortoiliac artery dissections should answer specific questions (Box 10-12). US can detect dissection flaps in the abdominal aorta, but cannot adequately evaluate the status of the major branch arteries. Both MRA and CTA are excellent modalities for evaluation of dissection in this vascular bed (Fig. 10-31). The 3-D data sets can be postprocessed on workstations to resolve complex anatomic issues.

Box 10-11   Etiologies of Abdominal Aortic and Iliac Artery Dissection

Atherosclerosis (extension thoracic aorta)
Marfan syndrome (extension thoracic aorta)
Penetrating atherosclerotic ulcer
Trauma
Fibromuscular dysplasia (iliac arteries)
Athletes (iliac arteries)
Iatrogenic
   Angiography/intervention
   Fogarty balloon embolectomy
   Clamp injury

Conventional angiography is usually indicated only in symptomatic patients prior to intervention. The diagnosis of aortic dissection is usually readily apparent on cross-sectional imaging studies. The stronger femoral pulse should be punctured (aortic dissections rarely extend beyond the common iliac arteries). Manipulation with a selective catheter may be required to find the true lumen. Midstream injection of contrast in the dissected abdominal aorta may not opacify both lumens unless fenestrations exist (Fig. 10-32). Sequential selective injection of both the true and false lumen, or repositioning of the catheter in the thoracic aorta proximal to the entry tear, is required in this situation. The lateral aortogram is particularly useful for evaluation of the visceral arteries.

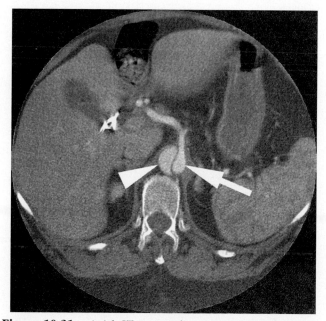

Figure 10-31   Axial CT scan with contrast at the level of the celiac artery origin in a patient with a type B dissection. The celiac artery is supplied by the smaller true lumen (arrow), rather than the larger false lumen (arrowhead).

The surgical management of symptomatic abdominal aortic dissection is resection of a small portion of the intimal flap, usually in the infrarenal aorta. A short aortic interposition graft may or may not be used as well. This creates a reentry point that decompresses the false lumen, allowing perfusion of the major branches that arise from the true lumen. Dissections isolated to the iliac arteries are treated surgically with bypass or placement of an interposition graft.

Occlusive symptoms of aortoiliac dissection can be effectively managed with percutaneous techniques. Compromise of blood flow may be due to compression of the true by the false lumen, involvement of the branch vessel by the dissection, or both. These complications can be relieved by percutaneous fenestration, stent placement, or stent-graft placement over the entry tear in the thoracic aorta (see Fig. 9-25). The initial step is detailed angiography to identify the extent of the dissection and the anatomy of the target branch vessels.

Percutaneous aortic fenestration is indicated when perfusion of the true aortic lumen is compromised by a distended false lumen. The essential components of the technique are identification of the true and false lumens, intravascular puncture through the dissection flap from one lumen to the other, and then balloon dilatation to enlarge the fenestration (Fig. 10-33). Careful review of CT or MR studies prior to the procedure helps to determine the orientation of the two lumens. Although it is sometimes possible to identify each lumen with direct cathcterization, sometimes only the true lumen can be accessed from a femoral approach. IVUS is a useful tool in these circumstances to localize the false lumen and guide the intervention. A long needle (such as one used for transjugular intrahepatic portosystemic shunts) is inserted through a long protective sheath to the desired point of fenestration. A short thrust is usually sufficient to cross the flap. Entry into the false lumen is confirmed by injection of contrast, followed by insertion of a guidewire. Puncture of the outer wall of the aorta is inconsequential, provided that the needle is simply withdrawn back into the aorta. The goal of the fenestration is to create a large communication between the two lumens, so large balloons with diameters equal to that of the aorta should be used. The final result is normalization of pressures in both lumens, with reexpansion of the true lumen, and improved perfusion of branch vessels.

Stent placement in a branch vessel is used to restore unimpeded flow from either the true or false lumen when the dissection flap extends into the vessel. The principles of stent placement in this setting are the same as for atherosclerotic occlusive disease. It is essential to be sure that satisfactory inflow from the aorta will be available after the stent has been placed (i.e., fenestration may also be necessary).

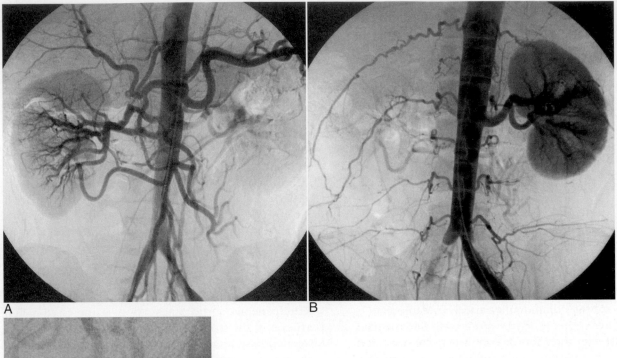

A   B

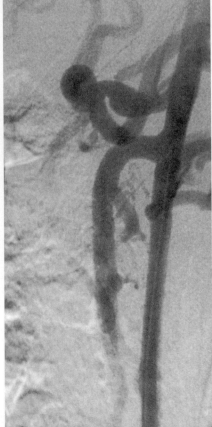

C

Figure 10-32 Abdominal extension of type B dissection. **A**, DSA true lumen aortogram in the anterior projection shows filling of the visceral arteries and right kidney. The left kidney and lumbar arteries are not visualized. **B**, DSA false lumen aortogram in the same projection. The left kidney and lumbar arteries are visualized, but the visceral arteries and right kidney are not. **C**, DSA true lumen aortogram in the lateral projection showing filling of the visceral vessels.

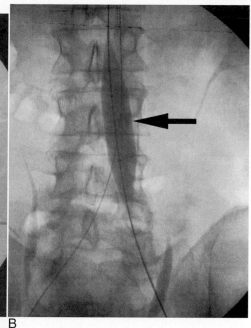

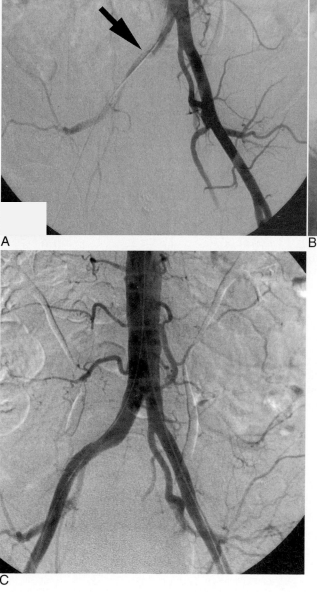

Figure 10-33   Percutaneous fenestration in a patient with type B dissection and right leg ischemia. **A**, DSA over the pelvis with injection into the compressed true lumen of the distal abdominal aorta showing minimal flow in the right iliac arteries (arrow). **B**, Using intravascular US guidance in the false lumen, a long sheathed needle was used to puncture the intimal flap from the true into the false lumen. A wire was advanced from the true to the false lumen and a 14-mm diameter balloon inflated across the fenestration (arrow) to enlarge the hole in the flap. **C**, DSA of the distal aorta after fenestration showing excellent filling of both sides of the pelvis. The patient had restoration of normal bilateral femoral pulses and relief of symptoms.

INFECTION

Native aortic infection presents with episodic fever, chills, and positive blood cultures. Mycotic pseudoaneurysm formation is associated with pain, distal embolization, or rupture. Patients may undergo an extensive evaluation for fever of unknown origin prior to arriving at the diagnosis of intravascular infection. Mycotic aneurysms of the native abdominal aorta can occur in

any location, but the supraceliac aorta is common. Organisms typically responsible for vascular infections are listed in Table 1-15.

Early in the infectious process of the native aorta the imaging findings may be subtle or absent. Rarely, gas may be observed in the vessel wall or lumen. Perivascular stranding representing an inflammatory process precedes aneurysm formation. Ultimately, the arterial wall is digested and a pseudoaneurysm forms. Typically, mycotic aneurysms have a lobulated, wild-looking appearance, with extensive surrounding soft tissue reaction and hematoma (see Fig. 1-34). Adjacent major branch vessel origins are often consumed by the infectious aneurysm.

Infection of aortic graft material may occur from hematogenous seeding, direct extension from adjacent abscesses, and erosion into gastrointestinal or genitourinary (usually the ureter) structures. Graft infection also presents with fever, chills, and positive blood cultures. In addition, drainage from surgical incisions (especially in the groin), graft thrombosis, gastrointestinal bleeding, and anastomotic pseudoaneurysms may occur. Gastrointestinal bleeding can occur from graft erosion into bowel (chronic occult lower tract blood loss) or rupture of a proximal anastomotic pseudoaneurysm into the duodenum (massive acute upper gastrointestinal bleeding). When graft infection manifests as anastomotic pseudoaneurysm, synchronous involvement of more than one anastomosis should be excluded. Rarely, vascular stents can become infected, resulting in a focal mycotic aneurysm as well as other characteristic symptoms of intravascular sepsis.

Infection of prosthetic graft material is suggested by perigraft fluid and/or air (see Fig. 1-35). Following aortic surgery, perigraft air should be reabsorbed within 2–3 weeks, and perigraft fluid within 2–3 months (see Fig. 10-15). Delayed appearance or persistence of perigraft fluid and air on CT or MRI are highly suggestive of infection. Soft-tissue stranding, lack of fat planes between graft material and bowel, graft thrombosis, and anastomotic pseudoaneurysms are also suggestive imaging findings. At conventional angiography the graft may appear completely normal, but intraluminal irregularities, focal anastomotic out-pouchings, and (very, very rarely) opacification of bowel may be seen (Fig. 10-34).

The treatment of native aortoiliac vessel or graft infection is surgical resection, bypass (through a sterile bed if possible), and antibiotics. Axillofemoral bypass with delayed aortic reconstruction, or direct vascular reconstruction with antibiotic-impregnated synthetic grafts, homograft, or autogenous femoral vein may be utilized.

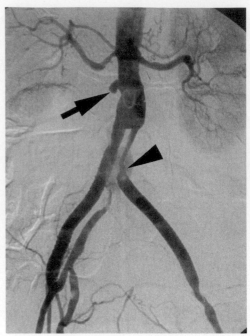

Figure 10-34 Aortoenteric fistula several years after aorto-bi-iliac (onlay) graft for occlusive disease. The patient presented with fever, septicemia, and occult blood in his stool. DSA aortogram reveals a small proximal anastomotic pseudoaneurysm (arrow) and collapse of the left limb of the graft (arrowhead) with an intraluminal filling defect.

of both limbs, with sudden return of one or more femoral pulses but persistent distal ischemia, may indicate fragmentation and distal embolization of a large aortic embolus. In contrast to embolic occlusion, thrombosis of a preexisting native arterial stenosis or a surgical graft is often preceded by a history of claudication and rarely results in critical ischemia owing to the presence of preexisting collaterals.

Patients with embolic occlusion of the aortoiliac arteries and profound ischemia have a surgical emergency. Imaging should be expedient and accurate, as rapid revascularization is essential to save limb and life.

EMBOLIC OCCLUSION

Acute aortoiliac arterial occlusion can be due to several different causes (Box 10-13). Embolic occlusion is sudden in onset in previously asymptomatic individuals, often resulting in profound ischemia. There is no associated chest or back pain to suggest a dissection. Over half of the patients with symptomatic arterial emboli will have a cardiac arrhythmia at the time of presentation. Over 20% of emboli lodge at the aortic bifurcation, resulting in bilateral lower-extremity ischemia. Smaller emboli may occlude one or both common iliac or common femoral arteries (see Table 1-13). Acute global ischemia

Box 10-13 Causes of Acute Aortic Occlusion

Embolus
Thrombosis of underlying stenosis
Dissection
Thrombosis of surgical graft
Hypercoagulable state
Trauma
Iatrogenic

Many patients undergo emergent surgical embolectomy without antecedent imaging as the delay would compromise limb viability. When the limbs are viable, CT/CTA or MRA can exclude an alternative diagnosis such as dissection, demonstrate the level of occlusion, and detect other evidence of emboli such as renal infarcts (Fig. 10-35). Conventional angiography demonstrates abrupt occlusion of the aorta or pelvic arteries by an intravascular filling defect, evidence of emboli and visceral arteries, and poor opacification of distal vessels with absence of developed collaterals. An axillary artery approach may be required when femoral pulses are absent, although the common femoral artery can be punctured with ultrasound.

There is little role for percutaneous techniques in patients with profound ischemia due to an embolus. When limbs are threatened but still viable, thrombolysis can be considered, although the risk of distal embolization during the procedure is high. In general, aortoiliac emboli are too large to be managed quickly and effectively with standard percutaneous techniques.

VASCULITIS

Aortoiliac occlusive disease is a well-recognized feature of Takayasu's arteritis. Patients are atypical in age and risk factors for atherosclerotic disease (see Table 1-5). The process is diffuse, involving the visceral, renal, and common iliac arteries. Patients may present with hypertension, symptoms of mesenteric ischemia, or claudication.

Aortic wall thickening with a narrowed lumen is evident on CT or MR, with wall enhancement by contrast. Aneurysms can also occur. The degree of wall calcification can be variable. At conventional angiography, long smooth stenosis of the aortoiliac arteries with extension into visceral and renal arteries is seen (Fig. 10-36).

Therapeutic options include surgical bypass, and, in some patients, angioplasty with stent placement. The lesions of Takayasu's arteritis are fibrotic and extensive, so it is unlikely that a normal arterial caliber will be achieved with percutaneous methods, especially in the abdominal aorta. Information on long-term results of stent placement is scant, but promising.

Radiation vasculitis can involve the aorta and iliac arteries. The type and location of tumor treated, as well as contributory risk factors such as smoking, influence the severity. Diffuse aortic stenosis can occur in children following radiation for abdominal tumors. Isolated iliac artery disease can be seen after pelvic irradiation for genitourinary malignancy.

Behçet's disease can present as multiple abdominal aortic aneurysms, but the thoracic aorta may also be involved (see Fig. 1-17). Patients have a characteristic

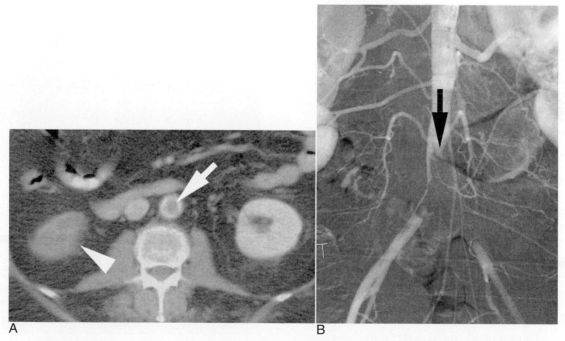

A   B

Figure 10-35   Acute embolic occlusion of the distal aorta. **A**, Axial contrast-enhanced CT scan showing a filling defect in the distal abdominal aorta (arrow) and lack of enhancement of the right kidney (arrowhead) consistent with multiple arterial emboli. **B**, DSA aortogram of a different patient showing embolic occlusion (arrow) of the distal abdominal aorta treated with surgical embolectomy. The source was cardiac.

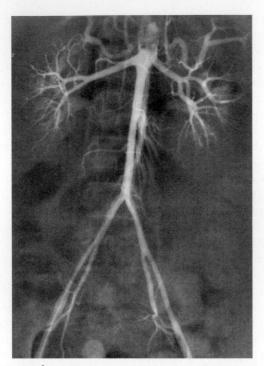

Figure 10-36 Angiogram showing the findings of Takayasu's arteritis of the abdominal aorta in a teenaged girl with aortic arch involvement. There is diffuse stenosis of infrarenal aorta and iliac arteries. This appearance is similar to that of hypoplastic aorta syndrome seen in middle-aged women in whom vasculitis work-up is negative.

constellation of clinical findings, including genital ulcers and uveitis.

MISCELLANEOUS

Hypoplastic aorta syndrome, also known as *abdominal aortic coarctation*, is believed to be a congenital disorder of unknown etiology and prevalence. Primarily found in young female patients, symptoms may not occur until middle age. Patients in this age group frequently have risk factors for atherosclerotic disease, such as smoking, diabetes, and hyperlipidemia. Atherosclerotic occlusive disease is frequently superimposed upon the already small aorta and iliac arteries in these patients. The angiographic appearance is striking, with a disproportionately small infrarenal abdominal aorta and iliac arteries. The differential diagnosis includes burned-out vasculitis (see Fig. 10-36), radiation injury, and neurofibromatosis. Visceral and renal artery involvement occurs when the lesion is centered in the mid portion of the abdominal aorta. Disease localized to the infrarenal aorta and common iliac arteries spares the visceral and renal arteries. Owing to the small caliber of the

arteries and diffuse disease, surgical bypass is the preferred therapy.

Neurofibromatosis is associated with diffuse narrowing of the abdominal aorta, with concurrent visceral and renal artery stenoses. At pathology, neurogenic cells are present in the media and adventitia. The appearance is similar to Takayasu's arteritis and hypoplastic aorta syndrome, with the exception that patients are much younger at presentation with other stigmata of neurofibromatosis (Fig. 10-37).

The iliac arteries are the third most common location for *fibromuscular dysplasia* (FMD) (Fig. 10-38). The typical patient is female, but older than those that present with renal artery FMD. Usually an incidental finding at angiography, patients may present with occlusive symptoms or, less often, spontaneous dissection. Occlusive symptoms respond well to angioplasty, and dissection can be treated with stent placement.

Iliac artery endofibrosis is a rare condition manifesting as unilateral or bilateral external iliac artery stenoses in young athletes (Fig. 10-39). The etiology may be linked to repetitive motion of the hip joint, such as during competitive cycling. The lesions are fibrotic in nature, and may produce a gradient only during exercise. Management is by behavior modification, stent placement, or surgical repair. Angioplasty alone is usually unsuccessful.

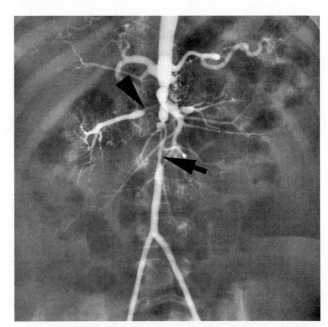

Figure 10-37 Abdominal aortic coarctation in a child with neurofibromatosis, hypertension, and diminished peripheral pulses. Aortogram showing renal artery stenosis (arrowhead) and diffuse narrowing of the infrarenal aorta (arrow). The celiac and superior mesenteric artery origins were also severely stenotic.

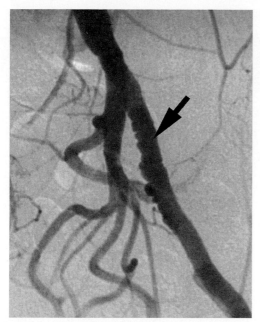

Figure 10-38   Fibromuscular dysplasia, medial fibroplasia type (asymptomatic) of the external iliac artery (arrow) in a middle-aged woman. The findings were bilateral.

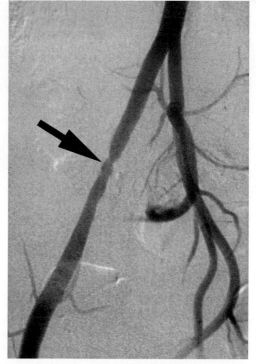

Figure 10-39   Iliac artery endofibrosis (arrow) in a young triathlete with right leg claudication.

TRAUMA

The majority of patients with out-of-hospital penetrating injuries to the abdominal aorta die immediately from exsanguination. Only 15% of patients are thought to survive long enough to undergo emergency surgery. Bleeding is contained in these patients by adjacent retroperitoneal tissues. The incidence of associated bowel or visceral organ injuries is high. Iatrogenic aortoiliac penetrating injury during spinal surgery may result in pseudoaneurysms or arteriovenous fistula and high-output cardiac failure (Figs. 10-40 and 10-41). Percutaneous treatment with an endograft is an elegant solution to these problems.

Blunt injury to the aorta can result in an intimal tear with dissection or thrombosis, but injuries to major branch vessels (especially the renal arteries) are more common (Fig. 10-42). Most injuries to the infrarenal aorta are caused by seat belts during car accidents. Associated colonic injury is almost universal in these patients.

Pelvic fractures can result in exsanguination from bleeding (both venous and arterial). Pelvic fractures can be grouped by the causative forces: (1) lateral compression; (2) anteroposterior compression; (3) vertical shear; and (4) combined mechanisms. A 3-cm diastasis of the symphysis pubis doubles the potential volume of the pelvis to 8 liters. The majority of patients with pelvic fractures are stabilized successfully with pelvic fixation

devices. Bleeding is controlled in this manner in 99% of patients with lateral compression injuries, which comprise 65% of all patients with pelvic fractures. Anteroposterior, vertical-shear, and combined-force injuries to the pelvis are less common but result in unstable injuries with bleeding unresponsive to pelvic fixation in 18-22% of cases.

Bleeding may be from fractured cancellous bone, or transected arterial and venous structures. A coagulopathic state induced by hypothermia or massive transfusion is a common complicating factor. Arterial injury

Box 10-14	Arteries Injured in Pelvic Fractures (decreasing order of frequency)
Superior gluteal	
Internal pudendal	
Obturator	
Inferior gluteal	
Lateral sacral	
Iliolumbar	
External iliac	
Deep circumflex iliac	
Inferior epigastric	

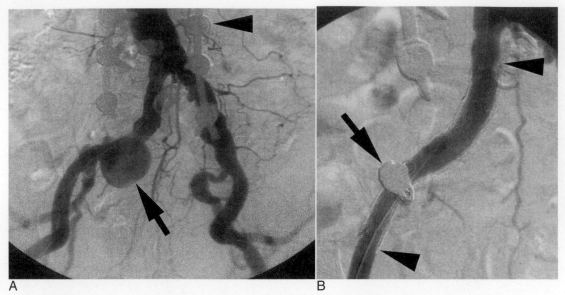

Figure 10-40 Posttraumatic common iliac artery pseudoaneurysm. **A,** New isolated saccular common iliac artery aneurysm (arrow) that appeared shortly after spinal surgery (arrowhead) consistent with an iatrogenic pseudoaneurysm. CT scan showed that the aneurysm arose from the back wall of the common iliac artery just proximal to the origin of the internal iliac artery. **B,** Successful exclusion of the aneurysm with a stent-graft (arrowheads). The internal iliac origin was occluded with coils prior to stent-graft placement (arrow) to prevent retrograde filling of the aneurysm.

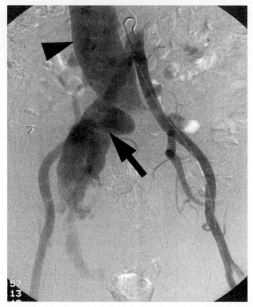

Figure 10-41 DSA of the pelvis showing a right common iliac artery to iliac vein fistula (arrow) in a patient who developed high-output cardiac failure following discectomy. Note the distended IVC (arrowhead) filled on aortic injection.

results from shearing of vessels against fixed ligamentous structures, avulsion of vessels attached to a displaced pelvic segment, or penetrating injury from a shard of bone (Box 10-14 and Fig. 10-43).

Peritoneal lavage or abdominal and pelvic CT with contrast is performed early in the evaluation of patients with pelvic fractures. If the lavage or the CT is positive for intraperitoneal hemorrhage, the patient proceeds to surgery. Only abdominal injuries are repaired, even if a large expanding retroperitoneal hematoma is discovered. Surgery in the confined space of the pelvic retroperitoneum is extremely difficult, decompresses the hematoma leading to increased blood loss, and may predispose surviving patients to infection. Pelvic fixation is performed externally in the ER or at the time of laparotomy. If the patient remains hemodynamically unstable, or has a transfusion requirement that exceeds 4-6 units of packed red blood cells in 24 hours, angiography is performed emergently.

Angiography in hemodynamically unstable patients with pelvic fractures should (1) rapidly evaluate potential sources of arterial bleeding, and (2) proceed expeditiously to embolization. Review of plain films and CT scans of the pelvis helps direct the initial angiogram. A pelvic arteriogram with a pigtail catheter positioned to fill the lower lumbar arteries should be performed to quickly determine the arterial anatomy and identify massive extravasation (see Fig. 1-28). Injuries that cause hemodynamic instability manifest angiographically as

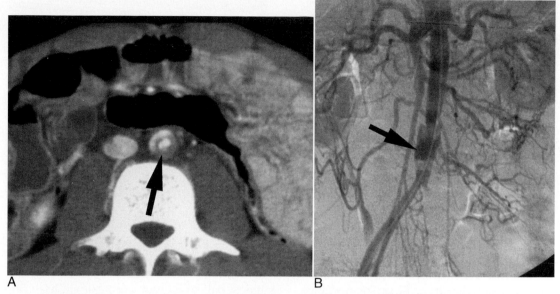

Figure 10-42 "Seat-belt injury" of the aorta in a young male involved in a high-speed motor vehicle accident, with absent left femoral pulse and a weak right femoral pulse. **A,** Axial contrast-enhanced CT showing an intimal flap in the aortic lumen (arrow) and partial thrombosis. **B,** DSA of the aorta shows the aortic transection (arrow) and occlusion of the left common iliac artery.

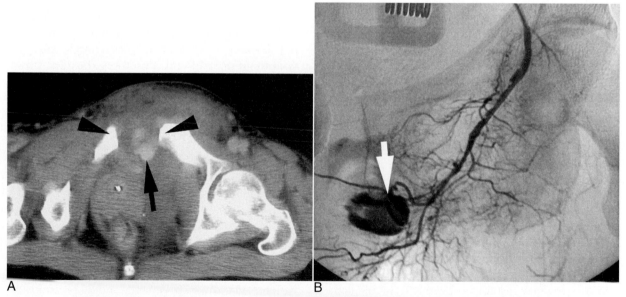

Figure 10-43 "Open book" pelvic fracture in a middle-aged male motorcycle rider occurring when he collided with an ambulance. He was hemodynamically stable but required aggressive fluid resuscitation despite application of a compression belt. **A,** Axial CT with contrast showing diastasis of the symphysis pubis (arrowheads) and extravasation (arrow) of contrast into a pelvic hematoma. **B,** Selective left internal pudendal DSA showing extravasation (arrow). This was embolized with Gelfoam pledgets. The right hypogastric artery was injected after embolization to confirm absence of cross-filling.

free extravasation, pseudoaneurysm, or large arterio-venous fistula. The absence of these findings on the flush pelvic injection does not exclude their presence. Selective bilateral internal and external iliac artery injections, with oblique views if necessary, should be performed as a routine. Recognition of important pelvic arterial anatomic variants such as replacement of the obturator artery to the inferior epigastric artery origin is critical. Extended filming over 20 seconds may be necessary to visualize pelvic arterial extravasation. The normal uterine blush in menstruating women and the bulbo-spongiosal stain at the base of the penis in males can be confused with extravasation.

The primary goal of embolization in patients with pelvic fractures is to quickly decrease or arrest the flow of arterial blood to the injured vessel. Supraselective catheterization should be used only in stable patients, to avoid unnecessarily prolonging the procedure. The longer the patient bleeds, the sicker he or she becomes.

Gelfoam (Upjohn, Kalamazoo, MI) cut into pieces to match the target vessel is an excellent choice for branch vessel embolization. Typical pledget dimensions range from 1-mm cubes to 1-mm × 2-mm × 5-mm rectangles. Small particles (Gelfoam powder or Ivalon) and alcohol should not be used. Embolization continues until extra-vasation is no longer visualized. Coils are useful when large vessels are transected, or in stable patients with pseudoaneurysms or arteriovenous fistulas when a precise embolization may be desired. Successful embolization is frequently clinically evident with sudden improvement in the patient's hemodynamic status. Careful completion angiography is important to exclude bleeding from a collateral source of blood supply (Fig. 10-44). Midline bleeding can be supplied from either internal iliac artery, and lateral bleeding may be supplied from lumbar, iliac circumflex, or profunda femoris artery branches as well as the internal iliac artery.

Most complications of percutaneous embolization in pelvic trauma are acceptable considering the alternative. Reflux of embolic material into the ipsilateral lower extremity can occur if the catheter is not well seated in the internal iliac artery. Emboli that lodge in the profunda femoris artery or other muscular branches are usually clinically silent. Occlusion of the superficial femoral or popliteal artery may result in a severely ischemic limb that requires urgent revascularization.

UTERINE ARTERY ANGIOGRAPHY AND EMBOLIZATION

The most common indication for selective uterine artery angiography is for embolization of symptomatic fibroids. Fibroids are common benign leiomyomatous neoplasms of the uterus that occur in women in their

Table 10-8   Classification of Fibroids by Location

Location	Definition
Submucosal	Protruding into endometrial cavity
Intramural	Within the myometrium
Subserosal	Based in the myometrium, but covered by parietal peritoneum
Pedunculated	Attached to uterus by small stalk
Cervical	Located in uterine cervix

reproductive years. Tumors may be single, small, multiple, or large (Table 10-8). Fibroids are vascular tumors that grow in size and increase in prevalence with age throughout a woman's reproductive life. Although almost half of women aged 40 will have fibroids, fewer than 20% will be symptomatic. The uterus may become so enlarged by fibroids that it fills the pelvis and distends the abdomen. The natural history of uncomplicated fibroids is involution following menopause. Leiomyosarcoma of the uterus is rare during reproductive years (<0.5% of rapidly growing fibroids), but should be suspected when fibroid enlargement occurs in a postmenopausal woman.

The indications for intervention are fibroids that cause heavy, prolonged periods (meno-metrorrhagia), pelvic pain, dyspareunia, miscarriages, and pressure symptoms on adjacent structures (bladder, bowel, and ureters). Pharmacologic treatment with GnRH analogues, which cannot be given indefinitely, results in temporary reduction in size, but fibroids will enlarge once medication is stopped. Conventional surgical procedures include hysterectomy and myomectomy, using open, laparoscopic, or hysteroscopic techniques.

Uterine artery embolization is an alternative approach to management of fibroids (Fig. 10-45). The basic principle is selective infarction of the fibroids with particulate embolic materials delivered directly into the uterine arteries. The indications are identical to those for surgery, although the procedure is not recommended when fibroids are pedunculated or largely submucosal. Young patients who desire pregnancy should be counseled that there can be a 2–5% incidence of premature menopause following the procedure. Patients should have a pelvic examination, endometrial biopsy (if the indication is bleeding), a PAP smear, and either an US or MR prior to the procedure. GnRH analogues should be stopped, if possible, for several weeks prior to the procedure. Currently, the procedure is not performed for nonfibroid causes of pelvic pain other than selected cases of adenomyosis. Embolization of massive fibroids prior to conventional surgery is also an accepted indication.

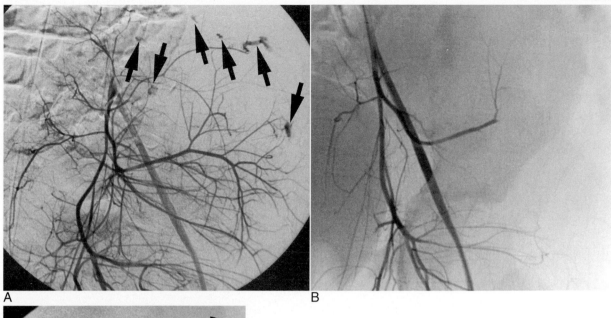

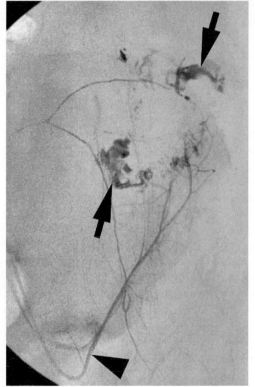

Figure 10-44   Young child with left iliac wing fracture and hypotension despite massive fluid resuscitation following a motor vehicle accident. **A**, DSA of left internal iliac artery injection showing numerous points of extravasation (arrows). **B**, Control angiogram following embolization with a spray of small Gelfoam cubes from the internal iliac artery trunk. There is cessation of bleeding from the hypogastric branches. However, the patient remained hemodynamically unstable. **C**, Selective injection of the deep circumflex iliac artery (arrowhead) showing continued extravasation (arrows) from collateral supply to the area of trauma. This was successfully embolized with Gelfoam pledgets.

On the day of the procedure a serum pregnancy test should be obtained, and a Foley catheter placed to keep the bladder empty. Preprocedural antibiotics and intravenous analgesics (narcotic and nonsteroidal) are administered prior to the embolization. An initial pelvic angiogram with a pigtail catheter positioned at the level of the renal arteries will show the pelvic circulation as well as the presence of enlarged gonadal arteries, one of the potential causes of clinical failure. The uterine arteries can be selected with an angled 5-French catheter (such as a Cobra), but spasm can be a problem so 4-French hydrophilic catheters or even 3-French microcatheters may be necessary (see Fig. 10-3). The choice of embolic material is a matter of operator preference, but

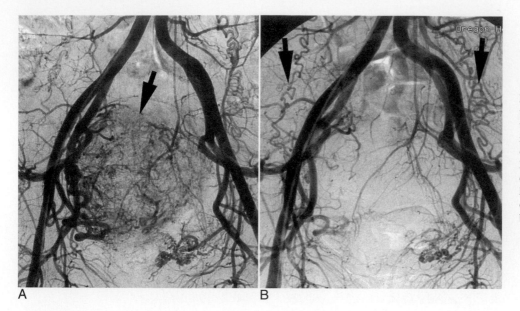

Figure 10-45 Fibroid embolization. **A**, DSA of the pelvis prior to embolization showing a large right-sided fibroid (arrow) with characteristic hypervascularity. **B**, Pelvic angiogram following bilateral embolization. The fibroid is no longer visible, although prominent ovarian arteries (arrows) are seen bilaterally.

permanent particles in the 300- to 700 μm diameter range (Ivalon or acrylic spheres) are generally used. Coil occlusion of the uterine artery is not necessary. Embolization is continued until there is sluggish flow in the uterine artery with elimination of the fibroid blush. Bilateral embolization is mandatory. This is usually accomplished by forming a Waltman loop or selecting the ipsilateral internal iliac artery with a recurved catheter, but bilateral femoral artery access may be required. Fluoroscopy should be kept to a minimum.

Patients experience severe pelvic cramping for 12–24 hours following the procedure, followed by gradually decreasing cramping for 7 days. Most patients are managed overnight in the hospital for pain, but can be sent home the next day. Severe complications are rare, but uterine infection requiring hysterectomy has been reported (Table 10-9). Embolized fibroids shrink on average 50–60% in volume, with relief of symptoms in 85–90% of patients (slightly more for bleeding and pain,

slightly less for bulk symptoms). Failures can be due to incomplete embolization, collateral supply from the gonadal or accessory uterine arteries, and coexistent pathology such as adenomyosis or endometriosis.

Pelvic embolization is sometimes required in women with vaginal bleeding following vaginal delivery, obstetric or gynecologic surgery, or from unresectable gynecologic tumors. Postoperative arterial bleeding is visualized as extravasation or a pseudoaneurysm at angiography, whereas postpartum and tumor bleeding usually is not seen. In fact, tumors may even appear relatively avascular.

The principles of angiographic evaluation for these types of gynecologic bleeding are the same as for pelvic trauma. Fortunately, these patients are generally not as unstable as patients with pelvic trauma. A pelvic angiogram followed by selective internal iliac injections should be obtained. Localized postoperative bleeding can be embolized with coils following general embolization principles. Postpartum bleeding from uterine atony or placental abnormalities can be managed with Gelfoam embolization of the uterine arteries. Small permanent particles, such as 300–500 μm, should be used to devascularize tumors. Since the bleeding sites are almost always in the mid-pelvis with the potential for shared blood supply, careful evaluation of both internal iliac arteries is necessary at completion.

Table 10-9 Complications of Fibroid Embolization	
Complication	**Incidence**
Premature menopause	2–5%
Expulsion of fibroid	<2%
Sepsis	<1%
Emergent hysterectomy	<1%
Death	<1%

PENILE ANGIOGRAPHY

The indications for penile angiography are the evaluation of impotence and trauma. Approximately 50% of males over the age of 40 experience some degree of

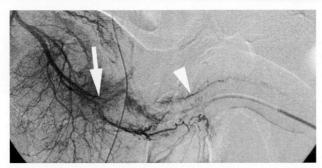

Figure 10-46   Vasculogenic (arterial) impotence following penile fracture. Selective right internal pudendal angiogram shows abrupt distal occlusion (arrow) with reconstitution of the deep cavernosal arteries via small collaterals (arrowhead). Similar findings were present on the left.

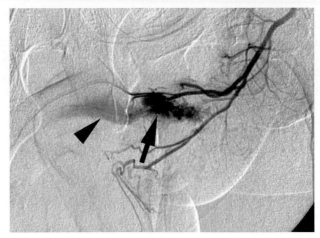

Figure 10-47   High-flow priapism following blunt perineal trauma in a skateboarder. Selective left internal pudendal angiogram showing extremely dense bulbar stain (arrow) with shunting into the corpora (arrowhead). This was successfully embolized through a superselective microcatheter with autologous blood clot.

erectile dysfunction. There are numerous possible causes, including neurologic, endocrine, pharmacologic, psychologic, and vasculogenic. The least common cause is vasculogenic, and should be pursued only after other etiologies have been excluded. There are two potential vascular causes of impotence, venous leak (inability to trap blood in the corpus cavernosum), and arterial insufficiency. Vasculogenic impotence has a venous etiology in one-third of cases, arterial in one-third, and combined venous and arterial in the remainder. Patients with venous leak tend to respond to well to pharmacologic therapies. Severe arterial insufficiency is more difficult to treat effectively, but in rare patients internal iliac artery angioplasty or microvascular bypass to the penis may be effective.

Duplex ultrasound of penile arterial flow in response to a pharmacologically induced erection can be used to screen for arterial insufficiency or venous leak. Dynamic cavernosometry and cavernosography can be used to diagnose a venous leak (see Chapter 13). When arterial insufficiency is suspected, angiography is indicated.

Prior to the angiogram, a Foley catheter is placed, and the patient is given an intracorporal injection of either prostaglandin E$_1$ or papaverine to induce an erection. The penile arteries in the flaccid state are contracted and difficult to opacify. Care should be taken to inject at 3 or 9 o'clock on the shaft of the phallus to avoid injury to the dorsal penile artery. In general, a little less is better than a little more, as too rigid an erection will compromise arterial flow. Pelvic angiograms in the anteroposterior projection and both obliques are obtained with the catheter at the aortic bifurcation to exclude correctable inflow disease of the common and internal iliac arteries. Selective internal pudendal arteriography is performed with a 5-French Cobra-2 or other visceral selective catheter (Figs. 10-4 and 10-46). Usually only one femoral access is required, and a Waltman loop is used to select

the ipsilateral internal pudendal artery. Filming in the anterior oblique with the phallus oriented towards the opposite hip provides visualization of the entire internal pudendal artery including the penile supply. Injection of 25 mg of tolazoline or 200 µg of nitroglycerin into the internal pudendal artery immediately prior to angiography (4-5 mL/s for 5 seconds) improves visualization. Bilateral angiograms should be obtained. Focal occlusion of the internal pudendal or common penile artery represents a correctable lesion.

Blunt and penetrating perineal trauma may result in an arteriovenous fistula of a cavernosal artery (Fig. 10-47). Clinically this presents as priapism, usually painful. When it is unresponsive to conventional measures, angiography and embolization may be warranted. Selective internal pudendal angiography is performed as described above. When a pseudoaneurysm or arteriovenous fistula is identified, embolization with a resorbable substance such as Gelfoam or autologous clot can be performed. Great care is needed not to confuse the normal bulbospongiosal stain with a vascular injury.

SUGGESTED READINGS

Abraham P, Saumet JL, Chevalier JM: External iliac artery endofibrosis in athletes. *Sports Med* 24:221-226, 1997.

Asensio JA, Forno W, Roldan G et al: Abdominal vascular injuries: injuries to the aorta. *Surg Clin N Am* 81:1395-1416, 2001.

Audet P, Therasse E, Oliva VL et al: Infrarenal aortic stenosis: long-term clinical and hemodynamic results of percutaneous transluminal angioplasty. *Radiology* 209:357-363, 1998.

Baum RA, Carpenter JP, Golden MA et al: Treatment of type 2 endoleaks after endovascular repair of abdominal aortic aneurysms: comparison of transarterial and translumbar techniques. *J Vasc Surg* 35:23-29, 2002.

Biffl WL, Smith WR, Moore EE et al: Evolution of a multidisciplinary clinical pathway for the management of unstable patients with pelvic fractures. *Ann Surg* 233:843-850, 2001.

Bosch JL, van der Graaf Y, Hunink MG: Health-related quality of life after angioplasty and stent placement in patients with iliac artery occlusive disease: results of a randomized controlled clinical trial. The Dutch Iliac Stent Trial Study Group. *Circulation* 99:3155-3160, 1999.

Brewster DC: Current controversies in the management of aortoiliac occlusive disease. *J Vasc Surg* 25:365-379, 1997.

Connolly JE, Wilson SE, Lawrence PL, Fujitani RM: Middle aortic syndrome: distal thoracic and abdominal coarctation, a disorder with multiple etiologies. *J Am Coll Surg* 194:774-781, 2002.

Cook RE, Keating JF, Gillespie I: The role of angiography in the management of haemorrhage from major fractures of the pelvis. *J Bone Joint Surg Br* 84:178-182, 2002.

Coulam CH, Rubin GD: Acute aortic abnormalities. *Semin Roentgenol* 36:148-164, 2001.

Darcy M: Complications of iliac angioplasty and stents. *Tech Vasc Intervent Radiol* 3:226-239, 2000.

Davis TP, Feliciano DV, Rozycki GS et al: Results with abdominal vascular trauma in the modern era. *Am Surg* 67:565-570, 2001.

Goodwin SC, McLucas B, Lee M et al: Uterine artery embolization for the treatment of uterine leiomyomata: midterm results. *J Vasc Interv Radiol* 10:1159-1165, 1999.

Gorich J, Rilinger N, Kramer S et al: Angiography of leaks after endovascular repair of infrarenal aortic aneurysms. *Am J Roentgenol* 174:811-814, 2000.

Grist TM: MRA of the abdominal aorta and lower extremities. *J Magn Reson Imaging* 11:32-43, 2000.

Kaufman JA, Geller SC, Brewster DC et al: Endovascular repair of abdominal aortic aneurysms: current status and future directions. *Am J Roentgenol* 175:289-302, 2000.

Koelemay MJ, Lijmer JG, Stoker J, Legemate DA, Bossuyt PM: Magnetic resonance angiography for the evaluation of lower extremity arterial disease: a meta-analysis. *JAMA* 285:1338-1345, 2001.

Lauterbach SR, Cambria RP, Brewster DC et al: Contemporary management of aortic branch compromise resulting from acute aortic dissection. *J Vasc Surg* 33:1185-1192, 2001.

Lederle FA, Wilson SE, Johnson GR et al: Immediate repair compared with surveillance of small abdominal aortic aneurysms. *N Engl J Med* 346:1437-1444, 2002.

Lee ES, Steenson CC, Trimble KE et al: Comparing patency rates between external iliac and common iliac artery stents. *J Vasc Surg* 31:889-894, 2000.

Lin PH, Chaikof EL: Embryology, anatomy, and surgical exposure of the great abdominal vessels. *Surg Clin N Am* 80:417-433, 2000.

Margolies MN, Ring EJ, Waltman AC, Kerr WS, Baum S: Arteriography in the management of hemorrhage from pelvic fractures. *N Engl J Med* 287:317-321, 1972.

Muller BT, Wegener OR, Grabitz K et al: Mycotic aneurysms of the thoracic and abdominal aorta and iliac arteries: experience with anatomic and extra-anatomic repair in 33 cases. *J Vasc Surg* 33:106-113, 2001.

Murphy TP, Khwaja AA, Webb MS: Aortoiliac stent placement in patients treated for intermittent claudication. *J Vasc Interv Radiol* 9:21-28, 1998.

Murphy TP: Technical aspects of aortoiliac interventions. *Tech Vasc Interv Radiol* 3:189-194, 2000.

Parker WH, Fu YS, Berek JS: Uterine sarcoma in patients operated on for presumed leiomyoma and rapidly growing leiomyoma. *Obstet Gynecol* 83:414-418, 1994.

Reyes R, Maynar M, Lopera J et al: Treatment of chronic iliac artery occlusions with guide wire recanalization and primary stent placement. *J Vasc Interv Radiol* 8:1049-1055, 1997.

Roth JW, Boyd CR: Recreational bicycling and injury to the external iliac artery. *Am Surg* 65:460-463, 1999.

Rubin GD: Techniques for performing multidetector-row computed tomographic angiography. *Tech Vasc Interv Radiol* 4:2-14, 2001.

Sawhney R, Kerlan RK, Wall SD et al: Analysis of initial CT findings after endovascular repair of abdominal aortic aneurysm. *Radiology* 220:157-160, 2001.

Scheinert D, Schroder M, Steinkamp H, Ludwig J, Biamino G: Treatment of iliac artery aneurysms by percutaneous implantation of stent grafts. *Circulation* 102(Suppl. 3): 253-258, 2000.

Siskin GP, Englander M, Roddy S et al: Results of iliac artery stent placement in patients younger than 50 years of age. *J Vasc Interv Radiol* 13:785-790, 2002.

Slonim SM, Miller DC, Mitchell RS et al: Percutaneous balloon fenestration and stenting for life-threatening ischemic complications in patients with acute aortic dissection. *J Thorac Cardiovasc Surg* 117:1118-1126, 1999.

Smith JC, Watkins GE, Taylor FC et al: Angioplasty or stent placement in the proximal common iliac artery: is protection of the contralateral side necessary? *J Vasc Interv Radiol* 12:1395-1398, 2001.

Spies JB, Warren EH, Mathias SD et al: Uterine fibroid embolization: measurement of health-related quality of life before and after therapy. *J Vasc Interv Radiol* 10:1293-1303, 1999.

Spies J, Niedzwiecki G, Goodwin S et al: Training standards for physicians performing uterine artery embolization for leiomyomata: consensus statement developed by the Task Force on Uterine Artery Embolization and the standards division of the Society of Cardiovascular & Interventional Radiology. *J Vasc Interv Radiol* 12:19-21, 2001.

Surowiec SM, Isiklar H, Sreeram S, Weiss VJ, Lumsden AB: Acute occlusion of the abdominal aorta. *Am J Surg* 176:193-197, 1998.

TransAtlantic Inter-Society Consensus (TASC): Management of peripheral arterial disease (PAD). *J Vasc Surg* 31:S1-S296, 2000.

Tetteroo E, van der Graaf Y, Bosch JL et al: Randomized comparison of primary stent placement versus primary angioplasty followed by selective stent placement in patients with iliac-artery occlusive disease. Dutch Iliac Stent Trial Study Group. *Lancet* 351:1153–1159, 1998.

Thompson RW, Geraghty PJ, Lee JK: Abdominal aortic aneurysms: basic mechanisms and clinical implications. *Curr Probl Surg* 39:110–230, 2002.

United Kingdom Small Aneurysm Trial Participants: Long-term outcomes of immediate repair compared with surveillance of small abdominal aortic aneurysms. *N Engl J Med* 346: 1445–1452, 2002.

van der Vliet JA, Boll AP: Abdominal aortic aneurysm. *Lancet* 349:863–866, 1997.

Vedantham S, Picus D, Sanchez LA et al: Percutaneous management of ischemic complications in patients with type-B aortic dissection. *J Vasc Interv Radiol* 14:181–194, 2003.

Walker WJ, Pelage JP, Sutton C: Fibroid embolization. *Clin Radiol* 57:325–331, 2002.

Visceral Arteries

JOHN A. KAUFMAN, M.D.

The arterial anatomy of the gastrointestinal tract, while constant in its basic pattern, is the most variable of any vascular bed. In addition, there is great diversity in the types of diseases that involve the gastrointestinal arteries and organs. Many visceral disorders, vascular and otherwise, can be treated effectively with endovascular techniques. As a result, visceral arterial diagnosis and intervention continues to be an important aspect of interventional radiologic practice.

NORMAL ANATOMY

Celiac Artery

The celiac artery arises from the anterior surface of the abdominal aorta at the level of the T12–L1 diskspace (Fig. 11-1). In the majority of individuals the inferior phrenic arteries arise from the aorta in close proximity to the orifice of the celiac artery. The celiac artery (also know as the celiac trunk) courses inferiorly under the posterior fibers of the diaphragmatic crura for a distance of 1.5–3 cm. There is frequently an indentation upon the superior aspect of the celiac artery caused by the fibers of the diaphragm (Fig. 11-2). This is exacerbated with expiration. Branches of the celiac artery supply the liver, spleen, stomach, and pancreas (Fig. 11-3). The first branch is usually the left gastric artery, arising from the superior wall of the celiac artery distal to the diaphragmatic crura. The left gastric artery supplies the fundus of the stomach and the gastroesophageal junction, and anastomoses with the right gastric artery (a branch of the hepatic arteries), and the short gastric arteries from the splenic circulation. Distal to the left gastric artery the celiac artery bifurcates into the common hepatic and splenic arteries. A large branch to the pancreas, the dorsal pancreatic artery, may arise from the celiac or the proximal hepatic or splenic arteries. This vessel supplies the body of the pancreas.

Conventional celiac artery anatomy is present in only 70% of individuals. A wide range of variants can occur (Table 11-1). An awareness of these variations and knowing where to look for celiac branches that may have

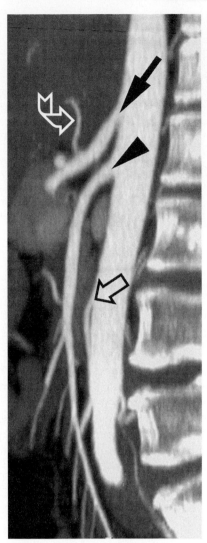

Figure 11-1   Lateral maximum-intensity projection (MIP) of an abdominal CTA (4-detector row) showing the origins of the celiac artery (solid arrow), superior mesenteric artery (SMA) (arrow-head), and inferior mesenteric artery (IMA) (open arrow). The left gastric artery (curved arrow) is visible arising from the superior wall of the celiac artery trunk.

anomalous origins are essential for visceral vascular imaging. Specific examples are provided in the following sections. As a rule, any of the celiac branches can arise independently from the aorta, or (with the exception of the left gastric artery) from the superior mesenteric artery (SMA). This is explainable because of the common embryology of the contents of the peritoneal cavity. For the same reason, celiac branches cannot arise anomalously from the renal arteries, as these organs are retroperitoneal in origin.

Liver (arterial supply)

The arterial circulation contributes roughly one-third of the blood supply to the liver, but nearly two-thirds of

Table 11-1   Celiac Artery Anatomy

	Incidence
Left gastric, splenic, common hepatic arteries from celiac trunk	70%
Above plus dorsal pancreatic artery from celiac trunk	10%
Splenic, common hepatic arteries from celiac trunk; left gastric from aorta	2%
Splenic, left gastric arteries only from celiac trunk	3%
Common hepatic, left gastric arteries only from celiac trunk	<1%
Celiacomesenteric trunk (shared origin celiac and superior mesenteric arteries)	<1%
All branches individually from aorta	<1%
Splenic artery from aorta	<1%
Splenic artery from superior mesenteric artery	<1%

the oxygen. Conversely, the portal vein supplies two-thirds of the blood volume, but only one-third of the oxygen (Table 11-2). The common hepatic artery arises from the celiac artery in over 95% of individuals. The terminal branches of this artery are the gastroduodenal and proper hepatic arteries (see Fig. 11-3). In a little over half of patients, the proper hepatic artery gives rise to the entire arterial supply of the liver. The proper hepatic artery continues for a short distance, and then divides into the left, middle, and right hepatic arteries. The left hepatic artery has a characteristic forked appearance that allows ready identification. The hepatic arteries are located anterior to the portal vein within the liver parenchyma.

The most common variants of hepatic arterial supply are replacement of part or all of the right hepatic artery from the SMA, or the left hepatic artery replaced to the left gastric artery (Fig. 11-4). These variants can occur in

Table 11-2   Hepatic Arterial Anatomy

	Incidence
All branches from common hepatic artery	55%
Right hepatic artery from superior mesenteric artery (SMA)	12%
Accessory right hepatic artery from SMA	6%
Left hepatic from left gastric artery	11%
Accessory left hepatic from left gastric artery	11%
Right hepatic from SMA and left hepatic from left gastric artery	2%
Common hepatic artery from SMA	2%
Common hepatic artery from aorta	2%
Right hepatic artery from celiac	<1%

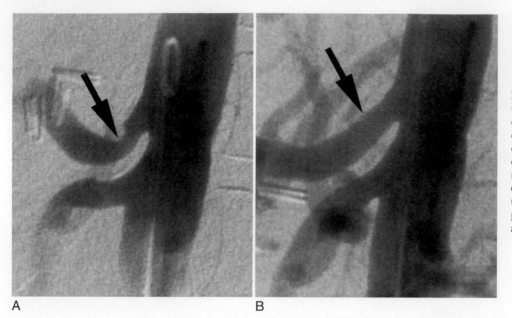

A   B

Figure 11-2 Crus impression upon the celiac artery. This is usually of no clinical significance. **A**, Lateral digital subtraction angiogram (DSA) of the aorta in expiration showing extrinsic compression on the superior aspect of the celiac artery (arrow) with post-stenotic dilatation. **B**, Repeat DSA in the same patient with inspiration showing absence of the stenosis (arrow).

isolation, or together. In general, 45% of patients have some variation in their hepatic arterial supply.

The cystic artery (to the gallbladder) is usually a branch of the right hepatic artery, although it may arise from the common hepatic, left hepatic, or even the superior mesenteric arteries (see Fig. 11-3).

Spleen

The spleen derives its blood supply from the celiac artery primarily via the splenic artery (see Figs. 11-3 and 2-21). This vessel courses posterior to the pancreas, and

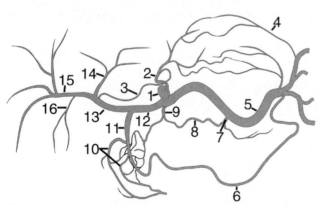

Figure 11-3 Anatomy of the celiac artery and its branches. **1**, Celiac trunk. **2**, Left gastric artery. **3**, Right gastric artery. **4**, Short gastric artery. **5**, Splenic artery. **6**, Gastroepiploic artery. **7**, Pancreatico-magna artery. **8**, Transverse pancreatic artery. **9**, Dorsal pancreatic artery. **10**, Superior pancreatico-duodenal arteries. **11**, Gastroduodenal artery. **12**, Common hepatic artery. **13**, Proper hepatic artery. **14**, Left hepatic artery. **15**, Right hepatic artery. **16**, Cystic artery.

anterior and superior to the splenic vein. The splenic artery is much longer than the hepatic artery, and frequently several millimeters larger in diameter. The splenic artery supplies many small twigs to the pancreas as well as the spleen. The splenic artery divides into multiple branches, usually in the hilum of the spleen but sometimes in a more proximal location.

Stomach

The stomach is uniquely well endowed with arterial blood supply (see Figs. 11-1 and 11-3). This is a key concept in the angiographic management of gastric bleeding. The fundus of the stomach is supplied primarily by the left gastric artery. This vessel is usually a branch of the celiac artery, but may arise from the aorta or the left hepatic artery. Additional blood supply is derived from the multiple small branches emanating from the hilum and upper pole of the spleen, the short and posterior gastric arteries. These arteries anastomose with the left gastric artery within the fundus of the stomach.

The body of the stomach is supplied by the gastroepiploic artery, which is located along the greater curvature of the stomach (see Fig. 11-3). This artery has origins from the gastroduodenal artery (where it is called the right gastroepiploic artery), and from the distal splenic artery (where it is called the left gastroepiploic artery). The lesser curvature of the stomach is supplied by branches from the left and right gastric arteries. The right gastric artery usually arises from the left or common hepatic arteries, and is a much smaller vessel than the left gastric artery.

The antrum and pylorus are supplied by the right gastroepiploic and right gastric arteries. In addition, the

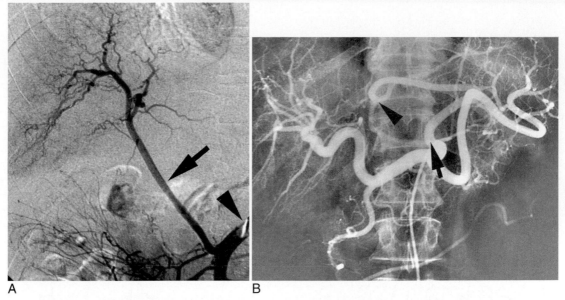

Figure 11-4   Hepatic arterial anatomic variants. **A**, Right hepatic artery replaced (arrow) to the SMA (arrowhead) in this patient with advanced cirrhosis. Note the characteristic corkscrew appearance of the intrahepatic arteries. **B**, Celiac angiogram showing the left hepatic artery replaced to the left gastric artery (arrow). The left hepatic artery has a characteristic forked appearance (arrowhead).

pancreatico-duodenal arteries (branches of the gastro-duodenal artery) provide blood supply to this part of the stomach.

Pancreas

The pancreatic blood supply is derived from both the celiac artery and the SMA. The head of the pancreas is supplied by the pancreatico-duodenal arteries (Figs. 11-3 and 11-5). These vessels are paired arteries anterior and posterior to the pancreatic head. They are further divided into superior and inferior vessels. The superior pancreatico-duodenal arteries arise from the gastroduodenal artery, while the inferior pancreatico-duodenal arteries arise from a common trunk off the proximal SMA.

The body of the pancreas is supplied by the dorsal pancreatic artery, usually a medium-size proximal branch of the splenic artery or the celiac artery (see Figs. 11-3 and 11-5). Less commonly, this vessel will arise from the common hepatic artery, the SMA, or the aorta. This is a small but important artery, as it can contribute to the blood supply of the transverse colon via an accessory or a replaced middle colic artery in 1–2% of patients. The pancreatico-duodenal arteries also supply the body of the pancreas through the transverse pancreatic artery.

There are numerous small arteries that arise directly from the splenic artery to supply the body and tail of the pancreas. These are termed, aptly, "small pancreatic arteries." The largest and most distal of these vessels is the pancreatica magna artery. All of these arteries

communicate with the transverse pancreatic artery. The left gastro-epiploic artery may provide small branches to the tail of the pancreas.

Superior Mesenteric Artery

There are usually four sources of arterial supply to the small bowel and colon: the gastroduodenal branches

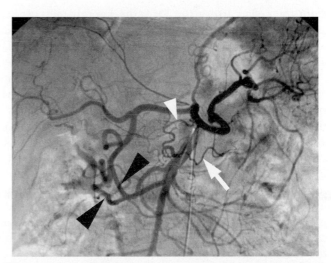

Figure 11-5   Enlarged pancreatico-duodenal arteries (black arrowheads) in a patient with occlusion of the celiac artery origin. The pancreatico-duodenal arteries are a collateral pathway between the SMA and the celiac artery. The dorsal pancreatic artery (white arrowhead) communicates with both the proximal SMA (via the Arc of Buhler) and the transverse pancreatic artery (white arrow).

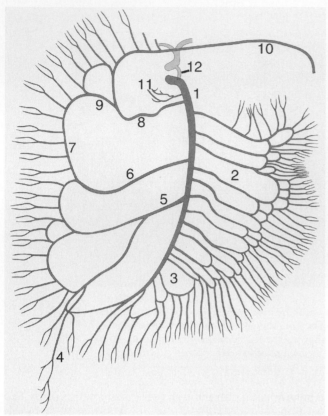

Figure 11-6 Drawing of conventional anatomy of the superior mesenteric artery. **1**, Superior mesenteric artery. **2**, Jejunal branches. **3**, Ileal branches. **4**, Appendicular artery. **5**, Ileocolic artery. **6**, Right colic artery. **7**, Marginal artery. **8**, Middle colic artery. **9**, Right branch of middle colic artery. **10**, Left branch of middle colic artery. **11**, Inferior pancreatico-duodenal arteries. **12**, Arc of Buhler.

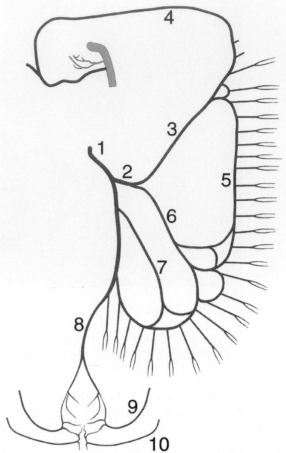

Figure 11-7 Drawing of the inferior mesenteric artery. **1**, Inferior mesenteric artery. **2**, Left colic artery. **3**, Ascending branch of left colic artery. **4**, Left branch of middle colic artery. **5**, Marginal artery. **6**, Descending branch of left colic artery. **7**, Sigmoid artery. **8**, Superior hemorrhoidal artery. **9**, Middle hemorrhoidal artery. **10**, Inferior hemorrhoidal artery.

from the celiac artery, the SMA, the inferior mesenteric artery (IMA), and the anterior divisions of the internal iliac arteries. The SMA supplies the duodenum, small bowel, and the colon as far as the splenic flexure (Fig. 11-6). The IMA supplies the left colon, sigmoid colon, and proximal rectum (Fig. 11-7). The internal iliac arteries provide supply to the rectum and anus (see Fig. 10-2). The vasculature of the bowel is, in essence, one long multi-tiered arcade. The most peripheral continuous vessel in this arcade runs along the mesenteric border of the bowel. In the colon, this vessel is usually well developed and termed the Marginal Artery of Drummond. The equivalent vessel in the small bowel is less prominent and unnamed. The classic areas of overlap (watershed areas) of the bowel vascular supply are the splenic flexure of the colon (Griffith's point) and the superior rectum.

The superior mesenteric artery arises from the anterior abdominal aorta 1–2 cm distal to the celiac artery (see Figs. 11-1 and 11-2). The SMA is typically 6–8 mm in diameter at its origin. The SMA passes behind the body of the pancreas and over the left renal vein, and runs

through the mesentery slightly to the right and posterior to the superior mesenteric vein (SMV). The first major branch of the SMA is either the inferior pancreatico-duodenal artery trunk or the middle colic artery. These two vessels may also arise conjointly. The middle of the SMA supplies the small bowel from the third portion of the duodenum to the terminal ileum through multiple branches that usually arise from the left border of the vessel. These are termed jejunal or ileal branches based upon the portion of small bowel that they supply. The right side of the artery gives rise to the right colic artery, which supplies the ascending colon. The SMA terminates in the ileocolic artery, which supplies the terminal ileum and the cecum. A small appendiceal artery may arise from the ileocolic artery or directly from the distal SMA. The middle and right colic arteries bifurcate at the mesenteric border of the colon; the right into ascending and descending branches, and the middle into right and left branches. Of particular importance is the left branch of the middle colic, as this artery anastomoses with the left colonic branches of the IMA.

In 1% of patients, the celiac artery and SMA share a common origin from the aorta. This is termed a celiaco-mesenteric trunk. The SMA frequently gives rise to an accessory or replaced right hepatic artery (20%), or less commonly a replaced proper or common hepatic artery (2%) (see Fig. 11-4). In fewer than 1% of patients, the splenic, transverse pancreatic, or dorsal pancreatic arteries may arise from the SMA. A persistent direct fetal communication between the celiac artery and the SMA, distinct from the dorsal pancreatic artery, occurs in fewer than 1% of patients and is termed the Arc of Buhler (see Figs. 11-5 and 11-6). A separate origin of some of the jejunal, ileal, or colic branches from the anterior surface of the aorta between the SMA and IMA, known as a "middle mesenteric artery," is extremely rare.

Interior Mesenteric Artery

The IMA arises from the left side of the anterior distal abdominal aorta at the level of the L3 vertebral body, approximately 2–3 cm above the aortic bifurcation (see Fig. 11-1). This artery is much smaller than the SMA in diameter, usually no more than 3 mm. The artery has a sharply caudal course through the sigmoid mesentery (see Fig. 11-7). The first branch of the IMA is the left colic artery, from which a large branch ascends through the mesentery to anastomose with the left branch of the middle colic artery at the splenic flexure. The blood supply of the sigmoid colon is provided by the IMA. The terminal branch of the IMA is the superior hemorrhoidal artery to the superior rectum. This is located in the center of the pelvis. On conventional angiography, the distal superior hemorrhoidal artery has a characteristic forked appearance, which distinguishes it from the straight median sacral artery. On a lateral view, the hemorrhoidal artery will be in the middle of the pelvis, whereas the median sacral artery lies close to the anterior surface of the sacrum. The remainder of the rectum is supplied by the middle and inferior rectal arteries, terminal branches of the anterior division of the internal iliac arteries.

KEY COLLATERAL PATHWAYS

With celiac artery stenosis or occlusion, the pancre-atico-duodenal arteries enlarge and provide collateral supply from the SMA (see Fig. 11-5). Similarly, the same circuit can provide collateral supply to the SMA from the celiac artery. In addition, transpancreatic primitive communications such as the Arc of Buhler can exist in some individuals.

The spleen receives collateral blood supply from the left gastric artery via the short gastric arteries, the right

gastroepiploic to the left gastroepiploic arteries, and omental collaterals (Arc of Barkow). Proximal splenic artery occlusion is usually well tolerated owing to the richness of this collateral bed.

Occlusion of the proper hepatic artery may result in the formation of small unnamed collateral arteries in the porta hepatis, as well as reversal of flow in the right gastric artery. The hepatic arteries anastomose within the liver parenchyma, so that proximal occlusion of a hepatic artery branch results in development of intra-hepatic collaterals (Fig. 11-8). This is an important consideration during embolization of intrahepatic bleeding.

When SMA stenosis or occlusion is present, collateral supply can be derived from the IMA as well as the celiac artery. The ascending branch of the left colic artery anastomoses with the left branch of the middle colic artery at the splenic flexure. The Arcade of Riolan is the medial, and the Marginal Artery of Drummond the lateral arcade in the mesentery of the left colon (Fig. 11-9). Unnamed retroperitoneal collaterals from the aorta to the SMA can develop in some patients.

In the setting of IMA occlusion, the anterior division of the internal iliac artery is a potential source of collateral blood supply to the left colon through the hemorrhoidal arteries. This pathway is extremely important in patients with IMA occlusion undergoing right hemi-colectomy, in which the anastomosis between the middle colic artery from the SMA and the left colic artery from the IMA is disrupted. In patients with intact collateral

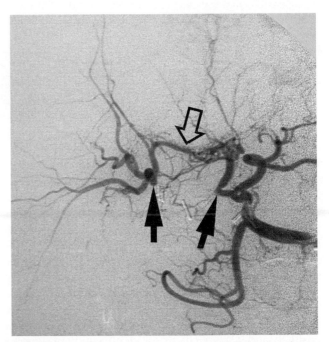

Figure 11-8   DSA of the hepatic artery showing intrahepatic collateralization (open arrow) around a right hepatic artery occlusion (black arrows).

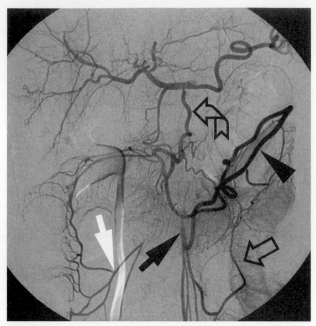

Figure 11-9 Filling of the celiac artery from the IMA (black solid arrow) via the dorsal pancreatic artery (open curved arrow) in a patient with SMA occlusion and celiac artery origin occlusion. IMA angiogram showing an intact Marginal Artery of Drummond (open arrow) and enlarged Arc of Riolan (arrowhead) filling the middle colic artery and ultimately branches of the ileocolic artery (white arrow) via the marginal arcade of the right colic artery.

pathways and chronic occlusive disease, a well-developed hypogastric collateral bed can supply the IMA, SMA, and celiac artery.

IMAGING

The proximal celiac artery and SMA are amenable to interrogation by ultrasound (color-flow and duplex US) in the majority of patients. The IMA is difficult to image in some patients owing to body habitus and the small size of the artery. The velocities and directions of flow within the celiac artery and SMA are essential elements of the study. Flow in the celiac artery, and its major branches, is usually low resistance. Peak systolic velocities in the celiac artery origin greater than 200 cm/s is indicative of at least 70% stenosis. The baseline waveform in the proximal SMA is high-resistance. A postprandial state induces a high-flow low-resistance waveform in the SMA. A peak systolic velocity ≥275 cm/s, and end-diastolic velocities ≥45 cm/s, have both been shown to be predictive of SMA stenosis. In expert hands, US has an 89% sensitivity and 92% specificity for identification of stenoses ≥70% of the SMA. Retrograde flow in the common hepatic artery is the best predictor of hemodynamically

significant celiac artery stenosis. US is less successful in the evaluation of distal branches of the SMA.

MR angiography with gadolinium has excellent sensitivity and specificity for visceral artery orificial and proximal disease (Fig. 11-10). Three-dimensional (3-D) acquisitions in the coronal plane, centered on the aortic bifurcation, will include the visceral arteries as well as the hypogastric artery origins. The ability to view vessel origins in multiple planes is useful when anatomy is complex or anatomic variants are present. Heavy calcification, metallic clips, and patient motion can cause artifacts. Small vessel disease is difficult to visualize with current technology. The lack of nephrotoxicity of gadolinium is an advantage compared to CT and conventional angiography.

CTA of the visceral arteries should begin with a noncontrast scan. Heavily calcified plaque in the visceral arteries can be overlooked on contrast-enhanced sequences. Image postprocessing is essential to evaluate the visceral arteries (Figs. 11-1 and 11-11). In addition to

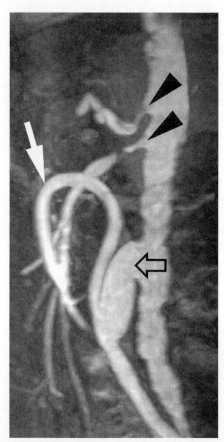

Figure 11-10 Lateral MIP of gadolinium-enhanced 3-D MRA in a patient with a bypass graft (solid white arrow) to the SMA arising from an onlay aortobifemoral graft (open arrow). The patient had chronic mesenteric ischemia due to celiac artery and SMA stenoses (arrowheads) and an occluded IMA.

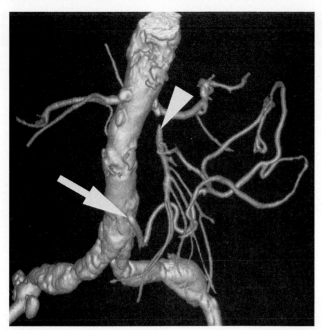

Figure 11-11   Volume rendering of CTA in a patient with celiac artery and SMA origin occlusion showing collaterals from the IMA (arrow) to the SMA (arrowhead).

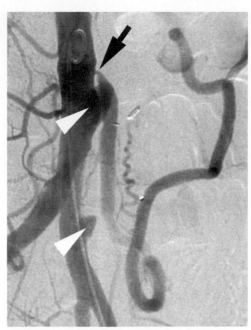

Figure 11-12   The origin of the IMA is seen best in a left posterior oblique projection. DSA aortogram showing a severe stenosis of the IMA origin (arrow). This patient has chronic mesenteric ischemia and two failed surgical bypasses. The stumps of the occluded grafts are visible arising from the distal abdominal aorta and left common iliac artery (arrowheads).

blood vessels, CTA provides valuable additional information about the perfusion of the visceral organs and bowel that can contribute to the diagnosis. For example, the status of the bowel wall is important in patients with suspected acute mesenteric ischemia.

Visceral angiography requires knowledge of a wide range of catheter shapes and guidewires. A quick fluoroscopic examination of the abdomen is useful in patients undergoing elective examinations with a history of recent oral or rectal contrast. Residual barium or gastrograffin in the colon may degrade the quality of the study. The best means of viewing the visceral artery origins is with a lateral aortogram. A pigtail catheter (4- to 7-French) should be placed with the tip at the T12–L1 vertebral interspace to visualize the celiac artery and SMA origins (see Figs. 11-2 and 10-8). A lower position (below the renal arteries) with a slight left posterior oblique angulations is necessary to view the IMA origin (Fig. 11-12). Selective catheters for the visceral arteries range from generic Cobra shapes to complex curves designed for specific branch vessels. In general, vessels that arise with angles 45–100 degrees from the aorta can be engaged with simple curved selective catheters (Table 11-3; see Figs. 2-10, 2-18, 2-19 and 2-20). When the artery arises at an acute angle, a recurved catheter that can be pulled into the orifice is the best choice. Review of prior CTA and MRA data when available can guide catheter selection. Visceral vessels are easily traumatized by catheters and guidewires, so gentle technique is required at all times.

Leading with the soft tip of a guidewire when pulling or pushing into a vessel limits spasm and the risk of dissection (see Fig. 4-27). Coaxial microcatheters are almost always necessary for selection of branch vessels for the reasons listed above (see Fig. 2-21).

The left gastric artery represents a specific challenge for selective catheterization when the vessel arises from its normal location. The Waltman loop, formed in the splenic or hepatic artery, was devised to catheterize this vessel (see Fig. 2-17). Once formed, the looped catheter is slowly pushed into the aorta, bringing the tip to the left gastric artery. In many cases a recurved pull-down catheter can be used to engage the left gastric artery. The catheter is pulled snuggly into the celiac artery so that the tip is advanced beyond the left gastric artery origin. Continued traction opens the catheter and withdraws the tip along the superior surface of the celiac trunk until the orifice of the left gastric artery is engaged. Occasionally, a left gastric artery that arises close to the origin of the celiac trunk can be selected directly with an angled catheter and a hydrophilic guidewire.

Celiac artery injections can be filmed in the anteroposterior projection (see Fig. 11-4B). Delayed filming is useful for visualization of the splenic and portal veins. The right anterior oblique projection is useful for selective common or proper hepatic artery injections to visualize the intrahepatic arteries. Complete coverage of the

Table 11-3   Injection Rates for Visceral Angiography

Artery	Typical Catheters	Injection (mL/s)/ (total volume)[a]	Filming
Celiac	Cobra-2, Celiac, Sos Omni	5–7/30–60	2–4/s × 10 s, then 1/s
Splenic	Cobra-2, Simmons-2	5–6/30–50	Same
Hepatic	Cobra-2, Celiac, Simmons-2	4–5/15–30	Same
Left gastric	Simmons-1, Left gastric, Cobra-2 (Waltman loop)	3–4/6–16	Same
Gastroduodenal	Cobra-2, Celiac	3–4/6–16	Same
SMA	Cobra-2, Celiac, Sos Omni	5–7/30–60	Same; may require two injections with overlapping upper and lower fields to include all of bowel
IMA	Sos Omni, Simmons-1	3–5/9–20	Same; for GI bleed, use left posterior oblique projection and include anal verge on film

[a] The higher injection rates are usually necessary for cut-film angiography.

SMA may require overlapping fields of view to ensure visualization of the splenic flexure and small bowel in the pelvis. Glucagon (1 mg intravenously) prior to injection of contrast decreases bowel motion artifact on DSA studies. Complete coverage of the IMA also frequently requires two injections to include both the splenic flexure and the anal verge. A left posterior oblique projection will open the sigmoid colon flexure.

ACUTE MESENTERIC ISCHEMIA

Acute mesenteric ischemia is one of the most potentially devastating visceral arterial emergencies. A variety of causative mechanisms have been described (Box 11-1). Over 50% of cases are due to embolic occlusion of the SMA, one-fifth are caused by thrombosis of a preexisting stenotic lesion, one-fifth occur during a period of low flow or hypotension (nonocclusive mesenteric ischemia), and 10% are due to mesenteric venous thrombosis.

Box 11-1   Etiologies of Acute Mesenteric Ischemia

Embolus (cardiac or aortic source)
Thrombosis existing atherosclerotic lesion
Dissection (aortic or localized to visceral artery)
Cholesterol embolization
Low-flow state (nonocclusive mesenteric ischemia)
Vasculitis
Iatrogenic (e.g., low placement of intraaortic balloon pump)
Mesenteric venous thrombosis

Acute occlusion of the SMA is tolerated poorly, even in the presence of a widely patent celiac artery and IMA with intact collaterals. Time is the primary determinant of survival for these patients. In most series, the mortality rate exceeds 80% without early and aggressive intervention. Delay in diagnosis equals death.

The classic presentation of acute intestinal ischemia is sudden onset of generalized abdominal pain out of proportion to the physical findings. This scenario is particularly suggestive of acute mesenteric ischemia of embolic origin in patients with cardiac dysrhythmias. The pain may also be subacute or stuttering in onset. Nausea, vomiting, and diarrhea are common subsequent symptoms. The white blood cell count may be elevated, but no laboratory test is specific for bowel infarction. Despite the severe abdominal pain, bowel sounds remain present and peritoneal signs are absent until the ischemia is advanced. The development of peritonitis heralds sepsis, shock, and onset of multi-organ system failure.

The patient's prior surgical history should be reviewed, with particular attention to the details of vascular reconstructions and bowel resections. The difficulty in imaging many patients with suspected acute mesenteric ischemia is that usually several other possible diagnoses are being considered at the same time. The plain film findings of early acute mesenteric ischemia are nonspecific. Gas in the bowel wall or portal vein indicates bowel infarction and is a late sign. Contrast-enhanced CT scan is an excellent initial imaging modality as it allows evaluation of arterial and venous structures, and the bowel wall. However, presence of barium in the colon from the CT can degrade subsequent angiograms.

Conventional angiography remains an essential diagnostic modality in suspected acute mesenteric ischemia. A lateral aortogram should be obtained first to inspect the celiac artery and SMA origins (Fig. 11-13). The classic

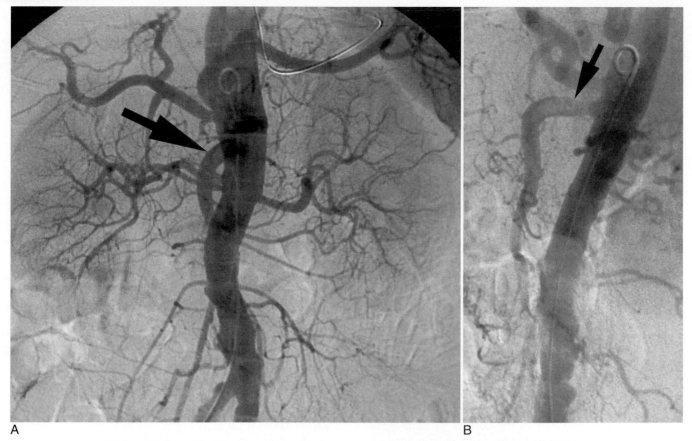

A   B

Figure 11-13   The lateral aortogram is the most useful view for visualizing the origins of the celiac artery and SMA. This patient had atrial fibrillation and acute simultaneous onset of abdominal pain and left leg ischemia. **A**, DSA aortogram in the anteroposterior projection. The visceral artery origins are obscured. (Arrow = SMA.) **B**, Lateral DSA aortogram showing a filling defect in the origin of the SMA (arrow).

findings of an embolus are contrast outlining a convex filling defect causing partial or complete luminal obstruction. An aortogram in the anteroposterior projection is valuable to assess the aorta and exclude associated renal artery emboli. Selective injection of the SMA to exclude peripheral pathology is mandatory if the origin is normal on the aortogram (Fig. 11-14). Celiac artery and IMA injections may be performed if the SMA is normal, but rarely are the culprit vessels.

Large emboli may lodge at the SMA origin. As many as 85% of emboli will then progress distally, usually stopping in the SMA just beyond the origin of the first mesenteric branch. These emboli result in profound ischemia, as major potential collateral pathways (either from the celiac artery via the pancreatico-duodenal arteries or the IMA via the middle colic artery) are obstructed. Simultaneous embolization to other organs is common. When the clinical examination and radiographic findings suggest that bowel remains viable, catheter-based intervention may be warranted. Thrombolysis has proven successful in

anecdotal cases, although a beneficial effect may not become apparent for several hours. Suction embolectomy using a large nontapered catheter can remove the embolus immediately (see Fig. 11-14). In most patients, emergent surgical embolectomy or bypass with resection of any portions of nonviable bowel is necessary.

Thrombosis of a previously symptomatic or asymptomatic visceral artery stenosis may cause acute ischemia if collaterals are poorly formed or nonexistent. This tends to occur during episodes of hemodynamic stress or derangement, such as during acute myocardial infarction or severe dehydration. A heavily calcified aorta or SMA on CT is indicative of underlying atherosclerosis. Thrombolysis (catheter-directed) with subsequent angioplasty and stent can be attempted when full-thickness bowel ischemia has not occurred. Surgical bypass with resection of any portions of nonviable bowel remains the standard therapy in acutely ill patients.

Nonocclusive mesenteric ischemia is best described as a syndrome of low flow in the SMA in the absence of

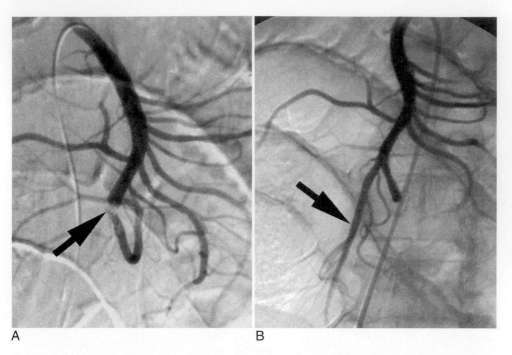

Figure 11-14 Aspiration thrombectomy of a distal SMA embolus. **A**, Selective DSA of the SMA in a patient with several days of intermittent abdominal pain, a normal physical examination, and small bowel wall thickening on CT scan. There is occlusion of the SMA by an embolus (arrow) distal to the right colic artery. **B**, DSA obtained following percutaneous aspiration thrombectomy during the same procedure showing reperfusion of the distal SMA (arrow).

a fixed lesion (Fig. 11-15). Most often associated with acutely ill patients on multiple vasopressor agents or digitalis, it can also be seen in the setting of cardiogenic shock and sepsis. Mortality is very high, usually from the precipitating conditions rather than the bowel ischemia. At angiography, vasoconstriction of the SMA and its branches, often with interposed areas of normal-caliber vessel, is characteristic. Injection of a vasodilator directly into the SMA, such as tolazoline or nitroglycerin, may break the spasm and can be used as a test. Direct infusion

of papaverine (0.5–1 mg/min) can be used to treat spasm until the patient stabilizes. There is little role for surgical intervention in these patients.

CHRONIC MESENTERIC ISCHEMIA

The symptoms of chronic mesenteric ischemia are completely different from those of acute ischemia. The onset is gradual, often months to years in duration.

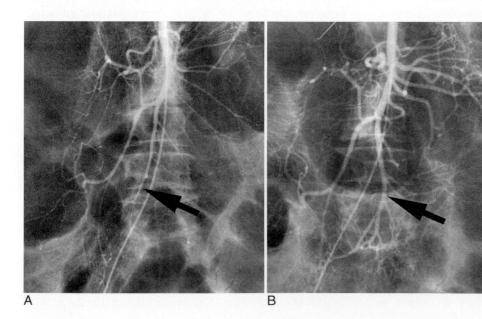

Figure 11-15 Nonocclusive mesenteric ischemia in a patient with abdominal pain following cardiac surgery. **A**, Selective SMA angiogram showing diffuse narrowing of all of the mesenteric vessels. For example, note the appearance of the ileocolic artery (arrow). **B**, Angiogram repeated after infusion of papaverine showing marked improvement in the caliber of the arteries (arrow).

Box 11-2 Risk Factors Associated with Chronic Mesenteric Ischemia

Age 50–70 years
Female:male ratio 3:2
Tobacco abuse
Generalized atherosclerosis
Hypertension
Chronic renal insufficiency
Diabetes
Past history of abdominal or vascular surgery

Postprandial pain is the defining symptom. Termed "intestinal angina," the pain occurs $\frac{1}{2}$–1 hour following a meal, is poorly localized, resolves after 2–3 hours, and may be associated with nausea, vomiting, or diarrhea. Patients usually report weight loss and fear of eating (Box 11-2). Progression to acute ischemia can occur if patients are left untreated.

Chronic stenosis or occlusion of at least two mesenteric arteries is usually necessary before symptoms develop (see Fig. 11-9). A number of conditions can be associated with chronic mesenteric ischemia (Box 11-3). Ostial atherosclerotic lesions may actually be aortic rather than visceral arterial plaque. Bulky, calcified intraluminal aortic plaque ("coral reef aorta") may cause physical obstruction of the visceral artery orifices (see Fig. 10-21). Although atherosclerosis is often limited to the proximal few centimeters of the vessels, symptomatic distal occlusive disease also occurs.

Median arcuate ligament syndrome is a somewhat controversial variant of chronic mesenteric ischemia that tends to occur in young, thin, female patients. The celiac artery is compressed by the median arcuate ligament, but the SMA and IMA are usually normal (see Fig. 11-2). The symptoms are typical of those of other forms of

Box 11-3 Etiologies of Chronic Mesenteric Ischemia

Atherosclerosis
Dissection
Vasculitis
Median arcuate ligament syndrome
Fibromuscular dysplasia
Thoracoabdominal aneurysm
Iatrogenic
Abdominal aortic coarctation

chronic mesenteric ischemia, with postprandial pain and even weight loss. Hemodynamically it is hard to explain the symptoms on the basis of ischemia when the SMA collateral pathways are intact.

The noninvasive evaluation of patients with suspected chronic mesenteric ischemia should exclude other diagnoses (such as pancreatic, bowel, or biliary pathology) as well as detect abnormal flow in the visceral arteries. As noted earlier in this chapter, US is an excellent modality provided the appropriate expertise is available. Careful interrogation of the visceral arteries is necessary to identify potentially confusing variant anatomy. Elevated fasting velocities, or a less than 20% increase in the SMA peak systolic velocity after eating, are useful diagnostic tests and for follow-up of interventions. Both CTA and MRA provide exquisite anatomic information about the visceral artery origins (see Figs. 11-10 and 11-11). Conventional angiography remains essential for preintervention planning and potential catheter-based therapy. In addition to the standard views, pressure gradients should be measured across any suspicious lesions.

The traditional therapy for chronic mesenteric ischemia is surgery. Transaortic endarterectomy, aorta-visceral bypass, and ilio-visceral bypass are common operations for atherosclerotic lesions (see Fig. 11-10). Relief of symptoms improves as the number of vessels revascularized increases; surgical mortality is approximately 5%, and 5-year graft patency approaches 80%. Median arcuate ligament syndrome is treated with division of the overlying diaphragmatic crura and sympathectomy, as well as celiac artery reconstruction when necessary.

Percutaneous therapy of ostial and proximal celiac artery and SMA stenoses has been employed primarily in atherosclerotic lesions, but is also successful in non-atherosclerotic etiologics such as Takayasu's disease. Angioplasty is rarely sufficient for ostial lesions; stent placement is almost always required (Fig. 11-16). The approach to these lesions is an important determinant of technical success. In many instances a femoral access works well for selecting the vessel and positioning devices. When the vessel origin has a steep downward angle from the aorta, an axillary artery access (usually left) facilitates selection of the vessel and manipulation across the lesion. Long 6- to 7-French sheaths that extend into the abdominal aorta provide stability during the procedure and allow injection of contrast to monitor the intervention. Short stents (usually balloon expandable for ostial lesions) should be used to avoid crossing into potential future surgical fields. The long-term results of stent placement in the celiac artery and SMA are encouraging with low morbidity, but large patient series have not been collected.

Percutaneous therapy of median arcuate ligament syndrome is rarely durable, as the primary problem is

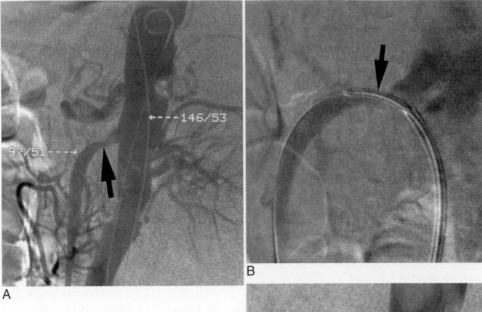

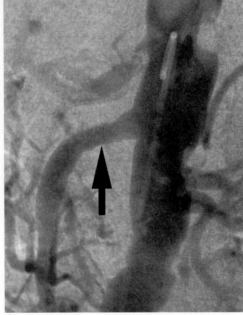

Figure 11-16 SMA stenosis treated with a stent in an elderly male with acute ischemic colitis in the splenic flexure during an episode of dehydration. The patient had a history of occasional postprandial abdominal pain after aortofemoral bypass graft for occlusive disease. **A,** Lateral DSA of the aorta showing a 60% proximal SMA stenosis (arrow) with a measured pressure gradient of 49 mmHg systolic. The celiac is not well visualized on this image but was severely stenotic, and the IMA was occluded. **B,** DSA during positioning of a balloon expandable stent (arrow) across the area of stenosis from a femoral approach. This was dilated to 7 mm. **C,** Lateral DSA of the aorta after stent placement. The gradient was 0 mmHg, and the angiographic appearance was excellent (arrow). The patient reported complete resolution of his postprandial pain.

extrinsic compression that is not addressed by an endovascular approach. Stent deformity or migration can occur owing to continuous extrinsic compression by the diaphragmatic crura.

GASTROINTESTINAL BLEEDING

Angiography for gastrointestinal (GI) bleeding was once a common study, often occurring at odd hours. Preventative pharmacologic therapy, endoscopic diagnosis and intervention, and improved medical interventions have vastly decreased the number of patients with this indication for angiography. However, the basic principles have not changed with time. When referred a patient with GI bleeding it is important to obtain several key pieces of clinical information (Box 11-4). This information determines the urgency, type, and sequence of diagnostic and therapeutic procedures. Be prepared to assume primary management responsibility for patients with GI bleeding, especially in the middle of the night.

Box 11-4 Key Clinical Information in Patients with Acute GI Bleeding

What orifices is the blood coming from?
Hemodynamically stable or unstable?
What resuscitative measures have been taken?
Nasogastric tube in place?
Has the patient been endoscoped?
Coagulopathy?
Prior gastrointestinal surgery?
What is treatment plan following localization of bleeding?
Foley catheter in place?

Box 11-5 Etiologies of Acute Upper GI Bleeding

Peptic ulcer
Gastritis
Portal hypertension (varices)
Mallory–Weiss tear
Marginal ulcer
Iatrogenic (post biopsy, percutaneous gastrostomy)
Arteriovenous malformation/angiodysplasia
Dieulafoy lesion
Tumor
Pseudoaneurysm
Hemobilia
Hemosuccous entericus
Pseudo-bleeding (swallowed blood from nasopharyngeal source)
Aortoenteric fistula

Acute GI Bleeding

Acute GI bleeding resolves spontaneously in 85% of patients. The first objective of management is therefore to stabilize the patient with fluid resuscitation, placement of large-bore venous lines, a Foley catheter in the urinary bladder, airway protection if necessary, and a nasogastric (NG) tube. Correction of deranged clotting studies should be performed aggressively, and transfusion of blood products should be initiated. Vital signs should be followed closely, and when there is continued evidence of bleeding, further diagnostic and therapeutic measures are indicated.

Localization of the source of the bleeding is critical, as it defines the therapeutic approach. By convention, the GI tract is divided by the Ligament of Treitz into upper and lower tracts. Bleeding is 5–8 times more common from the upper GI tract, typically from ulcers and gastritis. Lower GI bleeding is colonic in origin in 80% of patients, with one-third from the right colon, one-third from the transverse colon, and the remainder from the sigmoid colon and rectum. The most common etiology of colonic arterial bleeding in patients over age 50 is diverticulosis, followed by angiodysplasia (see Vascular Malformations below). In general, sources proximal to the Ligament of Treitz manifest clinically as hematemesis, and those more distal as melena or hematochezia. This is not a hard rule, and exceptions occur frequently. However, when the NG tube aspirate is positive for blood, an upper GI source is effectively ruled in (Boxes 11-5 and 11-6).

Patients with upper GI bleeding should undergo endoscopy as their initial diagnostic evaluation. A source can be identified in over 95%, and in many cases treated with electrocautery, injection sclerotherapy, or banding. Endoscopy in patients with lower GI bleeding is more difficult, particularly when bleeding is brisk (overall 70% success rate in identifying a bleeding source). Initial evaluation with a tagged red-blood cell (technetium[99m])

nuclear scan is helpful in these patients, as the study can detect bleeding at a rate of 0.1 mL/min. A higher rate of bleeding (0.5–1 mL/min) is required to visualize extravasation at angiography. The ability to localize bleeding to a particular segment of bowel can be as low as 50% with nuclear medicine examinations. In most centers, an angiogram is obtained following a positive bleeding scan unless localization is definitive. The likelihood of finding bleeding on an angiogram increases almost 10-fold when performed immediately after a positive bleeding scan

Box 11-6 Etiologies of Acute Lower GI Bleeding

Diverticulosis (most common etiology in older patients)
Hemorrhoids
Arteriovenous malformation/angiodysplasia
Post-endoscopic polypectomy (can occur as late as 14 days)
Inflammatory bowel disease (most common etiology in young adults)
Ischemic bowel
Portal hypertension (colonic, rectal, stomal varices)
Tumor
Vasculitis
Radiation colitis
Infection (especially immunocompromised host)
Small bowel/colonic ulcers
Aortoenteric and graft–enteric fistula
Meckel's diverticulum (children and young adults)

compared to angiograms obtained without prior positive bleeding scan. However, even in the best circumstances, angiograms are positive in only about 50% of patients. Contrast-enhanced multidetector row CT has promise as a noninvasive modality for diagnosis of GI bleeding, but is not yet widely used.

Angiography for acute GI bleeding should begin with selective injection of the vessel supplying the most likely source of bleeding based on all available clinical or historical data. The suspected level of bleeding within the GI tract determines which vessel to select: celiac artery for upper GI sources, IMA for sigmoid and rectum, SMA for small bowel and right colon. With occlusion of the IMA the SMA injection frequently suffices to evaluate the left colon and sigmoid. The anal verge must be included in the field of view on IMA injections. When bleeding is not identified on the first injection, selection of the next most likely artery is performed, and so on. A celiac injection should be included for lower GI bleeding when SMA and IMA injections are negative as the middle colic artery is replaced to the dorsal pancreatic artery in 1–2% of patients. Occasionally a hypogastric artery injection is necessary to exclude rectosigmoid bleeding when there is occlusion of the IMA.

Filming in GI bleeding studies should be rapid (3–6 frames/s) during the arterial phase, and then slower for the venous phase. Visualization of the portal phase is mandatory, as bleeding can be due to varices or mesenteric venous thrombosis. Intravenous glucagon decreases artifact from bowel gas on DSA examinations, an important source of artifacts. The use of CO_2 gas as a contrast agent has been reported to be extremely sensitive for depiction of GI bleeding. Flush aortography in patients with GI bleeding is rarely indicated.

The angiographic diagnosis of GI bleeding is based upon visualization of extravasation of contrast into the bowel lumen. The contrast should appear during the arterial phase, persist through the venous phase, and change with time (Fig. 11-17). False positives can be caused by preexisting barium in diverticula on cut-film examinations, bowel gas on DSA examinations, densely enhancing veins, hyperemic bowel due to inflammation, or adrenal blushes (Fig. 11-18). Digital images should be viewed in both subtracted and unsubtracted modes to confirm the diagnosis. Extravasated contrast pooling in the rugae of the stomach or the haustra of the bowel may look like a vein (the "pseudo-vein sign") (see Fig. 11-17). This "pseudo-vein" persists beyond the venous phase of the injection. False negative studies can result from injection of inadequate volumes of contrast, failure to include all of the injected vascular bed in the imaging field, and failure to select the appropriate arteries. Foley catheter drainage of the bladder improves visualization of the distal sigmoid and rectum.

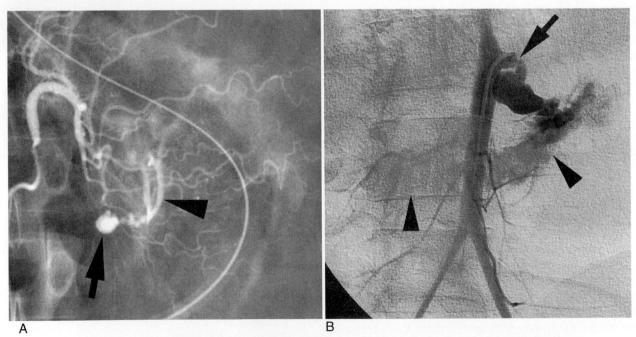

A   B

Figure 11-17   Angiographic demonstration of gastrointestinal bleeding. **A**, Selective left gastric angiogram showing bleeding of an antral ulcer (arrow) and tracking of contrast in the gastric rugae (the "pseudo vein sign") (arrowhead). **B**, Selective DSA of an aortoenteric fistula (arrow) showing opacification of the small bowel (arrowheads) in a patient with a necrotic retroperitoneal germ cell tumor and massive lower GI bleeding. (Image courtesy of Robert Sheley M.D. and Oliver Ochs M.D., Good Samaritan Hospital, Portland, OR.)

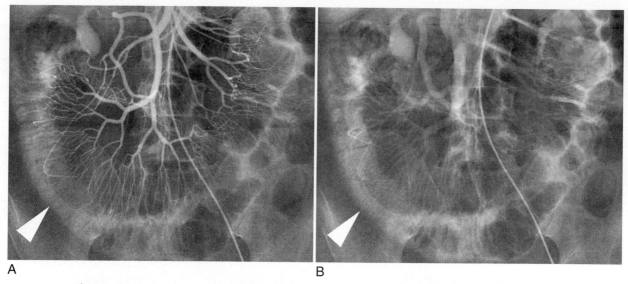

A   B

Figure 11-18   Crohn's disease. Inflammatory bowel diseases are common causes of lower GI bleeding in children and young adults. **A**, SMA angiogram showing splaying of the mesenteric arcades and hyperemic ileum (arrowhead). **B**, Portal venous phase from the same patient. There is no extravasation, but the small bowel remains densely staining (arrowhead) owing to inflammatory changes.

The therapy of GI bleeding depends upon the etiology and location. The management of variceal bleeding is discussed in Chapter 14. Cautery of upper GI peptic ulcers, vascular malformations, and angiodysplasias is effective in 85%, with the highest success rates reported for gastric lesions. Duodenal ulcers can be difficult to reach with an endoscope. Surgical therapy is required in only 2–5% of cases.

Catheter-based techniques for control of arterial GI bleeding are highly effective, safe, and rapid. The two basic techniques used for arterial bleeding are vasopressin infusion and embolization (Tables 11-4, 11-5 and 11-6).

Vasopressin (pitressin) is an anterior pituitary hormone that causes both smooth muscle constriction and water retention. Infused into the proximal SMA or IMA, it can control acute diverticular bleeding, post-polypectomy, and mucosal bleeding in up to 90% of cases, and half of the patients will never bleed again (Fig. 11-19). Vasopressin should not be used for patients with bleeding due to pseudoaneurysms, ischemic bowel, or arteriovenous malformations. Patients experience initial abdominal cramping due to smooth muscle constriction in the bowel, often accompanied by evacuation of any

Table 11-4	Intraarterial Vasopressin Therapy
Indications	Colonic and small bowel bleeding
Contraindications	Active myocardial ischemia, limb ischemia, bowel ischemia, uncooperative patient
Catheter location	Proximal SMA or IMA
Infusion	0.2–0.4 units/min
Protocol	Initiate at 0.2 unit/min; re-angio at 20–30 minutes to confirm cessation of bleeding; increase by 0.1 unit/min until bleeding controlled or maximum dose (0.4 units/min); infuse for 24 h; taper to normal saline over 12–24 h; pull catheter after 6–12 h no bleeding
Patient activity	Strict bedrest
Patient diet	Nil by mouth
Laboratory tests	Complete blood count and electrolytes every 12 hours
Troubleshooting	Is catheter still connected to pump? Is there a kink in the tubing? What is current dose? Has catheter become dislodged (check plain film or angio)

Table 11-5	Gastric/Duodenal Embolization for GI Bleeding
Indications	Ulcer, gastritis, Mallory–Weiss tear, pseudoaneurysm
Contraindication	Unidentified source of bleeding, inability to select artery
Catheter location	
Fundal bleed/gastroesophageal junction	Left gastric artery
Duodenal bleed	Gastroduodenal artery/inferior pancreatico-duodenal trunk
Preferred agents	Gelfoam pledgets, particles (500–900 μm), coils

Table 11-6	Colonic Embolization for GI Bleeding
Indication	Bleeding uncontrolled by vasopressin; bleeding not amenable to vasopressin therapy
Contraindications	Unidentified source of bleeding; ischemic bowel; inability to super-select bleeding artery
Catheter location	As close to bleeding site as possible
Preferred agents	Microcoils, Gelfoam pledgets

blood in the bowel. This should not be mistaken for continued bleeding. Although very effective, vasopressin therapy requires monitoring in an intensive care unit. Rare complications include cardiac or digital ischemia from vasoconstriction, or hyponatremia from water retention. Vasopressin can also be used for bleeding from gastritis, although embolization of the left gastric artery is preferred by most angiographers. Duodenal bleeding responds poorly to vasopressin because of the dual blood supply (celiac artery and SMA).

Embolization is commonly used for control of GI bleeding owing to the rapid and definitive results. The basic objective of embolization in GI bleeding is to decrease arterial pressure and flow to the point that hemostasis can occur, without creating symptomatic ischemia. In general, large particles, pieces of Gelfoam, or microcoils are used. The specific approach to embolization in the GI tract varies with the site of bleeding and the pathology. The rich collateral supply of the stomach allows embolization

with relative impunity. Although identification of a bleeding source prior to embolization is the rule, the left gastric artery can be embolized empirically in patients with endoscopically proven fundal or gastroesophageal junction lesions (Fig. 11-20). Conversely, bowel bleeding should only be embolized after super-selective catheterization confirms the precise site of extravasation, as there is a small risk of bowel infarction (Fig. 11-21). The duodenum represents a special situation, in that blood supply is from both the celiac artery and SMA. Following embolization, injections of both arteries should be performed to confirm control of bleeding.

Particulate embolic agents sized to occlude the target vessel are preferred in the gastrointestinal tract. In the left gastric artery, small Gelfoam cubes or large particles (up to 700–900 μm) are injected until stasis occurs. In duodenal bleeding a discrete feeding vessel may be identified which can be occluded with a coil. When necessary the gastroduodenal artery can be occluded with coils, although retrograde perfusion from the epiploic arteries is likely to occur. Bowel bleeding should always be embolized from the most selective position possible. If a super-selective position with a coaxial microcatheter cannot be achieved and operative therapy is indicated, the catheter can be left in position and methylene blue injected at the time of resection to outline the segment of bowel responsible for the bleeding. Alternatively, a coil can be placed as close as possible to the bleeding site which the surgeon can locate intraoperatively by palpation or transillumination of the mesentery.

Embolization is successful in over 90% of cases, with few instances of bowel ischemia. Rebleeding is reported to occur in 20% of patients. Great care to avoid nontarget

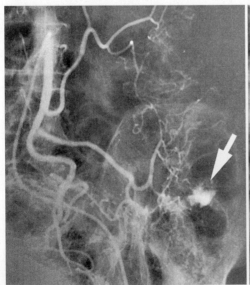
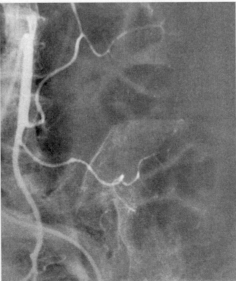

A   B

Figure 11-19 Management of lower GI bleeding with pitressin infusion. **A**, IMA angiogram showing extravasation (arrow) from a diverticulum. **B**, Repeat IMA angiogram after infusion of pitressin 0.2 U/min for 30 minutes shows typical vasoconstriction and cessation of bleeding. The patient was maintained on pitressin for 24 hours, then slowly weaned with no recurrence of bleeding.

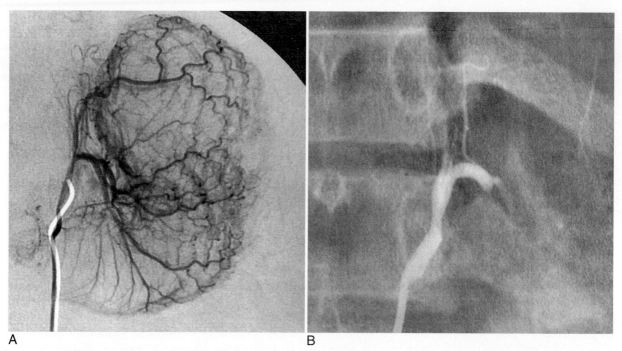

Figure 11-20   Embolization of left gastric artery with Gelfoam pledgets in a patient with diffuse fundal abnormality on endoscopy. **A**, Left gastric artery DSA showing hyperemic gastric fundus distended with thrombus but no extravasation. **B**, Injection in the left gastric artery following embolization with Gelfoam, showing truncation of the branches.

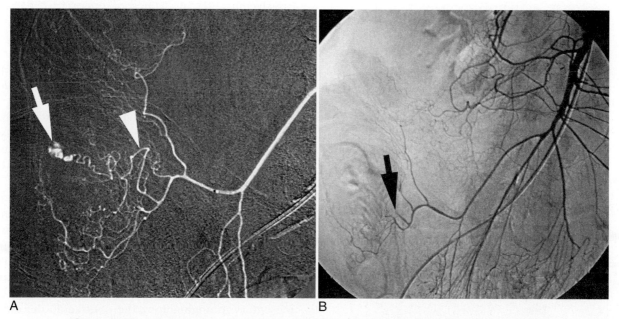

Figure 11-21   Embolization of colonic bleeding. **A**, Super-selective right colic angiogram through a microcatheter shows extravasation of contrast (arrow). The catheter was advanced into the small branch indicated by the arrowhead. Embolization was performed in this case with a few Ivalon particles, 500 μm in diameter. **B**, Completion SMA angiogram shows occlusion of the right colic branch (arrow) and cessation of bleeding. The patient had no further bleeding and no complications.

organ embolization is required. Patients undergoing bowel embolization should be monitored closely for evidence of ischemia. Delayed ischemic colonic strictures have been reported.

Chronic GI Bleeding

There are numerous causes of chronic GI bleeding (Box 11-7). Chronic GI blood loss can be characterized as occult or overt. Occult bleeding tends to be due to colonic malignancies, polyps, and small arteriovenous malformations, as well as gastroduodenal peptic disease. Chronic overt bleeding can be due to diverticulosis, pseudoaneurysms, and portal hypertension. Graft–enteric

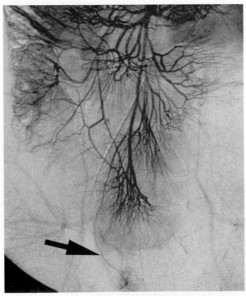

Figure 11-22 Demonstration of Meckel's diverticulum on selective DSA of the SMA. A characteristic Vitelline artery is seen (arrow) extending beyond the border of the normal ileum.

erosions should be considered in patients with prior abdominal aortic surgery and chronic GI bleeding of unknown etiology. Patients with chronic stomal bleeding and negative endoscopic examinations should be evaluated for occult portal hypertension and stomal varices (see Fig. 14-8).

Overall, failure to identify a bleeding source occurs in fewer than 5% of patients with chronic GI bleeding. The majority of lesions in these patients are colonic in origin. The evaluation includes upper and lower endoscopy, complete GI radiography, and nuclear medicine bleeding scans (including a Meckel's scan in young patients). The small bowel is the most difficult area to evaluate with these modalities.

A small percentage of patients will be referred for diagnostic angiography. Angiographic evaluation should be obtained only when all other studies are negative. Complete visceral angiography, with magnification views, should be performed. The lesions most often encountered are arteriovenous malformations and leiomyomas. Leiomyomas are discussed in the next section. Meckel's diverticula have a characteristic arterial supply, the Vitelline artery (Fig. 11-22). Treatment of most etiologies of chronic GI bleeding is surgical.

NEOPLASM

Bowel

Neoplasms of the bowel are usually diagnosed by noninvasive imaging modalities or endoscopy. Rarely, the diagnosis is made at angiography during work-up for GI bleeding. The most common lesion found angiographically is a small bowel leiomyoma or leiomyosarcoma (Fig. 11-23). Leiomyomas are found throughout the bowel; within the small bowel, the distribution of benign lesions is uniform, whereas malignant lesions are found more commonly in the ileum. Bleeding is usually due to erosion of overlying mucosa. Tumors may also be intramural or serosal. The angiographic appearance is distinctive – a densely staining vascular mass that persists through the venous phase.

Carcinoid tumors of the bowel have a unique angiographic appearance, but are rarely diagnosed in this manner. Slow-growing tumors arising from enterochromaffin cells, 20% of carcinoid tumors are found in the small bowel, of which 90% are located in the ileum. Although the actual lesion is usually small, the associated dense fibrotic response results in retraction of the mesentery. At angiography, the contractile deformity of the mesenteric arterial and venous structures is characteristic (Fig. 11-24). Carcinoid tumors release serotonin, which is metabolized by the liver unless metastases are present. The characteristic symptoms of flushing, hypertension, and diarrhea are indicative of liver metastases.

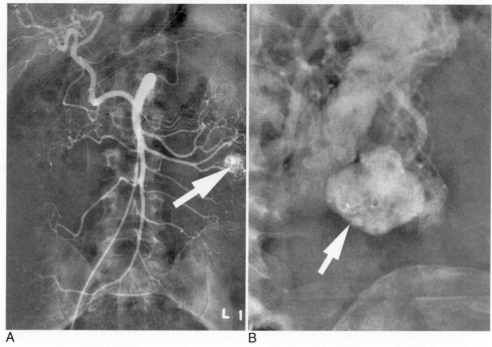

Figure 11-23 Angiographic appearance of small bowel leiomyoma in a patient with chronic lower GI bleeding. **A**, Selective SMA angiogram showing a densely staining mass in the left abdomen (arrow). Incidentally, the patient has a replaced right hepatic artery. **B**, Magnification view of the mass in the portal venous phase shows the persistent dense parenchymal stain (arrow) characteristic of leiomyomatous lesions.

A   B

Pancreas

Pancreatic neoplasms are almost always diagnosed and staged by CT, US, or MRI. The most common lesions are adenocarcinomas, although a variety of other primary and metastatic lesions can involve the pancreas. In selected instances, angiography is utilized to define preoperative anatomy, or to localize a small vascular lesion.

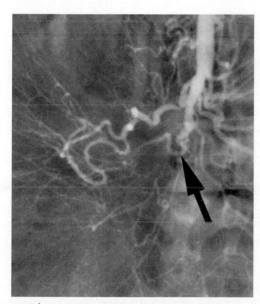

Figure 11-24 Selective SMA angiogram showing contraction of the mesentery and arterial occlusions (arrow) characteristic of fibrosis due to carcinoid.

Resectability of adenocarcinoma of the head of the pancreas is determined partially by the degree of vascular involvement, particularly the portal vein, hepatic artery, and SMA. Venous encasement is manifested by narrowing of the portal vein confluence in the region of the mass (see Figs. 1-26C,D). Occlusion and venous thrombosis can occur. Arterial encasement of the hepatic, splenic, or superior mesenteric artery is almost always a late finding, indicating an unresectable lesion. Thin-slice CT can supplant conventional angiography in most patients.

Islet cell tumors of the pancreas may be functioning (hormonally active) or nonfunctional. All islet cell tumors are slow-growing, so that malignancy is determined by the presence of local invasion and metastases. Patients are younger than those with adenocarcinoma (median age 53), with a better prognosis (up to 80% survival at 10 years for benign tumors). The most common functioning tumors are insulinomas, gastrinomas, and glucagonomas.

Large islet cell tumors are readily diagnosed by CT, MR, and US. Localization of small functioning lesions can be difficult. Thin-slice contrast-enhanced CT of the pancreas has been used very successfully to identify small lesions, which appear as densely enhancing masses. Intraoperative US is also used to confirm that presence of a lesion prior to resection. Islet cell tumors are usually hypervascular masses, but angiography is rarely required to localize lesions (Fig. 11-25).

Occult functioning islet cell tumors (insulinoma and gastrinoma) can be localized by sampling of the hepatic veins following selective arterial injections of a secretagogue. A catheter is placed selectively in the right

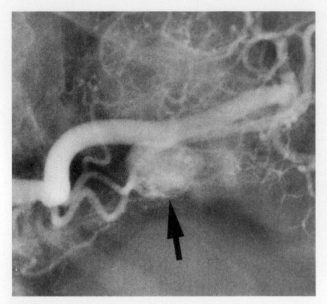

Figure 11-25 Typical hypervascular angiographic appearance of an islet cell tumor (arrow) in the body of the pancreas (in this case, insulinoma).

hepatic vein through a sheath in a peripheral vein. An arterial catheter is then used to select the gastroduodenal, splenic, SMA, and finally the proper hepatic arteries in sequence. Hepatic and peripheral venous blood is sampled after injection of an appropriate secretagogue into each artery (Table 11-7). An angiogram is obtained in each position as well. A rise in the hepatic vein concentration of the hormone after injection of the secretagogue helps to localize angiographically occult lesions to the head, body, or tail of the pancreas. The proper hepatic injection and angiogram is performed to exclude the presence of hepatic metastases.

Hepatic Neoplasms

Malignant

The most common hepatic malignancy in the United States is metastatic colon cancer. Almost 10% of all cancer deaths in this country are due to metastatic adenocarcinoma of the colon. In many parts of the world,

Table 11-7	Functioning Pancreatic Islet Cell Tumors	
Hormone	**Arterial Stimulant for Venous Sampling**
Insulin	Calcium chloride
Gastrin	Secretin

particularly Asian countries, hepatoma is the predominant hepatic malignancy. The major risk factors for hepatoma are chronic liver diseases such as cirrhosis and certain forms of hepatitis. One subtype, fibrolamellar hepatoma, occurs in younger patients with no apparent risk factors. Conventional angiography has a limited role in the diagnosis and staging of hepatic malignancy. CT, US, and MRI are excellent modalities for imaging liver tumors. Conventional angiography is used by some surgeons to define hepatic arterial anatomy prior to resection of tumors, although CTA and MRA can provide sufficient information in most cases.

The angiographic appearance of liver tumors depends on the vascularity of the lesion (Table 11-8). Hypovascular lesions can cause mass effect on adjacent vascular structures, defects in the parenchymal phase of the angiogram, or vascular encasement (Fig. 11-26). Vascular lesions may exhibit neovascularity, staining, shunting, and mass effect (Fig. 11-27). Arteriovenous shunting to the portal or hepatic veins, or the presence of tumor thrombus in the portal or hepatic veins, are highly suggestive of hepatoma (see Fig. 1-26B).

Although the diagnostic role of angiography in hepatic malignancy is limited, the therapeutic potential is great. Most primary and metastatic liver tumors derive the majority of their blood supply from the hepatic arteries. The dual nature of the hepatic blood supply allows arterial embolization to be performed safely. Furthermore, the direct delivery of a chemotherapeutic agent into the hepatic artery achieves a higher liver dose than could be administered peripherally.

Chemotherapeutic agents can be delivered as an infusion over several days or in larger single doses mixed with an embolic agent. Chemoinfusion is of uncertain value for patients with metastatic colon cancer, and rarely used for hepatomas. Arterial chemoembolization has been used most successfully to control hypervascular lesions such as hepatoma, metastatic carcinoid, metastatic ocular melanoma, and metastatic islet cell tumors. Although chemoembolization has been reported as curative in small hepatomas, this modality is usually considered an adjunct to surgery or a palliative measure, particularly for metastatic lesions.

Patients referred for hepatic chemoembolization should be evaluated for liver function (including coagulation studies), patency of the portal vein, portal hypertension, the presence of biliary obstruction, or malignant ascites. Hepatic failure or the presence of active liver infection are absolute contraindications to the procedure, as damage to some normal hepatic tissue is inevitable. Patients with indwelling biliary tubes or biliary obstruction are at increased risk of postembolization liver abscess. An occluded portal vein is considered a relative contraindication, as embolization of the hepatic artery could result in liver infarction. Patients should

Table 11-8   Angiographic Appearance of Malignant Liver Masses

Tumor	Vascularity	Angiographic Findings
Hepatoma	Vascular	Solitary or multifocal; neovascularity, parenchymal stain, arteriovenous shunting; hepatic and portal thrombus
Cholangiocarcinoma	Avascular	Venous and arterial encasement in porta hepatis
Metastatic adenocarcinoma (colon, pancreas, lung, etc.)	Avascular	Multiple; hypovascular area in parenchymal phase of angiogram; mass effect on adjacent blood vessels with large lesions; may have faint hypervascular rim with avascular center
Metastatic sarcoma, endocrine tumors, islet cell tumors, melanoma, renal cell carcinoma	Vascular	Multiple lesions; neovascularity, dense parenchymal stain; arteriovenous shunting unusual; portal and hepatic venous thrombus rare

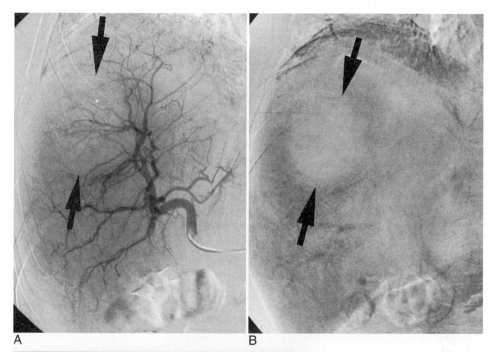

A   B

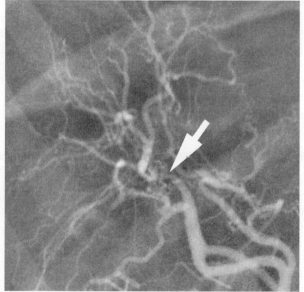

C

Figure 11-26   Angiographic appearance of two different avascular malignant lesions in the liver. **A**, Metastatic colon carcinoma: selective right hepatic DSA showing an area of hypovascularity (arrows) with splaying of surrounding vessels. **B**, Parenchymal phase from the same injection shows the hypovascular metastasis (arrows) with slight surrounding hyperemia believed to represent compressed normal liver tissue. **C**, Klatskin's tumor: selective hepatic angiogram showing arterial encasement (arrow) but no hypervascularity. (See Fig. 14-30 for an example of portal vein encasement in the same patient.)

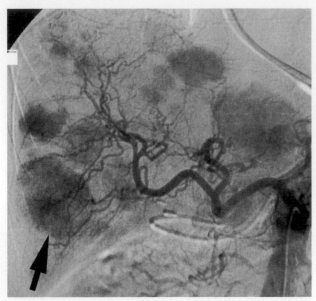

Figure 11-27 Angiographic appearance of hypervascular liver malignancy. Hepatic DSA, late arterial phase, in a patient with metastatic carcinoid (arrow). There are multiple lesions in the liver.

receive antibiotics (Gram-negative coverage), steroids, and antiemetics prior to the procedure.

There is no consensus on the best chemotherapeutic regimen or the best embolic agent. Drugs and dosages vary among institutions. At the Dotter Institute, Doxorubicin (50 mg) is used for hepatomas, and a combination of drugs (Cisplatinum (100 mg), mitomycin C (30 mg), and doxorubicin (30 mg)) are used for all other lesions. These agents are mixed with nonionic contrast and ethiodol for the embolization. Iodized oil is an excellent embolic agent for hepatoma, as it is selectively retained by the tumor cells (see Fig. 4-38). Gelfoam powder and small Ivalon particles (50–200 μm) may also used either in combination with or as a substitute for iodized oil. There is evidence that small particulate embolic agents alone are sufficient for metastatic neuroendocrine tumors. Yttrium[90]-loaded microspheres show promise as a beta-radiation emitting embolic agent for both hepatocellular carcinoma and metastatic adenocarcinoma. Scrupulous and gentle technique is necessary to avoid trauma to the access arteries, as arterial chemoembolization must be repeated several times for maximum benefit to the patient (Table 11-9).

Arterial chemoembolization can prolong life in patients with hepatoma and vascular metastases, with some centers reporting 1-year survival of 90%. The results with metastatic colon carcinoma are less encouraging using conventional chemotherapeutic agents, but are improved with Yttrium[90]-loaded microspheres. The symptoms caused by metastatic carcinoid tumor to the liver can be controlled with hepatic embolization in more than 90% of patients.

Table 11-9	Chemoembolization Technique
Preliminary angiography	Selective celiac artery and SMA with portal phase
Catheter placement	Proper hepatic (distal to gastroduodenal) or more selective; may need to select replaced hepatic arteries
Catheters	Coaxial microcatheter or 4-Fr hydrophilic catheter (minimizes spasm, risk of dissection); 5-Fr catheter used occasionally
Medications	Antibiotics for Gram-negative coverage; steroids; antiemetics; ± intraarterial heparin and nitroglycerin
Preparation of chemotherapy	Mix with nonionic contrast; transfer to sterile 10-mL syringe; emulsify with oil or particles using 3-way stopcock and additional syringe; judge volume of oil or particles by vascularity of lesion (typical total volume of combined embolic agents 10–15 mL) When using oil, will need metal stopcock
Delivery	1-mL aliquots using Luer-lock syringe
Endpoints	Sluggish flow in target hepatic artery
Special precautions	Face shields for operators and assistants Special disposal of syringes/catheters contaminated with chemotherapeutic agent

Fulminant hepatic failure or liver abcess formation occurs in fewer than 1% of patients undergoing chemoembolization. Nausea, abdominal pain, post-embolization syndrome, and measurable transient increases in liver enzymes are common. Risk factors for infection include biliary obstruction, indwelling biliary stents, and internal-to-external biliary catheters. Gallbladder infarction due to chemoembolization is rare.

Benign

A wide range of benign lesions are found in the liver (Box 11-8). As with malignant liver lesions, CT, MRI, and

---

Box 11-8   Benign Liver Masses

Simple cyst
Hemangioma
Adenoma
Focal nodular hyperplasia
Regenerating nodule
Abscess

US are usually diagnostic. Several of these lesions have characteristic angiographic appearances, but this modality is rarely necessary for diagnosis.

Hepatic cysts are present in at least 5% of individuals. Usually asymptomatic, they are avascular at angiography but may cause displacement of arterial and venous structures.

Hemangiomas are found in 7–20% of the adult population, more often in women than men, with a preponderance in the right lobe of the liver. Hemangiomas can vary in size and number. These lesions comprise large blood-filled spaces with little stromal tissue. Asymptomatic in the majority of patients, large hemangiomas can bleed spontaneously or cause mass effect. The angiographic appearance of hepatic hemangiomas is perhaps the most distinctive of all hepatic lesions: normal feeding arteries, with early pooling of contrast that increases and persists with time ("comes early and stays late") (Fig. 11-28).

Infantile hemangioendothelioma, though rare, is the most common benign hepatic tumor in infants. More frequent in females, patients present with hepatomegaly and high-output congestive heart failure in up to two-thirds of cases. The lesions are histologically benign; biopsy is not necessary unless the first appearance is after 1 year of age or atypical on imaging studies. Although lesions respond to steroids and alpha-interferon, embolization or surgical resection may be required. At angiography, recruitment of collateral arterial supply from phrenic, intercostal, abdominal wall, splenic, superior mesenteric, and renal arteries may be found (Fig. 11-29). Embolization with Gelfoam

pledgets or cyanoacrylate glue is frequently curative. Small particles should be avoided owing to shunting through the mass.

Hepatic adenomas are well-circumscribed encapsulated masses comprised of hepatocytes. These lesions are found in women of childbearing age, and are associated with oral contraceptive use. Spontaneous rupture with intraperitoneal bleeding can occur, particularly during pregnancy. The angiographic findings are a sharply defined hypervascular mass with enlarged feeding vessels (Fig. 11-30). This appearance is not unique, and hepatoma should be considered in the differential diagnosis.

Focal nodular hyperplasia is usually a solitary mass of hepatocytes, Kupfer cells, bile ducts, and connective tissue. Found most often in young women, the lesions are usually asymptomatic, with little propensity for bleeding or rupture. A hypervascular mass with a central scar ("spoke-wheel") is a characteristic imaging finding on CT, MR, and angiography (Fig. 11-31).

Hepatic abscesses can have a hypervascular rim of compressed and inflamed normal tissue surrounding a hypovascular center. Diagnosis by angiography is unusual.

Although not a focal mass lesion, peliosis hepatis is considered in this section as it is a benign condition with a distinctive angiographic appearance. Peliosis consists of cystic dilatations of the hepatic sinusoids that communicate with innumerable 1- to 3-mm diameter blood-filled spaces throughout the hepatic parenchyma. The cause is unknown, though associated with certain medications (steroids, oral contraceptive, tamoxifen) as well as AIDS, and the clinical course is usually benign.

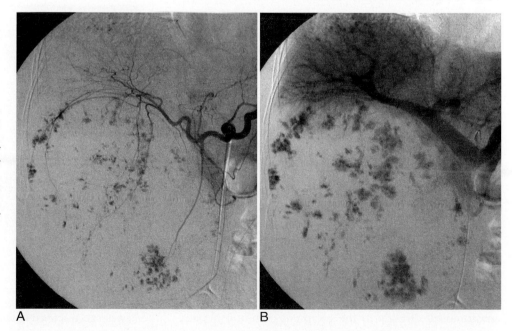

Figure 11-28   Giant hepatic cavernous hemangioma in a middle-aged woman. **A,** Celiac DSA showing a large liver mass with absence of neovascularity but multiple areas of fluffy staining. **B,** Image from the portal phase showing progressive increase in enhancement ("comes early, stays late") pathognomonic of cavernous hemangiomas.

A   B

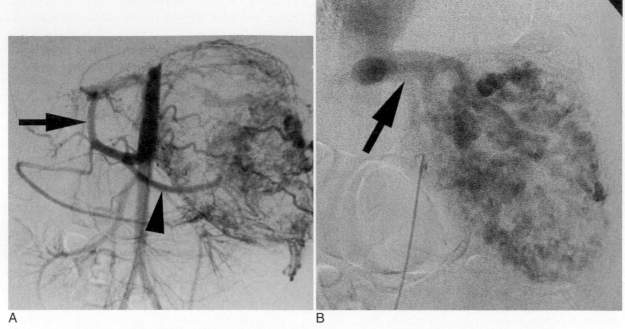

Figure 11-29 Infantile hepatic hemangioendothelioma causing high-output congestive heart failure in a week-old female. **A,** DSA aortogram showing a large shunting hypervascular mass supplied by the left hepatic artery (arrow), splenic artery (arrowhead), as well as numerous other collaterals. **B,** Later image from the same injection showing drainage through the left hepatic vein (arrow).

Complications such as portal hypertension and rupture have been reported. A distinctive diffuse patchy appearance of the liver parenchyma at angiography is produced by the lacunar spaces in the liver (Fig. 11-32).

LIVER TRANSPLANTATION

Liver transplantation is a curative procedure for patients with end-stage liver disease and small hepatomas (no more than three tumors, none greater than 3 cm in diameter). Current 5-year survival exceeds 50%, although the complication rates continue to be high.

The preoperative vascular imaging goals are largely directed at confirming vascular anatomy and patency of the hepatic arteries, the portal veins, and the inferior vena cava (IVC). In addition, a careful search for hepatic and extrahepatic malignancy is necessary. This work-up rarely requires conventional angiography, as US, CTA, and MRA can usually provide all required information. Once restricted to evaluation of recipients, the same evaluation is now applied to living related donors when available.

Imaging of the patient after liver transplant requires knowledge of the vascular anastomoses created during the transplant. Review of the surgical record or a conversation with the surgeon is the best way to get this information. For example, the donor celiac artery may be anastomosed directly to the recipient common hepatic

artery, or to the aorta. Portal vein and IVC anastomoses are usually end-to-end.

Vascular complications occur in 5–15% of liver transplants (Box 11-9). The presentation may be liver failure, breakdown of biliary anastomoses, or nonspecific. Duplex US is the primary modality used to evaluate the

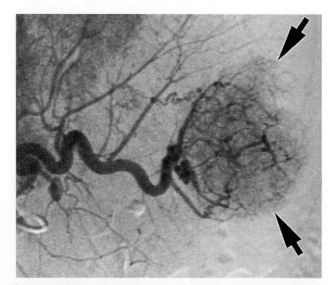

Figure 11-30 Hepatic DSA of proven hepatic adenoma (arrows) in the left lobe of the liver in a woman taking birth control pills. There is neovascularity and parenchymal staining of a well circumscribed lesion.

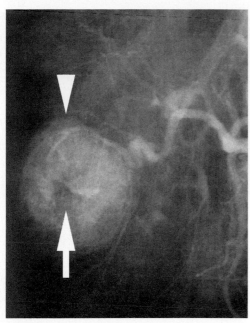

Figure 11-31   Hepatic angiogram of proven focal nodular hyperplasia (FNH) (arrowhead) showing the characteristic central scar (arrow).

treated with angioplasty and stent placement (Fig. 11-33). Thrombosis of a transplant artery can be treated with thrombolysis (Fig. 11-34).

In addition to arterial abnormalities, stenosis and thrombosis can occur in the portal vein, hepatic veins, and the IVC (see Chapters 13 and 14).

vasculature of the transplanted liver. Absence of flow in the hepatic artery, a waveform with slow or absent systolic upslope, or focal high velocity suggests stenotic complications. Anastomotic arterial pseudoaneurysms occur in 1–2% of patients. Angiography should be obtained to confirm and localize abnormalities detected by US. Transplant hepatic artery stenoses can be successfully

TRAUMA

Liver

Hepatic vascular trauma can result from penetrating or blunt injury. An important etiology is iatrogenic injury resulting from biopsies or interventional radiologic procedures. A classification system has been devised to describe the overall degree of hepatic injury (Table 11-10).

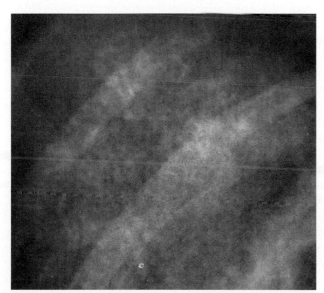

Figure 11-32   Angiogram showing peliosis hepatis in young woman taking birth control pills. There are innumerable small areas of hypervascularity throughout the right lobe of the liver.

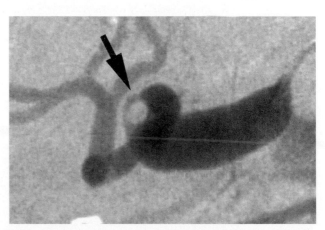

Figure 11-33   Stenosis of transplant hepatic artery. Selective hepatic artery DSA in a transplant patient with new onset of hepatic dysfunction showing a severe stenosis (arrow) in a tortuous segment of artery. This had minimal improvement with angioplasty and was successfully treated with a stent.

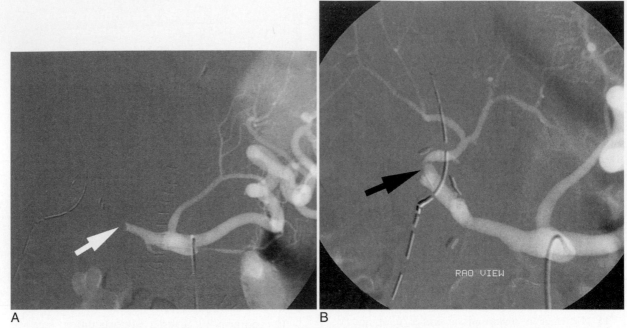

A   B

Figure 11-34   Thrombosis of a transplant hepatic artery treated with thrombolysis. **A**, Celiac DSA showing abrupt occlusion of the hepatic artery (arrow). **B**, Following thrombolysis with 500,000 U urokinase over 2 hours the hepatic artery is now patent with a visible kink (arrow).

Table 11-10	Liver Injury Scale of the American Association for the Surgery of Trauma
Grade	**Injury Description**
I	
Hematoma	Subcapsular, ≤10% surface area
Laceration	Capsular tear, ≤1 cm parenchymal depth
II	
Hematoma	Subcapsular, 10–50% surface area
	Intraparenchymal, ≤10 cm diameter
Laceration	1–3 cm parenchymal depth, ≤10 cm length
III	
Hematoma	Subcapsular, ≥50% surface area or expanding
	Ruptured subcapsular or parenchymal hematoma
	Intraparenchymal hematoma ≥10 cm or expanding
Laceration	>3 cm parenchymal depth
IV	
Laceration	Parenchymal disruption of 25–75% of hepatic lobe or 1 or 2 Couinard's segments within a single lobe
V	
Laceration	Parenchymal disruption of >75% of hepatic lobe or 3 Couinard's segments within a single lobe
Vascular	Juxtahepatic venous injuries (i.e., inferior vena cava or central hepatic veins)
VI	
Vascular	Hepatic avulsion

The overall mortality from liver trauma is approximately 10%. High-grade injury carries a mortality that exceeds 50% owing to hepatic vascular trauma and injury to other organs. The imaging modality most often used to evaluate patients with abdominal trauma is CT. Conventional angiography is rarely obtained for diagnosis, but often for therapy.

Hepatic vascular trauma can present as intraperitoneal bleeding, subcapsular hematoma, arteriovenous (hepatic or portal) fistula, hemobilia, pseudoaneurysm, and thrombosis (Figs. 11-35 and 11-36). Patients with known liver injury and persistent bleeding should undergo angiography with the intent to perform embolization. A thorough diagnostic angiogram should be performed, including as a minimum celiac artery, proper hepatic artery, and SMA injections with rapid initial filming and slower filming through the portal phase. Identification of the origin of the bleeding site may require super-selective injections in multiple projections. When evaluating a patient bleeding from a biliary drainage tube, it may be necessary to retract the tube briefly over a guidewire to unmask the injured vessel (Fig. 11-37). It is *critical* to leave the guidewire in place during diagnostic angiography, as reinsertion of the tube is the best means of acutely controlling bleeding.

The liver is rich in intrahepatic arterial collaterals. This is a critical concept when embolizing hepatic arterial lesions, as proximal occlusion may result in persistent bleeding from retrograde perfusion of the injury.

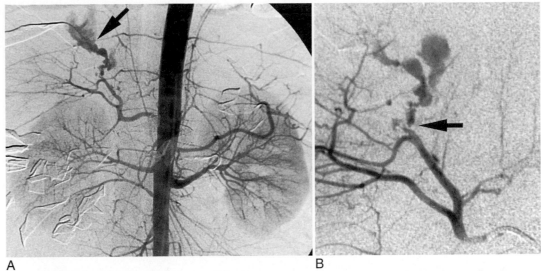

A   B

Figure 11-35   Arterial bleeding from traumatic laceration of the liver. The patient went directly from the emergency room to the operating room, but bleeding was uncontrollable. The patient was brought to angiography hypotensive with blood pouring from an open abdominal incision. **A**, DSA aortogram showing massive extravasation (arrow) in the right upper quadrant. The aortogram was obtained in this trauma patient because of the absence of any prior imaging. Note the generalized vasoconstriction of the visceral and renal arteries consistent with shock. **B**, Selective hepatic DSA showing extravasation from a right hepatic arterial transection (arrow). The objective of embolization in this setting is rapid control of bleeding to save the patient's life. This was successfully accomplished with coils and Gelfoam plugs.

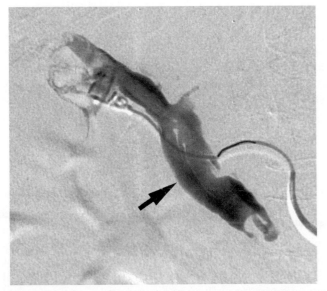

Figure 11-36   Patient with sudden onset of GI bleeding and right upper quadrant pain several months after hepatic laceration due to blunt trauma. Super-selective DSA of a branch of the right hepatic artery through a microcatheter shows opacification of the common bile duct (arrow).

Whenever possible, the artery on both sides of the abnormality should be occluded. Coils can be used for selective embolization, but particles may be necessary when injury is diffuse or selection is not possible owing to complex anatomy. The presence of a patent portal vein reduces the risk of liver infarction.

Spleen

The primary clinical manifestations of splenic injury are vascular (hemorrhage or infarction). Organ malfunction is not a clinical concern. Many splenic injuries can be managed conservatively with close observation, thus preserving the spleen and avoiding a laparotomy. This strategy is of particular importance in children, in whom the immunologic properties of splenic tissue are most desirable. A grading system has been devised to describe the extent of splenic injury to help determine management (Table 11-11). Grade I and II lesions are usually managed conservatively, although delayed rupture can occur in up to one-third of patients. More severely injured spleens usually require intervention owing to hemodynamic instability of the patient or ongoing bleeding.

The conventional treatment of severe splenic injury is splenectomy. Embolization is an alternative in patients with an injured but viable spleen (Fig. 11-38). The optimal technique has not been determined, but both

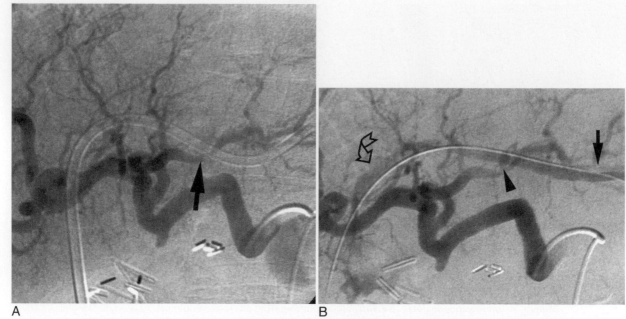

A   B

Figure 11-37   Patient with remote liver transplant and a left-sided biliary drainage tube and brisk, pulsatile bleeding from the tract during a routine catheter change. **A**, Hepatic DSA with the tube in place showing slight narrowing of the left hepatic artery (arrow), but no active extravasation. The gastroduodenal artery was ligated during the transplant surgery. **B**, Repeat DSA after removal of the tube *over a guidewire* showing a pseudoaneurysm (arrowhead), with extravasation into the bile ducts (curved arrow) and the parenchymal track of the tube (arrow). Coils were placed in the left hepatic artery on both sides of the pseudoaneurysm. The patient has since undergone numerous uneventful tube changes.

Table 11-11	Spleen Injury Scale of the American Association for the Surgery of Trauma

Grade	Injury Description
I	
Hematoma	Subcapsular, <10% surface area
Laceration	Capsular tear, <1 cm parenchymal depth
II	
Hematoma	Subcapsular, 10–50% surface area
	Intraparenchymal <5 cm diameter
Laceration	1–3 cm parenchymal depth not involving trabecular vessel
III	
Hematoma	Subcapsular >50% surface area or expanding
	Ruptured subcapsular or parenchymal hematoma
	Intraparenchymal hematoma >5 cm or expanding
Laceration	>3 cm parenchymal depth or involving trabecular vessels
IV	
Laceration	Laceration involving segmental or hilar vessels producing major devascularization (>25% of spleen)
V	
Laceration	Completely shattered spleen
Vascular	Hilar vascular injury which devascularizes the spleen

selective occlusion of sites of obvious vascular injury or proximal occlusion of the main splenic artery with coils have both been described. Theoretically, selective embolization addresses the point of injury, but risks focal infarction and splenic abscess. Embolization of the main splenic artery is thought to reduce bleeding by decreasing the arterial pressure in the splenic pulp, while avoiding splenic infarction due to collateral supply from the short gastric arteries. In some centers this practice has reduced the number of splenectomies required for splenic trauma.

Bowel

Bowel injury occurs in fewer than 5% of cases of blunt trauma to the abdomen, but is found in 80% of patients with aortoiliac artery injuries from blunt or penetrating trauma. Vascular injury such as thrombosis, arteriovenous fistula, pedicle avulsion, or transection can occur (Fig. 11-39). These injuries rarely require conventional angiography for evaluation or therapy.

VISCERAL ARTERY ANEURYSMS

Aneurysms of the visceral arteries are rare in comparison to aortic and iliac, femoral, and popliteal artery aneurysms.

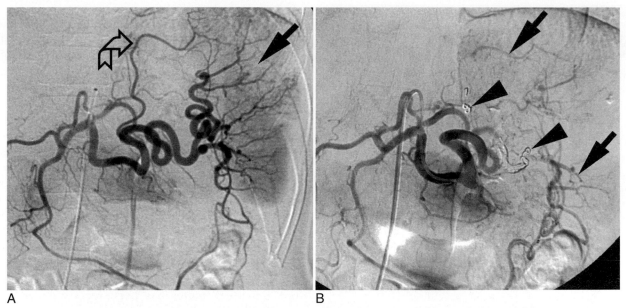

A   B

Figure 11-38   Splenic artery embolization for trauma in a patient with a fractured spleen following a motor vehicle accident. The objective of embolization in this stable patient is to decrease the overall splenic arterial flow but preserve viability of the organ. **A**, Celiac DSA showing the laceration of the upper pole of the spleen (arrow). There is an accessory upper-pole splenic artery (curved arrow) arising from the proximal main splenic artery. **B**, Following coil embolization of the distal main splenic artery and the accessory polar splenic artery (arrowheads), there is reconstitution of intrasplenic arteries (arrows) via the right gastroepiploic to left gastroepiploic and left gastric to short gastric arteries.

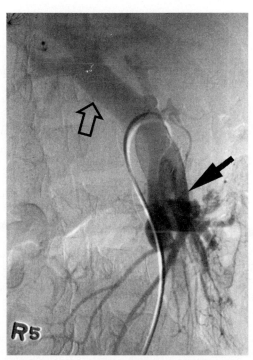

Figure 11-39   Subtracted image from an SMA angiogram (black arrow) following a stab wound to the abdomen, showing an arterioportal fistula (open arrow).

The most commonly affected arteries are the splenic, hepatic, and celiac, although multiple aneurysms have been found in one-third of patients in some series (Table 11-12). The etiology of the aneurysm has a great influence on whether it will be a true or false aneurysm (Box 11-10). Aneurysms related to degenerative processes, fibromuscular dysplasia (FMD), inherited disorders of the vascular wall, and vasculitis are true aneurysms unless they have ruptured. Aneurysms related to pancreatitis, infection, trauma, or surgery are always pseudoaneurysms.

Table 11-12   Visceral Artery Aneurysms

	Incidence
Splenic artery	60%
Hepatic artery	20%
Superior mesenteric artery	6%
Celiac artery	4%
Jejunal, iliac, colic arteries	4%
Pancreatico-duodenal arteries	2%
Gastroduodenal artery	2%
Inferior mesenteric artery	<1%

Box 11-10 Etiologies of Visceral Artery Aneurysms

Degenerative
Vasculitis
Pancreatitis
Trauma
Ehlers–Danlos syndrome
Fibromuscular dysplasia/segmental mediolytic
    arteriopathy
Mycotic
Behçet's disease
Iatrogenic (surgery, percutaneous interventions)
Celiac artery or SMA stenosis/occlusion
    (pancreatico-duodenal artery aneurysms)
Splenomegaly (splenic artery aneurysms)

The majority of these lesions are asymptomatic until first presenting with rupture. The indications for intervention in asymptomatic true aneurysms must be individualized to the patient and the artery involved. There are no set rules for management of these lesions. Pseudoaneurysms almost always require intervention, as the risk of rupture is high. The mortality of ruptured visceral artery aneurysms can be as high as 80%. Pseudoaneurysms due to pancreatitis are very amenable to embolization (Fig. 11-40).

Splenic artery aneurysms are four times more common in women than men (Fig. 11-41). Women with a history of multiple pregnancies are at highest risk. Splenic artery aneurysms are also frequently found in patients with massive splenomegaly and increased splenic arterial flow. Most splenic artery aneurysms are found incidentally, but patients may complain of epigastric, left upper quadrant abdominal, or back pain. The risk of rupture has not been quantified, but is highest in young patients (especially pregnant women) and the elderly. Rupture of true aneurysms is most often into the lesser sac or adjacent venous structures. Splenic artery pseudoaneurysms due to pancreatitis can rupture into a pancreatic pseudocyst, adjacent bowel or stomach, or the peritoneal cavity.

Intervention is probably warranted in any pregnant patient with a splenic artery aneurysm, or any symptomatic aneurysm. There are no firmly defined size criteria, but 2cm in diameter has been recommended as the threshold, especially in young women. In most cases surgical resection is performed, although percutaneous embolization can be very effective. Coils must be placed both distal and proximal to the aneurysm to effectively exclude it from arterial flow. Stent-graft placement is another option when the anatomy is suitable.

True aneurysms of the pancreatico-duodenal arteries are associated with increased collateral flow due to either celiac artery or SMA stenosis or occlusion. Rupture of these aneurysms can result in gastrointestinal bleeding,

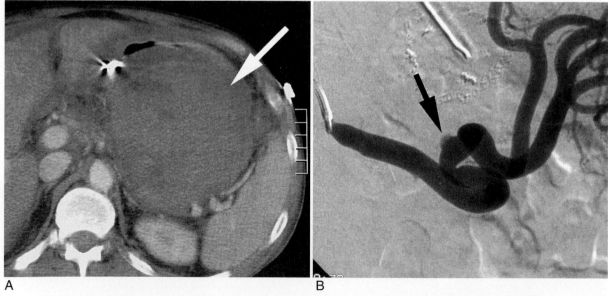

A   B

Figure 11-40   Splenic artery pseudoaneurysm due to necrotizing pancreatitis. **A**, CT scan showing huge hematoma (arrow) arising from the body of pancreas in a patient with acute abdominal pain and a drop in hematocrit level. **B**, Splenic artery DSA showing the pseudoaneurysm (arrow). The arterial abnormality is subtle compared to the CT finding. This was embolized by placing coils in the splenic artery distal and proximal to the pseudoaneurysm. The spleen remained well perfused by short gastric and gastroepiploic collaterals.

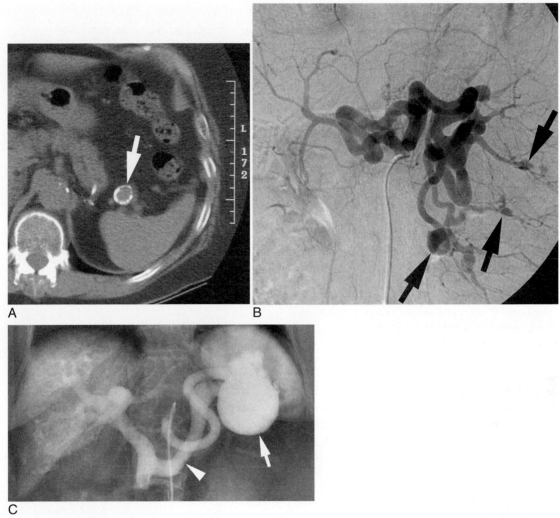

Figure 11-41   Splenic artery aneurysms. **A**, Noncontrast CT scan in an elderly female, showing a 2-cm diameter splenic artery aneurysm (arrow) with a calcified wall. **B**, Celiac DSA in a patient with massive splenomegaly, showing multiple small splenic artery aneurysms (arrows). **C**, Splenic artery angiogram in a patient with a massive splenic artery aneurysm (arrow) that has ruptured into the splenic vein (arrowhead) causing portal hypertension.

a large hematoma at the base of the mesentery, hypotension, and exsanguination (Fig. 11-42). Selective embolization with careful placement of coils on both sides of the aneurysm can be life-saving.

Mycotic aneurysms of mesenteric vessels are most often embolic in origin (Fig. 11-43). Cardiac valvular sources are typical, although paradoxical septic emboli have been reported.

FIBROMUSCULAR DYSPLASIA

The visceral arteries are vessels that are the sixth most frequently affected by FMD. Spontaneous dissection, focal aneurysm formation, and distal embolization can occur. The SMA, hepatic, and splenic arteries can be affected (Fig. 11-44). A rare variant of FMD known as segmental mediolytic arteriopathy presents as multiple small visceral artery aneurysms that mimic polyarteritis nodosa.

DISSECTION

Dissection of the visceral arteries is most often an extension of aortic dissection, but may be spontaneous, iatrogenic, or traumatic in origin. Symptomatic visceral artery compromise in aortic dissection occurs in approximately 6% of patients, with a 25–50% mortality at 30 days despite intervention. Up to 15% of acute deaths from aortic dissection are due directly or indirectly to mesenteric ischemia. MRA and CTA are highly

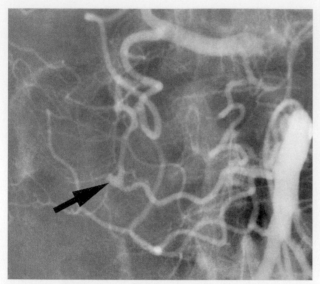

Figure 11-42   SMA angiogram showing an aneurysm (arrow) arising from an enlarged inferior pancreatico-duodenal artery in a patient with stenosis of the celiac artery origin. This patient presented with a spontaneous duodenal hematoma.

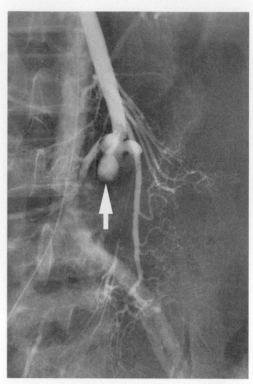

Figure 11-43   Mycotic SMA aneurysm in a patient with endocarditis and abdominal pain. Selective SMA angiogram showing a lobulated pseudoaneurysm (arrow) in the mid-SMA typical of a mycotic process.

sensitive and specific for diagnosis of aortic dissection and involvement of proximal visceral arteries (see Fig. 10-31). The celiac artery, SMA, and right renal artery are often supplied by the true lumen, whereas the left renal artery frequently arises from the false lumen (see Fig. 10-32). Compression of the true lumen and/or extension of the dissection into the visceral artery results in ischemia (Fig. 11-45). Surgical or stent-graft repair of the entry tear often results in improved perfusion of the visceral vessels (see Fig. 9-25). Surgical or percutaneous fenestration, sometimes with stent placement in the visceral artery, are alternative or additional approaches that result in a 60–70% survival at 5 years (see Fig. 10-33).

VASCULAR MALFORMATIONS

True vascular malformations of the liver, spleen, and pancreas are rare lesions, found in fewer than 1% of adults undergoing abdominal US. There is a strong association with the hereditary hemorrhagic telangiectasia (HHT) syndrome, but most often these are sporadic congenital lesions. In HHT, liver lesions may not be detected until many years after initial diagnosis of the syndrome. Liver malformations may be arterioportal or arteriovenous. The clinical presentation can be high-output congestive heart failure, portal hypertension, liver dysfunction, or biliary obstruction (Fig. 11-46). Ultrasound, CTA, and MRA are excellent modalities for diagnosis of liver arteriovenous malformations and distinction from shunting vascular tumors. Embolization has been successful in

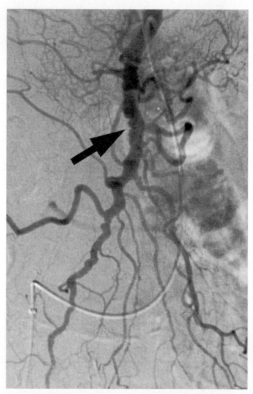

Figure 11-44   Fibromuscular dysplasia (FMD) of the SMA. Selective SMA DSA showing irregular beaded contour (arrow) of medial fibroplasia.

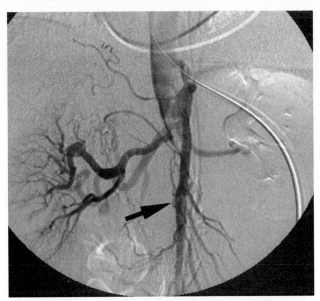

Figure 11-45 Visceral artery compromise due to thoracic aortic dissection extending into the abdomen. DSA in the true lumen, showing extreme compromise of the lumen and filling of the SMA (arrow), right kidney, and faint opacification of the common hepatic artery. Compare with Fig. 10-32.

controlling or averting congestive failure, but hepatic necrosis and death have been reported.

A wide variety of vascular lesions can affect the stomach, small bowel, and colon (Box 11-11). The typical presentation is gastrointestinal bleeding, either chronic or acute.

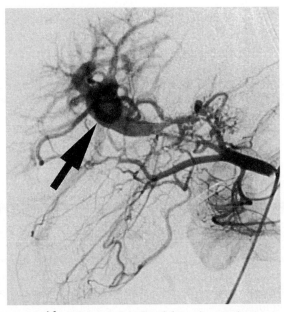

Figure 11-46 Congenital isolated hepatic arteriovenous malformation in an infant with congestive heart failure and hepatomegaly. The portal vein (arrow) is visualized on the celiac artery injection.

Box 11-11 Vascular Lesions Contributing to GI Bleeding
Vascular ectasia
Angiodysplasia
Hereditary hemorrhagic telangiectasia (GI bleeding in 15%)
CREST syndrome
Gastric antral vascular ectasia ("watermelon stomach")
Hemangioma
Isolated, sporadic (90%)
Intestinal hemangiomatosis
Blue rubber bleb syndrome (cutaneous and intestinal cavernous hemangiomas)
Klippel-Trenaunay Weber syndrome
Arteriovenous malformations
Dieulafoy lesion

CREST, calcinosis, Raynaud phenomenon, esophageal hypomotility, sclerodactyly, telangiectasia

Angiodysplasia is a common lesion consisting of dilated, thin-walled, submucosal veins, venules, and capillaries. They are frequently multiple, can be located anywhere from the stomach to the rectum, and are not associated with a systemic or generalized syndrome or disorder. Several segments of bowel may be affected synchronously, with the most common colonic location in the cecum. These are usually lesions of mature adults (usually 60+ years), without gender specificity. Angiodysplasia is now diagnosed most often at endoscopy, with treatment by cautery or injection. The classic angiographic appearance is vascular tuft or tangle with an early and dense draining vein (Fig. 11-47). Extravasation was classically reported in 10%, but is seen less frequently in current practice. Embolization of angiodysplasia has been reported, but surgical resection of lesions not amenable to endoscopic therapy remains the mainstay of therapy.

Gastric antral vascular ectasia ("watermelon stomach") is a rare lesion usually found in older women with iron deficiency anemia. Extensive submucosal venous dilatation in the antrum results in characteristic parallel red stripes. Diagnosis and therapy does not require angiography.

The Dieulafoy lesion is an abnormally large artery (1- to 3-mm diameter) close to the mucosal surface of the bowel. Originally described in the stomach in elderly patients (male to female ratio of 2:1), it is thought to account for 2–5% of acute upper GI bleeding. In modern series up to one-third of lesions are found in the colon, small bowel, and even the esophagus. Single lesions are typical. Dieulafoy lesions are usually diagnosed and treated at endoscopy, with mortality due to bleeding less

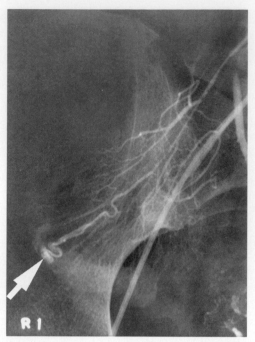

Figure 11-47   Angiogram showing right colonic angiodysplasia (arrow) with a small tuft of vessels and an early draining vein.

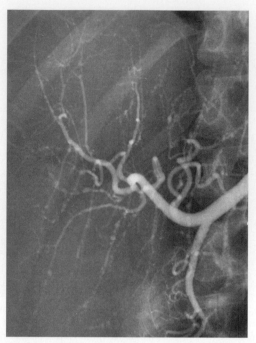

Figure 11-48   Celiac angiogram in a patient with polyarteritis nodosa, showing innumerable small aneurysms.

than 5%. When endoscopic management fails, angiographic localization of bleeding and embolization is usually successful.

Arteriovenous fistulas in the liver, spleen, pancreas, and bowel can occur after blunt or penetrating trauma, infection, or invasive procedures (see Fig. 11-39). In the liver communication may be with the hepatic or portal vein. Portal hypertension, variceal bleeding, and high-output cardiac failure may result from large fistulas. Endovascular treatment with embolization or small stent-grafts is frequently effective.

VASCULITIS

Polyarteritis nodosa is the most common vasculitis to affect the peripheral visceral arteries (Fig. 11-48). Stenoses and aneurysms may be found; the aneurysms are prone to rupture. Takayasu's arteritis can cause stenosis of the visceral artery origins.

HYPERSPLENISM

The syndrome of platelet sequestration and destruction by an enlarged spleen is termed hypersplenism. Primary hypersplenism is rare. Secondary hypersplenism can be due to portal hypertension, neoplasm, Gaucher's disease, or myeloproliferative disorders. More commonly symptomatic in children, hypersplenism also occurs in adults.

The conventional treatment of hypersplenism is correction of the underlying disorder or splenectomy. Although the latter is definitive, it is a major procedure that leaves the patient at risk for overwhelming sepsis from encapsulated bacteria. Partial embolization of the spleen (60–70% of the total parenchyma) will result in elevation of the platelet count and preservation of sufficient splenic pulp for maintenance of clinically relevant reticuloendothelial activity. Embolization should be with a permanent particulate agent from a distal position rather than proximal coil occlusion. Gelfoam pledgets soaked in antibiotics that provide coverage of both Gram-positive and Gram-negative organisms have also been used. Patients require pain control owing to infarction of splenic tissue, and broad-spectrum antibiotic prophylaxis for 7–10 days following the procedure.

Complete embolization (infarction) of the spleen is an alternative therapy for patients in whom splenectomy is required but high risk. An example would be a patient with a hostile abdomen and splenic vein occlusion and bleeding isolated gastric varices. Peripheral embolization and antibiotic coverage is necessary to prevent formation of a splenic abscess, which may occur in up to 40% of cases. In patients amenable to splenectomy, preoperative embolization with coils in the distal main splenic artery is beneficial when the spleen is huge, to limit blood loss.

Patients who undergo total splenic embolization should be immunized against encapsulated bacteria (*Pneumococcus, H. influenzae* type b, and

Meningococcus). When feasible, this should be performed 2-3 weeks prior to total embolization.

CIRRHOSIS

The primary symptomatic vascular abnormalities of cirrhosis are not arterial, but portal venous, and are discussed in detail in Chapter 14. Cirrhosis results in a small, nodular liver, often with hypertrophy of the left lobe. Ascites, splenomegaly, hepatofugal flow in the portal vein, and varices are usually present. Patients with cirrhosis have an increased incidence of hepatomas. The imaging diagnosis of cirrhosis is readily evident on US, CT, or MRI (see Chapter 14). Angiography is not performed to make this diagnosis, but the characteristic findings may be encountered during angiographic evaluation of the liver for other reasons. The arterial findings are an enlarged proper hepatic artery with corkscrew appearance of the intrahepatic arteries (owing to a small liver) and splenomegaly (see Fig. 11-4). During the venous phase varices and spontaneous portosystemic shunts may be seen, with diminished or even nonvisualized flow in the portal vein. Retrograde flow in the splenic and inferior mesenteric veins is indicative of portal hypertension. Rarely, in very severe portal hypertension with hepatofugal flow, hepatic artery injection will result in opacification of the portal vein even in the absence of a shunting intrahepatic mass.

SUGGESTED READINGS

Aina R, Oliva VL, Therasse E et al: Arterial embolotherapy for upper gastrointestinal hemorrhage: outcome assessment. *J Vasc Interv Radiol* 12:195-200, 2001.

Asensio JA, Forno W, Roldan G et al: Visceral vascular injuries. *Surg Clin N Am* 82:1-20, 2002.

Bandi R, Shetty PC, Sharma RP et al: Superselective arterial embolization for the treatment of lower gastrointestinal hemorrhage. *J Vasc Interv Radiol* 12:1399-1405, 2001.

Bodner G, Peer S, Karner M et al: Nontumorous vascular malformations in the liver: color Doppler ultrasonographic findings. *J Ultrasound Med* 21:187-197, 2002.

Brountzos EN, Critselis A, Magoulas D, Kagianni E, Kelekis DA: Emergency endovascular treatment of a superior mesenteric artery occlusion. *Cardiovasc Interv Radiol* 24:57-60, 2001.

Burrows PE, Dubois J, Kassarjian A: Pediatric hepatic vascular anomalies. *Pediatr Radiol* 31:533-545, 2001.

Carr SC, Mahvi DM, Hoch JR, Archer CW, Turnipseed WD: Visceral artery aneurysm rupture. *J Vasc Surg* 33:806-811, 2001.

Cognet F, Salem DB, Dranssart M et al: Chronic mesenteric ischemia: imaging and percutaneous treatment. *Radiographics* 22:863-879, 2002.

Covey AM, Brody LA, Maluccio MA, Getrajdman GI, Brown KT: Variant hepatic arterial anatomy revisited: digital subtraction angiography performed in 600 patients. *Radiology* 224:542-547, 2002.

Darcy M: Clinical management of gastrointestinal bleeding. In Murphy TP, Benenati JF, Kaufman JA eds: *Patient Care in Interventional Radiology*, SCVIR, Fairfax, VA, 1999.

Denys AL, Qanadli SD, Durand F et al: Feasibility and effectiveness of using coronary stents in the treatment of hepatic artery stenoses after orthotopic liver transplantation: preliminary report. *Am J Roentgenol* 178:1175-1179, 2002.

Edwards MS, Cherr GS, Craven TE et al: Acute occlusive mesenteric ischemia: surgical management and outcomes. *Ann Vasc Surg* 17:72-79, 2003.

Fishman SJ, Burrows PE, Leichtner AM, Mulliken JB: Gastrointestinal manifestations of vascular anomalies in childhood: varied etiologies require multiple therapeutic modalities. *J Pediatr Surg* 33:1163-1167, 1998.

Garcia-Tsao G, Korzenik JR, Young L et al: Liver disease in patients with hereditary hemorrhagic telangiectasia. *N Engl J Med* 343:931-936, 2000.

Gomes AS, Lois JF, McCoy RD: Angiographic treatment of gastrointestinal hemorrhage: comparison of vasopressin infusion and embolization. *Am J Roentgenol* 146:1031-1037, 1986.

Goueffic Y, Costargent A, Dupas B et al: Superior mesenteric artery dissection: case report. *J Vasc Surg* 35:1003-1005, 2002.

Harned RK, Thompson HR, Kumpe DA, Narkewicz MR, Sokol RJ: Partial splenic embolization in five children with hypersplenism: effects of reduced-volume embolization on efficacy and morbidity. *Radiology* 209:803-806, 1998.

Hastings GS: Angiographic localization and transcatheter treatment of gastrointestinal bleeding. *Radiographics* 20:1160-1168, 2000.

Horton KM, Fishman EK: Volume-rendered 3D CT of the mesenteric vasculature: normal anatomy, anatomic variants, and pathologic conditions. *Radiographics* 22:161-172, 2002.

Kasirajan K, O'Hara PJ, Gray BH et al: Chronic mesenteric ischemia: open surgery versus percutaneous angioplasty and stenting. *J Vasc Surg* 33:63-71, 2001.

Keller FS, Rosch J: Visceral and renal angiography. *Semin Interv Radiol* 17:29-71, 2000.

Kerr DJ, McArdle CS, Ledermann J et al: Intrahepatic arterial versus intravenous fluorouracil and folinic acid for colorectal cancer liver metastases: a multicentre randomised trial. *Lancet* 361:368-373, 2003.

Levine SM, Hellmann DB, Stone JH: Gastrointestinal involvement in polyarteritis nodosa (1986-2000): presentation and outcomes in 24 patients. *Am J Med* 112:386-391, 2002.

Llovet JM, Bruix J: Systematic review of randomized trials for unresectable hepatocellular carcinoma: chemoembolization improves survival. *Hepatology* 37:429-442, 2003.

Luscher TF, Lie JT, Stanson AW et al: Arterial fibromuscular dysplasia. *Mayo Clin Proc* 62:931-952, 1987.

Matsumoto AH, Angle JF, Spinosa DJ et al: Percutaneous transluminal angioplasty and stenting in the treatment of chronic mesenteric ischemia: results and longterm followup. *J Am Coll Surg* 194:S22-S31, 2002.

Meaney JF, Prince MR, Nostrant TT, Stanley JC: Gadolinium-enhanced MR angiography of visceral arteries in patients with suspected chronic mesenteric ischemia. *J Magn Reson Imaging* 7:171-176, 1997.

Meaney JF: Non-invasive evaluation of the visceral arteries with magnetic resonance angiography. *Eur Radiol* 9:1267-1276, 1999.

Mitchell AW, Spencer J, Allison DJ, Jackson JE: Meckel's diverticulum: angiographic findings in 16 patients. *Am J Roentgenol* 170:1329-1333, 1998.

Moore EE, Cogbill TH, Jurkovich GJ et al: Organ injury scaling: spleen and liver [1994 revision]. *J Trauma* 38:323, 1995.

Moneta GL: Screening for mesenteric vascular insufficiency and follow-up of mesenteric artery bypass procedures. *Semin Vasc Surg* 14:186-192, 2001.

Mozes MF, Spigos DG, Pollak R et al: Partial splenic embolization, an alternative to splenectomy: results of a prospective, randomized study. *Surgery* 96:694-702, 1984.

Norton ID, Petersen BT, Sorbi D et al: Management and long-term prognosis of Dieulafoy lesion. *Gastrointest Endosc* 50:762-767, 1999.

Orbuch M, Doppman JL, Jensen RT: Localization of pancreatic endocrine tumors. *Semin Gastrointest Dis* 6:90-101, 1995.

Parfitt J, Chalmers RT, Wolfe JH: Visceral aneurysms in Ehlers–Danlos syndrome: case report and review of the literature. *J Vasc Surg* 31:1248-1251, 2000.

Park WM, Gloviczki P, Cherry KJ et al: Contemporary management of acute mesenteric ischemia: factors associated with survival. *J Vasc Surg* 35:445-452, 2002.

Rha SE, Ha HK, Lee SH et al: CT and MR imaging findings of bowel ischemia from various primary causes. *Radiographics* 20:29-42, 2000.

Richard HM, Silberzweig JE, Mitty HA et al: Hepatic arterial complications in liver transplant recipients treated with pretransplantation chemoembolization for hepatocellular carcinoma. *Radiology* 214:775-779, 2000.

Salem R, Thurston KG, Carr BI, Goin JE, Geschwind J-FH. Yttrium-90 microspheres: radiation therapy for unresectable liver cancer. *J Vasc Interv Radiol* 13:S223-S229, 2002.

Sclafani SJ, Shaftan GW, Scalea TM et al: Nonoperative salvage of computed tomography-diagnosed splenic injuries: utilization of angiography for triage and embolization for hemostasis. *J Trauma* 39:818-825, 1995.

Schenker MP, Duszak R, Soulen MC et al: Upper gastrointestinal hemorrhage and transcatheter embolotherapy: clinical and technical factors impacting success and survival. *J Vasc Interv Radiol* 12:1263-1271, 2001.

Solomon B, Soulen MC, Baum RA et al: Chemoembolization of hepatocellular carcinoma with cisplatin, doxorubicin, mitomycin-C, ethiodol, and polyvinyl alcohol: prospective evaluation of response and survival in a US population. *J Vasc Interv Radiol* 10:793-798, 1999.

Song SY, Chung JW, Kwon JW et al: Collateral pathways in patients with celiac axis stenosis: angiographic-spiral CT correlation. *Radiographics* 22:881-893, 2002.

Sullivan KL: Hepatic artery chemoembolization. *Semin Oncol* 29:145-151, 2002.

Taourel PG, Deneuville M, Pradel JA, Regent D, Bruel JM: Acute mesenteric ischemia: diagnosis with contrast-enhanced CT. *Radiology* 199:632-636, 1996.

Waltman AC, Luers PR, Athanasoulis CA, Warshaw AL: Massive arterial hemorrhage in patients with pancreatitis: complementary roles of surgery and transcatheter occlusive techniques. *Arch Surg* 121:439-443, 1986.

Williams DM, Lee DY, Hamilton BH et al: The dissected aorta: percutaneous treatment of ischemic complications - principles and results. *J Vasc Interv Radiol* 8:605-625, 1997.

Zuccaro G: Management of the adult patient with acute lower gastrointestinal bleeding. American College of Gastroenterology. Practice Parameters Committee. *Am J Gastroenterol* 93:1202-1208, 1998.

Renal Arteries

JOHN A. KAUFMAN, M.D.

The kidneys receive almost 15% of the cardiac output, although they account for less than 5% of the total body mass. Obstructive arterial diseases of the kidney have both functional (such as decreased creatinine clearance) and hormonal (angiotensin-mediated hypertension) implications. There are few organs that have such a complex response to vascular disease and potentially rewarding results with intervention.

ANATOMY

Renal Arteries

The kidneys are paired organs that originate in the pelvis and ascend into the abdominal cavity in a retroperitoneal position. As each kidney travels cephalad it is supplied sequentially by a series of arteries from the aorta that regress spontaneously. Ultimately, each kidney is usually supplied by a single renal artery that originates from the aorta below the superior mesenteric artery (SMA) at roughly the L1–L2 diskspace in about two-thirds

of individuals. The right renal artery orifice is located on the anterolateral wall of the aorta, frequently quite close to the SMA origin. The right renal artery courses posterior to the IVC, and assumes a position posterior to the right renal vein in the retroperitoneum (Fig. 12-1). The left renal artery originates in a more lateral location, and courses through the retroperitoneum posterior to the left renal vein. An understanding of the typical locations of the renal artery orifices will avoid much frustration during selective angiography.

The renal artery is usually 4–6 cm in length and 5–6 mm in diameter. Each renal artery gives rise to a small proximal branch to the adrenal gland (the inferior adrenal arteries) and the renal capsule (Fig. 12-2). In the region of the renal pelvis the artery bifurcates into anterior and posterior divisions. The anterior division supplies the upper and lower poles and the anterior portion of the mid-kidney. The posterior division supplies primarily the posterior renal parenchyma, with supplemental supply to the upper and lower poles. The divisional arteries divide into segmental arteries (apical, upper, middle, lower, and posterior), which quickly give rise to the interlobar arteries. At the corticomedullary junction the interlobar arteries divide into the arcuate arteries. The terminal branches of the renal artery are the interlobular arteries, which ultimately supply the glomeruli.

Variations in number, location, and branching patterns of the renal arteries are present in over 30% of people. These vessels can enter the kidney through the hilum, or travel directly to a renal pole (termed a "polar artery") (Table 12-1). Supernumerary renal arteries can arise from the abdominal aorta and iliac (usually common) arteries. (see Fig. 10-8). Renal artery origins arising above the SMA origin are extremely rare. Congenital anomalies of renal position and conformation are often associated with aberrant locations of renal artery origins and supernumerary vessels. In particular, horseshoe kidney has a 100% incidence of multiple renal arteries. The fused

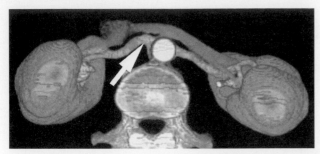

Figure 12-1 Volume rendering of CTA viewed in the axial projection showing the renal arteries and veins. The right renal artery origin (arrow) arises from the aorta more anteriorly than the left. Both renal arteries lie posterior to the renal veins.

Table 12-1 Renal Artery Anatomy

Description	Incidence (%)
Single renal artery bilaterally	55
Proximal bifurcation main renal artery	17
Polar branch directly from aorta	12
Two hilar arteries directly from aorta	12
Three or more hilar arteries directly from aorta	2
Multiple renal arteries, one kidney	32
Multiple renal arteries, both kidneys	10

lower poles of a horseshoe kidney, termed the isthmus, is trapped under the inferior mesenteric artery as the kidneys ascend out of the pelvis (Fig. 12-3). The isthmus can derive arterial blood supply from the distal aorta and iliac arteries.

The renal pelvis and proximal ureters are supplied by small branches of the interlobular, arcuate, and distal main renal arteries. The middle portion of the ureters are supplied by the gonadal arteries (see Fig. 10-1). The distal ureters are supplied by terminal branches of the internal iliac arteries, most notably the cystic artery.

Adrenal Arteries

The adrenal glands are retroperitoneal organs that receive their blood supply from the renal arteries, directly from the aorta, the inferior phrenic arteries, and rarely from the celiac artery or SMA. There are usually three adrenal arteries; the inferior, middle, and superior (see Fig. 10-1). In many instances these vessels are linked to capsular renal branches, and therefore are potential pathways for collateral blood supply to the kidney.

The inferior adrenal artery arises directly from the proximal renal arteries in two-thirds of people. The middle adrenal arteries are small vessels that usually arise directly from the aorta. These arteries are slightly more common

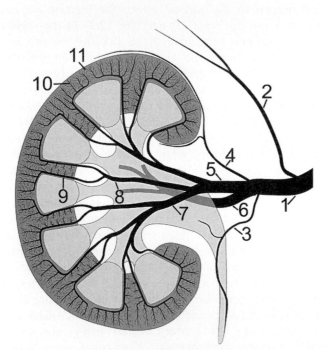

Figure 12-2 Drawing of typical renal artery anatomy. **1**, Main renal artery. **2**, Inferior adrenal artery. **3**, Ureteric artery. **4**, Capsular arteries. **5**, Anterior division. **6**, Posterior division. **7**, Segmental artery. **8**, Lobar artery. **9**, Interlobar artery. **10**, Arcuate artery. **11**, Interlobular artery.

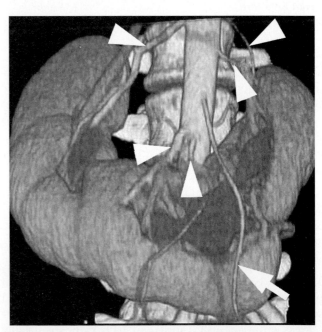

Figure 12-3 Volume rendering of abdominal CTA (4 detector row) showing a horseshoe kidney with multiple renal arteries (arrowheads). Note the inferior mesenteric artery (arrow) draped over the isthmus of the kidney.

on the left than the right. The origins of the middle adrenal arteries may be replaced to the celiac artery or SMA in 2–5% of patients. The superior adrenal arteries are constant branches of the inferior phrenic arteries. However, the origins of the inferior phrenic arteries are less predictable than their adrenal branches. These arteries arise from the aorta or the celiac artery in two-thirds of patients, but may also originate from the renal arteries or the left gastric artery.

KEY COLLATERAL PATHWAYS

The renal arteries are end arteries. In contrast to the colonic and hepatic vasculature, the intrarenal collateral pathways are poorly developed. In the presence of slowly progressive proximal renal artery stenosis, renal capsular, ureteral, adrenal, and other retroperitoneal arteries may enlarge sufficiently to provide enough collateral blood supply to keep the kidney alive, but not functioning normally (Fig. 12-4). Acute proximal occlusion of a previously normal renal artery results in profound ischemia owing to the inadequate preexisting collateral supply.

IMAGING

Renal Arteries

Ultrasound (US) is an excellent modality for imaging renal parenchyma, detection of nephrolithiasis, and hydronephrosis. The renal size should always be noted. Color-flow duplex US is required to image the renal arteries. Main renal arteries are reliably depicted in 95% of patients, but the detection of small accessory renal arteries is less accurate. The normal renal artery is a low-resistance vessel, with antegrade flow present throughout the cardiac cycle and a peak systolic velocity <180 cm/s (see Fig. 3-2). Evaluation of Doppler waveforms and velocities is required to identify stenoses (see next section, Occlusive Disease). The resistive index

$$[1 - (\text{end diastolic velocity} \div \text{maximum systolic velocity})] \times 100$$

is useful to estimate the underlying parenchymal disease of the kidney. Normal values should be less than 70; borderline increased resistance is 70–80; abnormal resistance is ≥80.

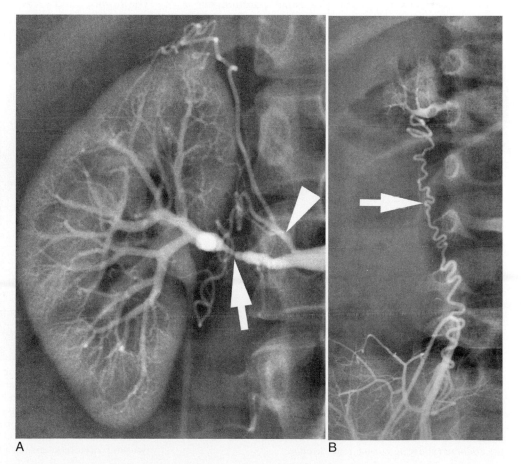

Figure 12-4 Renal artery collateral supply. **A,** Selective right renal angiogram of a young patient with hypertension due to fibromuscular dysplasia (probably intimal fibroplasia) (arrow) showing prominent capsular and peripelvic collaterals from the inferior adrenal artery (arrowhead). **B,** Selective injection of the right hypogastric artery showing retrograde flow in an enlarged ureteric artery (arrow) to the distal renal artery in a different child with renal artery stenosis. (Images courtesy of Frederick Keller M.D., Dotter Interventional Institute, Portland, OR.)

A

B

Nuclear medicine studies can provide functional information and infer the presence of occlusive vascular lesions. Occasionally, nuclear medicine studies are obtained in patients with renal masses or nonocclusive vascular lesions to assess renal function. A number of imaging agents are available, of which technetium^{99m} mercaptoacetyltriglycine (MAG3) is commonly used. A decrease in glomerular filtration of the agent, particularly following administration of an angiotensin-converting enzyme (ACE) inhibitor such as captopril, is highly suggestive of proximal renal artery stenosis.

CTA has a very high sensitivity and specificity for identification of renal arteries and detection of vascular pathology. A noncontrast scan should be obtained first to evaluate for nephrolithiasis, calcified renal artery lesions, and hyperdense renal masses such as hemorrhagic cysts. A thin-collimation breath-hold contrast-enhanced helical scan from the diaphragm to the common femoral arteries is required for a complete evaluation of the renal arteries. A good contrast bolus is essential. The celiac artery must be included in the study as hepato- or spleno-renal bypasses are surgical alternatives for treatment of proximal renal artery occlusive disease. The aorta is evaluated for concomitant occlusive or aneurysmal disease. The iliac arteries are included to detect accessory renal arteries and evaluate for occlusive disease that could impact treatment decisions. The renal parenchyma is inspected carefully for mass lesions. The presence of an adrenal mass in a hypertensive patient should raise the question of a pheochromocytoma or aldosteronoma (Conn's disease). When evaluating a patient as a potential donor for renal transplantation, a delayed scan is obtained for venous and collecting system anatomy.

Careful postprocessing of the 3-dimensional (3-D) volumes improves sensitivity for small accessory vessels.

Magnetic resonance (MR) imaging of patients with renal vascular disease involves both anatomic and flow sequences. In the future, physiologic information will also be obtained during MR imaging of the kidney. With current techniques, anatomic sequences provide information about renal size and the presence of masses. The most useful vascular sequence is a 3-D gadolinium-enhanced gradient echo breath-hold acquisition (Fig. 12-5). A coronal volume is used centered slightly posterior in order to encompass the renal artery as it courses through the retroperitoneum. The field of view should include from the celiac artery to the common femoral arteries to avoid overlooking an important accessory renal artery. Occasionally, a 3-D phase-contrast sequence is used in addition to the gadolinium acquisition when the severity of disease is unclear from the contrast-enhanced images. MRA is very sensitive and specific for ostial and proximal renal artery pathology. However, subtle FMD can easily be missed.

Conventional angiography is usually performed following noninvasive imaging of some type with the specific goal of intervention. Previous studies should be reviewed prior to the procedure. Conventional angiographic evaluation of the renal arteries begins with an aortogram. The number and location of renal arteries, and the condition of the ostia and proximal renal arteries, can be determined from this study. To perform the aortogram,

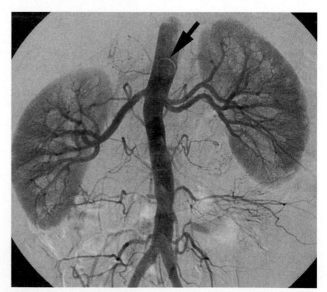

Figure 12-6   DSA of the abdominal aorta to evaluate the renal arteries. The catheter tip (arrow) is just proximal to the renal artery origins, and the x-ray tube has been angled slightly in the left anterior oblique projection. With the catheter in this position there is minimal opacification of potentially confusing mesenteric arteries. The field of view includes the proximal iliac arteries. There are two left renal arteries arising adjacent to each other from the aorta.

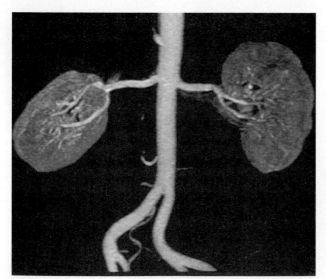

Figure 12-5   Coronal maximum intensity projection (MIP) of a gadolinium-enhanced 3-dimensional MR angiogram (3-D MRA) of the abdomen showing normal renal arteries.

a pigtail or other catheter designed for high-volume aortic injection is positioned with its tip just at or slightly above the renal arteries (Fig. 12-6). The x-ray tube should be obliqued in a slight left anterior oblique (LAO) projection to best visualize the renal artery origins. The most advantageous angle can be determined from review of prior imaging studies. An appropriate contrast injection (15–25 mL/s for 2 seconds) and rapid filming (3–6 frames/s) are necessary to obtain optimal images of the proximal renal arteries. The right renal artery can arise in a very anterior position, so that a steep left anterior oblique, or even a lateral view, may be necessary to visualize this renal artery ostium. Selective angiography is required to fully evaluate the branches of the renal artery and renal parenchymal masses. When multiple arteries are present to a single kidney, the junctional renal parenchyma typically has an irregular, indistinct contour (Fig. 12-7).

A wide variety of selective catheters can be used for renal angiography, but the basic choices are a curved selective catheter such as a Cobra-2, or a recurved catheter such as a Sos selective. The curved catheter shape is chosen when the renal artery arises at close to a 90-degree angle from the aorta, whereas a recurved catheter can be used to pull down into a renal artery that arises at an acute angle (see Figs 2-10 and 2-18 to 2-20). Rarely, a brachial approach is required to select a renal artery owing to a steep angle of origin, severe infrarenal aortic tortuosity, or aortoiliac occlusion. Injection rates of 5–6 mL/s for 2–3 seconds provide excellent opacification of intrarenal branches. Rapid filming (3–6 frames/s) is necessary. Oblique and craniocaudad oblique views are frequently required to optimally display the renal vasculature, but studies must be tailored to each patient (see Fig. 12-7). In general, an ipsilateral anterior oblique

presents the kidney *en face*. Administration of glucagon to reduce artifact from bowel motion on DSA may be helpful in some patients.

Adrenal Arteries

In most cases the adrenal glands can be evaluated for mass lesions using US, CT, or MRI. The need to visualize the arterial supply of the adrenals is rare, but the only way is with conventional angiography. The adrenal arteries are too small and variable in location to be reliably evaluated with noninvasive techniques. For the same reasons, selective angiography of the adrenal gland is also difficult. Flush injections of the abdominal aorta, and selective renal and phrenic arterial injections, will aid in identification of the inferior and superior adrenal arteries. The middle adrenal artery, which arises directly from the aorta, can be selected with a recurved catheter. Hand injections of contrast should be used, as rupture of the artery and adrenal infarction can occur. The normal adrenal gland appears as a dense wedged-shaped suprarenal stain.

RENAL ARTERY OCCLUSIVE DISEASE

There are many causes of obstructive lesions of the renal artery, but the most common are atherosclcrosis (90%) and fibromuscular dysplasia (FMD) (Box 12-1) The clinical manifestations of renal artery occlusive disease are hypertension, renal failure, or both. Although it is convenient to separate these clinical presentations for the purposes of discussion, this is not always possible in clinical practice.

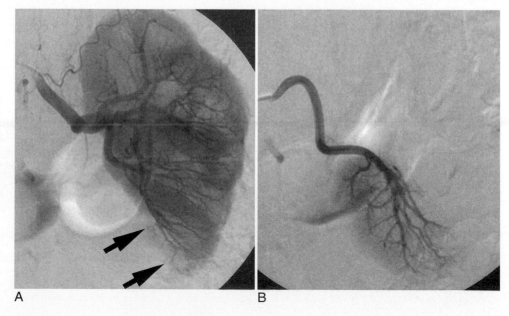

Figure 12-7   Selective renal artery DSA in a patient with accessory lower-pole renal artery. **A,** Selective injection of the main left renal artery shows an indistinct lower-pole margin (arrows). **B,** Selective injection of the lower-pole accessory renal artery shows the missing segment of the kidney.

A   B

Box 12-1   Causes of Renal Artery Stenosis

Atherosclerosis
Fibromuscular dysplasia
Dissection
Vasculitis
Neurofibromatosis
Developmental (abdominal aortic coarctation)
Compression of kidney by mass or hematoma
Iatrogenic

The majority (90–98%) of patients with elevated blood pressure have primary or essential hypertension. No structural lesions can be identified in these patients. Hypertension caused by a renal artery stenosis is termed "secondary hypertension," and accounts for only 1–5% of patients with hypertension. Most of these patients have some degree of primary hypertension as well. Nevertheless, these patients may benefit from treatment of the obstructing renal artery lesion. The mechanism of hypertension in renal artery stenosis is activation of the renin–angiotensin–aldosterone system (Box 12-2). The clinical presentation of patients is variable, but in general features severe hypertension that is extremely difficult to control (Box 12-3).

Patients with atherosclerotic renal artery stenoses are usually in their sixth decade or older, and are more likely to be male than female. The majority of patients with renal artery stenoses found at angiography are asymptomatic. Atherosclerotic stenoses are typically located within the first few centimeters of the origin of the renal artery. In the majority of patients the stenosis is at or within 1 cm of the origin. These lesions are caused by aortic plaque encroaching upon the origin of the vessel, and are termed "ostial stenoses" (see Fig. 4-3). Fewer than 10% of atherosclerotic lesions are truly confined to the renal artery proper (greater than 1 cm from the ostium). These are termed "proximal stenoses" (Fig. 12-8). In patients with severe atherosclerosis or longstanding hypertension, the smaller intrarenal branches may also be diseased (Fig. 12-9). Almost half of patients with atherosclerotic

---

Box 12-2   Renin–Angiotensin–Aldosterone System

Renin (kidney) → Angiotensinogen (liver) →
    Angiotensin I → Angiotensin II (lung) → Increased
    aldosterone secretion → Hypertension

Box 12-3   Clinical Signs of Renovascular Hypertension

Sudden-onset severe hypertension
Onset of hypertension <30 or >50 years of age
Sudden increased severity of hypertension
Hypertension unresponsive to, or poorly controlled by, triple drug therapy
Hypertension with rapidly progressive renal failure
Renal failure in response to ACE[a] inhibitors or angiotensin II-receptor blocking agents
Severe or uncontrolled hypertension in patients with generalized atherosclerosis
Episodes of recurrent severe hypertension and pulmonary edema
Hypertension with upper abdominal bruit over kidney

[a]ACE, angiotensin-converting enzyme.

---

renal artery stenosis will also have a lesion in the opposite renal artery.

Atherosclerotic renal artery disease is a progressive disorder, but predicting outcomes for individual patients is difficult. Some authors claim that up to 12–20% of atherosclerotic lesions that are >75% stenotic will proceed to occlusion within 1 year. However, this statistic is of questionable utility as many of these events are subclinical.

In contrast to atherosclerosis, hypertension due to renal artery FMD is found in young patients (third to fifth decade), and more commonly in females. Medial fibroplasia is the pathologic type present in 80% of patients with FMD, particularly in adults (Fig. 12-10; see also Fig. 1-11). The multiple small webs obstruct blood flow,

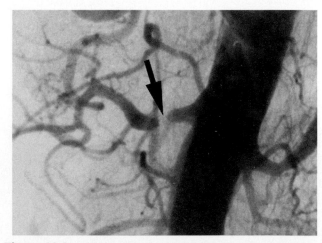

Figure 12-8   Atherosclerotic renal artery stenosis. Aortic injection (DSA) showing true proximal (>1 cm from the origin) renal artery stenosis (arrow). The tiny residual lumen is not seen on this nonselective injection.

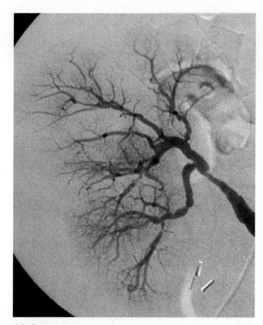

Figure 12-9   Selective right renal DSA of a transplant kidney showing focal severe stenosis of the main renal artery as well as diffuse disease of the small intrarenal branches and patchy parenchymal enhancement. The kidney had functioned well for 22 years after transplantation.

resulting in hypertension. Other forms of FMD result in stenoses in young patients and can be difficult to distinguish from disease such as Takayasu's arteritis and neurofibromatosis (see Fig. 12-4). Spontaneous intrarenal dissection is a rare form of FMD that presents with acute flank pain, hematuria, hypertension, and wedge-shaped renal infarcts on CT or MR (Fig. 12-11).

FMD of the medial fibroplasia type is usually located in the distal main renal artery, and extends into the first-order branches in 25% of patients. Over half of patients have bilateral disease, but when the disease is unilateral the right renal artery is involved in over two-thirds. The true rate of progression of FMD is unknown, but asymptomatic disease is common.

Other vascular causes of renovascular hypertension are less prevalent. Extension of an aortic dissection into the renal artery, vasculitis, neurofibromatosis, and compression of the renal parenchyma by a large subcapsular hematoma, can all result in hypertension (see Figs 10-32 and 10-37). The regional variations in etiologies of renovascular hypertension are striking; in India, Takayasu's disease is responsible for two-thirds of the cases of secondary hypertension.

Renal insufficiency on the basis of renal artery obstruction (ischemic nephropathy) is almost always the result of atherosclerosis. Renal artery stenosis or occlusion is thought to be the underlying etiology of 8–10% of patients requiring chronic hemodialysis. Bilateral renal artery stenosis is more likely to result in renal failure than

unilateral lesions, provided that the contralateral kidney is normal. This entity must be distinguished from nephrosclerosis caused by chronic poorly controlled hypertension. Renal failure due to FMD is unusual.

The choice of techniques used for diagnosis of renovascular disease is influenced by the clinical history. Young patients with normal renal function and suspected renal artery hypertension should undergo angiography, because subtle or peripheral FMD can be missed by noninvasive imaging modalities and treatment with balloon angioplasty can be performed at the same time. Adults with suspected renal vascular hypertension should first have at least one noninvasive test prior to angiography. When carefully performed, color-flow duplex ultrasound can detect renal artery stenosis (>60% reduction in diameter) with roughly 95% sensitivity and specificity. Multiple criteria exist for interpretation of duplex data, with no clear superiority of one over the other (Table 12-2). A resistive index under 80 is predictive of a positive outcome with renal revascularization. Both MRA and CTA have excellent sensitivity and specificity for detection of ostial and proximal renal artery stenosis (>90% in each category) (Fig. 12-12). Reduction in luminal diameter >75%, post-stenotic dilatation, and decrease in renal mass are indicative of hemodynamically significant disease. The reliable evaluation of small accessory renal arteries and intrarenal branches is not possible yet with these techniques. In patients with normal renal function, captopril scintigraphy has similar sensitivity and specificity but does not provide any anatomic information that can used for planning therapy.

The angiographic diagnosis of renal artery stenosis is suggested by the degree of luminal narrowing (50–75%), post-stenotic dilatation, slow flow distal to the lesion, the presence of collateral circulation, and decreased renal mass (see Figs 12-8 and 4-3). Delayed filming may be necessary to visualize a reconstituted artery distal to a proximal occlusion (Fig. 12-13). The location of the lesion (ostial or proximal) should be carefully determined, as well as the

Table 12-2   Duplex Criteria (Main Renal Artery) for Renal Artery Stenosis[a]

Stenosis	Renal Artery PSV (cm/s)	Renal Artery PSV/Aortic PSV
0%	<180	<3.5
<60%	≥180	<3.5
≥60%	≥180	≥3.5
100%	0	NA

[a]Resistive index of <80 is predictive of a favorable outcome following revascularization. PSV, peak systolic velocity; NA, not applicable owing to renal artery PSV of 0 cm/s.

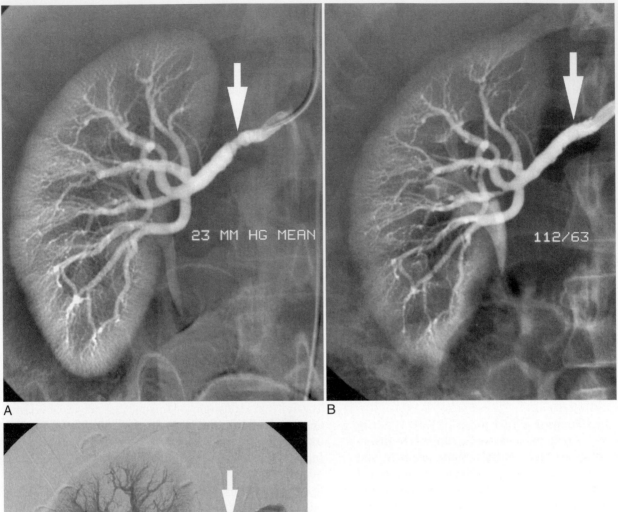

A

B

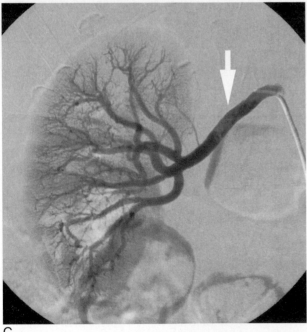

C

Figure 12-10 Renal artery FMD in a middle-aged woman with hypertension. **A**, Selective right renal artery DSA showing irregular beaded appearance (arrow) of medial fibroplasia in the proximal right renal artery. There was a 23-mmHg gradient across this lesion. **B**, Angiogram after angioplasty with a 6-mm diameter balloon. The artery has a normal diameter with typical postangioplasty irregularity of the intima (arrow). **C**, Selective angiogram obtained 4 years later shows a normal-appearing right renal artery (arrow).

extent of the disease. The best measure of the severity of stenosis is a systolic pressure gradient >10 mmHg between the aorta and the renal artery distal to the lesion. A normal gradient is conclusively normal, as is a very abnormal gradient. However, a catheter placed through a moderate lesion to measure pressure may

further decrease the cross-sectional area of the lumen and induce a gradient. Borderline gradients (10–15 mmHg) require careful assessment. Pressure-sensing guidewires may be useful in this situation.

Sampling of the hormone renin directly from the renal veins is occasionally helpful to establish the diagnosis of

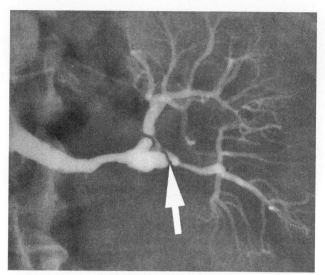

Figure 12-11   Selective renal angiogram of a middle-aged man with acute onset of left flank pain showing spontaneous intrarenal dissection (arrow) typical of FMD. The aorta was normal.

renal vascular hypertension and identify which kidney is responsible. A curved selective catheter (such as a Cobra-2) or a straight catheter with a tip deflecting wire can be used. A single side-hole should be punched near the tip of the catheter. Blood samples are obtained from each renal vein, and from the IVC above and below the renal veins. On the left, the catheter tip should be lateral to the orifice of the left gonadal vein. Samples need not be simultaneous, but closely spaced temporally. Renin levels from one kidney that are ≥1.5 times that of the

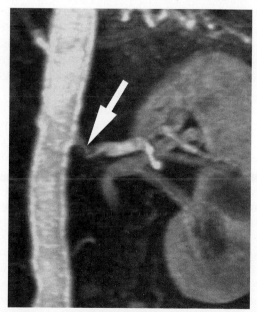

Figure 12-12   Coronal MIP of gadolinium-enhanced 3-D MRA showing left renal artery stenosis (arrow) in a patient with prior right nephrectomy.

Box 12-4   Indications for Intervention in Renal Artery Stenosis

Hypertension

Unilateral or bilateral stenosis
  Pressure gradient >10 mmHg
Atherosclerosis, FMD, Takayasu's, dissection
Severe hypertension (Box 12-3)

Azotemia

Bilateral stenosis[a]
  Pressure gradient >10 mmHg
Atherosclerosis, dissection
Rapidly progressive renal failure

[a]Unilateral renal artery stenosis is unlikely to cause renal failure when the contralateral kidney is normal.

contralateral kidney are indicative of renovascular hypertension. A rise in renin between the infra- and supra-renal IVC is further evidence of a renovascular hypertension. When multiple renal veins are present, samples should be obtained from each vein.

The indications for intervention in renal artery stenosis are slightly different for hypertension and ischemic nephropathy (Box 12-4). All symptomatic lesions that cannot be managed medically require intervention in patients with reasonable life expectancies. Asymptomatic lesions are generally not treated unless the kidney is solitary.

There are numerous surgical options for revascularization of the renal arteries (Box 12-5). Ostial and proximal atherosclerotic renal artery lesions are easier to deal with than distal main or segmental artery lesions. The overall mortality for surgical intervention is approximately 4%, with hypertension cured in 18%, improved in 71%, and unchanged or worse in 1%. In patients with renal failure, improvement can be expected in half of the patients, 39% remain unchanged, and 11% deteriorate.

Box 12-5   Surgery for Renal Artery Stenosis

Aortorenal bypass
Hepatorenal bypass (right kidney)
Splenorenal bypass (left kidney)
Aortorenal endarterectomy
Iliorenal bypass
Autotransplantation to pelvis
Nephrectomy

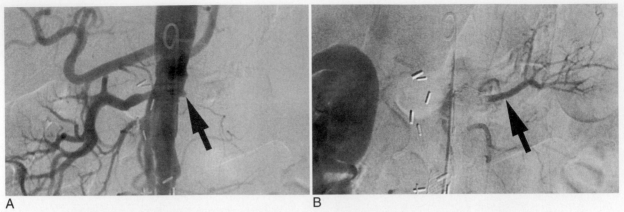

Figure 12-13   Delayed opacification of renal artery distal to an occluded stent. **A,** DSA of the aorta shows the stump of the occluded left renal artery (arrow). **B,** Late image from the same injection shows the distal renal artery reconstituted (arrow) through small retroperitoneal branches.

Angioplasty and stent placement are the percutaneous techniques used most often in treatment of obstructive lesions of the renal artery. These procedures should be approached in a careful, planned manner, as they can be among the most difficult arterial interventions. Patients scheduled for renal artery intervention for hypertension should stop or decrease longacting antihypertensive medications before the procedure if possible. Successful angioplasty or stent placement may lead to profound hypotension when drug effects persist after acute renal revascularization. Patients should be instructed to drink fluids until 2 hours prior to the procedure, at which time intravenous fluids should be initiated at a brisk pace. Some interventionalists administer a calcium-channel blocking agent such as oral nifedipine 10 mg prior to the procedure to prevent vasospasm. Patients with preexisting renal failure can be treated beforehand with a renal protective agent (see Table 2-5). An aortogram should be obtained in all cases; CO_2 gas or gadolinium can be used in patients with azotemia. Once the decision to intervene is made, syringes containing heparin (1000 U/mL) and nitroglycerin (100 μg/mL) are placed on the angiography table. A long curved 6- or 7-French sheath, or a 7- or 8-French curved guiding catheter, is inserted. The curve of the sheath or guide catheter is selected to match the angle of the renal artery as it arises from the aorta (see Fig. 2-22). Manipulation in the aorta should be minimized to decrease the risk of cholesterol embolization. Heparin (5000–10,000 units) is administered prior to selecting the renal artery. For ostial lesions, the image intensifier is angled to display the renal artery ostium in profile. A selective 5-French catheter appropriate for the configuration of the renal artery is used to find the renal artery origin. A gentle puff of contrast confirms catheter position. Ostial lesions are gently probed with a soft-tipped angled hydrophilic guidewire. Extremely tight ostial

lesions can sometimes be crossed only with micro wires. When using a pull-down catheter, leading with 1–2 cm of a Bentson guidewire will minimize the risk of subintimal dissection.

Once the selective guidewire has crossed the lesion, the catheter is advanced until it, too, has crossed the lesion. The guidewire is removed, blood is aspirated, and a small amount of contrast is injected, followed by 100–200 μg of nitroglycerin. When there is complete stasis of the intrarenal branches due to obturation of the lesion by the catheter, additional heparin can be delivered directly into the renal artery. A working wire is then carefully inserted. Typical working guidewires include the 0.035-inch 1.5-J Rosen, soft-tipped 0.035-inch stiff nitinol guidewires, or 0.014- to 0.018-inch guidewires with soft platinum or gold tips. A stiff guidewire may change the angle of the renal artery, facilitating the procedure (Fig. 12-14). Careful control of the guidewire at all times is critical to prevent spasm or dissection; straight guidewires can perforate the kidney.

The guiding catheter or sheath should be brought as close to the renal artery ostium as possible to provide added stability to the system. In addition, contrast can be injected through the sheath or guiding catheter to monitor the progress of the procedure. Ostial lesions almost always require stent placement, as the stenosis is caused by aortic rather than renal artery plaque. Predilatation with an undersized balloon facilitates positioning of the stent. The ideal stent design for renal artery ostia has not been determined, but most often a balloon-expandable stent is used. When required, the sheath or guiding catheter is advanced through the lesion before inserting the balloon-mounted stent to facilitate positioning. This maneuver minimizes the chance of the stent slipping off the balloon during positioning. Typical balloon diameters for renal artery ostia are 5–7 mm. Stent lengths

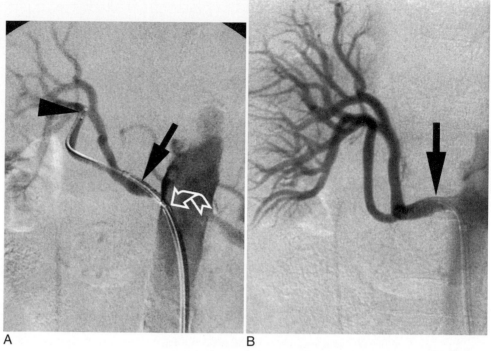

Figure 12-14   Guidewire straightening of a renal artery during stent placement. **A**, Control DSA obtained through the sheath (curved arrow) while positioning a balloon-mounted stent (arrow) across the ostial renal artery stenosis. A Rosen guidewire is in the posterior division (arrowhead). **B**, DSA after stent deployment and removal of the guidewire. Note the change in angle of the main renal artery (arrow) relative to the aorta compared to the previous image.

A   B

are usually 1.5–2 cm. The stent should be deployed so that it protrudes into the aorta a few millimeters in order to ensure adequate displacement of the aortic plaque (Fig. 12-15). "Flaring" the aortic end of the stent with a slightly larger balloon is cosmetically appealing but of unproven benefit.

Proximal renal artery atherosclerotic lesions – i.e., those that are located more than 1 cm from the aortic lumen – respond well to angioplasty alone. The indications for stents in these lesions are failed angioplasty (residual stenosis >30% or gradient >10 mmHg), an obstructing

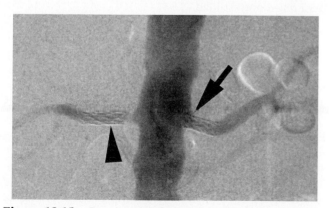

Figure 12-15   Proper and improper stent positioning. DSA after bilateral renal artery stent placement shows excellent position on the left with slight protrusion into the aortic lumen (arrow). The stent on the right ends within the renal artery (arrowhead). To completely cover the lesion, this stent should also extend to the aortic lumen.

postangioplasty dissection, recurrent stenosis, or recanalization of an occlusion. All of the same precautions described for intervention in ostial lesions should be exercised. A large branch in the vicinity of the stenosis can be protected by placing a 0.018-inch guidewire through the sheath or guiding catheter alongside the working wire and into the branch during the angioplasty. When the lesion occurs at a bifurcation of the renal artery, kissing balloons may be necessary (Fig. 12-16).

Renal artery FMD of the medial fibroplasia type responds well to simple angioplasty with excellent long-term results (see Fig. 12-10). There is less experience with other forms of FMD, but these lesions tend to be more fibrotic and elastic. Involvement of intrarenal branches commonly occurs with FMD, increasing the complexity of the procedure. However, as FMD tends to be found in young patients with normal iliac arteries and aortas, some of the technical aspects of the procedure can be less demanding than with atherosclerotic renal artery stenosis. FMD of segmental and smaller renal artery branches requires small-diameter balloons and 0.18-inch or smaller guidewires. Stents are rarely required to treat the medial fibroplasia form of FMD unless a dissection occurs.

Renal artery angioplasty and stent placement is a challenging procedure owing to the types and locations of lesions, the size of the vessels, and the angles between the aorta and the renal arteries. In addition, renal arteries are deep in the body, move with respiration, are poorly collateralized, and supply an organ that does not tolerate

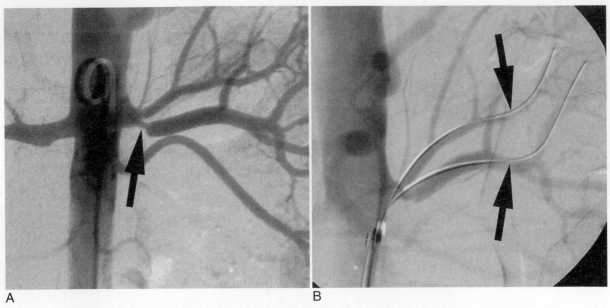

Figure 12-16 Early bifurcation of the left main renal artery with a proximal stenosis of the lower branch in a young patient with hypertension. **A**, DSA aortogram prior to angioplasty showing the proximal renal artery stenosis (arrow) that begins at the bifurcation of the renal artery. **B**, Aortic injection after angioplasty of the stenosis using the kissing technique (a small protective balloon in the upper artery and a 5-mm diameter balloon in the lower artery) showing the placement of the guidewires (arrows).

acute ischemia very well. In general, complications occur more frequently with stent placement (15% of patients) than with angioplasty alone (5–10% of patients) (Table 12-3). The lowest complication rates occur with angioplasty for FMD, and the highest with stent placement in patients with diffuse aortic and renal artery atherosclerosis. Hemodynamically significant angioplasty-induced renal artery dissection occurs in fewer than 5% of procedures, and can usually be treated with stent placement. The most severe complication, renal artery rupture, is

minimized when balloon sizes are carefully selected. Prompt recognition with reinflation of a balloon across the rupture is life-saving (Fig. 12-17). Once stabilized, either stent-graft placement or surgery can be considered. Complications may occur at any point during renal artery revascularization, and from balloons, stents, and even guidewires (Fig. 12-18). For this reason, meticulous attention to detail and technique is required throughout the procedure. Bilateral lesions, particularly in azotemic patients, can be treated several days apart in order to minimize contrast load.

The results of renal artery angioplasty must be considered separately for atherosclerosis and FMD. In addition the results for atherosclerotic lesions must be subdivided into proximal and ostial lesions, and hypertension must be considered differently than azotemia. The largest amount of data is available for patients treated for hypertension (Table 12-4). Angioplasty for FMD in patients with hypertension has the best results overall, with cure in almost 45% of patients in comparison to 10–15% of patients with atherosclerotic lesions. The results of angioplasty alone of ostial atherosclerotic lesions are poor. Metallic stents improve the technical and clinical outcomes in atherosclerotic disease, particularly for ostial lesions, but the clinical results are still less than that seen in angioplasty for FMD (Table 12-5). Unless complicated by a dissection, stents are not necessary for most forms of FMD.

Table 12-3 Complications of Renal Artery Angioplasty and Stents	
Complication	**Incidence (%)**
Death (30 days)	0.5
Renal artery rupture	<1
Renal artery thrombosis	<1
Cholesterol embolization (systemic)	1
Branch artery occlusion	3
Flow-limiting dissection	5
Renal failure	5
Puncture site[a]	5
Stent infection	Anecdotal

[a]Hematoma, pseudoaneurysm.

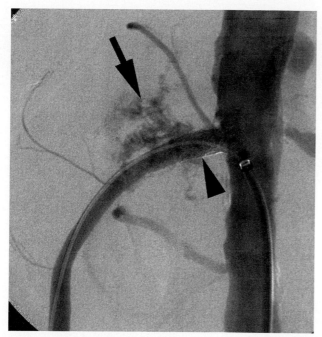

Figure 12-17   Renal artery rupture (arrow) during placement of a 6-mm diameter stent (arrowhead) in an elderly hypertensive female. This is a very rare complication, probably due to oversizing of the stent for this particular patient. After stent deployment the patient was hemodynamically stable and pain free; the rupture was only discovered on the completion angiogram. Note that the guidewire had been left in place until the final angiogram was obtained.

Angioplasty and stent placement for renal insufficiency has similar technical success rates as procedures performed for hypertension, but lower overall success rates (see Table 12-5). In patients with atherosclerotic lesions, normalization of serum creatinine is the exception,

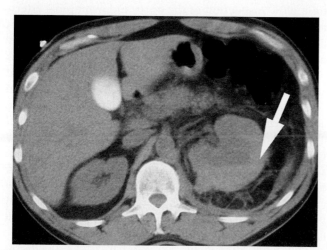

Figure 12-18   Renal capsular hematoma (arrow) presumably due to guidewire perforation of the kidney during angioplasty (same patient as Fig. 12-16). The patient developed flank pain several hours after the angioplasty.

Table 12-4	Results of Renal Artery Angioplasty in Hypertension	
Lesion	Technical Success (%)	Primary Clinical Success (%)[a]
Atherosclerosis (ostial)	40	50
Atherosclerosis (proximal)	85	70
Fibromuscular dysplasia[b]	90	85
Takayasu's arteritis	85	85[c]

[a]Hypertension improved or cured at 12 months.
[b]Primarily medial fibroplasia type.
[c]Limited number of patients.

with stabilization of renal function seen in approximately half of patients, improvement in about 20%, and continued deterioration in the remainder. The best clinical outcomes are in patients with bilateral proximal stenoses, serum creatinine <3.0 mg/dL, normal sized kidneys, and few comorbid diseases. The reason for these less impressive results in treatment of azotemia compared to hypertension is the multifactorial nature of renal insufficiency in these patients, who usually have diffuse atherosclerosis, diabetes, and chronic hypertension.

Intimal hyperplasia resulting in restenosis remains a major limitation of all renal artery interventions (percutaneous as well as surgical) (Fig. 12-19). Some degree of hyperplasia occurs after every intervention; therefore, the larger the initial postprocedural lumen, the better the long-term patency. When placing stents, the long-term results are best when the final diameter of the artery is 6 mm or more. Intimal hyperplasia leading to hemodynamically significant restenosis is seen in 10–15% of

Table 12-5	Results of Renal Artery Stents		
Lesion	Indication	Technical Success (%)	Primary Clinical Success (%)[a]
Atherosclerosis (ostial)	Hypertension	95	70
Atherosclerosis (proximal)	Hypertension	95	80
Atherosclerosis (ostial)	Azotemia	95	70
Atherosclerosis (proximal)	Azotemia	95	70

[a]At 12 months: Hypertension – cure or improved blood pressure control; Azotemia – stabilized or improved serum creatinine.

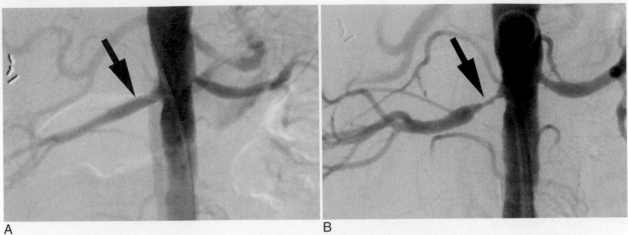

Figure 12-19   Recurrent stenosis of a renal artery stent due to intimal hyperplasia in a patient with hypertension. **A**, DSA after right renal artery stent placement (arrow) shows an excellent result. The patient had an excellent clinical response. **B**, DSA 6 months later – when the patient returned for evaluation of worsening hypertension – shows diffuse intimal hyperplasia causing stenosis within the stent (arrow). This was treated by placement of a second stent inside the first.

stents at one year. Covered stents, drug-eluting stents, brachytherapy, and distal protection devices are all being investigated to improve the outcomes of renal artery revascularization.

ACUTE RENAL ISCHEMIA

Acute occlusion of a normal main renal artery results in an ischemic kidney that must be revascularized within 60–90 minutes in order to preserve function ("warm ischemic time"). The normal kidney with normal vasculature has no collateral blood supply of clinical relevance. The most common etiology of acute occlusion in elderly patients is an embolus from a cardiac source, whereas trauma is usually the cause in the young (Box 12-6). Patients may complain of back pain, nausea, hematuria, and vomiting.

Box 12-6   Etiologies of Acute Renal Artery Occlusion

Embolus (cardiogenic)
Trauma
Aortic dissection
Spontaneous renal artery dissection
Iatrogenic
Hypercoagulable state
Thrombosis of existing stenosis
Thrombosis of renal artery aneurysm

Thrombosis of a chronic hemodynamically significant renal artery stenosis rarely results in immediate loss of the kidney. In most cases adequate collateral supply for renal preservation has developed prior to the occlusive event. Renal artery occlusion in these patients is frequently clinically silent.

The short warm ischemia time for kidneys precludes successful revascularization unless the patient happens to be undergoing surgery or angiography at the moment of occlusion. Nuclear medicine scans can be used to determine kidney perfusion in cases of suspected renal artery occlusion, but do not provide anatomic information when the etiology is unknown. CT or MRI with contrast allow inspection of the aorta and main renal artery, renal parenchyma, and adjacent soft tissue structures (see Fig. 10-35). Focal areas of abnormal perfusion may be seen in patients with peripheral arterial emboli, or main renal artery occlusion with patent accessory renal arteries (Fig. 12-20). CTA or MRA sequences may reveal aortic or renal artery dissection, evidence of multiple acute occlusions suggestive of emboli, or other structural abnormalities such as a renal artery aneurysm. At angiography, delayed filming well into the venous phase for both aortic injections and selective renal artery injections are necessary to detect distal reconstitution of the renal artery by collaterals (see Fig. 12-13). Both kidneys must be evaluated with selective injections, as bilateral renal artery emboli are found in almost a third of patients.

The management of acute renal artery occlusion depends on the etiology and timing. Occlusion due to dissection during angioplasty can be managed with stents if the true lumen can be entered distal to the dissection.

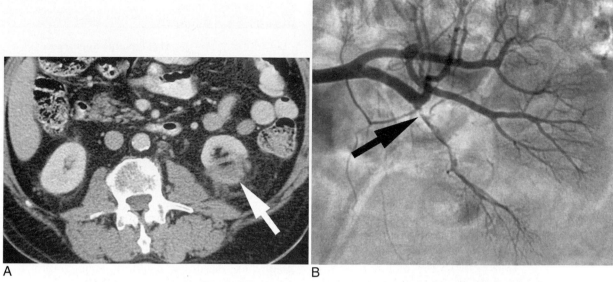

A   B

Figure 12-20   Focal renal infarction due to a small cardiac embolus. **A**, Axial CT image with contrast showing a focal area of inhomogeneous enhancement (arrow) with associated perinephric stranding in an elderly patient who had acute onset of left flank pain several days earlier. **B**, Selective left renal artery DSA showing a partially recanalized peripheral embolus (arrow).

Similarly, thrombosis during an intervention should be pursued aggressively with thrombolysis, mechanical displacement, or aspiration thrombectomy. Surgical revascularization may be necessary to avoid loss of the kidney.

RENAL ARTERY ANEURYSMS

Renal artery aneurysms are rare lesions, found in approximately 0.1% of patients undergoing angiography (Box 12-7). Nonspecific "degenerative" and FMD-related aneurysms are typically located at extraparenchymal locations and bifurcations of first- and second-order renal artery

branches in 90% of patients (Fig. 12-21). Aneurysms due to vasculitis (such as polyarteritis nodosa) or hematogenously disseminated infection occur in the peripheral intraparenchymal renal artery branches (see Fig. 1-14).

Degenerative aneurysms are symptomatic in fewer than 10% of patients, and fewer than 5% rupture (Fig. 12-22).

Box 12-7	Etiologies of Renal Artery Aneurysms

Fibromuscular dysplasia
Degenerative
Idiopathic
Vasculitis
    Polyarteritis nodosa (small arteries)
    Behçet's disease (large arteries)
Neoplasm (angiomyolipoma)
Trauma
Mycotic
Ehlers–Danlos syndrome
Iatrogenic (i.e., post-biopsy, angioplasty)

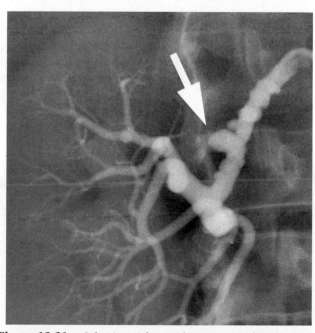

Figure 12-21   Selective right renal angiogram showing renal artery aneurysm (arrow) due to FMD (medial fibroplasia).

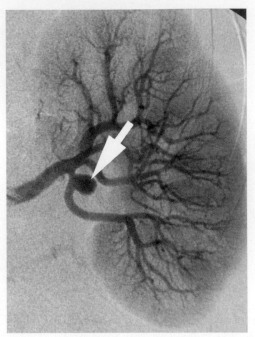

Figure 12-22 Degenerative renal artery aneurysm. Selective left renal DSA showing the typical appearance of a degenerative renal artery aneurysm (arrow).

The risk of rupture is increased when the diameter of the aneurysm is ≥2.0 cm, and in pregnant patients. Calcification of the aneurysm wall is believed to be somewhat protective. Rupture has a mortality rate of 10% in nonpregnant patients, but 55% in those who are pregnant. Other complications of renal artery aneurysms include spontaneous dissection, renal infarction due to emboli, hypertension due to compression of the renal artery, flank pain, and spontaneous arteriovenous fistula.

Large renal artery aneurysms may be detected by any of the cross-sectional imaging modalities. CT and MR allow assessment of the size of the aneurysm, presence of mural thrombus, and renal infarcts (see Fig. 3-16). Calcification of the aneurysm wall is believed to be a secondary rather than primary process. The other visceral

---

Box 12-8 Indications for Intervention in Renal Artery Aneurysms

Rupture
Size ≥2.0 cm
Renovascular hypertension
Expansion
Distal embolization
Symptomatic dissection
Flank pain
Woman of childbearing age/pregnancy

Table 12-6 Benign Renal Neoplasms

Lesion	Angiographic Appearance
Angiomyolipoma	Neovascularity, bizarre aneurysms, no shunting
Oncocytoma	Hypervascular mass, spoke-wheel appearance of arteries, central scar, no shunting
Adenoma	Sharply defined vascular mass, may have neovascularity, no shunting

---

arteries should be carefully inspected, as multiple aneurysms are present in a minority of cases. Small and intraparenchymal renal artery aneurysms require angiography for definitive diagnosis. Angiography may also reveal characteristic findings of FMD.

The indications for treatment of these rare and usually asymptomatic lesions must be individualized for each patient (Box 12-8). The traditional approach to extraparenchymal aneurysms is an attempt at surgical reconstruction, often requiring bench surgery.

Exclusion with small stent-grafts will be an attractive alternative in the future. Intraparenchymal aneurysms are managed with control of the underlying disease process or nephrectomy. Saccular aneurysms that have discrete necks can be treated with coil embolization in a fashion analogous to intracranial aneurysms.

NEOPLASM

A broad range of benign and malignant neoplasms can occur in the kidney (Tables 12-6 and 12-7). Although the

---

Table 12-7 Malignant Renal Neoplasms

Lesion	Angiographic Appearance
Renal cell carcinoma	Variable, but most often prominent neovascularity[a], mass effect, hypervascularity, shunting, +/− venous invasion
Transitional cell carcinoma	Neovascularity, mild hypervascularity, encasement; shunting unusual
Wilms' tumor	Hypo- or avascular mass, mild neovascularity, displacement, encasement
Lymphoma	Avascular mass, displacement of intrarenal branches
Metastatic carcinoma	Hypervascular (melanoma, sarcoma) Avascular (lung, breast, bowel)

[a]Avascular in 6%.

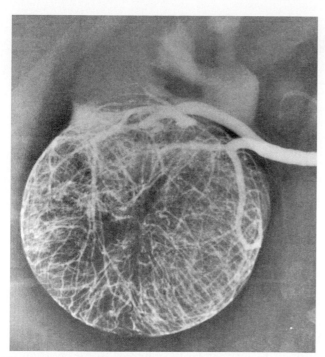

Figure 12-23 Renal oncocytoma in a patient with dual renal arteries. The mass is supplied entirely by the lower renal artery. Note the typical "spoke-wheel" pattern of neovascularity and the sharply defined borders of the mass. (Image courtesy of Frederick Keller M.D., Dotter Interventional Institute, Portland, OR.)

most common benign mass lesions of the kidney are simple renal cysts, the most common benign neoplasms are adenomas. Renal adenomas are usually small (<3 cm) tumors that can be histologically inseparable from well-differentiated renal cell carcinomas. They occur in the same population as renal cell carcinomas. Often found incidentally on cross-sectional imaging, the slow growth and lack of metastases suggests the benign nature of these lesions, but excision is usually performed.

Oncocytomas are sharply defined benign lesions that tend to be larger than adenomas, and more vascular. Similar lesions are found in endocrine and exocrine organs such as the thyroid and pancreas (Fig. 12-23). Definitive diagnosis requires excision.

Angiomyolipomas are hamartomatous lesions that contain fat, smooth muscle, and blood vessels (Fig. 12-24). The typical patient is a female aged 30–60 years. Multiple and bilateral lesions are found in up to 80% of patients with tuberous sclerosis. When small (<3 cm), these lesions are usually asymptomatic. Large lesions can extend outside the kidney. Acute spontaneous hemorrhage is a well-recognized complication of these lesions.

In adults, renal cell carcinomas comprise over 80% of all malignant renal masses, with transitional cell carcinoma of the pelvis (8–10%), nephroblastoma (Wilms' tumor) (5–6%), and miscellaneous sarcomas (2–3%)

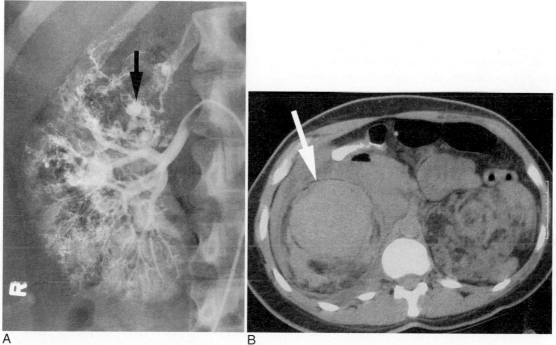

A   B

Figure 12-24 Renal angiomyolipomas. **A,** Selective right renal angiogram showing multiple hypervascular masses within the right kidney. The hypervascularity with aneurysms (arrow) is typical for angiomyolipoma. **B,** The same patient several months later after sudden onset of right flank pain. There is a large hematoma (arrow) arising from the upper-pole angiomyolipoma with associated retroperitoneal blood. The patient underwent successful embolization of the mass.

Table 12-8 Staging of Renal Cell Carcinoma

Stage	Definition	TNM
I	Tumor <2.5 cm confined by renal capsule	T1
	Tumor ≥2.5 cm confined by renal capsule	T2
II	Tumor extends beyond capsule or into ipsilateral adrenal gland but still within Gerota's fascia	T3a
IIIa	Renal vein involvement	T3b
	Renal vein and IVC involvement	T3c
IIIb	Lymph node involvement	
	Single node <2 cm	N1
	Single node >2 cm but <5 cm, or multiple nodes <5 cm diameter	N2
	Node >5 cm or fixed nodes	N3
	Juxtaregional nodes	N4
IIIc	Venous involvement plus nodal involvement	T3, 4; N1–4
IVa	Spread to contiguous organs (except ipsilateral adrenal)	T4a
IVb	Distant metastases	T4; M1

TNM, Tumor, Nodes, Metastases; IVC, inferior vena cava.

accounting for the remainder (Fig. 12-25). Renal cell carcinomas are more common in males than females, may be multiple when associated with von Hippel–Lindau disease, and are typically found in patients 40 years or older. A clinical grading system has been developed to describe renal cell carcinomas (Table 12-8). Tumor invasion of the renal vein or IVC in the absence of metastasis has a 5-year survival rate of approximately 50% in patients undergoing radical nephrectomy with complete removal of IVC thrombus.

Although Wilms' tumor is primarily a childhood lesion, a second peak incidence occurs in the sixth decade. As with renal cell carcinoma, this tumor is found more often in males than females.

The role of vascular imaging in the diagnosis of renal masses is limited, as cross-sectional imaging with US, CT, and MR can detect and characterize most lesions. A detailed discussion of the diagnostic features of renal masses is beyond the scope of this chapter. However, certain characteristic features are important to remember. Angiomyolipomas are distinctive because of the fat contained within the mass and the propensity for hemorrhage. Oncocytomas are hypervascular well-circumscribed masses, with central hypovascular area. Adenomas are smaller lesions, sharply defined with homogeneous enhancement. Venous invasion by any renal mass is highly indicative of malignancy, particularly renal cell carcinoma, although intravenous extension of angiomyolipoma has been reported. Venous invasion can be mimicked by inflow of unopacified blood from hepatic veins on CT; delayed images may be helpful to resolve this issue. Invasion of adjacent structures by a mass represents presumptive evidence of malignancy until proven otherwise. Lymphoma results in diffuse enlargement of the kidney without hypervascularity, whereas some portion of normal kidney is usually identifiable even with large malignant lesions.

Angiography is usually performed for intervention rather than diagnosis. An aortogram followed by selective injection of the renal arteries is required for complete staging of the arterial supply. Historically, selective intraarterial injection of 6–10 µg of epinephrine prior to contrast was used to constrict normal vessels so that the abnormal tumor vessels would be more evident. The availability of magnification DSA with rapid filming has limited the need for epinephrine renal angiography.

Occasionally it is necessary to perform IVC cavography and selective renal venography to exclude the presence of venous invasion. The origin of a retroperitoneal tumor is sometimes uncertain from cross-sectional imaging. Selective injection of renal and other visceral arteries can help identify the dominant arterial blood supply, and thus the organ of origin (see Fig. 1-25).

Angiographic intervention for benign neoplasms is unusual with the exception of angiomyolipomas that have bled spontaneously. Embolization of these masses with permanent particles or alcohol is an excellent alternative to resection. Careful follow-up with CT to confirm resorption of the hematoma and shrinkage of the mass is necessary. The uninvolved kidney should be studied as well to exclude multiple lesions.

The typical indication for angiographic intervention in renal cell carcinoma is preoperative embolization of the tumor (see Fig. 12-25). Large renal cell cancers, and those with venous invasion, can be difficult to resect owing to the extremely vascular nature of the mass. In these cases, embolization of the entire kidney prior to resection can reduce blood loss significantly. The timing

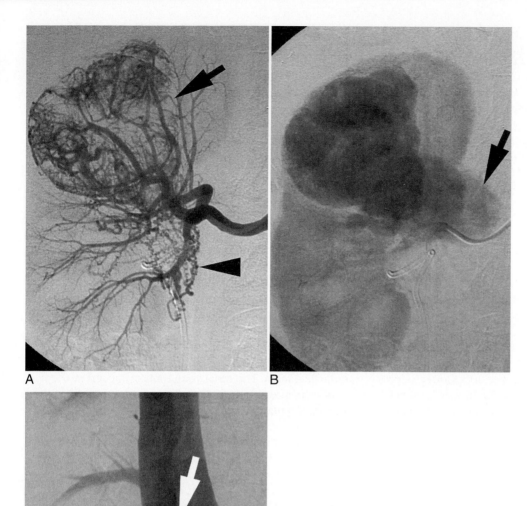

Figure 12-25   Renal cell carcinoma. **A,** Selective right renal artery DSA showing a hypervascular mass (arrow) with wild neovascularity in the upper pole of the kidney. There is hypertrophy of the peripelvic arteries (arrowhead) which provide collateral supply to the tumor. A ureteral stent is in place. **B,** Later image from the same angiogram showing extension of tumor thrombus into the right renal vein (arrow). The kidney was embolized first with Gelfoam pledgets and then coils in the distal main renal artery. **C,** Inferior vena cavogram of the same patient showing tumor thrombus (arrow) growing out of the right renal vein orifice. Note the coils in the distal main renal artery (arrowhead).

for embolization varies from one center to another, but is generally performed within 24 hours of the surgery. Embolization 4–6 weeks in advance was once advocated because of theoretical induction of an autoimmune response, but is now rarely practiced. The goal of embolization is devascularization of the tumor or kidney. For this reason, peripheral embolization is preferred. Small particles such as Ivalon, acrylic spheres, Gelfoam powder, or Gelfoam pledgets can be used. The choice of particle size should be based upon the presence of arteriovenous shunts and the rapidity desired for the embolization. Smaller particles will result in a longer procedure but a more peripheral embolization. Alcohol ablation using a balloon occlusion catheter for control in the main renal artery is favored by many interventionalists (Fig. 12-26). The volume of absolute alcohol required depends on the size and vascularity of the mass. At the termination of the embolization a few coils may be placed deep in the main renal artery. Coils placed in the proximal renal artery can be displaced into the aorta during surgical manipulation of the kidney. If coils are placed, the surgeon should be alerted to their presence.

RENAL TRANSPLANTATION

Evaluation of the renal vasculature is an essential component of the work-up of living donors, and frequently required when a transplanted kidney malfunctions or fails. The objectives of vascular imaging are different in each group. Vascular interventions are usually only necessary following transplantation.

The imaging of living renal donors is focused on detection of exclusionary vascular and parenchymal abnormalities or anomalies (Box 12-9). The left kidney is preferred by most surgeons because of the longer renal vein. In the past, when only open nephrectomy was performed, interest in the arterial anatomy was far greater than in the renal veins. However, with laparoscopic donor nephrectomy, information about renal vein anatomy is of great importance. Most centers rely heavily on CT/CTA

Box 12-9   Goals of Vascular Imaging of Renal Donors
Number of renal arteries Length of main renal arteries (preferred >2 cm) Quality of renal artery (presence of atherosclerosis or other pathology) Renal vein anatomy Quality of aorta

or MR/MRA, as these modalities provide information about renal parenchyma and the collection system in addition to the vascular structures (see Figs 12-3 and 12-5). Angiography is obtained when other imaging studies are unsatisfactory or unavailable. Flush aortography usually suffices with a slight left anterior obliquity, although the threshold for selective angiography should be low in this patient population.

Transplanted kidneys are usually placed in the recipient's iliac fossa. The renal vein is anastomosed to the iliac vein in an end-to-side fashion. Short saphenous or gonadal vein grafts may be necessary when the donor renal vein is inadequate. A variety of arterial anastomoses may be used, depending on the anatomy of the donor arteries and the recipient. Renal arteries of kidneys from living donors are usually anastomosed to recipient internal iliac artery in an end-to-end fashion, or end-to-side to the external iliac artery. Renal arteries from cadaveric donor kidneys may be anastomosed in similar fashions, or may include a portion of the donor aorta (termed a "Carrel patch"). This patch simplifies management of kidneys with multiple renal arteries, as the patch can be anastomosed directly to the external iliac artery rather than deal with each small artery separately. When performing imaging or interventions on renal transplants it is critically important to know the details of the surgery.

The indications for vascular imaging of the transplanted kidney include deterioration of renal function and hypertension. The goal of imaging in these patients is to find a correctable vascular cause of symptoms. In many cases there is already some degree of renal dysfunction, and patients are on nephrotoxic immunosuppressive drugs such as cyclosporine. For these reasons, the initial examination in most patients is US with duplex color-flow. In addition to vascular information, the collecting system and perinephric tissues can be examined as well. Alternatively, MRA has proven very useful in detection of arterial and venous abnormalities (see Fig. 3-16). This modality allows evaluation of the arterial inflow from the aorta to the renal artery, and the venous outflow from the kidney to the IVC. Angiography can be performed with nonionic contrast following pretreatment with renal

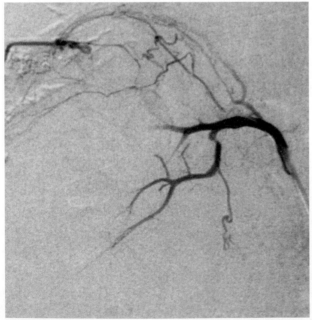

Figure 12-26   Typical angiographic appearance following alcohol embolization of a right kidney for tumor, showing branchless vessels with lack of parenchymal or tumor stain.

Table 12-9 Vascular Complications of Renal Transplantation

Complication	Incidence (%)
Renal artery stenosis	5-10
Renal artery thrombosis	1-2
Renal vein thrombosis	1-2
Post-biopsy pseudoaneurysm	1-2
Post-biopsy arteriovenous fistula	1-2
Anastomotic pseudoaneurysm	<1

protective agents, or alternative contrast agents such as CO_2 or gadolinium. Knowledge of the surgical anatomy helps determine the angiographic approach (contralateral femoral access is preferred when the anastomosis is to the internal iliac artery). Complex oblique views may be necessary to visualize the transplant artery.

Vascular complications occur in up to 15% of patients with renal artery transplants (Table 12-9). Acute renal artery thrombosis usually occurs within the first month of transplantation, and is associated with loss of the kidney in over 90% of patients owing to the lack of collateral supply to the transplanted kidney. Causes of thrombosis include technical factors related to the surgery, rejection, and postoperative hemodynamic instability. Late thrombosis is usually due to rejection or renal artery stenosis. Emergent surgical thrombectomy is usually required for renal salvage, although percutaneous mechanical techniques such as suction thrombectomy or thrombolysis may be indicated in selected cases.

Hemodynamically significant stenoses can also occur at any point in the arterial inflow to the kidney, including the common iliac artery (Fig. 12-27). Transplant renal artery stenosis usually occurs at the surgical anastomosis (Fig. 12-28; see also Fig. 3-16). Focal web-like stenoses immediately adjacent to the anastomosis are believed to be hyperplastic lesions related to the intraoperative placement of clamps. Extensive intrarenal artery stenoses are seen in chronic rejection, poorly controlled hypertension, diabetes, and atherosclerotic disease (see Fig. 12-9). Angioplasty with or without stent placement of transplant renal arteries has a technical success rate of approximately 90%, with a 1-year clinical success rate of approximately 75% for hypertension and 85% for renal function. When the stenosis is in a proximal inflow vessel, the long-term results are even better.

The presence of an anastomotic pseudoaneurysm should raise the suspicion of infection (Fig. 12-29). Pseudoaneurysms in the renal parenchyma are usually related to percutaneous biopsy. Patients may present with a retroperitoneal hematoma, hematuria, renal dysfunction, or a pulsatile mass. Embolization is the preferred treatment, as this allows maximal sparing of the renal

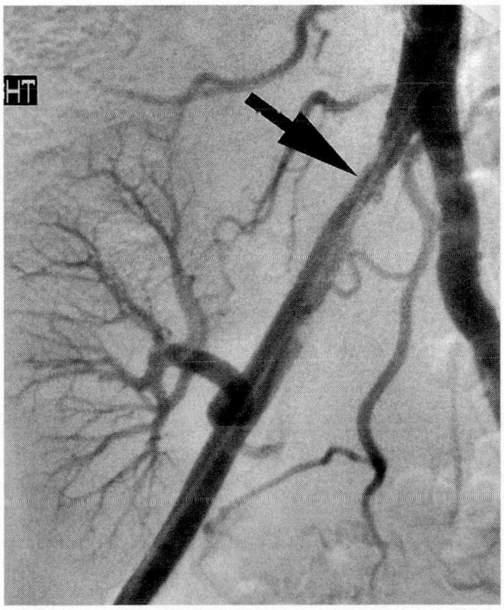

Figure 12-27 Common iliac artery (CIA) stenosis proximal to a renal transplant in a patient with new-onset hypertension. DSA of the pelvis shows focal right CIA stenosis (arrow) which produced a 46-mmHg gradient. The transplant renal artery was normal in other views. The gradient was eliminated after stent placement in the common iliac artery and the patient's hypertension resolved.

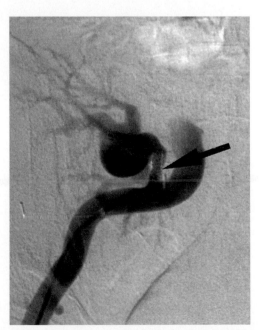

Figure 12-28 Stent placement (arrow) in a stenotic transplant renal artery. See Fig. 3-16 for preintervention images.

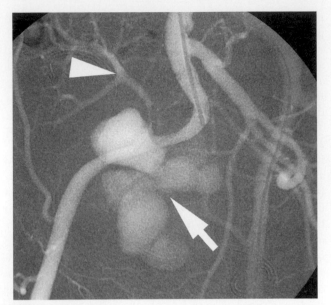

Figure 12-29 Mycotic pseudoaneurysm (arrow) of the arterial anastomosis of a transplanted kidney (arrowhead). The wild, multilobulated appearance is characteristic of mycotic pseudoaneurysms.

parenchyma (Fig. 12-30). This is important, as most of these patients are biopsied because of suspected rejection as manifested by deterioration of renal function. The use of super-selective 3-French coaxial catheters permits precise deployment of microcoils or glue near the origin of the pseudoaneurysm.

Arteriovenous fistulas in transplant kidneys are typically the result of percutaneous biopsies. These lesions may occur alone or in conjunction with a pseudoaneurysm. The treatment is the same as for pseudoaneurysms, with the goal to preserve as much renal parenchyma as possible.

Venous thrombosis occurs early within the post-transplant period. Patients present with renal dysfunction, pain, hematuria, and proteinuria. Loss of the transplanted kidney is common. Late renal vein stenoses are rarely diagnosed, but may respond to angioplasty or stent placement.

TRAUMA

The renal artery is injured in approximately 7% of penetrating abdominal wounds and in 4% of patients with major blunt trauma. The incidence of iatrogenic renal vascular trauma is not known, although it is thought to occur in as many as 2% of percutaneous nephrostomy

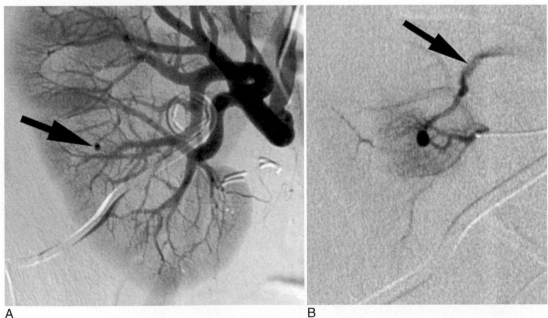

A   B

Figure 12-30 Iatrogenic renal artery injury in a transplant kidney. The patient presented with anuria and acute clot obstruction of the renal pelvis and ureter one day after a percutaneous renal biopsy. The bleeding persisted after percutaneous placement of a nephrostomy tube. **A**, Transplant renal artery DSA showing a small pseudoaneurysm (arrow) in the region of the biopsy. **B**, Super-selective DSA prior to embolization showing that there is also an arteriovenous fistula (arrow on vein).

Table 12-10   Renal Injury Scale

Grade	Definition	Description
I	Contusion	Hematuria without visible injury
	Hematoma	Subcapsular, stable, no parenchymal injury
II	Hematoma	Stable perirenal hematoma
	Laceration	<1.0-cm depth renal cortex, no urinary extravasation
III	Laceration	>1.0-cm depth renal cortex, urinary extravasation
IV	Hematoma	Laceration involves cortex, medulla, and collecting system
	Vascular	Main renal artery and/or vein injury, contained hemorrhage
V	Laceration	Shattered kidney
	Vascular	Avulsion of renal hilum with devascularized kidney

procedures. These patients present with brisk arterial bleeding from the nephrostomy tube tract during catheter exchanges, arterial bleeding into the collecting system, or in rare instances massive retroperitoneal hematoma. In cases of blunt trauma, almost 80% of injuries consist of renal contusions or small corticomedullary lacerations with an intact renal capsule. The renal capsule is disrupted in 17% of lacerations, of which 7% communicate with the collecting system. Renal pedicle disruption and/or fragmentation of the kidney occur in only 3% of cases. A classification scheme for blunt trauma to the kidney has been developed to facilitate management decisions (Table 12-10). Patients with grade I injuries are usually managed conservatively, whereas patients with grade V injuries frequently require surgery. Patients with intermediate grade injuries often require angiographic interventions.

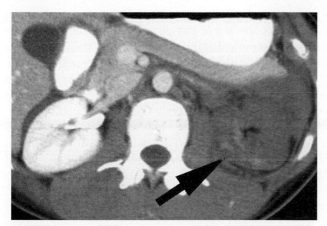

Figure 12-31   Traumatic left renal artery thrombosis after a motor vehicle accident (car + alcohol + tree). Axial CT image with contrast showing lack of perfusion of the left kidney (arrow) and a perinephric hematoma.

Patients with renal trauma are at risk of injury to multiple abdominal organs. CT scanning is the preferred imaging modality for these patients in most trauma centers. The grade of the renal injury can be established quickly in most patients, based on the CT findings. A nonenhancing renal artery and kidney indicates thrombosis of the main renal artery due to dissection or transection (Fig. 12-31). Active extravasation and pseudo-aneurysms may be seen in patients with fractured kidneys or penetrating trauma. Angiography is obtained when the diagnosis of a correctable vascular injury is uncertain, ongoing retroperitoneal bleeding that is amenable to embolization is suspected, or in patients with persistent hematuria (Fig. 12-32). Flush aortography is essential to determine the basic renal vascular anatomy and detect associated aortic, lumbar artery, and mesenteric artery injuries. Selective renal angiography is then performed to study the kidney. When evaluating a patient for suspected arterial injury related to percutaneous nephrostomy, temporary removal of the tube over a guidewire may be necessary to visualize the injury.

The full range of vascular injuries can be seen in patients with renal trauma (see Figs 12-30 through 12-32). Selective embolization of extravasation, pseudoaneurysms, and arteriovenous fistulas is efficacious and spares more renal parenchyma than would be possible with open repair. Permanent agents that can be precisely deposited, such as coils or glue, are used in most cases. The use of microcatheters allows super selective embolization. However, in cases of massive extravasation and a hemodynamically unstable patient, rapid control of hemorrhage is more important than maximizing preservation of renal tissue. Embolization is successful in controlling bleeding in more than 95% of patients.

In some circumstances main renal artery dissections and obstructive intimal flaps can be ameliorated with

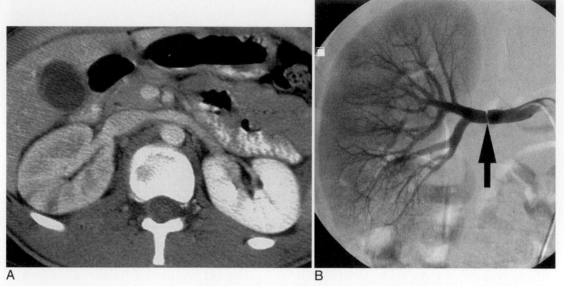

Figure 12-32   Focal intimal injury due to blunt trauma. **A**, Contrast-enhanced CT showing decreased enhancement of the right kidney relative to the left. **B**, Selective right renal DSA (an aortogram was obtained first) showing a focal circumferential intimal injury (arrow) in the main renal artery.

stents. The likelihood of preservation of renal function with surgical bypass or percutaneous recanalization of thrombosed renal arteries is very low.

ARTERIOVENOUS MALFORMATIONS AND FISTULAS

Congenital renal arteriovenous malformation (AVM) is rare in the general population, with an incidence of approximately 4 per 10,000 individuals. Arteriovenous fistulas (AVFs) are almost always acquired, although the patient may not recall a specific incident. Over 70% of AVFs are directly related to trauma or iatrogenic misadventures.

The majority of AVMs and AVFs are asymptomatic, and remain so throughout the life of the patient. Many post-traumatic AVFs close spontaneously. Symptomatic patients present with hematuria (72%), hypertension (more common with AVFs due to the "steal" phenomenon), and flank pain. Less common symptoms include high-output cardiac failure and spontaneous retroperitoneal hemorrhage.

Large lesions may be visible on CT or MR studies, but in general these examinations are most useful to exclude more common causes of hematuria, such as mass lesions or calculae. Angiography is required for the definitive diagnosis of renal AVMs and AVFs. Following flush aortography, selective angiography should be performed.

When extremely high-flow lesions are present, balloon occlusion angiography may be necessary to adequately visualize the lesion.

Percutaneous embolization with coils, glue, or alcohol is the preferred treatment for most symptomatic lesions (Fig. 12-33). Surgery for very large AVFs may be necessary when appropriate embolic agents are not available.

RENAL ABLATION

Intentional ablation of a functioning or nonfiltering but hormonally active kidney can be accomplished with transcatheter embolization provided that the renal artery is patent. Indications include intractable renal bleeding due to unresectable tumors, nephrotic syndrome with unmanageable proteinuria, and severe hypertension related to a nonfiltering kidney. Global embolization of the kidney with small particles or alcohol is usually effective. Placement of a few coils in the main renal artery without distal embolization may result in delayed reperfusion of the offending organ.

PHEOCHROMOCYTOMA

Pheochromocytoma is a functional adrenal tumor that can cause severe and unpredictable hypertension. These tumors are typically 2 cm or greater in size, and are

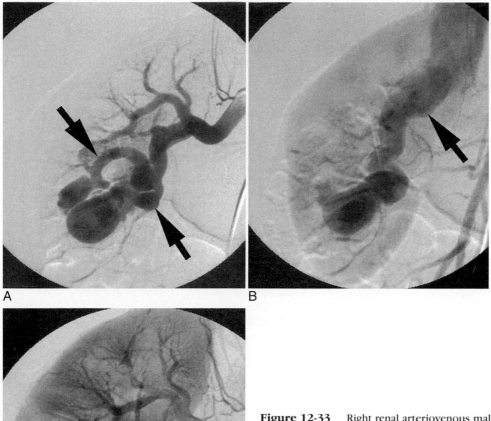

Figure 12-33   Right renal arteriovenous malformation in a teenage female presenting with intermittent gross hematuria and clot colic. **A**, Selective right renal DSA showing dilated lower-pole segmental renal arteries (arrows) with shunting to large veins through multiple small communications. **B**, Later image from the same injection showing dense opacification of the right renal vein (arrow). **C**, DSA following coil embolization (arrows) of the two large feeding arteries showing absent filling of the malformation.

diagnosed by CT, MRI, or ^{131}I-meta-iodobenzylguanidine (MIBG) nuclear medicine scans. Extraadrenal, metastatic, and bilateral pheochromocytomas are each found with an incidence of 10%. Adrenal pheochromocytomas secrete epinephrine and norepinephrine. Primary pheochromocytomas located outside the adrenal gland are termed "paragangliomas," are more likely to be malignant, and secrete only norepinephrine. Common extraadrenal locations are the renal hilum, the vicinity of the origin of the inferior mesenteric artery (Organ of Zuckerkandl), the bladder wall, and the posterior mediastinum.

Hypertensive crisis can be precipitated by contrast during angiography. Pretreatment with phenoxybenzamine (10 mg p.o. b.i.d. initially and increased to 20–40 mg p o b.i.d. until blood pressure is controlled), and careful procedural monitoring by an anesthesiologist is recommended whenever a patient with suspected pheochromocytoma receives iodinated contrast. Acute hypertensive crisis can be controlled with intravenous nitroprusside or 5 mg of phentolamine. Pheochromocytomas have a characteristic intense, prolonged parenchymal blush on arteriography (Fig. 12-34).

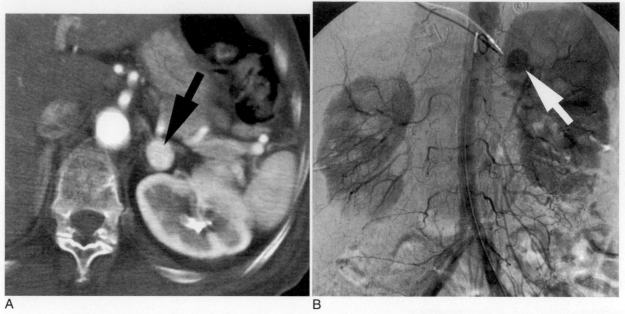

Figure 12-34   Pheochromocytoma in an elderly patient with severe hypertension. **A**, Axial image from contrast-enhanced CT scan showing what was thought to be a focal renal artery aneurysm (arrow) but is actually a densely enhancing adrenal mass. **B**, Late-phase DSA aortogram performed to evaluate the presumed renal artery aneurysm, showing a densely enhancing and staining left adrenal mass (arrow). The renal artery was normal. The angiogram was terminated after the first injection.

SUGGESTED READINGS

Bakal CW, Cynamon J, Lakritz PS, Sprayregen S: Value of preoperative renal artery embolization in reducing blood transfusion requirements during nephrectomy for renal cell carcinoma. *J Vasc Interv Radiol* 4:727-731, 1993.

Behar JV, Nelson RC, Zidar JP, De Long DM, Smith TP: Thin-section multidetector CT angiography of renal artery stents. *Am J Roentgenol* 178:1155-1159, 2002.

Bernstein MR, Malkowicz SB, Siegelman ES et al: Progressive angiomyolipoma with inferior vena cava tumor thrombus. *Urology* 50:975-977, 1997.

Blum U, Krumme B, Flugel P et al: Treatment of ostial renal-artery stenoses with vascular endoprostheses after unsuccessful balloon angioplasty. *N Engl J Med* 36:459-465, 1997.

Carlos RC, Dong Q, Stanley JC, Prince MR: MR angiography after renal revascularization: spectrum of expected anatomic results and postintervention complications. *Radiographics* 19:1555-1568, 1999.

Cocheteux B, Mounier-Vehier C, Gaxotte V et al: Rare variations in renal anatomy and blood supply: CT appearances and embryological background. A pictorial essay. *Eur Radiol* 11: 779-786, 2001.

Dinkel HP, Danuser H, Triller J: Blunt renal trauma: minimally invasive management with microcatheter embolization experience in nine patients. *Radiology* 223:723-730, 2002.

Dong Q, Schoenberg SO, Carlos RC et al: Diagnosis of renal vascular disease with MR angiography. *Radiographics* 19:1535-1554, 1999.

Golwyn DH, Routh WD, Chen MY, Lorentz WB, Dyer RB: Percutaneous transcatheter renal ablation with absolute ethanol for uncontrolled hypertension or nephrotic syndrome: results in 11 patients with end-stage renal disease. *J Vasc Interv Radiol* 8:527-533, 1997.

Goodman DN, Saibil EA, Kodama RT: Traumatic intimal tear of the renal artery treated by insertion of a Palmaz stent. *Cardiovasc Interv Radiol* 21:69-72, 1998.

Hagiwara A, Sakaki S, Goto H et al: The role of interventional radiology in the management of blunt renal injury: a practical protocol. *J Trauma* 51:526-531, 2001.

Halpern EJ, Mitchell DG, Wechsler RJ et al: Preoperative evaluation of living renal donors: comparison of CT angiography and MR angiography. *Radiology* 216:434-439, 2000.

Harden PN, MacLeod MJ, Rodger RS et al: Effect of renal-artery stenting on progression of renovascular renal failure. *Lancet* 349:1133-1136, 1997.

Henke PK, Cardneau JD, Welling TH et al: Renal artery aneurysms: a 35-year clinical experience with 252 aneurysms in 168 patients. *Ann Surg* 234:454-462, 2001.

Hohenwalter MD, Skowlund CJ, Erickson SJ et al: Renal transplant evaluation with MR angiography and MR imaging. *Radiographics* 21:1505-1517, 2001.

Ivanovic V, McKusick MA, Johnson CM et al: Renal artery stent placement: complications at a single tertiary care center. *J Vasc Interv Radiol* 14:217-225, 2003.

Kawashima A, Sandler CM, Corl FM et al: Imaging of renal trauma: a comprehensive review. *Radiographics* 21:557-574, 2001.

Kebebew E, Duh QY: Benign and malignant pheochromocytoma: diagnosis, treatment, and follow-up. *Surg Oncol Clin N Am* 7:765-789, 1998.

Klingler HC, Klingler PJ, Martin JK et al: Pheochromocytoma. *Urology* 57:1025-1032, 2001.

Lacombe M: Isolated spontaneous dissection of the renal artery. *J Vasc Surg* 33:385-391, 2001.

Lee W, Kim TS, Chung JW et al: Renal angiomyolipoma: embolotherapy with a mixture of alcohol and iodized oil. *J Vasc Interv Radiol* 9:255-261, 1998.

Mallouhi A, Rieger M, Czermak B et al: Volume-rendered multi-detector CT angiography: noninvasive follow-up of patients treated with renal artery stents. *Am J Roentgenol* 180: 233-239, 2003.

Moresco KP, Patel NH, Namyslowski J et al: Carbon dioxide angiography of the transplanted kidney: technical considerations and imaging findings. *Am J Roentgenol* 171:1271-1276, 1998.

Morris CS, Bonnevie GJ, Najarian KE: Nonsurgical treatment of acute iatrogenic renal artery injuries occurring after renal artery angioplasty and stenting. *Am J Roentgenol* 177: 1353-1357, 2001.

Murphy TP, Rundback JH, Cooper C, Kiernan MS: Chronic renal ischemia: implications for cardiovascular disease risk. *J Vasc Interv Radiol* 13:1187-1198, 2002.

Pantuck AJ, Zisman A, Belldegrun AS: The changing natural history of renal cell carcinoma. *J Urol* 166:1611-1623, 2001.

Perini S, Gordon RL, La Berge JM et al: Transcatheter embolization of biopsy-related vascular injury in the transplant kidney: immediate and long-term outcome. *J Vasc Interv Radiol* 9:1011-1019, 1998.

Radermacher J, Chavan A, Bleck J et al: Use of Doppler ultrasonography to predict the outcome of therapy for renal-artery stenosis. *N Engl J Med* 344:410-417, 2001.

Ramos F, Kotliar C, Alvarez D et al: Renal function and outcome of PTRA and stenting for atherosclerotic renal artery stenosis *Kidney Int* 63:276-282, 2003.

Rees CR: Stents for atherosclerotic renovascular disease. *J Vasc Interv Radiol* 10:689-705, 1999.

Ruggenenti P, Mosconi L, Bruno S et al: Post-transplant renal artery stenosis: the hemodynamic response to revascularization. *Kidney Int* 60:309-318, 2001.

Rundback JH, Gray RJ, Rozenblit G et al: Renal artery stent placement for the management of ischemic nephropathy. *J Vasc Interv Radiol* 9:413-420, 1998.

Rundback JH, Sacks D, Kent KC et al: Guidelines for the reporting of renal artery revascularization in clinical trials. American Heart Association. *Circulation* 106:1572-1585, 2002.

Rundback JH, Murphy TP, Cooper C, Weintraub JL: Chronic renal ischemia: pathophysiologic mechanisms of cardiovascular and renal disease. *J Vasc Interv Radiol* 13:1085-1092, 2002.

Safian RD, Textor SC: Renal-artery stenosis. *N Engl J Med* 344:431-442, 2001.

Schlansky-Goldberg RD: Renal transplantation. In Baum S ed: *Abram's Angiography*, 4th edn, Little Brown, Boston, 1325-1351, 1997.

Spinosa DJ, Isaacs RB, Matsumoto AH et al: Angiographic evaluation and treatment of transplant renal artery stenosis. *Curr Opin Urol* 11:197-205, 2001.

Takebayashi S, Hosaka M, Kubota Y et al: Transarterial embolization and ablation of renal arteriovenous malformations: efficacy and damages in 30 patients with long-term followup. *J Urol* 159:696-701, 1998.

Tikkakoski T, Paivansalo M, Alanen A et al: Radiologic findings in renal oncocytoma. *Acta Radiol* 32:363-367, 1991.

Tsuji Y, Goto A, Hara I et al: Renal cell carcinoma with extension of tumor thrombus into the vena cava: surgical strategy and prognosis. *J Vasc Surg* 33:789-796, 2001.

Urban BA, Ratner LE, Fishman EK: Three-dimensional volume-rendered CT angiography of the renal arteries and veins: normal anatomy, variants, and clinical applications. *Radiographics* 21:373-386, 2001.

van de Ven PJ, Kaatee R, Beutler JJ et al: Arterial stenting and balloon angioplasty in ostial atherosclerotic renovascular disease: a randomised trial. *Lancet* 353:282-286, 1999.

Verschuyl EJ, Kaatee R, Beek FJ et al: Renal artery origins: best angiographic projection angles. *Radiology* 205:115-120, 1997.

Yutan E, Glickerman DJ, Caps MT et al: Percutaneous transluminal revascularization for renal artery stenosis: Veterans Affairs Puget Sound Health Care System experience. *J Vasc Surg* 34:685-693, 2001.

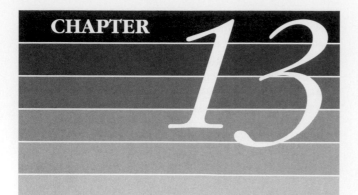

CHAPTER 13

Inferior Vena Cava and Tributaries

JOHN A. KAUFMAN, M.D.

The inferior vena cava (IVC) and its tributaries are frequent sites of vascular pathology. Diseases of the organs that have their venous drainage into the IVC may first become clinically apparent when the cava becomes involved. Imaging and intervention in the IVC are prominent components of current vascular and interventional radiology practice.

NORMAL ANATOMY

The IVC is formed by the confluence of the common iliac veins at the level of the L5 vertebral body (Fig. 13-1). In the abdomen, the IVC is usually located to the right of the midline and the aorta, anterior to the lumbar and lower thoracic spine. The IVC is a posterior structure for much of its course. The retrohepatic IVC resides in a groove or tunnel in the bare area of the liver encompassed posteriorly by suspensory ligaments of the liver and the diaphragm. The IVC exits the abdomen through a diaphragmatic hiatus, with a slight anterior course before draining through the inferoposterior wall of the right atrium. Frequently there is a membranous lip at the junction of the IVC with the right atrium, termed the "Eustachion valve" (Fig. 13-2). The supradiaphragmatic portion of the IVC is frequently intrapericardial.

The IVC typically has an oval shape in cross-section, but is easily deformed by adjacent abdominal or retroperitoneal masses. The average diameter of the infrarenal IVC is approximately 23 mm, although the intrarenal segment is usually slightly larger. The IVC is a valveless, elastic structure that responds to increased venous volume or pressure by dilatation, and decreased volume or increased intraabdominal pressure by collapsing. The dynamic nature of the IVC should always be considered when interpreting imaging studies or contemplating interventions.

The IVC is a single, right-sided structure in 97% of individuals (Table 13-1). The embryology of the IVC is complex in that the antecedent structures are paired and segmented. Anomalies of the IVC can be explained by aberrations of regression of these segments. The three pairs of fetal veins that become the IVC are the posterior cardinal, the subcardinal, and the supracardinal (see Fig. 13-1). The *posterior cardinal* veins normally involute completely, although persistence on the right results in a retrocaval right ureter. The *subcardinal* veins form the intrahepatic IVC, and contribute to the renal veins and suprarenal segment of the IVC. Regression of the right subcardinal vein results in azygos or hemiazygos continuation of the IVC (Fig. 13-3). The infrarenal IVC and the azygos veins are derived from the *supracardinal* veins. Duplication of the infrarenal IVC results from failure of regression of the left supracardinal vein, while a left-sided IVC results from regression of the right supracardinal vein (Fig. 13-4). When there is caval duplication, each iliac vein is usually isolated and drains through its own IVC, although communication at the normal level of the confluence may also occur. The left side of a duplicated IVC drains into the left renal vein,

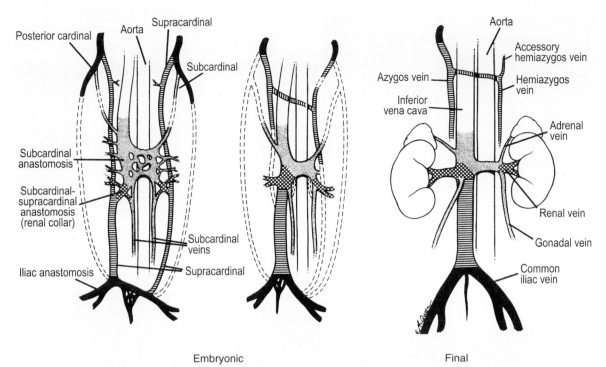

Figure 13-1   Development and normal anatomy of the inferior vena cava (IVC). (Reproduced with permission from Lundell L, Kadir S: Inferior vena cava and spinal veins. In (Kadir S ed): *Normal and Variant Angiographic Anatomy*, Saunders, Philadelphia, 1991.)

which then crosses the aorta in the normal location to join the right IVC, forming a normal single suprarenal IVC. When there is only a single left-sided IVC, both iliac veins drain into the IVC, which usually crosses the aorta at the level of the left renal vein to form a normally located suprarenal IVC (see Fig. 13-4). Thus, unless there

is an associated anomaly of the subcardinal veins, duplicated or left-sided IVCs usually revert to normal above the level of the renal veins.

The major tributaries of the IVC are the hepatic, renal, gonadal, and common iliac veins (see Fig. 13-1). Smaller tributaries include the lumbar, right adrenal, and phrenic veins. The common and external iliac veins are discussed in Chapter 16, and the hepatic veins in Chapter 14.

The most common pattern of renal vein anatomy is a single vein from each kidney, with the left renal vein passing anteriorly between the aorta and the SMA to join the IVC opposite the right renal vein at the level of the L2 vertebral body (see Fig. 12-1). The orifice of the normal left renal vein is anterior, while that of the right

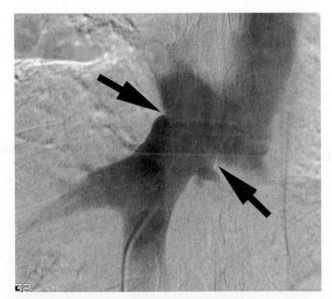

Figure 13-2   Digital subtraction venogram of the suprahepatic IVC showing the Eustachion valve (arrows).

Table 13-1	Anatomic Variants of the Inferior Vena Cava and Renal Veins
Variant	**Incidence (%)**
Duplicated IVC	1.0
Left-sided IVC	0.5
Absent IVC	0.1
Azygos/hemiazygos continuation of the IVC	0.5
Circumaortic left renal vein	7
Retroaortic left renal vein	3
Multiple right renal veins	28

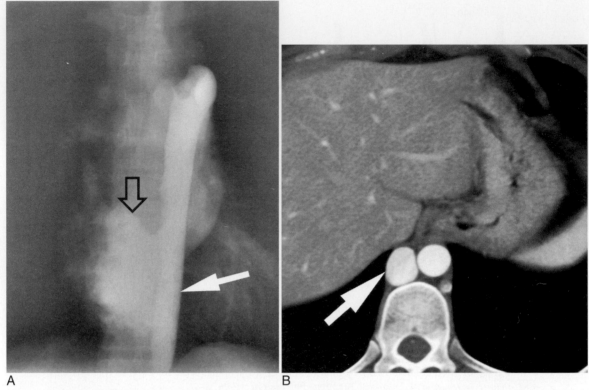

Figure 13-3   Hemiazygos and azygos continuation of the IVC. **A**, Venogram performed by injection in the IVC shows absence of the suprahepatic IVC and drainage via the hemiazygos vein (solid arrow) into a left-sided superior vena cava. Contrast is present in the right atrium (open arrow). **B**, Axial CT from another patient showing a dilated azygos vein (arrow) adjacent to the descending thoracic aorta and absence of the intrahepatic IVC.

is posterior. The right renal vein is shorter than the left, with average lengths of 3 cm and 7 cm, respectively (Fig. 13-5). Renal veins rarely have valves, but commonly connect to other retroperitoneal veins such as the lumbar, azygos, and gonadal veins. In patients with portal hypertension these connections may enlarge to allow drainage of portal blood from the splenic and short gastric veins into the left renal vein.

Variations in renal vein anatomy are present in almost 40% of individuals (see Table 13-1). This is due to the complex embryological relationships of the kidneys and the veins. In the fetus, the sub- and supracardinal veins form a web of veins that surround the aorta. As the kidneys rise out of the pelvis between the 6th and 9th weeks of gestation, they have a constantly changing vascular supply. Persistence of any of these venous elements may result in an anomaly, of which multiple right renal veins are the most common (28%) (Fig. 13-6). The next most common anomaly is a circumaortic left renal vein (5–7%), in which the left renal vein has both a preaortic and a retroaortic component. The latter may enter the IVC close to the level of the normal preaortic vein, or as low as the confluence of the iliac veins. In 3% of individuals

a single left renal vein passes behind (retroaortic) the aorta to reach the IVC.

The gonadal veins ascend from the pelvis anterior to the psoas muscle as companions of the gonadal arteries and the ureters. There are multiple small anastomoses between the gonadal veins and other retroperitoneal veins along the entire length of the vessels. This fact is crucial when considering gonadal vein interventions. The right gonadal vein drains into the anterior surface of the IVC just below, or at the level of, the right renal vein in most individuals (see Fig. 13-1). In fewer than 10% the right gonadal vein empties directly into the right renal vein. In the majority (>99%) of individuals the left gonadal vein empties into the left renal vein just before the renal vein crosses the aorta. Rarely, the left gonadal vein empties directly into the IVC. Usually, there is a valve present just at or below the orifice of the gonadal veins.

Four to five pairs of lumbar veins drain the vertebral column and the surrounding musculature. These veins empty into the posterolateral aspect of the IVC at the levels of the L4–L1 vertebral bodies. The lumbar veins anastomose with the ascending lumbar veins, paired structures that lie deep to the psoas muscles, parallel to the IVC (Fig. 13-7). The ascending lumbar veins originate from the superior aspect of the common iliac veins. In the thorax, the ascending lumbar veins become the azygos vein on the right and the hemiazygos vein on the left. The ascending lumbar veins interconnect with other retroperitoneal veins, such as the intercostal and renal veins.

The pelvic structures drain through veins that are named analogous to the arteries that supply the same anatomic structures. The superior gluteal, inferior gluteal, and obturator veins coalesce into the internal iliac veins, which drain into the common iliac vein. The visceral structures of the pelvis drain by the middle and inferior rectal (also known as hemorrhoidal), vesical,

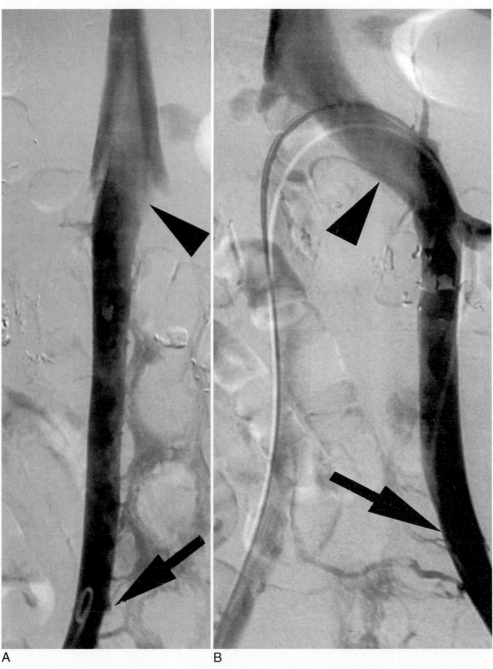

A   B

Figure 13-4   Anatomic variants of the IVC. **A**, Digital subtraction cavogram in a patient with a duplicated IVC. The catheter has been inserted from the right femoral vein. There is absent inflow from the left iliac vein (arrow), the IVC appears smaller than usual, and there is prominent inflow from the left renal vein (arrowhead). **B**, The same patient after catheterization of the left IVC (arrow) which empties into the left renal vein (arrowhead).   (*Continued*)

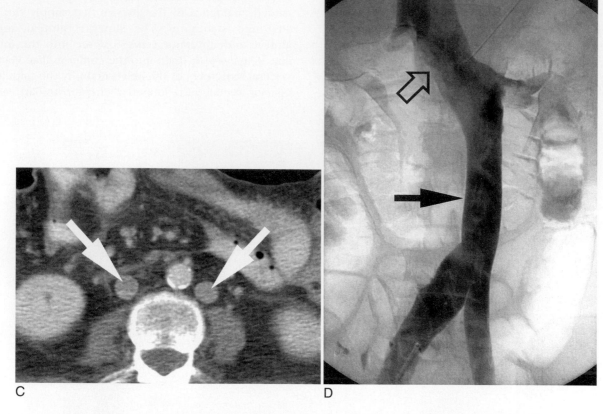

Figure 13-4   cont'd C, Axial CT scan from the same patient showing typical appearance of a duplicated IVC (arrows). **D**, Left-sided IVC (black arrow) that crosses to the right at the level of the left renal vein (open arrow).

uterine, vaginal, and prostatic veins. These veins are all interconnected with each other, so that precise labeling of structures is not always possible. In addition, the middle hemorrhoidal vein anastomoses with the portal venous system through the superior hemorrhoidal vein.

The venous drainage of the penis is through the deep dorsal and superficial dorsal veins. The deep vein drains to the crural, periprostatic, and ultimately internal iliac veins, whereas the superficial vein drains to the greater saphenous vein via the external pudendal vein (Fig. 13-8). The testicle drains initially into the pampiniform plexus, a complex of venous sinuses contained in the scrotum. This coalesces into the internal spermatic (gonadal) vein, which enters the renal vein on the left and the IVC on the right. Valves are usually present in these veins (see Fig. 13-1). Additional venous drainage is provided by branches to the external pudendal vein (and subsequently to the greater saphenous vein), the ductus deferens vein (and subsequently to the internal iliac vein), and the cremasteric vein (and subsequently to the external iliac vein). In addition, the internal spermatic vein may communicate with the portal and perirenal veins.

The internal spermatic vein is a single vessel in only about 50% of individuals.

The uterus has a prominent venous plexus that drains through the broad ligaments to the uterine veins. The uterine veins drain into the internal iliac veins. In pregnancy the uterine plexus dilates enormously. The uterine plexus communicates with the ovarian (gonadal) veins, which drain into the inferior vena cava at the level of the renal veins. Valves are present in 85% of left and 95% of right ovarian veins. In a manner analogous to the internal spermatic veins, the ovarian veins may be single or multiple, and have multiple communications with other retroperitoneal veins (Fig. 13-9).

The adrenal glands are each drained by a single vein in the majority of individuals. Both adrenal veins communicate with renal capsular and retroperitoneal veins. Multiple adrenal veins are the exception, but do occur. The right adrenal vein empties directly into the IVC about 2–4 cm above the right renal vein, usually at the level of the 12th rib (see Fig. 13-1). The orifice of the vein is located on the posterolateral wall of the IVC. Rarely a small accessory hepatic vein drains into the right adrenal

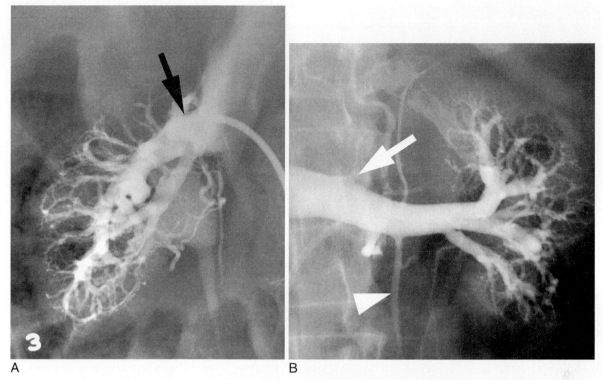

Figure 13-5   Normal conventional renal venograms. **A**, The right renal vein (arrow) is short with a caudal angulation. **B**, The left renal vein is long, crossing anterior to the aorta and posterior to the superior mesenteric artery to join the IVC. Note reflux of contrast into a normal-caliber left gonadal vein (arrowhead). The inferior adrenal vein (arrow) enters the superior aspect of the left renal vein.

vein, or vice versa. The left adrenal vein drains into the superior aspect of the left renal vein 3–5 cm from the IVC. The left inferior phrenic vein forms a common trunk with the left adrenal vein before it joins the renal vein. The location of the left adrenal vein is extremely constant, but in unusual cases the vein may drain directly into the IVC.

KEY COLLATERAL PATHWAYS

The collateral drainage of the IVC varies with the level of the occlusion. Infrarenal obstruction results in drainage of the lower extremities via ascending lumbar, paraspinal, gonadal, inferior epigastric, and abdominal wall veins (Fig. 13-10). Retrograde or obstructed flow in the internal iliac veins results in drainage through gonadal, ureteric, and the inferior mesenteric veins (the latter through anastomoses between the hemorrhoidal veins). Occlusion of the IVC between the renal and hepatic veins can be drained by all of the collateral routes described for infrarenal obstruction. In addition, the azygos and hemiazygos veins assume an important role, particularly for drainage of the renal veins. Obstruction at

the level of the suprahepatic IVC (above the hepatic vein orifices) results in collateral flow through all of the routes described, with the exception of the inferior mesenteric vein.

Renal vein obstruction on the right is drained via lumbar veins and the azygos vein (Fig. 13-11). The ureteric vein may also hypertrophy in these patients. Renal vein obstruction on the left is drained by the lumbar veins, hemiazygos vein, and the left gonadal vein.

The rich network of intercommunicating veins in the pelvis allows collateral drainage of occluded gonadal veins through transpelvic, ascending lumbar, and internal iliac veins. Obstruction of the adrenal veins results in drainage through small retroperitoneal collaterals such as renal capsular veins.

IMAGING

Evaluation of the IVC by ultrasound is inexpensive and readily available. The intrahepatic portion of the IVC can be consistently visualized. Duplex US can provide information about direction of flow. However, the depth of the vessel within the abdomen, bowel gas, and obesity

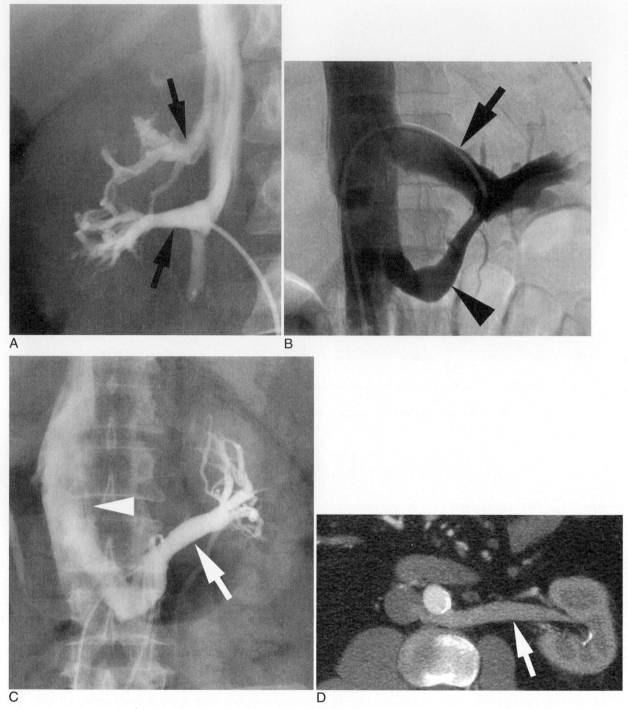

Figure 13-6   Anatomic variants of the renal veins. **A**, Conventional venogram showing multiple right renal veins (arrows). **B**, Digital subtraction study showing a circumaortic left renal vein with preaortic superior (arrow) and retroaortic inferior (arrowhead) components. **C**, Conventional venogram showing a retroaortic left renal vein (arrow) that courses caudad and posterior to the aorta before joining the IVC (arrowhead). **D**, Oblique reformatted CT image showing the anatomic relationships of a retroaortic left renal vein (arrow).

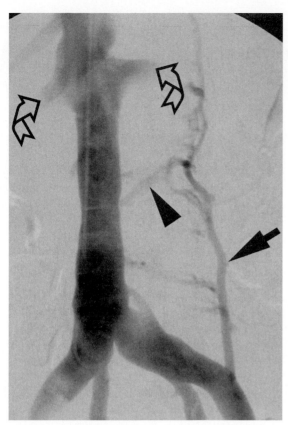

Figure 13-7   Digital subtraction cavogram performed from a jugular vein approach. The left ascending lumbar vein (arrow) communicates with a lumbar vein (arrowhead). There is reflux into the orifices of both renal veins (curved arrows).

makes imaging of the infrarenal IVC more difficult. Renal vein anatomy can be difficult to evaluate with US for similar reasons.

Imaging of the IVC with computed tomography is simple and highly accurate for most forms of pathology (see Fig. 13-4). For dedicated CT of the IVC, a triple phase study should be used consisting of a noncontrast scan, a helical arterial-phase acquisition during contrast injection, and a delayed acquisition (1–2 minutes) during the venous enhancement phase. Contrast can be injected through an upper-extremity vein. The collimation can be thicker than that used for arterial studies, as the venous structures are larger in diameter. The noncontrast scan is useful for detection of high-attenuation acute thrombus in tributary veins and the IVC. The late phase scan is necessary because mixing of opacified blood from the renal veins during the arterial phase can result in pseudo-filling defects. Variant IVC and renal vein anatomy is depicted with sensitivity and specificity that exceeds 95%, particularly when studies are viewed on postprocessing workstations that allow reconstruction in multiple planes (see Fig. 13-6).

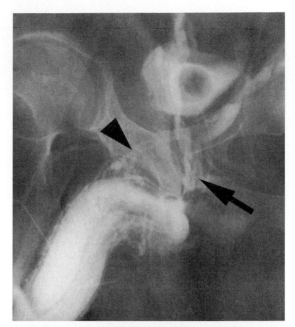

Figure 13-8   Cavernosogram showing drainage through deep (arrow) and superficial (arrowhead) veins.

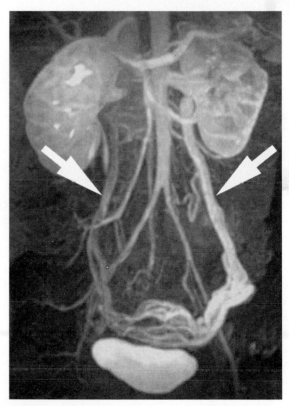

Figure 13-9   Maximum-intensity projection (MIP) of a gadolinium-enhanced 3-D MRA of a woman showing dilated ovarian veins (arrows). The direction of flow is retrograde in the left ovarian vein, across the pelvis through the uterine plexus, and antegrade in the right ovarian vein. This patient presented with chronic pelvic pain (see section Pelvic Congestion Syndrome). (Image courtesy of Barry Stein M.D., Hartford Hospital, CT.)

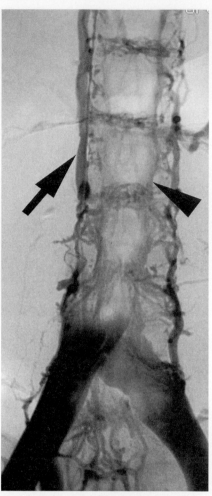

Figure 13-10 Digital subtraction cavogram of a patient with extrinsic compression of the IVC. There is filling of the paravertebral (arrow) and intravertebral (arrowhead) veins.

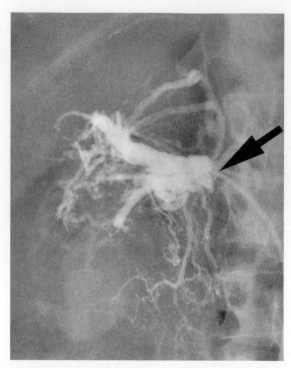

Figure 13-11 Conventional venogram showing a severely stenotic right renal vein orifice (arrow) and numerous retroperitoneal collateral veins.

Magnetic resonance imaging of the IVC and renal veins with venographic sequences (MRV) has similar accuracy, sensitivity, and specificity as contrast-enhanced CT. Anatomic sequences in at least two planes (axial and coronal) should be obtained, followed by flow sequences. Thick-sliced (5-mm) 2-dimensional time-of-flight (2-D TOF) sequences acquired in the axial plane with superior saturation provide excellent images, although slow or retrograde flow in obstructed segments will suffer from signal loss. Gadolinium-enhanced breath-hold 3-D acquisitions of the IVC in the coronal plane are not susceptible to signal loss. These sequences are similar to those used for evaluation of the abdominal aorta. Imaging of the venous system is accomplished by repeating the same sequence several times after the arterial phase (Fig. 13-12).

Cavography should be performed with a pigtail catheter positioned just at or slightly below the confluence of the common iliac veins (see Figs 13-4 and 13-7).

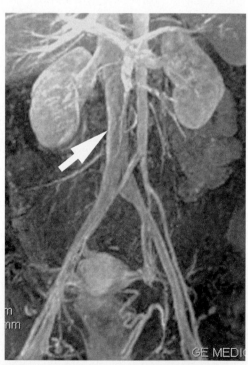

Figure 13-12 MIP of venous phase of gadolinium-enhanced 3-D MRA showing enhancement of the venous structures (arrow = IVC). (Image courtesy of Barry Stein M.D., Hartford Hospital, CT.)

When an abnormality is suspected higher in the IVC, the catheter can be repositioned at that level after the initial injection. Power injection of contrast (20–25 mL/s for 2 seconds) and rapid filming (3–4 frames/s) are necessary to adequately opacify the IVC. The projection most commonly obtained is anterior–posterior, but the lateral view can be very useful when evaluating for obstruction or intraluminal masses. In patients with renal insufficiency or contrast allergies, either gadolinium or CO_2 can be used. The major tributary veins are identified by inflow of unopacified blood, although reflux of contrast into these vessels can be seen (especially in patients with high right-sided heart pressures). Whenever the identity or location of a tributary vein is in doubt, selective injection with a visceral selective catheter should be performed. Alternatively, intravascular ultrasound (IVUS) with a low-frequency probe can be used to image the IVC and guide interventions. The major imaging IVUS landmarks of the IVC are the confluence of the iliac veins, the renal and hepatic veins, and the cavoatrial junction.

The renal veins have very high flow rates, which makes selective renal venography challenging. When the primary goals are localization of the renal veins or sampling, selective catheter shapes such as Cobra-2 or Simmons (1 for the right renal vein, 2 for the left) can be used. For diagnostic venography, catheters with multiple side-holes should be used so that large volumes of contrast can be injected without traumatizing the vein. A straight or pigtail catheter and a deflecting guidewire are a useful

combination for renal venography. When extensive filling of the intrarenal veins is required, injection of 10 μg of epinephrine into the renal artery will temporarily reduce venous outflow. Typical imaging parameters are contrast injection at 10–15 mL/s for 2 seconds, with rapid filming (3–4 frames/s) (see Fig. 13-5).

Selective gonadal venography is simplified by the consistent location of the left gonadal vein orifice in the left renal vein. A competent valve at the gonadal vein orifice can prevent selective placement of a catheter. The right gonadal vein orifice may be difficult to find in the IVC, particularly when the valve in the ostium is competent. When a femoral venous access is used, a Cobra-2 catheter or a straight catheter with a deflecting guidewire can be used to select the left gonadal vein, and a recurved catheter such as a Simmons-1 for the right. From a jugular approach, a Headhunter-1 or similar angled catheter can be used to select each vein. Many angiographers prefer a jugular venous access for gondal venography, particularly when an intervention is anticipated (Fig. 13-13). Hand injection of 5–15 mL of contrast is usually sufficient to opacify a normal gonadal vein. Higher volumes may be necessary in veins dilated due to incompetent valves. Shielding of the gonads is not possible in females.

Adrenal venography is usually only required to confirm catheter location during adrenal vein sampling (Fig. 13-14). A single side-hole is added near the tip of the catheter to facilitate aspiration of blood. The left adrenal vein is easily catheterized with a 5- or 6-French Simmons-2 or

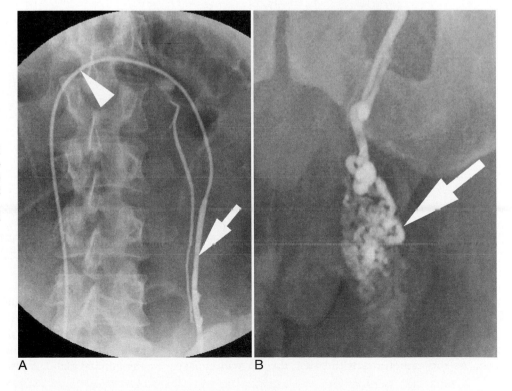

Figure 13-13   Selective left gonadal venogram in a patient with a varicocele. **A,** The left gonadal vein (arrow) has been selected from the right femoral approach (arrowhead). **B,** Digital image showing a distended pampiniform plexus (arrow).

A   B

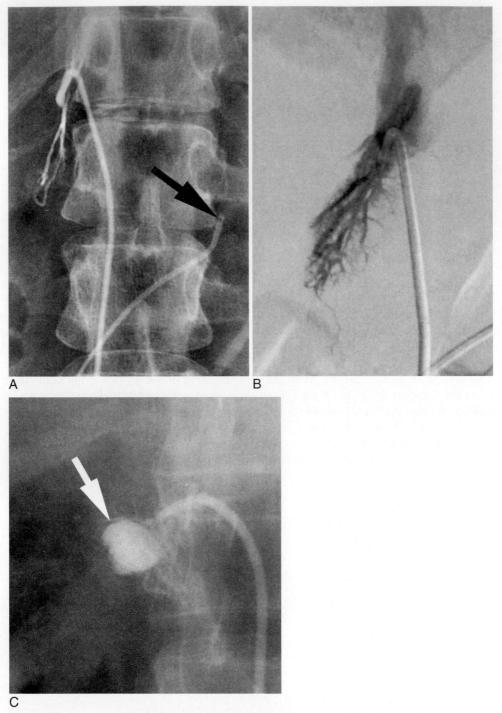

Figure 13-14   Adrenal venography. **A**, Unsubtracted digital image showing catheterization of both renal veins with injection of contrast on the right. Each catheter has a single side-hole (arrow) near the tip to facilitate sampling. **B**, Digital subtraction image showing a normal right adrenal gland. **C**, Extravasation (arrow) in the right adrenal gland due to overzealous injection of contrast. The patient had severe flank pain.

similar long recurved catheter. The tip of the catheter is placed in the left renal vein beyond the ostium of the left phrenic vein. The catheter is then slowly retracted so that the tip pushes against the superior wall of the renal vein. As the catheter is withdrawn, the tip will engage

the phrenic vein, and allow selection of the adrenal vein. On the right, a steeply angled 5- to 6-French catheter is used to find the right adrenal vein above the right renal vein. Small hepatic branches can be easily confused with the adrenal gland. A few milliliters of contrast should be injected slowly and gently to avoid rupture of the delicate adrenal veins. Patients will report a mild ache or sensation of fullness in the back with adrenal vein injections. This characteristic symptom can be used to help determine when the correct vein has been selected. The adrenal glands appear as well-defined wedge-shaped structures on venography. On the right, collateral drainage into a hepatic vein may be seen.

INFERIOR VENA CAVA OBSTRUCTION

The usual location (>90%) of caval occlusions is the infrarenal segment. Obstruction can be caused by intrinsic or extrinsic pathology (Box 13-1). The most common etiology of intrinsic obstruction is thrombosis, typically as an extension of iliac vein thrombus (Box 13-2). Isolated thrombosis of the IVC is unusual in the absence of a translumbar IVC line, an IVC filter, trauma, or surgery. Delayed thrombosis can occur following liver transplantation due to stenosis of the caval anastomoses.

Extrinsic compression of the IVC can be caused by tumor (including retroperitoneal or hepatic), adenopathy, aortic aneurysm, pericaval fibrosis, surgical ligation, and hepatic enlargement (see Fig. 13-10). In pregnant patients, positional obstruction of the IVC can caused by the enlarged uterus. This is usually relieved when the patient is in the left lateral decubitus position.

Box 13-1   Etiologies of Inferior Vena Cava Obstruction

Intrinsic

Thrombosis
Stenosis
Tumor:
    Primary
    Invasion from adjacent organ/retroperitoneum
Iatrogenic

Extrinsic

Enlarged liver:
    Hypertrophy
    Tumor
    Regenerating nodules
Compression by retroperitoneal mass:
    Adenopathy
    Tumor
    Aortic aneurysm
Pregnant uterus
Retroperitoneal fibrosis
Surgical ligation, clip
Abdominal compartment syndrome

Box 13-2   Risk Factors for Thrombosis of the Inferior Vena Cava

Hypercoagulable state
Instrumentation
Central venous access catheter (transfemoral or direct IVC)
Partial IVC interruption (filter or clip)
Surgery
Extrinsic compression
Tumor (primary IVC or invasion)
Chemotherapy

The symptoms of IVC obstruction vary with the rapidity of the occlusion, the status of collateral veins, and the flow within the venous system. Gradual occlusion of the IVC may be asymptomatic if the collateral veins are intact. Acute occlusion usually results in sudden onset of bilateral lower-extremity edema. The swelling subsides, sometimes completely, as collateral veins become recruited and enlarge. In some patients, sudden interruption of venous return from the lower extremities may result in hypotension. This rare complication is most likely to occur in a patient with an IVC filter that becomes acutely occluded by a large embolus. In patients with disrupted or thrombosed collateral veins, even gradual occlusion may cause symptoms. Exercise, or creation of a lower-extremity arteriovenous fistula, may unmask a previously asymptomatic obstruction by virtue of the increased venous flow.

On physical examination, the finding of bilateral lower-extremity edema and dilated abdominal wall veins should suggest occlusion of the IVC. Patients with long-standing IVC occlusion can develop typical venous stasis changes of the lower extremities, such as brawny discoloration of the skin, woody edema, and ulcers.

Obstruction of the IVC can be suggested on duplex US examination when there is stasis of flow, loss of the normal respiratory variation, or thrombosis of the iliofemoral veins bilaterally (Fig. 13-15). A blunted or absent Doppler response to Valsalva is suggestive of central occlusion when the finding is bilateral. Direct interrogation of the IVC may be possible, but it cannot be reliably performed in the infrarenal segment in all patients.

Cross-sectional imaging with CT and MR allows diagnosis of IVC obstruction as well as evaluation of the adjacent soft tissues for possible causes. Expansion of the IVC implies an intrinsic occlusion, whereas compression is almost always associated with an obvious mass lesion. High-attenuation material in the IVC on a noncontrast CT can be seen with acute thrombus. Enhancement of the wall of the IVC with a low-attenuation lumen after administration of contrast is diagnostic of an intrinsic

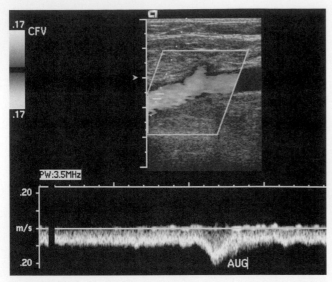

Figure 13-15   Duplex US showing indirect evidence of IVC occlusion. There is loss of respiratory and cardiac variation of flow at the common femoral vein, with preserved response to augmentation (AUG) by calf compression. These findings were bilateral. The level of obstruction could be in the iliac veins as well as the IVC. This is the same patient as Fig. 13-10.

Cavography actually provides less information about the etiology of an occlusion than US, CT, or MRI, but may be necessary to localize the pathology as intrinsic or extrinsic and determine the extent. Intraluminal occlusions have a characteristic appearance with contrast on both sides of a filling defect (Fig. 13-17). Extrinsic compression causes broadening or effacement of the lumen (see Fig. 13-10). Rarely, IVUS is required to make a conclusive diagnosis. Stenosis of the IVC can be evaluated with measurement of a pressure gradient across the lesion. In the supine patient the normal gradient should be less than 3 mmHg. When performing cavography in a patient with obstruction, contrast should be injected as close to the lesion as possible to avoid overestimating the extent of occlusion. Contrast injected in a remote location such as a femoral vein will preferentially opacify the collateral veins rather than the IVC. Patients should not be instructed to Valsalva during injection of contrast, as the IVC lumen may be artifactually obliterated by the transient increase in intraabdominal pressure.

Acute thrombosis of the IVC is usually linked to iliofemoral thrombosis or occlusion of an IVC filter by

occlusion (typically bland thrombus) (Fig. 13-16). Contrast may be visualized around an intraluminal filling defect at the proximal and distal extent of an occlusion, or with incomplete obstruction. Intraluminal tumor may enhance with contrast (see Tumors, below). The extent of an occlusion may be overestimated if stagnant blood caudad to an obstruction does not enhance with contrast.

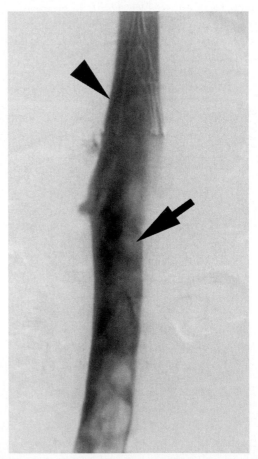

Figure 13-17   Digital subtraction cavogram showing thrombus extending to the level of the renal veins (arrow). A vena cava filter (arrowhead) was placed in the suprarenal IVC.

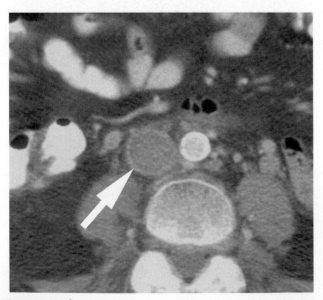

Figure 13-16   Axial CT scan showing a distended, thrombus-filled IVC (arrow) with enhancement of the vessel wall.

a massive embolus. Therapy for the IVC thrombus is frequently the same as for the lower-extremity deep venous thrombosis. Anticoagulation, elevation of the extremities, and compression stockings are the traditional medical treatments. Surgical thrombectomy is rarely indicated. Catheter-directed thrombolysis of iliofemoral veins and IVC thrombus can provide rapid relief of symptoms. (Venous thrombolysis is discussed in Chapter 16.) One of the goals of thrombolysis is the unmasking of underlying IVC pathology that may have precipitated the thrombosis (Fig. 13-18). There is a small risk (1%) of major pulmonary embolism (PE) during interventions for caval thrombus. Temporary IVC filters may have a role in selected patients as a preventative measure.

Symptomatic stenoses of the IVC or other occlusive lesion can be stented to prevent recurrent thrombosis.

A variety of stents have been used for this purpose, including both balloon-expandable and self-expanding. Stents with diameters in the range of 12–30 mm are required. The long-term results of IVC stents for benign stenoses have been excellent when large diameter stents can be placed.

Treatment of symptomatic extrinsic compression of the IVC should be directed, when possible, to the mass or lesion causing the compression. Resection of tumors, shrinkage of nodal masses with chemotherapy or radiation, or patience (especially in the case of compression of the IVC by a pregnant uterus) may resolve symptoms. Enlargement of collateral veins can result in sufficient decompression to satisfy many patients with uncorrectable retroperitoneal pathology. Anticoagulation or antiplatelet therapy should be instituted when possible.

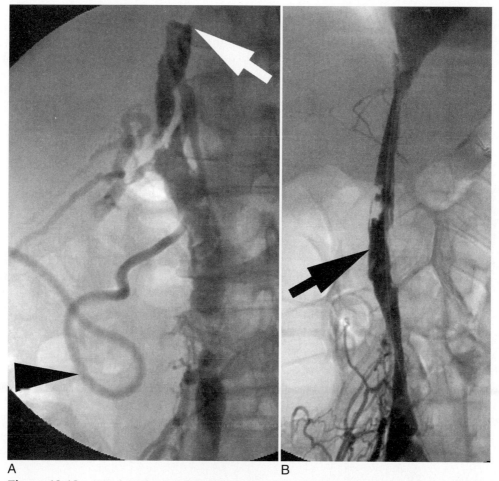

A   B

Figure 13-18   IVC thrombosis and stenosis due to a chronic indwelling translumbar IVC catheter. **A,** Two years after line placement the patient presented with leg swelling, a nonfunctional catheter, and renal insufficiency. Injection of the catheter (arrowhead) showed IVC occlusion (arrow) with extensive thrombosis. **B,** Digital cavogram after thrombolysis shows partial recanalization of the IVC (arrow). The patient underwent stent placement in the IVC and the right renal vein with resolution of the leg swelling and renal failure.   *(Continued)*

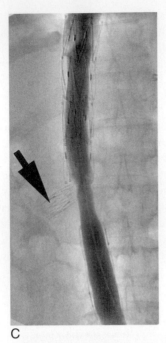

C

Figure 13-18   cont'd C, Digital cavogram 1 year after stent placement shows a patent IVC. The stent in the right renal vein (arrow) was patent on selective injection.

Surgical bypass of the IVC is reserved for unusual cases. Stent placement is an excellent option for patients with malignant or other terminal illnesses that seek an improvement in the quality of their remaining life (Fig. 13-19).

VENA CAVA FILTER PLACEMENT

Vena cava filters prevent thrombus from embolizing to the pulmonary circulation by trapping the thrombus in the vena cava. Filters do not prevent the formation of thrombus, enhance anticoagulation, or treat pulmonary embolism (PE) that has already occurred. The conventional treatment for deep venous thrombosis (DVT) and PE is anticoagulation. When patients with thromboembolic disease cannot be anticoagulated, or patients at high risk of developing DVT cannot be screened, monitored, or receive prophylaxis, filters are indicated. There is no role for filters in stable patients with thromboembolic disease who can be treated with anticoagulation (Box 13-3).

There are a large number of permanent vena cava filters available (Table 13-2 and Fig. 13-20). Several are designed to be removable (Fig. 13-21). All filters probably function equally well, so the criteria for selection of one device over another should be based upon availability, access routes, and vena cava anatomy. The low-profile

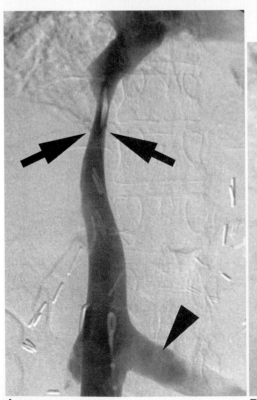

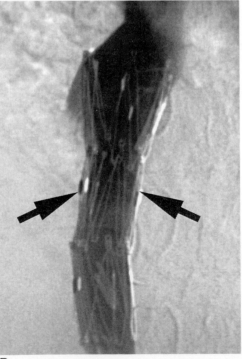

Figure 13-19   Intrahepatic IVC stenosis due to metastatic carcinoid tumor to the liver. The patient had tense bilateral lower-extremity edema. **A**, Digital cavogram showing compression of the intrahepatic IVC (arrows) and reflux into the left renal vein (arrowhead). There was a 22-mmHg gradient across the stenosis. **B**, Digital cavogram after placement of a 20-mm diameter Z-stent in the intrahepatic IVC (arrows). The gradient was reduced to 2 mmHg and the patient's edema resolved over the next few days.

A

B

Box 13-3 Indications for Vena Cava Filters

I. Classic

Documented deep vein thrombosis (DVT) and/or
pulmonary embolism (PE) with:

1. Absolute contraindication to anticoagulation
2. Documented progression of DVT or recurrent PE
   while anticoagulated
3. Complication of anticoagulation requiring
   termination of therapy
4. Failure of existing vena cava filter (recurrent PE)
   and continued contraindication to anticoagulation
5. Massive PE that requires surgical thrombectomy

II. Relative

Documented DVT and/or PE with:

1. Limited cardiac or pulmonary reserve
2. Unreliable patient
3. "Widow-maker" thrombus in vena cava
4. Patient that "falls a lot"

III. Prophylactic

No documented DVT or PE with:

1. High risk of developing DVT/PE (e.g., multiple
   trauma)
2. Past history of DVT and/or PE undergoing surgical
   procedure with high risk of postoperative DVT/PE

devices (Simon Nitinol and Recovery, Bard, Covington, GA; TrapEase and OptEase, Cordis Endovascular, Miami, FL; Vena Tech LP, B. Braun Medical, Bethlehem, PA) have the greatest flexibility in terms of the number of potential access sites. Only the Bird's Nest filter (Cook, Bloomington, IN) can be used when the caval diameter exceeds 35 mm. The Bird's Nest filter should be avoided in a suprarenal location as the wire mesh, which frequently prolapses during deployment, can extend up into the heart.

Removable filters can be classified as either temporary (must be removed) or optional (can be left in place as a permanent filter). Most temporary filters are attached to a catheter or wire that facilitates removal, but occupies a venous access site for 2–6 weeks. There is a 4–5% risk of access site infection and a 10–15% conversion rate to a permanent filter when these devices are used during lower-extremity deep venous thrombolysis. These filters can present a management dilemma when the time for removal has arrived if the filter is found to be full of trapped emboli. Optional filters, such as the Gunther Tulip (Cook), Recovery, and OptEase obviate this dilemma, in that the filter is "converted" to a permanent device by simply doing nothing. The window of retrievability was originally thought to be as short as 10 days for the Tulip and OptEase, but is probably closer to 4 weeks. The Recovery filter is potentially retrievable at any time. Early experience suggests that these devices are retrieved in over half of patients when used as a removable filter in a carefully selected population.

Table 13-2 Vena Cava Filters

Filter	Sheath Outer Diameter (Fr)	Access	Maximum Caval Diameter (mm)	Metal	MRI Artifact
24-F Greenfield	28	RFV, RIJ	28	Stainless steel wire	+++
Titanium Greenfield	15	RFV, RIJ	28	Titanium wire	+
12-F stainless steel Greenfield	15	RFV, LFV, RIJ, LIJ	28	Stainless steel wire	++
Bird's Nest	13.8	RFV, LFV, RIJ, LIJ	40	Stainless steel wire	++++
Vena Tech	12.9	RFV, LFV, RIJ	28	Phynox metal	++
Gunther Tulip[a]	10	RFV, LFV, RIJ, LIJ	30	Elgiloy	+
Vena Tech LP	9	RFV, LFV, RIJ, LIJ	28 (35 in Europe)	Phynox metal	+
Simon Nitinol	9	RFV, LFV, RIJ, LIJ, RSV, LSV, RAV, LAV	28	Nitinol wire	+
Recovery[a]	9	RFV, LFV	28	Nitinol wire	+
TrapEase	8.5	RFV, LFV, RIJ, LIJ, RAV, LAV	30	Nitinol hypotube	+
OptEase[a]	8.5	RFV, LFV, RIJ, LIJ, RAV, LAV	30	Nitinol hypotube	+

[a]Designed for percutaneous retrieval.

FV, femoral vein; IJ, internal jugular vein; SV, subclavian vein; AV, antecubital vein; R, right; L, left.

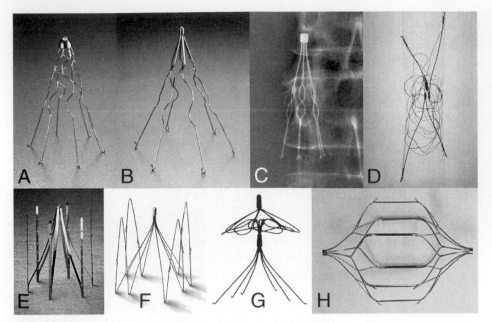

Figure 13-20   Examples of permanent IVC filters. **A**, Original 24-Fr Greenfield (courtesy Boston Scientific). **B**, Titanium Greenfield (courtesy Boston Scientific). **C**, The 12-Fr Stainless Steel Greenfield (courtesy Boston Scientific). **D**, Bird's Nest (courtesy Cook). **E**, Vena Tech (courtesy B. Braun Medical). **F**, Vena Tech LP (courtesy B. Braun Medical). **G**, Simon Nitinol (courtesy CR Bard). **H**, TrapEase (© Cordis Corporation 2003).

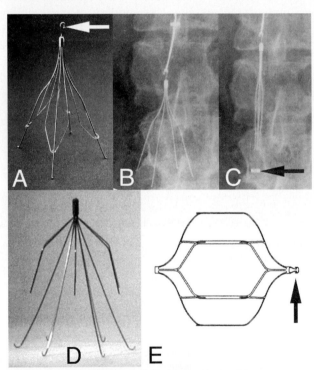

Figure 13-21   Optional vena cava filters. **A**, The Gunther Tulip has a 3- to 4-week window of retrievability (courtesy Cook). The hook at the apex of the filter (arrow) allows retrieval from a jugular approach with a snare. **B**, Digital image of a Gunther filter with the apical hook engaged with a snare prior to removal. **C**, The filter has been collapsed by advancement of a sheath (arrow). **D**, The Recovery filter, with an indefinite window of retrievability (courtesy CR Bard). The filter is retrieved using a proprietary grasping cone from a jugular approach. **E**, The OptEase variant of the TrapEase, with a 3- to 4-week window of retrievability (© Cordis Corporation 2003). The filter is retrieved by grasping the caudal hooks (arrow) with a snare from a femoral approach.

After determining the indication for the vena cava filter, a cavogram is performed to assess caval patency, anatomy, and dimensions. Injection of sufficient contrast (20–25 mL/s for a total volume of 40–50 mL) at the confluence of the iliac veins through a pigtail catheter will usually reflux a small amount of contrast into the iliac veins. The renal veins are identified as inflow of unopacified blood, although contrast may reflux into the origins in some patients. Digital subtraction imaging at 3–4 frames per second produces excellent images. A key anatomic variant is a duplicated IVC, which occurs in fewer than 1% of the population. When the pigtail catheter is placed from the right common femoral or the jugular vein, reflux of contrast into the left common iliac vein helps to exclude this anomaly as the left cava usually drains directly into the left renal vein. Multiple renal veins may also be present. Whenever in doubt regarding IVC anatomy, a selective catheter should be used to investigate further.

The level of the lowest renal vein should be identified. The filter delivery sheath is then inserted over a guidewire into the IVC, and the filter deployed with its apex just above or as close to the lower lip of the renal vein as possible (Fig. 13-22). The rationale for placement in this location is to minimize the potential deadspace above the filter should it become occluded with thrombus. If there is a long segment of infrarenal IVC between the filter and the renal veins, thrombus could form above the occluded filter and embolize. The high flow from the renal veins is thought to protect against this. When there is insufficient space below the renal veins owing to a short IVC or the presence of thrombus, the filter can be placed in the segment of IVC between the renal and hepatic veins

Table 13-3   Common Technical Problems During Insertion of Vena Cava Filter

Problem	Solution
Is the IVC too large?	If you ask the question, assume it is; use Vena Tech LP or Bird's Nest
Sheath kinks during filter delivery	Advance system as a unit by a few cm, then try to advance filter again
	Change to different device if kink persists
Legs cross after delivery	Unless grossly asymmetric, leave alone
	Gentle manipulation with catheter, but be careful not to dislodge or entangle the device
	Place second filter if unsuccessful or unwilling to manipulate
Filter fails to open	Cavogram to confirm location of device, exclude presence of thrombus in legs
	Place second filter
	Rarely, snare retrieval or reposition
Filter upside down	Retrieve if possible, or second filter central to first
	This does not happen with Bird's Nest or TrapEase
Filter entirely in wrong location	If no danger to patient, leave alone, and place second device
	If in heart, consider snare retrieval or surgery

(see Fig. 13-17). In the presence of a duplicated IVC, a filter should be placed in each IVC, or a single filter in the suprarenal location. When a mega cava is discovered (diameter >28–30 mm), the Vena Tech LP or Bird's Nest filter can be placed in the infrarenal IVC, or a filter of another design in each common iliac vein. After deployment of the filter a repeat cavogram is performed through the delivery sheath to document the final position of the device (Table 13-3).

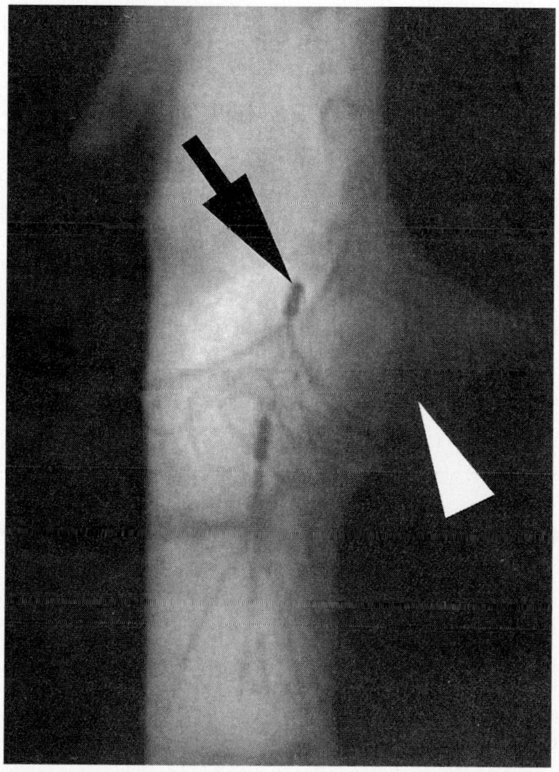

Filters can be placed in septic patients without fear of device infection. In pregnant patients in their first trimester, the entire procedure can be performed from a jugular approach if necessary to minimize radiation exposure. The classic teaching is to place the filter in the suprarenal location in pregnant women or women of childbearing age, but there is no objective evidence to support this practice. Rarely, patients with upper-extremity venous thrombosis will require a filter in the superior vena cava (SVC). In this situation, the filter should be oriented appropriately towards the heart (see Fig. 7-14). The TrapEase, OptEase, and the Bird's Nest should not be used in this location.

The outcomes of IVC filters are listed in Table 13-4. When a patient with a filter experiences a documented recurrent PE, the first step is to determine whether the patient can be treated with anticoagulation. Patients who can be anticoagulated require no further evaluation, but should be treated with a full course of therapy. Patients who cannot be anticoagulated require evaluation for the

Figure 13-22   Optimal infrarenal placement of a filter, here a Simon Nitinol (CR Bard) filter, in a patient whose renal veins enter the IVC at different levels. The filter apex (arrow) is at the orifice of the left renal vein (arrowhead).

Table 13-4   Outcomes of Inferior Vena Cava Filters

Outcome	Incidence (%)
Recurrent pulmonary embolism	5
Symptomatic complete IVC occlusion	5
Symptomatic insertion site thrombosis	2
Major filter migration (to heart, lungs, iliac veins)	<1
Filter fracture with clinical consequences	<1
Symptomatic perforation of adjacent structures	<1

origin of the PE. The discovery of new lower-extremity DVT, trapped thrombus in the filter, or thrombus extending above the filter suggests filter failure. In these situations a second device should be placed, usually inferior to the original filter unless thrombus extends above the first device or the IVC is thrombosed. In these instances the filter should be placed above the first, usually in the suprarenal IVC.

Other sources of emboli that should be considered when PE recurs in a patient with an IVC filter but no obvious lower-extremity source are the internal iliac, gonadal, renal, and upper-extremity veins. Management of emboli from the renal and gonadal veins may require a suprarenal filter. An SVC filter may be indicated to prevent further pulmonary embolism from upper-extremity DVT.

Symptomatic complete occlusion of the filter can be treated with anticoagulation or thrombolysis if the patient no longer has contraindications to these therapies. Otherwise, conservative measures such as elevation of the extremities and compression stockings are used. On very rare occasions IVC thrombosis after filter placement in the setting of extensive DVT (unilateral or bilateral) results in arterial ischemia (phlegmasia cerulea dolens) (see Chapter 16). A difficult problem to treat in patients who cannot be anticoagulated or undergo thrombolysis,

this usually occurs soon after initial filter placement in a hypercoagulable patient. Surgical venous thrombectomy and even amputation may be necessary, but the mortality rate is generally high.

The long-term outcomes of SVC filters is not known, as the majority of the patients reported in the literature have been extremely ill with short life expectancies.

TUMORS

Primary tumors of the IVC are rare, with fewer than 1 per 34,000 autopsies. They are almost always leiomyosarcomas. The most common location is the segment of IVC between the renal and hepatic veins (42%), followed by the infrarenal IVC (34%), and the intrahepatic IVC (24%). The tumors are mostly intraluminal, but extraluminal extension into the adjacent retroperitoneum is present in many cases (Fig. 13-23). Women are affected more often than men.

Invasion of the wall and lumen of the IVC by adjacent tumors should be distinguished from extension of tumor thrombus into the lumen. In the former case, the tumor grows through the wall of the IVC (Box 13-4). Tumor thrombus is an intraluminal extension of the mass

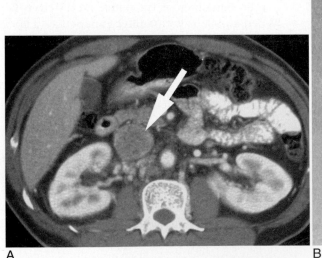

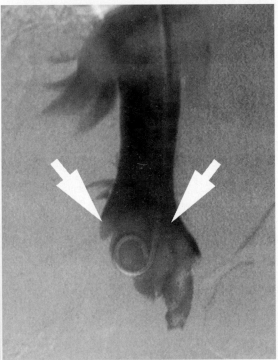

A   B

Figure 13-23   Primary leiomyosarcoma of the IVC. **A**, Axial CT image showing a heterogeneously enhancing mass expanding the IVC (arrow). The kidneys and renal veins were normal. **B**, Digital subtraction image obtained during transvascular biopsy of the mass, showing an intraluminal filling defect (arrows) expanding the IVC.

Box 13-4	Tumors that Secondarily Invade the IVC

Liposarcoma
Retroperitoneal leiomyosarcoma
Malignant fibrous histiocytoma
Cholangiocarcinoma
Hepatocellular carcinoma
Hepatic metastatic lesions
Pancreatic carcinoma
Duodenal carcinoma

without invasion of the wall of the IVC (Box 13-5; see also Fig. 1-25). Associated bland thrombus is common. The most common etiology of tumor thrombus is renal cell carcinoma (see Fig. 12-25). Up to 20% of patients with renal cell carcinoma have tumor thrombus in the renal vein, and 4–15% will have extension into the IVC. In the group of patients with tumor thrombus, 50% is located in the intrarenal IVC and 40% in the intrahepatic IVC. Tumor thrombus extension into the right atrium occurs in as many as 10% of these patients.

The clinical presentation of patients with IVC involvement by tumor varies with the degree and acuity of the obstruction, the type of tumor, and the extent of intracaval tumor or thrombus. Primary IVC tumors are generally advanced when they become symptomatic due to metastatic disease, iliofemoral thrombosis, or renal and hepatic vein obstruction. Secondary involvement of the IVC by malignancy and tumor thrombus is usually detected during work-up of the primary lesion. Pulmonary embolism, cardiac arrhythmias, and Budd–Chiari syndrome can occur with intracaval tumor thrombus.

Imaging of patients with IVC involvement by malignancy is focused on determining the origin and stage of the malignancy, localization of the level of IVC obstruction, and determination of the extent of intracaval thrombus or mass. CT and MRI are the preferred modalities for IVC imaging in these patients, as both the pericaval and intraluminal structures can be imaged. Expansion of the IVC with enhancing intraluminal tissue is consistent

Box 13-5	Sources of Tumor Thrombus in the Inferior Vena Cava

Renal cell carcinoma
Hepatocellular carcinoma
Pheochromocytoma
Adrenal carcinoma
Uterine sarcoma
Germ cell tumor

with tumor thrombus. Bland thrombus does not enhance with contrast. Leiomyosarcoma of the IVC with retroperitoneal extension may be indistinguishable from a primary retroperitoneal lesion with caval invasion.

Cavography is reserved for patients with inconclusive findings on cross-sectional imaging. Occasionally, intravascular biopsy is performed to confirm the nature of the intraluminal process. Some surgeons obtain preoperative embolization of renal cell carcinomas when there is associated intracaval tumor thrombus.

Therapy of primary IVC leiomyosarcoma is radical resection and replacement of the IVC with synthetic graft material when necessary. Operative mortality is as high as 13%, with a 5-year survival of only 28%. In patients with renal cell carcinoma, the presence of tumor thrombus in the IVC does not impact survival following nephrectomy and removal of the tumor. When the thrombus extends to or above the intrahepatic IVC, extensive surgical exposure of the IVC is required.

TRAUMA

The IVC and abdominal veins can be injured by penetrating or blunt trauma, surgery, or interventional procedures (Fig. 13-24). Though a low-pressure system, blood flow in the IVC and renal veins is substantial, with the potential for major blood loss. The IVC is injured in 2% of abdominal gunshot wounds. Over 50% of patients with caval injuries die prior to arrival at the hospital, as do up to 50% of those who survive to receive

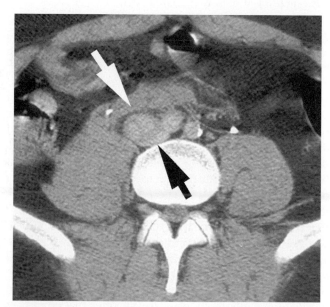

Figure 13-24   Traumatic laceration of the IVC due to blunt trauma, surgically repaired. Axial CT image showing an enlarged, irregular IVC (black arrow) and retroperitoneal hematoma (white arrow).

Box 13-6   Causes of Renal Vein Thrombosis

Hypercoagulable state
Membranous glomerulonephritis
Dehydration
Thrombosis of the inferior vena cava
Stenosis (transplant renal vein)
Extrinsic compression
    Retroperitoneal tumor
    Adenopathy
    Retroperitoneal fibrosis
Nephrotic syndrome
Tumor thrombus
    Renal cell carcinoma
    Adrenal carcinoma

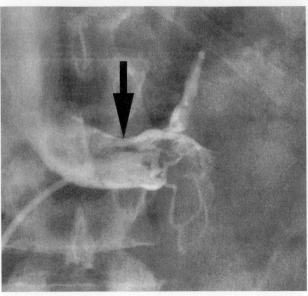

Figure 13-25   Renal vein thrombosis in a patient with membranous glomerulonephritis. Selective left renal venogram showing an intraluminal filling defect (arrow) with poor collateralization (compare with Fig. 13-11).

medical care. Multiple organ injuries are common in these patients, and 10% have associated major arterial injuries. The diagnosis is evident on CT scan, although cavography may be rarely required. Management is expectant whenever possible, as attempted surgical repair or ligation of the traumatized IVC is extremely difficult owing to the difficult exposure and diaphanous nature of the vessel wall. Most bleeding from the IVC will be tamponaded by surrounding structures. Owing to the 50% mortality rate from intraoperative exsanguination, surgery is reserved for patients with evidence of continued bleeding. Renal vein injuries are usually managed with ligation, which is tolerated well.

RENAL VEIN THROMBOSIS

Renal vein thrombosis may occur as an isolated event, as a result of a systemic disease, or in conjunction with IVC thrombosis (Box 13-6). Patients may be asymptomatic when occlusion is slowly progressive, as collateral drainage has sufficient time to enlarge (see Fig. 13-11). Acute venous occlusion results in renal dysfunction, back pain, and hematuria due to congestion and edema of the kidney (Fig. 13-25). These symptoms are similar to those caused by acute renal ischemia of arterial etiology. Extensive thrombosis can result in permanent ischemic damage to the kidney. Bland renal vein thrombus may be a source of pulmonary emboli. For this reason, careful identification of inflow of unopacified blood from the renal veins, indicating patent vessels, is critical when performing cavography prior to IVC filter placement.

US, CT, and MR are all useful imaging modalities in these patients, although CT has the disadvantage of requiring iodinated contrast. Variant renal vein anatomy may be difficult to detect by US in obese patients. An enlarged renal vein that lacks Doppler signal on duplex imaging or enhancement with contrast on CT or MR is conclusive for thrombosis. When the thrombus demonstrates enhancement with contrast, tumor thrombus should be suspected. MR imaging with anatomic and flow sequences provides excellent visualization of the main renal veins. Small renal veins with diminished or absent flow may be seen in patients with longstanding renal failure. When renal vein thrombus is detected, the kidney should be carefully inspected for tumor. Imaging of suspected renal vein thrombosis with CTA or MRA should also include an assessment of the renal arterial supply.

Renal venography is rarely required for diagnostic purposes alone. Venographic studies should begin with a cavogram, followed by selective injection of the renal veins. An intraluminal filling defect indicates acute thrombus. Webs, synechia, stenosis, and enlarged collateral veins connote chronic occlusion.

The conventional therapy of bland renal vein thrombosis in patients with stable renal function is anticoagulation. When anticoagulation is contraindicated, a suprarenal IVC filter should be placed. In patients with acute renal dysfunction due to renal vein thrombosis, thrombolysis with mechanical and pharmacologic techniques should be considered. Theoretically, combined renal vein and artery infusion of the thrombolytic agent maximizes delivery of the agent to the thrombus. Surgical thrombectomy may also be necessary, particularly when attempting to salvage a transplanted kidney.

RENAL VEIN VARICES

Renal vein varices are unusual lesions with a number of different potential etiologies (Box 13-7). Patients present with vague flank pain and hematuria. Varices are more common on the left than the right. Extrinsic compression of the left renal vein between the superior mesenteric artery and the aorta with the symptom complex described above is termed "nutcracker syndrome." Although there is disagreement about the verity of this condition, it is most often diagnosed in thin young women, particularly when there has been recent substantial decrease in weight.

Distended renal veins may be noted on US, CT, or MR studies. A careful search for an underlying cause is important. Venography reveals enlarged, tortuous hilar veins that drain into retroperitoneal veins (Fig. 13-26). The presence of high flow should suggest an arteriovenous malformation or arteriovenous fistula (see Fig. 12-33). A stenosis may be visualized at the orifice of the renal vein. A pressure gradient ≥2 mmHg is suggestive of renal venous hypertension due to outflow obstruction.

Treatment of renal vein varices varies with the etiology. Selective arterial embolization may be helpful

---

Box 13-7   Etiologies of Renal Vein Varices

Congenital venous malformation
Renal vein thrombosis
Obstruction of outflow ("nutcracker syndrome")
Spontaneous splenorenal shunt
Arteriovenous malformation
Arteriovenous fistula
   Intrarenal
   Aorta to left renal vein
Vascular renal tumor

---

or curative in patients with arteriovenous malformations or fistulas. Venous malformations are more difficult to treat, as they can be extensive with numerous points of communication with retroperitoneal veins. Tumor resection or chemotherapy usually resolves hematuria in patients with renal malignancies causing varices. The treatment of "nutcracker syndrome" is controversial, with little evidence to support stent placement within the left renal vein.

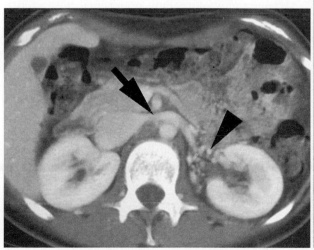

A

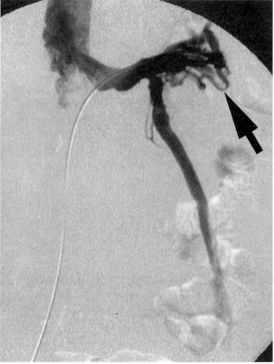

B

Figure 13-26   "Nutcracker syndrome" in a 17-year-old female with chronic pelvic pain. **A,** CT scan with contrast showing compression of the left renal vein (arrow) between the aorta and superior mesenteric artery and perirenal varices (arrowhead). **B,** Selective left renal venogram showing varices (arrow) and retrograde flow into the left gonadal vein. The pressure gradient between the IVC and the renal hilum was 7 mmHg.

PELVIC CONGESTION SYNDROME

Chronic pelvic pain is a perplexing and disturbingly frequent problem. An estimated 10 million women are affected, but an explanation can be found in fewer than half. The evaluation of these patients requires a thorough gynecologic work-up, including laparoscopy in most cases. A wide variety of gynecologic conditions can be responsible for chronic pelvic pain, including endometriosis, chronic infection, adhesions, fibroids, adenomyosis, and pelvic varicosities. Nongynecologic pathology can cause chronic pelvic pain as well. When dilated gonadal and periuterine veins are determined to be the etiology of the pain, the term "pelvic congestion syndrome" is applied. The symptoms of pelvic congestion syndrome include pelvic pain, dyspareunia, menstrual abnormalities, vulvar varices, and lower-extremity varicose veins. Symptoms are worse when standing, later in the day, with sexual arousal, and during menstruation. Dilated pelvic veins in the absence of symptoms is not considered pelvic congestion syndrome.

Reflux of blood in gonadal veins is the underlying etiology of pelvic varicosities in the majority of patients. Rarely, pelvic arteriovenous malformations or fistulas may be encountered. Valves are present at the orifices of the gonadal veins in 85% of women, but are incompetent in about 40% on the left and 35% on the right. Unimpeded reflux of blood into the pelvis results in distention and engorgement of the periuterine veins. Predisposing conditions include prior pregnancy, but may include "nutcracker syndrome," tubal ligation, and intrauterine devices. A subset of patients has reflux in the hypogastric veins as well. Pelvic congestion syndrome is uniformly a condition of women of child-bearing age.

Dilated gonadal and pelvic veins can be visualized with US, CT, and MRI (see Fig. 13-9). However, these studies are usually performed with the patient supine, which may underestimate the degree of venous distension. The normal diameter of the gonadal veins is ≤5 mm. When abnormal, the diameter can easily exceed 10 mm.

Gonadal venography remains the definitive diagnostic imaging modality. Ideally the patient should be studied on a tilting table. Flush cavography is not necessary prior to selection of the gonadal veins. As the left gonadal vein is more commonly affected than the right, and is also easier to catheterize, this vein should be addressed first. A left renal venogram should be obtained, as this will demonstrate reflux into the gonadal vein as well as any associated renal vein pathology. Competent gonadal vein valves are difficult to cross with a guidewire. Abnormal vein orifices tend to be patulous and easy to select. Injection into an abnormal gonadal vein will reveal retrograde flow into the pelvis and the uterine plexus of veins,

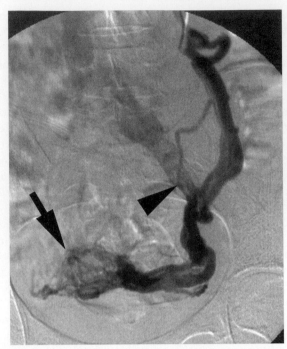

Figure 13-27   Digital subtraction left gonadal venogram in a patient with pelvic pain, showing filling of the uterine plexus (arrow) and drainage via the internal iliac vein (arrowhead).

with drainage through the hypogastric veins or through a contralateral normal gonadal vein (Fig. 13-27). In addition, washout of contrast is slow.

There is no effective medical management of pelvic congestion syndrome. Surgical management includes ligation of the ovarian veins via a laparoscope and hysterectomy. These procedures are effective in controlling symptoms in almost 75% of patients. However, as most patients with pelvic congestion syndrome are relatively young, embolotherapy represents an attractive alternative (Box 13-8).

Coils are the embolic agent used most often for gonadal vein occlusion. Some interventionalists also inject a sclerosing agent such as sotradecol. Access from either the femoral or jugular vein can be used, although the approach to the gonadal veins is antegrade with the latter. Recurved catheters and long curved guide catheters or sheaths are necessary when access is from the femoral vein (see Fig. 13-13). Gonadal venograms are obtained prior to embolization to confirm the anatomy and identify potential

---

Box 13-8   Indications for Ovarian Vein Embolization

Pelvic varicosities with:
- Chronic pelvic pain and otherwise negative work-up
- Dyspareunia and otherwise negative work-up
- Severe labial and perineal varicosities

sources of collateralization and variant anatomy. When the valve at the orifice of a gonadal vein is competent, the vein should not be embolized. Injection during the Valsalva maneuver or tilting the venography table in reverse Trendelenburg may be necessary to unmask reflux. The first coils should be placed at the level of sacroiliac joints. Coils should be deployed along the length of the vein in order to prevent collateralization from retroperitoneal veins (Fig. 13-28). In addition, this decreases the chance of spontaneous recanalization through the coiled segment. Spasm of the vein is common due to catheter manipulation, but can be reduced by injection of 150- or 200-μg aliquots of nitroglycerin. Multiple gonadal veins on the same side require embolization of each individual vessel.

Embolization reduces or eliminates symptoms in up to 80% of women. Patients may experience transient pelvic pressure or pain for a few days following the embolization, probably related to some degree of venous thrombosis in the pelvis. More serious complications are rare.

VARICOCELE EMBOLIZATION

Dilatation of the pampiniform plexus, termed a "varicocele," results from reflux of blood through incompetent gonadal vein valves in males. These are common lesions, found in 5-17% of males, with a left to right ratio of 10:1. When present, varicoceles are bilateral in fewer than 10%, and isolated to the right side in only 1-2%. Varicoceles are associated with pain, infertility, and testicular hypoplasia. The etiology of varicoceles is unclear, but this abnormality is rare in prepubertal males. Sudden onset of any varicocele or an isolated right varicocele should prompt imaging of the retroperitoneum to exclude an abdominal or renal mass. Varicoceles may cause infertility, pain, testicular atrophy, or scrotal enlargement. Varicoceles are more common than infertility in males, but sperm counts increase after treatment of the varicocele in 80% of appropriately selected patients.

The diagnosis of varicocele, unlike pelvic vein varicosities, is usually clinical. Patients present with a palpable scrotal abnormality that increases in size with Valsalva and diminishes in the supine position. Ultrasound is the preferred imaging modality when a subclinical varicocele is suspected (such as in an infertile male with a normal physical examination). The finding of a dilated pampiniform complex is diagnostic, with 2 mm being the upper limit of normal. Reflux may be noted with Valsalva using Doppler or color-flow imaging. MRI is also used for imaging of the scrotal contents. Venography is only performed as part of an embolization procedure (see Fig. 3-13).

There is no effective medical treatment for varicoceles (Box 13-9). As with pelvic congestion syndrome (see above), the goal of intervention is to interrupt the

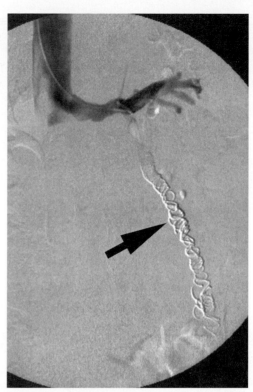

Figure 13-28   Digital subtraction venogram after embolization of the left ovarian vein for chronic pelvic pain. The coils extended from the pelvic brim to the renal vein.

internal spermatic vein in order to prevent retrograde flow of blood into the scrotum. Surgical or laparoscopic ligation of the internal spermatic vein can be performed at multiple levels – high retroperitoneal (Palomo), low retroperitoneal (Ivanissevich), and subinguinal (Marmar). The recurrence rate is approximately 10–20% following surgical ligation, usually due to collateral flow around the ligature, a missed additional internal spermatic vein, or a loose ligature.

Percutaneous embolization of the internal spermatic vein has many similarities to embolization of the ovarian vein. The initial technical features are identical in terms of access, selection of the veins, and venography. As is the case with pelvic congestion syndrome, embolization should not be performed when competent internal spermatic vein valves are found. Embolization with coils

---

Box 13-9   Indications for Internal Spermatic Vein Embolization
Varicocele with: • Infertility • Testicular hypoplasia • Pain

is preferred, although detachable balloons, sotradecol, and boiling contrast material have been described. The first coils are placed at the level of the inguinal canal, which usually corresponds to the superior pubic ramus. Multiple coils are then deposited along the entire length of the vein. Detachable balloons are expensive and have no real advantage over coils. Care must be exercised with liquid agents to avoid reflux to the scrotal level and subsequent thrombosis of the pampiniform plexus itself. In general, liquid agents are used as an adjunct after the initial coils have been placed to minimize the risk of reflux. When present, multiple internal spermatic veins should be individually embolized.

The results of embolization of internal spermatic veins are similar to surgery, with a technical success rate that exceeds 90%, and a recurrence rate that approaches 10%. Sperm counts improve in 80% of patients following successful embolization. Pampiniform swelling occurs in about 10%, and thrombosis in approximately 2%. Failures of embolization occur due to missed additional veins, collateralization from perirenal and retroperitoneal veins, and recanalization of occluded segments.

CAVERNOSOGRAPHY

Erectile dysfunction is a complex and frequently multifactorial problem. Veno-occlusive abnormalities are present in two-thirds of patients with vasculogenic impotence, and are the primary vascular cause of impotence in half of these. Failure to trap blood in the corpora results in failure to achieve erection.

Imaging of veno-occlusive abnormalities requires direct cavernosography with pharmacologic enhancement and measurement of intracavernosal pressures. The primary object of cavernosography is determination of the rate of venous leakage from the corpora. This is accomplished by measurement of pressures through an intracavernosal needle following injection of a pharmacologic relaxant (see Fig. 13-8) – either the infusion rate required to maintain a specified intracavernosal pressure (normal <10 mL/min at a pressure of 150 mmHg), or the rate of fall in pressure following cessation of the infusion (normal being 1.5 mmHg/s at a baseline pressure of 100 mmHg). Patients with venous leak tend to respond well to pharmacologic therapies such as prostaglandin E_1, papaverine, or sildenafil, which help trap blood in the corpora cavernosa. There is limited experience with venous ligation or percutaneous embolization.

ADRENAL VENOUS SAMPLING

Adrenal lesions rarely require catheter-based imaging for diagnosis. The majority of adrenal masses can be detected and evaluated with CT, MRI, or nuclear medicine studies. Masses of questionable etiology may be amenable to percutaneous CT-guided biopsy. The primary catheter-based procedure performed in patients with suspected adrenal pathology is venous sampling. These patients have confirmed endocrine disorders but require localization to an adrenal gland in order to guide surgery. Venous sampling should never be performed in order to make the diagnosis of an endocrine disease.

Aldosteronism

Aldosterone is a hormone secreted by the adrenal cortex that induces renal sodium retention and excretion of potassium. This is a normal response to renal artery stenosis, congestive heart failure, pregnancy, and cirrhosis, and is termed "secondary aldosteronism." Primary aldosteronism (Conn's syndrome) is hypersecretion of aldosterone by either an adrenal adenoma (two-thirds of cases) or bilateral idiopathic adrenal hyperplasia (one-third) (Box 13-10). Adenomas are bilateral in 2% of cases, and in fewer than 1% of cases an adrenal carcinoma is the source of the aldosterone.

A serum potassium <3.5 mEq/L in a patient with diastolic hypertension suggests Conn's syndrome. Additional laboratory investigation includes plasma renin activity, and 24-hour urine collections for sodium, cortisol, and aldosterone. Imaging of the adrenal glands is performed with CT or MRI. When a discrete or localized adrenal mass is not identified with certainty, adrenal venous sampling should be obtained. In many centers adrenal vein sampling is performed in all patients.

The patient should be systemically heparinized after obtaining access in both common femoral veins. Catheters are then positioned in both adrenal veins (see Fig. 13-14). Gentle contrast injections are the rule, as the adrenal veins are weak and prone to rupture. In some patients a 3-French microcatheter is necessary to engage the left adrenal vein. Samples should be obtained simultaneously from both adrenal veins and a peripheral (usually femoral) vein before and 15 minutes after administration of adrenocorticotropic hormone (ACTH, 0.25-mg bolus

---

Box 13-10   Symptoms of Primary Aldosteronism (Conn's Syndrome)

Diastolic hypertension
Hypokalemia
Hypernatremia
Hyperchlorhydria
Alkalosis

Table 13-5 Etiologies of Endogenous Cushing's Syndrome

Etiology	Mechanism	Incidence (%)
ACTH-secreting anterior pituitary tumor	Adrenal hyperstimulation	65
Adrenal adenoma or carcinoma	Independent secretion	20
Ectopic ACTH secretion by tumor	Adrenal hyperstimulation	15

followed by infusion of 0.15–0.20 mg/h). A clear understanding of the volume of blood needed for the samples, the types of tubes, and the handling requirements is important to perform the study correctly. Strict attention to labeling of the tubes is necessary so that right/left confusion does not occur with the results.

Samples are submitted for both aldosterone and cortisol, as it is assumed that the production of the latter is the same for both glands. The cortisol test helps to confirm that an adrenal vein has been sampled, to correct for dilution of right adrenal vein samples, and to distinguish between an adenoma and idiopathic adrenal hyperplasia. In patients with adenomas, the ratio of aldosterone/cortisol from the affected gland is high before and after ACTH, whereas the opposite gland is similar to the femoral vein samples at baseline and has a blunted response to stimulation. In patients with bilateral hyperplasia, there is no lateralization of ratios before or after ACTH. Some centers define lateralization as a ≥4:1 difference in ratios from side to side. Sampling provides diagnostic information in more than 95% of cases.

The treatment for a unilateral adrenal adenoma is surgical resection. Bilateral hyperplasia is usually managed medically, as adrenalectomy would result in adrenal insufficiency (Addison's disease). Transcatheter ablative techniques have been described but are not widely utilized.

Cushing's Syndrome

Cushing's syndrome is a distinctive clinical complex due to hypercortisolism (Box 13-11). The most common etiology is iatrogenic as a result of administration of glucocorticoids or adrenocorticotropic hormone (ATCH). Endogenous Cushing's syndrome has both central nervous system and peripheral etiologies (Table 13-5). The diagnosis is based on biochemical abnormalities. Urinary excretion of free cortisol is elevated, and plasma cortisol levels do not drop in response to a single dose of dexamethasone in patients with endogenous Cushing's syndrome.

Localization of the cause of Cushing's syndrome is of paramount importance in directing therapy. Patients with pituitary or ectopic sources of ACTH will have elevated serum levels. In general, the highest ACTH levels are found in patients with ectopic secretion. Patients with independently functioning adrenal masses have low serum ACTH levels as the pituitary mechanisms are intact. The contralateral adrenal gland is frequently atrophic.

Imaging of the adrenal glands in patients with Cushing's syndrome includes either a CT scan or MRI for detection of a mass. Selective catheterization of the adrenal veins for venous sampling for cortisol levels is occasionally required to confirm localization to the adrenal gland. Samples are obtained from both adrenal veins, the IVC above the adrenal veins, and below the renal veins. Stimulation is not required. The treatment of Cushing's syndrome due to unilateral adrenal abnormality is surgical resection. Catheter ablation of the adrenal gland has been described in a few patients.

SUGGESTED READINGS

Angle JF, Matsumoto AH, Al Shammari M et al: Transcatheter regional urokinase therapy in the management of inferior vena cava thrombosis. *J Vasc Interv Radiol* 9:917–925, 1998.

Aslam Sohaib SA, Teh J, Nargund VH et al: Assessment of tumor invasion of the vena caval wall in renal cell carcinoma cases by magnetic resonance imaging. *J Urol* 167:1271–1275, 2002.

Bass JE, Redwine MD, Kramer LA, Huynh PT, Harris JH: Spectrum of congenital anomalies of the inferior vena cava: cross-sectional imaging findings. *Radiographics* 20:639–652, 2000.

Bernstein MR, Malkowicz SB, Siegelman ES et al: Progressive angiomyolipoma with inferior vena cava tumor thrombus. *Urology* 50:975–977, 1997.

Box 13-11 Symptoms of Cushing's Syndrome

Hypertension	Peripheral edema
Muscle weakness	Glucose intolerance
Osteoporosis	Vascular fragility
Cutaneous striae	Hirsutism
Truncal obesity	Moon facies
Buffalo hump	Amenorrhea

Bonn J, Liu JB, Eschelman DJ et al: Intravascular ultrasound as an alternative to positive-contrast vena cavography prior to filter placement. *J Vasc Interv Radiol* 10:843-849, 1999.

Bower TC, Nagorney DM, Cherry KJ et al: Replacement of the inferior vena cava for malignancy: an update. *J Vasc Surg* 31:270-281, 2000.

Buckman RF, Pathak AS, Badellino MM, Bradley KM: Injuries of the inferior vena cava. *Surg Clin N Am* 81:1431-1447, 2001.

Butty S, Hagspiel KD, Leung DA et al: Body MR venography. *Radiol Clin N Am* 40:899-919, 2002.

Coakley FV, Varghese SL, Hricak H: CT and MRI of pelvic varices in women. *J Comput Assist Tomogr* 23:429-434, 1999.

Cornud F, Belin X, Amar E et al: Varicocele: strategies in diagnosis and treatment. *Eur Radiol* 9:536-545, 1999.

Decousus H, Leizorovicz A, Parent F et al: A clinical trial of vena caval filters in the prevention of pulmonary embolism in patients with proximal deep-vein thrombosis. *N Engl J Med* 338:409-415, 1998.

Dewald CL, Jensen CC, Park YH et al: Vena cavography with CO_2 versus with iodinated contrast material for inferior vena cava filter placement: a prospective evaluation. *Radiology* 216: 752-757, 2000.

Hines OJ, Nelson S, Quinones-Baldrich WJ, Eilber FR: Leiomyosarcoma of the inferior vena cava: prognosis and comparison with leiomyosarcoma of other anatomic sites. *Cancer* 85:1077-1083, 1999.

Kaufman JA, Waltman AC, Rivitz SM, Geller SG: Anatomical observations on the renal veins and inferior vena cava at magnetic resonance angiography. *Cardiovasc Interv Radiol* 18:153-157, 1995.

Kaufman JA, Geller SC, Bazari H, Waltman AC: Gadolinium-based contrast agents as an alternative at vena cavography in patients with renal insufficiency: early experience. *Radiology* 212:280-284, 1999.

Levy JM, Duszak RL, Akins EW et al: Inferior vena cava filter placement. American College of Radiology: ACR Appropriateness Criteria. *Radiology* 215:S981-997, 2000.

Maleux G, Stockx L, Wilms G, Marchal G: Ovarian vein embolization for the treatment of pelvic congestion syndrome: long-term technical and clinical results. *J Vasc Interv Radiol* 11: 859-864, 2000.

Matchett WJ, Jones MP, McFarland DR, Ferris EJ: Suprarenal vena caval filter placement: follow-up of four filter types in 22 patients. *J Vasc Interv Radiol* 9:588-593, 1998.

Millward SF, Oliva VL, Bell SD et al: Gunther Tulip retrievable vena cava filter: results from the Registry of the Canadian Interventional Radiology Association. *J Vasc Interv Radiol* 12:1053-1058, 2001.

Petersen BD, Uchida BT: Long-term results of treatment of benign central venous obstructions unrelated to dialysis with expandable Z stents. *J Vasc Interv Radiol* 10:757-766, 1999.

Razavi MK, Hansch EC, Kee ST et al: Chronically occluded inferior venae cavae: endovascular treatment. *Radiology* 214: 133-138, 2000.

Rosen MP, Schwartz AN, Levine FJ, Greenfield AJ: Radiologic assessment of impotence: angiography, sonography, cavernosography, and scintigraphy. *Am J Roentgenol* 157:923-931, 1991.

Shlansky-Goldberg RD, Van Arsdalen KN, Rutter CM et al: Percutaneous varicocele embolization versus surgical ligation for the treatment of infertility: changes in seminal parameters and pregnancy outcomes. *J Vasc Interv Radiol* 8:759-767, 1997.

Scultetus AH, Villavicencio JL, Gillespie DL: The nutcracker syndrome: its role in the pelvic venous disorders. *J Vasc Surg* 34:812-819, 2001.

Sheth S, Scatarige JC, Horton KM, Corl FM, Fishman EK: Current concepts in the diagnosis and management of renal cell carcinoma: role of multidetector CT and three-dimensional CT. *Radiographics* 21:S237-254, 2001.

Streiff MB: Vena caval filters: a comprehensive review. *Blood* 95:3669-3677, 2000.

Thornton MJ, Ryan R, Varghese JC et al: A three-dimensional gadolinium-enhanced MR venography technique for imaging central veins. *Am J Roentgenol* 173:999-1003, 1999.

Twickler DM, Setiawan AT, Evans RS et al: Imaging of puerperal septic thrombophlebitis: prospective comparison of MR imaging, CT, and sonography. *Am J Roentgenol* 169:1039-1043, 1997.

Tsuji Y, Goto A, Hara I et al: Renal cell carcinoma with extension of tumor thrombus into the vena cava: surgical strategy and prognosis. *J Vasc Surg* 33:789-796, 2001.

Venbrux AC, Chang AH, Kim HS et al: Pelvic congestion syndrome (pelvic venous incompetence): impact of ovarian and internal iliac vein embolotherapy on menstrual cycle and chronic pelvic pain. *J Vasc Interv Radiol* 13:171-178, 2002.

Zhang C, Fu L, Zhang G, Xu L et al: Ultrasonically guided inferior vena cava stent placement: experience in 83 cases. *J Vasc Interv Radiol* 10:85-91, 1999.

Zigman A, Yazbeck S, Emil S, Nguyen L: Renal vein thrombosis: a 10-year review. *J Pediatr Surg* 35:1540-1542, 2000.

Portal and Hepatic Veins

PETER J. BROMLEY, M.D., AND JOHN A. KAUFMAN, M.D.

End-stage liver disease is the tenth leading cause of death in the United States. Abnormalities of the portal and hepatic venous systems are common in this setting, with major metabolic and hemodynamic consequences. Mortality in these patients is closely linked to the consequences of chronic portal hypertension. Catheter-based techniques can effectively manage many of these conditions.

ANATOMY

Hepatic Segmentation

The distributions of the right and left hepatic arteries and portal vein branches are not accounted for by dividing the liver into right and left lobes using surface landmarks such as the ligamentum teres and falciform ligament. The most widely accepted schema is that proposed by Couinaud and modified by Bismuth (Fig. 14-1). The liver is divided into right and left halves by a plane that passes through the inferior vena cava (IVC) and the gallbladder fossa along the path of the middle hepatic vein. Each liver half is then further divided into four portions yielding a total of eight hepatic segments. The left-sided segments are numbered from 1 to 4 beginning with the caudate lobe. The right-sided segments are 5–8. Bismuth's modification divides segment 4 into 4a (superiorly) and 4b (inferiorly).

Vascular Anatomy

The portal venous system and hepatic veins are a paired network of valveless veins responsible for blood from all of the abdominal viscera, excluding the kidneys and adrenal glands. Before reaching the heart the blood collected by the tributaries of the portal vein passes through the hepatic sinusoids. After traversing the sinusoids, blood is collected in the hepatic veins and flows to the right atrium.

The portal vein is formed beneath the neck of the pancreas by the confluence of the splenic and the superior mesenteric veins and travels in the free edge of the gastrohepatic ligament (Fig. 14-2). The normal portal vein is about 8 cm in length and 10–12 mm in diameter. Upon reaching the liver hilum (porta hepatis) the portal vein bifurcates into right and left branches that ramify as they penetrate through the liver (Fig. 14-3). The portal vein bifurcation is extrahepatic in 40–48% of individuals but is generally surrounded by fairly dense fibrous connective tissue in the porta hepatis. A trifurcation of the main portal vein, resulting in absence of a right portal trunk, is encountered in about 11% of cases. Occasionally the left portal vein will provide a branch to a portion of the right lobe of the liver (4%), usually the anterior segments (V and VIII). The left portal branch is critical to the fetal circulation, receiving blood from the placenta via the left umbilical vein and delivering it across the liver to the IVC via the ductus venosus. The ductus venosus eventually atrophies and becomes the ligamentum venosum

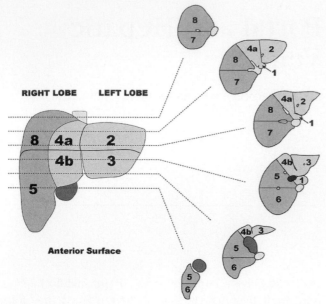

Figure 14-1 Drawing of hepatic segmentation. The right and left lobes are separated by a plane that passes through the inferior vena cava and the gallbladder fossa along the path of the middle hepatic vein. Segments 2 and 3 are separated from 4 by the ligamentum teres. The right-sided segments are numbered 5–8. The plane of the right hepatic vein separates the right posterior segments (6 and 7) from the right anterior segments (8 and 5). The superior segments (7 and 8 on the right and 4a and 2 on the left) are separated from the inferior segments (5 and 6 on the right and 4b and 3 on the left) by the planes of the right and left portal branches.

while the umbilical vein becomes part of the ligamentum teres. Persistence of the ductus venosus is very rare (Fig. 14-4). Valves are present in the portal vein *in utero* but rarely persist into adult life.

Blood in the portal system is collected from the gastrointestinal tract, pancreas, and the spleen by a network of major tributaries (see Fig. 14-2). The superior mesenteric vein (SMV) collects blood from the small bowel and the right colon (cecum to the mid transverse colon). Pancreaticoduodenal veins drain both into the SMV and directly into the main portal vein. The inferior mesenteric vein (IMV) collects blood from the left colon (mid transverse colon to rectum). The inferior mesenteric vein drains into the splenic vein in roughly two-thirds of individuals and in the remaining one-third enters the superior mesenteric vein at or just below the confluence. The splenic vein drains the spleen as well as portions of the stomach (short gastric veins) and pancreas. By convention, the terms "proximal" and "distal" in the venous system are based upon the normal direction of flow, with blood traveling from a proximal (peripheral) to a distal (central) location. The proximal splenic vein is therefore that portion closest to the spleen, whereas the distal portion is closest to the portal confluence.

The left gastric vein, or coronary vein, is a major draining vein of the stomach and lower esophagus. The coronary vein drains into the main portal vein in about two-thirds

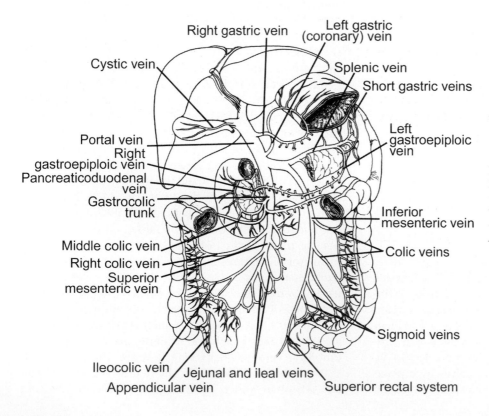

Figure 14-2 Drawing of portal and hepatic veins. (Reproduced with permission from Lundell C, Kadir S: The portal venous system and hepatic veins. In Kadir S ed: *Atlas of Normal and Angiographic Anatomy,* WB Saunders, Philadelphia, 1991.)

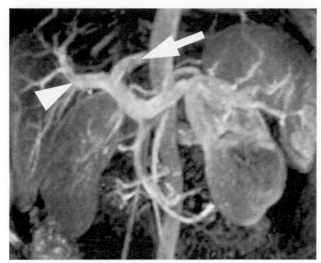

Figure 14-3   Gadolinium-enhanced 3-D MRA (maximum-intensity projection, MIP) of the abdomen showing a normal portal venous system. The main portal vein bifurcation into the right (arrowhead) and left (arrow) portal veins is well visualized. (Image courtesy of Barry Stein M.D., Hartford Hospital, CT.)

of individuals, and into the splenic vein in the remaining one-third.

The common bile duct and common hepatic artery lie with the portal vein in the gastrohepatic ligament. The portal vein, hepatic artery, and bile ducts continue together in the liver parenchyma in a grouping referred

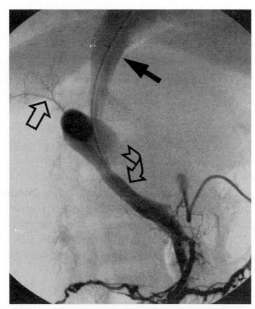

Figure 14-4   Patent ductus venosus. Digital subtraction angiogram (DSA) showing that the portal vein (curved arrow) communicates directly with the inferior vena cava (IVC) (straight arrow) through the ductus venosus. The intrahepatic portal veins are diminutive (open arrow).

to as "portal triads." There is actually a fourth element, the lymphatic ducts. The terminal branches of the portal vein join with the terminal branches of the hepatic artery to perfuse the hepatic sinusoids. Blood percolates through the sinusoids, where it is separated from the hepatocytes by a thin endothelial layer, and drains to the centrilobular hepatic veins. This forms the basic functional unit of the liver. The centrilobular veins join together forming sublobular veins that unite eventually to form the hepatic veins. The largest of the hepatic veins exit the posterosuperior surface of the liver and join the hepatic segment of the IVC just before it leaves the abdomen; usually about 2 cm below the right atrium. These are the right, middle, and left hepatic veins and are referred to by anatomists as the "upper group." The left and middle hepatic veins are oriented anterior and anterolateral (respectively) while the right hepatic vein typically has a lateral or posterolateral orientation (Fig. 14-5). The middle and left hepatic veins form a common trunk before joining the IVC in 65–85% of individuals. A second, lower group of hepatic veins arising from the caudate and right lobes are also present and vary in number. Large-caliber veins from the lower right lobe (inferior right hepatic veins) are seen in approximately 15% of individuals. These large veins are usually solitary but can be duplicated.

The quantity of blood flow in the portal vein is totally dependent on the perfusion of the spleen, pancreas, and gastrointestinal tract. After a meal, portal vein flow increases dramatically (postprandial portal hyperemia) as a consequence of increased perfusion of these organs. Portal blood flow normally represents approximately two-thirds of the total perfusion of the liver, with the remainder being made up by the hepatic artery. Normal portal blood flow is towards the liver (hepatopedal) but can be reversed. In cirrhosis, hepatic arterial inflow can be markedly increased to compensate for poor forward flow in the portal vein. As cirrhosis progresses and sinusoids are obstructed, the portal vein can become the outflow for the hepatic artery. This flow reversal is termed "hepatofugal" (literally, blood "fleeing" from the liver).

KEY COLLATERAL PATHWAYS

Two series of important collateral networks are recognized in the portal circulation. Portal-to-portal collaterals become apparent when focal occlusions develop within the portal circulation. Blood bypasses the occlusion but remains within the portal circulation. Three commonly encountered venous occlusions are in the splenic, portal, and SMV. When the splenic vein occludes, retrograde flow through the short gastric veins to the left gastric vein can occur (Fig. 14-6). Occlusion of the central SMV can result in collateral drainage through mesenteric, paraduodenal, and marginal veins. The collateral

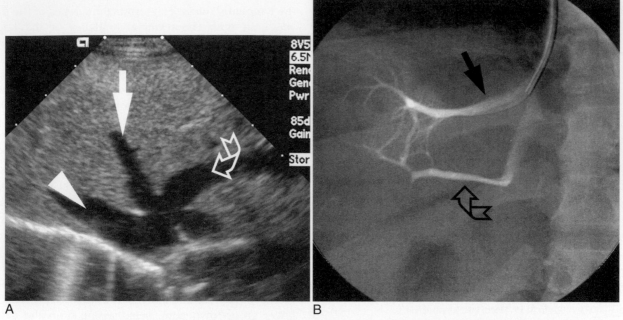

Figure 14-5   Hepatic vein anatomy. **A**, US showing the relationships of the hepatic vein orifices (arrowhead = right hepatic vein; straight arrow = middle hepatic vein; curved arrow = left hepatic vein. **B**, Inferior right hepatic vein. Injection of a somewhat small right hepatic vein (straight arrow) opacifies a second, lower right hepatic vein (curved arrow) that drains directly into the IVC.

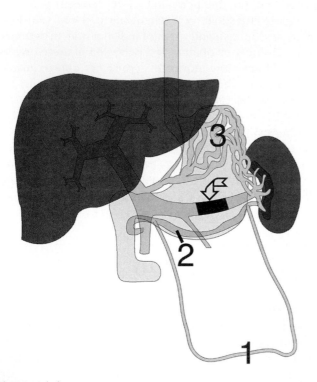

Figure 14-6   Drawing of collateral pathways to the portal vein in the setting of isolated splenic vein obstruction (curved arrow) in a patient with normal portal pressures. **1**, Omental vein to gastroepiploic vein or superior mesenteric vein (SMV). **2**, Gastroepiploic veins to SMV. **3**, Short gastric veins to coronary vein.

pathways for splenic vein and SMV occlusion are frequently submucosal, and therefore prone to bleeding into the gastrointestinal tract. Occlusion of the portal vein results in formation of a network of small veins in the gastro-hepatic ligament, termed "cavernous transformation" (Fig. 14-7). A small, residual, or recanalized main portal vein may exist within this network but can be difficult to identify.

Portal-to-systemic collaterals develop in the setting of portal hypertension and represent pathways for blood to escape the portal circulation and return to the systemic circulation (Fig. 14-8). Termed "varices," the majority of these pathways represent enlargement of preexisting small communications between the portal and systemic veins. Unusual portal-to-systemic collaterals can form following abdominal surgery. Both portal-to-portal and portal-to-systemic collaterals may be present in the same patient.

Obstruction of the main hepatic veins frequently results in intrahepatic collateralization to other hepatic veins. Provided that at least one hepatic vein remains patent, obstruction of main hepatic veins is usually well tolerated. Collateral drainage through capsular veins may also occur.

IMAGING

Transabdominal ultrasound (US) with Doppler interrogation is an excellent noninvasive means for evaluating

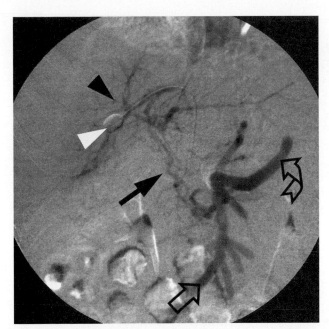

Figure 14-7   Cavernous transformation of the portal vein demonstrated on balloon occlusion (white arrowhead) wedged hepatic venogram using CO_2 gas as a contrast agent in a patient with known occlusion of the main portal vein. The only communication between the intrahepatic portal veins (black arrowhead) and the SMV (straight open arrow) and splenic vein (curved arrow) is through small periportal veins (straight solid arrow).

the patency of the portal vein, hepatic veins, and hepatic artery. Color-flow Doppler and power Doppler provide quick means for locating the vessels and confirming patency, with color-flow Doppler also providing directional information. Spectral Doppler should also be performed and the waveforms evaluated. Each vessel has a typical waveform (Fig. 14-9). The portal vein is a high-flow, low-pressure, low-resistance conduit characterized by a gentle phasic waveform with respiratory variation. The splenic and superior mesenteric veins have similar waveforms. Flow in the portal system increases dramatically after meals. The hepatic veins are characterized by a variable waveform influenced by right atrial contractions. The hepatic artery has a low-resistance arterial waveform. A structural evaluation of the liver should also be performed noting the overall size and echotexture of the liver, parenchymal masses (cystic or solid), and biliary dilatation. Ascites should be documented and qualitatively measured (minimal, moderate, large volume). Ultrasound can be technically very demanding depending on the patient's body habitus, ability to cooperate, and the severity of underlying liver disease.

Helical CT is an excellent modality for imaging the hepatic and portal veins. Furthermore, detection of mass lesions is highly sensitive. The 3-dimensional relationships of the vascular structures (notably the portal vein and hepatic veins) can be easily appreciated from the axial

CT images and postprocessed data (Fig. 14-10). Dedicated vascular spiral CT of the liver requires a minimum of two acquisition phases – hepatic arterial and portal venous. The first scan through the liver is obtained during the arterial phase of enhancement. Approximately 60 seconds from the initiation of the bolus the scan should be repeated to obtain the portal venous phase. Addition of preliminary noncontrast and delayed postcontrast images optimizes evaluation of the hepatic parenchyma for any mass lesion (quadruple phase examination). The arterial phase should be performed with thin effective collimation (2–5 mm) and overlapping slices to ensure longitudinal resolution adequate for the size of the hepatic artery. Wider collimation (5–7 mm) can be used for the portal venous phase and to cover the remainder of the abdominal contents if necessary.

MRI and MR venography (MRV) are also excellent tools for evaluating the portal venous system and hepatic veins, as well as the liver parenchyma. Basic T1- and T2-weighted sequences should be obtained in multiple planes for overall anatomic evaluation. The relatively slow and nonpulsatile flow in the portal venous system is well suited for MRV with time-of-flight (TOF) and phase-contrast (PC) techniques. However, the complex geometry of the vessels limits the utility of these sequences. Gadolinium-enhanced 3-dimensional gradient echo volume acquisitions, in both arterial and portal venous phases, provide dramatic angiographic images of these structures unaffected by signal loss due to complex or in-plane flow (see Fig. 14-3). Image postprocessing is an essential tool when interpreting hepatic and portal venous MRV.

Venographic evaluation can be performed by catheterization of the hepatic veins from either the femoral vein or internal jugular vein approaches. Femoral venous access is convenient if no other procedure is to be performed. A Cobra-type curved catheter can be used; however, a recurved catheter such as a Simmons-1 is very effective for engaging the hepatic veins from the femoral vein. Approach from the jugular vein is mechanically more advantageous, providing a direct line for the catheter into the hepatic vein. A multipurpose angled-tip catheter is generally effective in selecting the hepatic veins. The junction of the diaphragm with the right cardiac border represents a convenient fluoroscopic landmark for the hepatic vein orifices. The main trunk of the right hepatic vein is characteristically oriented in a lateral or slightly posterolateral direction while the middle and left hepatic veins are more anterior in orientation (see Fig. 14-5). A test injection of contrast should be performed by hand to ensure that the catheter tip is not wedged in a small hepatic vein branch. Some angiographers advocate the addition of a side-hole near the tip of the catheter to prevent an inadvertent wedged injection. A formal venogram can then be obtained by injecting

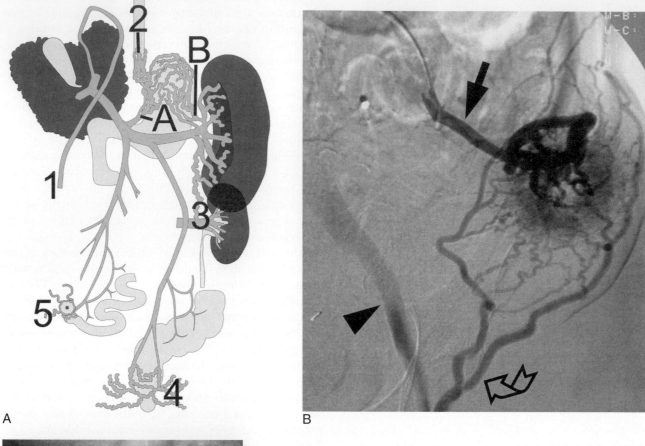

A

B

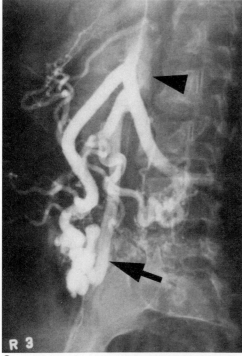

C

Figure 14-8 Portal-to-systemic collateral pathways. **A,** Drawing of portal-to-systemic collateral pathways. **1,** Recanalized umbilical vein (drains to anterior abdominal wall). **2,** Esophageal varices (drain to mediastinal veins), supplied by (A) retrograde flow in left gastric vein and (B) retrograde flow in short gastric veins. **3,** Splenorenal varices that drain through the retroperitoneum from the splenic vein to the right renal vein. **4,** Inferior mesenteric to hemorrhoidal vein varices. **5,** Portal-to-systemic collaterals at sites of prior abdominal or pelvic surgery (in this case an ileostomy). **B,** Stomal varices in a patient with portal hypertension and an ileostomy. DSA of injection in a mesenteric vein (straight arrow) shows dilated peristomal veins that drain to the abdominal wall veins (curved arrow) through innumerable small communications. The arrowhead points to the external iliac vein. **C,** Superior mesenteric venogram showing varices draining through retroperitoneal collaterals (arrow) to the IVC (arrowhead).

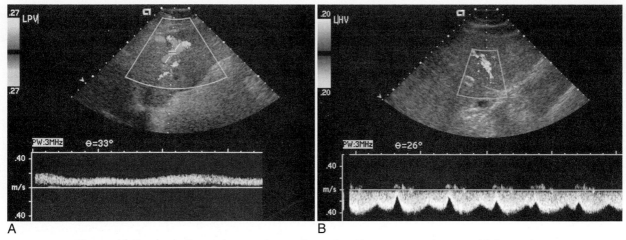

Figure 14-9   Normal Doppler waveforms of portal and hepatic veins. **A**, Normal left portal vein with monophasic hepatopedal flow. **B**, Normal left hepatic vein with triphasic hepatofugal flow.

contrast at a rate of 5-6 mL/s for a total of 15-18 mL during suspended respiration (Fig. 14-11).

Balloon-occlusion hepatic venography can be used to image the small hepatic veins and the portal vein (Table 14-1). An 8- to 11-mm diameter occlusion balloon is gently inflated with 2-3 mL of room air until the hepatic vein wall is circumferentially engaged (see Fig. 14-7). Room air is used instead of contrast to allow rapid deflation of the balloon. Standard iodinated contrast material or carbon dioxide (CO_2) gas can then be injected through the catheter by hand. In a normal liver the portal vein

will usually not be visualized since contrast will drain into other hepatic vein branches. With cirrhosis, opacification of the portal vein, and even retrograde flow, may be seen. Because of its extremely low viscosity, CO_2 gas easily traverses the hepatic sinusoids, providing superior opacification of the portal vein. When sinusoidal hypertension (discussed below) is present, the contrast will enter the portal vein and a portal venogram can be obtained. Aggressive injection of either iodinated contrast or CO_2 gas can result in hepatic fracture, a potentially lethal complication (Fig. 14-12).

Direct opacification of the portal system can be accomplished with a transhepatic approach analogous

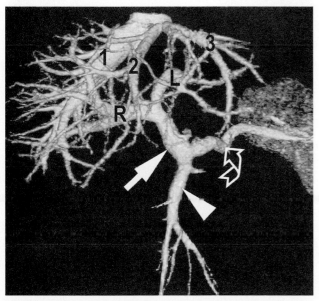

Figure 14-10   Volume rendering of portal and hepatic veins of the venous phase of a CTA. Arrowhead = SMV. Arrow = main portal vein. Curved arrow = splenic vein. R = right portal vein. L = left portal vein. 1 = right hepatic vein. 2 = middle hepatic vein. 3 = left hepatic vein.

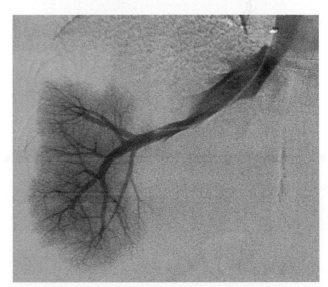

Figure 14-11   Normal free hepatic venogram showing typical ramification of the hepatic veins and a homogeneous liver parenchyma.

Table 14–1   Portal Venography

Technique	Catheter	Injection Rate	Notes
Wedged hepatic	Balloon occlusion	20 mL iodinated contrast 30–40 mL CO_2 gas	Hand injection
Transhepatic	Pigtail	12–15 mL for 36–45 mL	Transabdominal or transjugular access
Arterioportography	Visceral in SMA, celiac, or splenic artery	6–10 mL for 60–80 mL	Intraarterial priscoline and /or nitroglycerin[a] (SMA only)
Splenoportography	18-gauge needle in splenic pulp	10–20 mL	Hand injection

[a]Priscoline = 25–50 mg injected through the SMA catheter immediately prior to contrast injection. Nitrogylcerin = 200–300 μg prior to contrast injection. SMA, superior mesenteric artery.

to that employed during a transhepatic cholangiogram (Fig. 14-13). Local anesthetic is infiltrated into the skin and a narrow-gauge needle (typically 21-gauge) is advanced into the liver under fluoroscopic control. As the needle is slowly withdrawn, contrast is carefully injected with continuous fluoroscopic monitoring. The portal branches must be differentiated from hepatic arterial branches, which both flow in the same direction, although arterial flow is faster. Once a suitable portal vein radicle is opacified, a 0.018-inch guidewire can be introduced and the needle exchanged for a coaxial introducer set with a 4- or 5-French outer catheter. A 0.035-inch guidewire can then be inserted into the portal system and the introducer

set exchanged for a pigtail catheter positioned deep in the splenic vein or superior mesenteric vein. The same transhepatic tract can be used to insert larger instruments if interventions are to be performed. Depending on the size of the catheters used and the patient's coagulation status, it may be appropriate to embolize the tract with Gelfoam pledgets or stainless steel coils at the end of the procedure to reduce the risk of intraperitoneal bleeding.

Direct portal access can be obtained by using a special directional cannula introduced into a hepatic vein from the jugular vein (see below, Transjugular Intrahepatic Portosystemic Shunt). When performed correctly this

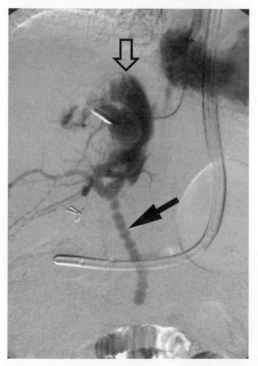

Figure 14-12   Liver laceration (open arrow) and contrast in the biliary duct (arrow) during wedged hepatic venogram with CO_2 gas.

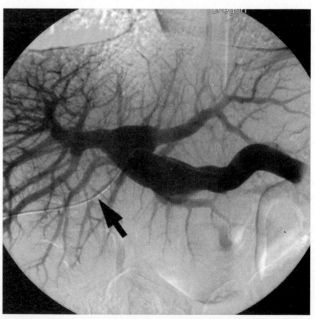

Figure 14-13   DSA portogram using a 5-Fr catheter (arrow) inserted transhepatically from the right midaxillary line. The patient had normal coagulation studies and no ascites. The transhepatic tract was embolized with Gelfoam pledgets at the termination of the procedure.

method avoids puncture of the liver capsule and thus reduces the risk of bleeding complications. The portal system can also be opacified by inserting a needle percutaneously into the splenic pulp and injecting either iodinated contrast or CO_2. This method, known as splenoportography, is rarely used. Lastly, percutaneous catheterization of a recanalized umbilical vein allows access to the left portal vein (Fig. 14-14).

Indirect opacification of the portal venous system can be achieved by arterioportography. Injection of the superior mesenteric artery (SMA) results in opacification of the mesenteric tributary veins, superior mesenteric vein, and portal vein as the contrast drains from the splanchnic capillary bed. The rate and density of opacification of these veins can be significantly improved by injecting a vasodilator such as priscoline or nitroglycerin through the arterial catheter immediately prior to the contrast injection (Fig. 14-15).

Injection of the celiac artery will also opacify the portal vein with blood draining from the spleen, stomach, and pancreas. Selective catheterization of the splenic artery will result in greater portal venous opacification (see Fig. 14-15). For selective splenic artery injections,

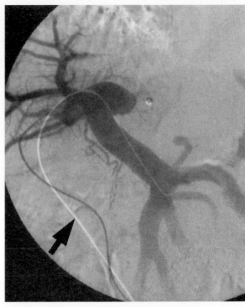

Figure 14-14 DSA portogram performed by retrograde catheterization of a recanalized umbilical vein (arrow). Subtraction artifact due to respiration results in a double image of the catheter.

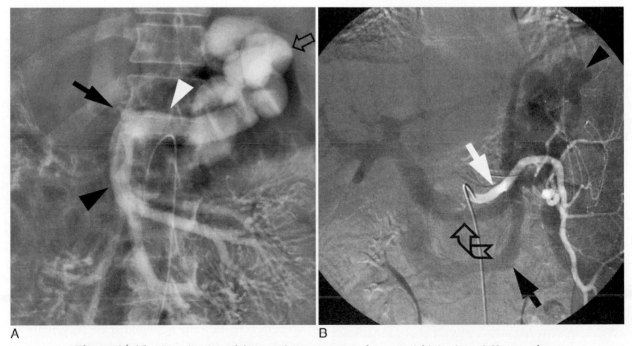

A   B

Figure 14-15 Visualization of the portal venous system from arterial injections. **A,** Venous phase image from a superior mesenteric artery (SMA) injection in a patient with hepatofugal flow in the portal vein. The SMV (black arrowhead) flows into the splenic vein (white arrowhead) which drains through large retroperitoneal varices (open arrow) to the left renal vein. There is absence of opacification of the portal vein (solid arrow) due to retrograde flow from the liver. **B,** Late DSA image from a splenic artery injection in a patient with portal hypertension masked to show the splenic artery (white straight arrow) in white and veins in black. The splenic vein (curved arrow) is patent as well as the portal vein. In addition, there is filling of retroperitoneal varices (arrowhead) with drainage into the left renal vein (black straight arrow).

volumes between 20 and 60 mL may be used depending upon the size of the spleen. Vasodilators are not of assistance in this vascular bed. This technique is less effective in the presence of congestive splenomegaly, which can significantly increase the transit time for contrast through the spleen.

PORTAL HYPERTENSION

Portal hypertension can be defined as an absolute portal venous pressure of greater than 10 mmHg. Elevated pressures can exist in the entire portal venous system, or in isolated segments. Mild portal hypertension may be occult, or manifest with characteristic clinical findings (Box 14-1).

In industrialized countries portal hypertension is most commonly encountered in patients with cirrhosis. The common diseases leading to cirrhosis and portal hypertension are alcoholic liver disease and chronic viral hepatitis (hepatitis B and C viruses) (Box 14-2). End-stage liver disease represents the tenth leading cause of death in the United States. In at least 50% of these patients alcohol is the most significant cause of liver failure. Patients in whom a cause cannot be identified are said to have "cryptogenic cirrhosis."

Not all patients with portal hypertension have cirrhosis. Cirrhosis refers to a specific histological finding of diffuse fibrosis and abnormal nodularity in the liver, resulting from chronic hepatocellular injury. The many causes of portal hypertension are organized into three categories based upon the level of obstruction: posthepatic, intrahepatic, and prehepatic (Box 14-3). Pathologists further divide the intrahepatic causes as presinusoidal, sinusoidal, and postsinusoidal on the basis of histological findings. The level of obstruction in alcoholic cirrhosis is primarily sinusoidal. In schistomasiasis, a common cause of portal hypertension in parts of Africa and South America, the obstruction is presinusoidal.

The pathophysiology of portal hypertension in cirrhosis is a combination of increased resistance to blood

---

Box 14–1 Physical Findings in Advanced Liver Disease

Ascites
Splenomegaly
Caput medusae
Spider nevi
Palmar erythema
Jaundice
Gynecomastia
Testicular atrophy

Box 14–2 Causes of Cirrhosis

Hepatocellular

Alcohol
Viral hepatitis (B, C, D)
Autoimmune
Metabolic
Steatohepatitis
Drugs/toxins

Cholestatic

Biliary obstruction
Primary biliary cirrhosis
Primary sclerosing cholangitis
Drugs/toxins

Venous Outflow Obstruction

Veno-occlusive disease
Budd–Chiari syndrome
Congestive heart failure
Constrictive pericarditis
Drugs/toxins

Adapted from Anand BS: Cirrhosis of liver. *World J Med* 171:110–115, 1999.

---

flow through the liver and an increased volume of blood flow through the splanchnic circulation. Fibrotic changes in the hepatic parenchyma increase the portal pressure by producing a relatively fixed component of increased resistance. More recently a dynamic resistive component has also been identified which involves abnormal vasoconstriction in prehepatic portal venules and in the sinusoids themselves. The rise in portal pressure resulting from increased intrahepatic resistance is then exacerbated by an increase in blood flow through the splanchnic capillary bed. This increased flow results from a generalized splanchnic arteriolar vasodilatation producing a hyperkinetic splanchnic circulation. The mechanisms by which the dynamic resistance and splanchnic vasodilatation are produced are multifactorial and incompletely understood. Abnormal regulation of vasoactive substances such as nitrous oxide (NO) and glucagon are felt to be important and thus represent potential mechanisms for pharmacological means to reduce portal pressure. Shunting of blood away from the liver directly into the systemic veins represents an additional means of reducing portal pressure. This occurs spontaneously in the form of numerous, characteristic portal-to-systemic collateral pathways (varices) or can be purposefully produced by surgical or radiological means. The spontaneous decompressive pathways are rarely sufficient to normalize the portal pressure.

Ascites is the most common complication of cirrhosis (Box 14-4 and Fig. 14-16). The development of ascites in cirrhotic patients marks a very significant prognostic

Box 14–3 Causes of Portal Hypertension

Prehepatic

Arterioportal fistulas
Portal vein thrombosis
Splenic vein thrombosis

Intrahepatic presinusoidal

Schistosomiasis
Sarcoidosis
Primary biliary cirrhosis
Toxins
Chronic hepatitis
Arterioportal shunting from hepatoma
Idiopathic portal hypertension
Myelofibrosis
Wilson's disease
Felty's syndrome

Intrahepatic sinusoidal

Alcohol abuse
Cirrhosis
Primary sclerosing cholangitis
Gaucher's disease
Myeloid metaplasia

Intrahepatic postsinusoidal

Veno-occlusive disease
Budd–Chiari syndrome

Posthepatic

Right heart failure
Constrictive pericarditis
Mitral valve disease
IVC obstruction

Box 14–4 Complications of Portal Hypertension

Ascites
Variceal hemorrhage
Hepatic encephalopathy
Congestive splenomegaly
Portal hypertensive gastropathy/colopathy
Hepatorenal syndrome
Hepatic hydrothorax
Hepatopulmonary syndrome

point in the progression of their liver disease. The 2-year survival after ascites develops is approximately 50%. Refractory ascites is defined as fluid overload that is unresponsive to a sodium-restricted diet and high-dose diuretic treatment or is associated with clinically significant complications of the diuretic therapy. Ascites refractory to maximal medical therapy is associated with a 12-month survival of only 25%. The pathogenesis of ascites is complex and multifactorial involving multiple hormonal pathways responsible for sodium and free water regulation. Nonetheless, sinusoidal hypertension is felt to be a critical factor in ascites development.

Varices are dilated, thin-walled veins (see Fig. 14-8). In portal hypertension, variceal blood flow is from the high-pressure portal system to the low-pressure systemic veins. Gastroesophageal varices are the source of gastrointestinal bleeding in 60–90% of patients with cirrhosis and portal hypertension. Other causes of bleeding include peptic ulcer, hemorrhagic gastritis, and Mallory–Weiss syndrome. Splenorenal varices can contribute to gastrointestinal bleeding if there are

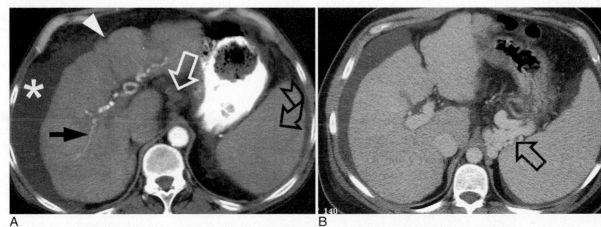

A   B

Figure 14-16   Imaging findings of portal hypertension on CT. **A**, Axial CT scan during the arterial phase of a patient with alcoholic cirrhosis, demonstrating many of the associated findings in portal hypertension – ascites (*), nodular contour of contracted liver (arrowhead), tortuous "corkscrew" arteries due to contraction of the liver parenchyma (straight closed arrow), gastroesophageal varices (straight open arrow), and enlarged spleen (curved arrow). **B**, Axial CT scan during the venous phase in a different patient, showing opacification of gastroesophageal varices (open arrow).

communications with the gastric mucosa via short gastric veins. Up to 90% of patients with cirrhosis will develop gastroesophageal varices, 25–35% of whom will bleed from these varices within 1 year of diagnosis. Of those who survive their first bleed, approximately 70% will rebleed, most within 6 months of the first hemorrhage. The mortality rate with each bleeding episode has been estimated to be 30–50%. One-third of all deaths in patients with cirrhosis and portal hypertension are the result of bleeding from gastroesophageal varices.

Hepatic encephalopathy is a neuropsychiatric condition that results from a combination of liver failure and portal-to-systemic shunting. Symptoms range from personality changes and sleep disturbance to coma (Table 14-2). Chemical substances produced in the intestine (likely by bacterial action) that are normally metabolized by a healthy liver are presumed to be responsible. Since portal-to-systemic shunting contributes to encephalopathy this condition can be worsened by surgical or radiological shunts performed to reduce portal pressure.

Congestive splenomegaly results from chronic venous congestion secondary to portal hypertension producing splenic enlargement and varying degrees of hypersplenism (thrombocytopenia being the most common manifestation). In a similar fashion, portal hypertensive gastropathy and portal hypertensive colopathy result from chronic venous congestion secondary to portal hypertension. These can lead to acute bleeding but more commonly cause chronic, low-grade blood loss associated with an iron-deficiency anemia.

"Hepatorenal syndrome" refers to renal failure in patients with advanced hepatic failure and portal hypertension, characterized by a very low glomerular filtration rate in the absence of other causes of renal impairment. These would include shock, sepsis, use of nephrotoxic drugs, or fluid loss such as from repeated vomiting or prolonged diarrhea. The syndrome has been estimated to occur in 10% of hospitalized patients with cirrhosis and ascites. The kidney is histologically normal but subject to abnormal vasoconstriction. The pathophysiology of the syndrome appears to be closely tied to the same abnormal regulation of sodium, free water, and arterial blood volume that contributes to ascites formation.

Hepatic hydrothorax is the accumulation of a significant volume of pleural fluid (usually >500 mL) in a patient with cirrhosis who has no cardiac or pulmonary disease that would otherwise account for the effusion. Other causes for effusion, including malignancy, should be ruled out before the diagnosis is established. Hepatic hydrothorax is usually right-sided and is thought to occur by the migration of fluid from the abdomen, across defects in the diaphragm. Ascites may or may not be present. In the latter situation, lymphatic fluid weeping from the bare area of the liver may be the source of the effusion. This condition is estimated to occur in 4–10% of patients with cirrhosis.

Hepatopulmonary syndrome is characterized by the triad of liver disease, hypoxemia due to right-to-left shunting, and intrapulmonary vascular dilations. The role of portal hypertension in this condition is controversial since investigations in experimental animals have indicated that portal hypertension is not a prerequisite for the development of the syndrome.

Portal hypertension, like the chronic liver diseases it typically results from, often remains clinically undetected until the late stages. Once clinically evident, the severity of disease is graded by the modified Child–Turcotte–Pugh scheme (Table 14-3).

Abnormalities found during cross-sectional imaging with CT, MRI, and US provide an opportunity for the interventionalist to diagnose portal hypertension (see Fig. 14-16). A small, nodular liver with associated varices and ascites is characteristic. The lateral segment of the left lobe of the liver may be hypertrophied in advanced cases. The diameter of the portal vein may be increased (>12 mm) in portal hypertension. On duplex color-flow US examination, hepatofugal flow in the portal vein, a recanalized umbilical vein, or the coronary vein is diagnostic (Fig. 14-17). The hepatic veins may have decreased, monophasic flow. The portal vein should be carefully inspected for thrombus.

The angiographic demonstration of portal hypertension can be accomplished with both visceral arterial and hepatic venous injections. Contraction of the liver, enlargement of the left lobe, and tortuous "corkscrew" appearance of the intrahepatic arteries are typical arterial findings (see Fig. 11-4A). Visualization of varices, retrograde flow in the inferior mesenteric vein, increased size of the portal vein, and hepatofugal flow on venous phase images are evidence of portal hypertension (see Fig. 14-15). Conventional hepatic venograms may reveal small hepatic veins with decreased flow in advanced cases. Wedged hepatic venograms demonstrate a patchy parenchymal stain, and opacification of the portal vein with hepatofugal flow (Fig. 14-18). These studies should be combined with free and wedged hepatic vein pressures.

Table 14–2	Hepatic Encephalopathy

Grade	Definition
I	Mild confusion, shortened attention span, sleep disorders, irritability, tremor
II	Lethargic or drowsy, variably oriented, personality changes, asterixis
III	Somnolent but arousable, confused, asterixis, positive Babinski sign
IV	Comatose, decerebrate neurological examination

Table 14–3   Child–Turcotte–Pugh Classification of Severity of Liver Disease in Cirrhosis

	Points[a]		
Variable	1	2	3
Encephalopathy (grade)	0	I–II	III–IV
Ascites	None	Mild	Moderate
Bilirubin (mg/mL)[b]	<2	2–3	>3
Albumin (g/dL)	>3.5	2.8–3.5	<2.8
INR	<1.7	1.7–2.3	>2.3

[a]Score obtained by adding up the total points: 5–6 = class A (well-preserved liver function); 7–9 = class B; 10–15 = class C (decompensated).
[b]Bilirubin points and values in patients with primary biliary cirrhosis: 1 = 1–4 mg/dL; 2 = 5–10 mg/dL; 3 = >10 mg/dL.
INR, international normalized ratio.

Determination of the portal pressure is useful in the diagnosis and treatment of portal hypertension. In most instances direct measurement of portal venous pressures is not practical. The most convenient method is to obtain hepatic sinusoidal pressure measurements using an occlusion-balloon catheter technique in combination with hepatic venography. This is analogous to evaluation of left heart pressures with pulmonary-artery wedged pressure measurements using a Swan–Ganz catheter. An occlusion balloon catheter is positioned in a hepatic vein but not inflated. A typical triphasic waveform should be observed on the transducer monitor and the mean pressure recorded (the free hepatic venous pressure, FHVP) (see Fig. 14-18). The occlusion balloon is then inflated with room air using a small (3-mL) syringe. Once the balloon is wedged the hepatic venous waveform will flatten and become monophasic. The wedged hepatic venous pressure (WHVP) is then measured.

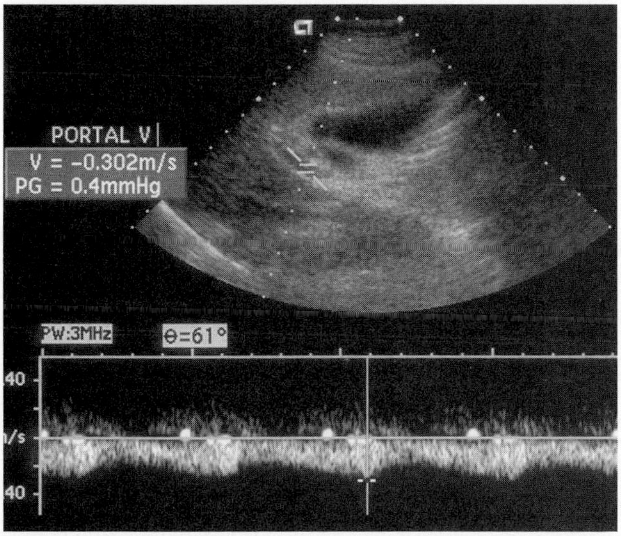

The intrahepatic portal pressure is expressed as the "hepatic vein pressure gradient" (HVPG) or "corrected sinusoidal pressure":

$$HVPG = WHVP - FHVP$$

The normal HVPG is less than or equal to 5 mmHg. An HVPG >5 mmHg is indicative of portal hypertension. An HVPG of 12 mmHg or higher is associated with the development of variceal hemorrhage (Table 14-4).

More invasive means can be used to obtain the absolute pressure in the portal vein by transhepatic puncture from either the jugular vein or right midaxillary line approaches. Similarly, direct percutaneous puncture of the spleen yields the splenic pulp pressure, which is indicative of the portal pressure. This latter method is rarely used today.

The initial management of patients with portal hypertension is with medical therapy (Table 14-5). Acute esophageal variceal bleeding can be controlled in 90% of patients with combined endoscopic and medical therapy. Dietary restriction and diuretic therapy can successfully control ascites in 90%. Patients with acute worsening

Figure 14-17 Duplex ultrasound of the portal vein shows hepatofugal flow (same patient as Fig. 14-15A).

Table 14–4   Hepatic Vein Pressure Measurements (Relative)

Level of Obstruction	FHVP	WHVP	HVPG
Prehepatic	Normal	Normal	Normal
Presinusoidal	Normal	Normal/slight increase	Normal/slight increase
Sinusoidal	Normal	Increased	Increased
Postsinusoidal	Normal	Increased	Increased
Posthepatic	Increased	Increased	Normal

FHVP, free hepatic vein pressure; WHVP, wedged hepatic vein pressure; HVPG, hepatic vein pressure gradient.

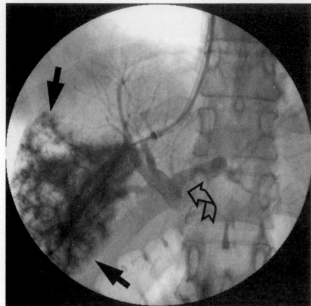

A

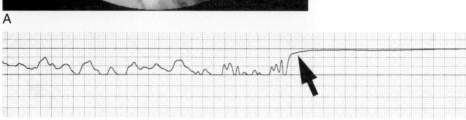

B

Figure 14-18   Demonstration of portal hypertension with hepatic venogram and pressure measurements. **A,** Balloon-occlusion wedged hepatic venogram using iodinated contrast in a patient with cirrhosis and portal hypertension. The hepatic parenchyma (straight arrows) has a patchy ("moth-eaten") appearance (compare with Fig. 14-13). In addition, there is opacification of the portal vein (curved arrow). **B,** Hepatic vein pressure tracing during free and wedged measurements using a balloon occlusion catheter. The free tracing (balloon deflated) has a low-pressure multiphasic waveform representative of the systemic venous system. With inflation of the occlusion balloon (arrow) the pressure rises and becomes monophasic, reflecting the portal venous pressure.

Table 14–5 Medical Therapy of Portal Hypertension	
Complication	**Medical Therapy**
Hepatic encephalopathy	Dietary protein restriction
	Oral lactulose therapy
Ascites	Dietary sodium restriction
	Diuretic therapy
	Large-volume paracentesis
Variceal hemorrhage	*Primary prevention:*
	Non-selective beta-blockers
	Acute hemorrhage:
	Volume resuscitation and management in an ICU setting
	Endoscopic sclerotherapy or variceal band ligation to control hemorrhage
	Vasoactive drugs (e.g., terlipressin, somatostatin, octreotide, beta-blockers, nitrates)
	Secondary prevention:
	Endoscopic sclerotherapy or variceal band ligation to obliterate gastroesophageal varices
	Nonselective beta-blockade
Hepatic hydrothorax	Dietary sodium restriction
	Diuretic therapy
	Large-volume paracentesis
	Thoracentesis

Table 14–6   Surgical Portal-to-Systemic Shunts

Type	Description
Total	Large diameter (15–25 mm) portocaval (end-to-side or side-to-side portal vein to IVC), mesocaval (side-to-side superior mesenteric vein to IVC), central splenorenal[a]
Partial	Small diameter (8–15 mm) side-to-side portocaval or mesocaval
Selective	Distal splenorenal[b]

[a]Spleen is removed and splenic vein is anastomosed end-to-side to left renal vein, diverting portal flow.
[b]Spleen is retained and splenic vein is anastomosed end-to-side to left renal vein so that only splenic venous flow is diverted from portal circulation.
IVC, inferior vena cava.

of hepatic encephalopathy should be evaluated for occult gastrointestinal bleeding and bacterial peritonitis. Protein restriction and lactulose are the mainstays of therapy.

Surgical creation of a portal-to-systemic venous shunt can lower portal pressure and address many of the complications of portal hypertension (Table 14-6). A total shunt, in which the entire portal flow is diverted into the systemic veins through a large (15- to 25-mm diameter) communication have >90% patency and minimal rebleeding. These shunts are associated with a 30–50% incidence of encephalopathy and often lead to an acceleration of underlying liver disease. Partial shunts use smaller anastomoses (8- to 15-mm diameter) in an attempt to reduce the portal–caval gradient to 12 mmHg while preserving hepatopedal flow. Lower incidences of both encephalopathy and liver failure have been reported with these procedures, with excellent control of bleeding. Selective shunts decompress only a portion of the portal system while preserving hepatopedal flow. The best known is the distal splenorenal shunt combined with ligation of the coronary and right gastroepiploic vein. Although effective in decompressing gastroesophageal varices and successful in maintaining forward flow to the liver in many cases, sustained sinusoidal hypertension with this shunt does not improve ascites.

Operative procedures such as interruption of the gastroesophageal and gastric veins, splenectomy, and esophageal transection and reanastomosis using staple devices can control bleeding in patients who are unsuitable for shunts. The ultimate surgical therapy for portal hypertension from chronic liver disease is liver transplantation; however, end-stage liver disease, not portal hypertension, is the indication for transplantation.

TRANSJUGULAR INTRAHEPATIC PORTOSYSTEMIC SHUNT

The transjugular intrahepatic portosystemic shunt (TIPS) procedure decompresses the portal venous system by the percutaneous creation of a low-resistance tract in the liver between the portal and hepatic venous systems. Conceived by Josef Rösch in 1969, TIPS became a useful clinical technique with the introduction of metallic stents in the late 1980s.

The TIPS procedure is of documented benefit and indicated in patients with variceal bleeding and ascites who have failed medical management (Boxes 14-5 through 14-7). This procedure has not yet achieved status as a first-line therapy owing to the frequency of stenosis in bare metal stents. Stent-grafts have vastly improved primary patency, which may lead to modification of indications for TIPS.

Patent portal and hepatic veins should be documented before TIPS is attempted. An ultrasound examination of the liver with Doppler interrogation of these veins is commonly used. Contrast-enhanced computed tomography or MRI with MRV of the liver can provide similar information. Cross-sectional imaging is also useful to exclude the presence of a mass lesion (cystic or solid) in the liver along the anticipated path of the shunt and to

Box 14–5   Indications for TIPS

Established

Acute hemorrhage from varices not responsive to medical therapy
Recurrent variceal hemorrhage not responsive to medical therapy (Child's B and C)
Refractory ascites
Refractory hepatic hydrothorax
Budd–Chiari syndrome

Promising

Portal hypertensive gastropathy
Hepatorenal syndrome
Hepatopulmonary syndrome

Box 14–6   Contraindications to TIPS

Absolute

Severe hepatic failure
Biliary sepsis
Isolated gastric varices with splenic vein occlusion
Severe left- or right-sided heart failure
Pulmonary hypertension

Relative

Cavernous transformation of the portal vein
Systemic infection
Severe hepatic encephalopathy
Biliary dilatation

---

evaluate for biliary dilatation (a relative contraindication to the procedure). When tense ascites is present, a large-volume paracentesis immediately prior to the procedure allows the liver to assume a normal position in the peritoneal cavity. The TIPS procedure is usually performed using conscious sedation in the elective setting. In critically ill patients with acute bleeding, intubation may be necessary for airway management. Intravenous antibiotics (usually a cephalosporin or other drug providing coverage for skin flora) are infused on call to the interventional suite. In elective cases, appropriate blood products should be transfused to keep the platelet count above 50,000 and the international normalized ratio (INR) below 1.8.

Several needle kits are available for TIPS procedures. All have several elements in common, including a long sheath that reaches from the jugular to the hepatic vein and a directional indicator on the hub of the needle or metal

---

Box 14–7   TIPS for Acute Bleeding: Questions to Ask

Has patient been endoscoped to confirm source of bleeding?
Where are the varices located?
Has endoscopic therapy been tried?
Is patient hemodynamically stable?
Is medical therapy optimized, including correction of coagulopathies?
Is the portal vein known to be patent (and by what imaging test)?
Is airway protection necessary to prevent aspiration of blood during the procedure?
Is patient a candidate for liver transplant?

---

cannula (Fig. 14-19). The two most commonly used kits are the Rösch–Uchida and Ring (Cook, Bloomington, IN). A kit designed specifically for use with CO_2 contrast is also available (Angiodynamics, Queensbury, NY). Although there are several choices for access kits, the core steps of the procedure are similar (Fig. 14-20 and Box 14-8).

The preferred access for introduction of the TIPS needle is the right internal jugular vein, although either internal or external jugular vein can be used. A left-sided approach actually facilitates catheterization of the right hepatic vein, but patients frequently experience chest discomfort during the procedure owing to the rigid devices in the mediastinum. Great care is necessary when advancing sheaths, metal cannulas, and needles through the heart. These maneuvers should be monitored fluoroscopically, even though they are performed over a guidewire, as lethal cardiac perforation has been reported.

The hepatic vein is usually selected with an angled catheter and a 3-J or angled hydrophilic guidewire (see Fig. 14-11). The catheter should be rotated lateral and slightly posterior to locate the right hepatic vein. Contrast injection is important to confirm the identity of the vein, especially in patients with small livers or massive ascites that displaces the liver and distorts venous anatomy. Inadvertent selection of an accessory hepatic vein or the right renal vein will result in procedural failure and possible severe complication. The choice of hepatic vein is dictated by anatomic considerations. In most patients the right hepatic vein is large, easily catheterized, and has a downward slope that accommodates the

---

Box 14–8   Basic Steps of the TIPS Procedure

Jugular vein access (usually right internal)
Catheterization of hepatic vein (usually right)
Wedged hepatic venogram (usually with CO_2 gas)
Puncture from hepatic vein to intrahepatic portal vein (usually right portal branch)
Portal venogram to confirm patency (especially splenic vein)
Measurement of pressure gradient between portal vein and inferior vena cava
Dilatation of parenchymal tract (8 mm × 3–4 cm balloon)
Deployment of stent-graft or stent (usually 10-mm diameter self-expanding)
Remeasure gradient (target is <12 mmHg)
Further dilatation of shunt or extension if necessary to reduce gradient
Embolization of varices (in patients with active variceal bleeding)
Completion portal venogram

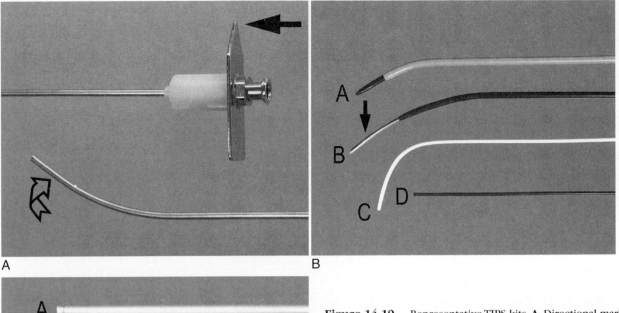

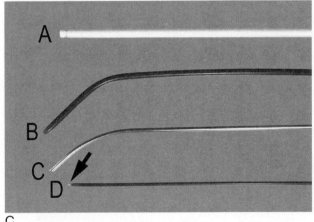

Figure 14-19   Representative TIPS kits. **A,** Directional marker (straight arrow) that indicates the direction of the tip of the needle or cannula (curved arrow). **B,** The Ring kit: (A) 9-Fr angled introducer sheath with dilator; (B) assembled 9-Fr angled needle guide catheter with the curved 16-gauge access needle (arrow) – portal vein access is achieved by direct puncture with this needle; (C) angled 5-Fr angiographic catheter; (D) straight 5-Fr Teflon catheter. **C,** The Rösch–Uchida kit: (A) straight 10-Fr introducer sheath; (B) 10-Fr angled catheter; (C) 14-gauge stiffening cannula for the 10-Fr angled catheter; (D) assembled 5-Fr catheter and 0.038-inch trocar stylet (arrow) – portal vein access is achieved by puncture with this assembly using the 10-Fr catheter and stiffening cannula to direct the thrust.

curved metallic elements of the TIPS kit. However, the middle hepatic vein is also large and can be easily confused with the right hepatic vein when viewed in the anteroposterior projection. The left hepatic vein is often smaller with an anterior course and almost perpendicular axis relative to the IVC.

The wedged hepatic venogram confirms patency of the portal vein, and provides a visual target for needle passes (see Figs. 14-7 and 14-18). In addition, the opacified hepatic parenchyma allows confirmation of the identity of the hepatic vein and localization of the border of the liver. This step is omitted with the Hawkins kit, as direct injection of CO_2 into the liver parenchyma through the access needle is used to opacify the portal vein.

The ideal location of the TIPS needle in the hepatic vein from which to start the puncture depends on specific patient anatomy. The target on the portal side is the right or left portal vein 2 cm or more peripheral to the bifurcation of the main portal vein (see Fig. 14-20).

Working through small portal branches can present technical challenges with respect to angulation and tortuosity of the final shunt, and puncture of the extrahepatic main portal vein can be associated with severe hemorrhagic complications. In most cases, punctures initiated from within 2–4 cm of the hepatic vein orifice are successful. Depending upon which hepatic vein is being used, the needle is rotated either anteriorly or posteriorly. The directional indicator on the hub of the needle or cannula provides useful directional information (Table 14-7).

Puncture with the Ring and Rösch–Uchida kits differ slightly. The 16-gauge modified Ross needle in the Ring kit is rotated and advanced at the same time. With the Rösch–Uchida kit the 14-gauge blunt metal cannula is rotated to engage the wall of the hepatic vein, after which the 0.038-inch flexible trocar and 5-French catheter assembly are thrust into the liver parenchyma. The needle should be advanced approximately 1 cm beyond the expected or known location of the portal vein. Aggressive thrusts may result in puncture of the liver capsule. The curve of the Ross needle and Rösch–Uchida cannula can be modified as needed, but the devices become difficult to advance through the sheath when the angles are too acute. The Ross needle is advantageous in hard livers, whereas the flexible Rösch–Uchida needle is easier to use when puncture at an acute angle is necessary. Periportal fibrosis, when present, produces a palpable "pop" when the portal vein is been entered.

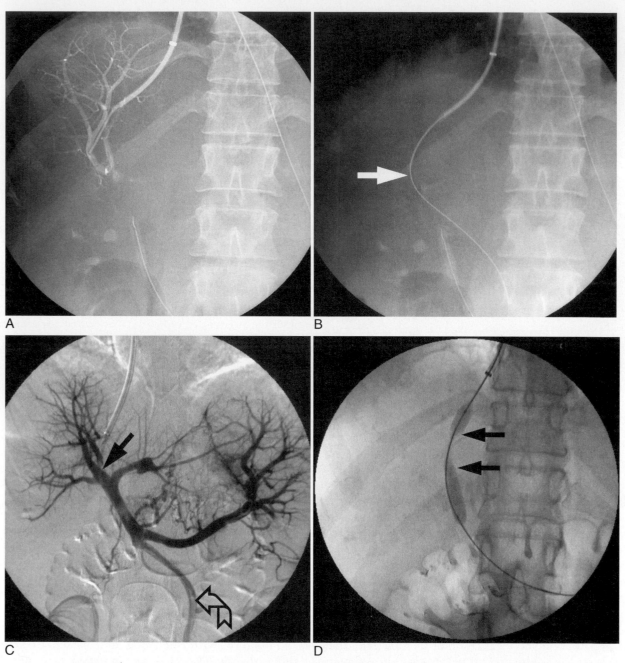

Figure 14-20   The transjugular intrahepatic portosystemic shunt (TIPS) procedure in a patient with recurrent variceal bleeding. **A**, Puncture of right portal vein branch from right hepatic vein. Identity of the portal vein is confirmed with contrast injection. **B**, Guidewire (arrow) advanced into the portal system. **C**, Portogram is obtained to confirm patency of the portal system. The catheter enters the right portal vein (arrow). Note the retrograde flow in the inferior mesenteric vein (curved arrow). The pressure gradient was then measured between the portal vein and IVC (23 mmHg). **D**, Balloon dilatation of the intrahepatic tract. The waist on the angioplasty balloon (arrows) identifies the length of the tract through the liver parenchyma between the right hepatic and portal veins.

(Continued)

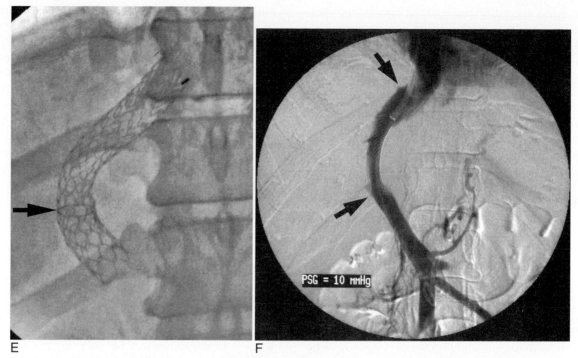

Figure 14-20   cont'd E, A self-expanding stent-graft (Viatorr, W.L. Gore, Flagstaff, AZ) was placed across the tract. The arrow indicates the marker between the bare distal rings of the stent in the portal vein, and the graft-covered portion of the stent in the liver parenchyma and hepatic vein. An angioplasty balloon was used to achieve full expansion. The pressure gradient between the portal vein and IVC was remeasured. **F**, Completion DSA portogram. Portal flow is diverted through the shunt with no filling of the intrahepatic portal veins. The stent spans from the right portal vein to the orifice of the right hepatic vein (arrows). Some filling of the intrahepatic portal vein is preferable, especially in patients who undergo TIPS for ascites. The final gradient was 10 mmHg.

The rotation of the needle or cannula should be maintained during all subsequent maneuvers. The natural tendency of the device is to orient itself to the hepatic vein, which moves the tip away from the portal vein. In addition, the operator should allow the puncture system to move slightly with inspiration and expiration, like a horseback rider in a saddle. When the device is held in a fixed position, the tip may migrate out of the portal vein as the liver moves up and down with each breath. Using a 10-mL syringe, the operator aspirates while slowly pulling the needle or catheter back. As soon as blood is freely aspirated, contrast is injected under fluoroscopic guidance. One of three structures will be visualized: the portal vein, the hepatic vein, or the hepatic artery. Hepatic arterial flow is hepatopedal and brisk, whereas portal flow is slower and either hepatopedal or hepatofugal. Hepatic veins flow towards the heart. If the portal vein is not opacified, another syringe can be attached and the aspiration maneuver continued until the hepatic vein is reached. The puncture is repeated varying the degree of rotation or starting location in the hepatic vein until the portal vein is found. Puncture of the hepatic artery within the hepatic parenchyma is usually inconsequential. Similarly, opacification of the biliary tree is typically without sequelae.

Once portal vein puncture has been confirmed, a guidewire is advanced into the main portal vein. A 0.038-inch Bentson or angled hydrophilic guidewire may be used. The former guidewire tends to prolapse down the main portal vein, whereas the latter allows directional control. When the guidewire remains in an intrahepatic portal vein, a 5-French hydrophilic Cobra-2 catheter can

Table 14-7	Needle Rotation during TIPS Puncture	
Hepatic Vein	**Portal Vein Target**	**Rotation of Needle**
Right	Right	Anterior
Middle	Right	Posterolateral
Middle	Left	Posteromedial
Left	Left	Posteromedial

be used to direct the guidewire into the main portal vein. Once the wire is deep in the portal system, the black outer guide for the Ring kit or Rösch–Uchida cannula can then be advanced over the wire into the portal vein. This provides maximum security when exchanging for a pigtail catheter. Pressure measurements are then obtained, followed by a portogram (preferably with the catheter in the splenic vein).

Dilatation of the transhepatic tract is the next step. This is the most painful part of the procedure for the patient so it is helpful to administer some additional analgesics prior to inflating the balloon. A stiff 0.035-inch Amplatz wire should be used for this and all other maneuvers. A noncompliant balloon, 8 mm in diameter and 3–4 cm in length is positioned across the transhepatic tract and the sheath is withdrawn. The balloon is inflated with dilute contrast under fluoroscopic visualization. The initial waist produced by the hepatic parenchyma will give way typically revealing two focal indentations on the balloon. These identify the length and location of the transhepatic tract since they represent the more resilient fibrous tissue surrounding the portal and hepatic veins. A digital spot film can be obtained and used as a reference for stent placement. For many years the standard stent was a self-expanding 10 mm × 68 mm Wallstent (Boston Scientific, Natick, MA), although nitinol stents are used with increasing frequency. Stent-grafts have replaced bare stents as the optimal device for the TIPS tract. These are usually covered with impermeable material (ePTFE) to prevent bile leaks into the tract, and are 8–12 mm in diameter. Once deployed, the 8-mm balloon is used to expand the stent in the tract. A venogram is performed with a pigtail catheter to document positioning and the pressure gradient across the shunt is determined. Additional stents or stent-grafts should be placed if the tract has not been adequately covered. If the pressure gradient has not dropped to 12 mmHg or less, then the entire tract should be dilated to 10-mm diameter. The stainless steel Wallstent can be overdilated to 12 mm if necessary. Nitinol-based stents and stent-grafts cannot be dilated beyond their predetermined maximum diameter. If the gradient is still not adequate, consideration should be given to creating a second (double-barrel) TIPS.

When the TIPS is performed to control acute bleeding, embolization of gastroesophageal varices should be performed. Stainless steel coils in the main trunk of the varix will suffice, but a more distal embolization will be obtained by preceding this with Gelfoam pieces soaked in sotradecol (Fig. 14-21). Sclerosis with 3–5 mL of absolute alcohol is also effective. However, most varices invariably recanalize.

Although internal jugular vein access is standard, TIPS procedures can be performed from the right external jugular or left jugular veins if necessary. A technique for performing a shunt from the femoral approach has also

been described for patients with aberrant anatomy. Mini-laparotomy with exposure of a mesenteric vein permits retrograde formation of the TIPS tract with puncture from the portal to the hepatic vein, rather than vice versa.

In some cases access to the portal vein by transhepatic puncture can be difficult. Percutaneous insertion of a wire or catheter into the portal system has been used to provide a target. This can be introduced from a transhepatic intercostal approach or via a recanalized umbilical vein when present (see Fig. 14-14). Metallic coils can be placed percutaneously next to the right portal vein under CT guidance just prior to TIPS. CT has also been used to place guidewires through the liver crossing the right portal vein and entering the IVC. The wire is snared from a jugular access and the shunt completed from that approach. Transabdominal ultrasound has been employed to guide portal vein puncture.

Direct puncture from the IVC through the caudate lobe to the main portal vein (DIPS – direct IVC-to-portal shunt) is an innovative alternative approach to TIPS (Fig. 14-22). An intravascular ultrasound probe in the IVC is used to guide the needle into the main portal vein, simplifying the most difficult and critical step of the procedure. A stent-graft is mandatory as extrahepatic puncture of the portal vein is common with this technique.

The complication rate from TIPS in experienced hands is under 5% with a mortality rate of less than 2% (Table 14-8). The most serious and potentially lethal

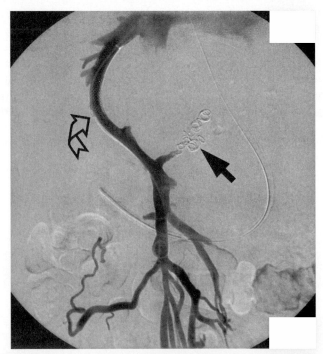

Figure 14-21   Completion DSA portogram with injection in the SMV following TIPS (curved arrow) for variceal bleeding shows coils occluding the left gastric vein (straight arrow).

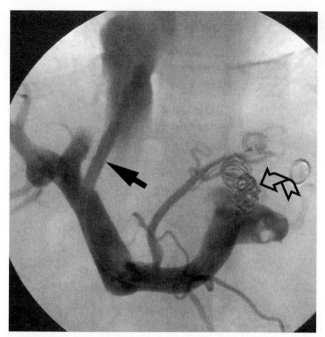

Figure 14-22 Completion DSA portogram following direct IVC-to-portal shunt (DIPS) with a stent-graft (straight arrow). Large retroperitoneal varices arising from the splenic vein were occluded with coils (curved arrow). (Image courtesy of Bryan Petersen M.D., Dotter Interventional Institute, Portland, OR.)

Table 14–8 Complications of TIPS Procedure	
Complication	**Incidence (%)**
Early	
Procedural mortality	<1
Intraperitoneal bleeding:	
Punctured liver capsule	5
Extrahepatic portal vein puncture	2
Hemobilia	2
Portal vein thrombosis	2
Stent migration/malplacement	2
Infection	2
Renal failure (contrast-induced)	5
Accelerated hepatic failure	1–5
Hemolysis	10
Worsened hepatic encephalopathy	20–30
Late	
Ascites, persistent requiring medical management	10–30
Recurrent variceal bleeding (bare stent)	15–25 (1 year)
Shunt stenosis (bare stent)	50 (1 year)

Adapted from Haskal ZJ et al. *J Vasc Interv Radiol* 12:131–136, 2001.

complications of TIPS are nearly all related to the transhepatic puncture. Peritoneal exsanguination can occur from perforation of an extrahepatic portion of the portal system or from hepatic arterial injury (in conjunction with transgression of the liver capsule). Hepatic artery injury may also prove fatal if it leads to occlusion; hepatofugal flow of portal blood before TIPS means that the liver may be entirely dependent on hepatic arterial supply after the procedure. The creation of an arterial–biliary fistula by combined bile duct and arterial injury can lead to significant hemobilia and/or biliary obstruction. Portal vein rupture has been described. Additional major early complications of TIPS creation include cardiac decompensation (from a combination of increased venous return through the shunt and elevation of right heart filling pressures), acceleration of liver failure, and precipitation or worsening of hepatic encephalopathy. Later on, the shunt may be subject to infection (bacterial or fungal) or malfunction (by thrombosis or stenosis). Rarely, stents may become dislodged and embolize to the heart or lungs. A transient hemolytic anemia has been described following TIPS. Careless manipulation of instruments in the right atrium can induce cardiac arrhythmias or perforate the atrium, causing cardiac tamponade.

TIPS creation is also subject to the same general group of complications associated with all percutaneous endovascular procedures. In particular, radiation-induced dermatitis has been described following very difficult and protracted cases.

The technical success rate for TIPS for variceal bleeding averages about 97% (range 89–100%) with hemostasis obtained in approximately 98% (range 97–100%). The benefit of concurrent embolization of varices during the TIPS procedure has not been proven, but is practiced widely. TIPS creation provides better long-term control of rebleeding compared to medical treatment (endoscopic interventions ± propanolol) when used as a preventative therapy. Rebleeding rates average 20% for TIPS (range 9–41%) versus 49% for medical therapy (range 23–61%). However, there is no proven survival benefit to TIPS with bare metal stents. In the setting of refractory ascites, TIPS results in elimination of ascites in 79% of shunt patients at 6 months compared to 24% of patients undergoing large-volume paracentesis. There is improved survival of patients with refractory ascites when treated with TIPS.

Shunt failure in the first 30 days is almost always secondary to acute thrombosis. This can be due to technical errors related to improper stent placement or shortening of an underexpanded Wallstent as it reaches its nominal diameter. Bile duct injury with leakage of bile and mucus into the shunt can also produce acute thrombosis (when bare metal stents or stent-grafts constructed from permeable fabric are used) (Fig. 14-23). Beyond 30 days, pseudointimal hyperplasia can produce either a focal stenosis at the hepatic vein end or narrowing of the parenchymal tract (the latter is limited to bare

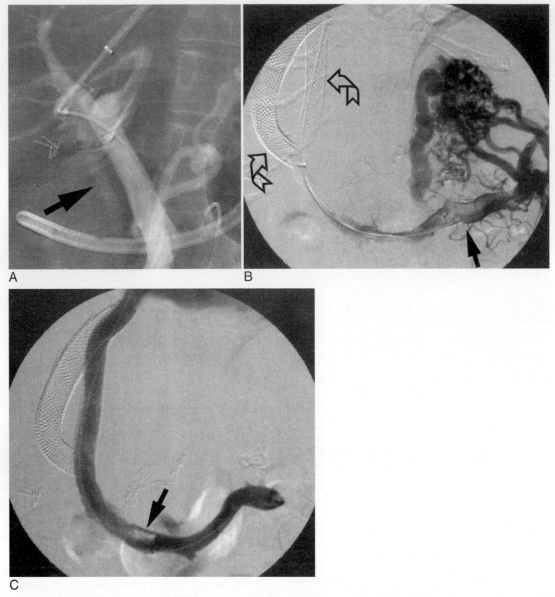

Figure 14-23 Bile duct injury during TIPS procedure is a predisposing factor for acute shunt occlusion when bare metal stents are used (same patient as Fig. 14-12). **A,** Unsubtracted image from the portogram obtained immediately after puncture of the portal vein. Faint opacification of the common bile duct (arrow) parallel to the portal vein is seen. The patient's TIPS thrombosed within a week. During attempted declotting, rethrombosis occurred instantaneously, so a second TIPS was then placed. Bare metal stents were used for both TIPS. **B,** The patient returned again within a week with thrombosis of the second TIPS and variceal bleeding. DSA portogram obtained after crossing one of the stents shows extensive thrombus in the portal venous system (straight arrow) and filling of retroperitoneal varices. There is no flow through either TIPS (curved arrows). **C,** TIPS rescue was achieved with a stent-graft placed within the medial shunt and thrombolysis. DSA portogram after 22 hours of thrombolytic infusion shows residual nonocclusive thrombus in the portal vein (arrow). Flow through the shunt is excellent.

metal stents). The hepatic vein stenosis can be treated with angioplasty and/or the placement of an additional stent. Care must be taken not to extend too far into the IVC with additional stents as this can complicate future liver transplant operation.

Late TIPS shunt dysfunction can be defined as stenosis or occlusion of the shunt resulting in recurrent elevation of the portal–systemic pressure gradient to >12 mmHg (Fig. 14-24). Recurrent variceal bleeding after TIPS is almost always secondary to shunt malfunction.

Unfortunately decreased function of the shunt is clinically silent until bleeding occurs or ascites reaccumulates. For bare metal stents, the reported 1-year primary patency of TIPS ranges from 25 to 66%. Primary assisted patency of 72–85% can be achieved at one year with bare stents by intervening when stenoses are identified. Restoring patency to shunts found to be occluded during follow-up yields a secondary patency rate of 86–99% at 1 year. Although there is little data available, in-tract restenosis is unusual with stent-grafts. One-year primary unassisted patency is dramatically improved with stent-grafts, approaching 80–90%.

Worsening of encephalopathy after TIPS occurs in 30%. Preexisting encephalopathy is a significant prognostic indicator. Other risk factors include increased age, hypoalbuminemia, and cirrhosis of nonalcoholic etiology. Fortunately, fewer than 10% of patients have mental status changes refractory to medical treatments. Options in these patients include diminishing the shunt diameter by placing a "shunt reducing" stent within the tract, shunt occlusion, or liver transplantation (Fig. 14-25). The same options apply to the occasional patient who develops rapidly deteriorating liver function after TIPS creation.

In order to identify shunt malfunction US can be used for shunt surveillance. An ultrasound study should be performed within 24 hours of TIPS creation with a bare metal stent to provide baseline measurements. When TIPS are created with some stent-grafts air trapped

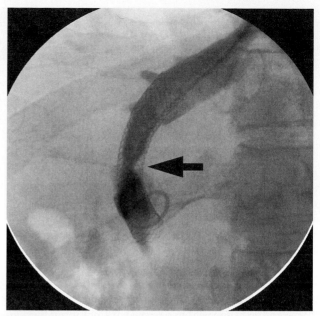

Figure 14-25   Reducing stent placed in a TIPS for hepatic encephalopathy. An hourglass-shaped stent-graft (arrow) was deployed in the TIPS tract, increasing the gradient from 4 mmHg to 14 mmHg.

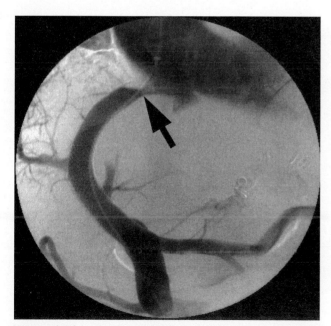

Figure 14-24   TIPS dysfunction due to stenosis in the hepatic vein. Portogram performed 6 months following initial TIPS procedure shows stenosis in the hepatic vein beyond the end of the stent (arrow).

in the graft material makes US impossible for 1–2 weeks. Follow-up examinations at 6 weeks, 3 months, and 6 months are then followed by examinations at 6-monthly intervals. A peak midshunt velocity of <50–60 cm/s has been used as an indicator of a hemodynamically significant stenosis.

Venography combined with pressure measurements represents the gold standard for assessing TIPS patency. This should be performed whenever a screening ultrasound suggests a stenosis or in the settings of recurrent bleeding or ascites. Because of the potentially fatal consequences of variceal hemorrhage in cirrhotic patients, some experts suggest surveillance venography every 6 months in patients treated for bleeding. With the wide acceptance of stent-grafts for TIPS, surveillance venography may not be necessary as often. An additional means to identify TIPS dysfunction may be the observation of recurrent varices during endoscopy.

HEPATIC VEIN OBSTRUCTION

In the nineteenth century, Budd and Chiari separately described thrombotic occlusion of the major hepatic veins, defining a clinical syndrome that now bears their names. Since then obstruction at a variety of levels have been included under the heading of Budd–Chiari syndrome (Box 14-9). Considered as a group, these disorders all have in common global obstruction of hepatic venous drainage. Symptoms usually do not develop provided that at least one hepatic vein is patent. Hepatic venous outflow obstruction leads to hepatic congestion and sinusoidal hypertension. Clinical findings include abdominal pain, hepatomegaly, and ascites (Box 14-10). Hepatocellular injury can progress rapidly to necrosis with high mortality, or more slowly, leading to cirrhosis. More than half of long-term survivors typically die from complications of portal hypertension (including bleeding from gastroesophageal varices) within 2 years. Patients with acute thrombotic occlusions may be hypercoagulable either from an underlying coagulation disorder, pregnancy, a malignancy, or oral contraceptive use. Not infrequently, however, no cause can be found (Box 14-11).

The characteristic cross-sectional imaging findings of Budd–Chiari syndrome include massive ascites, hepatomegaly, splenomegaly, slit-like or obliterated hepatic veins, intrahepatic hepatic vein to hepatic vein collaterals, and hepatic venous or IVC webs. Patients with chronic

Budd–Chiari syndrome may have hypertrophy of the caudate and atrophy of the right lobes of the liver, and gastroesophageal varices. On US, hepatic venous flow may be absent or dampened, with loss of transmitted atrial waves. Patchy, fan-shaped enhancement of the liver parenchyma with sparing of the caudate lobe is typical on contrast-enhanced CT or MRI (Fig. 14-26).

Venography for Budd–Chiari syndrome should include both cavography and selective hepatic venography. A pigtail catheter should be positioned in the suprarenal IVC with injection of 20-25 mL of contrast for a total volume of 40-50 mL. The intrahepatic IVC

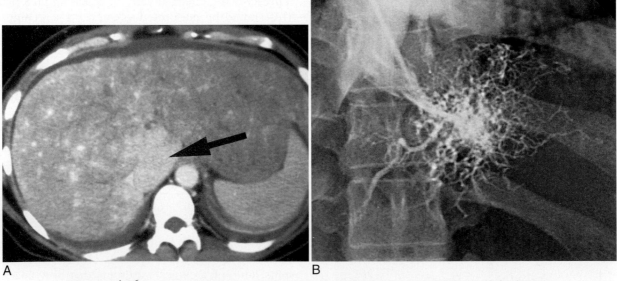

A   B

Figure 14-26   Classic appearance of Budd–Chiari syndrome due to thrombosis of the hepatic veins and venules. **A,** Contrast-enhanced CT scan showing patchy enhancement of the liver parenchyma with the exception of a hypertrophied caudate lobe (arrow). **B,** Digital left hepatic venogram showing the classic "spider-web" pattern. The recanalized and collateral branches of the hepatic vein have a deranged appearance.

Box 14–11   Risk Factors for Budd–Chiari Syndrome

Hypercoagulable syndromes
Oral contraceptives
Polycythemia
Connective tissue diseases
Paroxysmal nocturnal hemoglobinuria
Myelofibrosis
Pregnancy
Chemotherapy
Therapeutic irradiation
Liver transplantation (suprahepatic IVC)

Acute thrombotic occlusions of the main hepatic veins have been treated with thrombolytic agents administered both locally and systemically. Anticoagulation and correction of underlying stenotic lesions are important to ensure long-term success. Angioplasty and/or stenting of membranous webs or stenoses in the hepatic veins or IVC are frequently successful in relieving symptoms. Pressure gradients should be measured across hepatic vein or IVC webs (normal <2 mmHg) to determine whether intervention is necessary. TIPS creation has been used successfully to treat the massive ascites associated with hepatic venous outflow obstruction. Occlusion of the hepatic veins makes the procedure more complex, and swelling of the liver can distort portal venous anatomy. In comparison to patients with portal hypertension, the liver is enlarged, which requires longer stent tracts. Mesocaval shunt or liver transplantation may be necessary.

is frequently narrowed due to compression by the swollen liver parenchyma. Hepatic venous inflow may be absent when the level of obstruction is at the hepatic veins (Fig. 14-27). Obstructing webs may be identified in the suprahepatic IVC (Fig. 14-28). The classic venographic appearance of the hepatic veins in Budd–Chiari syndrome due to small vessel thrombosis is a spider-web-like network of small, unnamed collateral and recanalized veins draining directly into the IVC (see Fig. 14-26). Stenoses and webs in the hepatic veins may also be found.

PREHEPATIC VENOUS THROMBOSIS/OCCLUSION

Occlusions within the extrahepatic portal system are rare causes of portal hypertension. Although catastrophic widespread thrombosis of the portal system can occur, focal thromboses are more common and can be well tolerated for long periods. Portal vein thrombosis

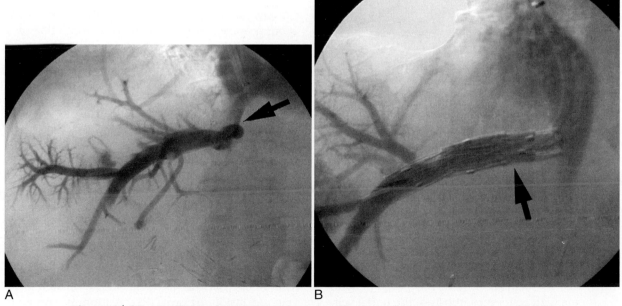

A   B

Figure 14-27   Budd–Chiari syndrome due to late hepatic vein stenosis in a liver transplant patient. **A,** At venography, only the right hepatic vein could be found. A focal stenosis is present at the orifice (arrow) with a 15-mmHg gradient. **B,** Following stent placement (arrow) the gradient was reduced to 2 mmHg. The patient had dramatic improvement of liver function.

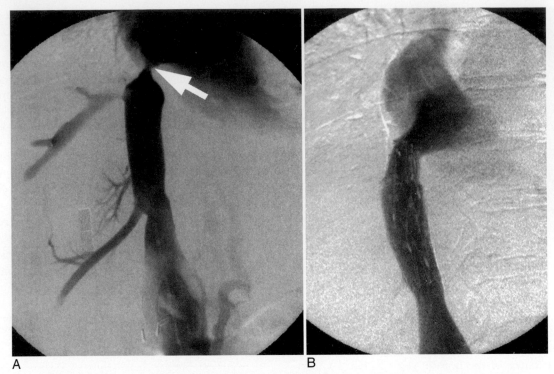

Figure 14-28   Budd–Chiari syndrome due to suprahepatic IVC stenosis in a patient with a liver transplant. **A**, DSA cavogram shows severe anastomotic stenosis (arrow) in the suprahepatic IVC and reflux into hepatic veins. The gradient was 12 mmHg across the stenosis. **B**, DSA cavogram after stent placement using 20-mm diameter Z-stents (angioplasty failed to reduce the gradient). The gradient was reduced to 0 mmHg. The hepatic vein reflux has disappeared.

and splenic vein thrombosis, in particular, can be clinically silent until bleeding develops from varices.

Portal Vein Thrombosis

Portal vein thrombosis is better tolerated than hepatic vein thrombosis because hepatic function tends to remain well preserved. Chronic portal vein thrombosis typically leads to an extensive system of dilated collateral channels in the gastrohepatic ligament and porta hepatis. This has been termed "cavernous transformation of the portal vein" and represents a network of portal-to-portal collaterals (see Fig. 14-7). Chronic hypertension in the splanchnic veins also leads to the formation of portal-to-systemic collaterals in these patients, notably gastroesophageal varices that can subsequently bleed. Although portal vein thrombosis often occurs in younger patients with hypercoagulable syndromes and normal livers, it can be superimposed on preexisting cirrhosis and portal hypertension, presumably due to stagnant flow in the portal system. Certain patients with acute thrombosis of the portal vein may benefit from endovascular recanalization of the portal vein using catheter-directed thrombolysis, mechanical thrombectomy, and/or stent placement. This has been described from transhepatic and trans-jugular approaches, the latter sometimes combined with TIPS creation. Chronic portal vein thrombosis with cavernous transformation, however, will not respond to thrombolysis and is considered a relative contraindication to TIPS placement.

Splenic Vein Thrombosis

Thrombosis of the splenic vein most commonly occurs as a result of recurrent pancreatitis, which is often associated with alcoholism. Other etiologies include pancreatic cancer, polycythemia vera, and hypercoagulable states. The short gastric veins become the major venous drainage of the spleen (see Fig. 14-6). Subsequently, acute upper gastrointestinal tract bleeding can occur from the resulting gastric varices. This is of particular importance because the clinical scenario may mimic variceal hemorrhage in cirrhotic patients. However, splenic vein thrombosis rarely results in esophageal varices. Patients bleeding from isolated gastric varices must be evaluated for splenic vein occlusion before TIPS creation is contemplated, since TIPS will not provide any benefit to these patients. Surgical splenectomy or splenic artery embolization are potential treatments options.

Mesenteric Venous Thrombosis

Superior mesenteric vein thrombosis often produces severe congestion in the affected segments of bowel, resulting in mesenteric ischemia. In stable patients without peritoneal signs, anticoagulation is generally the first line of therapy. Catheter-mediated thrombolysis has been attempted in selected cases using direct transhepatic access or indirect infusions through the SMA. Intestinal infarction, as suggested by the development of peritonitis, requires surgical intervention. Chronic occlusion of the superior mesenteric vein may result in formation of mesenteric varices and intestinal bleeding.

Post-transplant Portal Vein Stenosis

Portal vein complications occur in approximately 2% of patients undergoing liver transplantation. The donor portal vein is usually anastomosed to the recipient vein in an end-to-end fashion. Acute complications include portal vein thrombosis, kinks, and anastomotic strictures. Acute occlusion is frequently catastrophic with respect to viability of the transplant and requires urgent surgical revision. Intimal hyperplasia related to the anastomosis can result in late portal vein stenosis, which presents as presinusoidal extrahepatic portal hypertension.

US, CT/CTA, and MRI/MRV are excellent modalities for visualizing the portal vein anastomoses. Direct transhepatic access to the portal vein allows measurement of gradients across the area of stenosis, and treatment with stent placement. Embolization of the parenchymal tract in the liver with Gelfoam at the time of sheath removal prevents bleeding complications

NEOPLASM

Primary neoplasms of the portal and hepatic veins are extremely rare. Conversely, these veins are frequently involved by gastrointestinal tract malignancy.

Hepatoma has a characteristic ability to invade the portal vein and hepatic veins and propagate within the lumen. Care should be taken to exclude the presence of hepatoma in cirrhotic patients presenting with portal vein thrombosis. Hepatic arteriography or percutaneous image-guided biopsy may be needed to make the distinction between bland thrombus and tumor-thrombus in problem cases. Arterioportal shunting due to tumor can result in variceal bleeding (see Fig. 1-26B). The treatment for these patients is embolization of the tumor with permanent particles, rather than TIPS. Hepatoma may also invade the hepatic veins, with extension into the IVC and heart (Fig. 14-29).

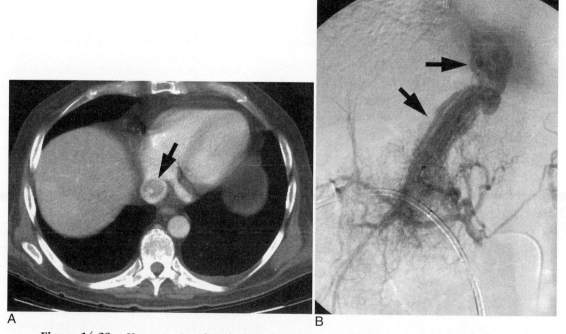

A   B

Figure 14-29   Hepatoma invading the hepatic vein. **A**, Contrast-enhanced CT scan at the level of the right atrium shows a filling defect in the IVC (arrow). **B**, Selective hepatic artery DSA shows a hypervascular mass invading the middle hepatic vein and extending into the IVC (arrows) with associated arteriovenous shunting. Note the typical "threads and streaks" in the tumor representing neovascularity.

Carcinoid tumor is a member of the neuroendocrine group of tumors and occurs most frequently in the right lower quadrant, either in the appendix or the terminal ileum. Although appendiceal carcinoid tumors are often benign, lesions in the terminal ileum are frequently malignant. A localized fibrotic reaction in the adjacent mesentery often occurs with carcinoid tumors and can obstruct the mesenteric veins (see Fig. 11-24).

Pancreatic adenocarcinoma characteristically obstructs the portal system by compression or malignant invasion of adjacent portions of the SMV, splenic vein, or portal vein (see Fig. 1-26C). Cholangiocarcinoma (Klatskin tumor) encases the portal vein producing stenoses in the intrahepatic portions of the portal vein (Fig. 14-30). Neoplastic enlargement of lymph nodes in the gastrohepatic ligament and porta hepatis can also lead to obstruction of the main portal vein.

TRANSJUGULAR LIVER BIOPSY

Transjugular liver biopsy is performed in patients with suspected diffuse parenchymal abnormalities such as cirrhosis when coagulopathy or ascites prevents safe performance of a percutaneous liver biopsy (Box 14-12). A platelet count less than 50,000 or an INR above 1.5 are considered contraindications to percutaneous liver biopsy. The amount of ascites sufficient to exclude the percutaneous route is less well defined, but certainly any volume of ascites that displaces the liver from the abdominal wall is of concern. The rationale for the technique is simple; jugular access can be safely obtained in the presence of coagulopathy, particularly with ultrasound

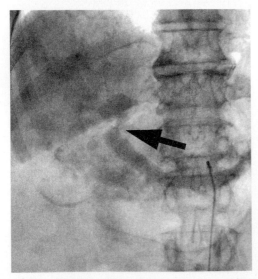

Figure 14-30 Venous phase image from a celiac artery angiogram showing stenosis of the intrahepatic portal vein (arrow) typical for encasement by cholangiocarcinoma (Klatskin tumor).

Box 14–12 Indications for Transjugular Liver Biopsy
Suspected hepatocellular disease Coagulopathy Ascites

guidance, and the biopsy needle never transgresses the liver capsule, thus eliminating the risk of intraperitoneal bleeding. Biopsy of liver masses is difficult with this technique.

Transjugular liver biopsy utilizes a system very similar to the Rösch–Uchida TIPS set but smaller in caliber. The biopsy needle is a modified version of the same core-biopsy devices routinely used for percutaneous organ biopsy (see Fig. 4-44). Jugular and right hepatic vein access is obtained as for TIPS. A hepatic venogram is performed to confirm the identity and patency of the vein. The assembled rigid guiding cannula system and introducer sheath is inserted over a guidewire into the right hepatic vein. The optimal location from which to perform the biopsy is within 3–4 cm of the IVC. Biopsy from more peripheral locations in the hepatic vein risks capsular perforation. The biopsy needle is then introduced through the guiding cannula. The tip of the cannula is rotated such that the needle will be directed in an anterior and caudal direction. The biopsy needle is then advanced a few millimeters into the hepatic parenchyma and the spring-loaded mechanism is fired, deploying the cutting needle and obtaining the biopsy. The biopsy needle is then removed and the sample inspected. An assistant should carefully hold the guiding cannula in the hepatic vein while the sample is retrieved from the biopsy device since respiratory motion will tend to displace the system from the hepatic vein. Additional samples can be obtained as required. After the procedure the patient should be monitored for 4 hours with frequent vital signs.

This technique is successful in obtaining hepatic tissue in at least 98% of cases and, in contrast to older transvenous techniques, yields samples of high diagnostic quality. Previous methods using a coring needle and suction, or grasping forceps, often produced crushed and/or fragmented specimens.

Capsular perforation is rare with this technique (2–6%), but bleeding complications can be fatal. Inadvertent renal biopsy has been described either by hepatic capsular perforation or unrecognized catheterization of the right renal vein. Hemobilia with biliary obstruction is another rare potential complication that may indicate intrahepatic vascular injury (Fig. 14-31). Patients who develop persistent abdominal pain following transjugular

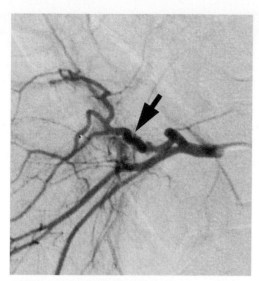

Figure 14-31   Arterial complication following transjugular liver biopsy. The patient developed abdominal pain and hemobilia following the biopsy. Selective right hepatic artery DSA showed irregularity of a right hepatic artery branch (arrow) and faint shunting into the portal vein. This was successfully embolized with coils.

liver biopsy should be evaluated with an abdominal CT followed by angiography as necessary.

SUGGESTED READINGS

Anand BS: Cirrhosis of liver. *World J Med* 171:110–115, 1999.

Blum U, Rössle M, Haag K et al: Budd–Chiari syndrome: technical, hemodynamic, and clinical results of treatment with transjugular intrahepatic portosystemic shunt. *Radiology* 197: 805–811, 1995.

Bosch J: Complications of cirrhosis: I. Portal hypertension. *J Hepatol* 32(S1):141–156, 2000.

Bradbury MS, Kavanagh PV, Becthold RE et al: Mesenteric venous thrombosis: diagnosis and non-invasive imaging. *Radiographics* 22:527–541, 2002.

Brountzos EN, Alexopoulou E, Koskinas I, et al: Intraperitoneal portal vein bleeding during transjugular intrahepatic portosystemic shunt: treatment with stent-graft placement. *Am J Roentgenol* 174:132–134, 2000.

Butterworth RF: Complications of cirrhosis: III. Hepatic encephalopathy. *J Hepatol* 32(S1):171–180, 2000.

Fishman EK: CT angiography: clinical applications in the abdomen. *Radiographics* 21:S3–16, 2001.

Garcia-Tsao GG, Groszmann RJ, Fisher RL et al: Portal pressure, presence of gastroesophageal varices and variceal bleeding. *Hepatology* 5:419–424, 1985.

Ginès P, Arroyo V: Hepatorenal syndrome. *J Am Soc Nephrol* 19:1833–1839, 1999.

Grace ND: Diagnosis and treatment of gastrointestinal bleeding secondary to portal hypertension. *Am J Gastro* 92:1081–1091, 1997.

Groszmann RJ, de Franchis R: Portal hypertension. In Schiff ER, Sorrell MF, Maddrey WC eds: *Schiff's Diseases of the Liver*, 8th edn, Lippincott-Raven, Philadelphia, 387–442, 1999.

Haskal ZJ, Rees CR, Ring EJ, Saxon R, Sacks D: Reporting standards for transjugular intrahepatic portosystemic shunts. Technology Assessment Committee of the SCVIR. *J Vasc Interv Radiol* 8: 289–297, 1997.

Haskal ZJ, Martin L, Cardella JF et al: Quality improvement guidelines for transjugular intrahepatic portosystemic shunts. SCVIR Standards of Practice Committee. *J Vasc Interv Radiol* 12:131–136, 2001.

Henderson JM: Surgical management of portal hypertension. In Schiff ER, Sorrell MF, Maddrey WC eds: *Schiff's Diseases of the Liver*, 8th edn, Lippincott-Raven, Philadelphia, 443–452, 1999.

Lazaridis KN, Frank JW, Krowka MJ, Kamath PS: Hepatic hydrothorax: pathogenesis, diagnosis, and management. *Am J Med* 107:262–267, 1999.

Little AF, Zajko AB, Orons PD: Transjugular liver biopsy: a prospective study in 43 patients with the quick-core biopsy needle. *J Vasc Interv Radiol* 7:127–131, 1996.

Lundell C, Kadir S: The portal venous system and heptic veins. In Kadir S ed: *Atlas of Normal and Angiographic Anatomy*, WB Saunders, Philadelphia, 1991.

Luketic VA, Sanyal AJ: Esophageal varices: II. TIPS (transjugular intrahepatic portosystemic shunt) and surgical therapy. *Gastroenterol Clin N Am* 29:387–421, 2000.

Madoff DC, Hicks ME, Vauthey J-N et al: Transhepatic portal vein embolization: anatomy, indications, and technical considerations. *Radiographics* 22:1063–1076, 2002.

Müller C, Schenk P: Hepatopulmonary syndrome. *Wien Klin Wochenschr* 111:339–347, 1999.

Ong JP, Sands M, Younossi ZM: Transjugular intrahepatic portosystemic shunt (TIPS): a decade later. *J Clin Gastroenterol* 30:14–28, 2000.

Otal P, Smayra T, Bureau C et al: Preliminary results of a new expanded-polytetrafluoroethylene-covered stent-graft for transjugular intrahepatic portosystemic shunt procedures. *Am J Roentgenol* 178:141–147, 2002.

Patel NH, Haskal ZJ, Kerlan RK eds: *Portal Hypertension: Diagnosis and Interventions*, 2nd edn, Society of Cardiovascular and Interventional Radiology, Fairfax, VA, 2001

Palmer BF: Pathogenesis of ascites and salt retention in cirrhosis. *J Invest Med* 47.183–202, 1999.

Petersen B: Intravascular ultrasound-guided direct intrahepatic portacaval shunt: description of technique and technical refinements. *J Vasc Interv Radiol* 14:21–32, 2003.

Ringe B, Lang H, Oldhafer KJ et al: Which is the best surgery for Budd–Chiari syndrome: venous decompression or liver transplantation? A single-center experience with 50 patients. *Hepatology* 21:1337–1344, 1995.

Rössle M: The transjugular intrahepatic portosystemic shunt. *J Hepatol* 25:224–231, 1996.

Rössle M, Ochs A, Gulberg V et al: A comparision of paracentesis and transjugular intrahepatic portosystemic shunting in patients with ascites. *N Engl J Med* 342:1701–1707, 2000.

Runyon BA: AASLD practice guidelines: management of adult patients with ascites caused by cirrhosis. *Hepatology* 27:264–272, 1998.

Russo MW, Zacks SL, Sandler RS, Brown RS: Cost-effectiveness analysis of transjugular intrahepatic portosystemic shunt (TIPS) versus endoscopic therapy for the prevention of recurrent esophageal variceal bleeding. *Hepatology* 31:358–363, 2000.

Sakorafas GH, Sarr MG, Farley DR, Farnell MB: The significance of sinistral portal hypertension complicating chronic pancreatitis. *Am J Surg* 179:129–133, 2000.

Sarfeh IJ: Partial vs total portacaval shunt in alcoholic cirrhosis: results of a prospective, randomized clinical trial. *Ann Surg* 219:353–361, 1994.

Saxon RR, Keller FS: Technical aspects of accessing the portal vein during the TIPS procedure. *J Vasc Interv Radiol* 8:733–744, 1997.

Uflacker R, Reichert P, D'Albuquerque LC et al: Liver anatomy applied to the placement of transjugular intrahepatic portosystemic shunts. *Radiology* 191:705–712, 1994.

Vargas HE, Gerber D, Abu-Elmagd K: Management of portal hypertension-related bleeding. *Surg Clin N Am* 79:1–21, 1999.

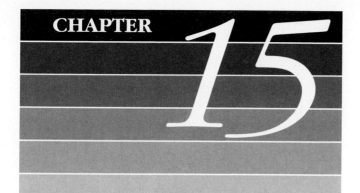

CHAPTER *15*

Lower-extremity Arteries

JOHN A. KAUFMAN, M.D.

The lower-extremity arteries are a common site for vascular diseases. The legs have a relatively large muscle mass, and a prominent role in basic daily activities such as walking. Lesions in this vascular bed produce troublesome symptoms at an early stage. Advanced disease frequently results in limb loss and decreased life expectancy. Interventions in the lower extremities are common, and increasing in frequency.

ANATOMY

The blood supply to the lower extremities can be roughly divided into runoff vessels (major conduits to the distal extremity) and muscular branches that supply the musculoskeletal structures. In most instances, the status of the runoff vessels is the primary clinical concern. However, in the presence of occlusion of the runoff vessels, the muscular branches become the principal source of collateral blood supply.

The common femoral artery (CFA) is the continuation of the external iliac artery. This vessel is usually 6–9 mm in diameter and 5–7 cm in length, with frequent and variable small, unnamed muscular branches. The CFA extends from the inguinal ligament to the origins of the superficial femoral (SFA) and profunda femoris (PFA) arteries just distal to the inferior margin of the femoral head (Fig. 15-1). Occasionally the artery will bifurcate while it is still anterior to the femoral head (termed a "high bifurcation") (Fig. 15-2). The CFA is contained within the femoral sheath, a continuation of the abdominal wall fascia. The sheath is funnel-shaped, with the broad base opening towards the abdomen. In addition to the artery, the sheath contains the femoral vein (medial to the artery) and the femoral canal (the most medial structure). The femoral nerve lies lateral to the femoral sheath, within the femoral triangle formed by the sartorius muscle laterally, the adductor longus muscle medially, the inguinal ligament superiorly, and the iliacus, psoas major, pectineus, and adductor longus muscles posteriorly.

The origin of the PFA has a lateral and posterior orientation relative to the SFA (see Fig. 10-9). The PFA provides proximal branches to the hip, the lateral and medial femoral circumflex arteries, before descending deep in the thigh adjacent to the medial edge of the femur. There are multiple branches from the PFA to the muscles of the thigh before it terminates above the adductor canal. These muscular branches anastomose with muscular branches of the SFA and popliteal arteries. Variations in the branching pattern and origin of the PFA are present in 40% of individuals. The most common

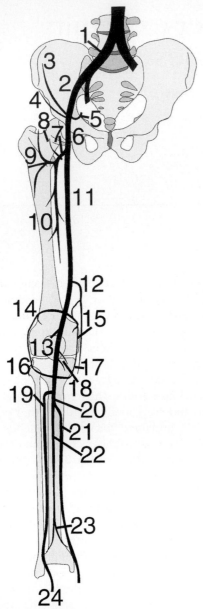

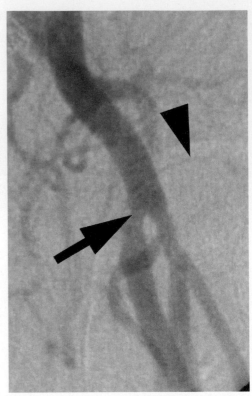

Figure 15-2   Digital subtraction angiogram (DSA) showing high bifurcation (arrow) of the left CFA anterior to the head of the femur. The arrowhead points to the top of the femoral head.

Figure 15-1   Drawing of lower extremity arteries. **1**, Common iliac artery (CIA). **2**, External iliac artery (EIA). **3**, Deep iliac circumflex artery. **4**, Superficial circumflex iliac artery. **5**, Inferior epigastric artery. **6**, Common femoral artery (CFA). **7**, Profunda femoris artery (PFA). **8**, Medial femoral circumflex artery. **9**, Lateral femoral circumflex artery. **10**, Descending branch of PFA. **11**, Superficial femoral artery (SFA). **12**, Descending genicular artery. **13**, Popliteal artery. **14**, Lateral superior genicular artery. **15**, Medial superior genicular artery. **16**, Lateral inferior genicular artery. **17**, Medial inferior genicular artery. **18**, Sural arteries. **19**, Anterior tibial artery. **20**, Tibio-peroneal trunk. **21**, Posterior tibial artery. **22**, Peroneal artery. **23**, Perforating branches to anterior and posterior tibial arteries. **24**, Dorsalis pedal artery.

The origin of the SFA from the CFA is anterior and medial to the PFA. The SFA runs beneath the sartorius muscle in the thigh, anterior to the femoral vein (Fig. 15-3). The artery passes through the adductor canal in the distal thigh, where it becomes the popliteal artery. The superficial femoral artery is usually 6–7 mm in diameter, with many unnamed muscular branches along its length. The last large medial branch is usually the descending or

variants are independent origins of one or both of the circumflex femoral arteries from the CFA or SFA.

The SFA is remarkable for the almost complete lack of variability in this vessel (rather boring for anatomists but appreciated by interventionalists) (Table 15-1).

Table 15-1   Anatomic Variants of the Lower-extremity Arteries

Variant	Incidence (%)
Two or more PFA branches from CFA	2
Persistent sciatic artery	0.025
Duplication of SFA	<0.001
High origin of a tibial artery	5
Peroneal origin from the anterior tibial artery	1
True popliteal artery trifurcation (no tibioperoneal trunk)	2
Hypoplastic posterior tibial artery	3.8
Hypoplastic anterior tibial artery	1.6
Hypoplastic anterior and posterior tibial arteries	0.2

CFA, common femoral artery; SFA, superficial femoral artery; PFA, profunda femoris artery.

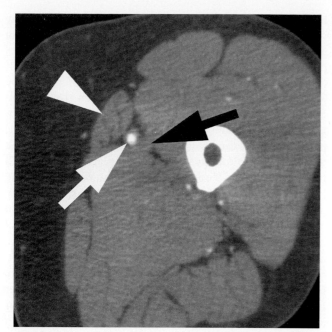

Figure 15-3 Axial CT image of the thigh during the arterial phase. The SFA (white arrow) lies beneath the sartorius muscle (arrowhead), slightly anterior and medial to the femoral vein (black arrow).

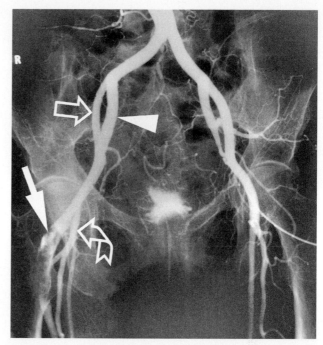

Figure 15-4 Persistent sciatic artery with aneurysmal degeneration. On the patient's right, the internal iliac artery (arrowhead) is enlarged, and the external iliac artery (open arrow) and CFA (curved arrow) are small compared to the left. The persistent sciatic artery (solid arrow) is aneurysmal and contains mural thrombus. The patient presented with distal embolization. Compare with the normal vascular anatomy on the left.

supreme genicular artery. The muscular branches of the superficial femoral artery are important collateral pathways in the setting of occlusive disease.

One of the few variants of SFA anatomy is a persistent sciatic artery (0.025%). This vessel is a normal fetal branch of the internal iliac artery that continues into the lower extremity posterior to the femoral head to supply the runoff vessels (Fig. 15-4). This artery usually regresses as the external iliac artery develops into the arterial supply of the lower limb. When persistent, the sciatic artery may terminate in the posterior thigh, in which case the runoff is through the SFA, or continue to the popliteal artery with a discontinuous or absent SFA. Persistent sciatic arteries are bilateral in 25% of patients. The posterior course of the artery renders it subject to repetitive trauma with aneurysm formation.

The popliteal artery is the continuation of the SFA from the adductor canal to the origins of the tibial vessels below the knee (see Fig 15-1). In clinical practice the joint line of the knee divides the artery into above-knee and below-knee segments. Although these are not official anatomic terms, the popliteal artery should always be described in this manner as the type of intervention and subsequent outcome are influenced by the level of disease.

The average diameter of the popliteal artery is 4–5 mm. The blood supply of the knee joint is provided by the superior and inferior (medial and lateral), and middle genicular arteries. These arteries are recognizable by their horizontal course around the knee. The posterior calf muscles are supplied by the vertically oriented sural arteries arising from the posterior aspect of the popliteal artery. The most common anatomic variation of the popliteal artery is a high origin of one or more of the tibial arteries. Usually, the popliteal artery bifurcates into the anterior tibial artery and the tibioperoneal trunk at the distal edge of the popliteus muscle. In 5% of individuals one of the tibial runoff vessels will have an origin from the popliteal artery above this level (Fig. 15-5).

The runoff vessels in the calf consist of the anterior tibial, posterior tibial, and peroneal arteries. The anterior tibial artery arises from the popliteal artery just distal to the popliteus artery. This vessel passes anteriorly through the interosseous membrane and then descends to the foot medial to the fibula in the anterior fascial compartment of the calf (Fig. 15-6). In fewer than 1% of individuals the peroneal artery will originate from the anterior tibial artery. The tibioperoneal trunk is a short artery of variable length that descends several centimeters beyond the anterior tibial artery origin before bifurcating into the posterior tibial and peroneal arteries. The posterior tibial artery courses deep to the soleus muscle to the medial malleolus. The peroneal artery descends to the ankle posterior and medial to the fibula. At the ankle, the peroneal artery terminates in a characteristic

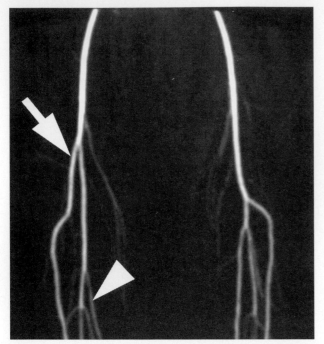

Figure 15-5   Coronal maximum-intensity projection (MIP) of a 3-dimensional gadolinium-enhanced MR angiogram (MRA) at the level of the knees, showing high origin of the right anterior tibial artery (arrow) and low origin of the right posterior tibial artery (arrowhead). Compare with the normal left tibial artery origins.

fork created by the anterior and posterior perforating branches (see Fig. 15-1). The posterior tibial and peroneal arteries are contained within the deep posterior fascial compartment of the calf.

The anterior and posterior tibial arteries continue into the foot in 95% of individuals, while the peroneal artery terminates above the ankle in an equal percentage. In roughly 5% of individuals one of the runoff vessels is absent. When one of the runoff tibial arteries is missing, the peroneal artery may continue into the foot.

There is much variability of the arterial supply to the foot, similar to the hand. Rather than memorize minutiae,

it is best to be familiar with the classical anatomy described below and use it as a basis when interpreting imaging studies. The anterior and posterior tibial arteries provide the bulk of the arterial supply to the foot (Fig. 15-7). The anterior tibial artery continues into the foot below the level of the ankle joint as the dorsalis pedis artery. The medial and lateral tarsal arteries are large branches that arise from the proximal dorsalis pedis artery. At the level of the proximal metatarsals the dorsalis pedis bifurcates into a deep plantar branch and the arcuate artery. The arcuate artery curves towards the lateral edge of the foot along the dorsal aspect of the metatarsal bone bases, supplying the dorsal metatarsal arteries to the distal foot before anastomosing with distal branches of the plantar arteries. The posterior tibial artery passes posterior and inferior to the medial malleolus, and then bifurcates into the medial and lateral plantar arteries. The lateral plantar artery is usually the larger of the two, with a course diagonally across the plantar aspect of the foot. The lateral plantar artery forms a second, deep plantar arch that supplies the plantar metatarsal arteries. This arch anastomoses with the deep plantar branch of the dorsalis pedis artery between the first and second metatarsals. The medial plantar artery travels inferior to the first metatarsal bone to supply the great toe.

KEY COLLATERAL PATHWAYS

The PFA is critically important in the collateral supply of lower-extremity arteries (Fig. 15-8). Occlusion of the CFA results in collateralization from the abdomen, pelvis, and the contralateral extremity to the PFA, which in turn reconstitutes the SFA (Box 15-1). These are the same collateral pathways that reconstitute the PFA when it is severely stenotic or occluded at its origin (Fig. 15-9).

Proximal occlusion of the SFA results in hypertrophy of PFA branches, which in turn reconstitute the SFA via muscular branches in the thigh (Fig. 15-10). This can be

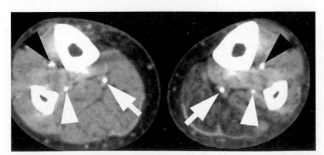

Figure 15-6   Axial CT image during the arterial phase at the level of the calf. Black arrowhead = anterior tibial artery. White arrowhead = peroneal artery. White arrow = posterior tibial artery.

Box 15-1   Collateral Pathways in Common Femoral Artery Occlusion

Lumbar artery $\Rightarrow$ circumflex iliac artery $\Rightarrow$ PFA $\Rightarrow$ SFA
Common iliac artery $\Rightarrow$ internal iliac artery $\Rightarrow$ PFA $\Rightarrow$ SFA
Contralateral PFA $\Rightarrow$ transpubic collaterals $\Rightarrow$ PFA $\Rightarrow$ SFA

SFA, superficial femoral artery; PFA, profunda femoris artery.

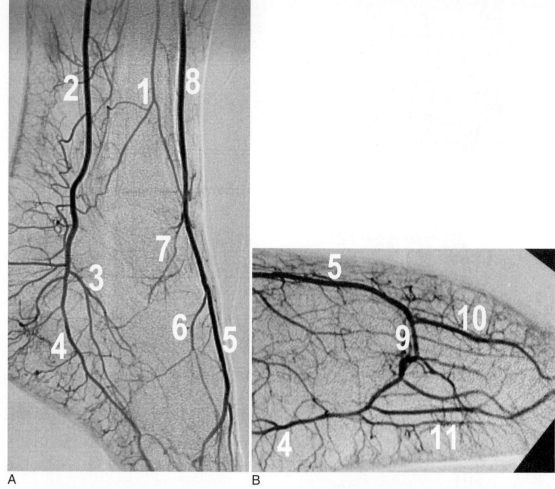

Figure 15-7   Pedal artery anatomy. **A**, Lateral DSA of the ankle and forefoot. **1**, Distal peroneal artery with anterior and posterior communicating branches. **2**, Posterior tibial artery. **3**, Medial plantar artery. **4**, Lateral plantar artery. **5**, Dorsalis pedis artery. **6**, Lateral tarsal artery. **7**, Medial tarsal artery. **8**, Anterior tibial artery. **B**, DSA of the forefoot. **4**, Lateral plantar artery. **5**, Dorsalis pedal artery. **9**, Arcuate artery. **10**, Dorsal metatarsal artery. **11**, Plantar metatarsal artery.

an extremely effective collateral pathway, so much so that patients may have palpable distal pulses. When the distal SFA is occluded, the descending trunk of the PFA provides collateral flow to the popliteal artery through the lateral genicular arteries. Occlusion of the above-knee popliteal artery can be collateralized from both the distal SFA (via the supreme genicular artery) and the PFA. In the presence of a below-knee popliteal artery occlusion, the sural and genicular arteries can reconstitute the tibial arteries (see Fig. 3-15C).

Occlusion of the tibioperoneal trunk and the proximal tibial arteries results in collateral supply from the sural and genicular arteries. Each of the tibial arteries has the potential to provide collateral supply to the others. The peroneal artery is the most common source of collateral supply, as it is frequently spared in occlusive disease and occupies a central location in the calf. At the

ankle the peroneal artery has a constant bifurcation that can collateralize to the distal anterior or posterior tibial arteries (see Fig. 15-7).

Occlusion of either the dorsalis pedis or posterior tibial artery distal to the medial malleolus is well tolerated if the plantar arches are intact. Occlusion of both the proximal dorsalis pedis and the infra-mallelolar posterior tibial artery is collateralized by tarsal and metatarsal arteries.

NONINVASIVE PHYSIOLOGIC EVALUATION

Evaluation of lower-extremity arterial occlusive disease requires determination of physiologic impact as well as imaging. The severity of an obstructive lesion does not

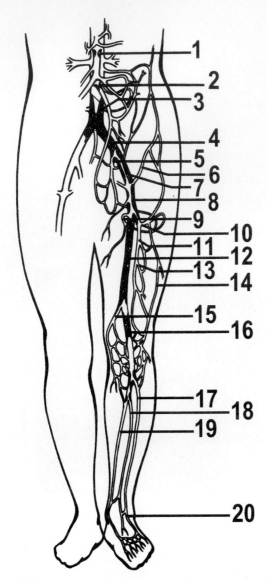

question. The lower extremities should be evaluated for skin integrity, capillary refill, temperature, and palpable pulses. In diabetics it is important to inspect between the toes for early skin breakdown and infection. The femoral, popliteal, dorsalis pedis, and posterior tibial arterial pulses should be checked in both legs, regardless of the laterality of symptoms.

The ratio of the systolic blood pressures of the ankle to the upper arm (the ankle–brachial index, ABI) is a basic measure of the status of the peripheral arteries. An appropriately sized blood pressure cuff and a Doppler ultrasound (US) probe are used to determine the systolic blood pressure at the ankle (dorsalis pedis or posterior tibial artery) and the brachial artery. The blood pressure in both arms should be obtained, and the

Figure 15-8 Diagram of collateral pathways to the lower-extremity arteries. Shaded areas are levels of obstruction. **1**, Superior mesenteric artery. **2**, Inferior mesenteric artery. **3**, Lumbar artery. **4**, CIA. **5**, Internal iliac artery. **6**, Deep iliac circumflex artery. **7**, EIA. **8**, CFA. **9**, Medial femoral circumflex artery. **10**, Lateral femoral circumflex artery. **11**, PFA. **12**, SFA. **13**, Second perforator. **14**, Descending branch of lateral femoral circumflex artery. **15**, Descending genicular artery. **16**, Popliteal artery. **17**, Anterior tibial artery. **18**, Peroneal artery. **19**, Posterior tibial artery. **20**, Dorsalis pedis artery. (Modified with permission from Kempczinski, RF: The chronically ischemic leg: an overview. In Rutherford RB ed: *Vascular Surgery*, 5th edn, WB Saunders, Philadelphia, 2000.)

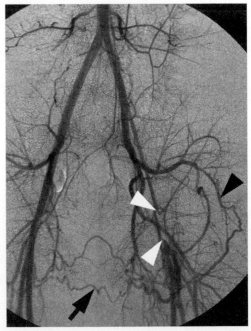

Figure 15-9 Collateralization around chronic left common femoral artery occlusion (white arrowheads) in an adolescent due to cardiac catheterization as an infant. The only symptom was leg-length discrepancy. There are well-developed collaterals from ipsilateral hypogastric branches (black arrowhead) and contralateral external pudendal arteries (black arrow).

always correlate with the severity of the symptoms. Noninvasive physiologic testing provides an objective measure of disease that can be used to follow patients and document outcomes of interventions (Box 15-2).

The most basic physiologic assessment is the physical examination. Important information can be obtained from the patient history and by examining the limb(s) in

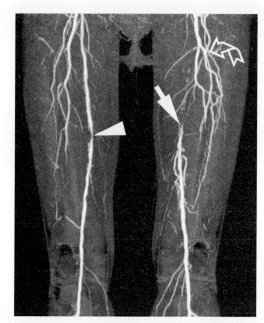

Figure 15-10   Collateralization of an SFA occlusion by enlarged PFA. Coronal MIP of a CT angiogram (CTA) showing an enlarged left PFA (curved arrow) that reconstitutes an occluded SFA in the mid-thigh (straight arrow). Note the focal SFA stenosis (arrowhead) on the right.

highest used to calculate the ratio. Ratios slightly greater than 1.0 are typical in normal individuals. In patients with occlusive disease, the ABI correlates roughly with the extent of disease and degree of ischemia (Table 15-2). This is a simple test that can be performed at the bedside or the procedure table before and after an intervention.

The ABI can be falsely elevated in diabetics with noncompressible vessels due to calcific medial sclerosis. The digital arteries are not as severely affected by this process. In these patients toe pressures are an important indicator of the severity of occlusive disease. The normal systolic blood pressure in the toe is >50 mmHg,

with a toe–brachial index ≥0.6. Toe pressures below 30 mmHg are incompatible with healing of ulcers or surgical incisions.

One of the major limitations of the ABI is that it does not provide any information about the level of the obstruction. A useful and simple modification is to obtain blood pressures at three or four different levels in the leg ("segmental limb pressures"). A Doppler probe is positioned over a pedal artery as cuffs over the thigh, calf, and ankle are inflated and deflated. The pressure at which signal reappears in the foot is noted as each cuff is deflated. Appropriately sized cuffs are used for each segment of the leg. The variability in limb circumference of the leg results in slightly higher pressure measurements with the thigh cuffs, especially in obese patients. In addition, diabetics may have falsely normal pressure measurements for reasons noted above. A drop in pressure of more than 20–30 mmHg at any level suggests hemodynamically significant occlusive disease in that vascular segment. In addition, a difference in pressures from side to side of more than 20 mmHg indicates occlusive disease at that level or proximal in the affected limb.

Segmental limb pressures are frequently combined with Doppler waveform analysis of arterial flow at each level (Fig. 15-11). This greatly enhances the utility of the study by providing an assessment of flow in addition to pressure. A Doppler probe is used to obtain a waveform from the vessel. Changes in the shape and amplitude of the waveform reflect increasing severity of disease (Fig. 15-12). Precise identification of the insonated vessel is essential for accurate testing.

Common noninvasive examinations for peripheral vascular disease are volume and photoplethysmography. These techniques measure the global perfusion of the extremity by recording the minute changes in the volume

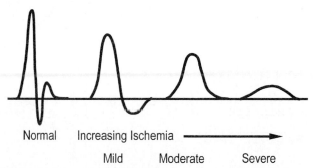

Figure 15-11   Schematic of changes in lower-extremity arterial Doppler waveforms with different levels of ischemia. Note that the normal pattern is triphasic (high peripheral resistance). (Adapted with permission from Rholl K, Sterling K, Jones CS: Noninvasive vascular diagnosis in peripheral vascular disease. In Kaufman JA, Hartnell GA, Trerotola SO eds: *Noninvasive Vascular Imaging With Ultrasound, Computed Tomography, and Magnetic Resonance*. Society of Cardiovascular and Interventional Radiology, Fairfax, VA, 1997.)

Table 15-2	Resting Ankle–Brachial Indices	
ABI	**Severity of Disease**	**Typical Symptoms**
≥0.95	None	None
0.75–0.95	Mild, single segment	None, claudication
0.5–0.75	Moderate	Claudication
0.3–0.5	Moderate severe, usually multilevel	Severe claudication
<0.3	Critical, multilevel or acute occlusion	Rest pain, tissue loss

ABI, ankle–brachial index (ratio of ankle systolic blood pressure and brachial systolic blood pressure).

of the extremity that occur throughout the cardiac cycle. The terms "volume plethysmographic recordings" (VPRs) or "pulse volume recordings" (PVRs) are essentially interchangeable. A series of blood pressure cuffs are applied to the extremity, and sequentially inflated to 60–65 mmHg. The pressure in the cuff changes slightly as the volume of blood changes with systole and diastole. These changes are displayed as a waveform (Fig. 15-13). Abnormalities in the waveform indicate occlusive disease in the vascular segment proximal to the cuff. For example,

an abnormal tracing at the thigh is not caused by SFA disease, but disease in the aorta, common iliac artery, or common femoral artery.

The plethysmographic waveform can be analyzed for both contour and amplitude. The contour of the waveform is determined by the status of the arterial blood supply. As the degree of stenosis becomes more severe, the dicrotic notch is lost and the overall slope is flattened. The amplitude of the waveform reflects the underlying muscle mass. Fat and bone are relatively avascular,

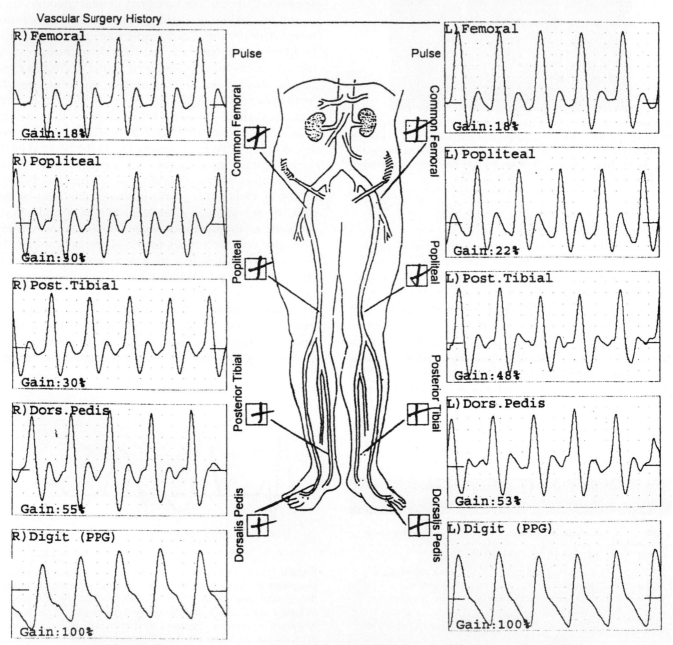

Figure 15-12 Normal and abnormal lower-extremity Doppler waveforms. **A,** Normal examination showing excellent waveforms and pressures at all levels. The pedal waveforms typically lose the triphasic pattern. *(Continued)*

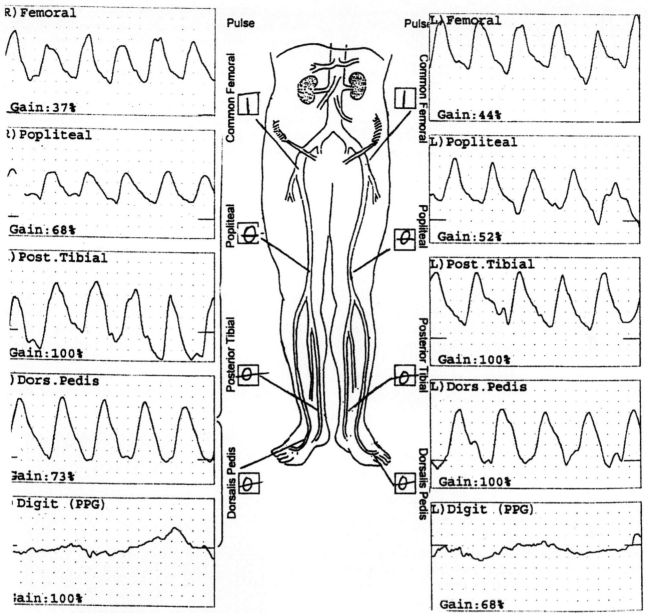

Figure 15-12   cont'd B, Examination in a patient with severe ischemia. The arm/thigh blood pressures ratios were 0.53 on the right and 0.43 on the left, indicating bilateral inflow disease. The arm/calf pressure indices dropped to 0.35 on the right and 0.28 on the left, indicative of bilateral SFA disease as well. The ankle/brachial index (ABI) was 0.28 on the right and 0.24 on the left. The waveforms are barely biphasic proximally, and essentially flat in the toes. These findings are consistent with severe bilateral multilevel disease.

and contribute little to the change in volume during the cardiac cycle. This explains why the amplitude increases slightly at the calf in normal individuals owing to the lower amount of adipose tissue. Photoplethysmography can be used in the evaluation of vasospastic disorders by testing before and after temperature stimuli.

Knowledge of the patient's past surgical history and body habitus are important when interpreting plethysmography. Medial sclerosis does not affect plethysmography, but patient motion will degrade the study.

Patients with claudication but normal pulse examinations, segmental pressures, and plethysmography should undergo exercise testing. Occlusive lesions that are well compensated at rest may be unmasked by hyperemia created in the distal muscular bed during exercise. Testing is performed before and after walking on a treadmill at a grade of 10–12 degrees for 5 minutes at 1.5–2 miles per hour. The time to onset and features of the symptoms are recorded. Normally, the ABI remains unchanged or even increases with exercise, and the

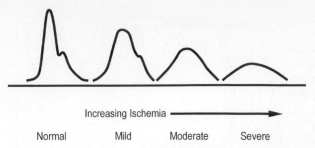

Increasing Ischemia ⟶

Normal   Mild   Moderate   Severe

Figure 15-13 Schematic of volume plethysmographic waveforms in relationship to degree of inflow disease. As disease progresses, the waveform becomes blunted and diminished in amplitude. (Adapted with permission from Rholl K, Sterling K, Jones CS: Noninvasive vascular diagnosis in peripheral vascular disease. In Kaufman JA, Hartnell GA, Trerotola SO eds: *Noninvasive Vascular Imaging With Ultrasound, Computed Tomography, and Magnetic Resonance*. Society of Cardiovascular and Interventional Radiology, Fairfax, VA, 1997.)

amplitude of the volume recording increases with preservation of the contour. An abnormal response indicates hemodynamically significant occlusive disease.

IMAGING

A wide variety of imaging modalities can be applied to the lower-extremity arteries. Availability of a technique at a particular institution depends upon the presence of appropriate equipment and expertise. Regardless of the imaging modality, it is essential to know the patient's symptoms, past surgical history, and results of noninvasive testing prior to performing and interpreting a study.

Color-flow Doppler US can be used to image the lower-extremity arteries and surgical bypass grafts. A variety of criteria have been promoted to categorize occlusive lesions (Table 15-3). Careful inspection of each abnormal vascular segment with gray-scale, color, and Doppler US is necessary to precisely localize abnormalities. Bypass grafts are particularly well suited to US imaging when they are superficial in location.

Table 15-3 Duplex Criteria for Native Lower-extremity Arterial Stenosis

Stenosis	PSV (sample value)	Poststenotic turbulence
None	Normal (100 cm/s)	None
<50%	<2 × normal (<200 cm/s)	Minimal
50–75%	2–4 × normal (>200 cm/s)	Moderate
76–99%	>4 × normal (≥400 cm/s)	Severe
100%	No flow	Not applicable

PSV, peak systolic velocity.

MR angiography (MRA) can detect luminal stenoses >50% in the lower-extremity arteries with sensitivity and specificity that exceed 95%. The first technique to produce reliable imaging was 2-dimensional time-of-flight (2-D TOF) MRA. This appeared to have the ideal quality of imaging blood flow rather than contrast enhancement, so that timing issues were nonexistent. However, overestimation of stenoses, saturation of in-plane flow, and the long time ($1\frac{1}{2}$–2 hours) needed for a complete examination were among several serious limitations (see Fig. 3-14). The initial enthusiasm for 2-D TOF MRA in the extremities has subsided as techniques for dynamic gadolinium-enhanced 3-dimensional (3-D) acquisitions have improved. Stepping table technology permits true gadolinium-enhanced MRA runoffs. Bolus chase or multiple injections of gadolinium (usually no more than 30–40 mL in total) provide excellent images from the renal arteries to the ankle (see Fig. 3-15). In the foot, small vessel size and prominent venous enhancement can be a limitation of contrast-enhanced MRA unless dedicated pedal imaging is performed (Fig. 15-14). An entire runoff from the renal arteries to the foot can now be acquired in less than 30 minutes.

CT angiography (CTA) of the lower-extremity arteries has become a clinical reality with multirow detector

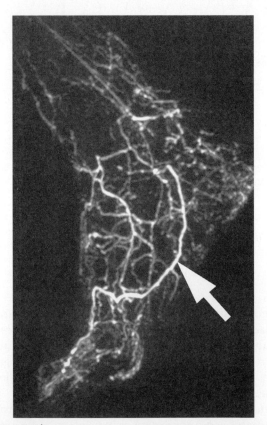

Figure 15-14 Dedicated 3-dimensional (3D) gadolinium-enhanced MRA of the foot in a patient with severe tibial artery disease demonstrates a patent lateral plantar artery (arrow).

(MDCT) technology. As the number of rows increases (16+), the imaging of lower-extremity arteries improves. Nominal section thickness of 1–3 mm results in a 20–30 second scan duration to image from the renal arteries to the calf (see Fig. 15-10). Contrast is injected at 3–5 mL/s for a total volume of approximately 150 mL, although the volume may decrease as the number of detector rows increases. A scan delay of 15–20 seconds is usually sufficient. Opacification is generally excellent from the renal to the tibial arteries. Venous enhancement, calcification, and small vessel size are limitations in the calf and foot, but can be overcome by focused examinations (Fig. 15-15).

The role of conventional angiography in the diagnosis of lower-extremity arterial disease has changed substantially with the improvement in noninvasive imaging techniques. Angiography was once obtained uniformly in all patients prior to surgery or intervention. Increasingly, angiography is becoming a secondary imaging modality to resolve results of conflicting noninvasive tests, or to confirm an abnormality prior to percutaneous intervention.

Angiographic evaluation of the lower extremities includes, as a minimum, the aortic bifurcation to the ankle. In most patients an abdominal aortogram is performed prior to imaging the lower extremities, particularly when renovascular or visceral artery occlusive disease is suspected (see Fig. 10-8). Pelvic arteriography can be performed with a pigtail catheter just proximal to the aortic bifurcation. Anteroposterior and bilateral oblique views should be obtained whenever iliac artery pathology is suspected (see Fig. 10-9). Typical parameters are 8–10 mL/s of contrast injected for 2–3 seconds, and an exposure rate of 2–4/s for digital subtraction angiography (DSA) and 1 film per second for cut film. Pressure gradients should be obtained across any stenosis (either pull-down with a straight catheter when ipsilateral, or pull-back when contralateral).

Positioning of the legs is an important consideration during runoff angiograms. The legs should be held as close together and as stationary as possible, without tight straps or tape that could compress vessels and created artifactual occlusions. The latter is most likely to occur at the ankles and feet. The optimum positioning of the feet varies among departments, but it is not critical as dedicated foot imaging can and should always be added when indicated.

Bilateral lower-extremity runoffs are obtained with the catheter at the aortic bifurcation using two basic strategies. The simplest and most reliable is stationary overlapping DSA down the legs. Small (10–20 cc) contrast injections are performed with imaging at 1 frame/s until all vessels are fully opacified. Rapidly filling normal arteries and slowly filling reconstituted arteries are both easily imaged. The overall volume of contrast necessary is dependent upon the severity of disease; as the length and number of occlusions increase, more contrast is needed to opacify reconstituted distal vessels. However, the ability to postprocess images greatly enhances the value of this approach.

The second basic approach is to image a long, continuous contrast injection at sequential overlapping levels as it progresses down the extremity. Although less overall contrast is typically used compared to stationary runs, the likelihood of underfilling of a segment of vessel is greater. Images are acquired in either subtracted or unsubtracted modes, and with either physician-activated or programmed changes in table position (Fig. 15-16). Both versions require setting parameters for changes in the table position, imaging technique, as well as careful patient positioning. Physician-activated change in table position (termed "bolus chase") is based upon real time assessment of vascular opacification. A timing run at the knees should be obtained before the runoff so that hyperemia can be induced if one leg is much slower than the other. Images can be acquired as either subtracted or unsubtracted digital angiograms. A standard contrast injection can be used (such as full-strength or diluted low osmolar contrast at 6–10 mL/s for 10–12 seconds). Less popular is the programmed table-stepping technique, in which the change in position is automated to occur after preselected duration of filming at each level. When programmed stepping is used a certain amount of time must elapse following initiation of the contrast

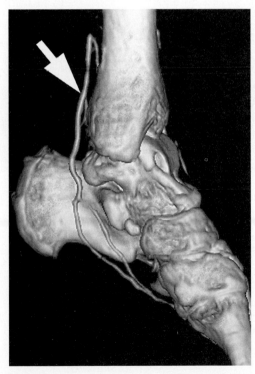

Figure 15-15 Volume rendering of a CTA at the level of the foot showing a reconstituted distal posterior tibial (arrow) and plantar arteries.

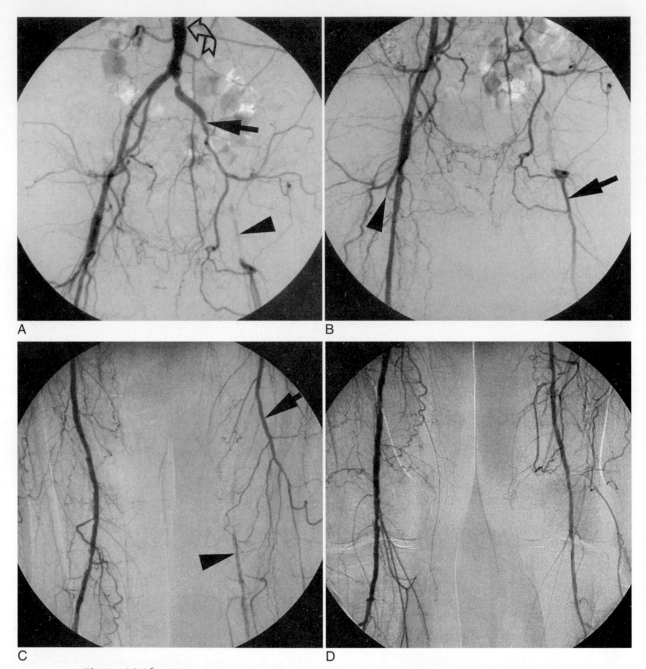

Figure 15-16   Bilateral lower-extremity runoff using bolus-chase DSA technique. Each level is carefully programmed to have several centimeters of overlap with the previous level. The levels were changed during the acquisition by the angiographer who monitored arterial opacification on a live image during the injection. Contrast was diluted to two-thirds strength and injected at a rate of 10 mL/s for a total duration of 10 seconds. **A**, Station 1 – Pelvis: A pigtail catheter (curved arrow) is positioned in the distal abdominal aorta. There is occlusion of the left EIA (straight arrow). The left CFA (arrowhead) is faintly reconstituted by the iliac circumflex vessels, whereas the left PFA is well visualized owing to collaterals from the left internal iliac artery. **B**, Station 2 – Groin: The left SFA is occluded with an enlarged left PFA (arrow). On the right, the descending trunk of the PFA (arrowhead) is occluded. Note the overlap with the preceding station and the decreased density of contrast on the left due to CIA occlusion. **C**, Station 3 – Thigh: The left PFA (arrow) reconstitutes the distal left SFA (arrowhead). Contrast density on the left is diminished compared to the right owing to multiple levels of proximal obstruction. **D**, Station 4 – Knees: The popliteal arteries are patent with mild diffuse disease.   (*Continued*)

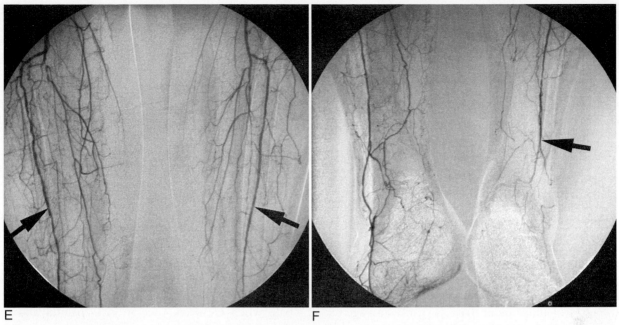

Figure 15-16   cont'd E, Station 5 – Proximal calves: There is anterior tibial artery runoff bilaterally (arrows), with diffuse disease on the right. The posterior tibial and peroneal arteries are occluded bilaterally. **F**, Station 6 – Distal calves: The anterior tibial artery on the left is occluded at the ankle (arrow), but on the right continues into the foot.

injection before imaging in order to ensure adequate filling of the arteries. This is termed the "delay." The optimum way to determine the delay is to image over the knee while injecting 10 mL of contrast through the catheter. The time required for contrast to appear at the knee joint, minus 2–3 seconds, is the filming delay.

When there is a great disparity in the delay between legs, or if the delay is longer than 12 seconds, then reactive hyperemia should be used. Reactive hyperemia effectively reduces the delay to 6–7 seconds in almost all patients. This simple maneuver is performed by inflation of a blood pressure cuff to a suprasystolic pressure at the ankle for 2–3 minutes. Contrast is injected immediately after release of the cuffs.

Selective single-limb angiography provides excellent filling of vessels with less dilution of contrast. The inflow vessels should first be examined with pelvic (or aortic and pelvic) arteriography. Subsequently, when the access is from the ipsilateral CFA, a 5-French straight multiple side-hole or a tightly recurved end-hole catheter can be withdrawn into the external iliac artery. When the access is from the contralateral CFA an end-hole catheter can be positioned over the aortic bifurcation in the common or external iliac artery. Stationary DSA runs with injections of 4 mL/s for 2 seconds each is a quick technique that produces excellent images (see Fig. 15-7).

The origins of the SFA and PFA are usually viewed best from an ipsilateral anterior oblique projection (see Fig. 10-9). These views should be obtained when the vessel origins are not clearly seen in anteroposterior projections. Additional oblique and even lateral views of specific abnormalities are not usually obtained, but can be important to accurately grade stenoses particularly in the tibial arteries where overlying bone can obscure vessels or create subtraction artifacts (Fig. 15-17).

Whenever there is pathology present in the foot, dedicated views are necessary. A single lateral view that includes the malleolus to the toes is usually sufficient, although an anteroposterior projection may be necessary for specific indications (see Fig. 15-7). Positioning the catheter tip in the external iliac artery or SFA maximizes the delivery of contrast to the foot. The foot should be carefully taped in position (with special attention to delicate skin and pressure points). Hyperextension of the foot should be avoided to prevent artifactual occlusion of the dorsalis pedis artery (Fig. 15-18). In the presence of extensive proximal occlusive disease it is important to use reactive hyperemia, prolonged image acquisition, and injection of full-strength low-osmolar contrast at 5 mL/s for 4–6 seconds.

CHRONIC OCCLUSIVE DISEASE

There are many causes of peripheral arterial occlusions (Box 15-3). This section will focus on atherosclerotic

Box 15-3   Etiologies of Chronic Peripheral Vascular Occlusions

Atherosclerosis
Thromboangiitis obliterans (Buerger's disease)
Popliteal entrapment syndrome
Adventitial cystic disease
Radiation
Vasculitis
Ergotism
Trauma
Chronic embolism

disease, as this is the most common chronic pathology encountered in lower-extremity arterial circulation.

The prevalence of atherosclerotic peripheral arterial disease increases with age from 3% of individuals aged 40–59 to 20% of adults older than 70 years. Until age 65, men are affected more often than women. Fewer than half of people with atherosclerotic peripheral arterial disease are symptomatic, most commonly with pain upon ambulation (claudication). A much smaller percentage

have rest pain, tissue loss, or gangrene. Smoking, diabetes, hyperlipidemia, homocystinemia, advanced age, ethnicity, and hypertension are important risk factors.

The symptoms of chronic peripheral arterial occlusive disease are related to the level of the occlusion and the presence of comorbid conditions such as diabetes. Symptoms are typically manifested in the limb segment distal to the occlusive process. The usual complaint is claudication, which is consistently described by patients as onset of muscular tightening or cramping with exertion. This should resolve with rest within minutes. Patients may also report nonspecific leg weakness and numbness with exercise that also resolves with rest. As chronic ischemia progresses, skin changes such as scaling, hair loss, and atrophy occur. Advanced disease is manifested as rest pain, ulceration, and tissue necrosis (critical ischemia). Rest pain is aggravated by elevation of the extremity, and relieved when the limb is dependent. The foot may be noticeably red when dependent, and pale when elevated. Ulceration is painful and usually occurs in the distal forefoot or between the toes. Severe ischemic changes can develop in diabetics in the presence of palpable pedal pulses, owing to extensive microvascular pathology. In order to facilitate communication

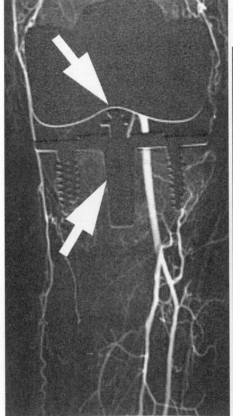

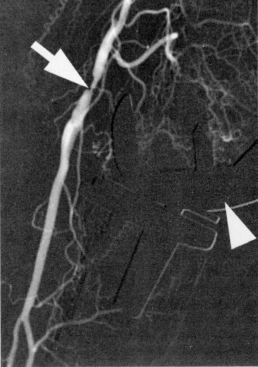

Figure 15-17 Importance of careful limb positioning and multiple views during angiography. Popliteal artery stenosis obscured by total knee prosthesis. **A**, DSA in the anteroposterior projection showing the above-knee popliteal artery obscured by the knee prosthesis (arrows). **B**, Lateral view of the same patient showing a focal stenosis (arrow) in the above-knee popliteal artery that was treated successfully with angioplasty. The arrowhead points to the knee prosthesis.

A   B

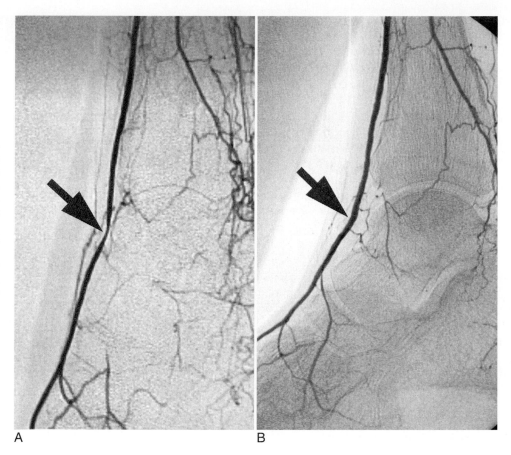

Figure 15-18 Artifactual stenosis of dorsalis pedis artery due to positioning of the foot ("ballerina sign"). **A,** Lateral DSA of the foot in plantar flexion ("en pointe" like a ballerina) showing focal stenosis (arrow) of the dorsalis pedis artery. **B,** The angiogram was repeated with the foot in neutral position. The dorsalis pedis stenosis is now gone (arrow). This same artifact can also be caused by tight straps or tape on a limb.

A   B

about patients with peripheral vascular disease, the classification devised by Rutherford and associates should be used (Table 15-4).

Not all ulcers are ischemic in nature. Diabetics with severe neuropathy can develop ulceration over pressure points such as the metatarsal head. Venous ulcers are distinguished from lesions due to arterial insufficiency by their typical location around the ankles and associated manifestations of chronic venous stasis (see Chapter 16).

Atherosclerotic peripheral arterial occlusive disease is a marker of systemic atherosclerosis. Approximately 65%

Table 15-4   Rutherford Categories of Chronic Limb Ischemia

Grade	Category	Clinical Description	Objective Criteria[a]
0	0	Asymptomatic	Normal treadmill or reactive hyperemia test
	1	Mild claudication	Completes treadmill test; ankle pressure after exercise >50 mmHg but at least 20 mmHg lower than brachial pressure
I	2	Moderate claudication	Between categories 1 and 3
	3	Severe claudication	Cannot complete treadmill test; ankle pressure <50 mm Hg after exercise
III	4	Ischemic rest pain	Resting ankle pressure <40 mmHg; flat or barely pulsatile ankle or metatarsal pulse volume recording; toe pressure <30 mmHg
III	5	Minor tissue loss; nonhealing ulcer, focal gangrene with diffuse pedal ischemia	Resting ankle pressure <60 mmHg; flat or severely dampened ankle or metatarsal pulse volume recording; toe pressure <40 mmHg
	6	Major tissue loss extending above trans-metatarsal level; functional foot unsalvageable	Same as category 5

[a]Treadmill test is 5 minutes at 2 mph on a 12-degree incline.

of patients with lower-extremity arterial disease will have abnormal cardiac stress tests, and 25% will have carotid artery stenoses >70%. The underlying cause of death in 60% of patients with peripheral vascular disease is a cardiac event. A diagnosis of peripheral vascular disease confers a mortality rate that is almost treble that of age-matched controls (Table 15-5).

The distribution of lower-extremity atherosclerosis is symmetric in almost 80% of patients, although the severity of the lesions may not match (Box 15-4). Involvement of adjacent segments is common, with combined iliac artery and SFA disease in 46%, and femoropopliteal and tibial disease in 38%. The iliac arteries are diseased in 46% of patients with SFA and popliteal stenoses. There are several well-recognized patterns of distribution of disease, including: normal inflow with severe infrapopliteal artery disease in patients with diabetes and renal failure; isolated distal aortic and bifurcation disease in middle-aged females; and ileofemoral disease in smokers (Fig. 15-19; see also Fig. 10-23).

Limb loss is one of the most clearly defined measures of outcome in peripheral vascular disease. Only 12% of symptomatic patients will require amputation within 10 years of diagnosis, or roughly 1% of claudicants per year. Diabetes and continued smoking result in higher rates of amputation. Symptomatic peripheral vascular disease remains stable or even improves in three-quarters of patients.

The management of the majority of claudicants is conservative. Lifestyle modification (cessation of smoking being the most important), exercise programs, and control of comorbid diseases are frequently successful in stabilization or slight improvement of symptoms in patients able to comply. A 6-month trial of conservative therapy is usually required before considering more aggressive treatment. Unfortunately, few medications have been shown to conclusively improve claudication symptoms, although cilostazol can increase walking

Box 15-4 Typical Locations for Atherosclerotic Stenosis in the Lower Extremities

Superficial femoral artery in Hunter's Canal
Common iliac artery
Popliteal artery at joint line
Tibioperoneal trunk
Origins of tibial arteries

distance by up to 50% in some patients. Aspirin and other antiplatelet drugs reduce overall risk of cardiovascular events, but have little impact on claudication symptoms. Patients with progressive symptoms or who are severely limited by their claudication are considered early for revascularization procedures. Patients with critical ischemia (rest pain, tissue loss, and gangrene) more often require aggressive intervention to preserve the limb. As a general rule, healing of an ischemic foot ulcer will not occur in the absence of a pulse in at least one pedal artery.

Physiologic testing is relatively inexpensive and has a major role in the diagnosis and follow-up of patients with symptomatic peripheral vascular disease. True claudicants can be separated from patients with limb pain due to spinal stenosis and osteoarthritis. Progression of disease can be documented objectively, as well as the results of interventions. Exercise testing should be obtained in any patient with suspected claudication who has a normal or near-normal study at rest.

The decision to pursue imaging in a patient with peripheral vascular disease is dependent upon the management plan. Owing to the expense and potentially invasive nature of the imaging studies, these examinations should not be obtained unless a patient requires revascularization. The history, physical examination, and results of physiologic testing are sufficient to diagnose peripheral vascular disease in almost all patients.

The most experience with noninvasive imaging has been with US and MRA. The sensitivity and specificity for occlusive lesions are reported to exceed 95% for both modalities. In patients with renal insufficiency, allergy to iodinated contrast, and severe multilevel disease, MRA and US are excellent choices for imaging. MRA is particularly useful in imaging the lower-extremity runoff of patients with infrarenal occlusions, as both the arterial inflow and outflow can be visualized (see Fig. 10-24). The degree of a focal arterial stenosis is often overestimated on MRA, and metal in vascular clips or joint prostheses can create susceptibility artifacts that obscure vascular segments. US does not reliably image aortic and iliac inflow, but can quantify flow through abnormal areas. In the future, CTA may be used routinely to evaluate lower-extremity arterial disease.

Table 15-5 Survival in Patients with Peripheral Vascular Disease

Parameter	(%)
5-year survival, all patients	70
10-year survival, all patients	50
15-year survival, all patients	30
5-year survival, claudication managed conservatively	87
5-year survival, claudication requiring surgery	80
5-year survival, limb-threatening ischemia treated with surgery	48
5-year survival, reoperation for limb-threatening ischemia	12

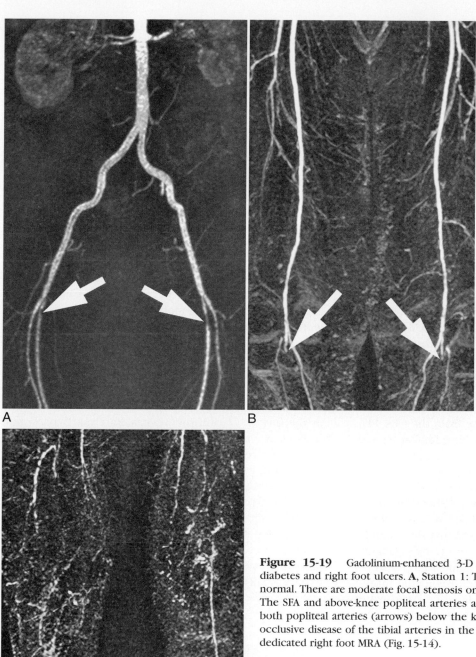

A

B

C

Figure 15-19 Gadolinium-enhanced 3-D MRA runoff in a patient with severe diabetes and right foot ulcers. **A**, Station 1: The abdominal aorta and iliac arteries are normal. There are moderate focal stenosis on the proximal SFAs (arrows). **B**, Station 2: The SFA and above-knee popliteal arteries are patent. However, there is occlusion of both popliteal arteries (arrows) below the knee joint. **C**, Station 3: There is extensive occlusive disease of the tibial arteries in the calf. A patent plantar artery was seen on dedicated right foot MRA (Fig. 15-14).

Conventional angiography remains crucially important in the evaluation of patients with symptomatic peripheral vascular disease. Angiography is indicated when a percutaneous intervention is highly probable based upon noninvasive testing, or when discrepant results have been obtained. Surgical bypass can be performed on the basis of high-quality US, MRA, or CTA.

Percutaneous access for angiography in patients with severe occlusive disease or prior surgery can be challenging. Posterior plaque on the common femoral artery is common, and can impede insertion of a guidewire. Patients with prior surgery or angiograms may have scarring of the soft tissues that actually prevents advancement of a catheter. Continued pushing leads to a kink in the guidewire (see Fig. 2-44). In this situation, overdilatation of the tract by 1 French size over a stout guidewire is necessary before placement of the catheter. The presence of an aorto-bifemoral bypass graft can also complicate the initial access (see Fig. 2-32). When femoral access cannot be obtained, translumbar or axillary puncture may be required. Patients with prior distal surgical bypass procedures can require additional views for a complete study. Surgical anastomoses frequently have a flared appearance ("the hood" of the graft) related to the manner in which the graft is attached to the native vessel (Fig. 15-20). Distal bypasses may arise from the CFA, PFA, SFA, or even the popliteal artery. The proximal anastomosis is usually on the anterior wall of the vessel when the origin is the CFA, PFA, or SFA; filming in a steep anterior oblique projection may be necessary for adequate visualization. Distal anastomoses vary in orientation depending upon the target vessel. The course of the bypass graft may be similar to the native artery or extraanatomic. Careful attention to coning and positioning during the angiogram is necessary to avoid inadvertently excluding a portion of the graft. When there is a severe stenosis in the mid or distal portion of the graft, contrast injected proximal to the graft may not opacify the stagnant column of blood in the graft. This "pseudo occlusion" should be suspected when a definite meniscus is not seen at the origin of the graft, or a pulse is known to be present in the nonvisualized bypass. Selective injection into the graft is necessary to determine the status of the graft in these cases.

The most common surgical interventions in patients with chronic occlusive disease are various bypass procedures. A number of surgical conduits have been investigated, but autogenous vein and polytetrafluoroethylene (PTFE) have proven the most successful. In general, synthetic grafts are used only when bypass is to the above-knee popliteal artery. Autogenous vein (usually the greater saphenous) is preferred for more distal bypass. Veins may be harvested from either leg, or constructed from available lengths of arm veins. An *in situ* saphenous vein graft is created by fashioning proximal and distal arteriovenous anastomoses without removing the vein from the leg. Intraluminal cutting devices are used to destroy the intervening vein valves, and all side branches are carefully obstructed or ligated. The size of the vein at the anastomosis site approximates that of the artery. Reversed saphenous vein grafts are first harvested from the leg, followed by ligation of branches. The vein is then tunneled through the soft tissues in reverse orientation, so that the smaller (formerly most peripheral) end is at the common femoral artery, and the larger (formerly most central) end is at the distal anastomosis. Local endarterectomy procedures alone or in combination with distal bypass are sometimes utilized, especially for lesions of the common femoral artery and PFA origin.

Perioperative mortality for peripheral vascular bypass is 2–5%, largely due to cardiac events. Early graft thrombosis (within 30 days) due to technical errors, such as kinking or a retained valve, or a hypercoagulable state occurs in 2–7%. Intimal hyperplasia is the cause of most graft failures between 3 months and 2 years. In synthetic grafts this occurs at the anastomoses or at sites of clamp placement on native vessels. In addition to these locations, intimal hyperplasia can occur anywhere within a vein graft, but usually the sites of former valves, branch vessels, or vein-to-vein anastomoses. Graft failure after 2 years is usually the result of progression of disease in the inflow or outflow vessels. Rarely, a bypass graft (especially vein) will remain patent despite occlusion of the native inflow. Graft infection and anastomotic pseudoaneurysms are additional complications. The overall results of surgical bypass grafts are listed in Table 15-6. Long-term rates of limb salvage and patient survival are best when the indication for surgery is claudication rather than critical ischemia.

Graft surveillance with US is believed to be important to prevent thrombosis and extend the life of the bypass. A fall in the ABI of 0.15–0.2, or identification of a

Table 15-6   Results of Lower-extremity Surgical Bypass

Procedure	5-year Primary Patency (%)
Femoral to popliteal artery bypass	
Synthetic above knee	60
Synthetic below knee	30
Saphenous vein above knee	75
Saphenous vein below knee	75
Femoral to tibial artery bypass	
Synthetic	14
Saphenous vein	75
Femoral to pedal artery bypass	
Saphenous vein	55

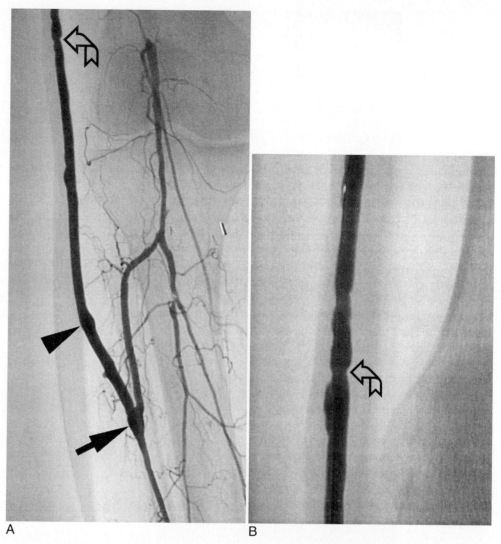

Figure 15-20 DSA of reversed saphenous vein graft from the CFA to the right anterior tibial artery. The course of the graft is posterior and lateral to the knee joint in an extraanatomic location in order to facilitate anastomosis to the anterior tibial artery. **A**, There is focal stenosis in the graft (curved arrow). Note the normal appearance of the vein valves (arrowhead) and the flared surgical anastomosis (straight arrow) to the anterior tibial artery. **B**, DSA following angioplasty of the stenosis with a 6-mm balloon shows improved appearance (curved arrow) and small associated dissection. This is a typical angiographic result following angioplasty of these fibrotic lesions.

A   B

hemodynamically significant stenosis at any point in the graft, should prompt further imaging. Focal stenoses can be treated with percutaneous or surgical patch angioplasty (see Fig. 15-20). Long-segment lesions are best managed with graft revision or insertion of a jump graft around the stenotic area. Thrombolysis of an acutely thrombosed graft may unmask an underlying stenosis, although no lesion is found in up to a third of cases. When the graft crosses the knee joint and no stenosis is found after thrombolysis, flexion and stress views should be obtained to exclude kinking or external compression.

SFA and Popliteal Angioplasty and Stents

Percutaneous intervention for occlusive disease of the infrainguinal arteries has a long history; the first percutaneous angioplasty ever was performed in the leg (see Fig. 4-1). A wide variety of technologies have since been applied to this vascular bed, including angioplasty, stents, stent-grafts, mechanical atherectomy, and laser

atherectomy. The latter two technologies appear to have no advantage in outcomes over angioplasty, and will not be discussed further.

Occlusive disease of the SFA and popliteal artery can be effectively treated with angioplasty when the stenoses or occlusions are focal (<5 cm in length) (Box 15-5; see also Fig. 4-6). Stenoses and occlusions of almost any length can be attempted, but the results in the past have been less satisfactory as the length and number of lesions increase. Long occlusions can be treated with subintimal angioplasty (Fig. 15-21). A short trial of catheter-directed thrombolysis to reduce the length of the occlusion or convert it to a stenosis can be used when fresh appearing thrombus is present. Drug-eluting stents hold promise for use in long-segment recanalization of the SFA and popliteal artery.

The most direct approach to infrainguinal interventions is from an antegrade puncture in the ipsilateral CFA, as this provides the greatest mechanical advantage and permits use of standard length materials. Antegrade access

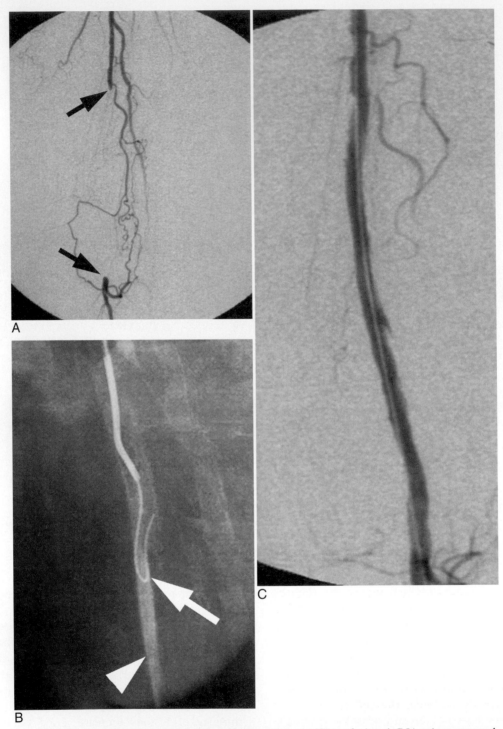

Figure 15-21   Subintimal recanalization of a long-segment SFA occlusion. **A**, DSA prior to recanalization showing the occluded SFA (arrows) reconstituting below the adductor canal. **B**, Spot film during recanalization showing the guidewire forming a "J" (arrow) in the subintimal space. Note the stagnant subintimal contrast (arrowhead). **C**, DSA after re-entry into the distal lumen and angioplasty showing excellent flow. (Images A and C courtesy of David Spinosa M.D., University of Virginia, Charlottesville, VA. Image B courtesy of Peter Bromley M.D.)

Box 15-5 TransAtlantic Inter-Society Consensus (TASC) Recommendations for Femoropopliteal Interventions (2000)[a]

Lesion type A: Endovascular is treatment of choice

1. Single stenosis <3 cm of SFA or POP (unilateral/bilateral)

Lesion type B: Endovascular frequently used but insufficient scientific evidence

2. Single stenosis or occlusion 3–5 cm in length, not involving the distal popliteal artery
3. Heavily calcified stenosis up to 3 cm in length
4. Multiple lesions, each <3 cm in length (stenoses or occlusions)
5. Single or multiple lesions to improve inflow for distal bypass

Lesion type C: Surgical treatment used more often but insufficient scientific evidence

6. Single stenosis or occlusion >5 cm in length
7. Multiple stenoses or occlusions, each 3–5 cm in length, ± heavy calcification

Lesion type D: Surgery is treatment of choice

8. Complete CFA, SFA, or POP (including proximal trifurcation) occlusions.

[a] These recommendations are likely to change in favor of catheter-based interventions as stent-grafts, drug-eluting stents, and pharmacologic adjuncts become scientifically evaluated.

SFA, superficial femoral artery; CFA, common femoral artery; POP, popliteal artery.

is frequently not possible owing to patient obesity, or undesirable when the lesion is high in the SFA. A 30- to 45-cm flexible sheath placed over the aortic bifurcation from the contralateral CFA provides a stable platform for most interventions. However, exchange length guidewires and balloons with long shafts will be necessary. Typical balloon diameters for the SFA are 5–7 mm, and 4–6 mm for the popliteal artery. Standard 0.035-inch guidewires and balloons on 5-French shafts can be used. The tight 1.5-mm "J" on the tip of the 0.035-inch Rosen guidewire prevents inadvertent selection of a tibial artery during the procedure, but can create intimal trauma if excessive motion occurs. Self-expanding bare metal stents or stent-grafts are used when angioplasty yields a suboptimal result (Fig. 15-22). Balloon-expandable stents should not be used in the SFA or popliteal artery, as they are subject to compression by external forces. Stent-grafts may allow percutaneous treatment of long-segment disease or occlusions, but placement across

points of flexion should be avoided with first-generation devices (Fig. 15-23). Intravascular brachytherapy and drug-eluting stents may significantly improve long-term patency of SFA interventions.

Careful monitoring of guidewire tip position during SFA interventions will reduce the risk of spasm in distal vessels. Intraprocedural heparin (3000–5000 U), nitroglycerin, and antiplatelet drugs should be used. An overnight course of anticoagulation or antiplatelet therapy is used by many interventionalists, particularly when long-segment disease is treated or runoff is poor. As a minimum, patients should be discharged on aspirin 80–360 mg/day for life unless contraindicated. In addition, an oral platelet inhibitor such a clopidogrel 75 mg q.d. for 2–6 months may be beneficial.

The most common complications of SFA and popliteal interventions are intraprocedural thrombosis, occlusive dissection, and distal embolization. The overall rate of complications is less than 5% in most centers, but increases with the extent of preexisting disease, complexity of the procedure, and duration. Intraprocedural thrombosis or embolization can be managed with thrombolysis or suction thrombectomy. Dissections are effectively treated with stent placement. Anticoagulation, gentle catheter and guidewire manipulation, and careful attention to guidewire and device positions will minimize injury to the SFA or distal vessels.

The technical success rate for percutaneous SFA and popliteal interventions is greater than 95% for stenoses and 85–90% for occlusions. The lower rate in occlusions is due to occasional failures to cross the lesion. Pressure gradients as a definition of technical success are usually not employed in SFA and popliteal artery angioplasty. The degree of residual stenosis (<30%), qualitative assessment of flow, return of palpable distal pulses, or an ABI measured on the procedure table are used to determine the procedural endpoints.

The reported long-term patencies of SFA and popliteal angioplasty are not equal to those of surgical bypass, but few true comparative studies have been performed (Table 15-7). Furthermore, the best measure of outcome may be functional rather than lesion patency. The data

Table 15-7 Results of Superficial Femoral and Popliteal Artery Angioplasty and Stents

Procedure	Indication	Primary Patency at 3 Years (%)
Angioplasty (stenosis)	Claudication	62
Angioplasty (stenosis)	Limb salvage	43
Angioplasty (occlusion)	All	40
Stent placement, SFA	All	65

on stents and stent-grafts is even more limited. However, as devices and techniques improve, percutaneous intervention is likely to become the preferred treatment option for many patients.

Tibial Artery Angioplasty and Stents

Angioplasty of the tibial arteries is performed less often than in the SFA or popliteal artery. The indications are usually limb salvage in the setting of critical ischemia with impending or ongoing tissue loss, or preservation of runoff distal to a bypass graft. Tibial artery occlusive disease is rarely isolated, but frequently occurs in conjunction with SFA and popliteal artery disease. Almost three-quarters of patients undergoing tibial artery angioplasty are diabetics.

The optimal approach to tibial artery angioplasty is antegrade from the ipsilateral CFA. When this is not possible, use of a long flexible sheath placed over the aortic bifurcation from the contralateral CFA is necessary to provide stability and allow contrast injections. When working over the bifurcation all guidewires must be exchange length (260 cm or longer) and balloons mounted on 100- to 120-cm shafts. Typical balloon diameters for tibial arteries are 2–4 mm (Fig. 15-24). These small vessel balloons are mounted on sub-4-French shafts, and typically require 0.018-inch or smaller guidewires. Lesions at the origins of the tibial arteries can be angioplastied safely using "kissing balloons" or a safety wire (Fig. 15-25). Stents are rarely used in this vascular bed, but when required can be balloon-expandable or self-expanding coronary stents.

Intraprocedural thrombosis is of greater concern with tibial artery intervention than SFA or popliteal artery. Patients should be well anticoagulated with heparin (ACT >250) during the procedure, and antiplatelet drugs

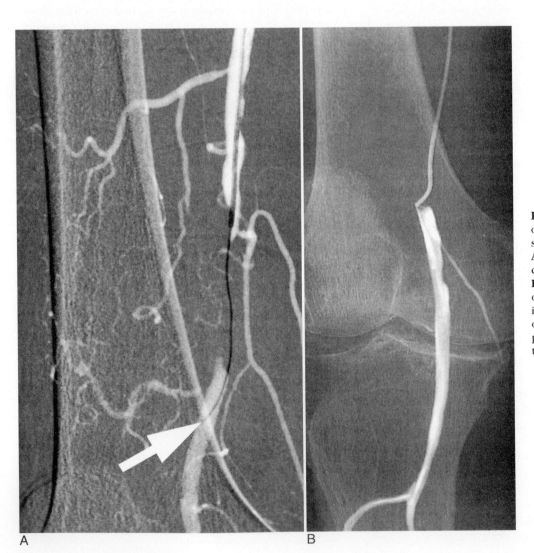

A   B

Figure 15-22 Recanalization of a short SFA occlusion with a stent (same patient as Fig. 1-6). **A**, DSA after lesion has been crossed with a guidewire (arrow). **B**, A 5-Fr catheter was advanced over the wire through the lesion into the popliteal artery. Injection of contrast confirms intraluminal position of the catheter distal to the occlusion.   *(Continued)*

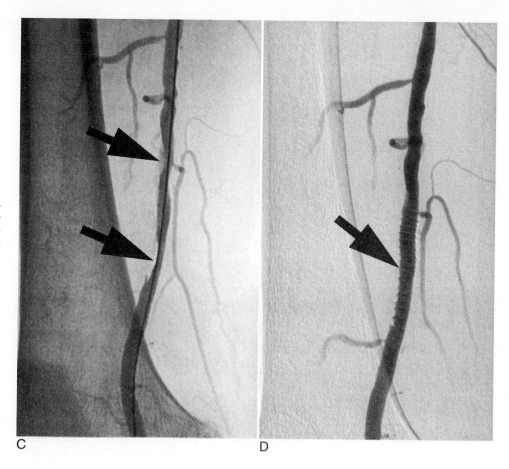

Figure 15-22   cont'd C, DSA following angioplasty showing residual stenoses (arrows). **D**, DSA following placement of a bare metal stent (arrow).

C   D

should be considered. Liberal use of intraarterial nitroglycerin is important to prevent spasm in these small vessels. Distal embolization occurs in fewer than 2% of patients.

The published literature on tibial artery angioplasty is scant in comparison to more proximal lesions. The technical success approaches 95%, particularly for focal, limited disease in native vessels that have in-line runoff to the foot. Occlusions, stenoses of bypass graft anastomoses, and lesions in vessels with poor runoff have a lower technical success. Limb salvage is a more accurate measure of outcome than lesion patency, as most tibial angioplasties are performed for this indication (Table 15-8).

ACUTE LIMB ISCHEMIA

The acute, profoundly ischemic limb is a surgical emergency. Cell death begins after 4 hours of total ischemia, and is irreversible after 6 hours. Urgent revascularization is therefore necessary, or limb loss will result. The clinical presentation can be summarized as the "five Ps" (Box 15-6). These symptoms reflect the greater sensitivity of nerves and muscle to ischemia than

skin and subcutaneous tissues. The mortality of patients with acute limb ischemia is almost 25% despite aggressive intervention, with amputation in 20% of those that survive.

There are numerous causes of acute limb ischemia (Box 15-7). A major diagnostic goal is the distinction between primarily embolic versus thrombotic occlusion (Table 15-9). Embolic occlusions tend to result in profound ischemia owing to the absence of developed collaterals (see Fig. 1-32). Thrombosis of a preexisting stenosis is generally tolerated better as the collateral circulation is already established.

Table 15-8   Results of Tibial Artery Angioplasty

Parameter	Result (%)
Technical success	95
Limb salvage at 1 year	80
Limb salvage at 2 years	75
Limb salvage at 3 years	65
Limb salvage at 2 years, no continuous runoff to foot	50

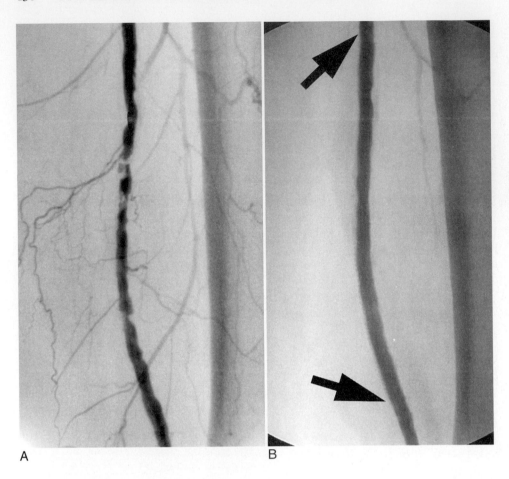

A   B

Figure 15-23   Long-segment SFA stenoses treated with ePTFE-covered stent graft. **A**, DSA showing multiple stenoses in the distal SFA. Note the small muscular branches arising from the SFA. **B**, DSA following angioplasty and placement of a stent-graft (W.L. Gore, Flagstaff, AZ). The multiple small branches seen in the previous image are no longer present (arrows).

A classification system has been devised for describing the degree of acute limb ischemia (Table 15-10). This classification is different from the one for patients with chronic ischemia, as the clinical presentation and outcomes are different. For example, tissue loss and gangrene are late findings of ischemia, but paralysis and sensory loss indicate acute hypoxia of nerves and muscle.

Patients presenting with acute limb ischemia should be heparinized immediately. This prevents propagation of thrombus and has a beneficial mild vasodilatory effect.

The history of onset of symptoms frequently suggests the etiology of the occlusion. Examination of all of the peripheral pulses is important to gauge the presence of peripheral vascular disease or multiple emboli. The electrocardiogram may provide an important clue regarding

---

Box 15-6   The Five "P"s of Acute Limb Ischemia

Pulseless
Pain
Pallor
Paresthesia
Paralysis

Box 15-7   Etiologies of Acute Limb Ischemia

Embolic
Trauma
Thrombosis of atherosclerotic stenosis
Thrombosis of surgical bypass graft
Thrombosis of degenerative popliteal aneurysm
Popliteal artery entrapment or cyst with thrombosis
Iatrogenic
Dissection
Vasospasm
Venous thrombosis (phlegmasia cerulea dolens)
Low-output cardiac state

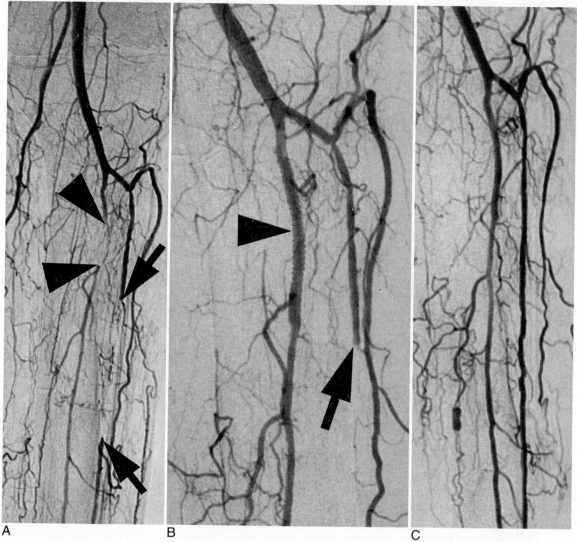

A   B   C

Figure 15-24   Tibial artery reconstruction in a patient with critical foot ischemia. **A**, DSA showing short occlusion of the proximal peroneal artery (arrowheads) and longer occlusion of the anterior tibial artery (arrows). The posterior tibial artery is occluded. **B**, DSA after recanalization of the peroneal artery occlusion with 2.75-mm diameter coronary stents (arrowhead). The anterior tibial artery occlusion (arrow) was then crossed with a guidewire. **C**, DSA after balloon angioplasty of the anterior tibial artery occlusion.

Table 15-9   Differentiating Features of Acute Arterial Occlusion

	Embolic	Thrombotic
Identifiable source of emboli	Frequent	Rare
Preexisting claudication	Rare	Frequent
Physical examination	Normal proximal and contralateral pulses	Evidence of peripheral vascular disease in ipsilateral and contralateral limb
Degree of ischemia	Frequently profound	Frequently threatened but viable
Imaging findings	Normal vessels with abrupt occlusion (sometimes multiple), frequently at major bifurcation of vessel, no collaterals, menicus sign	Diffuse atherosclerotic disease, well developed collaterals, usually mid-vessel occlusion

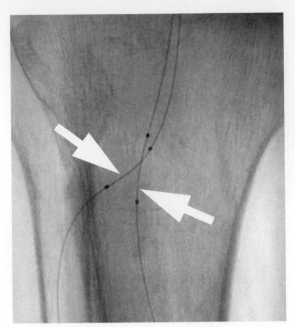

Figure 15-25 Spot film showing positioning of angioplasty balloons (arrows) for kissing balloon angioplasty of anterior tibial and tibio-peroneal artery origin stenoses.

the etiology of the occlusion (looking specifically for atrial arrhythmias or prior myocardial infarction).

The decision to obtain an imaging test is based upon the clinical status of the limb and the probable etiology of the occlusion. Patients with critically ischemic limbs due to a presumed embolus or graft thrombosis should proceed directly to surgical exploration, as the delay required to obtain imaging may jeopardize the ability to salvage the extremity. Intraoperative angiography can be performed in patients with profound ischemia when visualization of distal runoff is necessary. Patients with less threatened limbs, and extensive underlying vascular disease or a complex vascular surgical history, benefit from preoperative imaging.

Imaging with MRA and CTA can provide diagnostic information in cooperative patients. The reason that these modalities are not considered first in many patients is that current therapeutic vascular procedures are not routinely feasible with CT or MR guidance. Conventional diagnostic angiographic studies have the option of becoming therapeutic interventions such as thrombolysis or aspiration thrombectomy.

The angiographic evaluation of a patient with acute limb ischemia should be tailored to the clinical situation. Standard catheters, guidewires, and injection rates can be used. Percutaneous access should be planned to support a possible intervention. In patients with suspected embolic disease, an aortogram may reveal silent emboli to renal or visceral branches, or pathology such as an aneurysm or large ulcerated plaque. As a minimum, imaging should include from the aortic bifurcation to below the level of the occlusion. Oblique views of the pelvis may demonstrate emboli in the hypogastric arteries, thus confirming the nature of the occlusion. A dedicated, but reasonable effort should be made to image the reconstituted vessels distal to the occlusion in order to facilitate planning of interventions. However, in patients with poor collaterals this may be difficult or impossible.

Surgical intervention remains the first consideration in the therapy of acute critical limb ischemia. Thrombectomy with Fogarty balloon catheters through limited CFA or popliteal artery incisions is an effective method to relieve acute obstruction. This can be accomplished with local anesthesia. Balloon catheters can also be passed in a retrograde manner into the pelvic inflow arteries. When embolectomy is unsuccessful in restoring sufficient flow for limb viability, bypass surgery can be performed. Fasciotomy may be necessary in patients who develop compartment syndrome (especially anterior calf) following surgery. Surgical interventions result in limb salvage in 75-90% of patients, and a 30-day mortality of 10-15%. However, embolectomy is frequently incomplete,

Table 15-10 Clinical Categories of Acute Limb Ischemia						
			Physical Examination		**Doppler Signals**	
Category	Definition	Prognosis	Sensory Loss	Muscle Weakness	Arterial	Venous
I	Viable	Not immediately threatened	None	None	+	+
II	Threatened					
	a. Marginally	Salvageable with prompt treatment	Minimal (toes)	None	Occasional +, frequently –	+
	b. Immediately	Salvageable with immediate treatment	More than toes, rest pain	Mild to moderate	Rare +, usually –	+
III	Irreversible	Major permanent tissue loss	Anesthetic	Paralysis	–	–

particularly in the tibial and pedal arteries, and may result in intimal injury.

Percutaneous interventions in appropriate patients are indicated when emergent revascularization is not required to salvage a viable extremity. The objectives of thrombolysis are to rapidly restore flow and identify underlying lesions that can be corrected percutaneously or with surgery. Pharmacologic thrombolysis, mechanical thrombolysis, and aspiration thrombectomy are useful techniques in both embolic and thrombotic occlusions (see Fig. 4-21). Occlusions less than 14 days old are amenable to pharmacologic and mechanical thrombolysis. Mechanical thrombectomy devices are very useful for rapid restoration of flow, but certain devices may result in trauma to normal endothelium when used in native vessels or vein grafts. Pharmacologic thrombolysis and/or anticoagulation are frequently necessary for optimal results. Aspiration thrombectomy should be considered for acute (<48 hours) occlusions (see Fig. 4-26).

Thrombolysis and mechanical thrombectomy successfully restore antegrade flow in over 95% of patients provided that the occlusion can be crossed with an infusion catheter or thrombectomy device. Causes of failure include severe coexistent inflow or outflow disease, organized thrombus, or large atheromatous emboli. Long-term limb preservation with thrombolysis and surgery is identical to surgical therapy alone, but mortality may be lower owing to fewer cardiovascular complications.

BLUE TOE SYNDROME

Spontaneous rupture of atheromatous plaque can result in distal embolization of cholesterol crystals, atheromatous debris, thrombus, and platelet aggregates (Table 15-11). The estimated incidence is 0.03% in hospitalized patients. Emboli are believed to be large in approximately 40% of patients, and may present as acute limb ischemia (see previous section). In 60% of patients the emboli are small or even microscopic, measuring 200 μm or less in diameter. Lower-extremity microembolization

presents with sudden onset of painful, localized red-purple discolorations of one or more toes (thus the name "blue toe syndrome") (see Fig. 1-33). The region of discoloration may contain interlaced areas of discoloration and normal skin, known as livedo reticularis. Patients with microembolization frequently have intact pedal pulses, although combined micro- and macro-embolization occurs in 16% of patients overall. Embolization may be spontaneous, or following endovascular procedures or surgical manipulation. Extensive, friable aortic plaque is a known (but unquantified) risk factor.

The distribution of emboli may suggest the location of the source. Unilateral extremity symptoms usually indicates an in-line source (common iliac artery or distal), especially when recurrent. Bilateral limb involvement is suggestive of an aortic source. When renal failure occurs synchronously with the lower-extremity symptoms, a thoracic aortic source with concurrent cholesterol embolization of the kidneys should be suspected.

The imaging of patients with atheroembolism is directed at identification of a source. When the thoracic aorta is suspected, transesophageal echocardiography (TEE), CTA, and MRA are sensitive noninvasive modalities. Diffuse or localized plaque, ulcerations, or aneurysms are suspicious lesions in this setting, but it is often difficult to be conclusive. When an abdominal aortic source is suspected, CTA and MRA can be used in search of similar pathology. Unfortunately, a "smoking gun" lesion may never be identified with certainty.

Angiography is obtained when noninvasive studies are inconclusive, or a pulse deficit is present. When the patient has unilateral embolization the catheter should be inserted from the contralateral CFA. An irregular or severe stenosis, ulcerated plaque, or aneurysm may be found (Fig. 15-26). Intraluminal filling defects will not be seen in patients with microembolism, as the occlusions are in vessels below the limits of resolution of the angiogram. Thus, a normal angiogram does not rule out atheroembolism.

Patients who do not receive definitive treatment will have recurrent embolization in up to 90% of cases within 5 years. A crucial component of the care of these patients is exclusion of the embolic source from the arterial circulation. Traditionally, surgical excision or bypass has been the standard therapy. Surgical treatment of aortic lesions is associated with a 4% overall 30-day mortality, and a 10% incidence of intraoperative embolization. Surgery for peripheral arterial sources carries much lower risk. Percutaneous exclusion of aortic lesions with stent-grafts, and treatment of iliofemoral artery lesions with angioplasty and stent placement have been utilized with success. Interestingly, these procedures have not generally been associated with an acute periprocedural atheroembolism. The long-term outcomes of percutaneous interventions for atheroembolism are not known.

Table 15-11	Sources of Atheroemboli
Source	**Percentage of All Atheroemboli**
Aortic or iliac stenosis	47
Aortic or iliac aneurysms	20
Upper-extremity stenosis and aneurysm	14
Lower-extremity stenosis	12
Degenerating synthetic graft	7

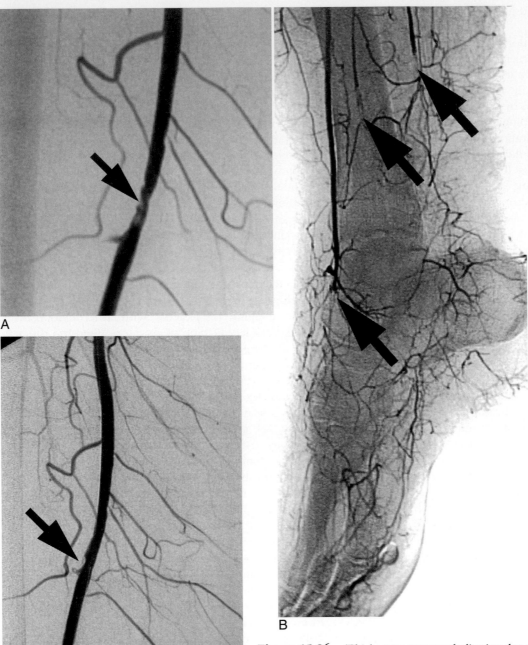

Figure 15-26 Tibial artery macroembolization due to an ulcerated SFA stenosis. **A,** Magnified view of SFA DSA showing a focal stenosis with an irregular surface (arrow). **B,** DSA of the ankle and foot showing embolic occlusions of all three tibial arteries (arrows). **C,** DSA of the SFA lesion following angioplasty shows marked improvement in the appearance of the lumen (arrow). Repeat distal angiography showed no new emboli related to the angioplasty. The patient was maintained on anticoagulation and antiplatelet therapy.

ANEURYSMS

Aneurysms of the lower-extremity arteries are less common than those of the abdominal aorta. There are numerous etiologies of peripheral aneurysms, but degenerative (true aneurysms) and iatrogenic (pseudoaneurysms) are the most common (Box 15-8). Degenerative popliteal artery aneurysms are slightly more common than CFA aneurysms, and occur in patients with demographics typical of degenerative aneurysms. Over 70% of patients with degenerative peripheral aneurysms have concurrent abdominal aortic aneurysms (AAA), although curiously only 3% of patients with AAA have peripheral aneurysms. Aneurysms in otherwise normal young patients or the SFA, PFA, and tibial arteries are rare, and should prompt evaluation for an unusual etiology such as Ehlers–Danlos syndrome (Fig. 15-27).

Popliteal Artery Aneurysm

Popliteal artery aneurysms are bilateral in 60–70%, with a male to female ratio of about 15:1, and association with concomitant CFA aneurysms in approximately 40%. Almost three-quarters of patients with bilateral popliteal artery aneurysms will also have abdominal aortic aneurysms (AAA). The etiology is degenerative in over 90%. Mural thrombus is common. Patients are usually asymptomatic, with a popliteal artery pulse on physical examination that feels generous. Distal pulses may be diminished or reduced. Rarely, a pulsatile mass will be appreciated. Both limbs should be examined for abnormal pulses. The entire popliteal artery may be aneurysmal, but focal aneurysms most often involve the vessel above the joint line.

The most feared complications of popliteal artery aneurysms are thrombosis (40%), distal embolization of mural thrombus (25%), and compression of adjacent veins (10%) (see Fig. 1-7). The typical presenting symptoms of popliteal aneurysms are related to distal ischemia rather than the aneurysm itself. Rupture is the least common complication of true popliteal artery aneurysms, reportedly occurring in approximately 2%.

Imaging of patients with suspected popliteal artery aneurysms should always include the abdominal aorta and both popliteal arteries. The calcified wall of the aneurysm may be visible on plain radiographs. US is an excellent initial diagnostic modality for patients with suspected popliteal artery aneurysms. The average diameter of the popliteal artery is 8 mm in patients with AAA. The presence of mural thrombus in a large popliteal

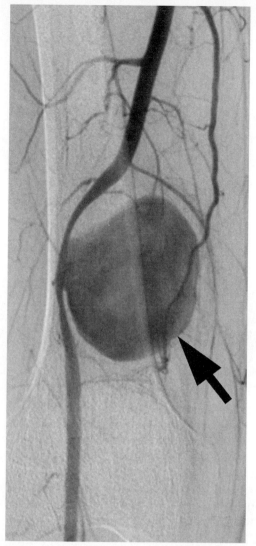

Figure 15-27   One of many peripheral pseudoaneurysms (arrow), in this case in the above-knee popliteal artery, that occurred over a period of 3 years in a middle-aged male with Ehlers–Danlos type IV. The patient eventually died from a ruptured iliac artery several years later.

artery is diagnostic of an aneurysm. A proportionally large popliteal artery in the setting of diffuse arteriomegaly does not constitute an aneurysm. The entire length of the popliteal artery and the contralateral popliteal artery should always be studied. MRA (gadolinium-enhanced) and CTA can detect the aneurysm as well as image the tibial runoff (Fig. 15-28). Angiography is useful for accurate delineation of the runoff prior to intervention, but can fail to detect aneurysms that are noncalcified and lined with mural thrombus.

Popliteal artery aneurysms require treatment before development of symptoms. Almost half of patients with asymptomatic aneurysms will develop distal ischemia within 5 years. Surgical excision and bypass is recommended for all symptomatic aneurysms and asymptomatic

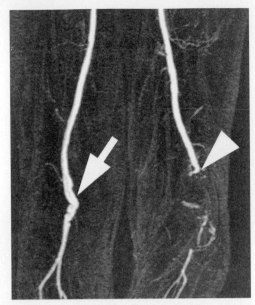

Figure 15-28   Coronal MIP of gadolinium-enhanced 3-D MRA of a patient with acute onset of left calf claudication. There is abrupt proximal occlusion of the left popliteal artery (arrowhead) with distal reconstitution. On the right there is a patent right popliteal artery aneurysm (arrow). An ultrasound confirmed a thrombosed popliteal artery aneurysm on the left that was bypassed surgically.

aneurysms that exceed 2 cm in diameter. Thrombolysis of an acutely thrombosed popliteal artery aneurysm can be beneficial for recovery of distal runoff. Stent-grafts may have a role in percutaneous treatment of popliteal artery aneurysms in selected patients, but kinking and device fracture due to joint motion are a concern with early generation devices.

Common Femoral Artery Aneurysm

True aneurysms of the CFA are usually degenerative in origin, whereas most pseudoaneurysms are related to angiographic procedures or surgical anastomoses. The clinical course of degenerative aneurysms is not well understood, but thrombosis in up to 15%, distal embolization in up to 10%, and rupture in 1–5% have been reported. Patients present with groin pain, a pulsatile mass, or compression of adjacent nerves or veins. Degenerative aneurysms are found most often in elderly males, and are bilateral in over 70%. The normal common femoral artery averages about 9 mm in diameter in adults. A diameter of 2 cm is therefore considered an aneurysm, and 2.5 cm an indication for intervention (Fig. 15-29). The imaging modality that is used most often to evaluate the CFA for aneurysms is US. In postoperative patients an important distinction is the difference between the generous hood of a graft and an aneurysm; diameter >2 cm and the presence of mural thrombus are helpful clues that an aneurysm is present. When a

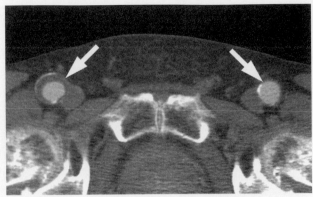

Figure 15-29   Contrast-enhanced CT showing bilateral degenerative CFA aneurysms (arrows) in a patient with an AAA. The aneurysm on the right is lined with mural thrombus.

degenerative or anastomotic aneurysm is found, MRA or CTA should be obtained to evaluate the aortic and pelvic vessels for additional aneurysms. Angiography may be required for complex lesions, or when distal embolization is suspected. When possible it is best to avoid access through a CFA aneurysm or pseudoaneurysm as compression can be difficult.

Postcatheterization false aneurysms occur in up to 5% of patients undergoing cardiac catheterization when arterial closure devices are not utilized. The incidence is less than 1% in most interventional radiology practices. Patients present with groin or retroperitoneal hematomas, groin pain, a pulsatile mass, and a new bruit within 24–48 hours of the procedure (see Fig. 3-7). Patients with large groin hematomas may harbor pseudoaneurysms despite the lack of a palpable pulsatile mass. The artery of origin may be the CFA, SFA, or PFA. Groin pseudoaneurysms (especially small) thrombose spontaneously in more than 90% of patients, but rupture can occur in up to 3%. Treatment with US-guided compression, or (preferably for both the patient and physician) US-guided thrombin injection, can effectively obliterate up to 90% of puncture-related pseudoaneurysms. Patients with Ehlers–Danlos syndrome and Behçet's disease are at particularly high risk of development of puncture-site pseudoaneurysms.

Anastomotic pseudoaneurysms occur in 3% of all femoral surgical anastomoses (see Fig. 3-19). The rate of complication (rupture, distal embolization, and thrombosis) is low when the diameter of the anastomotic aneurysm is less than 2 cm. Graft degeneration and infection are potential etiologies in this setting, so discovery of one anastomotic pseudoaneurysm should prompt evaluation of all anastomoses of the graft.

Persistent Sciatic Artery Aneurysm

The embryology of persistent sciatic arteries is described above in the Anatomy section of this chapter.

Aneurysmal degeneration complicates 40% of persistent sciatic arteries. These aneurysms occur distal to the sciatic notch, probably as a result of repetitive trauma to the superficially located anomalous vessel. Patients present with thrombosis, distal embolization, or a mass lesion in the buttock, but rupture is rare. The rate of limb loss is almost 18% in symptomatic patients.

The diagnosis of asymptomatic persistent sciatic artery is usually made during preintervention imaging in patients with claudication. On MRA and CTA the SFA is hypoplastic or absent, while the internal iliac artery is enlarged and continues into the posterior thigh through the greater sciatic foramen to the popliteal artery. Aneurysms can be large, calcified, and filled with thrombus, and have been confused with soft tissue neoplasms by the unwary (see Fig. 15-4). At angiography, a large posterior branch of the internal iliac artery is seen continuing into the thigh, often with a small external iliac artery and CFA.

The treatment of persistent sciatic artery aneurysms has classically been surgical excision or exclusion with restoration of in-line runoff to the popliteal artery. Stent-graft treatment of selected patients may be feasible, but device fracture due to external compression is a risk.

ARTERIOMEGALY

Arteriomegaly is a distinct condition of unknown etiology in which there is diffuse ectasia of the aorta, iliac, and femoropopliteal arteries (Fig. 15-30). As many as a third of patients will also have focal, discrete aneurysms superimposed on generalized ectasia, especially of the femoral and popliteal arteries. Most common in men, this condition has been reported in up to 5% of patients undergoing imaging for aortic aneurysms.

TRAUMA

The extremities are the site of injury in one-third of all civilian patients with vascular trauma. The predominant mechanisms are penetrating and blunt trauma. Penetrating trauma is more common in urban locations, whereas blunt injury is more prevalent in rural settings. The rate of limb loss with major injuries is less than 15%, but dysfunction due to associated bone and nerve injury occurs in about a quarter of the remaining patients.

Penetrating Trauma

Penetrating trauma from projectiles, stabbing devices, or bone fragments can cause a spectrum of vascular injuries (see Table 1-12). In civilian populations bullets are responsible for 64%, knives for 24%, and shotgun pellets in 12% of penetrating injuries.

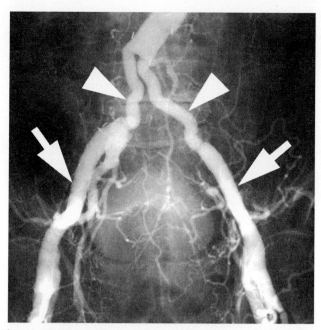

Figure 15-30   Pelvic angiogram of an elderly male with arteriomegaly. The patient was 5 feet 6 inches tall. The patient had previously undergone aorto-bi-iliac graft placement (arrowheads) for AAA. The diameter of the limbs of the surgical graft is 12 mm. The external iliac (arrows) and CFAs dwarf the large surgical graft. The patient also had diffusely large SFAs and bilateral popliteal artery aneurysms.

The initial evaluation and management of a patient with penetrating extremity trauma should focus initially on diagnosis and treatment of lethal truncal or head injuries. Once these issues have been addressed, the mechanism of injury to the extremity should be ascertained if possible. The wound should be examined for bleeding, expanding hematoma, or other "hard" signs of vascular injury (Box 15-9 and Fig. 15-31). A complete

---

Box 15-9   Signs of Vascular Injury

Hard

Active arterial hemorrhage
Thrill or bruit
Expanding hematoma
Extremity ischemia
Pulse deficit

Soft

Adjacent fracture
Adjacent nerve injury
Stable hematoma
Delayed or decreased capillary refill
History of hypotension or bleeding
Extensive soft tissue injury

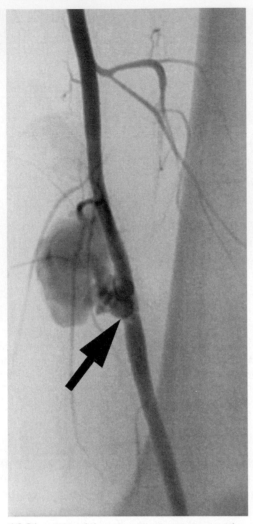

Figure 15-31   DSA of the extremity in a patient with a gunshot wound to the medial thigh and an expanding hematoma. Distal pulses were intact. There is a pseudoaneurysm (arrow) of the SFA at the adductor canal.

pulse examination with determination of an ABI is crucial. In patients with a normal ABI (>1.0) and a normal physical examination, the incidence of vascular injury is 9%, of which almost all are minor (such as small nonobstructing intimal flaps) or confined to branch vessels. The incidence increases to 20% in patients with soft signs of injury or an ABI less than 1.0 (assuming baseline normal arteries). Patients with a pulse deficit, neurologic deficit, or shotgun injury have a 40% incidence of vascular injury (Fig. 15-32).

Angiography was at one time performed emergently on every patient presenting with a penetrating injury in the vicinity (within 1 cm of the expected course) of a major runoff vessel. The overall positive rate for clinically important vascular injuries was less than 10%. Imaging of patients with penetrating extremity trauma is now reserved for those with clinical findings suggestive of injury.

With the exception of shot gun injuries, asymptomatic patients with normal pulses do not require imaging regardless of the proximity of the injury to a major runoff vessel. These patients are observed for 12-24 hours, and then released if the examination remains normal. Conversely, patients with a profoundly ischemic limb or active hemorrhage from the wound should proceed directly to surgery. Stable patients with viable limbs but a diminished ABI or clinical signs of vascular injury are suitable candidates for imaging.

The use of US has been investigated extensively as a diagnostic tool in this patient population. The sensitivity and specificity for major vascular injury are reported to each exceed 95%, provided that a skilled sonographer performs and interprets the study. When patients are undergoing CT for evaluation of head or truncal injury, continuation of the scan through the area of interest may identify an injury. However, angiography remains a very useful examination in these patients, and catheter-based therapy such as stent-graft placement or embolization may be feasible. Entry and exit wounds should be identified prior to the study to ensure that the entire region at risk is included in the imaging field. At least two views are necessary to exclude subtle intimal injuries. When a pulse deficit is present the entire runoff should be imaged.

The treatment of penetrating injuries varies with the type and extent of the injury. Small intimal flaps and arteriovenous fistulas frequently heal spontaneously. Injuries to branch vessels can be effectively managed with coil embolization. Open repair is the standard treatment for major injuries to the SFA or popliteal artery, although small stent-grafts may have a role in the SFA. Injury to a single tibial artery can be managed with coil occlusion or ligation if appropriate, but open reconstruction is recommended when more than one artery is traumatically occluded.

Knee Dislocation

Knee dislocations receive special consideration in terms of the potential for vascular injury. The massive force required to create this injury, coupled with the fixed position of the popliteal artery in relation to the knee joint, results in arterial injury to 30–40% of dislocations. Posterior dislocations have the highest risk of vascular injury. Popliteal artery occlusion is tolerated poorly in normal individuals owing to the sparse collateral supply to the lower leg. A delay more than 8 hours in diagnosis and therapy of an occlusive arterial injury results in an amputation rate of 86%.

The physical examination should focus on the integrity of the distal pulses and the presence of hard signs of vascular injury. Only 2% of patients with entirely normal vascular examinations before and after reduction of the knee will have a vascular injury. However, a low

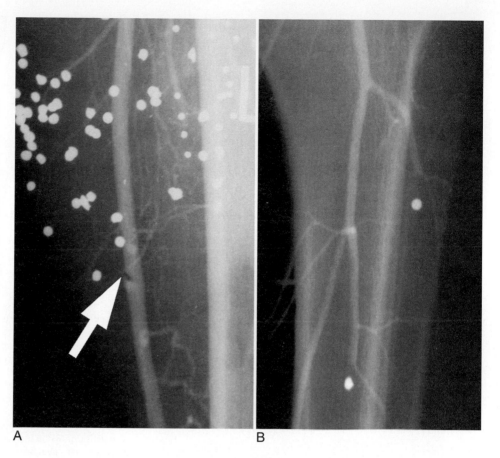

Figure 15-32 Patient with diminished dorsalis pedis pulse following shotgun injuries to the thigh. **A**, Magnified view of SFA angiogram showing an intimal flap (arrow) in the proximal SFA. There are numerous lead pellets in the surrounding soft tissues. **B**, Magnified view of the proximal tibial arteries showing intraluminal pellets occluding the anterior tibial and peroneal arteries. The lead pellets entered the SFA through the proximal injury and became emboli.

A

B

threshold for imaging should be maintained when the physical examination is not absolutely satisfactory. Patients with an ischemic limb should proceed directly to surgery.

Angiography remains the imaging modality most often utilized in these patients. Multiple views, including a lateral or steep oblique, should be obtained. Typical findings include small intimal tears, spasm, and thrombosis (Fig. 15-33). Small and nonocclusive lesions are managed conservatively.

VASCULITIS

The most prevalent large vessel inflammatory-type disease of the lower extremities is Buerger's disease. The lower extremities are affected by Buerger's disease more often than the upper extremities. More than 60% of patients will present with intermittent claudication, and 46% will have ischemic ulcers. Buerger's disease should be suspected in any patient presenting with symptoms of peripheral vascular disease before the age of 45. There is a strong association with tobacco abuse and male gender. The pathology of Buerger's disease is discussed in Chapter 1.

Patients with Buerger's disease frequently have severe symptoms of peripheral vascular disease; rest pain is a presenting complaint in 80%. Noninvasive testing usually indicates obstruction at the infrapopliteal level. There are no characteristic findings at MRA or CTA that distinguish Buerger's disease from conventional atherosclerosis other than the distribution of the disease. The conventional angiographic findings are striking (Box 15-10; see also Fig. 1-16). Cessation of smoking is crucial to arrest progression of disease, and intense wound care is required to heal ulcers. Amputation is depressingly common, as reconstructive surgical or endovascular therapies are usually not feasible owing to the lack of distal runoff vessels.

Box 15-10 Angiographic Findings in Buerger's Disease

Extensive involvement of medium and small arteries
Segmental disease and occlusion with intervening normal segments
Sparing of CFA, SFA, and popliteal arteries
"Corkscrew" collaterals in vasa vasorum

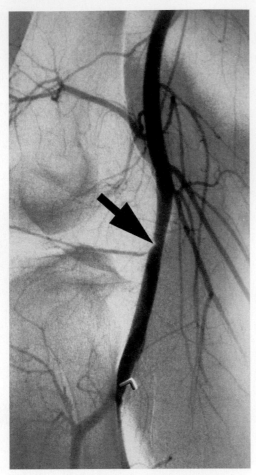

Figure 15-33   Subtracted image from an angiogram of the popliteal artery in an athlete with transient diminished distal pulses after a knee dislocation. This small intimal flap (arrow) arising at the joint line was managed with 6 months of anticoagulation.

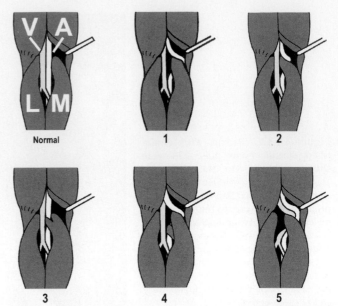

Figure 15-34   Schematic of popliteal artery entrapment (see Table 15-12). V = Popliteal vein. A = Popliteal artery. L = Lateral head of gastrocnemius muscle. M = Medial head of gastrocnemius muscle. **1**, Type I: Medial deviation of popliteal artery around normal gastrocnemius muscle. **2**, Type II: Aberrant lateral insertion of the medial head of the gastrocnemius. **3**, Type III: Aberrant lateral slips of medial gastrocnemius muscle. **4**, Type IV: Entrapment by popliteus muscle or fibrous band. Artery shown medial to medial head of gastrocnemius muscle in this case. **5**, Type V: Entrapment of both popliteal artery and vein. (Adapted with permission from Andrews, RT: Diagnostic angiography of the pelvis and lower extremities. *Semin Interv Radiol* 17:71–111, 2000.)

Other large vessel vasculitides are rare in the lower extremities, but include Behçet's disease, AIDS-related vasculitis, and systemic lupus erythematosus.

POPLITEAL ARTERY ENTRAPMENT

Two forms of popliteal artery entrapment have been described: functional and anatomic. The normal anatomic relationships of the popliteal artery as it exits the popliteal fossa is to pass between the heads of the gastrocnemius muscle and posterior to the popliteus muscle (Fig. 15-34). Patients with functional entrapment syndrome have normal anatomy but hypertrophy of the plantaris and other calf muscles which compress the neurovascular structures in the lower popliteal canal during exercise. The arteries remain normal in these patients despite repetitive compression. In patients with anatomic entrapment, the popliteal artery has a different relationship to these muscles, which results in muscular compression of the artery with exercise (Table 15-12). This leads first to adventitial thickening and fibrosis, followed by aneurysm formation, thrombosis, and distal embolization.

Popliteal artery entrapment syndrome presents as calf and foot claudication during activity. The incidence is thought to be less than 0.2%, and is bilateral in 25% of affected patients. Functional entrapment presents in women twice as often as men at a mean age of 24, with less severe claudication than in patients with anatomic abnormalities. Patients are usually highly trained athletes, particularly runners. The resting ABIs are almost always normal in this group. Anatomic popliteal artery entrapment tends to occur in males (70%), at a mean age of 43 (but as early as the second decade), with severe claudication. The resting ABI is abnormal in 30%, indicative of fixed occlusive disease.

Imaging with MRI and MRA may reveal an abnormal artery as well as an aberrant relationship to the muscles in the popliteal fossa in patients with anatomic entrapment (Table 15-13). The tibial vessels should be included in the examination on the affected side. The contralateral popliteal artery should always be imaged to detect

Table 15-12 Types of Anatomic Entrapment Syndrome

Type	Characteristics
I	Medial deviation of popliteal artery around normal medial insertion of gastrocnemius muscle
II	Aberrant lateral insertion of the medial head of the gastrocnemius muscle causes medial deviation of popliteal artery
III	Aberrant lateral slips of medial gastrocnemius muscle entrap normally situated popliteal artery
IV	Popliteus muscle or fibrous band entraps popliteal artery; the artery may also pass medial to medial head of gastrocnemius muscle in some cases
V	Entrapment of both popliteal artery and vein by medial head of the gastrocnemius muscle

asymptomatic entrapment. Conventional angiography is highly sensitive for entrapment, but does not provide information about specific muscular abnormality. When the popliteal artery is normal on initial images, bilateral stress views with the foot in dorsiflexion (such that the gastronemius is contract against resistance) are mandatory in any young patient studied for claudication (Fig. 15-35). Thrombolysis prior to surgery may recover tibial arteries occluded by emboli.

ADVENTITIAL CYSTIC DISEASE

Adventitial cystic disease is a rare disorder of the adventitia in which a focal accumulation of mucinous fluid compresses the arterial lumen. This entity should be considered in the differential diagnosis of patients presenting with unexplained popliteal artery occlusion, as 82% of cases have been reported in the popliteal

Table 15-13 Imaging Findings of Popliteal Artery Entrapment

Finding	Anatomic	Functional
Popliteal aneurysm (poststenotic)	+	−
Segmental occlusions (popliteal and/or tibial artery)	+	−
Medial deviation of the popliteal artery	+	−
Muscular anomalies in popliteal fossa	+	−
Compression of popliteal artery with stress maneuvers (active plantar flexion, dorsiflexion)	+	+
Hypertrophied normal muscles with normal popliteal artery	−	+

artery (Box 15-11). Patients are typically males in their fourth or fifth decade who present with claudication. The imaging findings are characteristic, with extrinsic compression of the mid-portion of the popliteal arterial lumen by a cystic mass (see Fig. 1-40). US, CTA, and MRI with MRA sequences are elegant techniques for imaging the cystic mass and the arterial compression. Surgical excision and bypass is the preferred treatment, as cyst aspiration always results in recurrence.

ERGOTISM

Ergot alkaloids are used for treatment of migraine headaches (ergotamine tartrate), for prophylaxis of deep vein thrombosis (dihydroergotamine), and for illicit recreation (lysergic acid diethylamide). An α-adrenergic blocking agent, ergotamine stimulates smooth muscle contraction. Excessive use of ergot alkaloids results in ergotism, with gastrointestinal, neurologic, and vascular symptoms. Patients tend to be younger than would be typical for atherosclerotic disease, with demographics that closely resemble those of the population with migraine headaches. Diffuse vasospasm, more commonly of the lower-extremity than upper-extremity arteries, results in symptoms of peripheral vascular disease. The aorta, carotid arteries, mesenteric vasculature, and retinal arteries may be affected as well. Untreated, patients may develop tissue loss and even gangrene.

At conventional angiography the stenoses are long, smooth, and in unusual locations. The typical findings of atherosclerosis are usually absent. Remarkably, cessation of the ergot use may result in complete reversal of the occlusive lesions (see Fig. 1-31).

RECONSTRUCTIVE SURGERY

Patients with nonhealing lesions of the extremity related to trauma or infection frequently undergo reconstructive surgical procedures that require tissue transfers. In addition, the proximal fibula is utilized in

Box 15-11 Etiologies of Popliteal Artery Occlusion

Atherosclerosis
Embolus
Thrombosis of degenerative aneurysm
Trauma
Popliteal artery entrapment
Adventitial cystic disease

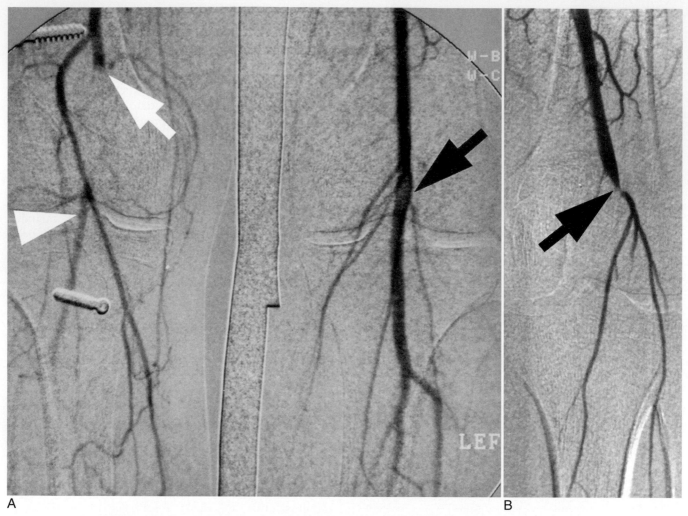

A   B

Figure 15-35   Popliteal artery entrapment in a young male athlete with bilateral exercise-induced claudication, suddenly much worse on the right. **A**, Angiogram showing acute occlusion of the above-knee right popliteal artery (white arrow) with reconstitution (white arrowhead) at the joint line via a middle genicular artery. The left popliteal artery has a subtle lateral deviation (black arrow). **B**, Angiogram of the left popliteal artery with plantar flexion against resistance shows occlusion (arrow). At surgery, type II entrapment was found bilaterally with a thrombosed poststenotic aneurysm on the right.

some patients as a vascularized bone graft. Preoperative vascular imaging is obtained in these patients to detect anatomic variants, exclude inflow occlusive lesions, and delineate donor or recipient vessels. This is particularly important in elderly patients in whom the inflow and tibial arteries may be abnormal.

The exact surgical plan should be understood in order to provide appropriate images. When the leg is the donor site, images of the recipient site may be required as well. MRA is used in many centers for this purpose, but conventional angiography remains important for this indication. Biplane views of the areas of interest are useful to fully delineate vascular anatomy.

ARTERIOVENOUS MALFORMATIONS

The lower extremities are the most common location for congenital arteriovenous malformations (see Chapter 1). Arteriovenous malformations may be located in and involve any structure in the lower extremity, including skin, muscle, bone, and joints (see Fig 1-22). In the pelvis, the bladder, reproductive organs, and bowel may be involved. Lesions that cause pain, deformity, bleeding, and high-output cardiac failure can sometimes be managed with transcatheter embolization techniques. Hemangiomas may require direct puncture for effective treatment.

Cross-sectional imaging with MRI is useful to determine the extent of the lesion. Embolization of the nidus is essential for effective treatment, but sometimes these are multiple and inaccessible. Common embolization agents include glue, other polymers, and alcohol (see Fig 4-37). Small particles should be avoided whenever large shunts are suspected. Coils have a high failure rate due to distal reconstitution around proximal occlusions. Pain control, anti-inflammatory medications including steroids, and frequent neurologic examinations are important immediately after the procedure. Compartment syndrome, nerve dysfunction, skin and muscle necrosis, and pelvic organ dysfunction can occur with embolization. Patients should be carefully counseled that embolization controls, but does not cure, the lesion, and that multiple procedures may be necessary over their lifetime.

SUGGESTED READINGS

Abou-Sayed H, Berger DL: Blunt lower-extremity trauma and popliteal artery injuries: revisiting the case for selective arteriography. *Arch Surg* 137:585–589, 2002.

Andrews RT: Diagnostic angiography of the pelvis and lower extremities. *Semin Interv Radiol* 17:71–111, 2000.

Brountzos EN, Malagari K, Gougoulakis A et al: Common femoral artery anastomotic pseudoaneurysm: endovascular treatment with hemobahn stent-grafts. *J Vasc Interv Radiol* 11:1179–1183, 2000.

Diwan A, Sarkar R, Stanley JC, Zelenock GB, Wakefield TW: Incidence of femoral and popliteal artery aneurysms in patients with abdominal aortic aneurysms. *J Vasc Surg* 31:863–869, 2000.

Dorros G, Jaff MR, Dorros AM, Mathiak LM, He T: Tibioperoneal (outflow lesion) angioplasty can be used as primary treatment in 235 patients with critical limb ischemia: five-year follow-up. *Circulation* 104:2057–2062, 2001.

Drescher P, Crain MR, Rilling WS: Initial experience with the combination of reteplase and abciximab for thrombolytic therapy in peripheral arterial occlusive disease: a pilot study. *J Vasc Interv Radiol* 13:37–43, 2002.

Duda SH, Tepe G, Luz O et al: Peripheral artery occlusion: treatment with abciximab plus urokinase versus with urokinase alone: a randomized pilot trial (the PROMPT Study). *Radiology* 221:689–696, 2001.

Hafez HM, Woolgar J, Robbs JV: Lower-extremity arterial injury: results of 550 cases and review of risk factors associated with limb loss. *J Vasc Surg* 33:1212–1219, 2001.

Hiatt WR: Medical treatment of peripheral arterial disease and claudication. *N Engl J Med* 344:1608–1621, 2001.

Hiatt WR: Pharmacologic therapy for peripheral arterial disease and claudication. *J Vasc Surg* 36:1283–1291, 2002.

Hollier LH, Stanson AW, Gloviczki P et al: Arteriomegaly: classification and morbid implications of diffuse aneurysmal disease. *Surgery* 93:700–708, 1983.

Ikezawa T, Naiki K, Moriura S, Ikeda S, Hirai M: Aneurysm of bilateral persistent sciatic arteries with ischemic complications: case report and review of the world literature. *J Vasc Surg* 20:96–103, 1994.

Jahnke T, Andresen R, Muller-Hulsbeck S et al: Hemobahn stent-grafts for treatment of femoropopliteal arterial obstructions: midterm results of a prospective trial. *J Vasc Interv Radiol* 14:41–51, 2003.

Kandarpa K, Becker GJ, Hunink MG et al: Transcatheter interventions for the treatment of peripheral atherosclerotic lesions: I. *J Vasc Interv Radiol* 12:683–95, 2001.

Kasirajan K, Gray B, Beavers FP et al: Rheolytic thrombectomy in the management of acute and subacute limb-threatening ischemia. *J Vasc Interv Radiol* 12:413–421, 2001.

Levy JM, Duszak RL, Akins EW et al: Thrombolysis for lower-extremity arterial and graft occlusions. American College of Radiology Appropriateness Criteria. *Radiology* 215:S1041–1054, 2000.

Lofberg AM, Karacagil S, Ljungman C et al: Percutaneous transluminal angioplasty of the femoropopliteal arteries in limbs with chronic critical lower limb ischemia. *J Vasc Surg* 34:114–121, 2001.

Mahmood A, Salaman R, Sintler M et al: Surgery of popliteal artery aneurysms: a 12-year experience. *J Vasc Surg* 37:586–593, 2003.

Matchett WJ, McFarland DR, Eidt JF, Moursi MM: Blue toe syndrome: treatment with intra-arterial stents and review of therapies. *J Vasc Interv Radiol* 11:585–592, 2000.

Nehler MR, Mueller RJ, McLafferty RB et al: Outcome of catheter-directed thrombolysis for lower-extremity arterial bypass occlusion. *J Vasc Surg* 37:72–78, 2003.

Olin JW: Thromboangiitis obliterans. *Curr Opin Rheumatol* 6:44–49, 1994.

Oliva VL, Denbow N, Therasse E et al: Digital subtraction angiography of the abdominal aorta and lower extremities: carbon dioxide versus iodinated contrast material. *J Vasc Interv Radiol* 10:723–731, 1999.

Ouriel K: Peripheral arterial disease. *Lancet* 358:1257–1264, 2001.

Rholl K, Sterling K, Jones CS: Noninvasive vascular diagnosis in peripheral vascular disease. In Kaufman JA, Hartnell GA, Trerotola SO eds: *Noninvasive Vascular Imaging With Ultrasound, Computed Tomography, and Magnetic Resonance.* Society of Cardiovascular and Interventional Radiology, Fairfax, VA, 1997.

Rose SC: Noninvasive vascular laboratory for evaluation of peripheral arterial occlusive disease: I. Hemodynamic principles and tools of the trade. *J Vasc Interv Radiol* 11:1107–1114, 2000.

Rose SC: Noninvasive vascular laboratory for evaluation of peripheral arterial occlusive disease: II. Clinical applications: chronic, usually atherosclerotic, lower-extremity ischemia. *J Vasc Interv Radiol* 11:1257–1275, 2000.

Rose SC: Noninvasive vascular laboratory for evaluation of peripheral arterial occlusive disease. III. Clinical applications: non-atherosclerotic lower-extremity arterial conditions and upper-extremity arterial disease. *J Vasc Interv Radiol* 12:11–18, 2001.

Roth SM, Bandyk DF: Duplex imaging of lower-extremity bypasses, angioplasties, and stents. *Semin Vasc Surg* 12: 275–284, 1999.

Rubin GD, Schmidt AJ, Logan LJ, Sofilos MC: Multi-detector row CT angiography of lower-extremity arterial inflow and runoff: initial experience. *Radiology* 221:146–158, 2001.

Rutherford RB, Baker D, Ernst C et al: Recommended standards for reports dealing with lower-extremity ischemia. *J Vasc Surg* 26:517–538, 1997.

Saha S, Gibson M, Magee TR, Galland RB, Torrie EP: Early results of retrograde transpopliteal angioplasty of iliofemoral lesions. *Cardiovasc Interv Radiol* 24:378–382, 2001.

Saxon RR, Coffman JM, Gooding JM, Natuzzi E, Ponec DJ: Long-term results of ePTFE stent-graft versus angioplasty in the femoropopliteal artery: single center experience from a prospective, randomized trial. *J Vasc Interv Radiol* 14:303–311, 2003.

TransAtlantic Inter-Society Consensus (TASC): Management of peripheral arterial disease (PAD). *J Vasc Surg* 31:S1–296, 2000.

Turnipseed WD: Popliteal artery entrapment. *J Vasc Surg* 35:910–915, 2002.

Uflacker R: Arteries of the lower extremities. In Uflacker R: *Atlas of Vascular Anatomy: an Angiographic Approach*, Williams & Wilkins, Baltimore, 1997.

Visser K, Hunink MG: Peripheral arterial disease: gadolinium-enhanced MR angiography versus color-guided duplex US: a meta-analysis. *Radiology* 216:67–77, 2000.

Visser K, Kuntz KM, Donaldson MC, Gazelle GS, Hunink MG: Pretreatment imaging workup for patients with intermittent claudication: a cost-effectiveness analysis. *J Vasc Interv Radiol* 14:53–62, 2003.

de Vries SO, Visser K, de Vries JA et al: Intermittent claudication: cost-effectiveness of revascularization versus exercise therapy. *Radiology* 222:25–36, 2002.

Walsh DB, La Bombard E: Lower-extremity bypass using only duplex ultrasonography: is the time now? *Semin Vasc Surg* 12:247–251, 1999.

Lower-extremity Veins

JOHN A. KAUFMAN, M.D.

Venous pathology is eight times more common in the lower extremities than arterial disease. Conversely, the range of clinically important venous pathology in the lower extremities is relatively narrow, with thrombotic disorders and valvular insufficiency comprising more than 95%. There are an estimated 2,000,000 new cases of deep venous thrombosis (DVT) each year in the United States. Complications of venous thromboebolism are thought to be responsible for 15% of in-hospital deaths. Severe chronic venous stasis with ulceration is thought to affect 3–8% of the adult population, and cost the healthcare system over $1 billion each year. Venous diseases are one of the most important areas of diagnosis and intervention in current practice of interventional radiology.

ANATOMY

The pelvic veins consist of the external, internal, and common iliac veins. The external iliac vein begins at the inguinal ligament and ends at the merger with the internal iliac vein (Fig. 16-1). This vein is the direct continuation of the drainage of the lower-extremity blood, with small contributions from the anterior abdominal wall through the inferior epigastric veins, and from the

pelvis through circumflex iliac and pubic veins. The right external iliac vein is initially located medial to the external iliac artery, but crosses posterior to this vessel before it is joined by the internal iliac vein. The left external iliac vein remains medial to the artery throughout its length. The external iliac vein may have a single valve.

The external and iliac veins join at roughly the level of the sacroiliac joints to form the common iliac veins. This occurs deep in the pelvis, so that the common iliac veins are angled both anteriorly and cranial. The common iliac veins do not have valves. The right common iliac vein has a vertical course posterior to the right common iliac artery. The left common iliac vein is located medial to the left common iliac artery. In order to join the inferior vena cava on the right, the left common iliac vein passes underneath the right common iliac artery and anterior to the S1 or L5 vertebral body (see Fig. 13-12). This frequently results in broadening of the left common iliac vein, and sometimes functional compression. The confluence of the common iliac veins forms the inferior vena cava (IVC).

The venous structures of the lower extremities are divided into superficial and deep systems, linked by perforating veins (see Fig. 16-1). The perforating veins direct blood from the superficial into the deep system (Fig. 16-2). All veins of the lower extremity normally have valves. In contrast to the upper extremities, the deep veins of the lower extremity are the dominant drainage pathway.

The common femoral vein (CFV) is formed by the confluence of the femoral and deep femoral veins. This vein lies within the femoral sheath medial to the common femoral artery (Fig. 16-3; see also Fig. 2-27). The major tributaries of the CFV are the femoral vein (FV) and profunda femoris vein (PFV). The smaller tributaries include the greater saphenous vein, and the medial and lateral circumflex femoral veins.

The FV extends from the groin, where it is joined by the PFV, to the adductor canal. This vein is frequently

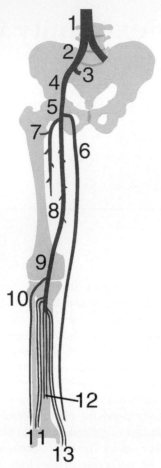

Figure 16-1   Drawing of lower-extremity veins. **1**, Inferior vena cava (IVC). **2**, Common iliac vein (CIV). **3**, Internal iliac vein (IIV). **4**, External iliac vein (EIV). **5**, Common femoral vein (CFV). **6**, Greater saphenous vein (GSV). **7**, Profunda femoris vein (PFV). **8**, Femoral vein (FV). **9**, Popliteal vein (PV). **10**, Lesser saphenous vein (LSV). **11**, Anterior tibial veins (ATV). **12**, Peroneal veins (PerV). **13**, Posterior tibial veins (PTV).

referred to as the "superficial femoral vein" or "SFV" because of its anatomic proximity to the superficial femoral artery. However, this nomenclature can cause confusion when trying to distinguish between deep and superficial veins in the extremity, so the term "femoral vein" will be used in this text. The FV lies slightly deep and lateral to the superficial femoral artery in the thigh (see Figs 16-3 and 15-3). This vein is duplicated or complex in up to 20% of patients (Fig. 16-4). The adductor canal in the thigh marks the transition of the FV to the popliteal vein. The PFV runs alongside the profunda femoris artery, draining the same muscles that are supplied by this artery. In approximately half of individuals the PFV communicates directly with the popliteal vein at the level of the adductor canal.

The popliteal vein is formed from the confluence of the tibial veins in the upper third of the calf. In relation

to the anterior surface of the leg, the popliteal vein lies posterior to the popliteal artery. In relation to the skin of the popliteal fossa (the posterior surface of the knee joint) it is more superficial (see Fig. 16-3). This vein is duplicated or complex in 35% of the population. In addition to the tibial veins, the gastrocnemius and lesser saphenous veins drain into the popliteal vein.

The deep veins of the calf are paired structures that parallel each of the three tibial arteries (see Figs 16-1 and 16-3). The posterior tibial and peroneal veins are larger than the anterior tibial veins owing to the larger muscle mass of the posterior and medial compartments. The posterior tibial vein is a continuation of the venous structures of the plantar surface of the foot, whereas the anterior tibial veins drain the dorsal aspect of the foot. The peroneal vein originates at the level of the ankle. The posterior tibial and peroneal veins are joined by deep muscular branches from the soleus veins in the calf, and perforating branches from the superficial veins. The tibial veins reside in the same fascial compartments as their companion arteries.

The primary components of the superficial veins of the leg are the greater and lesser saphenous veins (see Figs 16-1 and 16-2). Both vessels lie within the subcutaneous fat of the lower extremity superficial to the fascial layers of the muscles. The location and caliber of these veins contributes to their desirability as conduits for arterial bypass surgery. The greater saphenous vein has its origins in the veins along the medial edge of the foot. At the ankle the vein becomes the greater saphenous, which ascends along the medial aspect of the leg to join the CFV below the inguinal ligament. The greater saphenous vein communicates with the deep system along its entire length through small perforating veins. These veins are of great importance as they drain the saphenous vein into the deep system, where venous return to the heart is assisted by the pump-like action of muscular contraction and relaxation around the veins. Disruption of the valves in the perforating veins allows blood to drain out of the deep into the superficial system, which contributes to varicose veins (dilated, tortuous superficial veins). The greater saphenous vein receives tributaries from the medial and lateral accessory saphenous veins, and variably from the inferior epigastric and external pudendal veins, just before joining the CFV.

The lateral edge of the foot drains into the lesser saphenous vein, a small vessel that ascends along the posterior midline of the calf in a groove between the medial and lateral bodies of the gastrocnemius muscle. The lesser saphenous vein joins the popliteal vein at or just below the knee joint. In some patients the lesser saphenous vein also communicates with medial branches of the greater saphenous vein through the Vein of Giacomini (see Fig 16-2).

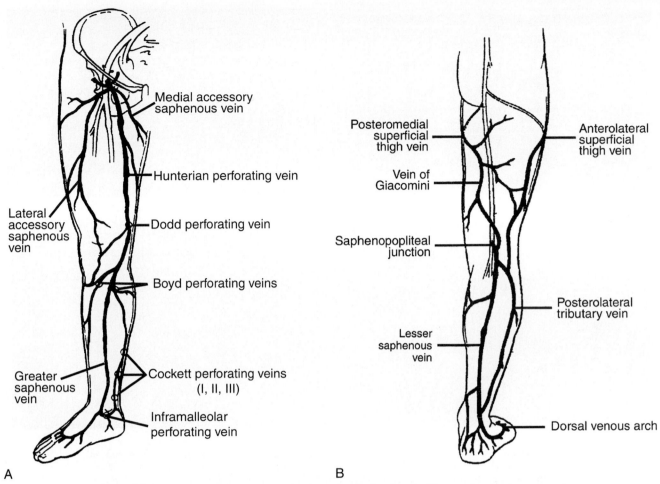

Figure 16-2   Drawings of the superficial veins of the leg. **A**, The greater saphenous vein with tributary and perforating veins. **B**, Posterior superficial veins. (Modified with permission from Bergan JJ: Varicose veins: treatment by surgery and sclerotherapy In Rutherford RB ed: *Vascular Surgery*, 5th edn, WB Saunders, Philadelphia, 2000.)

KEY COLLATERAL PATHWAYS

The deep system of the lower extremity provides collateral drainage for the superficial, and vice versa. The drainage afforded by just one system alone is frequently sufficient to avoid swelling and discomfort in a prolonged upright posture. Obstruction of the CFV and external iliac vein results in drainage through the profunda femoral veins to the internal iliac veins via gluteal and other pelvic veins (Fig. 16-5). In addition, drainage through the ipsilateral abdominal wall veins and across the perineum to the contralateral CFV can occur.

Occlusion of one internal iliac vein results in drainage through the contralateral vessel. When both vessels are occluded, venous drainage through ascending lumbar, gonadal, and even inferior mesenteric veins can occur. Isolated occlusion of one common iliac vein results in retrograde flow in the ipsilateral internal iliac vein with cross-pelvic collateralization to the contralateral internal iliac vein. Occlusion of both the common and external iliac veins results in drainage through the pubic, inferior epigastric, and lumbar veins (Fig. 16-6). Additional collateral drainage by lumbar, paraspinal, and other retroperitoneal veins can also occur. Occlusion of both common iliac veins is functionally identical to obstruction of the infrarenal IVC.

IMAGING

Ultrasound (US) is the primary imaging modality for the lower-extremity venous system. The procedure carries virtually no risk, can be successfully performed in the majority of patients, and provides both anatomic and functional data. Massive obesity, severe edema, external orthopedic hardware, and large areas of abnormal skin can limit the study. The venous system from the tibial

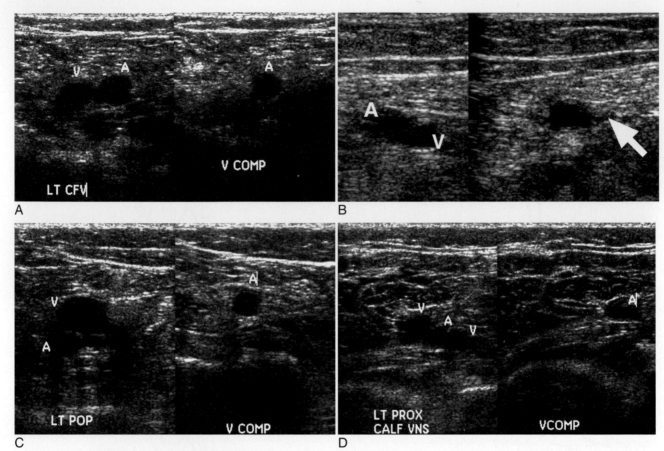

Figure 16-3 Anatomic relationships of the lower-extremity veins and arteries demonstrated on ultrasound. **A,** The CFV (V) lies medial to the common femoral artery (A) in the femoral canal. When the ultrasound probe is used to apply pressure over the vein (VCOMP) the normal low-pressure vein collapses but the high-pressure artery remains visible. LT = left. **B,** In the thigh, the femoral vein (V) travels lateral and deep to the superficial femoral artery (A). With compression, the normal vein collapses (arrow). **C,** The popliteal vein (V) lies more superficial to the artery (A) in relationship to the posterior surface of the knee (the popliteal fossa). With compression the normal vein collapses so that only the artery is visible. **D,** The paired tibial veins (V) are parallel to the single tibial artery (A). With compression the veins collapse so that only the artery is visible.

veins to the proximal common femoral vein can be imaged with a 5- to 7.5-MHz linear transducer (see Fig. 16-3). Lower-frequency transducers may be required in large patients and for the iliac veins. Superficial veins, such as the greater saphenous vein, can be imaged with a 10-MHz transducer. Imaging of the pelvic veins with ultrasound is inconsistent owing to the depth and tortuosity of the vessels.

A complete examination involves visualization of all portions of the venous system from the iliac veins to the ankle. The US transducer is used to compress the infra-inguinal veins; this is not possible in the pelvis. Color-flow and Doppler evaluation can determine patency and flow direction. The walls of the vein should coapt with gentle pressure (see Fig. 16-3). Noncompressibility is diagnostic of an intraluminal abnormality, usually a thrombus (Table 16-1). The normal response to Valsalva is cessation

Table 16-1 US Appearance of Intraluminal Venous Filling Defects

Etiology	US Appearance
Acute thrombus	Expanded vein, hypoechoic lumen, noncompressible vein
	Flow absent or around margins of filling defect
Chronic thrombus	Contracted vein, lumen partially or completely filled with hyperechoic material
	May have flow though center of lumen or small channels
Valve leaflet	Thin, linear, usually paired structure with mobile free margins in center of lumen

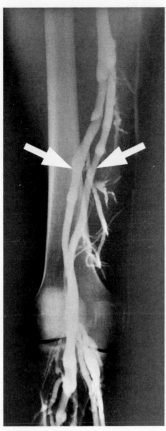

Figure 16-4   Contrast venogram showing duplicated popliteal and femoral veins (arrows).

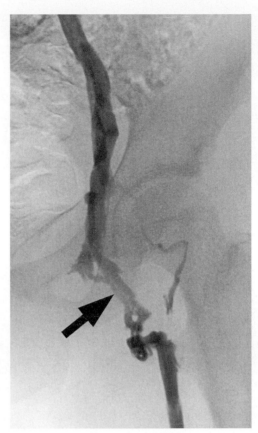

Figure 16-5   Digital subtraction venogram showing chronic occlusion of the left CFV with collateral drainage through inferior gluteal veins (arrow). The patient had a cardiac catheterization as a child.

of flow; a blunted response indicates proximal obstruction, and retrograde flow indicates valvular insufficiency (Fig. 16-7; see also Figs 3-5 and 13-15). The patency of nonvisualized segments can be inferred by imaging the Doppler signal central to the area of interest while gently squeezing the calf ("augmentation") (see Fig. 3-4). A sudden increase in velocity or flow is the expected normal response.

The femoral and popliteal veins can be imaged with the patient supine or in slight reverse Trendelenburg (head up, foot down). A tourniquet at the knee, or dangling the calf over the edge of the examination table, may be required to optimally visualize the calf veins.

Diameter measurements and mapping of the superficial veins are frequently performed prior to harvest for surgical bypass. The course of the saphenous veins and the major branch points should be marked on the skin with indelible ink.

MR venography (MRV) of the lower-extremity veins using 2-dimensional (2-D) time-of-flight (TOF) or contrast-enhanced 3-dimensional (3-D) gradient-echo techniques can be used to image the lower extremity and pelvic veins. The results with 2-D TOF sequences in depiction

of anatomy and detection of lower-extremity thrombosis have been excellent (Fig. 16-8). A superior saturation band with slice thicknesses of 5–8 mm are used. Complex flow patterns in the pelvis frequently result in signal loss in the external iliac veins as they enter the pelvis, and at the confluence with the internal iliac veins. Contrast-enhanced sequences are helpful in this setting to resolve diagnostic issues. Anatomic sequences are useful when venous compression by an adjacent mass is suspected.

The low cost and ready availability of US limits the need for MRV in the majority of patients with lower-extremity venous disease. MRV is useful in the evaluation of venous malformations, congenital abnormalities of venous anatomy, and suspected isolated pelvic deep vein thrombosis.

Lower-extremity CT venography (i.e., infusion of contrast via a foot vein) is feasible with multidetector row technology, but this technique has found little clinical application in daily practice. In general, lower-extremity venous imaging with CT is performed by imaging during the venous phase of a conventional injection of contrast. Arterial enhancement is therefore always present, which can make identification of weakly opacified small veins

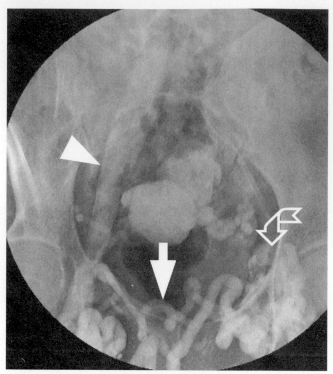

Figure 16-6 Chronic occlusion of the left CFV, EIV, and CIV. Contrast injected in the left leg (curved arrow) crosses the pelvis through pubic collaterals (arrow) to the right iliac veins (arrowhead). The density in the center of the pelvis is in the gastrointestinal tract.

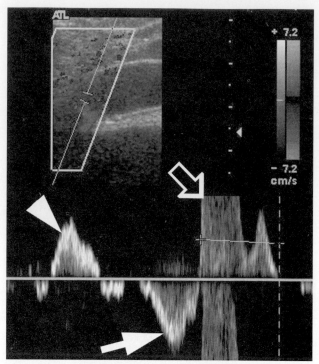

Figure 16-7 Duplex US showing retrograde flow in the GSV due to venous valvular insufficiency. Flow above the line is retrograde, and below the line antegrade. With a gentle cough in the upright position there is retrograde flow (arrowhead) in the GSV. Compression of the calf (augmentation) results briefly in antegrade flow (closed arrow), followed by rapid (note the aliasing) and prolonged retrograde flow (open arrow).

difficult. In the absence of an iodinated blood-pool contrast agent, routine venous imaging of the lower extremities with CT will not readily supplant US. CT is an excellent choice when compression of iliac veins by a pelvic mass is suspected as the etiology of lower-extremity swelling.

Conventional contrast venography is performed infrequently, but remains an important and definitive imaging modality in lower-extremity venous disease. The usual indications for ascending venography are suspected DVT with equivocal or negative noninvasive imaging, chronic venous diseases, and rarely venous mapping. Ascending venography is performed with the patient on a tilting procedure table oriented for a reverse Trendelenburg position. A block is placed under the foot of the leg opposite to the side under study. This allows the patients to support their weight on the normal leg when the table is tilted. A 21-gauge or smaller butterfly needle or intravenous catheter is inserted into a vein on the dorsum of the foot and secured in place. Ideally, the tip of the needle should be oriented towards the toes, but most of the time one is satisfied with any usable access. Finding a vein can be a challenge in patients with edematous feet. Application of gentle pressure with a thumb or two fingers can displace the edema and reveal a usable vein in these patients.

The contrast used should be 30% iodine low-osmolar or a dilute high-osmolar agent such as Conray 43. The contrast is loaded into three or four 50-mL syringes. The table is tilted head-up 30–60 degrees with all weight-bearing on the opposite leg of interest. A tourniquet is

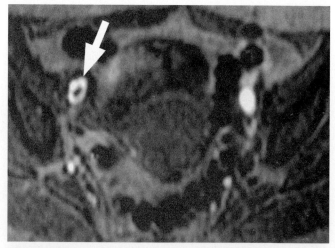

Figure 16-8 Axial image from a 2-dimensional time-of-flight (2-D TOF) MR venogram showing nonocclusive thrombus in the right external iliac vein (arrow).

placed around the ankle to force contrast into the deep system. Hand injection is used in order to control the amount of contrast in the veins during the study. The initial injection of 5–10 mL of contrast is watched fluoroscopically as it exits the needle (Fig. 16-9). At the same time the patient is questioned regarding pain at the injection site. The injection is stopped for obvious extravasation or persistent pain.

Filling of the venous system is monitored by intermittent fluoroscopy during continuous hand injection of contrast. The calf veins will be opacified in most patients with 50–80 mL of contrast. Images are obtained in three projections (anteroposterior and both obliques) using a large field of view coned side-to-side. Magnification views should be obtained of any area of question. Digital subtraction venography is usually not performed as contrast clears too slowly from the veins, resulting in poor image quality on subsequent images. When the study is performed for varicose veins, a radiopaque ruler is positioned adjacent to the leg. Tourniquets are used at the mid-calf and knee to compartmentalize the superficial veins and allow identification of retrograde flow from the deep system through incompetent perforating veins.

The contrast is followed as it ascends the leg. The saphenous vein, when opacified, should be included on the films. Unopacified inflow from muscular veins and the profunda femoris vein can mimic intraluminal filling defects and dilute the contrast density. The iliac veins are filled by compressing the femoral vein, repositioning the table so that the patient is either flat or in mild Trendelenburg, then releasing the femoral vein compression. The contrast-filled leg will then empty into the iliac veins, and proximal IVC.

Once the study has been completed the foot is connected to an infusion of sterile saline or 5% dextrose solution. A minimum of 150–200 mL is infused to flush the contrast from the leg before removing the needle. Traditionally, an abdominal film is obtained after each venogram to evaluate renal excretion and contours.

Venography is a safe procedure, but it requires 100–150 mL of contrast per limb. The overall complication rate is currently lower than 5%. The use of low-osmolar contrast has greatly reduced the incidence of phlebitis (thought to be due to the injurious effect of high-osmolar contrast on the venous endothelium) and the risk of tissue necrosis from extravasation of contrast. Patients with renal insufficiency, contrast allergy, and ischemic extremities should not undergo ascending venography if alternative diagnostic modalities are available.

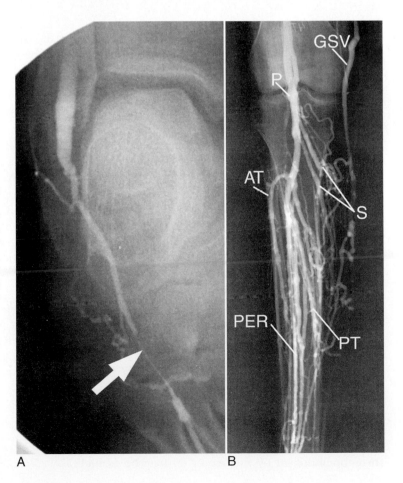

Figure 16-9   Conventional venogram performed with the patient tilted 50 degrees and bearing weight on the left leg. **A,** Initial image during injection of an intravenous catheter in a lateral foot vein (arrow) confirms absence of extravasation. **B,** Anterior view of the calf shows filling of the anterior tibial (AT), posterior tibial (PT), and peroneal (PER) veins. Sural (S) veins drain directly into the popliteal vein (P). The GSV is also filled. The complete study included two opposing oblique views of the calf.   *(Continued)*

A   B

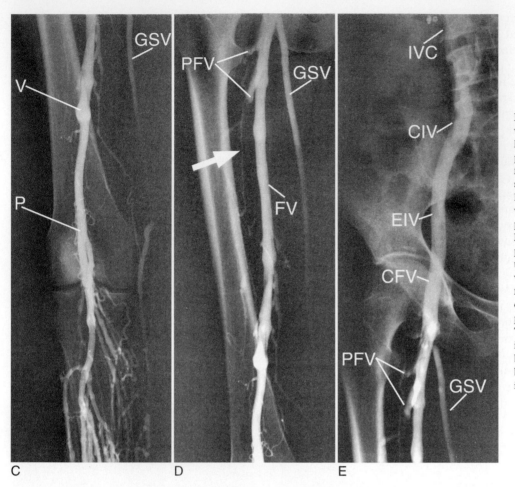

Figure 16-9   cont'd C, Anterior view of the popliteal vein. Note the large valve (V) in the above-knee portion of the vein. The GSV is also filled. **D**, Anterior view of the thigh showing the femoral vein (FV). Drainage of some deep muscular veins (arrow) faintly opacify the profunda femoris vein (PFV). **E**, Anterior view of the groin and pelvis showing the insertion of the GSV into the common femoral vein (CFV), known as the sapheno-femoral junction. The valves at the origin of the PFV are competent, preventing retrograde opacification. The external (EIV) and common iliac veins (CIV) are well visualized, but contrast in the IVC is attenuated by inflow from the left common iliac vein.

Descending venography is indicated for the evaluation of venous valvular incompetence. The patient is placed on a tilting table and the groin of the leg of interest prepared as for a conventional femoral vein puncture. Using standard techniques, a 5-French straight multi-side-hole catheter or dilator is inserted with the tip in the external iliac vein. The table is tilted with the head elevated to 60 degrees, and 15–20 mL of contrast is injected. In normal patients the contrast will flow slowly towards the heart. In patients with incompetent valves the contrast will reflux to the level of a normal valve (Fig. 16-10). Spot films are obtained, with special focus on the most distal extent. When patients cannot be tilted, filming is performed during Valsalva maneuver. The degree of reflux is graded according to the distance from the injection site (Table 16-2).

ACUTE DEEP VEIN THROMBOSIS

Thrombosis of the deep veins of the lower extremity is thought to occur in adults with a yearly incidence of 1.6 per 1000. The cumulative risk of developing venous thromboembolism by the age of 80 may be as high as 11% in males. Acute DVT is rare in children. The coagulation pathway is discussed in Chapter 1. A number of conditions are believed or known to predispose patients to development of DVT (Box 16-1). Nonocclusive thrombus is believed to form first in an area of slow flow in a valve cusp, followed by central propagation and occlusion (Fig. 16-11).

The calf veins are involved in almost 90% of cases of DVT at the time of first presentation, with concurrent extension to the thigh in 50% and the pelvis in 25%. When untreated, calf vein DVT will progress centrally in

Grade	Definition
0	No reflux
1	Reflux to mid-thigh in femoral vein
2	Reflux to above-knee popliteal vein
3	Reflux to below-knee popliteal vein or proximal tibial veins
4	Reflux to distal calf or ankle

Table 16-2   Grading of Venous Reflux

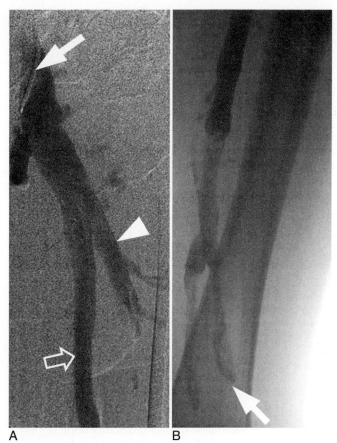

A   B

Figure 16-10   Descending venography showing reflux to the adductor canal. **A**, Digital subtraction image of the upper thigh. The contrast has been injected into the left CFV through a catheter (arrow). There is reflux into both the PFV (arrowhead) and FV (open arrow). The study was performed with the patient tilted upright at 60 degrees. **B**, Spot film of the lower thigh showing retrograde flow of contrast to the level of the above-knee PV (arrow) (grade 2 reflux).

approximately a quarter of patients. Thrombosis limited to the iliac vein is unusual (<3%), and is usually related to a pelvic mass, May–Thürner syndrome (see below, Chronic Venous Obstruction), extension of internal iliac vein thrombus, or CFV thrombosis.

The consequences of DVT can be acute (lower-extremity swelling, pulmonary embolism, and lower-extremity arterial insufficiency) or chronic (venous reflux, varicosities, and stasis changes). The most common acute symptom that has major mortality is pulmonary embolism (PE), which occurs in 20–30% of patients with DVT. In addition, clinically silent PE is common, with positive nuclear medicine scans or pulmonary CT in almost 50% of patients with DVT. The risk of PE is higher with proximal thrombus (extending above the popliteal vein), but PE also occurs in approximately 10% of patients with isolated calf DVT. Chronic venous disease

(discussed in the next section) occurs in 30% of patients within 5 years of their first episode of thrombosis.

The clinical diagnosis of DVT is suggested by symptoms of leg swelling, pain, tenderness on deep palpation, erythema, and pain on dorsiflexion of the foot ("Homan's sign"). Unfortunately, the accuracy of these clinical clues as independent indicators of DVT is widely accepted to be in the vicinity of 50%. Assessment of patient risk factors improves the positive predictive value of the physical examination for DVT. Many other common conditions can cause symptoms similar to acute DVT, such as heart failure, trauma, chronic venous insufficiency, and cellulitis. For these reasons further diagnostic evaluation is necessary to establish the diagnosis.

Lower-extremity arterial insufficiency due to extensive DVT can present in two forms (Table 16-3). Phlegmasia alba dolens, in which the limb is swollen, pale, with diminished pulses, is believed to be due to arterial spasm in response to iliofemoral thrombosis. Phlegmasia cerulea dolens reportedly can occur in up to 6% of cases of DVT, with a strong association with malignancy (Fig. 16-12). The mechanism of ischemia in these patients is arterial collapse due to massive tense edema in the presence of extensive venous thrombosis – in essence a compartment syndrome involving the entire limb. Venous gangrene and amputation complicates more than 50% of cases of phlegmasia cerulea dolens.

Measurement of serum D-dimer, a degradation product of fibrinolysis, can be used as an initial screening test for

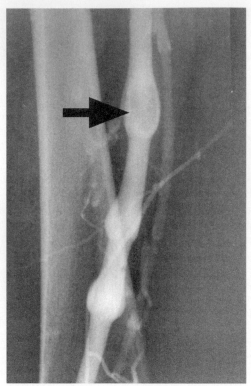

Figure 16-11 Venogram showing nonocclusive thrombus in a FV valve cusp (arrow).

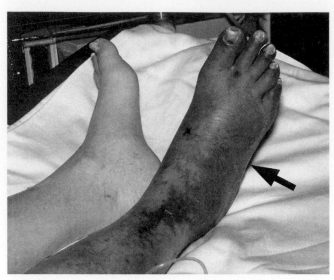

Figure 16-12 Photograph of a patient with phlegmasia cerulea dolens of the right foot. Note the edema and discoloration of the foot (arrow). Subdermal bleeding and skin blisters are also common.

the presence of thrombus. A normal D-dimer level has a 97% negative predictive value, but a positive test can result from thrombus anywhere in the body. Nevertheless, imaging remains essential in the diagnosis of DVT.

The most widely applied imaging modality for detection of lower-extremity DVT is ultrasound (Box 16-2). A noncompressible vein is the single most reliable criteria for the presence of thrombus, provided that the examination is adequate (Fig. 16-13). The sensitivity and specificity for US are both greater than 95% for detection of thrombus in the popliteal vein and above in patients

with symptoms of DVT. The sensitivity and specificity are both closer to 80% for calf DVT in asymptomatic patients. Small thrombi, particularly those limited to valve cusps or perforating veins, are easily missed by US. Great care must be taken to ensure that duplicated femoral or popliteal veins are not overlooked by US, as thrombus in one moiety of a duplicated vein segment can occur.

The low cost, low risk, and wide availability of US for DVT has resulted in relaxation of the indications for venous imaging. The number of studies for DVT has increased 10-fold since the introduction of US compared to the number when venography was the only available test. The rate of positive studies is lower than 10% in many institutions, particularly those with large trauma populations in whom surveillance US is performed on

Table 16-3	Clinical Presentation of Lower-extremity Venous Thrombosis
Category	**Findings**
Superficial thrombophlebitis	Erythema, palpable cord in saphenous or other superficial vein, limited edema
Deep venous thrombosis	Edema, pain, distended superficial veins, warm extremity
Phlegmasia alba dolens	Pale, cool extremity with weak or absent pulses; usually transient
Phlegmasia cerulea dolens	Cyanotic, cool, painful, pulseless extremity; limb loss likely

Box 16-2 Ultrasound Criteria of Acute Deep Venous Thrombosis

Absolute

Noncompressible, hypoechoic vein (frequently expanded)

Adjunctive

Intraluminal filling defect on color flow

Absent color-flow signal in lumen despite augmentation

Absent Doppler signal from lumen despite augmentation

Absent respiratory variation

Absent response to Valsalva

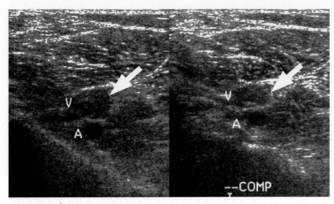

Figure 16-13 US appearance of deep venous thrombosis (in this case the popliteal vein). The vein (V, arrow) does not compress (COMP). The artery (A) is slightly flattened with compression, indicating application of sufficient pressure with the transducer.

a regular basis. This has resulted in investigations to optimize utilization of US, particularly in the study of calf veins, asymptomatic extremities, and patients with persistent symptoms despite negative initial US examinations. In general, the fewer the risk factors for and symptoms of venous thrombosis, the lower the positive rate of US examinations.

Detection of acute DVT by MRV has excellent sensitivity and specificity (both >95%). The expense, length of the examination, and relatively limited availability (compared to US) has prevented routine use of this test. The introduction of blood-pool agents may substantially change the utilization of MRV for detection of DVT.

On CT images, venous thrombosis appears as either intraluminal high density on noncontrast scans, or low density with enhancement in the vein wall on contrast studies. Thrombus in a lower-extremity vein is occasionally noted during the venous phase of pelvic CT obtained

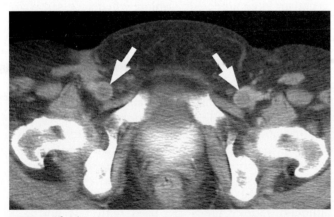

Figure 16-14 Axial image from contrast-enhanced CT performed to look for a postoperative abscess, showing enlarged CFV bilaterally (arrows) with low-attenuation centers and enhancement of the vein wall. These findings are diagnostic of acute thrombosis.

for other indications (Fig. 16-14). The addition of a scan of the pelvis and legs following pulmonary CT angiography (CTA) for PE reveals DVT in 10% of patients.

Conventional venography remains the most sensitive and specific examination for acute DVT, though it is used infrequently owing to the small risk of complications, increased cost relative to US, and patient discomfort. The most reliable venographic finding is an intraluminal filling defect outlined by contrast (Box 16-3 and Fig. 16-15). When the defect is smooth and fills a normal sized or enlarged vein, the thrombus is acute (<7 days) in age. When the filling defect is contracted, irregular, and the vein is smaller than normal, the thrombus is chronic (Fig. 16-16). However, both acute and chronic DVT can coexist in the same patient and in the same venous segment. Nonvisualization of a vein implies thrombosis, but without visualization of an actual filling defect the diagnosis cannot be made with certainty (Fig. 16-17). In this situation the absence of collateral veins and varicosities is suggestive of an acute thrombus, but this finding should be corroborated with a cross-sectional imaging modality if necessary. Venography is no longer used routinely for diagnosis of DVT (Box 16-4).

The primary treatment of acute DVT is anticoagulation. The purpose of anticoagulation is to prevent formation of new thrombus while the existing thrombus undergoes thrombolysis by endogenous means. Heparin in either unfractionated or low-molecular-weight preparations are used to initiate therapy, followed by oral coumadin or low-molecular-weight heparin for chronic therapy. The duration of therapy is 3–6 months with a target international normalized ratio (INR) of 2–3 (when coumadin is used). Some degree of patency of thrombosed venous

---

Box 16-3 Venographic Findings in Acute and Chronic Deep Venous Thrombosis

Acute

Smooth concentric intraluminal filling defect outlined by thin rim of contrast
Occlusion of vein with convex superior or inferior contour with few collaterals

Chronic

Irregular eccentric intraluminal filling defect, sometimes string-like
Transverse webs
Narrowed, irregular lumen
Absence of valves
Absence of filling of deep veins with prominent collateral veins and varicosities
Rarely, calcified thrombus

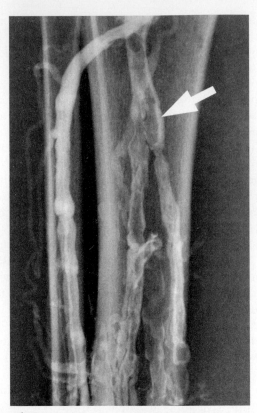

Figure 16-15   Classic venographic appearance of thrombosis, with contrast outlining a central filling defect (arrow). There is thrombus in the posterior tibial and peroneal veins.

Box 16-4   Indications for Lower-extremity Venography in Patients with Suspected DVT

Negative ultrasound with high index of suspicion
Indeterminate or inadequate ultrasound with high index of suspicion
Conflicting results of serial ultrasound examinations
Acute symptoms superimposed upon chronic
Ultrasound not feasible due to dressings, wounds, hardware

segments is restored in over 80% of patients by 6 weeks, with complete resolution of thrombus in up to 50% over time. The aggregate risk of a bleeding complication at an INR of 2–3 is 3–5%. After completion of treatment, recurrent DVT occurs in 3–10%, with the higher rates in patients with defined or occult risk factors. Vena cava filters are not indicated in the treatment of uncomplicated DVT unless the patient cannot be anticoagulated, has sustained a massive PE, or lacks the cardiopulmonary reserve to tolerate a PE.

The risk of symptomatic PE during initiation of therapy is approximately 5%. Failure of therapy as defined by propagation of thrombus occurs in 6–10%. Approximately 2% of patients receiving unfractionated heparin experience a drop in platelets (heparin-induced thrombocytopenia, HIT); this complication is less common with low-molecular-weight heparin. In severe cases of HIT patients develop widespread vascular occlusions due to platelet aggregation, and hemorrhage (disseminated intravascular coagulation, DIC).

Superficial thrombophlebitis (thrombus limited to the saphenous vein or its tributaries) is usually managed with elevation, compression stockings, and local heat when limited to small segments of vein. Anticoagulation is recommended by some when the upper thigh is involved, as extension into the CVF (and therefore conversion to DVT) occurs in up to 11%.

Surgical therapy for acute DVT is reserved for patients with impending or full-blown phlegmasia cerulea dolens. Iliofemoral thrombectomy, with or without creation of an arteriovenous fistula, has a 4% or lower mortality and a clinical success rate of approximately 80%. Fasciotomies are frequently necessary in patients with phlegmasia cerulea dolens. Despite fair long-term results, surgical thrombectomy is infrequently performed in the United States.

Catheter-directed thrombolysis for extensive lower-extremity DVT is very successful in rapidly restoring venous patency, and may reduce damage to venous valves. This technique has replaced surgical thrombectomy in many centers; many more patients currently undergo thrombolysis than would have been operated upon in the past. The indications for thrombolysis are not well defined, but typically patients have extensive, symptomatic iliofemoral DVT of less than 14 days' duration. Access for thrombolysis can be achieved from a number of locations, but most interventionalists prefer to puncture a posterior tibial or popliteal vein on the affected side using US guidance. The thrombosed vein is easier to negotiate in an antegrade fashion; when accessed retrograde from a jugular vein or contralateral CFV the valves can impede catheter placement. Multi-side-hole catheters must be placed across the entire length of the thrombus. A triaxial system can be constructed with infusion through a 5- or 6-French sheath at the access site, a 5-French infusion catheter in the middle segment, and a 3-French infusion catheter extending to the most central portion of the thrombus (Box 16-5 and Fig. 16-18). Patients receive systemic anticoagulation during the thrombolysis, but lower levels are used when the thrombolytic agent is one of the tissue plasminogen activators (t-PA). Infusion for 2 and rarely 3 days may be required with urokinase, although shorter times are used with t-PA and r-PA (Table 16-4). Patients should receive aspirin or other antiplatelet drugs during the procedure, and be maintained on chronic anticoagulation afterwards. Symptomatic PE

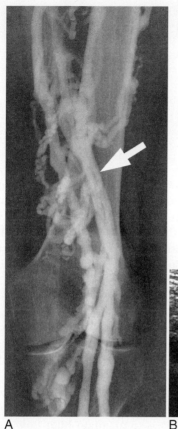

A

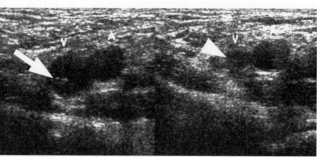

B

Figure 16-16 Chronic changes following deep venous thrombosis. **A**, Venogram showing varicosities and a linear filling defect in the above-knee popliteal vein (arrow). **B**, US of a different patient showing an echogenic structure in the CFV (arrow). With compression, the vein does not completely disappear owing to the postphlebitic synechia in the lumen.

is rare during lysis, but fatal PE was reported in 1 of 473 cases enrolled in an American registry. Bleeding complications are more frequent (6–25%) but usually consist of hematomas.

The initial results of catheter-directed thrombolysis for acute DVT are promising, with complete lysis of thrombus in up to one-third, and >50% lysis in half. Clinical success is observed in over 70% of patients, with patency maintained at 1 year in almost two-thirds. Stents are frequently required in the iliofemoral segment when patients with chronic disease are treated or the thrombosis is on the left (presumed due to underlying May–Thürner syndrome). The long-term benefits of thrombolysis are improved quality of life, venous patency, and preserved venous valvular function.

Box 16-5 Principles of Venous Thrombolysis

Fresh thrombus will lyse quickest

Infuse agent over entire length of thrombus

Establish flow quickly: consider mechanical thrombectomy first, then thrombolysis

Anticoagulate during infusion (low dose with tissue plasminogen activators)

Platelet inhibitors (aspirin or glycoprotein IIB/IIIA agents)

Stents frequently required in patients with chronic disease

Long-term anticoagulation

CHRONIC VENOUS OBSTRUCTION

Venous obstruction, rather than valvular incompetence, is the underlying etiology of chronic lower-extremity swelling in almost 10% of patients. The most common etiology of chronic obstruction is prior DVT (Box 16-6). Patients present with extremity swelling and thigh pain with exercise, termed "venous claudication." Clinical signs of valvular incompetence may be present, but non-pulsatile, distended varicosities that do not decompress with elevation are characteristic of outflow obstruction. In addition, patients may have abdominal and perineal venous distension, with a bluish tinge to the leg.

Patients with May–Thürner (also known as Cockett's) syndrome may present with chronic symptoms or acute thrombosis. The underlying abnormality is compression of the left common iliac vein between the right common

Table 16-4   Thrombolytic Agents for Venous Thrombolysis

Agent	Total Hourly Dose	Heparin Hourly Dose	Duration
Urokinase	100,000–150,000 U	800–1200 U	48 hours
rt-PA	0.5–1 mg	500 U	24–48 hours
r-PA	0.5–1 U	500 U	24–48 hours
TNK-t-pa	0.25–0.5 mg	500 U	24–48 hours

iliac artery and the lumbosacral spine (Fig. 16-19; see also Fig. 13-12). The typical patient is in the second to fourth decade, with a female to male ratio of 3:1. Three venographic stages have been described: asymptomatic compression of the left common iliac vein with no filling of collaterals and a pressure gradient ≤2 mmHg; intraluminal webs or "spurs"; and thrombosis.

The imaging of patients with chronic venous obstruction is directed at determination of the level of occlusion and detection of correctable underlying causes. US is excellent for imaging the lower extremity, but less useful

in the pelvis. Analysis of Doppler waveforms in response to respiratory maneuvers infers the status of the iliac veins. Both CT and MR are excellent modalities for evaluation of the pelvic veins and surrounding soft tissues. Venous obstruction from extrinsic compression by lymph nodes, aneurysms, masses, and even the distended bladder can occur (Fig. 16-20). Ascending venography, performed from either the foot (for obstruction of the extremity veins) or CFV (for obstruction in the iliac veins) is used to confirm inconclusive results of other studies or prior to interventions.

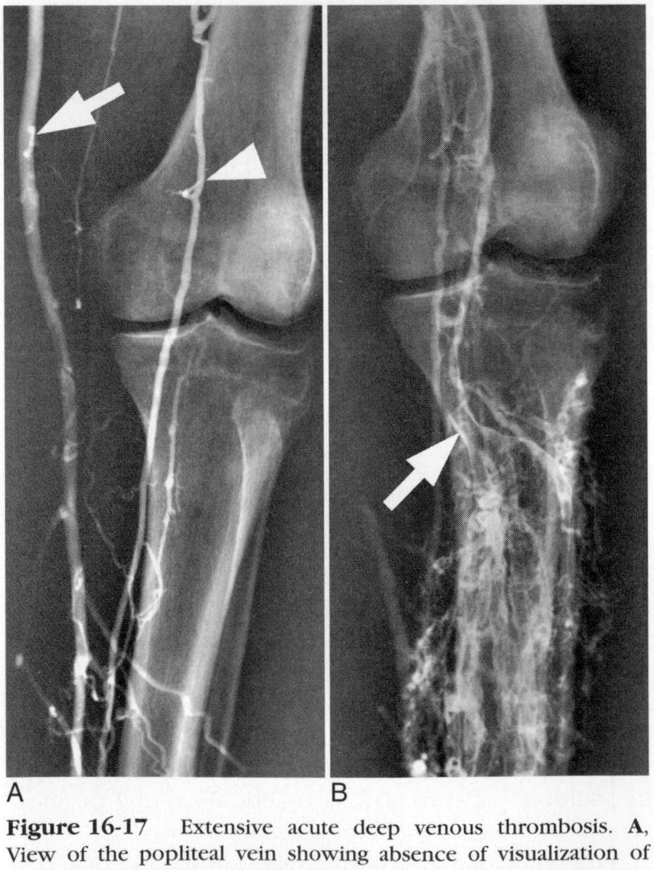

Several surgical procedures have been devised for iliac vein occlusion, including femoral-to-femoral venous bypass and CFV-to-IVC bypass with or without creation of a small arteriovenous fistula in the groin. The purpose of the fistula is to maintain high flow rates through the graft. Clinical improvement has been reported in about 75% of these patients, with similar graft patencies. Results reported for May–Thürner syndrome have been better than those for chronic thrombosis. Surgical bypass for femoral and popliteal vein occlusion has met with poor results.

Endovascular reconstruction of occluded venous segments with metallic stents is usually feasible provided that the occlusion can be crossed with a guidewire. Both antegrade and retrograde approaches should be attempted. The jugular approach provides excellent leverage for crossing common iliac vein occlusions. A trial

A   B

Figure 16-17   Extensive acute deep venous thrombosis. **A,** View of the popliteal vein showing absence of visualization of deep veins and filling of the GSV (arrow) and lesser saphenous vein (arrowhead). **B,** With continuing injection of contrast there is delineation of thrombus in all of the deep veins of the calf as well as the popliteal vein (arrow).

Box 16-6   Etiologies of Chronic Obstruction of Lower-extremity Veins

Deep venous thrombosis
Trauma
Irradiation
Retroperitoneal fibrosis
Neoplasm
Arterial aneurysms
Cysts (e.g., Baker's cyst in popliteal fossa)
Muscular entrapment (e.g., type 5 popliteal artery entrapment)
May–Thürner syndrome

of thrombolysis can be beneficial in patients with chronic thrombosis, but most interventionalists will stent primarily. Self-expanding stents should be sized 2–3 mm larger in diameter than the normal diameter of the vein (Fig. 16-21). Patients should be anticoagulated for 3–6 months after successful recanalization. The 1-year patency of iliac vein stents when the infrainguinal veins are patent is 90%. Long-term results in the femoral veins have not been as promising. Provided that the procedure can be performed safely, an attempt at endovascular reconstruction should precede surgery in most patients.

CHRONIC VENOUS VALVULAR INSUFFICIENCY

Incompetent valves in superficial, deep, and perforator veins results in venous hypertension in the lower extremity. Over 25% of the adult population has a detectable abnormality related to this process, most often varicose veins or telangiectasias. In 3–8% of the population chronic venous insufficiency results in swelling, pain, hyperpigmentation, dermatitis, and ulceration. Venous ulceration occurs in 3.5 per 1000 per year in patients older than 45 years, and is recurrent in 75%.

Box 16-7   Etiologies of Venous Valvular Incompetence

Genetic
Past history of deep or superficial vein thrombosis
Female gender
Parity
Prolonged standing

The etiology of the valvular incompetence is multifactorial (Box 16-7). The pathophysiology of the skin changes is not completely understood, but it is linked to the high venous pressures. Venous pressures may rise to over 80 mmHg at the ankle in patients with severe disease. The volume of refluxed blood is also important in development of symptoms. Although the initial abnormality is located at the venous valve, the end organ that is damaged is the skin with the subcutaneous tissues. A classification has been developed to describe patients with chronic venous diseases (clinical class, etiology, anatomy, and pathology (CEAP), Table 16-5). A complex modification (Venous Severity Scoring) has been proposed that includes the degree of disability,

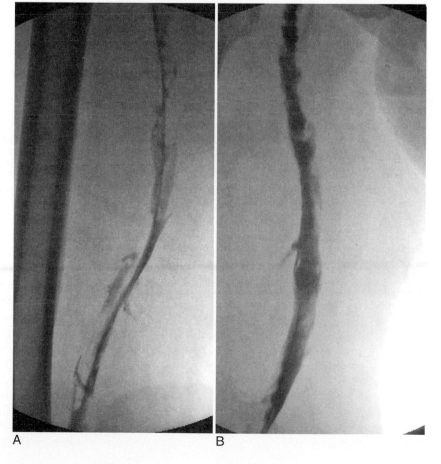

Figure 16-18   Lower-extremity venous thrombolysis for acute deep venous thrombosis. **A**, Venogram of the thigh obtained after puncture of the posterior tibial vein using US guidance. There is extensive thrombus that was continuous from the tibial veins to the IVC. A guidewire has been advanced into the IVC. **B**, After passage of a mechanical thrombectomy device there has been substantial reduction in the volume of thrombus, but antegrade flow was still absent.   *(Continued)*

A   B

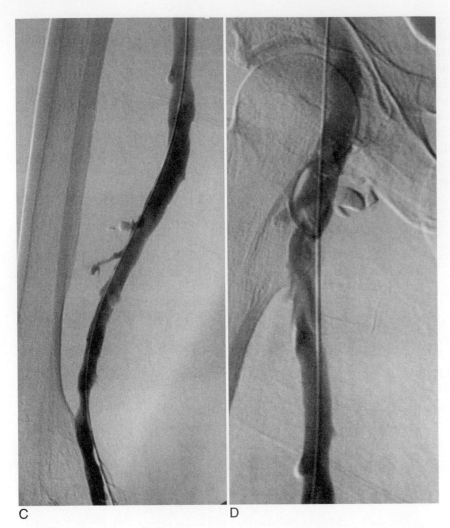

C   D

Figure 16-18 cont'd **C**, After catheter-directed thrombolysis there is excellent antegrade flow with only minimal filling defects in the FV. **D**, View of the groin showing a patent CFV.

severity of symptoms, and location and type of venous abnormality.

Telangiectasias and reticular ("spider") veins (CEAP 1) are so common that they are considered by many to be normal manifestations of aging. Incompetent small perforator veins result in dilatation of the subdermal venous network. Telangiectasias are flat, red blemishes that blanch on pressure with slow return of color. When return of color is brisk, or the lesion is pulsatile, an arteriovenous malformation should be suspected. Reticular veins are small, superficial, thin-walled veins that lie close to the surface of the skin.

Varicose veins (CEAP 2) are dilated, tortuous superficial veins that distend when the patient is upright and can cause aching. Rarely, varicose veins can rupture resulting in major hemorrhage. The dilated veins collapse and symptoms improve with elevation of the extremity. Valvular incompetence in the greater saphenous vein contributes to over 75% of varicosities, with isolated perforating vein incompetence accounting for the remainder.

Edema (CEAP 3) due to chronic venous stasis indicates severe venous hypertension. Without intervention, there is a high likelihood of progression to permanent damage to the skin.

The characteristic skin changes of venous insufficiency (CEAP 4) are thickening, scaling, and brownish

Class	Description
	Table 16-5 CEAP Classification of Chronic Venous Disease
0	Normal
1	Telangiectasias or reticular ("spider") veins
2	Varicose veins
3	Edema
4	Skin changes (pigmentation, venous eczema, lipodermatosclerosis)
5	Skin changes as above with healed ulceration
6	Skin changes as above with active ulceration

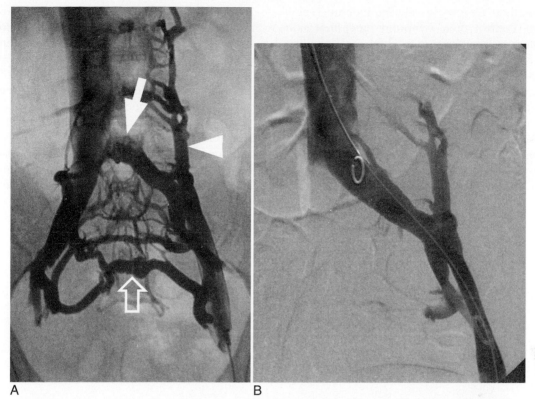

A   B

Figure 16-19   Venographic appearance of May–Thürner syndrome. The patient is a 21-year-old woman with chronic left leg swelling. **A,** Digital venogram obtained by injection of the left EIV showing an attenuated left CIV (closed arrow), with drainage via cross-pelvic collaterals (open arrow) to the right iliac system, and the ascending lumbar vein (arrowhead). **B,** After angioplasty of the left CIV and placement of a 14-mm diameter self-expanding stent there is excellent antegrade flow with absent filling of collateral veins. The patient has a belly-button ring that is projected over the iliac vein.

discoloration. There is almost always associated edema, and patients report itching and burning sensations. The color changes are largely irreversible.

Lower-extremity venous ulcers (CEAP 5,6) are the most severe manifestation of venous valvular insufficiency. These lesions must be distinguished from arterial, traumatic and diabetic ulcers in order to initiate appropriate therapy. Venous ulcers are shallow, irregular, associated with charactcristic skin changcs, and arc located in the medial aspect of the supramalleolar region. Incompetence of the deep and perforating veins, with or without saphenous vein reflux, is present in more than 80% of these patients. Isolated saphenous vein reflux is unusual in patients with advanced disease (skin changes and/or ulceration).

Imaging of patients with chronic venous insufficiency is aimed at determining the location and extent of reflux. Ultrasound with Doppler and color flow is highly sensitive and specific (both >95%) for valvular incompetence. Identification of incompetent perforating veins is 80% sensitive but very specific. The examination is performed in a fashion identical to that for DVT, with the addition of maneuvers to induce flow reversal. These include tilting the table in reverse Trendelenburg, Valsalva, and compression techniques. Segmental evaluation is important to localize the abnormal veins. Reversal of flow that lasts less than 0.5 seconds is normal. Flow reversal for 0.5–2 seconds is suggestive of valvular incompetence, while reversal for longer than 2 seconds is diagnostic (see Fig. 16-7). Dilated, incompetent perforating veins underlying venous ulcers may also be identified by US.

Contrast venography currently has a limited role in the diagnostic evaluation of patients with chronic venous disease. Conventional ascending venography may be performed prior to intervention to localize incompetent perforating veins when US has been unsuccessful. A radiopaque ruler should be placed adjacent to the leg to permit precise localization of the venous abnormality. Descending venography can localize reflux and define the extent when US is unsatisfactory (see Table 16-2 and Fig. 16-10).

The therapy of venous insufficiency varies with the clinical findings and the symptoms. There is currently no satisfactory method to reverse valvular incompetence. Many patients control their symptoms and limit skin changes by wearing compression stockings and avoiding prolonged standing. Ulcerations require aggressive local care including debridement, medicated dressings, surgical ligation of underlying incompetent perforating veins, and skin grafts.

Patients seek treatment for varicose veins for a variety of reasons (Box 16-8). The traditional treatments include surgical removal of the thigh portion of the greater saphenous vein, division of incompetent perforating veins, and excision of abnormal vein clusters (phlebectomy)

when feasible. Ligation of the saphenofemoral junction and stripping of the saphenous vein is included in over three-quarters of surgical procedures for chronic venous insufficiency. Surgical interventions result in ulcer healing in almost 90% of patients. Recurrence of varicosities after saphenous vein stripping has been reported to be as high as 29%. Surgical reconstruction or transplant of venous valves has been unsuccessful unless performed in specialized centers.

Interventional radiology has a rapidly enlarging role in the treatment of chronic venous insufficiency. Catheter-based techniques for ablation of the greater saphenous

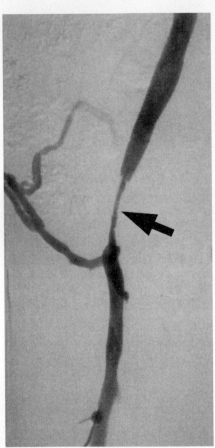

A

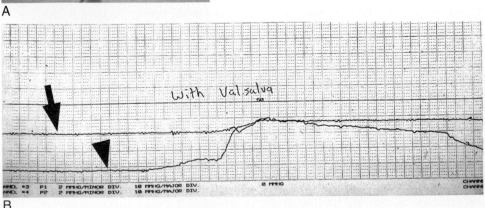

B

Figure 16-20   External iliac vein obstruction due to enlarged lymph nodes in a patient with metastatic cervical carcinoma. The patient had chronic right leg swelling. **A**, Digital venogram showing stenosis of the EIV (arrow). **B**, Simultaneous pressures measured in the IVC (arrowhead) and right CFV (arrow). There is elevated baseline pressure in the CFV. With Valsalva, the IVC pressure rises to meet the CFV pressure.

(Continued)

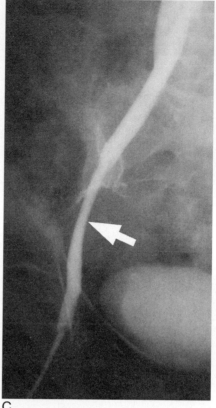

C

Figure 16-20   cont'd **C**, Venogram after stent placement in the EIV (arrow). **D**, Simultaneous pressure measurements from the IVC and right CFV now show identical, superimposed tracings.

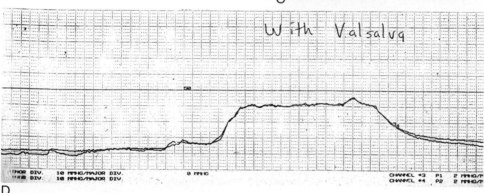

D

<table>
<tr><td>NOR DIV.</td><td>10 MMHG/MAJOR DIV.</td></tr>
<tr><td>NOR DIV.</td><td>10 MMHG/MAJOR DIV.</td></tr>
</table>

With Valsalva

0 MMHG

CHANNEL #3 P1   2 MMHG/*
CHANNEL #4 P2   2 MMHG/*

Box 16-8 Indications for Intervention for Varicose Veins

General appearance
Aching pain
Leg heaviness
Leg fatigue
Superficial thrombophlebitis
External bleeding
Edema
Ankle hyperpigmentation
Skin changes
Venous ulcer

vein offer an effective percutaneous alternative to venous stripping. Laser and radio-frequency (RF) ablation have been used with success for this purpose. The common components of the procedure are careful patient selection and evaluation. (Treatment of varicose veins is almost always elective and frequently motivated primarily by cosmetic concerns.) Mapping of the superficial varicosities with US is essential to determine the patency and competency of the greater and lesser saphenous veins, the major superficial draining veins, and the perforating veins. The status (especially the patency) of the deep venous system is also documented. In addition, the extremity should be examined for evidence of arterial disease, infection, and active venous ulceration.

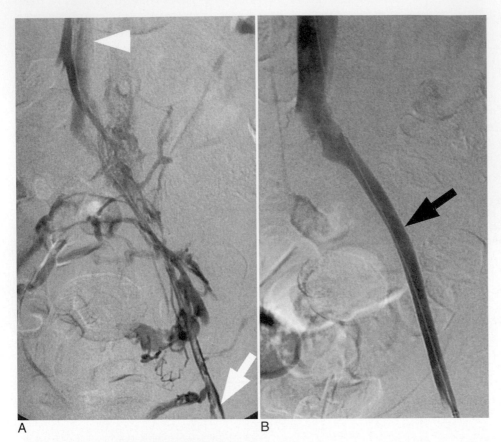

A   B

Figure 16-21   Recanalization of chronic left CIV and EIV occlusion (same patient as Fig. 16-7). **A**, Digital venogram from injection into the left CFV shows a narrowed vein with an intraluminal filling defect consistent with chronic thrombosis (arrow), but no obvious EIV or CIV (arrowhead = IVC). **B**, A hydrophilic guidewire and an angled catheter were used to negotiate through the occluded iliac veins, followed by angioplasty and self-expanding stent placement. There is now excellent flow through the stents (arrow).

Historical evidence of hypercoagulable syndromes, central venous obstruction, and occluded or absent deep veins should prompt reassessment of the need and type of intervention. Most practices obtain a photographic record of the limb prior to treatment.

Prior to treatment the course of the greater saphenous vein is reconfirmed with US. The leg is sterilely prepared and draped, and percutaneous venous access is obtained with US guidance and a micropuncture needle. The usual site of entry is just above or below the knee joint. When access is below the knee, there is an increased risk of injury to the saphenous nerve resulting in sensory loss over the medial upper calf. A long vascular sheath is then advanced to the saphenofemoral junction over a guidewire using US guidance. The ablation device is then positioned in the sheath with the tip in the greater saphenous vein approximately 1 cm proximal to the saphenofemoral junction (Fig. 16-22). Dilute local anesthetic is then infiltrated along the course of the greater saphenous vein using US guidance and multiple punctures. Termed "tumescent anesthesia," this critical step ensures patient comfort during the ablation and minimizes potential damage to surrounding structures by providing a physical barrier (Fig. 16-23).

Once adequate anesthesia has been achieved, the device is activated and withdrawn through the vein. The device should never be activated in the common femoral vein. The device is turned off before withdrawing through the soft tissues and skin to avoid local burns and nerve damage. A compression stocking is applied and the patient ambulates immediately.

This procedure is performed on an outpatient basis, frequently in clinics or private offices. The technical success rate is reportedly greater than 95%, with fewer

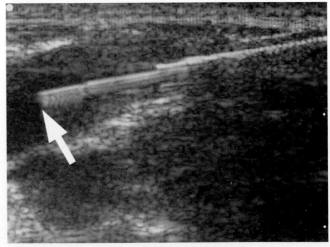

Figure 16-22   US image showing a laser probe (arrow) in the GSV. The probe is never activated in the CFV. (Image courtesy of Angiodynamics, Queensbury, NY.)

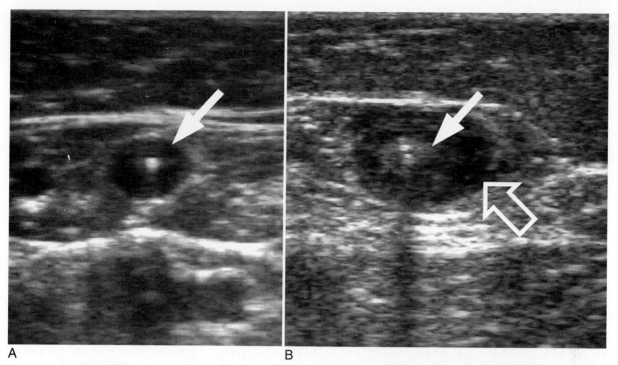

A   B

Figure 16-23   Tumescent anesthesia. This is a critical step in the procedure. **A**, Axial US image of the GSV (arrow) with a laser probe in place. The bright object in the center of the vein is the probe. **B**, Axial image after infiltration of dilute lidocaine around the GSV. The vein (solid arrow) is now compressed around the catheter by the large volume of surrounding anesthetic (open arrow). (Images courtesy of Robert Min M.D., NYC, NY.)

than 10% recurrences at 2 years (Fig. 16-24). Deep venous thrombosis occurs in fewer than 1% of patients, and nerve injury in fewer than 5%.

Localized small varicosities, telangiectasias, and reticular veins can be effectively treated with injection of sclerosing agents (Box 16-9). When the greater saphenous vein is incompetent, this should be treated first in order to achieve the most durable results with sclerotherapy. A small syringe is used to inject 0.5–1 mL of sclerosant directly into the vein through a 25-gauge or smaller needle. The small needle eliminates the need for local anesthetic. Entering the skin at an angle of about 30 degrees, slight negative pressure is applied to the syringe plunger. As soon as a flash of blood is seen, the sclerosant is gently injected. Blanching of the telangiectasias or reticular veins indicates an intravascular injection. Varices should be compressed proximal and distal to the injection site to retain the sclerosant in the vessel. The injection is stopped immediately if the patient complains of pain or there is obvious local extravasation. The most commonly used agent worldwide is polidocanol 0.25–0.5%, but this drug is not approved for this indication in the United States. Local ulceration, pain, and hyperpigmentation can occur, especially with concentrated sclerosants. Anaphylactic reactions have occurred with sodium morrhuate and sodium tetradecyl sulfate.

Percutaneous replacement of venous valves is a promising experimental technique that may relieve venous hypertension in a nondestructive manner. A number of materials for construction of valves have been described (Fig. 16-25). The valves are typically mounted in a metallic stent and delivered with imaging guidance.

SEPTIC THROMBOPHLEBITIS

The definition of septic thrombophlebitis is pus and infected thrombus within the venous lumen. Almost all cases are acquired secondary to intravascular devices such as central venous catheters and pacemakers. The causative organism is *Staphylococcus aureus* in over

Box 16-9   Sclerosing Agents

Sodium tetradecyl sulfate
Polidocanol
Sodium morrhuate
Hypertonic saline
Polyiodinated iodine

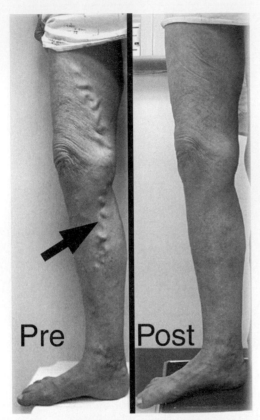

Figure 16-24   Pre- and post-treatment images of a patient who underwent percutaneous endoluminal laser ablation of the greater saphenous vein for varicosities. A distended, rope-like GSV (arrow) can be clearly seen on the pretreatment photo (Pre). One month after treatment there is dramatic improvement (Post).

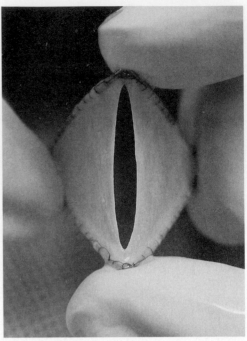

Figure 16-25   Venous valve that can be delivered percutaneously through a catheter. The valve is constructed of a biomaterial that gradually remodels into a structure that appears identical to a native valve. (Image courtesy of Dusan Pavcnik M.D., Ph.D, Dotter Interventional Institute, Portland, OR.)

50% of reported cases. The incidence is far lower than catheter or pacemaker pocket infections. Patients present with bacteremia, sepsis, pain over the affected vein, and sometimes purulence at the catheter insertion site. The finding of venous thrombosis, intraluminal gas, and extensive perivascular inflammatory changes are suggestive imaging findings. Removal of the device (with cultures of the intravascular portion), antibiotics, and rarely surgical thrombectomy are the standard treatment. Anecdotal cases of successful treatment with thrombolysis have been described.

KLIPPEL–TRENAUNAY AND PARKES–WEBER SYNDROMES

Klippel–Trenaunay syndrome is a congenital but not heritable syndrome (Table 16-6). The incidence of this rare syndrome is similar in males and females. In addition to the lower extremity, the pelvis, abdomen, and upper limb can be involved. A characteristic finding is hypoplasia or absence of the deep veins with persistent lateral embryonic and sciatic veins (Fig. 16-26). Lymphatic and digital anomalies may also occur. Documentation of the status of the deep veins is mandatory before considering intervention for varicosities. The optimal imaging modality for the diagnosis of Klippel–Trenaunay syndrome and the determination of the extent of the venous vascular abnormalities is MRV. Conventional venography is useful when other imaging studies are inconclusive.

Parkes–Weber syndrome is even more rare than Klippel–Trenaunay syndrome. Patients have similar findings, with limb hypertrophy, atypical varicosities, and port wine stains. The critical difference is the presence of a high-flow arteriovenous malformation (AVM). The AVM can cause major local complications such as bleeding and ulceration, as well as high-output cardiac failure. Embolization of the AVM may control symptoms.

VENOUS MALFORMATIONS

Venous malformations are congenital lesions distinct from acquired varicosities (see Chapter 1). Venous malformations are soft, nonpulsatile, and decompress when the patient is prone. Superficial lesions can present with bleeding, limb discoloration, local thrombosis, and pain with ambulation. Deep lesions may present only as limb swelling without visible external abnormalities. The arterial pulse examination is normal. MRI is an excellent

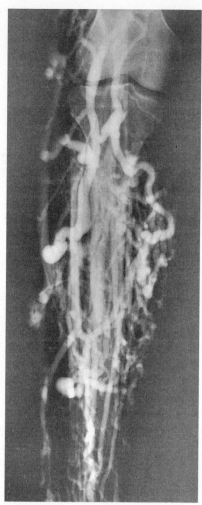

Figure 16-26   Venogram of the calf of a 12-year-old boy with Klippel–Trenaunay syndrome. The deep veins of the calf are atretic and valveless, and there are extensive, dilated superficial veins.

imaging modality for diagnosis and delineation of the extent of the lesion. Angiography demonstrates normal arteries with faint or absent opacification of the lesion; venography, especially with direct puncture of the malformation, allows diagnosis and treatment (see Fig. 1-23). Sclerosis with alcohol is effective in the management

Table 16-6   Klippel–Trenaunay Syndrome

Feature	Incidence (%)
Capillary malformations ("port wine stain")	98
Atypical varicosities, hypoplasia or absence of deep veins	72
Bony and/or soft tissue hypertrophy	67
All three features	63
Two features	37

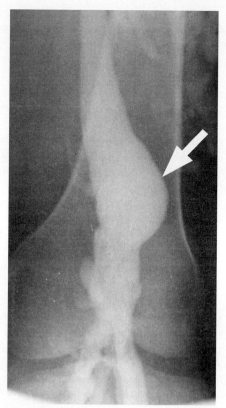

Figure 16-27   True popliteal vein aneurysm (arrow). There was no history of trauma or deep venous thrombosis.

of these lesions. General anesthesia, injection of limited volumes of alcohol with fluoroscopic guidance, and multiple treatments are usually necessary. Skin necrosis, nerve and muscle dysfunction, and cardiac arrhythmia can occur.

VENOUS ANEURYSMS

True venous aneurysms are rare lesions. Congenital venous aneurysms are focal dilatations of otherwise normal-diameter veins. Aneurysms can develop in the outflow veins of patients with arteriovenous fistulas and malformations. Posttraumatic venous pseudoaneurysms have also been described. Congenital aneurysms are most commonly found in the superficial veins, the internal jugular veins, and the deep veins of the lower extremities (Fig. 16-27). Complications include thrombosis, PE, and even rupture. Treatment with surgical excision has been recommended for symptomatic aneurysms.

SUGGESTED READINGS

Aldridge SC, Comerota AJ, Katz ML et al: Popliteal venous aneurysm: report of two cases and review of the world literature. *J Vasc Surg* 18:708–715, 1993.

Bergan JJ, Kumins NH, Owens EL, Sparks SR: Surgical and endovascular treatment of lower extremity venous insufficiency. *J Vasc Interv Radiol* 13:563-568, 2002.

Berry SA, Peterson C, Mize W et al: Klippel–Trenaunay syndrome. *Am J Med Genet* 79:319-326, 1998.

Borsa JJ, Patel NH: The venous system: normal developmental anatomy and congenital anomalies. *Semin Interv Radiol* 18:69-82, 2001.

Breugem CC, Maas M, Reekers JA, van der Horst CM: Use of magnetic resonance imaging for the evaluation of vascular malformations of the lower-extremity. *Plast Reconstr Surg* 108:870-877, 2001.

Comerota AJ, Throm RC, Mathias SD, Haughton S, Mewissen M: Catheter-directed thrombolysis for iliofemoral deep venous thrombosis improves health-related quality of life. *J Vasc Surg* 32:130-137, 2000.

Fraser JD, Anderson DR: Deep venous thrombosis: recent advances and optimal investigation with US. *Radiology* 211:9-24, 1999.

Golledge J, Quigley FG. Pathogenesis of varicose veins. *Eur J Vasc Endovasc Surg* 25:319-324, 2003.

Gottlieb RH, Voci SL, Syed L et al: Randomized prospective study comparing routine versus selective use of sonography of the complete calf in patients with suspected deep venous thrombosis. *Am J Roentgenol* 180:241-245, 2003.

Helsted M, Vilmann P, Jacobsen B, Christoffersen JK: Popliteal venous aneurysms with or without pulmonary embolism. *Eur J Vasc Surg* 5:333-342, 1991.

Kasirajan K, Gray B, Ouriel K: Percutaneous AngioJet thrombectomy in the management of extensive deep venous thrombosis. *J Vasc Interv Radiol* 12:179-185, 2001.

Katz DS, Loud PA, Bruce D et al: Combined CT venography and pulmonary angiography: a comprehensive review. *Radiographics* 22:S3-24, 2002.

Merchant RF, DePalma RG, Kabnick LS: Endovascular obliteration of saphenous reflux: a multicenter trial. *J Vasc Surg* 35:1190-1196, 2002.

Mewissen MW, Seabrook GR, Meissner MH et al: Catheter-directed thrombolysis for lower-extremity deep venous thrombosis: report of a national multicenter registry. *Radiology* 211:39-49, 1999.

Min RJ, Khilnani NM: Lower-extremity varicosities: endoluminal treatment. *Semin Roentgenol* 37:354-360, 2002.

Min RJ, Khilnani N, Zimmet SE: Endovenous laser treatment of saphenous vein reflux: long-term results. *J Vasc Interv Radiol* 14:991-996, 2003.

O'Sullivan GJ, Semba CP, Bittner CA et al: Endovascular management of iliac vein compression (May–Thürner) syndrome. *J Vasc Interv Radiol* 11:823-836, 2000.

Patel NH, Stookey KR, Ketcham DB, Cragg AH: Endovascular management of acute extensive iliofemoral deep venous thrombosis caused by May–Thürner syndrome. *J Vasc Interv Radiol* 11:1297-1302, 2000.

Polak JF, Fox LA: MR assessment of the extremity veins. *Semin Ultrasound CT MR* 20:36-46, 1999.

Porter JM, Moneta GL: Reporting standards in venous disease: an update. *J Vasc Surg* 21:635-645, 1995.

Prandoni P, Bilora F, Marchiori A et al: An association between atherosclerosis and venous thrombosis. *N Engl J Med* 348:1435-1441, 2003.

Rabinov K, Paulin S: Roentgen diagnosis of venous thrombosis in the leg. *Arch Surg* 104:134-144, 1972.

Raju S, Owen S, Neglen P: The clinical impact of iliac venous stents in the management of chronic venous insufficiency. *J Vasc Surg* 35:8-15, 2002.

Ridker PM, Goldhaber SZ, Danielson E et al: Long-term, low-intensity warfarin therapy for the prevention of recurrent venous thromboembolism. *N Engl J Med* 348:1425-1434, 2003.

Roebuck DJ, Howlett DC, Frazer CK, Ayers AB: Pictorial review: the imaging features of lower limb Klippel–Trenaunay syndrome. *Clin Radiol* 49:346-350, 1994.

Rutherford RB, Padberg FT, Comerota AJ et al: Venous severity scoring: an adjunct to venous outcome assessment. *J Vasc Surg* 31:1307-1312, 2000.

CHAPTER 17

Image-guided Percutaneous Biopsy

MICHAEL J. LEE, M.D.

Percutaneous image-guided biopsy has gained wide popularity. It can be used to establish the identity of superficial or deep masses in many parts of the body. Advances in cytopathologic techniques, the ability to precisely guide needles to various locations in the body using CT and sonography, and the safety of fine-needle biopsy, have led to widespread acceptance of biopsy procedures by clinicians. The vast majority of biopsies are performed to confirm suspected malignancy, particularly in a patient with a known primary tumor. In addition, many biopsies are performed in oncologic patients with residual masses after therapy to determine whether such a mass represents residual viable tumor or necrotic tissue.

In the early years of image-guided percutaneous biopsy, most biopsies were obtained with thin needles (20–22 gauge). These needles obtain a cytologic aspirate which is sufficient to confirm or refute a diagnosis of malignancy, but which often is not able to provide a specific histologic diagnosis. More recently, there has been a tendency to use spring-activated cutting needles (biopsy guns) to obtain core biopsies. The advantage of core biopsy needles is that cores of tissues retain the organization of the lesion and often allow precise histologic diagnosis of tumor type if the lesion is malignant, and may confidently allow the diagnosis of benignity if the lesion is benign.

PATIENT PREPARATION

The vast majority of image-guided biopsies can be performed on an outpatient basis. The clinician should obtain routine partial thromboplastin time (PTT), prothrombin time (PT), and platelet levels in all patients undergoing chest or abdominal biopsies or biopsy of any deep-seated lesion. If the lesion to be biopsied is superficial, such as in the neck, coagulation studies are not required, as direct pressure will achieve hemostasis if bleeding occurs. If the patient is receiving a nonsteroidal anti-inflammatory drug such as aspirin, either defer the procedure for 10 days or, depending on where the lesion is, perform a fine-needle biopsy given that the likelihood of bleeding (in the absence of any abnormality in pro-thrombin time, partial thromboplastin time, or platelet count) as a result of aspirin alone is very low. Most biopsies can be performed under local anesthesia without the use of sedo-analgesia. Exceptions include biopsies in pediatric patients and biopsies of deep lesions such as pancreatic masses or retroperitoneal masses. In addition, if the patient is apprehensive, sedo-analgesia may be required. The combination of midazolam and fentanyl is the most advantageous for achieving conscious sedation. A loading dose of 1–2 mg of midazolam with 50–100 μg of fentanyl, given intravenously, is appropriate. Doses can then be titrated against the patient's level of anxiety throughout the procedure. Monitor patients with a pulse oxymeter, and vitacuff for blood pressure measurements. A nurse should monitor the patient during the procedure so that the operator can concentrate solely on the biopsy.

BIOPSY TECHNIQUE

Needle Choice

Fine-needle biopsies are obtained with 20- to 25-gauge needles (Table 17-1 and Fig. 17-1). There are a wide variety of needle types and needle tip designs on the market. Broadly, fine-gauge needles can be divided into those with a sharp beveled tip (e.g., Chiba or spinal needles for simple aspiration) or those with a modified, tissue cutting tip (see Table 17-1). The advantage of using a needle with a cutting tip is that a core of tissue may be obtainable with this needle type. The author's personal preference is the Turner needle for all fine-needle biopsies. Advantages of fine-needle biopsy include the ability to

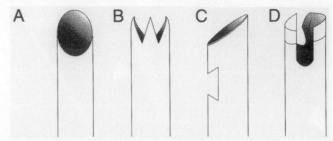

Figure 17-1 Turner (**A**), Franseen (**B**), Westcott (**C**), and E-Z-EM (**D**) needles. The Turner needle has a 45-degree bevel which provides a cutting edge. The Franseen needle has a three-pronged tip. The Westcott needle has a side-cutting trough near its end. The E-Z-EM needle has a trough cut in the tip of the needle. Despite the various appearances of these needles there are no data to suggest any one needle yields consistently better samples. The author tends to predominantly use the Turner needle.

traverse bowel without ill effect, and the likelihood of inducing hemorrhage when sampling vascular lesions is minimal. In the author's practice, fine-needle biopsy is performed on virtually all lung biopsies, all neck biopsies, and in abdominal biopsies where the patient has a known primary with liver or other lesions that are thought to be metastases (Box 17-1).

Large-gauge needle biopsies (14- to 19-gauge) are almost universally performed with a spring-activated, modified trucut system (Box 17-2). There are many of these on the market, of variable gauge, throw length, and design (Fig. 17-2). Most are disposable needle systems, although there are some systems, such as the Bard biopsy gun, which can be used over and over with disposable needles. This is the least expensive option as once the gun is bought only the needles need to be replaced. The author's preference is for a nondisposable biopsy gun and disposable 18- and 20-gauge needles. The advantages in using these devices are: that they are easy to use and can be held with one hand, which is particularly important when biopsies are being performed under ultrasound guidance; and the tissue obtained is of almost uniform consistency in size and amount. This is a major advantage over unautomated large-gauge biopsy

Table 17-1 Fine-gauge Biopsy Needles

Name	Description	Company
Turner	45-degree bevel tip to provide cutting edge	Cook, Bloomington, IN
Franseen	Three-pronged needle tip like "teeth"	Cook, Bloomington, IN
Westcott	Slotted 2.2-mm opening, 3 mm from needle tip	Becton–Dickinson, Rutherford, NJ
E-Z-EM	Trough cut in needle tip	E-Z-EM Inc., Westbury, NY

Box 17-1 Fine-needle Biopsy (20- to 25-gauge)

Proper technique more important than needle type
Can traverse bowel if necessary
CT or sonographic guidance
Nonaspiration technique for vascular lesions
Coaxial or tandem technique can be used
Often sufficient when known primary neoplasm present

Box 17-2 Large-gauge Core Biopsy (14- to 19-gauge)

Spring-activated modified trucut needle preferable
Advantages include ease of use, consistent tissue obtained, decreased pain
Can be inserted in tandem with fine-gauge needle
Must not traverse bowel
Use if lymphoma suspected or failed fine-needle biopsy

systems where the consistency of the tissue obtained is directly related to the operator's skill; because of the automated mechanism used in taking the biopsy, the biopsy procedure is fast and the biopsy needle system does not remain in the patient for long. Anecdotally, this appears to decrease the amount of pain experienced by the patient compared to the conventional large-gauge biopsy systems. In general, large-gauge automated needle biopsies are performed in patients in whom there is no known primary tumor, where there is a possibility of lymphoma, or the biopsy is a repeat after a failed fine-needle biopsy (see Box 17-2).

In recent years this distinction between large-gauge biopsy and fine-needle biopsy has become blurred because of the development of 20-gauge automated trucut needles. These 20-gauge needles are in the "fine needle" category but obtain a core of tissue like any other trucut needle. These needles are now used more and more frequently, particularly where an experienced cytopathologist is not present for the biopsy procedure.

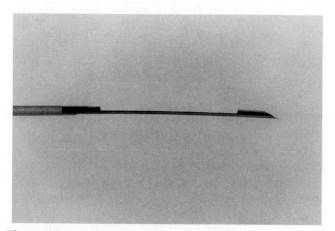

Figure 17-2   Schematic showing the end of an automated trucut needle. A trough is apparent in the end of the needle. A core of tissue which conforms to the length and depth of the trough is obtained when this needle is used. The core of tissue is cut by the outer needle sliding down over the trough and capturing the specimen.

Image Guidance

Computed tomography and sonography are the two main image guidance modalities used for biopsy procedures. Although magnetic resonance interventional systems have arrived in clinical practice, their role in performing routine biopsies is limited by cost and lack of widespread availability. The choice between CT and sonography is largely guided by clinician preference and the nature, size, location, and site of the lesion. All neck and soft tissue lesions, most liver lesions, large abdominal masses, and some pancreatic lesions can be biopsied under sonographic guidance. Mediastinal lesions, most pancreatic, retroperitoneal, adrenal and pelvic lesions, and some liver lesions are biopsied under CT guidance. The relative advantages and disadvantages of CT and sonography are shown in Table 17-2.

Sonography

Where possible, sonography should be used for image guidance because it provides continuous real-time needle visualization. There are many commercially available biopsy guides which can be fitted to existing ultrasound transducers which will direct the needle into the path of the ultrasound beam. The author prefers to use a free-hand approach with the needle inserted through the skin into the plane of the ultrasound beam. The free-hand technique offers more flexibility in that needle position and angle adjustments can be made as the biopsy is being performed to correct or realign the needle path if necessary.

The transducer can be covered with a sterile sheath using sterile KY-jelly as an acoustic coupling agent. Alternatively, the transducer can be sterilized by painting the surface with betadine. The author's unit tends to sterilize the probe without using a sterile cover. The skin is cleansed with betadine and the lesion located in the center of the ultrasound beam. The shortest and safest path to the lesion is chosen. The needle is aligned with the ultrasound beam and inserted through the anesthetized skin and subcutaneous tissues towards the lesion to be biopsied. With proper alignment of the needle within the

Table 17-2 Image Guidance

	CT	Sonography
Continuous needle visualization	No	Yes
Learning curve	Short	Long
Cost	Moderate	Low
Portable	No	Yes
Expediency	Slow	Fast
Ionizing radiation	Yes	No

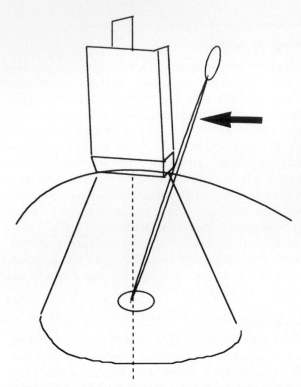

Figure 17-3 Schematic showing correct technique for free-hand ultrasound-guided biopsy. The probe is maneuvered so that the lesion lies in the center of the ultrasound beam. The needle (arrow) is then inserted at the short end of the transducer, and with proper alignment in the ultrasound beam, the entire needle shaft should be visible at all times.

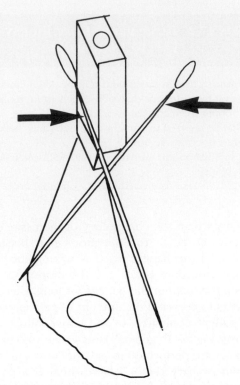

Figure 17-4 Schematic showing incorrect alignment. If the needle (arrows) is inserted at an angle to the direction of the ultrasound beam, the full length of the needle will not be seen and the biopsy will be difficult to perform. Proper alignment of the needle in the plane of the ultrasound beam is mandatory for correct visualization of the needle.

plane of the ultrasound beam, the entire length of the needle shaft should be visualized at all times (Fig. 17-3). If the entire needle is not visible, some malalignment of the needle with the ultrasound beam exists (Fig. 17-4). This can be corrected by rechecking the alignment of the needle with the central beam of the transducer. A slight jiggling or in-and-out motion of the needle will help to visualize the needle (Fig. 17-5). When experience is gained with sonographically guided freehand biopsy methods, this becomes a very rapid and reliable method of guiding biopsy needles to the target in question.

Sonographic guidance can be problematic in obese patients because the echogenic needle can be hard to visualize in the echogenic soft tissues. Obviously, lesions located within bones, or deep to bone or bowel, cannot be biopsied owing to lack of visualization of the lesion.

Computed Tomography

CT can be used to guide biopsy needles to virtually any area of the body. It provides excellent visualization of the lesion to be biopsied and allows accurate identification of organs between the skin and the lesion. CT is

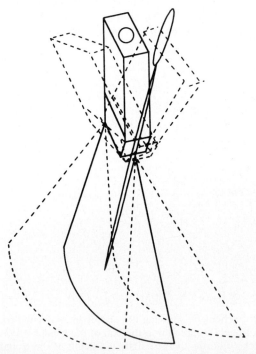

Figure 17-5 Visualization of the needle is aided by a gentle rocking movement of the transducer and a slight to-and-fro jiggling motion of the needle.

particularly suited to guiding biopsy of deep lesions within the body such as retroperitoneal, pelvic, thoracic, and musculoskeletal lesions. The learning curve associated with CT-guided biopsies is generally shorter than that associated with sonographically guided biopsies and it has therefore become a popular guidance modality. Scans through the region of interest are first performed with either a commercially available grid system (EZ-EM, Westbury, NY) or a home-made grid system placed on the patient's skin. Commercially available grid systems contain multiple lead lines constructed in a grid pattern. Alternatively, a home-made phantom can be constructed by taping together approximately ten 15-cm lengths of 4- or 5-French catheters at 1-cm intervals. The home-made grid fulfils the same function as the commercially available systems.

On the CT image that gives the best view of the lesion, a safe access route is chosen and the distance to the lesion marked on the image. The patient is then brought to the table position where the biopsy is to be performed and the skin site marked using the grid on the patient's skin and the centering laser light beam in the CT gantry. The needle is inserted to the predetermined depth and location. Scans are taken at the level of the needle entry site to determine the location of the needle. The tip of the needle is readily recognized by a black streak artifact that occurs at the needle tip (Fig. 17-6). If the needle is not in an appropriate position, further needles can be inserted and scanned (using the first needle as a guide for adjusting the trajectory of further needles) until an appropriate position within the lesion is obtained.

Compared to sonography, the lack of real-time visualization with CT guidance is a limiting factor. The recent

introduction of CT fluoroscopy with helical and multi-slice CT scanners has attempted to redress this balance. However, CT fluoroscopic units will undoubtedly make CT guidance a much more viable – albeit more expensive – option for biopsies.

Performing the Biopsy

Fine-needle Aspiration Biopsy (FNAB)

A 10-mL syringe is applied to the hub of the needle that has been inserted into the lesion, and suction is applied. In general, 3–5 mL of suction is appropriate for most biopsies. If the lesion is vascular, such as a thyroid lesion or some liver lesions, minimal (1–2 mL) suction is appropriate. Larger amounts of suction may cause considerable quantities of blood to be aspirated into the syringe. For more scirrhous lesions such as pancreatic tumors, 5–10 mL of suction may be required. While suction is applied, the needle is moved quite firmly in a to-and-fro motion through the lesion for approximately 10–15 seconds or until blood appears in the hub of the needle. Suction is released while the needle is being removed to prevent aspiration of cells along the needle track that may confuse the cytologic interpretation of the sample. Ideally, a cytologic technician should be available to handle the specimen and a cytopathologist should be in attendance to render a preliminary report. The biopsy procedure can then be guided by the initial cytopathologist's report. If insufficient tissue is available for interpretation, more samples are taken up until a diagnosis is reached. If after four or five samples have been obtained a diagnosis is still not forthcoming, a large-gauge core biopsy sample should be obtained.

Nonaspiration Fine-needle Biopsy

In some situations, it is more advantageous to perform a nonaspiration fine-needle biopsy. The nonaspiration technique is particularly valid for hemorrhagic organs such as the thyroid and occasionally hemorrhagic lesions within the liver. Using the nonaspiration technique, the needle is inserted into the lesion and again multiple to-and-fro motions through the lesion are performed until either blood appears in the hub of the needle or 15 seconds have elapsed. The needle is then removed. No syringe is used in the nonaspiration technique. The hypothesis is that cells advance into the needle lumen by capillary action.

This technique has not found widespread acceptance, although it is useful, in combination with aspiration cytology, for biopsy of thyroid lesions.

Coaxial versus Tandem Technique

Using the coaxial technique, a single needle is placed in the periphery of the lesion and a smaller, longer needle is placed through the initial needle to biopsy

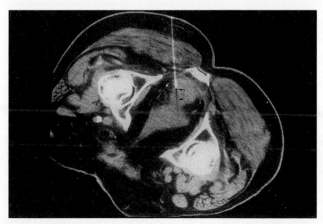

Figure 17-6   CT-guided biopsy of a presacral transgluteal mass illustrating the black streak artefact that occurs when the CT slice passes through the needle tip. A transgluteal approach has been used to biopsy this presacral mass. Streak artifact (arrows) can be seen at the tip of the needle. If this is not visualized, the CT slice has not passed through the needle tip.

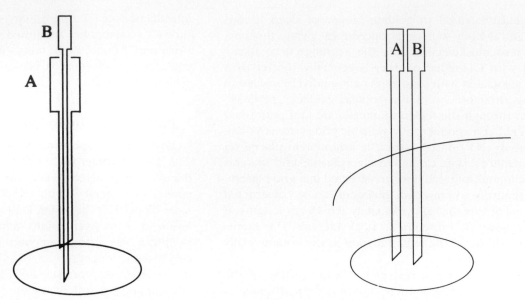

Figure 17-7   Schematic showing (*left*) the coaxial and (*right*) the tandem techniques. For the coaxial technique, a needle (A) is inserted down to the anterior edge of the lesion. A thinner, longer needle (B) is placed through the first needle and samples are taken from the lesion using the insert needle. In this way multiple specimens can be taken from the lesion without making separate punctures. Additionally, the larger needle can be manipulated at the skin so that it points in different directions for sampling different parts of the lesion. Using the tandem technique, a single needle (A) is first guided into the lesion and remains untouched throughout the biopsy. Other needles (B) are inserted in tandem to the first or reference needle (A) to obtain biopsies from the lesion. The subsequent needles do not have to be specifically guided into the lesion, when the first needle is used as a reference.

the lesion (Fig. 17-7). Using the Turner biopsy needle system, a 23-gauge needle will pass through a 20-gauge needle and a 22-gauge through a 19-gauge. The coaxial technique has several advantages in that only one puncture is made into the organ, reducing the propensity for hemorrhage or other complications. Multiple tissue samples can be obtained through the first needle. Lastly, precise needle placement is required only for the first needle.

Using the tandem technique, a 22-gauge needle is placed into the lesion and used as a reference needle (see Fig. 17-7). This reference needle then stays within the lesion until the end of the procedure. Further needles are inserted in tandem to the reference needle and are placed to the same depth and follow the same trajectory as the reference needle. This technique is useful for CT-guided biopsies where multiple fine-needle samples can be obtained without precisely localizing each subsequent needle that is passed.

In the main, the coaxial and tandem techniques are primarily used with CT guidance. With real-time sonographic guidance, the author's unit generally takes a sample with a single needle, and guides subsequent needles into the lesion as required. Because of the flexibility of sonography and continuous real-time visualization, the tandem and coaxial techniques are rarely necessary.

However, they are useful when using CT guidance so that further needle passes do not require precise CT monitoring, which is cumbersome and time consuming.

ABDOMINAL BIOPSY

Liver

Computed tomography or ultrasound can be used to guide liver biopsies, depending on clinician preference. The author prefers to use ultrasound where possible, as it is less cumbersome, is faster, and employs real-time guidance (Fig. 17-8). In experienced hands, ultrasound can be used to biopsy the vast majority of liver lesions. For lesions that are high in the liver, near the diaphragm, the patient is placed in a right anterior oblique position. By scanning obliquely in the intercostal space, it is usually possible to visualize the lesion and guide needles into it (Fig. 17-9). Occasionally, if a lesion near the dome of the diaphragm is not visible by sonography, a transpleural or transpulmonary route under CT guidance may be the only approach possible (Fig. 17-10). When biopsying peripheral lesions on the edge of the liver, it is best to try to traverse some normal liver before entering the lesion. This is particularly true when

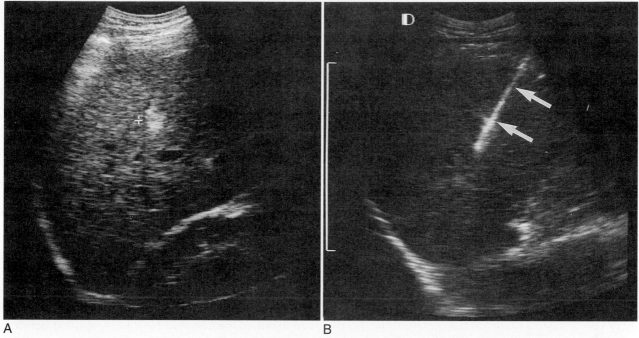

A   B

Figure 17-8   A patient with hepatitis B and a hyperechoic lesion seen on an annual screening ultrasound. **A,** Small (1.5-cm) hyperechoic lesion is seen in the right lobe of the liver. An MR study was performed to exclude the presence of a hemangioma. **B,** Using appropriate free-hand ultrasound technique, the lesion was biopsied using first fine needles and then an 18-gauge automated trucut needle. Note the full length of the needle (arrows) can be seen with appropriate ultrasound technique. This proved to be an area of fibrosis and did not represent a hepatocellular carcinoma.

performing a large-gauge needle biopsy. The rationale behind this practice is that by traversing normal liver first there will be a "safety zone" to tamponade any possible bleeding. In general, when biopsying a liver lesion it is best to biopsy the edge of the lesion; this avoids any potential necrotic areas in the centre of the lesion (Fig. 17-11).

Liver biopsy for diffuse liver disease has become an increasing part of the service provided by interventional radiologists. Traditionally, these biopsies were performed by clinicians without any image guidance. Although generally a safe procedure, complications such as pneumothorax, hemothorax, and indeed failure to obtain liver tissue occurred in patients with slightly abnormal

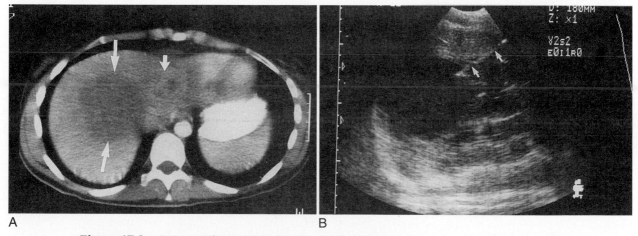

A   B

Figure 17-9   Patient with a previous history of melanoma and lesions present in the liver. **A,** CT scan showing a large lesion (large arrows) high up near the dome of the diaphragm. A smaller lesion is noted in the left lobe (small arrows) of the liver. **B,** Using an intercostal approach with the patient in the right anterior oblique position, the lesion was easily sampled. A 22-gauge needle (arrows) can be seen entering the lesion. The biopsy confirmed a melanoma metastasis.

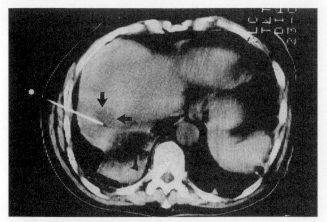

Figure 17-10   Transpulmonary biopsy of a small lesion near the dome of the diaphragm using CT guidance. A solitary lesion (arrows) was seen in this patient with a previous history of cancer. The lesion measured 2.5 cm but could not be seen well with ultrasound. A transpulmonary CT-guided approach was therefore used to biopsy this lesion which proved to be a colorectal metastasis. This approach is rarely used but can be used if there is no other means of obtaining a biopsy specimen.

anatomy. Many interventional radiologists are now performing these biopsies under ultrasound guidance. Most of the biopsies are performed on an outpatient basis. The author's unit uses ultrasound to locate the right lobe of the liver and obtain samples under suspended respiration using 18-gauge automated core biopsy needles. A point in the mid-axillary line is chosen overlying the right lobe of the liver and local anesthetic infiltrated into the skin. The liver capsule is also infiltrated with local anesthetic; this can be painful, and the patient should be warned and asked not to move. Take two 18-gauge samples while the breath is held in expiration.

Tell the patient that some right shoulder tip pain may develop after the procedure (it occurs in about 10-20% of such biopsies).

Pancreas

Pancreatic biopsy can be performed under ultrasound guidance if the lesion is visible. More often than not, the lesion may not be optimally visualized under ultrasound, and CT guidance is used (Fig. 17-12). The stomach is avoided if possible, but if impossible, the stomach can be punctured with 20- or 22-gauge needles to access the pancreas. Many pancreatic cancers are associated with some surrounding pancreatitis, so that on a noncontrast CT scan the tumor may appear larger and biopsy of the area around the tumor may lead to a false negative biopsy. The accuracy of CT-guided pancreatic biopsy can be increased by performing a contrast-enhanced scan before the biopsy to precisely locate and map the tumor.

Pancreatic carcinomas are often very scirrhous and up to 10 mL of suction may have to be applied before cells are obtained. If appropriate specimens are not obtained after three or four passes, a large-gauge core biopsy may be required. This can be performed with the biopty gun or other automated biopsy system. When a fluid-filled pancreatic lesion such as a cystic tumor is encountered, it is vitally important not to transgress the colon with a small-gauge needle en route to the lesion. This may convert a sterile mass into an abscess (Box 17-3).

Kidney

Renal biopsies are performed infrequently as most solid renal masses require surgical removal. Biopsies are performed if there is a suggestion of lymphoma or renal

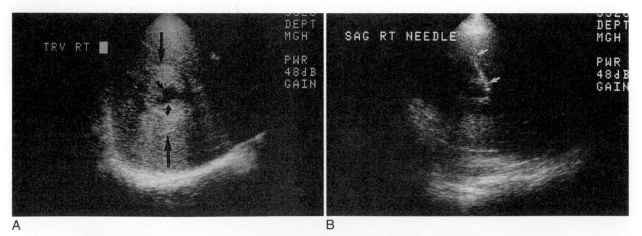

Figure 17-11   Biopsy of a necrotic liver lesion in a patient with colon cancer. **A**, Ultrasound showed a 4-cm lesion (arrows) in the right lobe of the liver. Central necrosis (small arrows) is seen in the center of the lesion. **B**, Biopsy of the edge of the lesion is mandatory in this situation because if the center is biopsied an unrepresentative sample will be obtained. The needle (arrows) can be seen in the edge of the lesion.

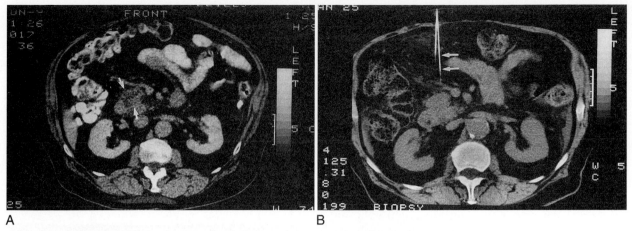

A   B

Figure 17-12   Patient presenting with mild jaundice and a 20-lb weight loss. **A**, Dynamic CT through the head of the pancreas prior to biopsy revealed a small mass (arrows) in the uncinate lobe of the pancreas. **B**, Using the tandem technique, needles (arrows) were placed into the abnormal area and biopsies were performed. The patient proved to have a pancreatic carcinoma.

Box 17-3   Pancreatic Biopsy
Pancreatic Biopsy CT guidance often necessary Stomach avoided if possible Accuracy improved by giving intravenous contrast Maximal suction often necessary Do not traverse colon en route to a cystic lesion

metastatic disease. Complex renal cysts may also occasionally require aspiration. Renal lesions can be biopsied under ultrasound or CT guidance (Fig. 17-13). With ultrasound guidance, either a posterior or posterior oblique approach can be used. With CT guidance, a posterior approach is generally used. In general, core biopsies are needed for renal masses as sufficient tissue to differentiate metastases from primary tumors or to subtype lymphoma is required.

More recently, nephrologic renal cortical biopsies are performed under ultrasound guidance in many centers. Ultrasound guidance is used to obtain core biopsies from both native and transplant kidneys. The lower pole is

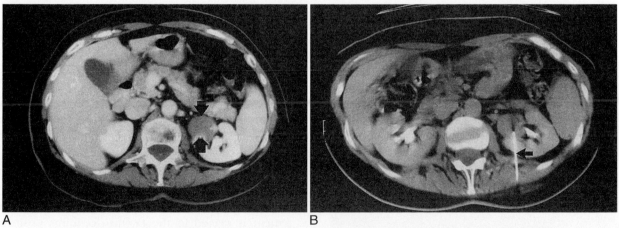

A   B

Figure 17-13   Patient with lymphoma and a renal mass discovered on a routine follow-up CT. **A**, A nonenhancing mass (arrows) was noted on the dynamic CT. The patient was referred for biopsy rather than surgical removal because of the possibility that the mass represented recurrent lymphoma. **B**, A CT-guided biopsy was performed using a posterior approach. A 22-gauge needle (arrow) was inserted into the lesion and used as a reference. Multiple cores where then obtained from the lesion using 18-gauge automated biopsy needles. The lesion proved to be recurrent lymphoma.

chosen for these biopsies and an 18-gauge automated core biopsy needle guided into the lower pole. Biopsies are not performed in hydronephrotic systems, and it is important to avoid the renal hilum with the biopsy needle. Ultrasound guidance for nephrologic biopsy substantially reduces the complication rate when compared to blind biopsy.

Adrenal Glands

The need for adrenal biopsy has fallen dramatically with the recent introduction of lipid-sensitive imaging techniques for differentiating benign from malignant adrenal masses. Because of their position, high up in the retroperitoneum, the adrenal glands can pose problems for biopsy in that a direct posterior approach will often pass through lung.

Adrenal lesions are predominately biopsied under CT guidance, although occasionally, if the adrenal mass is large, ultrasound guidance can be used (Fig. 17-14). There are a number of methods for performing the biopsy under CT guidance. These include the right lateral trans-hepatic approach (see Fig. 17-14) (right adrenal gland), the left anterior transhepatic approach (left adrenal), the angled posterior approach, and the lateral decubitus approach. The right transhepatic and left transhepatic approaches are direct routes to the right and left adrenal glands, respectively. The right transhepatic approach passes through the right lobe of the liver and into the right adrenal gland. The left transhepatic approach passes through the left lobe of the liver and into the left adrenal gland. The patient lies supine on the CT in both approaches. The angled prone approach takes advantage of Pythagoras' theorem to place a needle angled from a subcostal approach into the lesion (Fig. 17-15). The lateral

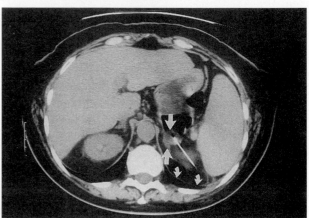

A

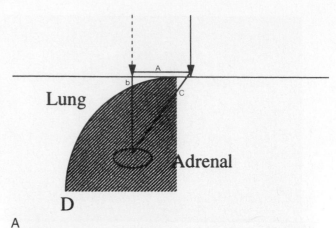

B

Figure 17-15   The angled prone approach to adrenal gland biopsy. **A**, Schematic showing the angled prone approach. (D) represents the diaphragm, the shaded area represents the abdominal cavity and the white area above the diaphragm represents the lung. The broken arrow represents the direct posterior approach to the adrenal lesion. Note that this would pass through lung parenchyma. The solid arrow represents the biopsy site to be used for the angled approach which does not pass through lung parenchyma. Using the angled approach, the distance to the lesion can be calculated by using Pythagoras's theorem. This states that the square of the hypotenuse (C) is equal to the sum of the squares of the other two sides (A, B). This applies only for a right-angled triangle. Knowing distances A and B, the distance to the lesion using the angled approach can be calculated using Pythagoras's theorem. The needle is inserted at a 45-degree angle. **B**, Example of an angled prone approach in this patient with a left adrenal lesion (large arrows). An angled prone approach had to be used because of intervening lung (curved arrows). Note that scans through the lesion using this approach will only show the distal half of the needle. Angling the CT gantry may help to visualize the whole length of the needle.

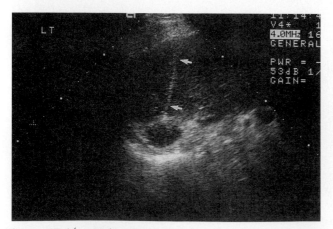

Figure 17-14   Right adrenal mass biopsy using a right lateral transhepatic approach. Under ultrasound guidance the adrenal mass was biopsied using a transhepatic approach. The needle (arrows) can be seen entering the adrenal lesion. The adrenal mass proved to be a small metastasis from a non-small-cell lung cancer.

decubitus approach works on the principle that when a patient is placed in the lateral decubitus position, the underlying lung expands less than the overlying lung. The patient is placed in a lateral decubitus position with the side containing the adrenal lesion placed nearest the table top (Fig. 17-16). A direct posterior approach can then be used, as the intervening lung will usually no

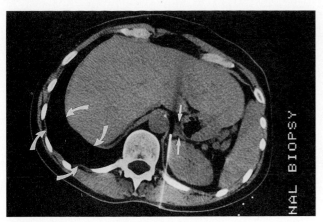

Figure 17-16   Lateral decubitus approach to the adrenal gland. In this patient, using a lateral decubitus position, a direct posterior approach was used to biopsy the adrenal lesion (arrows) because the intervening lung becomes hypovolemic and no longer is in the path of the needle. Note that the uppermost lung has hyper-expanded (curved arrows).

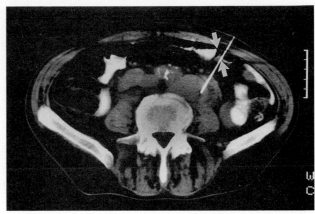

Figure 17-17   CT-guided anterior approach to the retroperitoneum. A lymph node mass was noted at the level of the aortic bifurcation in this patient with cervical cancer. A posterior approach was not possible because the iliac crest and transverse process denied a good access route. An anterior transabdominal approach was used with a 20-gauge needle placed into the lesion for sampling. The needle has passed through a loop of small bowel (arrows). No complications were encountered and the biopsy was positive for metastatic spread from cervical cancer.

longer be present. The lateral decubitus approach is used predominately in the author's unit as it means that a direct posterior approach can be used for adrenal biopsy.

Retroperitoneum

Retroperitoneal masses are generally biopsied under CT guidance. A posterior approach is usually used, passing either through or alongside the psoas muscle. If an anterior approach is used, thin-gauge needles are used because often many structures lie within the path of the needle (Fig. 17-17). Using a posterior approach, large-gauge needles can be used (Fig. 17-18). Occasionally in thin individuals retroperitoneal masses can be visualized with sonography using a posterior approach and the psoas muscle as an acoustic window. It is always worth checking whether the retroperitoneal mass can be seen with sonography. If it is visible, the biopsy can be performed under ultrasound guidance.

Prostate

There has been an explosion in the number of prostate biopsies performed since the introduction of the PSA (prostate-specific antigen) test in the late 1980s. While a level of up to 4 ng/mL is taken to be within normal limits, unfortunately a level greater than 4 ng/mL does not specifically imply cancer. The PSA level rises with benign prostatic hyperplasia (BPH) as well as with cancer, and many older men will have abnormal PSA levels. However, it can be said that the likelihood of cancer increases, the higher the PSA. This is particularly true when the PSA level is greater than 10 ng/mL. To address

the nonspecificity of a raised PSA level, PSA density has been introduced. This entails measuring gland volume and correlating gland volume with the PSA level. This latter measure reflects an attempt to correlate the PSA level with the amount of BPH. Unfortunately, measuring gland volume by transrectal ultrasound is also problematic so that many men end up having prostate biopsies.

There are two methods of performing prostate biopsy: transrectal (Fig. 17-19) and transperineal. Ultrasound guidance using a transrectal probe is used for both; but in the transperineal route the needle is placed through the skin of the perineum, while in the transrectal route the

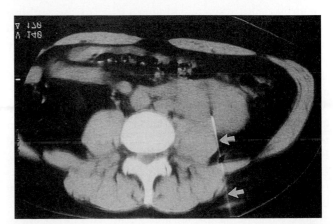

Figure 17-18   A posterior approach was used in this patient with a large retroperitoneal mass which proved to be metastatic cancer. A 20-gauge needle (arrows) is seen within the lesion. Using this needle as a guide, multiple large-gauge core samples were obtained for pathologic analysis.

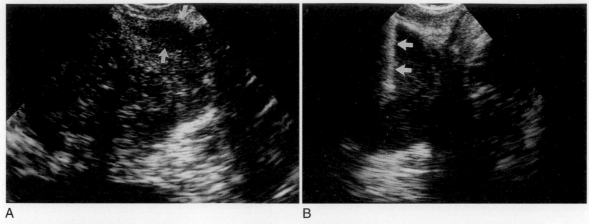

A   B

Figure 17-19 Transrectal ultrasound-guided prostate biopsy. **A**, Transrectal ultrasound of the prostate shows a focal hypoechoic nodule (arrows) in the peripheral gland in this patient with a raised PSA level. **B**, An 18-gauge core biopsy is obtained through the nodule using an automated trucut needle (arrows). Random samples were also taken from other parts of the prostate gland.

needle is passed through the rectal wall. Proponents of the transperineal route claim a lower infection rate. However, the transperineal route is more cumbersome, requires local anesthesia, and takes more time. The author prefers the transrectal route because it is faster, requires no local anesthesia, and with appropriate antibiotic coverage the infection rate is minimal.

Using the transrectal route, either eight or ten quadrant biopsies are performed with an 18-gauge automated needle system. The patient is placed in the decibutus position and the prostate imaged. Hypoechoic lesions in the peripheral gland are biopsied if present, even though only 20–30% of these are malignant. The author's unit uses an end-firing transrectal ultrasound probe. There are many such probes on the market with most of the major ultrasound manufacturers having transrectal ultrasound probes. It is important to biopsy the four quadrants of the prostate to reduce sampling error (in the author's unit we usually do 8–10 biopsies). Biopsies are obtained in the axial plane avoiding the midline area of the prostate where the urethra lies. No local anesthesia is used but all patients receive antibiotic prophylaxis. The antibiotic regimen we use consists of oral ciprofloxacin 500 mg b.i.d. starting the day before the procedure and continuing for 3 days after the procedure (i.e., 5 days in total). The patient also receives 80 mg of gentamycin intramuscularly in the buttock just before the biopsy. Using the latter antibiotic regimen, the author's unit has had only three episodes of sepsis in over 1000 prostate biopsies. The patient is allowed home after the procedure when he has passed some urine. It is important to ask the patient to pass urine before leaving the department to ensure that clot retention which may lead to bladder obstruction does not occur. The patient is instructed to expect hematuria and/or blood in the ejaculate for

24 hours and instructed to return to the emergency room if he is unable to pass urine or develops a fever.

Special Considerations

Biopsy of Pelvic Lesions

Masses in the pelvis can be approached using a variety of different access routes. These include the transrectal and transvaginal routes, which use ultrasound guidance, and the transgluteal approach through the greater sciatic notch and the presacral approach through the gluteal cleft, which use CT guidance. An anterior approach is occasionally possible (Fig. 17-20). The route chosen depends to a large extent on what the clinician

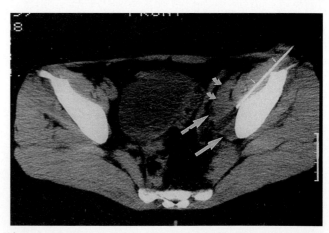

Figure 17-20 Anterior CT-guided biopsy of a pelvic lymph node, using an anterior approach. The lymph node mass (large arrows) is seen adjacent to the external iliac vessels (curved arrows). An anterior approach through the ilioposas muscle was used to avoid the iliac vessels. A needle (short arrows) can be seen parallel with the iliac bone down to the lesion. The lesion proved to be metastatic cancer.

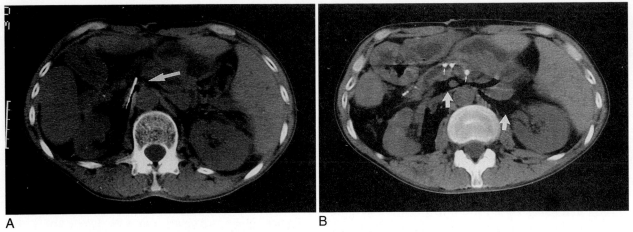

Figure 17-21   CT-guided celiac ganglion to block, in a patient with chronic pancreatitis and severe intractable pain. **A**, A single 20-gauge needle was inserted from a posterior approach and placed close to the celiac axis (arrow). Air was injected to ensure good diffusion throughout the retroperitoneum. **B**, CT section lower down shows the injected air (large arrows) bathing the retroperitoneum. Note the pancreas situated anteriorly with multiple areas of calcification (small arrows). Thirty milliliters of 90% alcohol was injected into the retroperitoneum for celiac ganglion block. The patient had temporary relief of pain but the pain recurred 6 months later.

prefers and is comfortable with. In general, practice at the author's unit has evolved such that we predominantly perform transvaginal and transrectal US-guided biopsy as opposed to transgluteal biopsy.

A transgluteal route was used extensively before transrectal and transvaginal US-guided biopsy became possible. The transgluteal route involves placing the patient prone on the CT table and passing a needle from the buttock through the greater sciatic foramen into the deep pelvis. Care is taken to avoid the sciatic nerve which passes close to the ischial tuberosity. The needle is therefore passed as close as possible to the coccyx.

With the advent of endocavitary ultrasound probes, access to pelvic lesions is now possible via the transvaginal and transrectal routes. Most endocavitary probes have a needle guide through which a needle can be passed into the lesion. When using the transvaginal approach the posterior fornix is infiltrated with local anesthetic and a 20- or 22-gauge needle passed into the lesion. Similarly, the rectal wall can be infiltrated with local anesthetic before passing a needle through the rectal wall. If needed, 18-gauge core samples can be obtained using an automated biopsy device. The access routes for pelvic biopsy are discussed in more detail in Chapter 18.

Celiac Ganglion Block

Celiac ganglion block has traditionally been performed by anesthetists under fluoroscopic guidance. It is a procedure that is ideally suited to CT guidance, as the precise location of the celiac axis, and therefore the celiac ganglia, can be determined. Either one or two

20-gauge needles can be placed on either side of the celiac axis using an anterior or posterior approach. A test injection of air or contrast is performed to ensure that good diffusion of air or contrast occurs around the aorta and bathes the retroperitoneum between the celiac axis and superior mesenteric artery (Fig. 17-21). Twenty to forty milliliters of 95% alcohol is then injected through the needle into the retroperitoneum.

Patients with pancreatic cancer or other malignancies in the upper abdomen respond very well to celiac axis ablation with a 70–80% response rate. Patients with chronic pancreatitis respond less well (50–60% response rate) (Box 17-4).

Lymphoma

Image-guided biopsy of suspected lymphoma deserves special mention. Not only is it necessary to differentiate lymphoma from carcinoma, but it is also necessary to differentiate Hodgkin's from non-Hodgkin's lymphoma and subtype the Hodgkin's or non-Hodgkin's lymphoma. Treatment regimens may differ substantially

---

Box 17-4   Celiac Ganglion Block

CT guidance preferred
One or two needles placed adjacent to celiac axis
20–40 mL of alcohol injected
Patients with pancreatic cancers respond best
Patients with chronic pancreatitis respond less well

depending on the lymphoma subtype. Although it may be possible to subtype lymphomas on fine-needle aspirates alone, it is prudent to take some large-core biopsies if lymphoma is suspected. Two or three 18-gauge core biopsy samples will generally ensure that the cytopathologist has enough tissue to render a diagnosis and to subtype.

Aftercare

Most abdominal biopsies are performed as outpatient procedures. After the procedure is finished the patient is taken to a nursing observation area and vital signs are recorded every 15 minutes for 2 hours in patients who have had fine-needle biopsies and for 3–4 hours in patients who have had a large-gauge needle biopsy. An exception to the latter are patients who have had prostate biopsies, who can leave as soon as they pass urine after the procedure.

All patients are instructed to rest at home after the biopsy and are given an instruction leaflet detailing the procedure performed, symptoms that may herald complications, and contact numbers for the interventional radiology department. If serious problems occur, patients are instructed to go to the nearest emergency department.

Complications of Abdominal Biopsy

Complications related to fine-needle abdominal biopsy are rare. Deaths have been reported in the literature, and mortality rates from three large studies (of 66,397, 10,766, and 16,381 biopsies) showed mortality rates of 0.008%, 0.018%, and 0.031%, respectively. The first two studies were European whilst the third was North American. Deaths in these studies were mostly due to hemorrhage after liver biopsy, while the next major cause of death was pancreatitis after pancreatic biopsy. Anecdotally, it is apparent that biopsy of normal pancreatic tissue dramatically increases the risk of pancreatitis developing. Stated alternatively, it is imperative to be absolutely sure that a pancreatic mass exists before biopsying the pancreas (Fig. 17-22).

With liver biopsy, the complication rate can be reduced by avoiding the biopsy of a hemangioma. Hemangiomas can be characterized with either liver magnetic resonance imaging or nuclear scintigraphy, and the need for biopsy is thus avoided. In addition, superficial liver lesions should not be punctured directly; rather, the needle should be angled obliquely to pass through some normal intervening liver tissue which theoretically should tamponade any bleeding. Other measures to reduce the number of complications from liver biopsy include the correction

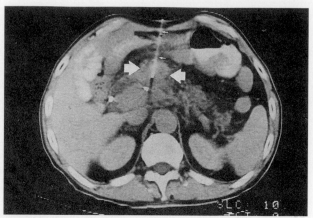

Figure 17-22 CT-guided pancreatic biopsy. This patient had two previous biopsies at another institution for a suspected pancreatic mass. Some peripancreatic inflammation was present at the time the patient underwent another pancreatic biopsy for possible pancreatic tumor. The needle (small arrows) can be seen entering the suspected mass (large arrows) in the pancreas. The biopsy revealed no malignant cells. The patient developed acute severe pancreatitis and remained in hospital for 35 days post-biopsy. The patient eventually made a complete recovery and follow-up imaging revealed no mass in the pancreatic head. It was likely that the initial mass may have represented an area of focal pancreatitis. Note also some areas of calcification in the head of the pancreas which would support this.

of any bleeding diathesis and/or plugging the biopsy track with gelfoam after performing the biopsy in patients with bleeding diathesis. Alternatively in patients with a bleeding diathesis, a transjugular liver biopsy can be performed (Box 17-5).

Abdominal Biopsy Results

Image-guided biopsy has a reported accuracy of 70–100%, depending on the abdominal location biopsied. Accuracy rates in the retroperitoneum tend to be a little lower than in the liver and other locations in the abdomen. This is mainly related to the fact that biopsy of lymphomas in the retroperitoneum decreases the accuracy.

Box 17-5 Steps to Reduce Complications
Avoid biopsying liver hemangiomas
For superficial liver lesions, traverse normal liver parenchyma
Correct bleeding diathesis
Plug the biopsy track with gelfoam if bleeding diathesis, or consider a transjugular liver biopsy
Do not biopsy 'normal' pancreas

CHEST AND MEDIASTINAL BIOPSY

Percutaneous biopsy of the chest is often required for peripheral lung masses or for central masses that have had a negative bronchoscopy. In general, masses that involve lobar or segmental bronchi on chest radiography or computed tomography suggest the presence of an endobronchial component and these nodules are best approached and biopsied at bronchoscopy. Conversely, bronchoscopy is less likely to yield a specific cytologic diagnosis in peripheral nodules and these are best approached percutaneously. Possible metastatic lung lesions are also best approached percutaneously. Occasionally, sufficient tissue can be obtained from a suspected benign nodule to confirm benignity and avoid thoracotomy.

Similarly, mediastinal masses can be biopsied using percutaneous biopsy techniques. Contraindications to thoracic biopsy are relative and include severe chronic obstructive pulmonary disease where pneumothorax may not be well tolerated, bleeding diathesis, and pulmonary hypertension. In general, the therapeutic and prognostic significance of obtaining a diagnosis must be weighed against the patient's condition. The biopsy technique can also be modified to reduce possible complications if any of the above factors are present.

Technique

Patient Preparation

Informed consent is obtained from the patient, and in particular the possible complication of a pneumothorax is discussed. For the vast majority of lung biopsies, intravenous sedation or analgesia is not required. The procedure can be performed safely and without causing patient discomfort under local anesthesia. Occasionally, if the patient is very restless or anxious, a small dose of intravenous midazolam can be given. It is important to enlist the patient's help for the procedure and careful explanation of breathing instructions should be performed and practised.

Image Guidance

Large lung lesions can be biopsied quickly and inexpensively using fluoroscopic guidance. Preferably a fluoroscopic unit with a C-arm should be used so that needle position can be confirmed on both frontal and lateral projections.

Sonography can be used for pleural-based nodules which are often easily visualized with high-frequency 5- or 7-MHz transducers (Fig. 17-23). Sonographically guided biopsy is then performed in a similar fashion to sonographically guided abdominal biopsy. CT is used for all mediastinal biopsies, lesions which are not visible or

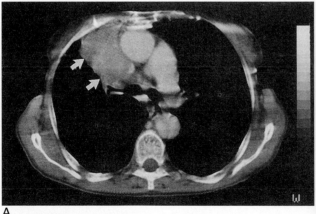

A

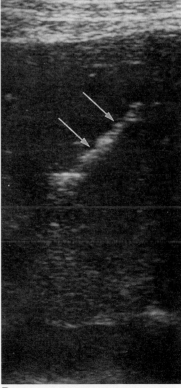

B

Figure 17-23 Ultrasound-guided biopsy of right upper lobe lung mass. **A,** CT scan shows a large right upper-lobe lung mass (arrows) with some associated loss of volume. Because the mass abuts the pleural surface, a US-guided biopsy was performed. **B,** An 18-gauge core biopsy needle was used to obtain a sample from the mass under ultrasound guidance. The needle (arrows) can be seen within the mass. This proved to be a primary lung cancer.

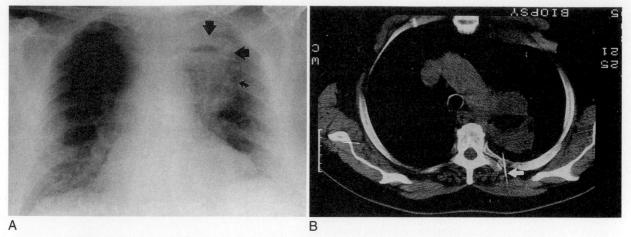

Figure 17-24 CT-guided biopsy of a necrotic lung lesion after two failed fluoroscopically guided biopsies. **A,** Plain chest radiograph showing a cavitating lesion in the left upper lobe (large arrows) with associated hilar adenopathy (curved arrows). Two previous fluoroscopic biopsies failed to obtain representative tissue because only necrotic cells were obtained. **B,** A CT-guided biopsy was performed using a coaxial technique. A 20-gauge needle (arrow) was placed in the periphery of the lesion and 23-gauge needles were used to obtain samples from the posterial wall of the lesion. The lesion proved to be a squamous cell carcinoma.

poorly visible on fluoroscopy, for small lesions less than 1 cm where documentation of needle position in the lesion is required, for fluoroscopically guided biopsies that have failed on at least two occasions, and for large necrotic lesions where biopsy of the wall is mandatory to obtain appropriate cytologic tissue after a failed fluoroscopic biopsy (Fig. 17-24).

Needle Choice

Similar to abdominal biopsy, many of the same fine needles can be used for chest biopsy. The author's preference is the Turner cutting needle (Cook, Bloomington, IN). Many authors prefer the Wescott side-cutting needle for chest biopsy, but there seems little to choose between these needles. For large pleural-based lesions or for mediastinal lesions (especially if lymphoma is suspected), a spring-activated modified trucut 18- or 20-gauge needle biopsy system can be used. The risk of pneumothorax is low for these lesions that abut the pleural surface. In addition, there has been a recent trend towards biopsying more deep-seated pulmonary lesions with 20-gauge spring-activated core biopsy needles. The 20-gauge caliber minimizes the risk of pneumothorax while maximizing tissue gain. At present, the author's unit reserves the option of using 20-gauge core biopsy needles for failed fine-needle biopsies.

Performing the Biopsy

Fluoroscopic Guidance

Generally, the shortest route (that traverses the least number of pleural surfaces) to the lesion is chosen. For lesions in the anterior half of the lung the patient is placed supine, and for lesions in the posterior half of the lung the

patient is placed prone. It is important to identify fissures adjacent to lung lesions, since crossing a fissure means that three pleural surfaces are crossed instead of one. Fluoroscopy is used to identify the lesion to be biopsied and a position on the skin directly over the lesion is marked. The skin is then prepared with betadine and infiltrated with 1% lidocaine. Lidocaine is infiltrated into the soft tissues down to, but not puncturing, the parietal pleura.

The biopsy needle is then inserted and advanced in 2- to 3-cm increments using a sterile forceps, under fluoroscopic guidance, in suspended respiration. When the biopsy needle traverses the parietal pleura the patient will often experience a short-lived painful feeling. The patient should be warned of this beforehand and asked not to move when it happens. The patient is instructed to stop breathing while needle advances are being made. Rather than taking a full inspiration or expiration during which the needle can deviate quite substantially, the patient is instructed to take shallow breaths and not to cough or move during the procedure. As the lesion is entered, there may be increased resistance to advancing the needle, however this is variable and lateral fluoroscopy should be performed to confirm needle position before sampling. If the needle is noted to be deviating away from the lesion, it can be withdrawn and the needle path readjusted. However, it is important not to withdraw the needle through the pleural surface. The risk of pneumothorax is increased by the number of pleural punctures. Therefore, if possible it is important to make as few pleural punctures as possible.

For large lesions (≥ 2.5 cm), the author's unit uses a 22-gauge Turner needle to obtain samples. A 10-mL syringe is attached to the needle hub after the stylet is removed in suspended respiration. With 3–4 mL of suction

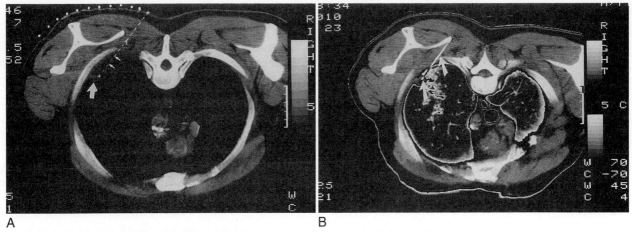

Figure 17-25   Coaxial biopsy for a small peripheral lung lesion. **A,** A 1.5-cm lung lesion (large arrows) is situated posterolaterally, covered by the scapula. A posteromedial approach (small arrows) was used to avoid the scapula. This tangential approach is often better for sampling small peripheral lung lesions than a direct approach. **B,** A 20-gauge needle (arrows) was inserted into the lesion and 23-gauge needles were used to obtain multiple samples from the lesion. The lesion proved to be a small metastatic deposit.

applied, vigorous in–out motions of the needle are performed to obtain a sample. The suction is released and the needle is withdrawn and given to a cytopathologic technician in attendance. One or two drops of the aspirated fluid are smeared on glass slides and the remainder is washed into a solution of formalin. If a cytopathologist is in attendance, an answer can be obtained immediately as to whether or not a second pass is necessary. If a cytopathologist is not in attendance, a second pass with a 22-gauge needle is made for insurance. For smaller lesions (< 2.5 cm), or lesions that are difficult to approach, a coaxial technique can be used. A 20-gauge Turner needle is placed in the superficial edge of the lesion and a longer 23-gauge Turner needle is placed through the 20-gauge needle and samples obtained. The 20-gauge needle is left *in situ* and two or three samples can be obtained with the 23-gauge needle without repuncturing the pleura. Finally a further sample can be taken with the 20-gauge needle before removing it.

CT Guidance

For CT-guided lung biopsies, the coaxial technique (see Fig. 17-7) is preferentially used. Advantages are the fact that the lung parenchyma at the puncture site can be clearly visualized, and structures such as blebs and bullae can be avoided. Additionally, unaerated portions of lung abutting the pleural surface can be visualized and used as an access route to the lesion. This is particularly true of a collapsed or consolidated lung. If an area of unaerated lung is used as an access route to perform the biopsy, a pneumothorax will not occur. In most cases, it is best to use a direct approach to the lesion. The only exception to this is for small peripheral lesions. In this situation it may be difficult to puncture the lesion directly and more than one puncture may be necessary, thus increasing the

risk of pneumothorax. A tangential approach which allows room for needle course adjustment can be used in this situation (Fig. 17-25).

Lidocaine 1% is used to infiltrate the skin and subcutaneous tissues down close to the parietal pleura. The hypodermic needle used for lidocaine administration is then scanned to check needle course alignment with the lesion to be biopsied. The coaxial needle is introduced and inserted in increments of 2–3 cm with suspended respiration.

The needle course can be adjusted by withdrawing the needle to the periphery of the lung (taking care not to withdraw the needle outside the pleura) and adjusting the direction of the needle to puncture the lesion. Needle course adjustment can also be aided by patient inspiration or expiration, depending on the location of the needle in relation to the lesion. Additionally the bevel on the needle can be used to steer the needle somewhat toward the lesion, particularly if small adjustments are necessary. The outer coaxial needle is inserted 2–3 mm into the superficial edge of the lesion to be biopsied so that it has some purchase within the lesion during coaxial biopsies.

When the outer coaxial needle is in position, the insert needle is used to obtain multiple biopsies from the lesion. In the author's unit, a 10-mL syringe is attached to the insert needle and, with one hand holding the coaxial needle, a vigorous to-and-fro motion with the insert needle is used to obtain biopsy specimens (see Fig. 17-25; Box 17-6).

Mediastinal Biopsy

CT guidance is used for all mediastinal biopsies in the author's unit so that vascular structures can be avoided. It is important to perform a contrast-enhanced CT before performing any mediastinal biopsy to ensure that one is not dealing with an aneurysm or other vascular abnormality and to delineate the position of all mediastinal vessels. Anterior mediastinal masses are best approached using an anterior parasternal approach (Fig. 17-26). It is important, too, to avoid the internal mammary artery and vein which course in a parasternal location approximately 1 cm lateral to the sternum. The needle is inserted lateral to the internal mammary artery and vein and angled medially, or occasionally the needle is inserted medial to the internal mammary artery and vein. If necessary, the mediastinum may be widened by an injection of sterile saline. This is usually accomplished by first placing a 22-gauge needle into the anterior mediastinal fat and injecting saline to distend the anterior mediastinum. With the mediastinum distended, large-gauge cutting needles can be inserted into the anterior mediastinum without crossing adjacent lung parenchyma.

For masses in the posterior mediastinum and carinal area, a paravertebral approach can be used. The paravertebral space can be distended by inserting a 22-gauge needle into the paravertebral space and distending this

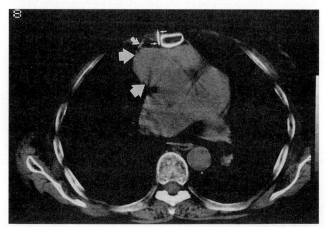

Figure 17-26   CT-guided mediastinal mass biopsy. A patient presented with an anterior mediastinal mass (large arrows) thought to be consistent with lymphoma. A dynamic CT scan was first performed to delineate the position of all vessels in the mediastinum. An anterior mediastinal approach was used. A 20-gauge needle was used as a reference (small arrows). The internal mammary artery and vein (curved arrow) were avoided using this approach. Multiple 20-gauge core samples were obtained with an automated needle system placed in tandem to the initial 20-gauge reference. The mass proved to be a non-Hodgkin's lymphoma.

with isotonic saline. In this way, large-gauge needles can be placed into the posterior mediastinum without crossing lung parenchyma.

Aftercare and Complications

Place the patient in the puncture-site-down position with the biopsied site dependent for 2 hours. The puncture-site-down position helps to decease the amount of air leakage at the biopsy site because the weight of the lung itself helps to oppose the two pleural layers. After 2 hours an erect chest x-ray is obtained. If no pneumothorax is present at this time, the patient is discharged. If a small pneumothorax is present at 2 hours and the patient is asymptomatic, a further chest x-ray is taken at 4 hours. If the pneumothorax has resolved, the patient is discharged. If the pneumothorax is small and remains stable, the patient is discharged but must return the next day for a further chest radiograph. If the pneumothorax is moderate or large, or if the patient is symptomatic, the patient is admitted to hospital and the pneumothorax treated. Depending on the size of the pneumothorax and the patient's symptoms, treatment can consist of simple aspiration, insertion of a small-gauge pneumothorax catheter and Heimlich valve, or insertion of a catheter with connection to an underwater seal. In the author's unit, simple aspiration with an 18-gauge cannula inserted into the second intercostal space is usually attempted first. If the pneumothorax recurs or symptoms deteriorate, a chest tube is inserted and connected to an underwater seal.

Pulmonary hemorrhage with or without hemoptysis rarely causes problems. For minor amounts of hemoptysis, patient reassurance is all that is necessary. If hemoptysis is moderate, the patient can be placed in the lateral decubitus position with the biopsied lung dependent to prevent aspiration of blood into the contralateral lung. The hemoptysis usually subsides within a few hours.

Air embolism is a rare complication of thoracic fine-needle aspiration biopsy (FNAB). Air embolism results when there is communication between a pulmonary vein and atmospheric air. Air embolism may be facilitated by leaving the needle open to the air while the needle is in the chest, or by deep breathing or coughing by the patient. Treatment includes administration of 100% oxygen, placing the patient in the left lateral decubitus position, with the head down (to prevent cerebral air embolism), and/or transfer to a hyperbaric unit.

Results

Sensitivity of FNAB for diagnosing neoplastic lung lesions ranges from 70 to 97%. A negative result often leads to a repeat biopsy, with positive results being obtained in as many as 35–45% of patients undergoing repeat biopsies.

In addition, the sensitivity of FNAB in determining cell type in primary bronchogenic carcinoma is high. Correlation between the FNAB, cytologic diagnosis, and eventual histologic diagnosis varies between 80 and 90%.

NECK BIOPSY

Sonographically guided needle biopsy of thyroid nodules, cervical lymph nodes, and parathyroid glands is a highly accurate (90–100% accuracy) and safe technique for differentiating benign from malignant conditions. High-frequency (7–10 MHz) transducers are required and biopsies are performed using 22- to 25-gauge hypodermic needles. The author finds that it is best to lie the patient supine on a stretcher with the neck extended. The operator sits on a chair at the head of the patient's stretcher facing the ultrasound monitor, which is placed as near as possible to the operator (Fig. 17-27). Using this setup you can perform the biopsy and watch the ultrasound monitor more easily than in other positions.

Hypodermic needles are preferred for neck biopsy as they pass through tissues easily and cause less patient discomfort in the neck. Because the thyroid is a vascular organ, minimal amounts of suction are applied to the needle to obtain samples. Alternatively, samples can be

taken without using any suction using the nonsuction technique. The author's practice is to take a sample with a 25-gauge needle (Becton–Dickinson, Rutherford, NJ) using the suction technique, and then to take a second sample using the nonsuction technique. Usually, core needles are not required for biopsying neck lesions.

Cervical lymph nodes smaller than 1 cm can be biopsied using sonographic guidance (Fig. 17-28). In patients with previous thyroid cancer, it is useful to send samples for markers of thyroid cancer as well as for cytologic analysis. If the patient has a previous history of papillary

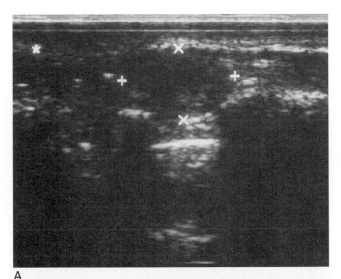

A

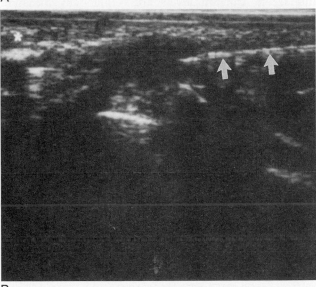

B

Figure 17-28 Ultrasound-guided neck lymph node biopsy in a patient with previous partial thyroidectomy for papillary thyroid cancer. **A**, Follow-up sonogram 2 years after surgery showed a 1-cm lymph node in the neck. **B**, Biopsy was performed using a 25-gauge hypodermic needle and ultrasound guidance with a 7-MHz probe. The needle (arrows) can be seen entering the lymph node and a diagnosis of recurrent papillary cancer was made.

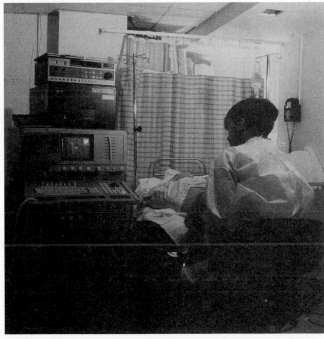

Figure 17-27 Room setup for neck biopsy. Room setup is important for facilitating appropriate ultrasound-guided neck biopsy. The patient lies supine on the stretcher with the neck hyperextended and feet towards the US machine. The operator sits at the patient's head facing the US monitor. An assistant is required to work the US machine. In this way, the biopsy procedure can be performed more easily than with other room arrangements.

or follicular cancer, a sample can be sent for thyroglobulin analysis. If the patient has a history of medullary cancer, a sample can be sent for calcitonin evaluation. The needle used to take the cytology sample is simply rinsed with 1 mL of saline into a sterile tube and sent to the endocrine laboratory for calcitonin or thyroglobulin analysis. In patients with metastatic lymph nodes, the thyroglobulin will be dramatically elevated if the patient had a previous history of papillary or follicular cancer, and calcitonin is dramatically elevated in patients with prior histories of medullary carcinoma. This is a useful method of differentiating benign from malignant lymph nodes if cytology is unhelpful.

In patients with hyperparathyroidism secondary to a parathyroid adenoma, the adenoma can be ablated under ultrasound guidance using 95% alcohol. Depending on the size of the parathyroid adenoma, a small (1–2 mL) volume of absolute ethanol is injected into the gland under sonographic visualization. Parathyroid hormone and serum calcium levels are sequentially measured after ablation. This is a useful technique for managing hyperparathyroidism in patients who are unfit for surgery (Box 17-7).

SUGGESTED READINGS

Bernardino ME: Automated biopsy devices: significance and safety. *Radiology* 176:615–616, 1990.

Bernardino ME: Percutaneous biopsy. *Am J Roentgenol* 142:41–45, 1984.

Brandt KR, Charboneau JW, Stephens DH et al: CT- and US-guided biopsy of the pancreas. *Radiology* 187:99–104, 1993.

Bernardino ME, McClellan WM, Phillips VM et al: CT-guided adrenal biopsy: accuracy, safety and indications. *Am J Roentgenol* 144:67–69, 1985.

Boland GW, Lee MJ, Mueller PR et al: Efficacy of sonographically guided biopsy of thyroid masses and cervical lymph nodes. *Am J Roentgenol* 161:1053–1056, 1993.

Charboneau JW, Reading CC, Welch TJ: CT- and sonographically guided needle biopsy: current techniques and new innovations. *Am J Roentgenol* 154:1–10, 1990.

Fornari F, Civardi G, Cavanna L et al: Complications of ultrasonically guided fine-needle abdominal biopsy: results of a multicenter Italian study and review of the literature. *Scand J Gastroenterol* 24:949—955, 1989.

Kattapuram SV, Rosenthal DI: Percutaneous biopsy of skeletal lesions. *Am J Roentgenol* 157:935–942, 1991.

Kinney TB, Lee MJ, Filomena CA et al: Fine-needle biopsy: prospective comparison of aspiration versus nonaspiration techniques in the abdomen. *Radiology* 186:549–552, 1993.

Lee MJ, Hahn PF, Papanicolaou NP et al: Benign and malignant adrenal masses: CT distinction with attenuation coefficients, size and observer analysis. *Radiology* 179:415–418, 1991.

Lee MJ, Mueller PR, vanSonnenberg E et al: CT-guided celiac ganglion block with alcohol. *Am J Roentgenol* 161:633–636, 1993.

Lee MJ, Ross DS, Mueller PR et al: Fine-needle biopsy of cervical lymph nodes in patients with thyroid cancer: a prospective comparison of cytopathologic and tissue marker analysis. *Radiology* 187:851–854, 1993.

Lee MJ, Mueller PR, Dawson SL et al: Measurement of tissue carcinoembryonic antigen levels from fine-needle biopsy specimens: technique and clinical usefulness. *Radiology* 184:717–720, 1992.

Livraghi T, Damascelli B, Lombard C, Spagnoli I: Risk in fine needle abdominal biopsy. *J Clin Ultrasound* 11:77–81, 1983.

McNicholas MJ, Lee MJ, Mayo-Smith WW et al: An imaging algorithm for the differential diagnosis of adrenal adenomas and metastases. *Am J Roentgenol* 165:1453–1459, 1995.

Moore EH: Technical aspects of needle aspiration lung biopsy: a personal perspective. *Radiology* 208: 303–318, 1998.

Shepard JO: Complications of percutaneous needle aspiration biopsy of the chest: prevention and management. *Semin Interv Radiol* 11(3):181–186, 1994.

Silverman SG, Mueller PR, Pfister RC: Hemostatic evaluation before abdominal interventions: an overview and proposal. *Am J Roentgenol* 233–238, 1990.

Silverman SG, Mueller PR, Pinkney LP et al: Predictive value of image-guided biopsy: analysis of results of 101 biopsies. *Radiology* 187:715–718, 1993.

Silverman SG, Lee BY, Mueller PR, Cibas ES, Seltzer SE: Impact of positive findings at image-guided biopsy of lymphoma on patient care: evaluation of clinical history, needle size and pathological findings on biopsy performance. *Radiology* 190:759–764, 1994.

Smith ED: Complications of percutaneous abdominal fine-needle biopsy. *Radiology* 178:253–258, 1991.

Weisbrod GL: Transthoracic percutaneous fine-needle aspiration biopsy in the chest and mediastinum. *Semin Interv* 8(1):114, 1991.

Weisbrod GL: Transthoracic percutaneous lung biopsy. *Radiol Clin N Am* 28:647–655, 1990.

Weiss H, Duntsch U, Weiss A: Risiken der feinnadelpunktion: ergebnisse einer umfrage in der BRD (DEGUM-Umfrage). *Ultraschall Med* 9:121–127, 1988.

Welch TJ, Sheedy PF, Johnson CD et al: CT-guided biopsy: prospective analysis of 1000 procedures. *Radiology* 171:493–496, 1989.

CHAPTER 18

Percutaneous Abscess and Fluid Drainage

MICHAEL J. LEE, M.D.

Percutaneous drainage is now the accepted technique for draining abscesses in most body locations. This situation has evolved over the last ten to fifteen years because of precise imaging localization of fluid collections, improved methods of percutaneous drainage, and improved antibiotic regimens. Initially, percutaneous abscess drainage (PAD) was reserved for those collections that were unilocular with a clear access route and without evidence of fistulous communication. This situation has completely changed over the last 10–15 years and it is now the procedure of choice for drainage of a wide number of more complicated abscesses including multilocular collections, abscesses with fistulous communications, pancreatic abscesses, hematomas, enteric abscesses, splenic abscesses, and abscesses in difficult anatomic locations such as in the deep pelvis and subdiaphragmatic areas. Lung abscesses, mediastinal abscesses and pleural empyemas are also amenable to percutaneous drainage.

Indeed, percutaneous abscess drainage is one of the major minimally invasive advances in patient management. When compared with surgical exploration, particularly in critically ill patients or in postoperative patients, the rapid imaging localization and percutaneous treatment of abscesses has played a major role in decreasing the morbidity and mortality associated with surgical exploration. Additionally, the role of the interventional radiologist in treating these patients is extremely gratifying, in that patients usually recover quite quickly as soon as the infected material has been drained.

ABDOMINAL FLUID COLLECTIONS

Patient Preparation

Any correctable abnormalities such as coagulopathies and fluid electrolyte imbalances should be corrected prior to abscess drainage. The patient should receive prophylactic intravenous antibiotics as determined by blood culture results. If blood cultures are negative, then an appropriate broad-spectrum antibiotic regimen such as gentamycin, ampicillin, and metronidazole (or any other appropriate broad-spectrum coverage, recommended by your local infectious disease personnel) should be used.

Detection and Localization

Without doubt, computed tomography (CT) is the most appropriate modality for the detection and localization of intra-abdominal fluid collections. Sonography may be helpful in detecting upper abdominal collections such as subdiaphragmatic collections, paracolic collections, or collections in solid viscera such as the liver and spleen. However, ultrasound suffers from its inability to penetrate gaseous interfaces. This is a particular problem in patients with intra-abdominal abscesses as many will have an associated ileus. Naturally, this is particularly problematic in the postoperative patient. CT is therefore the preferred imaging modality for the identification of intra-abdominal abscesses. The other advantage of CT is that an appropriate access route can be planned because all of the adjacent organs can be visualized.

One of the disadvantages of CT is that loculation may be difficult to visualize on CT scans, as often the septa are of the same density as the adjacent fluid and cannot be seen. Septation and loculation are much more easily identified by sonography. It is important also that patients have appropriate bowel opacification with gastrograffin where possible. This is important because unopacified bowel may be difficult to differentiate from an abdominal abscess. Additionally, appropriate bowel opacification is necessary for planning the access route to make sure that small or large bowel is not traversed with a catheter when draining the abscess.

It is important to realise that neither sonography nor CT can predict whether a collection is infected or uninfected (unless there is air present). Collections have to be sampled and Gram stain and culture obtained before this determination can be made (Box 18-1).

For pleural space collections, plain films and sonography are often sufficient to demonstrate the entire fluid collection. With multiloculated empyemas, mediastinal abscesses, and lung abscesses, CT is necessary for full delineation of the abscess cavity.

Technique

Catheter Types

There are various catheters available for drainage. These include sump designs and nonsump designs. Sump catheters have double lumens and are particularly suited for intra-abdominal abscesses. The outer lumen in the sump catheter is designed to prevent side-holes from becoming blocked when the catheter is adjacent to the wall of an abscess cavity. Twelve- to 14-French sump catheters are suitable for most intra-abdominal abscesses (Boston Scientific, Natick, MA) (Fig. 18-1). Larger (16- to 28-French)

Box 18-1   Abscess Detection

CT is the preferred imaging modality
Appropriate bowel opacification is mandatory
Sonography can be useful for solid-organ abscess
  detection
Sonography is best for identification of loculation
Imaging cannot predict whether a collection is infected
  or uninfected

catheters will be required in specific circumstances such as for pancreatic abscesses, hematomas, or where the abscess cavity contents are extremely viscous (see Fig. 18-1). Nonsump catheters are used in the chest. Generally these catheters have large side-holes to permit appropriate drainage. Catheters inserted in the chest also tend to be larger (16- to 30-French) because kinking occurs commonly with smaller catheters because of respiratory excursion which compresses the catheter against adjacent ribs.

Locking pigtail catheters (8- to 10-French) are used in specific circumstances such as when draining lymphoceles and seromas, or when draining deep pelvic abscesses transrectally or transvaginally. It is important to use locking catheters when using the transvaginal or transrectal route as any abdominal straining may dislodge a nonlocking catheter.

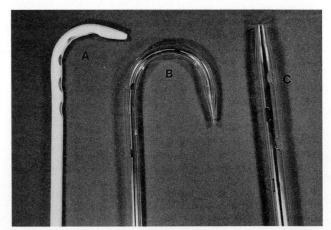

Figure 18-1   Various catheters used for abscess drainage. **A**, 14-Fr sump catheter (Boston Scientific, Natick, MA). **B**, 16-Fr nonsump catheter (Cook, Bloomington, IL). **C**, 24-Fr nonsump drainage catheter (Cook, Bloomington, IL). The sump catheter comes in 12- or 14-Fr sizes and is the predominant catheter used by the author for abdominal abscess drainage. The 16- and 24-Fr catheters are used for empyema drainage and for abscesses in the abdomen that need larger catheters placed.

Image Guidance

The decision whether to drain an abscess under ultrasound or CT guidance is based largely on the location of the abscess, the size of the abscess, and operator preference. Most pleural fluid collections or empyemas can be drained under ultrasound guidance, as can hepatic abscesses, subphrenic abscesses, paracolic abscesses, and some of the larger, more central intra-abdominal collections. However, from a practical point of view many abdominal abscesses are detected by CT scanning and therefore it is often easier to drain the abscess under CT guidance at the time of diagnosis. In addition, some abscesses absolutely require CT guidance, such as retroperitoneal and iliopsoas abscesses, deeply located abscesses, small abscesses, or abscesses which are not visible by ultrasound.

Diagnostic Fluid Aspiration

Diagnostic fluid aspiration is often requested to determine whether a fluid collection detected by either CT or sonography is infected or uninfected. It is important to plan the access route carefully so that bowel is not transgressed en route to the collection. This is to ensure that a potentially sterile collection is not contaminated by a diagnostic aspiration. Generally a 20-gauge needle is used for diagnostic aspiration. This can be performed under ultrasound or CT guidance, provided a safe access route is visible. Two to three milliliters of fluid are aspirated and specimens sent to the bacteriology laboratory for Gram stain and culture. If fluid cannot be obtained with a 20-gauge needle, an 18-gauge needle is placed in tandem to the 20-gauge needle into the fluid collection. Failure to aspirate fluid through this 18-guage needle usually means that the cavity contents are very viscous. Fluid can usually be aspirated in small amounts if rapid to-and-fro motions with the 18-gauge needle are performed. Alternatively, 1–2 mL of sterile saline can be injected into the cavity and reaspirated for the purpose of Gram stain and culture.

If the sample obtained is pus, a catheter should be placed straight away. If the specimen obtained is not pus and it is unclear whether it is infected or not, either wait for the result of the Gram stain or place a catheter. Some interventional radiologists prefer to wait for the result of the Gram stain. It is the practice in the author's unit to place a drain in the vast majority of abdominal collections, particularly if the patient is sick and has a high fever. One can then await the result of the Gram stain and culture. If these are negative, the catheter can be removed after 48 hours (Box 18-2).

It is important for the interventional radiologist to be able to interpret Gram stain results because the result may directly affect decision making. A Gram stain that has abundant bacteria and white cells indicates an abscess. A stain that yields bacteria without white cells may be consistent with colonic contents. The CT scan

Box 18-2 Diagnostic Fluid Aspiration

Do not transgress colon
18-gauge needle if no fluid obtained with 20-gauge
Inject and reaspirate saline if no fluid with 18-gauge needle
If pus obtained, place a catheter

should be reviewed to confirm that the suspected abnormality does represent an abscess and not unopacified colon and that the aspiration needle did not traverse the colon. Alternatively, it may mean that the patient is immunnocompromised and cannot mount a leukocyte response. It is not uncommon, with the modern use of antibiotics, that a Gram stain may show white cells without bacteria, indicating a so-called sterile abscess. These collections should however be drained (Box 18-3).

Drainage Procedure

It is now routine to perform the drainage procedure under either ultrasound or CT guidance at the initial time of localization of the intra-abdominal fluid collection. An appropriate access route is chosen that allows a clear route to the collection without passing through adjacent structures.

There are two basic methods of draining an abscess or fluid collection. In the first of these, the Seldinger technique is used. An 18-gauge long-dwell sheath is placed in the cavity and a 0.038-inch guide wire is coiled within the cavity. Alternatively, a one-stick system using a 22-gauge needle and 0.018-inch guidewire can be used (Neff set, Cook, Bloomington, IN). The track is dilated with fascial dilators to two French sizes larger than the catheter to be placed. The catheter is then inserted over a stiff guidewire into the collection. It is important to coil the catheter within the collection so that all of the sideholes are within the collection. Initially, when using the Seldinger technique the needle, long-dwell sheath, and wire were placed into the abscess cavity under CT or ultrasound guidance and then the patient was moved to fluoroscopy to complete the procedure. When experience is gained, it is possible to perform the entire

Box 18-3 Gram Stain Interpretation

Abundant bacteria and white cells indicates an abscess
Bacteria without white cells indicates immunocompromise or needle through colon
White cells without bacteria indicates a sterile abscess

procedure under CT or ultrasound guidance. However, the Seldinger technique can be a relatively blind procedure without using fluoroscopy, and for this reason the author prefers to use the trocar technique where possible.

The tocar technique (Fig. 18-2) consists of placing a reference needle into the abscess cavity. A catheter with a sharp stylet is inserted alongside the localizing needle into the collection in a single stab. It is important to leave the reference needle *in situ*, as the catheter can be directed along the exact trajectory of the localizing needle. Adequate dissection of the skin and subcutaneous tissues with a standard surgical forceps is necessary for this procedure. You will usually feel a "give" when the

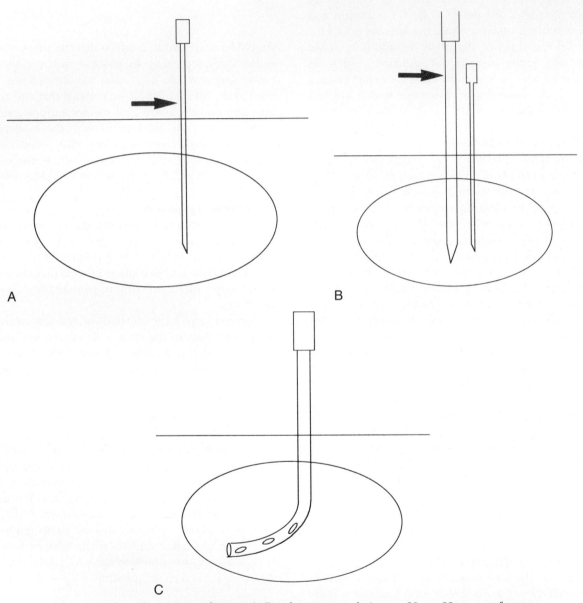

Figure 18-2 The trocar technique. **A,** For the trocar technique a 20- or 22-gauge reference needle (arrow) is placed into the abscess after first planning an appropriate access route. The abscess is reimaged to confirm the location of the needle within the abscess cavity and fluid aspirated for Gram stain and culture. **B,** The catheter to be placed (arrow) is then trocared into the cavity alongside the reference needle. Adequate skin dissection with a sterile forceps must be performed before catheter insertion. When the abscess cavity is entered a "give" will be felt. Confirmation that the catheter is in the abscess cavity can be obtained by withdrawing the stylet and aspirating pus. **C,** After confirming that the catheter is in the abscess cavity, the catheter is pushed forward into the cavity while withdrawing the trocar. The reference needle is then removed. The abscess cavity is completely aspirated and irrigated with normal saline until the aspirate comes back clear. At the end of the procedure the abscess cavity is reimaged to ensure that there are no undrained areas or loculations.

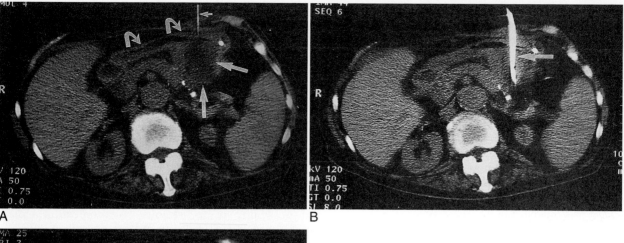

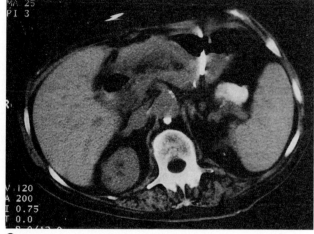

Figure 18-3   Trocar technique example. **A,** Patient with a pancreatic abscess (large arrows) referred for percutaneous drainage. The 20-gauge reference needle (small arrow) can be seen passing through the stomach (curved arrows) and into the abscess. Pus aspirated confirmed the location of the tip of the needle in the abscess. **B,** A 12-Fr sump catheter (arrow) was trocared into the abscess cavity alongside the needle and the needle then removed. This image was obtained after aspiration of the cavity contents. The cavity is now collapsed. **C,** Further CT scan 4 days later shows no residual abscess cavity. The drainage through the catheter was less than 10 mL per day and the catheter was removed.

cavity is entered. Once the catheter is felt to be in place, the central stylet is removed and the catheter aspirated to confirm that the catheter is in the cavity. Once pus or fluid is aspirated, the catheter can be coiled in the cavity by disengaging and withdrawing the trocar and pushing the catheter forward (Fig. 18-3).

When the catheter is secure within the cavity, the cavity contents are completely aspirated. This is best performed using a closed system with a three-way stopcock and drainage bag. In this way the cavity contents can be completely aspirated and drained into the drainage bag. When the cavity is completely aspirated, the cavity is irrigated with sterile saline until the aspirate returns clear. This is to ensure that most of the debris and more viscous contents, if present, will also be drained.

There are many available methods for securing the catheter to the skin, ranging from simply suturing the catheter to the skin, to using commercially available catheter fixation devices. The author's unit uses an ostomy disk (Hollister) placed on the skin over the catheter (Fig. 18-4). A piece of tape is placed round the

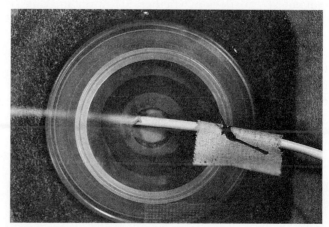

Figure 18-4   Catheter fixation. In this example, the tape placed around the catheter can be seen sutured to a Hollister ostomy disc with a 3/0 silk suture. The ostomy disc is fixed to the patient's skin at the catheter exit site.

catheter and the tape is then sutured to the ostomy disk. This system works quite well for catheter fixation, and if there is any pericatheter leakage the ostomy disk usually protects the surrounding skin. If ostomy disks are not available, the tape placed around the catheter can be sutured directly to the patient's skin or one of the commercially available fixation devices can be used.

It is imperative to repeat the imaging after evacuation of the cavity contents to make sure that the cavity is completely evacuated and that there is not another loculation present. If there is an undrained area, placement of a second or more catheters to completely drain the abscess cavity will be required because the patient will not defervesce if pus is left behind (Box 18-4).

Aftercare

It is vitally important that the interventional radiologist becomes actively involved in patient management when a drainage catheter is placed. It is not acceptable to place a catheter and abdicate on the clinical responsibility of looking after the catheter and the patient's abscess. Respect by clinical colleagues is also gained by this approach and increased referrals to the interventional radiology service usually ensues. Interventional radiologists are the best people to look after abscess drainage catheters as they have usually inserted the catheter and know most about the abscess type, size, consistency of the fluid content, and loculation. It is mandatory that daily ward rounds are made on each patient with an indwelling catheter. During these ward rounds, the skin site, catheter and connections, the amount of drainage, clinical wellbeing, changes in white cell count, and fever are assessed. With daily ward rounds and careful observation, the interventional radiologist can decide whether follow-up imaging or intervention is required, and when the catheter should be removed.

Virtually all catheters are left to gravity drainage on the ward and fluid output is recorded by the nursing staff. It is important that the catheter be irrigated 3-4 times daily, with 10-mL aliquots of sterile saline to prevent clogging. This is usually performed by the nursing staff, but if there is any question of catheter patency, the catheter should be irrigated by the interventional radiologist on ward rounds to ensure patency.

The endpoint of catheter drainage is dependent on a number of factors. Primarily these are clinical factors such as clinical wellbeing, defervescence, reduction in white cell count, and decreased catheter drainage to less than 10-15 mL per day. It is not necessary to perform follow-up imaging on simple collections, particularly if the patient is recovering. Imaging endpoints include disappearance of the collection on repeat imaging and/or a reduction in size of the cavity on a contrast abcessogram. In general, abscessograms are rarely performed unless the possibility of a fistulous communication exists. Resumption of appetite is another good clinical criterion for successful drainage. When some or all of these criteria are met, the catheter is withdrawn. Usually for simple collections that drain quickly and successfully, the catheter can be simply removed. For more complicated abscesses or those that take longer to resolve, the catheter is best withdrawn over a number of days, as with surgical drains. It is always preferable to do this than have to redrain the abscess (Box 18-5).

Specific Abscess Drainages

Enteric Abscesses

Abscesses complicating appendicitis, diverticulitis, or Crohn disease are referred to as enteric abscesses. A complicating abscess in these conditions makes immediate surgery extremely difficult and may make multistage surgery, with its associated cost and discomfort, a reality for these patients. In these circumstances, percutaneous drainage, in combination with appropriate antibiotic therapy, can be used to effectively drain the abscess and resolve sepsis. Elective one-stage surgery can then be performed at an appropriate interval after resolution of sepsis.

Drainage of diverticular abscesses can often avoid two- or three-stage surgery and convert the surgical procedure to an elective one-stage operation. The three-stage operation was in use before the general availability

---

Box 18-4 Draining an Abscess

Plan access route to avoid intervening organs
Seldinger or trocar technique used
Aspirate cavity and irrigate with saline until aspirate
  is clear
Repeat imaging to ensure no undrained locules

Box 18-5 Endpoints for Catheter Removal

Improvement in clinical wellbeing and resumption of
  appetite
Defervescence and normalization of white cell count
Catheter drainage <10-15 ml daily
Disappearance or reduction in size of collection on
  repeat imaging

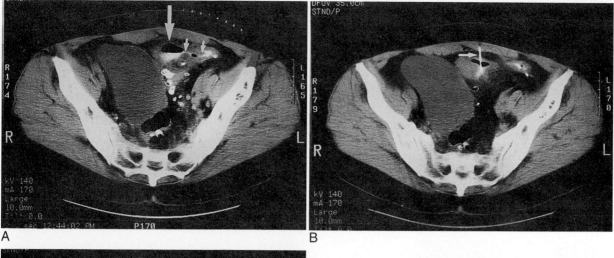

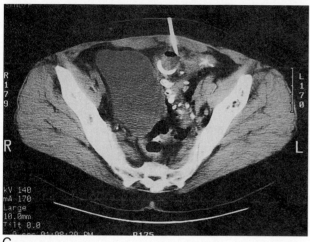

Figure 18-5   Patient with acute diverticulitis, high white cell count, fever, and marked tenderness in the left lower quadrant. **A**, Abdominal CT scan shows pericolonic inflammatory stranding in the sigmoid colon consistent with acute diverticulitis and an abscess (large arrow) with a fistulous communication (small arrows) to the sigmoid colon. **B**, A reference needle (arrow) was placed into the abscess cavity and rescanned to document appropriate position. **C**, A 10-Fr catheter was trocared into the abscess cavity and coiled in the abscess. The catheter remained *in situ* for 10 days until drainage had decreased to less than 10 mL per day. The small fistulous track closed spontaneously. The patient went on to have elective one-stage surgery 2 months later.

of antibiotics. The three-stage operation consisted of initial surgical abscess drainage and colostomy, a resection of the diseased colon and reanastamosis, and lastly a revision of the colostomy. In general, surgeons will now resect the diseased segment and any small associated abscess (less than 5 cm in diameter) and do a primary anastamosis. PAD is used for draining the larger abscesses to permit elective one-stage surgery (Fig. 18-5). Success rates of between 80 and 90% have been quoted for PAD of diverticular abscesses, permitting single-stage surgery.

Periappendiceal abscesses result from a walled-off appendiceal perforation. Drainage of the periappendiceal abscess and appropriate antibiotic therapy usually permits elective appendicectomy in 4-6 weeks. Indeed, there is some debate in the surgical literature regarding whether interval appendicectomy is actually necessary or not. Success rates of 90-100% have been quoted for PAD in periappendiceal abscesses.

Abscesses complicating Crohn disease occur in approximately 12-25% of patients at some point in their disease course. Crohn abscesses are difficult to manage and PAD is useful in temporizing patients with enteric communication prior to definitive surgery (Fig. 18-6). Alternatively, PAD can be curative if there is no enteric communication. Enterocutaneous fistulas resulting from percutaneous drainage in patients with Crohn abscesses have not been reported to date. Success rates for abscess drainage in Crohn disease range from 70 to 90%.

It is important to use CT as both the diagnostic and therapeutic guiding modality in these patients with enteric abscesses. Good bowel opacification is necessary for secure diagnosis and for planning the access route for drainage. These abscesses occur in close proximity to bowel loops, and CT is mandatory to ensure that small or large bowel is not traversed by the catheter during drainage (Box 18-6).

Abscess-Fistula Complex

Fistulization to collections can occur from various structures including the pancreatic duct, bile duct, urinary

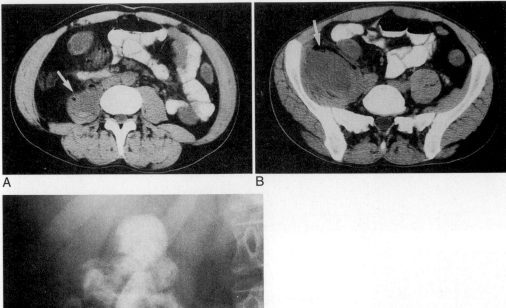

Figure 18-6   Patient with Crohn disease and an ilipsoas abscess with a fistulous communication to the cecum. **A**, Fluid collections with air (arrow) can be seen in the psoas muscle. **B**, Abscess also extends into the iliacus muscle (arrow). **C**, Because of continuous output from the drain inserted, an abscessogram was performed which showed clear fistulous communication (arrow) with the diseased segment of the cecum and terminal ileum. The patient improved with drainage but the fistulous communication did not heal. The patient eventually went to surgery for definitive resection of the terminal ileum and right hemicolectomy. The abscess drainage helped to temporize the patient prior to surgery.

system, and bowel. The commonest abscess fistula complex is the enteric abscess with fistulous communication to the small or large bowel. Principles of treatment are the same for all abscesses associated with fistulas. Therefore enteric abscesses associated with fistulous

communication will be discussed as they are the prototypical abscess–fistula complex.

The index of suspicion for fistulous communication should always be high when managing enteric abscesses. Persistent high outputs (>100 mL/day) or an increase in output after 3–4 days of drainage indicates the presence of a probable fistula. This can be confirmed with an abscessogram. Fistulas are designated as high-output if drainage is greater than 200 ml per day. In these high-output abscess–fistula complexes the communication is usually with small bowel. Management principles include draining the abscess, proximal diversion of bowel contents, and bowel rest. Abscesses associated with fistulas also take longer to heal (often 3–6 weeks for high-output fistulas) and this should be communicated to the referring physician and to the patient. Proximal diversion of bowel contents can be achieved by nasogastric suction and also by

---

Box 18-6   Enteric Abscess Drainage

Abscesses associated with Crohn disease, diverticulitis, and appendicitis fall in this group
Abscess drainage generally allows elective one-stage surgery
CT best for abscess localization and access route planning
Good bowel opacification is mandatory

placing a catheter through the fistulous track into the bowel (Figs 18-7 and 18-8). The catheter placed in the fistulous track is left *in situ* for approximately 10–14 days to allow a mature fibrous track to form. When catheter output recedes to less than 30–40 mL per day the catheter can be slowly withdrawn. With high-output fistulas it is important to monitor and correct electrolyte and fluid losses from the small bowel to speed fistula healing. Patients with high-output fistulas are usually fed parenterally.

In patients with low-output fistulas from the colon, drainage of the associated abscess with bowel rest is often sufficient for complete healing of the fistula. As might be expected, low-output abscess–fistula complexes usually heal successfully with percutaneous drainage. High-output fistulas do less well. It is useful to clamp the abscess catheter before removing it for 2–3 days in patients with high-output fistulas. If a CT scan after 2–3 days of catheter clamping shows no evidence of recurrence, the catheter can be removed.

Other factors that influence successful drainage and fistula healing include the presence of distal obstruction, the health of the bowel at the fistula site, and the immune status of the patient. In the presence of distal obstruction fistulas will not heal. Similarly, if the bowel at the fistula site is diseased (e.g., affected by Crohn disease or malignancy), the fistula is unlikely to heal. Additionally, if the patient is immunocompromised, fistula healing will be delayed. Quoted success rates for successful resolution of abscesses associated with fistulas vary from 66 to 82% (Box 18-7).

Subphrenic Abscess

The vast majority of subphrenic abscesses are postoperative, often resulting from pancreatic, gastric, or biliary surgery. Anatomically, they are located in a difficult position with the pleural attachment often making an extrapleural access route a technical challenge. The pleura is attached at the 12th rib posteriorly, 10th rib laterally, and 8th rib anteriorly. Traditionally, these abscesses were drained using a subpleural or extrapleural approach. This involved angling an 18-gauge sheath needle or 22-gauge single-stick needle up under the rib cage and into the collection under ultrasound guidance and using fluoroscopic guidance to dilate a track over a stiff wire and place the catheter (Fig. 18-9).

It has become apparent that an intercostal approach can be used in selected cases without a major increase in the complication rate, and the author's unit now uses this route for the vast majority of subphrenic abscesses. It is likely that the two pleural surfaces are firmly adhesed by the time of drainage because of the adjacent abscess, making pneumothorax or empyema unlikely with an intercostal approach. However, it is prudent when draining these abscesses intercostally to

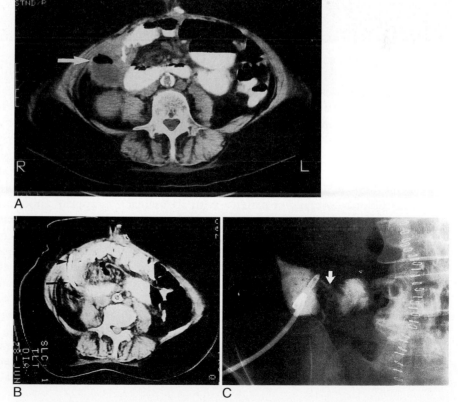

Figure 18-7   Abscess–fistula complex in a patient with fevers and a recent right hemicolectomy. **A,** Abdominal CT scan shows an extraluminal collection with an air-fluid level (arrow) in the right paracolic gutter adjacent to the anastamotic site. **B,** A 14-Fr sump catheter (arrows) was placed into the abscess collection. It was noted on the day after insertion that the drainage had increased to greater than 100 mL per day and a fistulous communication was suspected. **C,** An abscessogram was performed which confirmed a fistulous communication (arrow) to the bowel. Because the fistulous communication was small, a catheter was not placed through the fistulous track. The fistulous track closed spontaneously after 9 days. During this time the patient had a nasogastric tube placed and was fed parenterally. The catheter was then removed.

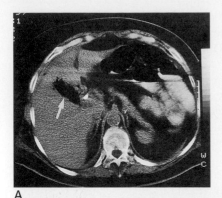

Figure 18-8   Patient with a biliary leak after laparoscopic cholecystectomy. **A**, CT scan showing an air collection (arrows) in the gallbladder fossa. Further air fluid levels were noted around the liver and in the right paracolic gutter. **B**, Endoscopic retrograde cholangiopancreatography documented a fistulous communication (arrows) between a small right-sided bile duct with the gallbladder fossa and the abscess cavity, into which a catheter had been placed. A stent was placed in the bile duct to divert bile away from the fistula. **C**, A total of three catheters were placed to drain all of the abscesses in the right upper quadrant. A combination of stent insertion to divert bile and the abscess drainage allowed the fistula to heal spontaneously within 14 days. The abscess drainage catheters were removed at this stage. The stent was removed 2 months later.

A

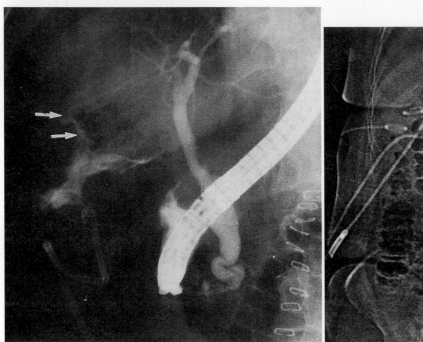

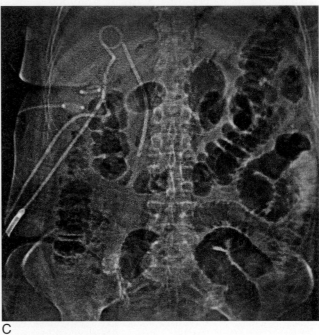

B   C

go through the lowest intercostal space possible that gives access to the abscess (Fig. 18-10). Quoted success rates for PAD of subphrenic abscesses lie between 80 an 90%.

Hepatic Abscess

Pyogenic hepatic abscess is rare since the improvement in antibiotic coverage of patients with abdominal

sepsis. In earlier days, most hepatic abscesses occurred secondary to bowel infections such as diverticulitis and appendicitis. Now, most hepatic abscesses are secondary to liver or biliary surgery. PAD of hepatic abscess is very successful and should be curative in over 90% of cases. Many hepatic abscesses at presentation appear loculated, have multiple septations, or portions may even appear solid on imaging. However, it is worthwhile placing a catheter in all hepatic abscesses, as almost all such abscesses respond dramatically to PAD (Fig. 18-11). Access can be intercostal or subcostal depending on the location of the abscess. Some interventionalists advocate needle aspiration alone for hepatic abscesses. The author prefers to place catheters for larger abscesses and use needle aspiration for smaller abscesses.

Renal Abscess

Renal abscesses can result from the liquefaction phase of focal bacterial nephritis or they can be hematogenous

---

Box 18-7   Abscess–Fistula Complex

Diagnosed by catheter outputs <100 mL/day
High output fistula >200 mL/day
Managed by abscess drainage, proximal bowel
    diversion, and bowel rest
Fistula healing influenced by distal obstruction,
    integrity of bowel at fistula site, and immune status

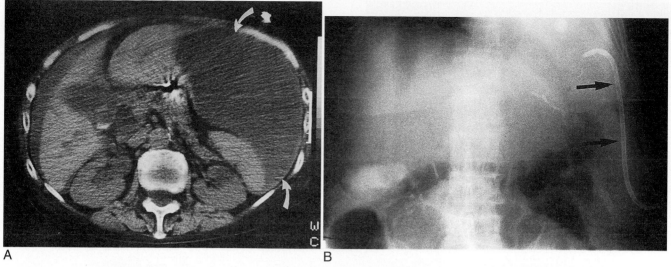

Figure 18-9   Patient with large left subphrenic abscess. **A**, Elderly patient presented with abdominal pain and fever and, on abdominal CT examination, had a large (arrows) left subphrenic fluid collection. It ultimately proved to be caused by a perforated colon. The subphrenic collection is pushing the spleen posteriorly and the collection also extended down to just below the costal margin laterally. Note the patient also has gallstones. **B**, Plain film of the abdomen shows a sump cathether (arrows) which was inserted from a lateral approach using ultrasound guidance and trocar technique. Because the abscess collection was so large and extended below the costal margin, it was relatively straightforward to use a subcostal approach. The collection ultimately proved to be fecal material and the patient eventually proceeded to surgery for a resection of the diseased colon after the patient's condition improved with abscess drainage.

in origin. The hematogenous type are cortical in location whereas those resulting from focal bacterial nephritis are medullary. Either type can break through into the perinephric space resulting in perinephric extension. Small intrarenal abscesses often respond to appropriate antibiotics. Larger intrarenal abscesses, perinephric abscesses, or small intrarenal abscesses not responding to antibiotics require drainage. Drainage can be performed under ultrasound or CT guidance. Locking catheters should be used if possible.

Infected urinomas are drained in a similar fashion. If there is a persistent communication with the urinary collecting system or obstructive uropathy, a percutaneous nephrostomy will be required to divert urine from the urinoma. If there is no communication, simply draining the urinoma should be sufficient.

Cure rates of 60–94% have been reported for PAD of renal and perirenal abscesses.

Retroperitoneal Abscess

Retroperitoneal abscesses usually locate in the iliopsoas compartment and can have varied etiologies ranging from acute spinal osteomyelitis, to Crohn disease or hematogenous spread. These abscesses will require CT guidance for drainage because of the deep location. If the abscess involves the psoas muscle in the abdomen and the iliacus in the pelvis, it is often sufficient to place

a catheter in the iliacus muscle as there is extensive communications between the iliacus and psoas muscles.

A catheter is first placed in the iliacus muscle and pus aspirated. If on the postprocedure CT scan the psoas component has also resolved, another catheter may not be necessary. If the psoas component has not fully resolved, another catheter will be necessary (Fig. 18-12). This is best done under fluoroscopic guidance, using the same puncture site as that used for the catheter in the iliacus abscess. The existing catheter is removed over a guidewire and a second guidewire inserted and manipulated up into the psoas muscle. Twelve- to 14-French catheters are then placed over each guidewire, one catheter in the iliacus abscess and the second in the psoas abscess.

Between 80 and 90% success rates have been reported for PAD of iliopsoas abscesses.

Splenic Abscess

There has always been a reluctance on the part of interventional radiologists to drain splenic abscesses. This is because the spleen is a highly vascular organ and there is a propensity for causing massive haemorrhage. However, over recent years the author's unit has drained a number of splenic abscesses. Careful attention to technique is important so that the catheter traverses the minimal amount of normal splenic tissue en route to the abscess. CT guidance is preferable for precise

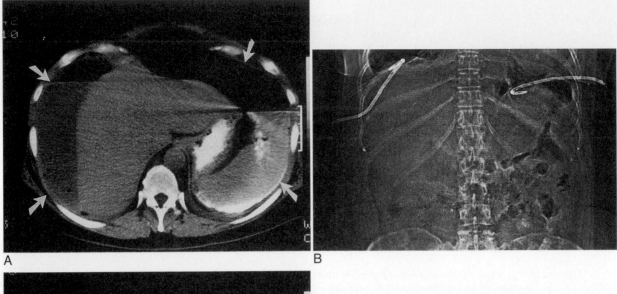

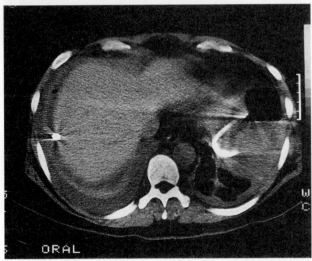

Figure 18-10   Patient with a leaking enterocolic anastomosis causing bilateral subphrenic abscesses. **A**, CT scan in the postoperative stage showed two large subphrenic abscesses (arrows). The subphrenic abscess on the left contains gastrograffin. These were drained using 14-Fr sump catheters and trocar technique. **B**, Topogram from a CT examination performed 5 days later to assess the adequacy of drainage shows the right subphrenic abscess catheter placed between the 9th and 10th ribs, which was the lowest intercostal space available for puncture of the subphrenic abscess. On the left side the drainage catheter is inserted between the 8th and 9th ribs. Undoubtedly, both of these catheters are transpleural but no complications developed from using this approach. It is important to use the lowest intercostal space possible to insert the catheter in order to reduce the complication rate. **C**, CT scan 5 days later shows catheters *in situ* with good drainage of both abscess cavities. The patient eventually made an uneventful recovery without recourse to surgery.

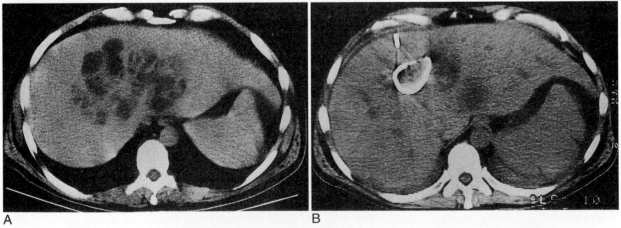

Figure 18-11   Patient with multilocular hepatic abscess. **A**, CT examination shows a multiloculated abscess in patient with high fevers. **B**, Using ultrasound guidance, a 14-Fr sump catheter was trocared into the collection and, despite the loculation present, a dramatic response was achieved. Approximately 100–200 mL of pus was aspirated initially and the catheter was left *in situ* for 7 days. The combination of catheter drainage and appropriate antibiotic therapy resulted in a successful abscess drainage. A repeat CT examination after 5 days of drainage shows the abscess catheter *in situ* with marked diminution in size of the abscess cavity.

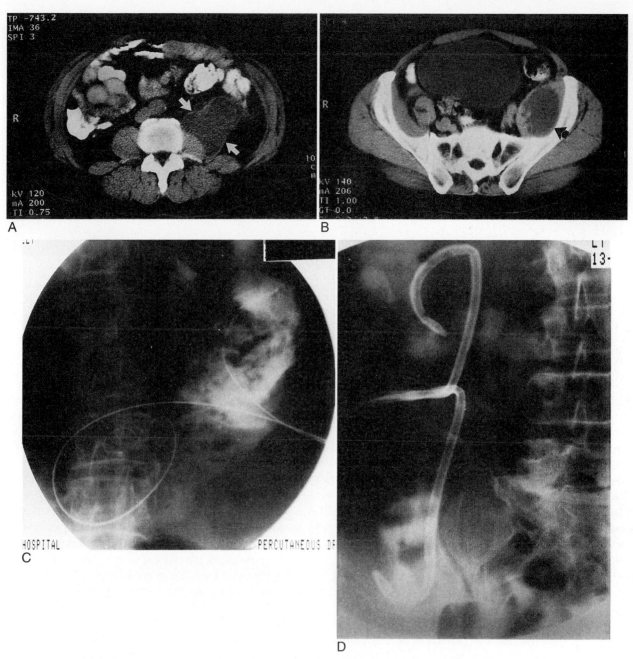

Figure 18-12   Patient with large iliopsoas abscess. **A**, CT examination just below the level of the kidney shows a large fluid collection (arrows) in or adjacent to the left psoas muscle. **B**, CT image of the pelvis shows the iliacus component (arrow). A single catheter was placed but this was not sufficient to drain the abscess and the patient remained febrile. Two days later the patient returned to the radiology department and two catheters were placed. **C**, The existing catheter was moved over a guidewire and an 8-Fr feeding tube was placed over the wire into the collection. A second super-stiff 0.038-inch wire was then placed through the feeding tube. One wire was manipulated into the iliacus component of the collection and the second wire manipulated up into the psoas component. **D**, Two 14-Fr sump catheters were placed over each wire for adequate drainage. The patient settled after the second catheter was placed and the abscess drainage was ultimately successful.

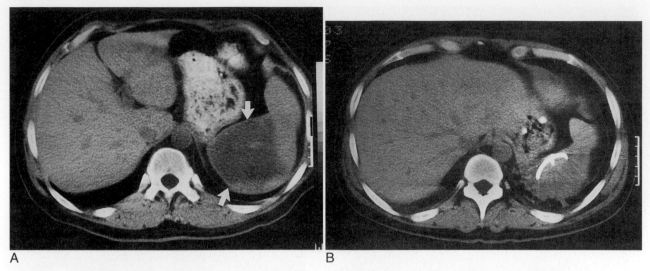

A

B

Figure 18-13 Immunocompromised patient with fever and high white cell count. **A**, CT image shows a large splenic abscess (arrows). **B**, A 10-Fr catheter was trocared into the abscess using ultrasound and fluoroscopic guidance and 100 mL of pus aspirated. A repeat CT scan shows the abscess catheter *in situ* with almost complete resolution of the abscess. The catheter remained *in situ* for 5 days until the abscess had resolved. No complications were encountered.

localization of the abscess and careful planning of the access route. Small 8- to 10-French catheters are used because of the vascular nature of the spleen (Fig. 18-13). Experience with splenic abscess drainage is limited, but it should no longer be a taboo organ for PAD (Box 18-8).

Pancreatic Collections

Pancreatic pseudocyst, abscess, and necrosis can be drained percutaneously, endoscopically, or surgically with varying results.

Pancreatic Pseudocyst

Not all pancreatic pseudocysts require drainage, and indications for percutaneous drainage are shown in Box 18-9. The commonest reasons for drainage include pain or the possibility of infection. The access route is usually transperitoneal. CT guidance is preferable

because the precise relationship of the pseudocyst with surrounding organs can be seen clearly. Usually an 8- or 10-French catheter will suffice for drainage. This can be placed using the Seldinger or trocar technique. The author prefers to use a trocar technique and avoid intervening organs if possible (Fig. 18-14). If it is not possible to avoid the stomach, then a transgastric approach is used. Indeed, the approach is chosen for patients who seem unlikely to tolerate a tube for long periods of time or who have a pancreatic duct communication.

A catheter is placed for some days and the patient then brought to the interventional suite. A nasogastric tube is inserted and the stomach inflated with air. The pseudocyst is filled with contrast and a 12-French vascular sheath is placed into the pseudocyst after removing the percutaneous catheter. Using lateral screening, a 10- or 12-French double biliary stent is placed between the pseudocyst and the stomach (Fig. 18-15). This internalizes drainage for patients who might not tolerate a

---

Box 18-8 Miscellaneous Abscess Drainage

An intercostal approach can be used for many subphrenic abscesses

Multilocular liver abscesses are often cured by catheter placement

In iliopsoas abscesses, a single catheter in the iliacus component may drain the entire abscess

Splenic abscesses can be drained with small catheters (8–10 French)

Box 18-9 Indications for Pseudocyst Drainage

Size >5 cm
Enlargement over time
Pain
Suspected infection
Biliary/GI obstruction

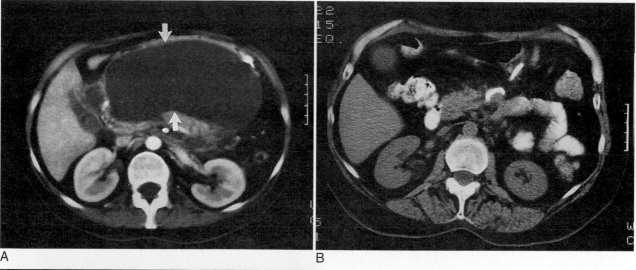

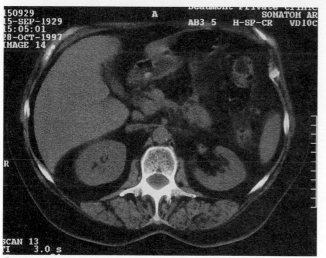

Figure 18-14   Percutaneous drainage of a large pseudocyst. **A**, Image from a CT examination of patient with a large pseudocyst (arrows) causing upper abdominal pain and discomfort. A 10-Fr catheter was trocared into the collection using an access route which did not pass through the stomach or any other intervening organs. **B**, Image from CT scan taken 10 days later shows the catheter within the pseudocyst cavity. The pseudocyst has collapsed. However, patient was still draining 100–150 mL of fluid per day. At this stage, octreotide was administered to the patient subcutaneously every day for a period of 3 weeks. Catheter output slowly decreased and at the end of 6 weeks of drainage catheter output had decreased sufficiently to warrant catheter removal. **C**, Image from a further CT examination performed 6 months after drainage shows no recurrence of the pseudocyst.

percutaneous catheter for a long time. The author has been using this approach increasingly. The stent can be removed endoscopically after 3–4 months.

The relationship of the pseudocyst with the pancreatic duct will determine the length of drainage to a large extent. If there is communication with the pancreatic duct, the duration of drainage will be prolonged for often up to 6–8 weeks. The duration of drainage can be decreased by the use of somatostatin or its analogue octreotide. These peptides serve to decrease the secretion of pancreatic juice and accelerate pseudocyst resolution. If there is communication and the downstream pancreatic duct is obstructed by a stricture or stone, pseudocyst drainage will not be successful unless the downstream obstruction is relieved (Fig. 18-16).

Modern percutaneous drainage should be successful in up to 90% of pancreatic pseudocysts (Table 18-1). Drainage can be lengthy, often taking up to 2–3 months

(particularly if communication with the pancreatic duct exists) and this should be explained to the patient (Box 18-10).

Pancreatic Abscess

Drainage of pancreatic abscess is a challenge for interventional radiologists. Patients with pancreatic abscess have severe acute pancreatitis and usually have a severe systemic illness. In addition, pancreatic abscesses are often multilocular and the contents are usually very viscous, requiring large catheters (14- to 26-French) for drainage.

CT is the preferred guidance modality, because these patients will have an associated ileus, making ultrasound guidance difficult. Catheters that are 16-French or smaller can be trocared into the collection under CT guidance. Catheters larger than 16-French will ultimately require placement using the Seldinger technique and fluoroscopic guidance, after initial placement of the

Table 18-1   Differentiation of Abscess from Infected Necrosis

	Abscess	Infected Necrosis
Onset	>4 weeks	1–2 weeks
Contents	Pus	Solid debris
Morbidity	++	+++++
Mortality	10–20%	15–50%
Therapy	PAD	Debridement

Box 18-10   Pancreatic Pseudocyst Drainage

Access route avoids stomach if possible
Communication with pancreatic duct prolongs drainage
Duration of drainage decreased by octreotide
Drainage may be unsuccessful if downstream pancreatic duct obstruction

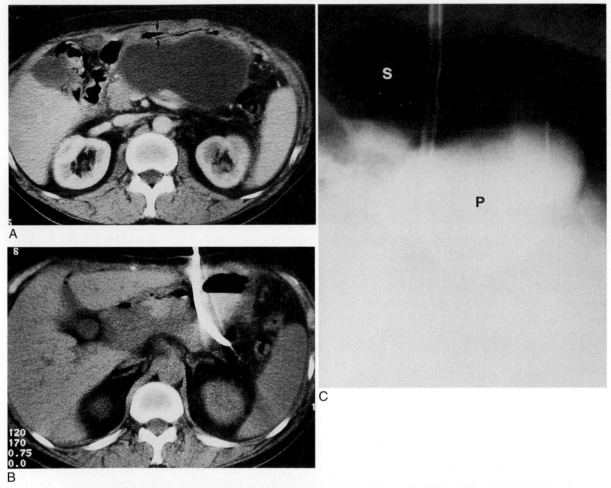

Figure 18-15 Transgastric stent placement for pseudocyst drainage. A 44-year-old man presented with a large pseudocyst 3 months after a bout of acute pancreatitis. The patient did not want an external tube. ERCP had shown communication between the pancreatic duct and the pseudocyst. **A**, CT shows the large 10-cm pseudocyst in the lesser sac, behind the stomach (arrows). **B**, Using CT guidance, a 12-Fr catheter was trocared into the pseudocyst. **C**, A nasogastric tube was placed, and the stomach (S) filled with air. Contrast material was injected into the pseudocyst (P). Lateral screening shows the catheter in the pseudocyst, which contains contrast material. *(Continued)*

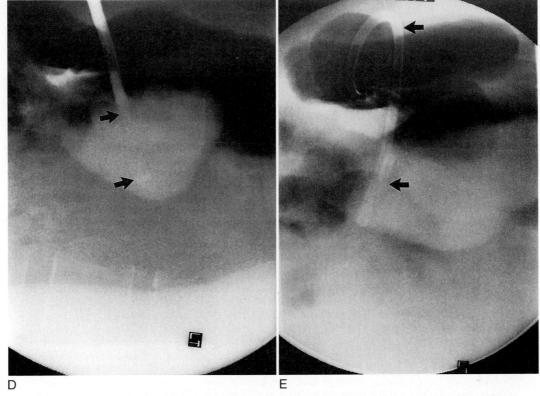

D   E

Figure 18-15   cont'd D, The 12-Fr catheter was removed and a 12-Fr vascular sheath (arrows) was placed. **E,** A 5-cm 10-Fr double pigtail stent (arrows) was placed through the vascular sheath with its distal end in the pseudocyst, and proximal end in the stomach. The stent was removed 3 months later, and follow-up imaging at 1 year has shown no evidence of recurrence.

needle and guidewire under CT guidance. In many cases more than one catheter will be required because of very viscous cavity contents and/or multiloculation. Vigorous irrigation and careful monitoring of the patient is also necessary. Repeat CT scans should be performed if the patient is not defervescing or improving. Larger catheters or multiple catheters may have to be placed depending on the size of residual collections. It is best to place large catheters (20- to 30-French) in patients with pancreatic abscess to achieve the best chance of success (Fig. 18-17).

There has been much confusion in the literature between pancreatic abscess and necrosis. Undoubtedly, in many series the lack of distinction between pancreatic abscess and infected necrosis has made the interpretation of pancreatic abscess results difficult. Success rates for drainage of pancreatic abscess vary from 32 to 80%. However, even if percutaneous drainage ultimately fails, a significant positive effect can be achieved, in that the patient may be temporized for surgery. In other words, the patient's condition may be considerably improved prior to surgery from the percutaneou drainage.

Pancreatic Necrosis

As opposed to pancreatic abscess, pancreatic necrosis occurs early in the course (<2 weeks) of severe acute

pancreatitis (Table 18-2). It is diagnosed by dynamic contrast-enhanced CT as an area of absent perfusion in the pancreas. It is of critical importance to differentiate sterile from infected necrosis. This differentiation cannot be made clinically, because sepsis indicators can be raised in patients with both sterile and infected necrosis.

Table 18-2   Pseudocyst: Percutaneous Drainage Results

Author	Patients	Success (%)
Gerzof	11	90
Colhoun	10	100
Hancke	18	100
Torres	15	67
Matzinger	12	67
Grosso	43	76
vanSonnenberg	101	90
D'egidio	23	96
Sacks	7	88
Anderson	22	59
Burnweit	13	39
Lang	12	70

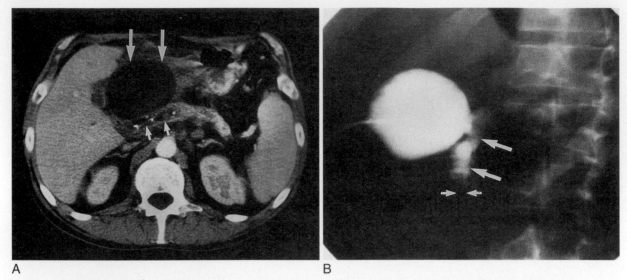

Figure 18-16   Failed pseudocyst drainage. **A,** Image from CT examination in a patient with chronic pancreatitis and a pseudocyst. CT image shows a pseudocyst (large arrows) anterior to the head of the pancreas, a dilated pancreatic duct (small arrows), and some areas of calcification within the pancreatic duct. The patient had upper abdominal pain and discomfort and was referred for drainage. **B,** It was decided to drain the pseudocyst under ultrasound and fluoroscopy. The initial needle inserted under ultrasound guidance was used to opacify the pseudocyst. This showed communication with a dilated pancreatic duct (large arrows). The downstream duct near the ampulla contained a stone (small arrow) which was causing the dilatation. Because of the downstream obstruction it was decided that percutaneous drainage was not feasible, and the patient was referred for a cystenterostomy. This procedure was successful and the patient had no further symptoms.

Moreover, both groups of patients are usually critically ill. Patients with infected necrosis require immediate surgery (necrosectomy). The necrotic tissue usually requires scooping out by hand and has been likened to "dogmeat". Because of the nature of the contents in necrotic cavities, pancreatic necrosis is generally not suitable for percutaneous drainage. Occasionally, if the necrotic contents have liquefied, percutaneous drainage may be attempted. Large-bore 24- to 26-French catheters will be required for effective drainage. A number of authors have recently proposed "minimally invasive necrosectomy" as an alternative to open necrosectomy. This is similar to percutaneous nephrolithotomy, in that a 30-French sheath is placed into the area of necrosis using CT and fluoroscopic guidance. The patient is then brought to the operating room, where necrotic fragments are removed through the sheath with the aid of a rigid endoscope and graspers. The cavity is then irrigated. A large-bore catheter is left in place, so that more treatments can be performed if required.

The principal goal of interventional radiology in patients with pancreatic necrosis is to differentiate sterile from infected necrosis. This is done by percutaneous sampling of the necrotic area. Sampling is carried out with a 20-gauge needle under CT guidance (Fig. 18-18). It is of paramount importance not to introduce bacteria into a potentially sterile necrotic area. Therefore, it is vital to use CT to guide needle placement and to plan the access route so that the colon and intervening organs are avoided. If nothing can be aspirated with a 20-gauge needle, 2–3 mL of sterile saline can be injected and reaspirated. The aspirate is sent for Gram stain, and aerobic and anerobic cultures.

Pelvic Abscess

Drainage of pelvic abscesses deserves special consideration because of the many different and evolving access routes available. Abscesses in the pelvis are surrounded by the pelvic bony ring and can be difficult to access. There are many different access routes, including anterior transperitoneal, transgluteal, presacral, transvaginal, and transrectal. The anterior transperitoneal route is suitable for a minority of pelvic collections and these tend to be located anteriorly underneath the anterior abdominal wall.

Transgluteal Access

The transgluteal route is the traditional method of draining deep pelvic abscesses. CT guidance is used, and with the patient placed prone on the CT table a 20-gauge needle is placed into the abscess. A CT scan confirms the position and ensures that the needle is close to the sacrum and not near the sciatic nerve which exits behind the ischial tuberosity. A catheter is trocared alongside the 20-gauge needle, through the greater sciatic foramen and into the

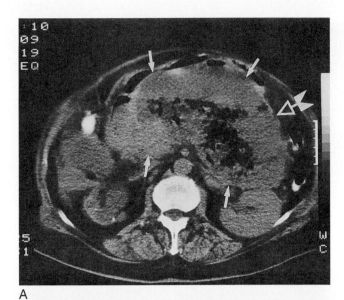

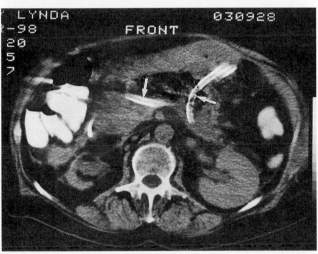

Figure 18-17   Percutaneous drainage of a pancreatic abscess. **A**, Patient with a large pancreatic abscess (arrows) containing air. The patient was quite sick and required immediate drainage. An access route (large arrow) was available from an anterolateral approach which avoided the bowel. Two 14-Fr catheters were trocared into the collection under CT guidance using this approach. **B**, Because of the size of the collection, the 14-Fr catheters were upgraded to 20-Fr the next day to provide adequate drainage. This was done under fluoroscopic guidance using dilators to dilate up both tracts. A CT image taken 5 days later shows almost complete collapse of the abscess cavity. Two 20-Fr abscess catheters (arrows) can be seen within the abscess cavity. Catheters remained *in situ* for 4 weeks and the patient made an uneventful recovery.

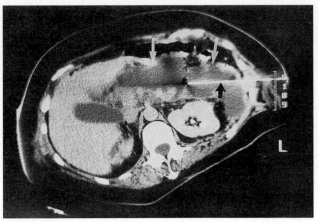

Figure 18-18   CT guided aspiration of pancreatic necrosis. Image from a CT examination shows an extensive area of pancreatic necrosis (white arrows) in a sick patient with possible infected necrosis. A lateral approach was used for needle aspiration that avoided the colon. A 20-gauge needle (black arrow) was inserted into the collection and multiple areas sampled within the collection. Samples were sent for Gram stain and culture. There was no evidence of infection in this patient and the pancreatic necrosis was treated conservatively. This large area of pancreatic necrosis eventually evolved into a pseudocyst and the patient was treated by the surgical creation of a cystgastrostomy 6 months after the bout of acute pancreatitis.

there are usually no sciatic nerve problems. Occasionally, temporary leg pain occurs but this usually resolves within 24–48 hours. The advantage of the transgluteal route is that large (12- to 16-French) catheters can be placed.

Presacral Access

The presacral route can be used for collections in the presacral space, but not for collections elsewhere in the pelvis. The patient lies prone on the CT table and a needle is placed into the presacral collection. The needle is placed through the gluteal cleft underneath the coccyx. The needle is then tracked parallel to the sacrum and angled up into the collection. Needle position can be confirmed by doing a scannogram and then scanning through the level of the needle tip as seen on the scannogram. This approach has limited applications but is useful for presacral collections in patients who have had abdominoperineal resections.

Transvaginal and Transrectal Access

These two routes have been gaining in popularity for draining abscesses in the rectouterine or rectovesical pouches. They are the most direct routes to abscesses in the deep pelvis and permit truly dependent drainage. The author's unit now tends to use the transvaginal route in females and the transrectal route in males.

Sonographic guidance is used for transvaginal catheter placement. The author uses an Acuson (Mountain View, CA) unit with a 7-MHz endocavitary probe. The endocavitary probe is fitted with a 9-French peel-away sheath (Cook) which is attached to the probe by rubber bands

abscess cavity. The access route should stay as close as possible to the sacrum to avoid the sciatic nerve which exits through the greater sciatic foramen close to the ischial tuberosity (Fig. 18-19). This route requires adequate sedation as many fascial planes are crossed and there can be significant pain. If the catheter is close to the sacrum

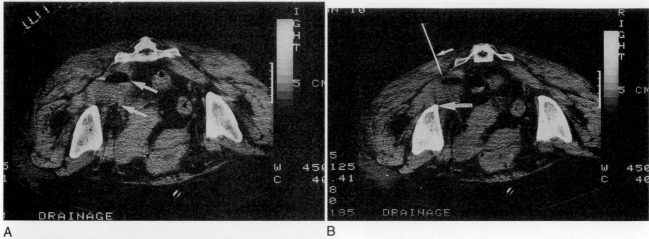

A

B

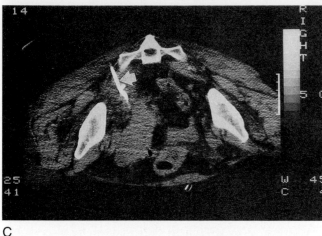

C

Figure 18-19 Transgluteal drainage of a pelvic abscess associated with acute diverticulitis. **A**, Abscess (large arrows) adjacent to the right pyriformis muscle. Note the markers (small arrows) on the skin surface used to pick an appropriate skin access site. **B**, A 20-gauge needle (arrow) was inserted into the collection using an approach that stayed close to the coccyx. It is important to keep the needle and catheter close to the coccyx to avoid the sciatic nerve which exits just behind the ischial tuberosity (large arrow). **C**, A 10-Fr catheter (arrow) was trocared into the collection and the collection decompressed. The abscess was successfully treated using the transgluteal approach.

(Fig. 18-20). The probe with the attached sheath is placed into the vagina and the abscess localized. Local anesthetic is injected into the vaginal wall adjacent to the collection with a 20-gauge 20-cm needle (Chiba) and an 8-French pigtail catheter trocared into the cavity. Locking catheters should be used when using both the transvaginal and transrectal access routes, because non-locking catheters can dislodge with straining, coughing, or any increase in abdominal pressure.

CT, fluoroscopy, or sonography can be used to place transrectal catheters. The author prefers to use sonography and a similar technique to that described for transvaginal drainage (Fig. 18-21). Advantages and disadvantages of transrectal and transvaginal drainage versus transgluteal are shown in Table 18-3.

Special Considerations

Hematoma

Drainage of hematoma is usually indicated only if the hematoma is infected. Most sterile hematomas will resolve spontaneously and do not require therapy. Infected hematomas that have liquefied are relatively

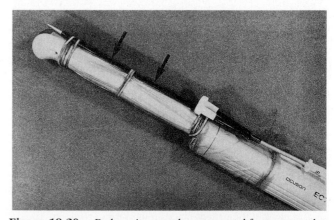

Figure 18-20 Endocavitary probe setup used for transrectal or transvaginal drainage. A 9-Fr peel-away sheath (arrows) is fitted to the probe in the same position as the probe's needle guide would be attached. It is attached to the probe by rubber bands and then covered with a further condom. The 9-Fr peel-away sheath is used to guide needles and catheters into pelvic collections for aspiration and drainage. An 8-Fr catheter can be trocared through the 9-Fr peel-away sheath into pelvic collections using either a transvaginal or transrectal approach.

Table 18-3 Endocavitary versus Transgluteal Approach to Pelvic Abscess		
	Transgluteal	**Endocavitary**
Catheter size	10–16 Fr	8–10 Fr
Catheter fixation	Good	Poor
Guiding modality	CT	US
Procedural pain	High	Low
Sciatic nerve damage	Yes	No
Procedure time	Moderate	Short
Efficacy	>90%	>90%

easy to drain. Acute organizing hematomas are almost impossible to drain percutaneously because they contain solid blood clot rather than fluid. It is therefore important to determine whether or not the collection is infected. Aspiration of the hematoma will yield the answer. It is usually necessary to use an 18-gauge needle to retrieve some fluid for Gram stain and culture. If it is difficult to obtain fluid with an 18-gauge spinal needle then the haematoma is usually not amenable to percutaneous drainage (Fig. 18-22). If the hematoma is organizing and infected, it is often not possible to drain percutaneously. If the hematoma is of mixed density, it may be possible to drain the fluid contents and then use a thrombolytic agent such as urokinase to lyse the clot. Early results with thrombolytic agents are promising in this regard.

Sclerosis

Occasionally, some collections (such as hepatic and renal cysts and lymphoceles) may require sclerosis because of recurrence or persistence despite long-term drainage. Lymphoceles are the classic example of collections that tend to recur and may take a long time to drain completely, because of persistent leakage from small lymphatics. Many different agents are available for sclerosis. The commonest agents used are tetracycline, ethanol, bleomycin, and betadine. The author's unit uses betadine for sclerosing abdominal collections. It is important to delineate the cavity by injecting contrast through the catheter before starting sclerosis to ensure that there is no communication to bowel, ureter, or other organs. Betadine is instilled to a total of three-quarters the size of the cavity. The betadine remains in the cavity for 1 hour, during which the patient turns every 15 minutes into supine, prone, and both decubitus positions. The betadine

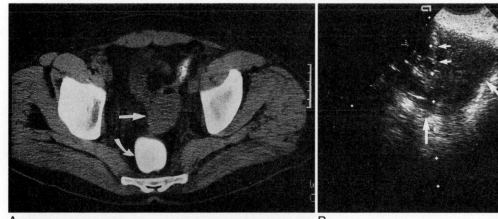

A   B

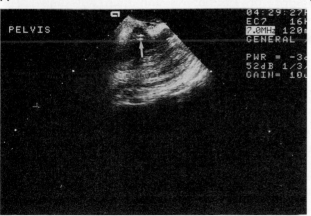

C

Figure 18-21 Transrectal drainage of a pelvic abscess in a patient who had recently been operated on for a perforated appendicitis. **A**, Image from a CT examination shows the abscess cavity (straight arrow) anterior to the rectum (curved arrow). **B**, A transrectal drainage was performed. The collection (large arrows) can be seen adjacent to the endocavitary probe. After first infiltrating the wall with local anesthetic, the 20-guage needle (small arrows) has been inserted through the rectal wall to get a sample for microbiology. **C**, An 8-Fr catheter was trocared through the rectal wall into the abscess cavity and the contents of the abscess cavity evacuated. The catheter (arrow) can be seen within the collapsed abscess. The catheter was left *in situ* for 3 days, after which time it was removed and the patient made an uneventful recovery.

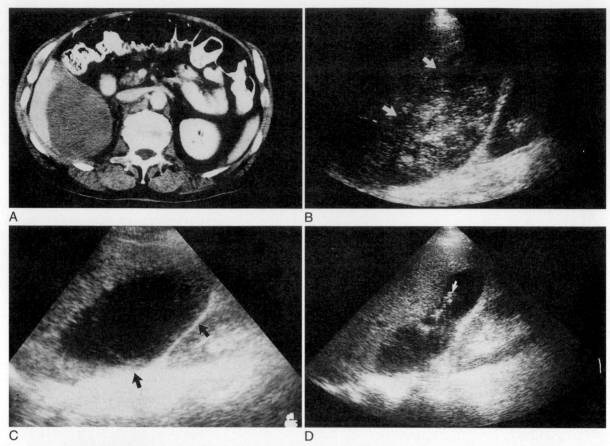

Figure 18-22 Drainage of an infected haematoma in a patient with signs of abdominal sepsis after a cholocystectomy. **A,** CT examination shows a collection of high density in Morrison's pouch. This was felt to be consistent with a hematoma. **B,** Ultrasound at the same time showed the collection (arrows) to be of mixed echogenicity. An 18-gauge needle inserted into the collection yielded some clot but no-free flowing fluid. At this time it was decided that the collection was not amenable to percutaneous drainage. The patient was placed on antibiotics but low-grade fevers continued. **C,** Five days later the patient returned for ultrasound examination, at which time the fluid collection (arrows) had liquefied. A 14-Fr catheter was trocared into the collection for decompression. **D,** The catheter (arrow) has been inserted and the cavity is being decompressed. The patient defervesced and the hematoma was completely evacuated over a period of 5 days.

is then reaspirated. If the collection is small (<5–10 cm) a single session may be sufficient. If the collection is large (>10 cm), or if the collection has recurred after a single-session injection of sclerosant, sclerosis is repeated, on a daily basis, for 7–10 days (Fig. 18-23). This can be performed as an outpatient. The collection will decrease in size over this time period necessitating a lesser volume of sclerosant. Finally, the catheter can be withdrawn when the collection has receded.

Thrombolysis-assisted Drainage

In circumstances where the contents of a collection are particularly viscous, thrombolysis with urokinase can help decrease the drainage duration and may help to achieve a complete cure. Urokinase has been used successfully in drainage of pleural empyemas, abdominal abscesses, and hematomas. There is no significant deleterious effect on serum coagulation with the use of intracavitary urokinase. In the author's unit the protocol consists of instilling 85,000 units of urokinase, followed by 10 mL of sterile saline into the collection. The catheter is clamped for 15 minutes and then unclamped. The process is repeated every 8 hours, up to a time limit of 48 hours.

Amebic Abscess and Echinococcal Cyst Drainage

Amebic abscesses are treated medically and usually do not require percutaneous drainage. In some circumstances PAD may be necessary particularly if the abscess fails to respond to medical therapy. Some authors have also advocated PAD for abscesses greater than 8–10 cm, abscesses with signs of pleural or peritoneal leakage, and abscesses that occur in the left lobe of the liver which have a greater likelihood of intrathoracic rupture with potentially serious consequences. PAD is usually curative within a few days.

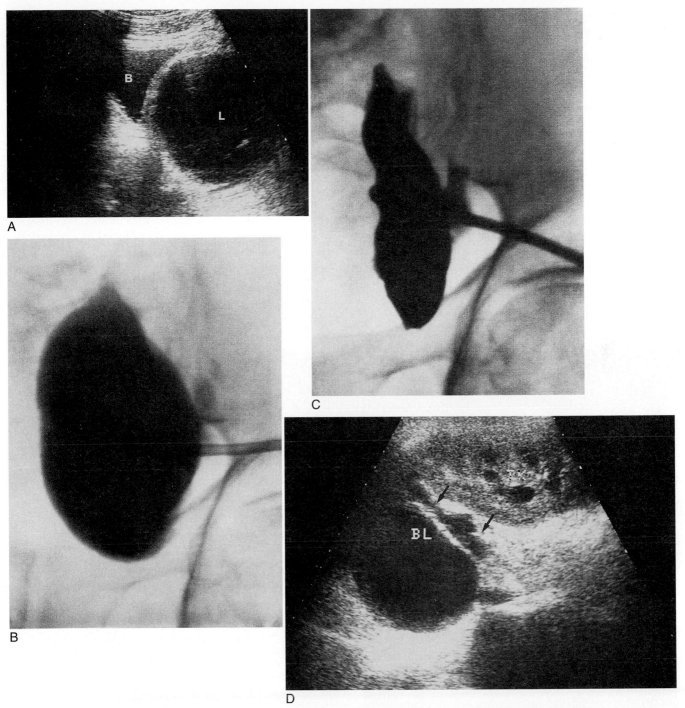

Figure 18-23   Patient with a lymphocele after renal transplantation. The lymphocele was marsupialized into the peritoneal cavity but recurred. **A**, Axial ultrasound image through the pelvis shows the bladder (B) which is pushed to the right by a large fluid collection (L) consistent with a lymphocele. This lymphocele was also causing ureteric compression and hydronephrosis. **B**, The lymphocele was drained percutaneously using ultrasound guidance and a 12-Fr catheter was inserted into the collection. On this contrast study no communication was noted between the lymphocele and the ureteric system. The volume of the cavity was 200 mL, so 150 mL of betadine was instilled into the cavity on a daily basis for 7 days. **C**, Contrast material injected on the eighth day shows that the cavity has markedly reduced in size and the catheter was removed at this stage. **D**, Follow-up ultrasound examination performed 2 months after sclerosis shows the bladder (BL) and transplant kidney (TK) with a small residual collection (arrows) between the two. Note that the hydronephrosis is now resolved in the transplant kidney. The sclerosis was ultimately successful and the graft was not compromised.

Echinococcal cysts or abscesses were traditionally considered unsuitable for percutaneous drainage because any leakage of cyst contents into the peritoneal cavity could potentially cause anaphylactic shock. However, there are now many reports of successful PAD in these patients without the development of anaphylaxis. The cysts can also be sclerosed with alcohol to prevent recurrence.

Complications

Complications during percutaneous abscess drainage are rare and can be minimized with appropriate planning of the access route and daily supervision of the catheter after insertion. Reported total complication rates lie between none and 10%. Minor complications such as pain can be avoided by routine use of sedoanalgesia and adequate local anesthesia during catheter placement. It is not unusual for catheter drainage of an abscess to induce a bacteremia because abscess walls are highly vascular. It is important to ensure that the patient has appropriate broad-spectrum antibiotic coverage before performing the abscess drainage. If the patient is not, then start the patient on intravenous ampicillin, gentamycin, and metronidazole before the procedure. When Gram stain and culture results become available, the antibiotic regimen may be changed according to sensitivities. Two deaths have been reported due to septicemia and disseminated intravascular coagulation after catheter placement for abscess drainage, and although this is not a common occurrence, it can be prevented by appropriate antibiotic coverage.

As with all interventional procedures, bleeding can occur but its frequency can be reduced by correction of any coagulopathy before the procedure. Bleeding may also be more likely when draining abscesses in vascular organs such as the liver or spleen (Fig. 18-24). Use of a small sized catheter may help minimize bleeding

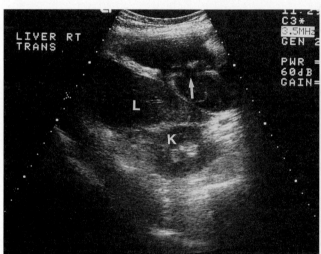
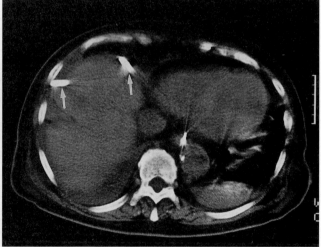

A

B

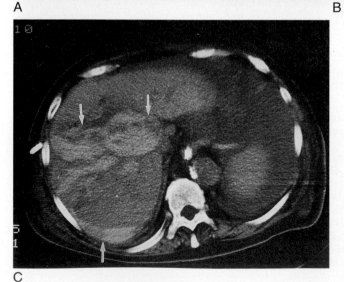

C

Figure 18-24 Elderly patient presented with a perforated gallbladder and a right subphrenic abscess. This patient developed a large hepatic hematoma after catheter drainage. **A**, Initial ultrasound examination shows a perforated gallbladder (arrow) with a collection anterior to the gallbladder. A further collection was noted in the right subphrenic space. Liver (L) and kidney (K) can also be seen. **B**, A 10-Fr catheter was inserted into the collection anterior to the gallbladder and a 12-Fr catheter trocared into the right subphrenic collection. CT image 3 days later shows the 12-Fr catheter (arrows) in the right subphrenic space with almost complete drainage of the right subphrenic collection. On the fourth day the patient developed acute respiratory distress and a pulmonary embolus was suspected. The patient was started on anticoagulation therapy but became over-anticoagulated. Two days after starting anticoagulant therapy the patient became acutely hypotensive and had a large drop in hematocrit. **C**, A repeat CT scan on the sixth day showed a large intrahepatic hematoma in the right lobe of the liver (arrows), presumably related to anticoagulation and percutaneous catheter drainage of the right subphrenic abscess. The patient settled with conservative management and stabilized. Unfortunately the patient died 12 days later from acute respiratory distress syndrome.

problems, particularly in the spleen. Vascular laceration may also occur from needles or catheters used to access abscesses. If the vessel is small, the bleeding will usually stop spontaneously. Occasionally, a larger catheter may have to be inserted to tamponade the bleeding. If this does not work, angiographic embolization may be required.

Percutaneous abscess drainage may be complicated by bowel perforation from being transfixed by a needle or catheter. If the bowel has been transfixed by a needle only, there will usually be no sequelae. However, if a catheter has been placed through the bowel en route to the abscess, the situation is slightly more complex. Recognition of enteric communication is usually evident after the catheter has been in place, in that small bowel contents usually drain through the catheter. The catheter can be left in place for 10 days, after which a mature fibrous track should form around the catheter. By this time, the abscess should have healed and the catheter can be removed. Any leakage from the bowel can then pass into the fibrous track and there will not be free communication with the peritoneal cavity. The percutaneous track will usually close over within 12–24 hours, provided there is no distal obstruction. However, if the patient develops signs of peritonitis after catheter transfixation of bowel, then surgical intervention may be required immediately. This complication can usually be prevented by careful planning of access routes and ensuring adequate opacification of the bowel when draining abscesses under CT guidance.

Most complications occurring during percutaneous abscess drainage can be managed conservatively by the interventional radiologist. However, it is also true that most complications that do occur can be prevented by close attention to the technique of abscess drainage. The anatomic location of the abscess, preprocedural broad-spectrum antibiotic coverage, careful planning of the access route, sedoanalgesia, and careful postprocedural catheter care should all help to reduce abscess drainage complications. Delayed catheter problems such as kinking, blockage, and dislodgement can be managed expeditiously by performing daily ward rounds and anticipating or dealing with problems as they arise (Box 18-11).

THORACIC FLUID COLLECTIONS

Aspiration and drainage of thoracic fluid collections follow similar principles to those for abdominal collections. Ultrasound guidance is used for guiding needles and catheters into the majority of pleural fluid collections. CT is required as the guidance modality for draining mediastinal and lung abscesses.

PLEURAL FLUID COLLECTIONS

Diagnostic Thoracentesis

Pleural effusions are divided into transudates and exudates based on aspirated fluid characteristics (Table 18-4). Common causes of transudates and exudates are shown in Box 18-12. Transudates result from decreased oncotic pressure or from changes in hydrostatic pressure with congestive heart failure being the most common cause. Exudative effusions are most commonly malignant or infective in nature with other causes being less frequent.

The two main indications for diagnostic thoracentesis are to exclude malignancy or infection in the pleural space. The evaluation of parapneumonic effusions is an important use of diagnostic thoracentesis because some of these parapneumonic effusions will progress to form empyemas and require drainage.

There are three stages in the formation of empyemas described by Light and associates. The first or exudative stage occurs when a focus of infection contiguous to the pleura promotes a pleural effusion. Lactate dehydrogenase (LDH) levels are raised above 200 IU/L, but pH, glucose, and polymorphonuclear leukocytes levels are normal. Appropriate antibiotic therapy is usually all that is required to treat this exudative stage. The second or fibrinopurulent stage occurs when the effusion is colonized by bacteria. Glucose and pH levels fall (glucose ≤40 mg/dL or 2.2 mmol/L, pH ≤7.0) and catheter drainage is required to prevent progression to the third stage.

Box 18-11   Minimizing Complications of PAD

Ensure appropriate broad-spectrum antibiotic coverage before PAD
Use adequate sedoanalgesia
Correct any coagulopathy
Use adequate bowel opacification for CT
Perform daily rounds on the patient after PAD

Table 18-4   Differentiation of Transudates from Exudates

	Exudates	Transudates
Pleural fluid protein	>3 q/dL	<3 q/dL
Pleural:serum protein	>0.5	<0.5
Pleural fluid LDH	>200 IU	<200 IU
Pleural:serum LDH	>0.6	<0.6

Box 18-12   Common Causes of Transudates and Exudates

Transudates

Congestive cardiac failure
Cirrhosis
Nephrotic syndrome
Peritoneal dialysis
Constrictive pericarditis

Exudates

Malignancy
Infected parapneumonic effusion/empyema
Tuberculous effusion
Pulmonary infection
SLE
Rheumatoid
Dressler syndrome
Pancreatitis
Trauma

Box 18-13   Empyema Stages

In the exudative stage (LDH >100 IU/L, normal pH, glucose, and WBC count) antibiotics are usually curative

In the fibrinopurulent stage (glucose ≤40 mg/dL, pH ≤7.0) catheter drainage is required

In the third stage a pleural peel forms which requires surgical decortication

---

In the third stage, fibrin is deposited in the form of a pleural peel which is usually not amenable to percutaneous therapy. Surgical drainage and decortication are usually required for this stage (Box 18-13).

Technique

Patients are placed sitting on the side of a stretcher facing away from the operator. Ultrasound is used to locate the pleural effusion and a 22-gauge needle is inserted into the pleural fluid collection immediately above the adjacent rib. Needle entry should be performed above the rib to avoid the neurovascular bundle. Thirty to 50 mL of fluid are aspirated and routinely sent for Gram stain and culture, total protein, LDH, glucose, and cytology. If there is any indication of infection, fluid is also sent for pH. Ultrasound-guided thoracentesis is a highly effective procedure. Difficulties may arise in patients with small amounts of fluid or ventilated patients where access may be limited.

Pleural Biopsy

Not infrequently, diagnostic aspiration may not yield a diagnosis and pleural biopsy will be required. This can be performed percutaneously or thoracoscopically. The advantage of thoracoscopic biopsy is that the pleura can be visualized and areas of abnormality specifically biopsied. Percutaneous biopsy is more often negative owing to sampling errors. However, against this pleural biopsy is less invasive than thoracosopic biopsy. Percutanoeus biopsy with a large-gauge cutting needle is the procedure of first choice when a pleural mass or thickening is present. However, institutional preferences

may dictate whether percutaneous or thorascopic biopsy is performed in patients with pleural effusions and a negative diagnostic thoracentesis.

Technique

Cope or Abrams needles can be used to biopsy the pleura. The author prefers the Cope needle system which consists of (1) a short blunt open-ended cannula; (2) a sharpened, 45-degree angle, open-ended trocar; (3) a solid 45-degree stylet which fits into the cannula; and (4) a reverse-bevel cutting-edge needle (Fig. 18-25). The first

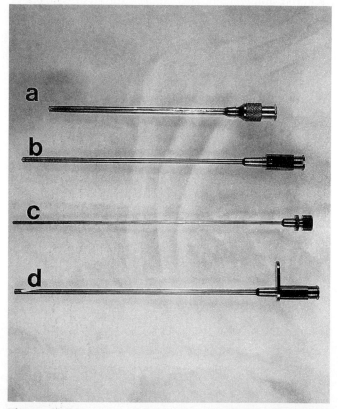

Figure 18-25   Cope pleural biopsy needle system. The needle system consists of four components: (**a**) a short open-ended outer cannula; (**b**) an open-ended trocar with a 45-degree angle tip; (**c**) a solid stylet; and (**d**) the Cope needle itself which has a reverse-bevel cutting edge.

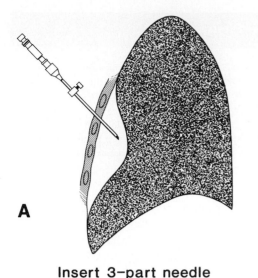

A Insert 3–part needle

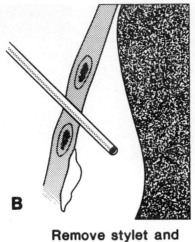

B Remove stylet and inner cannula

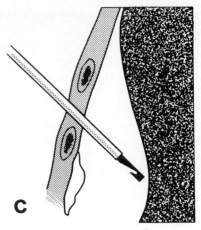

C Insert "hook" needle

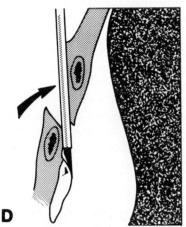

D "Hook" pleura

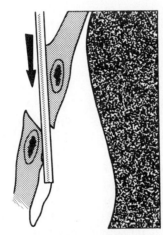

E Cut pleura with outer cannula

Figure 18-26 Schematic illustrating a pleural biopsy. **A,** The cannula, trocar, and stylet are fitted together and inserted into the pleural space. **B,** The stylet and trocar are removed. **C,** The Cope needle is inserted. **D,** The Cope needle and outer cannula are maneuvered using the rib as a fulcrum so that the Cope needle is adjacent to the pleura. The needle system is then withdrawn until the hook engages the pleura. **E,** Once the pleura is engaged, the outer cannula is advanced over the Cope needle to capture the piece of pleura. The Cope needle is then withdrawn and the trocar and stylet placed back through the outer cannula in case other pleural biopsies are required. (Reproduced with permission from Mueller PR, Saini S, Simeone JF et al: Image-guided pleural biopsies: indications, technique, and results in 23 patients. *Radiology* 169:1–4, 1988.)

three parts are inserted as a unit into the pleural fluid and the stylet and trocar removed (Fig. 18-26). The cutting needle is inserted beyond the tip of the short outer cannula and the needle is then withdrawn at a steep angle, using the rib as a fulcrum until resistance is encountered. Resistance indicates that the pleura has been engaged. The outer cannula is inserted over the needle to shear the core sample within the cutting needle, which is then withdrawn. The outer cannula is left *in situ* and the stylet and trocar are reinserted to seal the pleural space. Specimens are sent for both microbiological and cytological examination.

Therapeutic Thoracentesis

The principal indication for therapeutic thoracentesis is to relieve chest discomfort and dyspnea in patients with malignant pleural effusions. This procedure can be performed as an outpatient in the vast majority of patients.

Technique

There are many different methods used to perform therapeutic thoracentesis, including using a large-gauge needle, an intravenous cannula, or a small catheter. The author prefers the catheter technique using a 7-French catheter (Electro-catheter Corp., Rathway, NJ) with multiple side-holes which is trocared into the pleural space. It is connected by a three-way stopcock and tubing to a sterile 1-liter vacuum bottle which drains fluid from the chest. This can be changed when full. Usually a total of 2–3 L is removed in any one procedure. If severe coughing, dyspnea, or chest pain develop, the rate of fluid removal can be slowed and titrated against the patient's symptoms. If symptoms persist the catheter is clamped and a chest radiograph obtained to check for a pneumothorax.

In patients with malignant pleural effusions, occasionally the lung does not expand when fluid is removed; the underlying lung appears to be noncompliant. The cause of this is uncertain but it may be related to lymphangitis carcinomatosa which is microscopic in nature. This phenomenon (a "vacuthorax") does not have any clinical symptomatology and does not require treatment even when large. If treated with chest tube insertion the lung will usually not reexpand.

Pleurodesis

Malignant effusions often recur following therapeutic thoracentesis and may require pleurodesis for effective palliation. The sclerosing agent is injected into the pleural space and is designed to irritate the pleura so that the visceral and parietal pleura become fixed and prevent the reaccumulation of fluid. A number of sclerosing agents are available, with the most commonly used being doxycycline, bleomycin, or talc. Talc is generally instilled into the pleural space by surgeons in the operating room under general anesthesia. Doxycycline and bleomycin can be administered percutaneously. Tetracycline was originally used for pleurodesis but is no longer made by the manufacturer; doxycycline has been substituted. Doxycycline is administered in doses of 1–2 g dissolved in 100 mL of normal saline on three consecutive days. Bleomycin pleurodesis is performed in one session using 60 IU dissolved in 50 mL of 5% dextrose as a single dose. It has been shown by Belani and associates that bleomycin is the most cost-effective therapy for pleurodesis, even though initially more expensive than doxycycline.

Technique

Before pleurodesis, the pleural effusion needs to be drained almost dry for maximal sclerosant effect. Small catheters tend to kink in the pleural space and therefore larger (16- to 24-French) catheters are preferred. The catheter is connected to 20-cm negative wall suction using an underwater-seal pleural drainage system. Although the aim is to drain the effusion completely, this is frequently not possible with most malignant effusions. Therefore, a compromise position is reached such that, when the chest tube output has fallen below 100 mL per day, sclerotherapy is performed. If sclerotherapy is performed with chest tube drainage above 100 mL per day, the pleurodesis is more likely to fail.

After the agent is injected, the catheter is clamped for 1 hour and the patient is rolled every 15 minutes from supine to right lateral decubitus to prone to left lateral decubitus positions. This ensures efficient distribution of the sclerosing agent throughout the pleural space. The chest tube is then unclamped and the sclerosant

> **Box 18-14 Pleurodesis**
>
> Agents used include talc, doxycycline, and bleomycin
> Bleomycin is most cost-effective
> Pleurodesis performed when chest tube drainage is
>   <100 mL/day
> After pleurodesis the chest tube is placed on
>   underwater seal for 24 hours and then removed

allowed to drain through the chest tube. The tube is then placed on underwater seal drainage for 24 hours, and if a chest radiograph performed at that time shows no pneumothorax, the tube is removed (Box 18-14).

Empyema Drainage

Parapneumonic effusions that are complicated based on Light's criteria (described previously) require drainage. In addition, any diagnostic thoracentesis that yields pus or has a positive Gram stain or culture requires drainage.

It is logical to use image-guided catheter drainage for loculated empyemas as opposed to blind surgical techniques which are based on the chest radiograph as a reference. Not infrequently, blind empyema drainage results in a tube being placed in the pleural space outside the loculated empyema. Precise catheter placement with image guidance should be the first choice for loculated empyema drainage.

Technique

Ultrasound is the preferred image guidance modality as it is fast, efficient, and portable. The patient is positioned in a similar position to either a diagnostic or therapeutic thoracentesis. The skin position is marked over the mid-point of the loculated fluid collection. The skin is infiltrated with local anesthetic and incised with a #11 scalpel blade. Deep blunt dissection with a forceps considerably helps with tube placement and should be performed routinely. Large catheters are mandatory for empyema drainage to prevent tube clogging and kinking; 16- to 24-French catheters can be used, but the author prefers catheters larger than 20-French, particularly to reduce the effect of kinking which often happens with smaller catheters because of the effect of respiratory excursions pressing the catheter against the adjacent rib. The smaller catheters can usually be inserted using a trocar technique, while larger catheters are best inserted using the Seldinger technique (Fig. 18-27). The larger catheters can be inserted solely under ultrasound guidance by the Seldinger technique, but if the operator is uncomfortable with this, the patient can be brought to fluoroscopy and a combination of ultrasound and fluoroscopy used. After catheter insertion, the catheter is

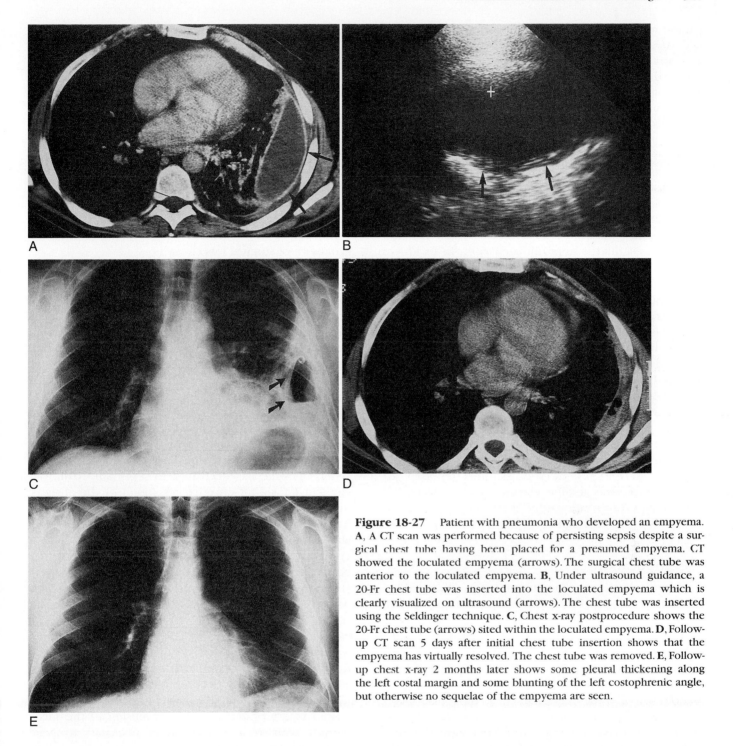

Figure 18-27   Patient with pneumonia who developed an empyema. **A**, A CT scan was performed because of persisting sepsis despite a surgical chest tube having been placed for a presumed empyema. CT showed the loculated empyema (arrows). The surgical chest tube was anterior to the loculated empyema. **B**, Under ultrasound guidance, a 20-Fr chest tube was inserted into the loculated empyema which is clearly visualized on ultrasound (arrows). The chest tube was inserted using the Seldinger technique. **C**, Chest x-ray postprocedure shows the 20-Fr chest tube (arrows) sited within the loculated empyema. **D**, Follow-up CT scan 5 days after initial chest tube insertion shows that the empyema has virtually resolved. The chest tube was removed. **E**, Follow-up chest x-ray 2 months later shows some pleural thickening along the left costal margin and some blunting of the left costophrenic angle, but otherwise no sequelae of the empyema are seen.

stitched to the skin and connected to an underwater-seal pleural drainage system. Close daily supervision of the patient and catheter should be performed by the interventional team.

Although the patient may be followed up by chest radiography, the author prefers CT scanning to evaluate the adequacy of drainage, particularly if the collection

has been loculated. The catheter can be removed if the patient is afebrile and drainage has decreased to less than 10–15 mL per day. Loculated empyemas or more complex collections may require multiple catheters for complete drainage and/or the use of intrapleural urokinase to lyse fibrinous septae and hemorrhagic components. The author's unit routinely uses urokinase if the patient remains febrile and there is residual fluid identified on follow-up imaging. Eighty-five thousand units are injected through the indwelling catheter which is clamped for 1–2 hours and then restored to suction. This is repeated every 8 hours for a total of 4–6 treatments. If urokinase treatment fails then open surgical drainage is usually indicated.

Results

Ultrasound-guided diagnostic thoracentesis is a low-risk procedure which can be successfully performed in up to 97% of patients. In patients with proven malignant effusions, the yield from cytological examination of aspirated pleural fluid is approximately 50%. In exudative effusions remaining undiagnosed after thoracentesis, a pleural biopsy may be performed. Pleural biopsy is highly specific for either tuberculosis or malignancy, with sensitivities of 90% and 68%, respectively. Pleural biopsy is particularly useful when tuberculosis is suspected, but less useful when malignancy is suspected.

Belani and associates, in a metanalysis of the literature, reported overall success rates for pleurodesis with tetracycline, bleomycin, and talc of 68.1%, 74.9%, and 94.1%, respectively. However, bleomycin proved to be the most cost-effective treatment overall.

The overall success rate for percutaneous drainage of empyema from reported series is 77%, which compares favorably to the 32–71% success rates reported for conventional surgical tube placement. It is likely that the overall success rate can be increased by the use of urokinase in selected patients.

Complications

Complications are uncommon with image-guided pleural intervention. Pneumothorax rates for US-guided thoracentesis vary from none to 3%, which compares favorably with the pneumothorax rates of 3–20% associated with blind aspiration. The author's unit has reported a pneumothorax rate of 7.5% in 350 consecutive patients who underwent therapeutic thoracentesis, with approximately 3% of these requiring chest tube placement. Re-expansion pulmonary edema has been reported by others as a result of rapid evacuation of pleural fluid, but in practice this is an extremely infrequent occurrence and the author's unit routinely aspirates 2–3 L of fluid in one treatment session. Complications reported with image-guided drainage of empyemas are uncommon and quoted to be less than 2%.

Pneumothorax is a common complication with all of the various pleural and lung interventions. Interventional radiologists should be familiar with the techniques of image-guided treatment of pneumothorax as detailed in Chapter 17.

LUNG AND MEDIASTINAL ABSCESSES

Primary lung abscesses are rare. When they do occur, they are most commonly due to aspiration or as a consequence of primary specific pneumonias due to organisms such as *Klebsiella*, *Pseudomonas*, or *Staphylococcus*. Secondary lung abscesses may result from septic emboli or obstructing bronchogenic neoplasms. Percutaneous drainage of lung abscesses is rarely required, as about 80–90% of patients respond to antibiotic therapy. For those lung abscesses that do not respond to antibiotic therapy, percutaneous abscess drainage is a valuable procedure both for abscess decompression and the avoidance of surgical lobectomy.

Although percutaneous drainage of lung abscesses can be performed under fluoroscopy, the author prefers to use CT guidance for placement of the initial needle into the abscess cavity. Small 8- or 10-French locking catheters are used for drainage. These can be placed either by trocar or Seldinger technique. It is important to repeat the CT scan after drainage to ensure that there are no undrained locules, and careful monitoring of the catheter after the procedure is necessary. The abscess contents are aspirated after the catheter has been inserted and the catheter is connected to an underwater-seal pleural drainage system. As with pleural empyema, CT is best used to evaluate the adequacy of drainage. When drainage has decreased to less than 10 mL per day and CT shows effective resolution of the abscess, the catheter can be removed. Success rates of 80–90% have been described for percutaneous drainage of lung abscesses.

Mediastinal abscesses are very uncommon, but may occur after cardiothoracic operations. Drainage of these abscesses follows the same principles as for mediastinal biopsy. Because of the proximity of vascular and mediastinal structures, these abscesses require very precise guidance and are best drained under CT control with the Seldinger technique. After the initial needle is placed, the patient is brought to fluoroscopy for track dilatation and catheter insertion. As with mediastinal biopsy, careful planning of the access route to avoid the internal mammary artery and vein and distension of the mediastinum with sterile saline may be necessary to avoid pneumothorax.

SUGGESTED READINGS

Acunas B, Rozanes I, Celik L et al: Purely cystic hydatid disease of the liver: treatment with percutaneous aspiration and injection of hypertonic saline. *Radiology* 182:541–543, 1992.

Balthazar EJ, Freeny PC, vanSonnenberg E: Imaging and intervention in acute pancreatitis. *Radiology* 193:297–306, 1994.

Belani CP, Eiranson TR, Arikan SR et al: Cost-effectiveness analysis of pleurodesis in the management of malignant pleural effusion. *J Oncol Manag* Jan/Feb:24-34, 1995.

Bennett JD, Kozak RI, Taylor MB. Deep pelvic abscesses: transrectal drainage with radiologic guidance. *Radiology* 185: 825-828, 1992.

Boland GW, Lee MJ, Dawson SL et al: Percutaneous abscess drainage: complications. *Semin Interv Radiol* 11:267-275, 1994.

Boland G, Lee MJ, Silverman S et al: Review: Interventional radiology of the pleural space. *Clin Radiol* 50:205-214, 1995.

Casola G, vanSonnenberg E, Neff CC: Abscesses in Crohn disease: percutaneous drainage. *Radiology* 163:19-22, 1987.

Casola G, vanSonnenberg E, D'Agostino HB et al: Percutaneous drainage of tubo-ovarian abscesses. *Radiology* 182:399-402, 1992.

Eisenberg PJ, Lee MJ, Boland GW et al: Percutaneous drainage of a subphrenic abscess with gastric fistula. *Am J Roentgenol* 162:1233-1237, 1994.

Gazelle GS, Haaga JR, Stellato TA et al: Pelvic abscesses: CT-guided transrectal drainage. *Radiology* 181:49-51, 1991.

Hovsepian DM: Transrectal and transvaginal abscess drainage. *J Vasc Interv Radiol* 8:501-515, 1997.

Kerlan RK, Jeffrey RB, Pogany AC, Ring EI: Abdominal abscess with low-output fistula: successful percutaneous drainage. *Radiology* 155:73-75, 1985.

Lahorra JM, Haaga JR, Stellato T et al: Safety of intracavitary urokinase with percutaneous abscess drainage. *Am J Roentgenol* 160:171-174, 1993.

Lambiase RE, Deyoe L, Cronan JJ et al: Percutaneous drainage of 335 consecutive abscesses: results of primary drainage with 1-year follow-up. *Radiology* 184:167-179, 1992.

Lambiase RE: Percutaneous abscess and fluid drainage: a critical review. *Cardiovasc Interv Radiol* 14:143-157, 1991

Lambiase RE, Cronan JJ, Dorfman GS et al: Postoperative abscesses with enteric communication: percutaneous treatment. *Radiology* 171:497-500, 1989.

Lee MJ: Non-traumatic abdominal emergencies: imaging and intervention in sepsis. *Eur Radiol* 12:2172-2179, 2002.

Lee KS, IM JG, Kim YH et al: Treatment of thoracic multiloculated empyemas with intercavitary urokinase: a prospective study. *Radiology* 179:771-775, 1991.

Lee MJ, Saini S, Brink JA et al: Interventional radiology of the pleural space: diagnostic thoracentesis, therapeutic thoracentesis, pleural biopsy, and pleural sclerosis. *Semin Interv Radiol* 8:23-28, 1991

Lee MJ, Saini S, Brink JA et al: Interventional radiology of the pleural space: management of thoracic empyema with image-guided catheter drainage. *Semin Interv Radiol* 8:29-35, 1991.

Lee MJ, Rattner DW, Legemate DA et al: Acute complicated pancreatitis: redefining the role of interventional radiology. *Radiology* 183:171-174, 1992.

Lee MJ, Wittich GR, Mueller PR: Percutaneous intervention in acute pancreatitis. *RadioGraphics* 18:711-724, 1998.

Light RW: Parapneumonic effusions and empyemas. *Clin Chest Med* 6:55-61, 1985.

Light RW, Macgregor ML, Luchingser PC et al: Pleural effusions: the diagnostic separation of transudates from exudates. *Ann Intern Med* 77:507-513, 1972.

Light RW, Erozan YS, Ball WC: Cells in the pleural fluid: their value in differential diagnosis. *Arch Intern Med* 132:854-860, 1973.

Martin EC, Karlson KB, Fankuchen EJ et al: Percutaneous drainage of postoperative intraabdominal abscesses. *Am J Roentgenol* 138:13-15, 1982.

Moore AV, Zuger JH, Kelley MJ: Lung abscess: an interventional radiology perspective. *Semin Interv Radiol* 8:36-43, 1991.

Moulton JS, Moore PT, Mencini RA: Treatment of loculated pleural effusions with transcatheter intracavitary urokinase. *Am J Roentgenol* 153:941-945, 1989.

Mueller PR, Saini S, Wittenbeurg J et al: Sigmoid diverticular abscesses: percutaneous drainage as an adjunct to surgical resection in 24 cases. *Radiology* 164:321-325, 1987.

Neff CC, vanSonnenberg E, Casola G et al: Diverticular abscesses: percutaneous drainage. *Radiology* 163:15-18, 1987.

Position Paper of the American Thoracic Society adopted by the ATS Board of Directors, June 1988: Guidelines for thoracentesis and needle biopsy of the pleura. *Am Rev Respir Dis* 140: 257-258, 1989.

Position Paper, Health and Public Policy Committee, American College of Physicians: Diagnostic thoracentesis and pleural biopsy in pleural effusions. *Ann Intern Med* 103:799-802, 1985.

Rattner DW, Legemate DA, Lee MJ et al: Early surgical debridement of symptomatic pancreatic necrosis is beneficial irrespective of infection. *Am J Surg* 163:105-111, 1992.

SCVIR Standards of Practice Committee: Quality improvement guidelines for adult percutaneous abscess and fluid drainage. *J Vasc Interv Radiol* 6:68-70, 1995.

Shepard JO: Complications of percutaneous needle aspiration biopsy of the chest: prevention and management. *Semin Interv Radiol* 11:181-186, 1994.

vanSonnenberg E, Mueller PR, Ferrucci JT: Percutaneous drainage of 250 abdominal abscesses and fluid collections: I. Results, failures and complications. *Radiology* 151:337-341, 1984.

vanSonnenberg E, Mueller PR, Ferrucci JT: Percutaneous drainage of 250 abdominal abscesses and fluid collections: II. Current procedural concepts. *Radiology* 151:343-347, 1984.

vanSonnenberg E, Wittich GR, Casola G et al: Periappendiceal abscesses: percutaneous drainage. *Radiology* 163:23-26, 1987.

vanSonnenberg E, D'Agostino HB, Casola G et al: US-guided transvaginal drainage of pelvic abscesses and fluid collections. *Radiology* 181:53-56, 1991.

vanSonnenberg E, D'Agostino HB, Casola G et al: Percutaneous abscess drainage: current concepts. *Radiology* 181:617-626, 1991.

vanSonnenberg E, Wroblicka JT, D'Agostina HB et al: Symptomatic hepatic cysts: percutaneous drainage and sclerosis. *Radiology* 190:387-392, 1994.

Walters R, Herman CM, Neff R et al: Percutaneous drainage of abscesses in the postoperative abdomen that is difficult to explore. *Am J Surg* 149:623-626, 1985.

Watkinson, AE, Adam A: Complications of abdominal and retroperitoneal biopsy. *Semin Interv Radiol* 11:254–266, 1994.

Weisbrod GL: Transthoracic percutaneous fine-needle aspiration biopsy in the chest and mediastinum. *Semin Interv Radiol* 8:1–14, 1991.

Westcott JL: Percutaneous catheter drainage of pleural effusion and empyema. *Am J Roentgenol* 144:1189–1193, 1985.

Zerbey AL, Dawson SL, Mueller PR: Pleural interventions and complications. *Semin Interv Radiol* 11:187–197, 1994.

CHAPTER 19

GI Tract Intervention

MICHAEL J. LEE, M.D.

Over the last number of years the role of the radiologist in GI tract intervention has mushroomed with the advent of percutaneous gastrostomy and more recently esophageal and colorectal stenting. These new procedures, coupled with the older procedures of GI stricture dilatation, have made GI tract intervention an important area of visceral intervention. Additionally, these procedures are predominantly performed under fluoroscopic guidance so that they can be performed in almost all radiology departments.

PERCUTANEOUS GASTROSTOMY

Surgical gastrostomy was first proposed in 1837 and successfully performed in 1876. It was not until almost a century later that Gauderer reported the endoscopic placement of a gastrostomy tube under local anesthesia.

The technique of radiologic gastrostomy quickly followed in 1983 and since then there have been numerous papers describing and refining the technique.

Indications

Percutaneous gastrostomy is predominantly performed for patients who need prolonged nutritional support. These include patients with neurologic disease (degenerative CNS disease, cerebral vascular accidents), head, neck and esophageal carcinoma, swallowing disorders, and esophageal strictures. Chronic conditions such as cystic fibrosis and congenital heart disease may also require a percutaneous gastrostomy. Occasionally, a percutaneous gastrostomy or gastrojejunostomy may be placed for bowel decompression. Indications for this include malignant small bowel obstruction or patients with prolonged ileus from major abdominal operations.

Contraindications

Contraindications are divided into absolute and relative (Box 19-1). Absolute contraindications include colonic interposition, total gastrectomy or severe uncorrectable coagulopathy, and extensive gastric varices. In patients with relative contraindications, the procedure may be technically more demanding and require more careful planning but is usually possible.

Technique

Patient Preparation (Box 19-2)

Informed consent is obtained before the procedure, usually from a relative or from the patient, if possible. The referring clinician is asked to pass a nasogastric (NG) tube on the evening prior to the procedure and administer 300 mL of an oral barium suspension. The barium

---

Box 19-1 Contraindications to Percutaneous Gastrostomy

Absolute

Gastric varices
Total gastrectomy
Uncorrectable coagulopathy

Relative

Ascites
Partial gastrectomy
Overlying colon
Coagulopathy
Inability to pass a nasogastric tube

Box 19-2 Pregastrostomy Requirements

Informed consent (usually from a relative)
Nasogastric tube placement
300 mL oral barium the evening prior to the procedure
Intravenous access

---

serves to delineate the relationship of the transverse colon to the stomach on the day of the procedure (Fig. 19-1). Occasionally, in patients with esophageal strictures it may not be possible for the referring team to place an NG tube. In this situation, in the author's unit we place the NG tube under direct fluoroscopic visualization at the time of the percutaneous gastrostomy. It is usually possible to place an NG tube even through tight strictures by first using a 5-French angiographic catheter and a hydrophilic wire. Once the stricture is crossed, the hydrophilic wire can be exchanged for a superstiff wire and an NG tube placed in the stomach.

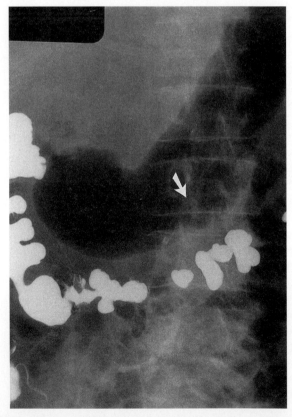

Figure 19-1 Patient referred for percutaneous gastrostomy. Barium given the night before delineates the colon which can be seen clearly separated from the stomach. The stomach is distended with air via the nasogastric tube (arrow). Colonic opacification is important so that it can be avoided during percutaneous gastrostomy.

Ask the referring team to place an intravenous cannula for sedoanalgesia and to fast the patient from midnight of the evening before the procedure. If, the barium that has been given has not reached the colon by the following day, there are a number of options available. Sometimes, the transverse colon may be visible on supine fluoroscopy without recourse to any other technical maneuveres to demonstrate the colon. If the colon is not visible, air can be insufflated via a rectal tube to demonstrate the colon. Alternatively, if lateral fluoroscopy is available the stomach is distended and a forceps is placed at the skin entry site and the location of the skin entry site vis-à-vis the stomach is ascertained. Usually the stomach is directly underneath the anterior abdominal wall with no intervening bowel loops. When the position of the colon is ascertained, the stomach is distended with air via the NG tube.

The author's unit does not routinely use a paralytic agent such as glucagon unless gastric peristalsis becomes a problem. Neither do we routinely give antibiotic prophylaxis. Some authors mark the position of the left lobe of the liver using ultrasound. We have not done this and have not had any hepatic complications in over 500 procedures. Usually, once the stomach is fully distended the entry site will be well below the left lobe of the liver. In general, the puncture site should be lateral to the rectus sheath to avoid the superior epigastric artery. Sometimes, it may not be possible to do this depending on the orientation and size of the stomach, and in this case a midline puncture is chosen. A combination of midazolam and fentanyl are used in small amounts for sedoanalgesia.

Gastropexy

The author's unit performs a gastropexy routinely in all patients. The advantages and disadvantages of this are discussed later. Gastropexy fixes the anterior wall of the stomach to the anterior abdominal wall and prevents guidewire buckling into the peritoneal cavity and early or late intraperitoneal leakage. Gastropexy is performed using "T" fasteners (Boston Scientific, Natick, MA) (Fig. 19-2). With the stomach maximally inflated, the puncture site into the stomach is chosen midway between the superior and inferior margins of the inflated stomach just proximal to the incisura. The puncture site is marked on the skin and subcutaneous injections of local anesthesia are given at the puncture site and at the four corners of a 2.5-cm square around the puncture site. A slotted 18-gauge needle is used to insert four "T" fasteners at the corner of this square. The "T" fasteners consist of a metal "T" bar attached to a Nylon suture which is attached to a cotton wool pledget. The Nylon suture runs through the cotton wool pledget, and between the cotton wool pledget and the distal end of the suture there are two small metal cylinders which are freely mobile on the suture (see Fig. 19-2).

The "T" fasteners are loaded on the slotted 18-gauge needle. The 18-gauge needle is attached to a partially saline-filled syringe and the stomach is punctured at the four corners of the 2.5-cm square. When air is aspirated, the tip of the slotted 18-gauge needle lies in the stomach. The syringe is removed and the stylet is used to push the "T" fastener out of the needle and into the stomach. The stylet and needle are removed and gentle tension on the external

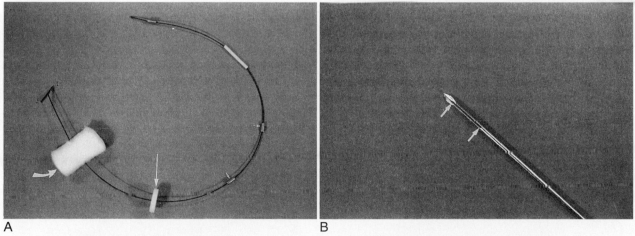

A   B

Figure 19-2   T-fastener gastropexy device. **A,** The T-fastener consists of a metal "bar" (T) attached to a Nylon suture which has a dental pledget (curved arrow), plastic ring washer (straight arrow), and two small metal cylinders (small arrows). The T-fastener is inserted into the end of the slotted needle which is inserted into the stomach. The T-fastener is dislodged using the stylet that comes with the set. The cotton wool pledget lies on the anterior abdominal wall and the metal cylinders are crimped on the Nylon suture using a surgical forceps while maintaining tension on the suture. This helps to fix the stomach to the anterior wall. **B,** Close-up of the end of the slot of the slotted needle showing the slot (arrows) in the end of the needle into which the T-fastener fits.

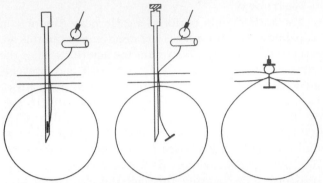

Figure 19-3 Illustration showing T-fastener gastropexy. The slotted needle containing the T-fastener is inserted into the stomach and the T-fastener pushed out of the needle using the stylet. Tension on the suture then opposes the T-fastener against the anterior abdominal wall which pulls the stomach up to the anterior abdominal wall. By crimping the metal cylinder on the suture the stomach is fixed to the anterior abdominal wall.

nylon suture opposes the stomach wall to the anterior abdominal wall (Fig. 19-3). The stomach is fixed in position by crimping the metal cylinders around the suture using a sterile forceps. When all four "T" fasteners are *in situ* the gastrostomy tube is placed (Fig. 19-4).

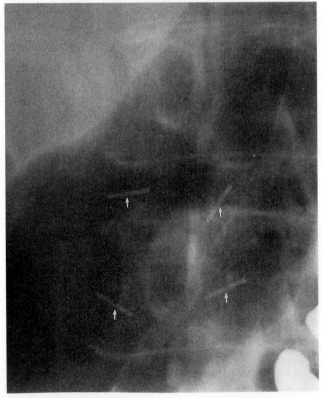

Figure 19-4 T-fastener gastropexy. Four T-fasteners (arrows) have been inserted at the corners of a 2.5-cm square to fix the stomach to the anterior abdominal wall. The gastrostomy tube can now be inserted.

Box 19-3   Gastrostomy: Key Points

Keep stomach optimally distended by air at all times
T-fastener gastropexy optional
Angle gastrostomy track toward pylorus
14- to 16-French tube placed
Gastrojejunostomy performed if history of hiatus
   hernia, reflux, or aspiration

Gastrostomy Tube Placement (Box 19-3)

The proposed site of entry for the gastrostomy tube (in the center of the "T" fastener square) is now anesthetized and a 3- to 4-mm transverse incision is made and dissected with a blunt forceps. The slotted needle that was used for the gastropexy is now used to puncture the stomach, and a 0.035-inch superstiff guidewire inserted so that it coils in the stomach lumen. The author tends to angle the puncture site towards the pyloric canal or antrum, so that if the gastrostomy needs to be converted to a percutaneous gastrojejunostomy in the future, the angle of the track will facilitate this (Fig. 19-5). It is important to keep the stomach inflated during gastropexy and gastrostomy tube placement. Complications are more likely to be encountered if the stomach is not maximally inflated at all times. Successive fascial dilators can be used to dilate the percutaneous track. The track is dilated to a size that is 1- to 2-French larger than the catheter

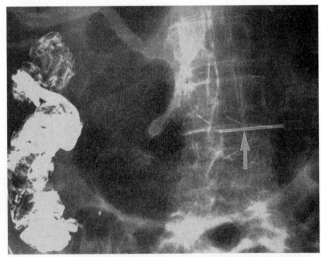

Figure 19-5 Gastrostomy tube angle of entry. The hypodermic needle (arrow) shows the approximate angle of entry of the gastrostomy tube into the stomach. The needle is inserted towards the pylorus at a 45-degree angle; if conversion of the tube to a gastrojejunostomy is required at a later date, the track will be angled towards the pylorus.

to be inserted. A 14- to 18-French gastrostomy catheter (Cook, Bloomington, IN) is placed through a peel-away sheath into the stomach. The peel-away sheath is usually provided with the gastrostomy tube. The guidewire is removed and contrast injected to confirm the intraluminal position of the gastrostomy tube. Although the percutaneous track may be angled towards the antrum, the gastrostomy tube will usually end up in the fundus of the stomach (Fig. 19-6). This is because the fundus is more posterior and more capacious than the gastric antrum. The NG tube is removed at the end of the procedure and the patient returned to the ward.

Aftercare

Begin tube feeding after 12–24 hours. Gastrostomy tubes should be flushed thoroughly after each feeding to prevent clogging. This is particularly important after the administration of crushed tablets through the tube. If clogging occurs, it can be treated by gentle flushing with hot water to dissolve impacted material. The "T" fasteners are cut at 2 to 5 days and allowed to fall into the stomach. This is simply performed by cutting the Nylon suture underneath the cotton wool pledget on the anterior abdominal wall.

In the author's unit we generally do not fix gastrostomy catheters to the skin as there is usually an internal fixation device on the catheter that prevents catheter dislodgement. The catheter entry site is simply covered with a sterile dressing. Suturing of the catheter to the skin may cause skin irritation and skin breakdown particularly if there is any leakage around the tube.

Special Considerations

Is Gastropexy Necessary?

Many authors do not routinely perform a gastropexy when a percutaneous gastrostomy tube is being placed. Gastropexy was devised to emulate surgical gastropexy which is used prior to placing surgical gastrostomy tubes. There is a lot of debate as to whether routine use of gastropexy devices is necessary. The literature would indicate that routine use is probably not necessary. There are many large series in the literature that describe percutaneous gastrostomy without gastropexy without any increase in complications. The theoretical advantages of using gastropexy are that larger catheters can be placed *de novo*, catheters and guidewires do not buckle into the peritoneal cavity, peritoneal leakage of gastric contents is less likely, and the catheter can be replaced if it is inadvertently pulled out soon after the procedure.

We recently performed a prospective randomized study involving 90 consecutive patients referred for percutaneous radiological gastrostomy (PRG) placement. Forty-eight patients underwent T-fastener gastropexy,

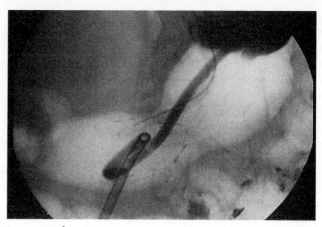

Figure 19-6   Gastrostomy tube insertion. After tract dilatation the catheter is inserted through a peel-away sheath and then locked in position. The catheter placed has a pigtail retention device (Cook, Bloomington, IN) which keeps the catheter in place. Even though the gastrostomy track is angled towards the pylorus, the tip of the tube usually ends up in the fundus of the stomach as this is the most dependent portion of the stomach.

while 42 underwent PRG without gastropexy. In four of the 42 patients (9%) from the nongastropexy group, serious technical difficulties were encountered with misplacement of the gastrostomy tube in the peritoneal cavity in two patients. This was discovered on injecting contrast material at the end of the procedure. T-fastener gastropexy was performed, and the procedure completed radiologically in 2 patients. In another patient the procedure was completed successfully without T-fastener gastropexy. In the remaining patient, it was decided to repeat the procedure on the following day. However, the patient underwent endoscopic placement of a gastrostomy tube the following day. In the gastropexy group, five patients experienced pain at the gastrostomy site, which was relieved by removing the T-fasteners. This would suggest that the placement of large-bore gastrostomy tubes (greater than 14-French) may cause problems without performing gastropexy. However, it is very much up to the operator's preference whether or not gastropexy is performed.

There are some situations where the use of a gastropexy device is important. This would include patients with ascites in which gastropexy combined with regular paracentesis is necessary to prevent tube dislodgement from the stomach.

CT Guidance

The author occasionally uses CT guidance for percutaneous gastrostomy in patients with no safe percutaneous access route to the stomach by means of standard fluoroscopic guidance, in patients in whom an NG tube cannot be placed owing to esophageal obstruction, and in patients with very scaphoid abdomens in which the stomach is tucked up underneath the rib cage. In addition, CT is often used in patients who have failed percutaneous endoscopic gastrostomy because of poor transillumination from the stomach to the anterior abdominal wall. In the latter situation, CT is often prudent to outline the relationships of the stomach to the anterior abdominal wall. Also, in patients with previous gastric surgery CT guidance may be necessary to place the tube. It needs to be emphasized that CT guidance is used in a minority of patients and the routine use of CT is unwarranted.

If CT guidance is used, the patient is placed supine on the CT table and a radiopaque grid placed on the anterior abdominal wall overlying the stomach. When the stomach is located, a safe path is chosen to place the initial needle. If an NG tube has not been placed in the stomach and the stomach is not distended, it may be possible to distend the stomach somewhat by giving carbonated granules to the patient before the CT procedure. If NG tube placement is not possible, or carbonated granules cannot be given, a 22-gauge Chiba needle is placed into the stomach and contrast injected to confirm an intraluminal position. Air is then injected, through the 22-gauge needle to distend the stomach. An 0.018-inch guidewire is placed through the needle into the stomach and a 5-French introducer sheath is placed over the guidewire with a final exchange made for a 0.038-inch "J" guidewire. The patient is then moved to fluoroscopy for the remainder of the procedure (Fig. 19-7).

Although CT guidance is necessary only in a minority of patients, it solves the anatomic or other impediments that make patients unsuitable for fluoroscopically guided gastrostomy.

The Postoperative Stomach

A previous subtotal gastrectomy is considered a relative contraindication to percutaneous gastrostomy. However, a number of techniques have been described to place gastrostomy tubes percutaneously in these patients. One of the problems with patients who have Bilroth 11 procedures or gastrojejunostomies is that air insufflated into the stomach almost immediately passes into the small bowel. In these patients it is useful to give glucagon or hyoscine butyl bromide to paralyse the stomach and small bowel. In general, the procedure can be performed under fluoroscopy. Lateral fluoroscopy is helpful to assess the position of the stomach remnant vis-à-vis the anterior abdominal wall. Giving barium prior to the procedure will help localize the colon. If a safe access is visualized then the procedure is carried out under fluoroscopy. If not, CT guidance is used (see Fig. 19-7). Some authors have described the placement of a large balloon into the stomach remnant – the balloon is inflated and direct puncture of the balloon is used to obtain initial percutaneous access. In the author's unit we use a technique similar to that used for a standard gastrostomy. Cephalocaudal angulation of the x-ray tube can help substantially in accessing a small stomach that lies subcostally. Sometimes the body of the stomach can be entered directly with a needle, on other occasions the efferent small bowel loop is punctured and the catheter tip ultimately positioned in the gastric remnant.

In general, gastric remnants that have previously been operated on are relatively fixed in the abdomen owing to postoperative fibrosis and adhesions. "T" fasteners are therefore not generally used. Once access to the stomach

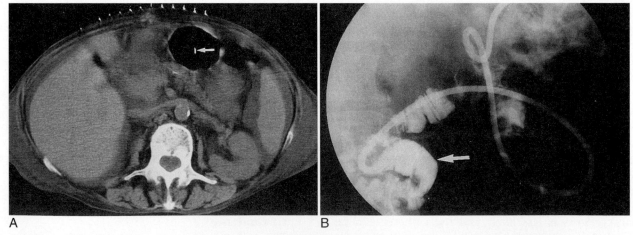

A   B

Figure 19-7   CT-guided gastrostomy tube placement in a patient with a previous Bilroth II gastrectomy. **A**, CT was used to guide the initial needle placement because of the small stomach remnant. The stomach was distended with air using a nasogastric tube with the aid of glucagon to decrease peristalsis. A needle (arrow) was placed into the stomach under CT guidance and the patient moved to fluoroscopy. **B**, After track dilatation the gastrostomy tube was placed into the efferent limb of the gastroenteric anastomosis. Contrast injection at the end of the procedure shows the catheter tip (arrow) located distally in the efferent limb.

Table 19-1   Technical Success and Complications Associated with Percutaneous Gastrostomy in Adults

Author	Year	Patients	Technical Success (%)	Complications (%)		Procedure-related Mortality (%)
				Major	Minor	
O'Keefe	1989	100	100	0	15	0
Saini	1990	125	99	1.6	9.5	0
Halkier	1990	252	99	1.6	4.4	0.8
Hicks	1990	158	100	6	12	2
Bell	1995	519	95	1.3	2.9	0.4
Ryan	1997	316	99	1.9	3.2	0.3

is gained with a one-stick needle system, the track is dilated and a 12- to 14-French nephrostomy type catheter is placed in the gastric remnant.

Results

Technical success rates of 98–100% have been reported in several large series describing percutaneous gastrostomy (Table 19-1). In one meta-analysis of the literature by Wollman and associates, the average success rate of percutaneous gastrostomy tube placement was 99.2% in a combined series of 837 patients (Table 19-2). This compares favorably with a 95.7% success rate for placement of percutaneous endoscopic gastrostomy tubes and 100% for surgical gastrostomy tube placement. By and large, percutaneous gastrostomy has become a widely accepted technique for gastrostomy tube placement and compares favorably with the endoscopic technique. The advantage of percutaneous gastrostomy over other techniques includes the ability to perform a percutaneous gastrojejunostomy at the time of initial tube placement, conversion of existing gastrostomy tubes to gastrojejunostomy tubes, and the ability to perform a gastrostomy in those patients with esophageal strictures through which an endoscope cannot pass.

Complications

Complications are described as major or minor as in the surgical literature. Minor complications include dislodged or leaking tubes and superficial wound infections requiring skin care. Major complications include wound-related problems (major infection, septicemia, etc.), aspiration, peritonitis, other gastrointestinal complications (perforation, hemorrhage), and dislodgement of the tube (Fig. 19-8) requiring a repeat procedure. From Wollman's meta-analysis of the literature, the complication rate for percutaneous gastrostomy is quite low in these categories. The complication rates can be seen in Table 19-2. Additionally, complication rates in two of the largest series in the radiologic literature are also quite low. In the series by Bell and associates, a major complication rate of 1.3% was seen in a total of 519 gastrostomy procedures; the minor complication rate was 2.9% (see Table 19-1). The major complication rate included four patients with peritonitis, two with hemorrhage requiring blood transfusion, and one with external leakage of gastric contents. In a second series by Ryan and associates, a major complication rate of 1.9% was seen in 316 consecutive patients with a minor complication rate of 3.2% (see Table 19-1).

Table 19-2   Comparison of Radiologic, Endoscopic and Surgical Gastrostomy [a]

Gastrostomy method	Patients	Technical Success (%)	Complications (%)		Procedure-related mortality (%)
			Major	Minor	
Radiologic	837	99.2	5.9	7.8	0.3
Endoscopic	4194	95.7	9.4	5.9	0.5
Surgical	721	100	19.9	9.0	2.5

[a]From Wollman BD, Agostino HB, Walus Wigle et al: Radiologic, endoscopic, and surgical gastrostomy: an institutional evaluation and meta-analysis of the literature. *Radiology* 197:699–704, 1995.

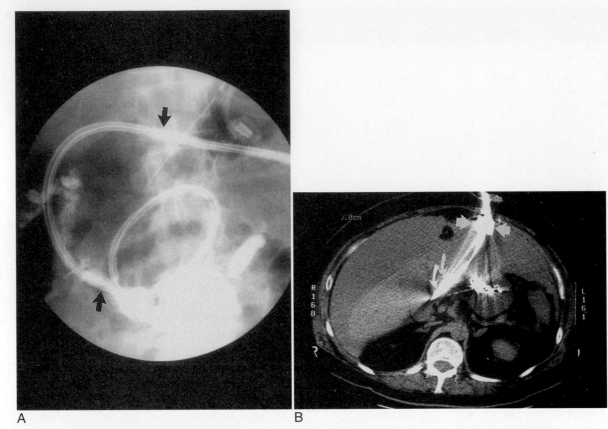

Figure 19-8   Gastric tube dislodgement with leakage of gastric contents into the peritoneal cavity in a patient with malignant ascites. **A**, A gastrojejunostomy tube (arrows) was placed for drainage of the small bowel which was partially obstructed. **B**, Twenty-four hours later the patient complained of severe abdominal pain and had peritoneal signs. A CT scan performed shows a moderate amount of ascites within the peritoneal cavity. Note the retention balloon device (large arrows) on the gastric catheter lying underneath the anterior abdominal wall. The retention device of the gastrostomy catheter had pulled out of the stomach because of the weight of the ascites pressing on the stomach wall. The remainder of the gastrostomy catheter (curved arrows) remains within the stomach. It is important if performing percutaneous gastrostomy in a patient with ascites to drain the ascites on a regular basis to prevent this happening. This patient was bought to the operating theater where it was noted that the four T-tacks had pulled through the stomach wall and were tying under the anterior abdominal wall. There was a 2-cm necrotic area in the anterior wall of the stomach which was repaired. (Reproduced with permission from McFarland EG, Lee MJ, Boland GW et al: Gastropexy breakdown and peritonitis after percutaneous gastrojejunostomy in a patient with ascites. *Am J Roentgenol* 164:189–193, 1995.)

Procedure-related complications can be minimized by careful attention to detail. Prior opacification of the colon and avoiding the location of the superficial epigastric artery can help avoid colonic perforation and hemorrhage, respectively. Adequate gastric distension at all times is mandatory to avoid losing access to the stomach during the procedure. Performing a gastropexy may help to decrease the incidence of guidewire buckling and dislodgement of the gastrostomy tube into the peritoneal cavity. Postprocedural complications such as tube clogging and dislodgement can generally be managed conservatively. Adequate grinding of pills and tablets before administration will help to decrease the incidence of tube clogging. Clogged tubes can be opened with either high-pressure syringes, heated water, or carbonated beverages.

If the tube remains clogged, the tube can often be opened up by passing a guidewire down through the tube.

If the tube becomes dislodged it is important to have the patient return to the interventional suite as soon as possible. The percutaneous track will often close over within 24–48 hours depending on the maturity of the track. If the patient comes to the interventional suite soon after catheter dislodgement, it is usually possible to regain access to the stomach using a combination of a Kumpe catheter and hydrophilic wire. A new catheter can then be placed. The referring clinician should be advised to replace the tube if it does fall out at night or over a weekend so that the percutaneous track is kept open until a new tube can be placed the following morning. The patient is not fed through the replaced tube until it is checked or replaced.

Wound infection may occur with any percutaneous procedure. Management depends on the extent. Minor edema can be treated with frequent dressing changes and wound cleansing. More significant cellulitis requires antibiotic therapy.

Leak of gastric contents around the tube is a rare phenomenon. However, when it does occur it may lead to marked skin irritation, infection, and skin breakdown. The combination of wound toilet, application of an antacid solution around the stoma, and upsizing the tube all help to control the skin irritation and breakdown. Occasionally, none of these procedures work and the tube may have to be removed, particularly if the skin breakdown is severe (Box 19-4).

New Departures in Percutaneous Gastrostomy

Placement of Endoscopic Catheters

Recently, modifications of the percutaneous gastrostomy technique have been employed. Unfortunately, existing gastrostomy catheters are either derived from "abscess drainage" catheters or "Foley"-type balloon catheters. Both are associated with the long-term complications of catheter clogging and/or dislodgement. Because of this, some authors have embarked upon the placement of the more robust endoscopic gastrostomy tubes using a percutaneous approach. In general, the "pull" type endoscopic gastrostomy catheters are used. The stomach is punctured and a guidewire is placed in the stomach. A 5 French angiographic catheter is placed over the guidewire and used to cannulate the esophagus. The catheter and guidewire are brought out through the mouth. If you are unable to cannulate the esophagus from below, a snare can be used to pull the guidewire out of the stomach and into the esophagus and out through the mouth. The "pull" type endoscopic gastrostomy catheter is then pulled from the mouth down through the esophagus and out through the anterior abdominal wall. A "pull" type gastrostomy tube is more secure and durable, and is less likely to occlude than radiologic counterparts. Disadvantages include seeding of metastases from oropharyngeal or esophageal tumors, the

potentially risk of infection, and the procedure requires two operators.

Primary Button Gastrostomy Placement

Button gastrostomy catheters have been widely used in the pediatric population where the low-profile nature makes them esthetically pleasing. A major disadvantage of the "button"-type catheter is the fact that a mature track of at least 3 months is advised before insertion of a gastrostomy button. The author's unit has recently embarked upon primary button gastrostomy catheter placement using a percutaneous technique.

There are two types of retaining device used in button gastrostomy catheters. One type uses the "mushroom" retaining device (Abbott Laboratories, Abbott Park, IL) while the second uses "a balloon" ("Cubby" – Corpak, Wheeling, IL; and "Mic-Key" – Ballard Medical Products, Draper, UT) (Fig. 19-9). Unfortunately, we have not been able to place the "mushroom"-type button without having a mature track. The balloon retention gastrostomy button we have placed in over a hundred patients.

Fourteen-, 16- or 18-French gastrostomy button catheters can be placed radiologically. The patient preparation is similar to standard gastrostomy catheter insertion. T-fastener gastropexy is mandatory for primary button gastrostomy catheter insertion. Accurate measurement of the track length is essential for button placement. When the stomach has been punctured and a superstiff guidewire placed, the track length can be measured by using an angioplasty balloon catheter, which is inflated

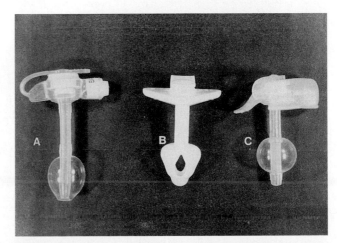

Figure 19-9   Image showing three different button gastrostomy catheters. **A** and **C** are examples of the "balloon retention" type gastrostomy button, while **B** is a "mushroom" type retention gastrostomy button. Traditionally, these buttons were placed in mature tracks; i.e., tracks that were in place for at least 6 weeks. The "balloon retention" type buttons can be placed *de novo* by percutaneous means using a gastropexy. We have not been able to place the "mushroom" type button *de novo*. (A, MIC-KEY gastrostomy button, Ballard Medical Products, Draper, UT; B, Abbott Laboratories, Abbott Park, IL; C, Cubby button, Corpak, Wheeling, IL.)

Box 19-4   Avoiding Complications

Prior colonic opacification
Regular paracentesis if ascites present
Optimal gastric distension during procedure
T-fastener gastropexy allows a more controlled
    procedure
Avoid superficial epigastric artery

within the stomach and pulled back until it abuts the anterior abdominal wall. The operator then holds the shaft of the catheter between the thumb and forefinger at skin level. The balloon catheter is then deflated and the balloon is withdrawn over the guidewire until it is fully visible. The balloon is then reinflated and the distance between the proximal end of the balloon and the operator's thumb and forefinger is measured to give the track length. In general, a button is chosen that is 5 mm longer than the track length measured (buttons vary in length from 2 to 5 cm). The slightly longer button is to account for changes in patient position, which may require extra adjustment of catheter length.

Alternatively, the track can be measured using the guidewire technique. The latter involves placing an angiographic catheter over the guidewire and into the stomach. Lateral screening is necessary to measure the track length using this method. The guidewire is pulled back until the end of the guidewire is flush with the anterior wall of the stomach. A kink is made in the guidewire, at the catheter hub. The guidewire is then pulled back until the distal end of the guidewire is at the skin site. Another kink is made in the guidewire at the hub of the catheter. The distance between the two kinks in the guidewire equates to the track length.

The track can be dilated using either the balloon catheter or serial fascial dilators. To place a 14-French button the track is dilated to 18-French; to place a 16-French button the track is dilated to 20-French; and to place an 18-French button the track is dilated to 22-French. When the track is dilated, a small fascial dilator is placed through the button and loaded on the guidewire (6-French dilator for a 14-French button; 7-French dilator for a 16-French button; and 8-French dilator for 18-French button). Abundant sterile jelly is used to lubricate the button, which is then pushed through the track into the stomach. The balloon is inflated with 5 mL of saline, the guidewire is removed, and the dilator is pulled back into the button before contrast material is injected to confirm an intragastric position (Fig. 19-10).

The advantages of button catheters are many, with the most significant being the avoidance of catheter clogging due to the short tube length. Also, the low-profile nature means that confused patients cannot grip the catheter

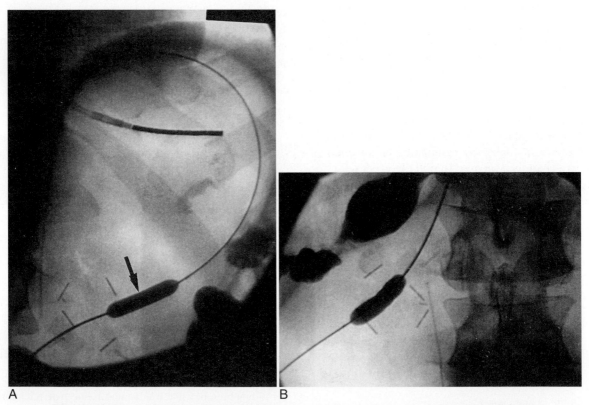

A   B

Figure 19-10   Gastrostomy button placement in a patient with neurologic disease. **A**, T-fastener gastropexy has been performed. A 6-mm balloon (arrow) was used to measure track length by inflating the balloon in the stomach and pulling it back against the stomach wall. The balloon catheter is gripped between the operator's thumb and forefinger at the skin, the balloon is deflated, removed from the stomach, and reinflated. The distance between the operator's thumb and forefinger on the shaft and the proximal end of the inflated balloon yields the rack length. **B**, The balloon catheter is then used to dilate the percutaneous track.   *(Continued)*

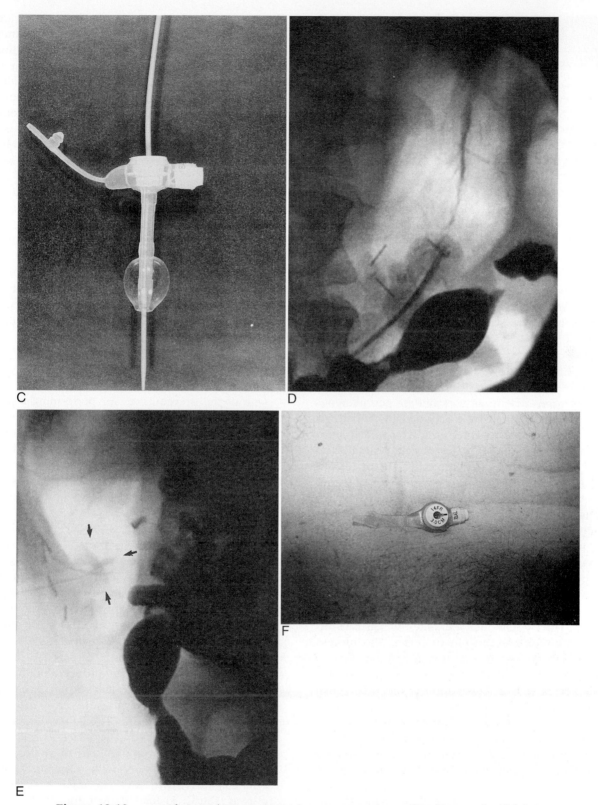

Figure 19-10   cont'd C, A 14-Fr gastrostomy button, mounted on a 6-Fr dilator and well lubricated, was inserted into the stomach over the superstiff guidewire. **D,** The dilator is pulled back into the shaft of the button, and contrast material injected to confirm an intragastric position. **E,** Lateral screening shows the stomach filled with air and the button balloon (arrows) present within the stomach lumen. **F,** The low-profile nature of the inserted button can be seen in this image of the patient's abdomen after removal of T-fasteners.

Box 19-5   Percutaneous Gastrostomy Modifications

Standard radiologic gastrostomy tubes have poor long-term patency

Pull-type PEG tubes can be placed percutaneously

Balloon retention button gastrostomy catheters can be placed *de novo*

T-fastener gastropexy required for button gastrostomy

---

sufficiently to remove it. The main disadvantage is that because it is a balloon retention device the balloon eventually bursts. On average the balloon lasts 3–6 months. The button devices can be simply replaced at the patient's bedside with a similar balloon retention button device. Alternatively, a "mushroom" type button can be placed because of the mature track (Box 19-5).

PERCUTANEOUS GASTROJEJUNOSTOMY

There is some debate as to whether percutaneous gastrojejunostomy should be performed in all patients as opposed to a percutaneous gastrostomy. The main indication for a percutaneous gastrojejunostomy is a previous history of reflux or aspiration. In one study comparing percutaneous gastrostomy to percutaneous gastrojejunostomy, scintigraphy was used to detect gastroesophageal reflux and determine whether gastrostomy tubes caused reflux. Patients were evaluated over 2 years with scintigraphic studies immediately before and 1 week after percutaneous gastrostomy. In almost half the patients at least one scintigraphic study was positive for reflux. Importantly, no causal relationship was noted between the presence of the gastrostomy tube and reflux. This would indicate that the gastrostomy tubes per se do not appear to incite reflux. The interesting point from this study was that a high number of patients (46%) referred for percutaneous gastrostomy had evidence of reflux. This supports the theory that gastrojejunostomy tubes should be placed *de novo* in many patients. However, it is difficult to say from this study whether the reflux was significant or not. Some authors do prefer to insert percutaneous gastrojejunostomy tubes *de novo*. The author prefers to place gastrostomy tubes initially unless there is a history of aspiration, if there is a large hiatus hernia, or if the patient's pulmonary status is such that an episode of aspiration could not be tolerated. If any of the above situations exist, a gastrojejunostomy tube is placed *de novo*.

Percutaneous gastrojejunostomy can be more technically challenging and tedious because the gastrostomy catheter has to be negotiated past the pylorus and duodenum into the jejunum. While this is often straightforward, it can be difficult in some patients. Additionally, a totally different feeding regimen is used for jejunal as opposed to gastric tubes. With gastric tubes feedings are usually of the bolus variety. For nursing staff, bolus tube feedings are more convenient as less time is spent monitoring feeding. In addition, for the patient who is active, bolus feeding intrudes minimally on a patient's lifestyle. Bolus feeding cannot be used for jejunal tubes as severe diarrhea will ensue. A slower drip feeding is used for jejunal tubes. This leads to more prolonged feeding times and increased nursing care. Jejunal feeding is also more of an intrusion on the patient's lifestyle. Indeed, some nursing homes are slow to accept patients on continuous feeding as opposed to bolus feeding. For these reasons, the author's unit tends not to place percutaneous gastrojejunostomy tubes *de novo*. However, once the decision is made to place a percutaneous gastrojejunostomy tube, the procedure is not dissimilar to percutaneous gastrostomy tube placement.

Technique

One of the prerequisites for performing a percutaneous gastrojejunostomy tube placement is the angulation of the percutaneous track. It is vitally important to angle the track towards the pylorus to facilitate passage of a guidewire and eventual passage of the tube towards the pyloric canal. Failure to do this may result in catheter and guidewire buckling up into the fundus of the stomach.

The procedure followed is similar to that of percutaneous gastrostomy initially. The stomach is distended and a gastropexy performed. The needle is then inserted through the chosen point of entry into the stomach and angled towards the pylorus. At this stage a 0.035-inch "J" guidewire is passed through the needle towards the pylorus. A Kumpe catheter is placed over the guidewire and the guidewire removed. A small amount of contrast is injected through the Kumpe catheter to outline the pyloric canal, duodenal cap, and descending duodenum. A 0.035-inch hydrophilic guidewire is then used in conjunction with the Kumpe catheter to negotiate the pyloric canal and duodenum. The guidewire and Kumpe catheter are placed beyond the ligament of Treitz in the proximal jejunum, and the hydrophilic guidewire is exchanged for a 0.035-inch superstiff guidewire (Meditech, Watertown, MA). The track is dilated and a peel-away sheath is loaded over the guidewire down towards the pylorus. The peel-away sheath also helps to direct the catheter through the pylorus and into the jejunum. The author's unit uses a similar catheter to that used for percutaneous gastrostomy, except that the catheter is longer, but has a similar self-retaining proximal pigtail (Cook Inc., Bloomington, IN). When the catheter is placed contrast is injected to confirm the jejunal location and the peel-away sheath is removed (Fig. 19-11).

Results and Complications

Percutaneous gastrojejunostomy is associated with a high technical success rate similar to that of percutaneous gastrostomy. However, the success rate is slightly lower because of occasional technical problems in cannulating the pylorus. Bell and associates, in a large series, reported a 2.8% failure rate because of inability to catheterize the pylorus.

The complications associated with percutaneous gastrojejunostomy are similar to those reported for percutaneous gastrostomy. Duodenal perforation has been reported as a distinct complication of percutaneous gastrojejunostomy but this is rare.

CONVERSION OF PERCUTANEOUS GASTROSTOMY TO GASTROJEJUNOSTOMY

More and more frequently, the author's unit is asked to convert existing gastrostomy tubes to gastrojejunostomy

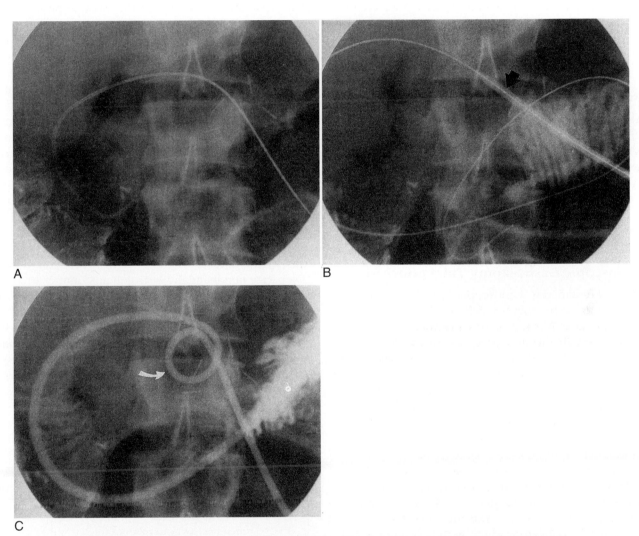

Figure 19-11   Placement of a percutaneous gastrojejunostomy tube in a patient with a history of reflux and aspiration. **A**, A Kumpe catheter (Cook, Bloomington, IN) (arrow) is used to cannulate the pylorus with the aid of a 0.035- or 0.038-inch guidewire. Track angulation towards the pylorus is important to facilitate this maneuver. When the Kumpe catheter is in the jejunum the guidewire is exchanged for a 0.038-inch superstiff guidewire (Boston Scientific, Nadic, MA) and the percutaneous track dilated. **B**, The gastrostomy catheter (arrow) is inserted through a peel away sheath over the guide wire and into the jejunum. **C**, An injection of contrast medium at the end of the procedure shows the retention loop of the catheter (curved arrow) in the stomach with the catheter tip in the jejunum distal to the ligament of Treitz.

tubes in patients who aspirate or who are not able to tolerate gastric feeding. There are a number of factors to consider before converting one of these tubes.

The first consideration is whether the existing tube was inserted radiologically, endoscopically, or surgically. The second consideration is the length of time between initial tube placement and the request for conversion. For some radiologic and endoscopic tubes, a mature track may not have had time to form between the stomach and the anterior abdominal wall. In this situation, there is a risk of disrupting the track or losing access during attempts at conversion to a percutaneous gastrojejunostomy tube. A further consideration is the size of the existing tube. Generally, surgically and endoscopically placed gastrostomy tubes may be larger than radiologically placed tubes. The catheter you intend placing must be of a size that will take up most of the percutaneous track, otherwise leakage of gastric contents may be a problem.

Radiologic Gastrostomy Tube Conversion

At our institution, percutaneous gastrostomy tubes placed by us will have had "T" fasteners placed and the percutaneous track is usually angled towards the pylorus. This facilitates easy conversion of the gastrostomy tube to a percutaneous gastrojejunostomy tube. Use of "T" fasteners means that even if the track is immature, the conversion can still be performed as access to the stomach will not be lost.

Endoscopic Gastrostomy Tube Conversion

Most percutaneous endoscopic gastrostomy (PEG) tubes have inner bumpers which are designed to hold the tube in place. It is not usually possible to pull these bumpers through the percutaneous track. You can cut the endoscopic tube flush with the skin and allow the inner portion with the bumper to fall into the stomach. Alternatively, the PEG tube can be left *in situ* and a new percutaneous gastrojejunostomy tube inserted through a new track. The author prefers to cut the percutaneous endoscopic gastrostomy tube at the skin and allow the inner bumper to fall into the stomach. One of the downsides in using this approach is that occasionally the inner bumper may cause symptoms of GI obstruction. In the author's experience this happens rarely, but this complication has been reported in the literature. One of the other problems that can be found with PEG tubes is that the percutaneous track is often angled towards the fundus of the stomach, making it difficult to redirect the track towards the antrum. The use of a large 15- or 16-French peel-away sheath and dilator has been helpful in this regard (Fig. 19-12). Over a wire placed in the stomach, the 16-French peel-away sheath is placed and the track angled towards the antrum by applying pressure to

the peel-away sheath. The guidewire is then redirected towards the pyloric antrum. Once this is done, the dilator is removed, leaving the peel-away sheath and guidewire *in situ*. A Kumpe catheter and glidewire are then used to negotiate the pyloric canal, and the procedure is then performed in a similar fashion to percutaneous gastrojejunostomy.

Surgical Conversion to Percutaneous Gastrojejunostomy

The success of surgical gastrostomy conversion to percutaneous gastrojejunostomy depends on the type of surgical procedure used to place the gastrostomy tube. The common procedure is the Stamm procedure in which, through a laparotomy incision, a portion of the mid-gastric body is opened and a Mallecot or Foley-type catheter is placed. Concentric purse-string sutures are placed around the catheter and tightened around the gastrostomy tube. The tube is then delivered externally through a separate stab incision in the anterior abdominal wall. The stomach is pulled up to the anterior abdominal wall and sutured to it with a number of interrupted sutures. The other technique described is that of a Witzel gastrostomy. In this procedure a long subcutaneous tunnel is fashioned around the external portion of the tube. This tunnel is directed towards the fundus of the stomach. In the author's experience, if a Witzel gastrostomy has been performed, it is virtually impossible to convert to a percutaneous gastrojejunostomy. In this situation, it is best to start *de novo* and perform a separate percutaneous gastrojejunostomy.

It is usually possible to convert surgical gastrostomy tubes to percutaneous gastrojejunostomy tubes if the Stamm technique has been used. Again, similar to PEG tube conversion, a 16-French sheath is used to re-angle the track towards the antrum. When this is done the gastrojejunostomy tube is placed as with the PEG conversion (Box 19-6).

Box 19-6   Gastrostomy to Gastrojejunostomy Conversion

Cut PEG tubes at skin level
15/16-French peel-away to redirect track toward pylorus
Kumpe catheter and hydrophyllic guidewire placed in jejunum
Gastrojejunostomy catheter placed over superstiff guidewire
Witzel surgical gastrostomy not possible to convert
Stamm surgical gastrostomy can be converted

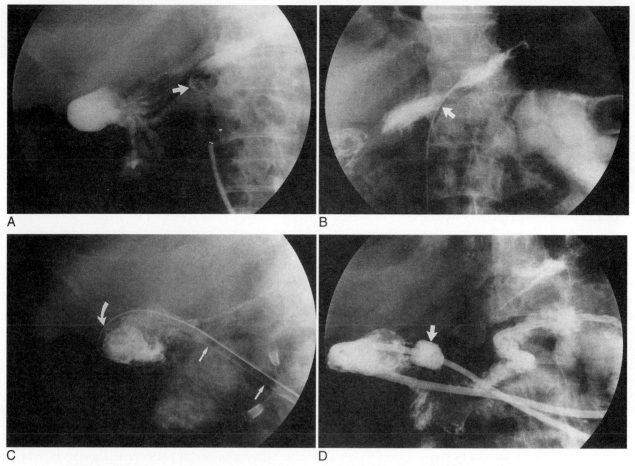

Figure 19-12   Conversion of an endoscopically placed gastrostomy tube to a gastrojejunostomy tube. **A**, Contrast injection through the endoscopically placed gastrostomy tube shows the tube and balloon retention device (arrow) present within the stomach lumen. **B**, The tube was removed and a Kumpe catheter inserted into the stomach. Note the track angulation (arrow) toward the fundus of the stomach. **C**, A 16-Fr peel-away sheath (straight arrows) was placed into the stomach and used to redirect the percutaneous tract toward the pylorus. A Kumpe catheter (curved arrow) was used to cannulate the pylorus and a 0.038-inch superstiff guidewire was manipulated into the proximal jejunum. **D**, A gastrojejunostomy catheter was placed through the peel-away sheath with the tip placed into the proximal jejunum. Note the balloon retention device (arrow) on this catheter.

Results

In a study of 63 patients by Lu and associates, conversion of surgical gastrostomy to percutaneous gastrojejunostomy was successful in 83%. The success rate for conversion of PEG tubes to percutaneous gastrojejunostomy tubes was slightly lower at 78%, while conversion of percutaneous gastrostomy tubes to percutaneous gastrojejunostomy tubes had a success rate of 100%. Failures with surgical tubes and PEG tubes were related to the inability to redirect the percutaneous track towards the pyloric antrum. Recoil of the guidewire into the fundus of the stomach invariably occurred in these patients and pyloric cannulation was not possible. In these patients a *de novo* percutaneous gastrojejunostomy tube had to

be placed. The 100% success rate for conversion of percutaneous gastrostomy tubes to percutaneous gastrojejunostomy tubes reflects the fact that "T" fasteners are used at the author's institution and that the percutaneous track is angled towards the pylorus on initially placing gastrostomy tubes.

COMPARISON OF PERCUTANEOUS, ENDOSCOPIC, AND SURGICAL GASTROSTOMY

Percutaneous gastrostomy performed radiologically has the lowest rate of major complications as well as the lowest procedural mortality when compared with percutaneous endoscopic gastrostomy and surgical gastrostomy. However, it has been estimated that percutaneous gastrostomy accounts for 35% of all gastrostomies in academic institutions, decreasing to 18% in community practices. This is partially due to the fact that percutaneous gastrostomy was described after the percutaneous endoscopic gastrostomy technique, but it also reflects the lack of access to patients by interventional radiologists.

In a meta-analysis of 5752 patients (837 percutaneous gastrostomy procedures, 4194 percutaneous endoscopic gastrostomy procedures, and 721 surgical procedures) significant differences in rates of successful tube placement between percutaneous endoscopic gastrostomy and percutaneous gastrostomy techniques were seen (95% versus 99.2%, $p < 0.01$). A smaller difference was seen between percutaneous gastrostomy and surgical gastrostomy. Significant differences ($p < 0.01$) in the procedural mortality rate between all three techniques were also seen, with percutaneous gastrostomy having the lowest procedural mortality rate (percutaneous gastrostomy 0.3%, percutaneous endoscopic gastrostomy 0.53%, surgical gastrostomy 2.5%). The 30-day mortality rate was similar for all three gastrostomy techniques and ranged from 7 to 14%. This reflects the underlying debility of many of these patients referred for gastrostomy procedures rather than the efficacy of the procedure itself. Major complications occurred less frequently after percutaneous gastrostomy (5.9%) versus percutaneous endoscopic gastrostomy (9.4%), and surgical gastrostomy (19.9%).

Other points to consider are that percutaneous endoscopic gastrostomy offers diagnostic capabilities that are not available with percutaneous gastrostomy. In other words, the stomach can be inspected endoscopically during the percutaneous endoscopic gastrostomy procedure and abnormalities recorded and/or treated. The rate of abnormal findings seen during PEG procedures has varied from 10 to 70.1% in the literature. The most common are inflammation or ulceration of varying degrees of severity. However, almost none of the abnormalities is as serious as an unexpected cancer.

It seems that percutaneous gastrostomy and percutaneous endoscopic gastrostomy are both viable, minimally invasive techniques for performing gastrostomy and both should be preferred over surgical gastrostomy. They are both quick and easy to perform and associated with fewer complications than surgical gastrostomy. However, percutaneous gastrostomy is associated with significantly fewer major complications, lower rates of tube complications, and slightly higher rates of successful tube placement. The advantage of percutaneous gastrostomy over other techniques includes the ability to perform gastrojejunostomy at the time of initial tube placement, conversion of existing gastrostomy tubes to gastrojejunostomy tubes, and the ability to perform gastrostomy in those patients who are unsuitable for PEG tube placement (Box 19-7).

Box 19-7   Advantages of Radiologic Gastrostomy over PEG

Fewer major complications
Lower rates of tube complications
Higher technical success rate
Gastrojejunostomy is technically easier
Gastrostomy performed in patients unsuitable for PEG

DIRECT PERCUTANEOUS JEJUNOSTOMY

Direct percutaneous jejunostomy is infrequently performed but has some well-recognized indications. The most common indication is when gastrojejunostomy tube conversion is not appropriate or has failed in a patient who is aspirating. A unique indication for direct percutaneous jejunostomy is the replacement of a prematurely dislodged surgical jejunostomy tube.

Technique

Direct percutaneous jejunostomy can be performed under fluoroscopic or CT guidance. Hallisey and Pollard described the fluoroscopic technique and reported on the largest number of patients. In their technique, a jejunal loop in the left upper quadrant is identified by air insufflation through a nasogastric tube. A direct puncture of the distended loop is then performed with a 17-gauge needle under fluoroscopic guidance. Contrast material is injected once the needle is in position, and when intraluminal position is confirmed a 0.035-inch hydrophilic guidewire is introduced along with a 5-French hydrophilic catheter. An anchoring procedure with Cope sutures or "T" fasteners is then performed to hold the jejunum up to the anterior abdominal wall. Dilatation of the tract is performed followed by placement of a 14-French locking pigtail catheter.

Ultrasound or CT guidance can also be used for jejunal catheter placement. Using ultrasound or CT, a safe path to a proximal jejunal loop can be chosen and in particular the colon can be avoided. Additionally, it is important not to traverse more than one jejunal loop. The author tends to place a 0.018-inch wire in the jejunal loop after first puncturing the jejunal loop with a 22-gauge needle. The patient is then transferred to fluoroscopy and "T" fasteners are inserted followed by tract dilatation and tube placement.

Results and Complications

The total number of patients in whom direct percutaneous jejunostomy has been performed is small and the reported technical success rates have varied from 60 to 100%. Hallissey and Pollard reported the largest series of 13 patients with a successful outcome in 11 of 13 patients. Complications are similar to those described for percutaneous gastrostomy.

PERCUTANEOUS CECOSTOMY

Cecostomy has been a standard surgical technique since 1710 when it was first described. It is usually performed through an open surgical procedure but more recently it has been performed laparoscopically. Percutaneous cecostomy is a novel alternative to the surgical technique. The method used is similar to that for percutaneous gastrostomy. Percutaneous cecostomy can be performed under local anesthesia and intravenous sedoanalgesia as opposed to the surgical technique which is usually performed under general anesthesia.

Indications

Cecal dilatation of greater than 10 cm is associated with a significant risk of perforation. If perforation occurs, there is an associated mortality of up to 50%. Therefore, it is prudent to decompress the at-risk cecum quickly and effectively. The main indication for colonic decompression is colonic pseudo-obstruction or the so-called Ogilvie's syndrome. Colonoscopic decompression has been used for this condition and can be successful in up to 70% of cases. However, patients who do not respond to colonoscopic decompression will require cecostomy. Other indications for percutaneous cecostomy include cecal dilatation proximal to a distal large bowel obstruction, and cecal volvolus.

Before a percutaneous cecostomy is planned, it is important to make sure that there is no evidence of bowel necrosis or perforation. If there are clinical signs of perforation or bowel necrosis, then surgical exploration and appropriate surgical therapy is warranted.

Technique

Access Route

The author's unit uses an anterior transabdominal approach to the cecum. This is an intraperitoneal approach, as might be expected. An extraperitoneal approach has been described. This involves using a posterior access route and using CT guidance. The potential advantage of this approach is that if there is any leak it will be extraperitoneal. However, the right peritoneal reflection often extends in a deep posteromedial direction behind the cecum, which leaves only a small portion of the cecum that is extraperitoneal. It can be difficult to be sure that a catheter inserted from a posterior approach

is in fact extraperitoneal. For this reason, and because the anterior approach is more straightforward, the anterior approach is preferred.

Cecopexy

The author uses "T" fasteners to perform a cecopexy which fixes the anterior wall of the cecum to the anterior abdominal wall and helps to prevent leakage into the peritoneal cavity. This is an important part of percutaneous cecostomy and, while it may be optional for the percutaneous gastrostomy technique, it should be performed during percutaneous cecostomy. The patient is placed in a supine position on the table and the midpoint of the distended cecum is chosen as the needle entry site. "T" fasteners are inserted at the corners of a 2-cm square around the needle entry site as previously described for percutaneous gastrostomy. When the "T" fasteners are *in situ*, they are fixed with gentle traction on the suture (Fig. 19-13).

Cecostomy Catheter Insertion

Using a 14- to 16-French gastrostomy catheter (Cook, Bloomington, IN), the cecum is punctured at the needle entry site with the slotted needle used for "T" fastener insertion. A 0.038-inch superstiff wire is inserted into the cecum and manipulated up the ascending colon. The percutaneous track is dilated with serial fascial dilators and a 14- to 16-French gastrostomy catheter is placed through a peel-away sheath (see Fig. 19-13).

Aftercare

The catheter is left to gravity drainage and attached to a bag. Frequent flushing with 50–100 mL of normal saline every 2–4 hours is very helpful in breaking down solid fecal material and also in preventing catheter blockage. Cecostomy catheters require close supervision from the interventional radiology team and daily rounds are required to detect any catheter malfunction, pericatheter leakage, or intraperitoneal leak (Box 19-8).

Box 19-8 Percutaneous Cecostomy: Key Points

Do not perform if signs of bowel ischemia/perforation
Anterior transabdominal approach and fluoroscopic guidance
T-fastener cecopexy mandatory
14- to 16-French catheter placed
Frequent catheter irrigation with 50–100 mL of saline
Close catheter supervision mandatory

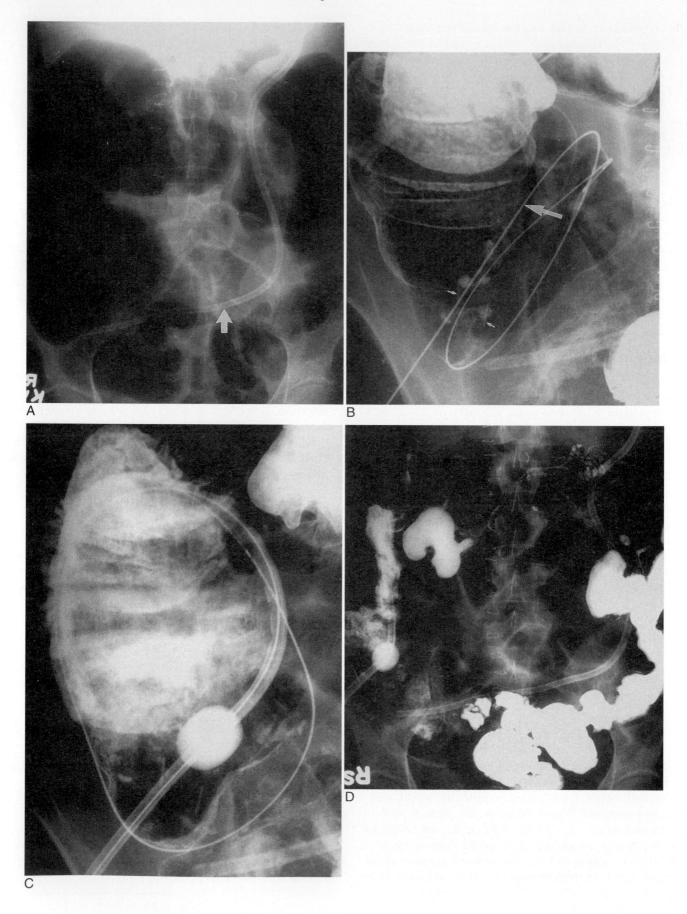

				Guidance		
First Author	**Year**	**Patients**	**Indication**	**Modality**	**Approach**	**Complications**
Quinn	1997	1	Volvolous	CT	IP	None
Maaga	1987	1	Pseudo-membranous colitis	CT	EP	None
VanSonnenberg	1990	5	Ogilvies	CT (1) Fl (4)	IP	Pericatheter leak in one
Morrison	1990	2	Miscellaneous	Fl	IP	None
Masterson	1991	1	Ogilvies	US	EP	Septicemia
Salim	1991	28	Distal bowel obstruction	None	IP	None
Maginot	1993	1	Ogilvies	Fl	IP	Abdominal wall sepsis

Table 19-3 Literature Experience with Percutaneous Cecostomy[a]

[a]Modified from Varghese JC, Lee MJ: Percutaneous cecostomy. *Semin Interv Radiol* 4:351-354, 1996.
CT, computed tomography; Fl, fluoroscopy; IP, intraperitoneal; EP, extraperitoneal.

Results

There have been a total of just 39 percutaneous cecostomy procedures reported in the literature, all technically successful. The main indication for cecostomy was Ogilvie's syndrome. In all cases, the catheters have functioned well with good cecal decompression. Catheters have remained *in situ* for between 24 hours and 1 month. Most authors have used fluoroscopy for guidance, with occasional use of CT. One author used no imaging guidance, which cannot be recommended (Table 19-3).

Complications

Complications reported in the literature are few and include one patient with a pericatheter leak of fecal material, another patient with a septicemia postprocedure, and a third patient with abdominal wall sepsis. In this latter patient, multiloculated abscesses formed in the anterior abdominal wall due to fecal contamination along the catheter track. This patient eventually died from sepsis and multiorgan failure. Potential complications are many and include catheter dysfunction, pericatheter leakage, fecal peritonitis, sepsis, and cecal trauma during the procedure (see Table 19-3). With close attention to detail many of these complications can be minimized. The use of "T" fasteners should theoretically help to prevent fecal peritonitis and pericatheter leakage. Placement of large-bore catheters (greater than 12-French) and frequent irrigation with normal saline should reduce the incidence of catheter blockage.

Overall percutaneous cecostomy is an effective method for decompression of the cecum and is associated with a low complication rate provided close attention is paid to technique.

RADIOLOGIC MANAGEMENT OF GI TRACT STRICTURES

Benign GI Strictures

Strictures of the GI tract have traditionally been treated by surgical techniques which have been associated with unacceptably high morbidity and mortality. More recently, endoscopic and interventional radiologic procedures are rapidly becoming accepted as an

Figure 19-13 Percutaneous cecostomy in a patient with ovarian cancer and encasement of the sigmoid colon causing colonic obstruction. The patient was debilitated and a poor surgical risk. **A**, Plain film of the abdomen shows considerable colonic distension with the cecum measuring 15 cm. One staple line is noted on the anterior abdominal wall and a long nasogastric decompression tube (arrow) is noted within the small bowel. However, this did not decompress the colon. **B**, Using an anterior approach, two T-fasteners (small arrows) were placed into the cecum and the T-fastener needle was then used to puncture the cecum and a 0.038-inch Ring guidewire placed (large arrow). **C**, A 14-Fr gastrostomy catheter with retention balloon was then placed into the cecum through a peel-away sheath. **D**, Plain film of the abdomen obtained 2 days later shows decompression of the colon from the cecostomy tube. Regular irrigation with 50 mL of saline was performed every 4-6 hours to facilitate drainage of cecal contents. After a week of cecostomy tube drainage the patient returned to theater for a colostomy.

effective method for dealing with this frustrating clinical problem. Esophageal stenoses are the most common strictures which present for treatment. However, gastric, duodenal, and colorectal strictures may also be amenable to balloon dilatation.

Balloon Dilatation of Esophageal Strictures

Bougienage has been performed for centuries for esophageal stricture dilatation. This involves the use of an instrument with a round, oval tip which is inserted through the stricture and progressively stretches the stricture to achieve the desired lumen. This procedure is now performed endoscopically and most of the bougies used can now be passed over a guidewire. These devices have one major disadvantage compared with balloon dilatation – they produce significant longitudinal shear forces on the stricture and on the normal esophagus (Fig. 19-14). These shear forces can lead to perforation or mucosal tears. On the other hand, balloon dilatation, which involves passing a small balloon catheter over a guidewire, produces radial stretch forces only without any element of longitudinal shear. Theoretically, this should decrease the risk of mucosal tear or perforation.

Technique

If a recent barium swallow is not available, then a barium swallow should be performed to assess the size and location of the stricture. The author's unit generally performs this on the day prior to the procedure. On the day of the procedure the patient is placed in a decubitus position and a mouthpiece placed in the mouth. A transoral route is preferred for this procedure. A topical anesthetic spray is applied to the back of the throat to reduce the gag reflex. We then use a 5-French angiographic catheter and a hydrophilic guidewire to enter the esophagus under fluoroscopic control. The guidewire and catheter are manipulated down to a level just above the stricture. A small amount of contrast is injected at this stage to outline the proximal end of the stricture. The guidewire and catheter are then manipulated through the stricture and down into the stomach. The guidewire is then changed for an exchange length stiff wire (180 cm or 260 cm).

Depending on the stricture, start with a 10- or 12-mm diameter balloon. The goal is a luminal diameter of 20-mm. However, it is prudent to start with a smaller balloon and, if this is well tolerated, then a 15-mm followed by a 20-mm diameter balloon can be used. However, if the patient experiences significant discomfort with a 10-mm or 12-mm balloon, the session is terminated for that day. The balloon is left inflated for 1–2 minutes until the "waist" disappears (Fig. 19-15).

The author's unit does not do an immediate esophagogram after the procedure but prefers to wait for 6–12 hours. If the patient experiences significant pain during the procedure, we inject some nonionic contrast material to make sure there is no mucosal tear or frank perforation. Otherwise the patient returns to the ward and is kept fasting until the esophagogram is performed 4–6 hours later. If the esophagogram is performed immediately after dilatation, the stricture often appears similar to the predilatation stricture. This is because of acute

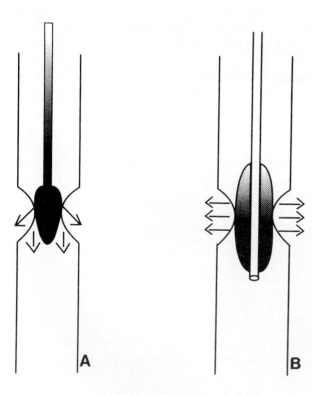

Figure 19-14 Schematic showing the difference between a bougie dilatation and balloon dilatation. **A**, Bougie dilatation produces longitudinal sheer stress as shown by the arrows. This is more likely to perforate the esophagus. **B**, Balloon dilatation on the other hand produces radial forces which are less likely to perforate the esophagus.

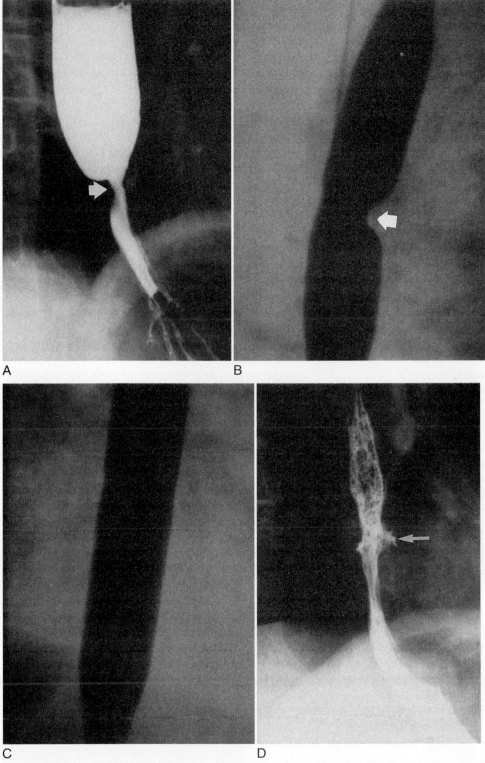

Figure 19-15 Patient with a recurrent benign esophageal reflux stricture referred for balloon dilatation. **A,** Esophagogram performed prior to the procedure shows a tight stricture (arrow) in the distal esophagus. **B,** The stricture was negotiated with a 5-Fr angiographic catheter and guidewire. Initially 12-mm and 15-mm balloons were used to dilate the stricture. Minimal effect was noted with these. A 20-mm balloon was placed and a waist (arrow) was clearly seen on the balloon. **C,** The balloon was inflated until the waist had disappeared and the balloon remained inflated for 2 minutes. **D,** Esophagogram the following day shows a good result with decompression of the esophagus. There was a little intramural tear and contrast present in the esophageal wall (arrow). The patient was asymptomatic and remained fasting for a further 2 days at which time the small intramural tear had healed.

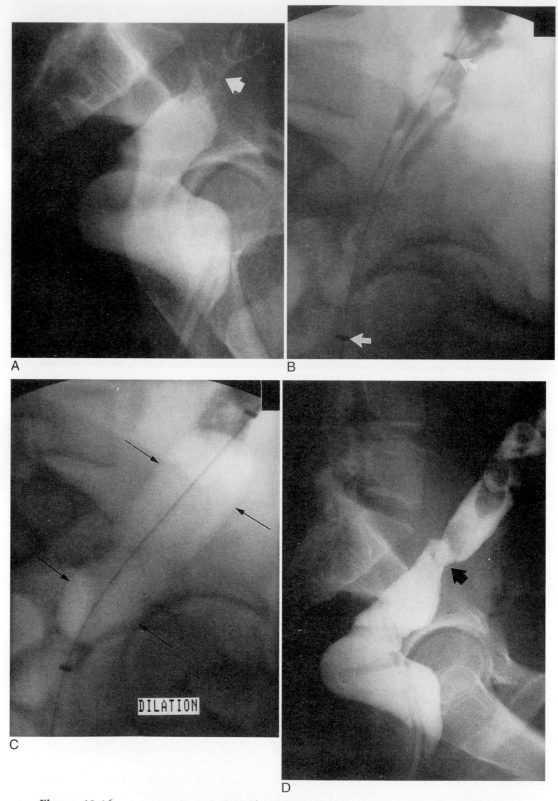

Figure 19-16   Anastamotic rectosigmoid stricture dilatation in a patient who underwent a sigmoid resection for diverticulitis complicated by the development of a stricture at the anastomosis. **A**, The patient presented with constipation and partial colonic obstruction and had a barium enema performed. The barium enema showed a tight stricture (arrow) at the rectosigmoid anastomosis. **B**, Using a combination of midazolam and fentanyl for sedoanalgesia, a balloon dilatation was performed. The stricture was negotiated using a Kumpe catheter and a 0.035-inch guidewire.

(Continued)

Box 19-9 Benign Esophageal Stricture Dilatation

Esophagogram before procedure
Start with 10- to 12-mm balloon
Eventual goal is 20-mm balloon
Keep fasting after procedure
Esophagogram next morning
Metal stents – caution!

muscular spasm induced by the dilatation. A technical success rate of 90–95% should be expected with appropriate dilatation. Approximately 70% of patients remain asymptomatic for 2 years following dilatation.

Some authors have developed retrievable metallic stents particularly for use in patients with benign strictures. The stents have hooks at the proximal end which can be grasped using an endoscope and the stent removed. In general, the stent can be removed only within 3 months after insertion. These stent designs may have a limited role to play in patients with benign esophageal strictures where recurring problems are common (Box 19-9).

Gastric and Duodenal Strictures

Strictures of the gastric antrum, pylorus, and duodenum can also be dilated. Twenty- to 30-mm balloons are usually necessary for successful dilatation in these locations. The balloon used in the author's unit is the rigiflex balloon (Boston Scientific, Natick, MA). These strictures are often more technically challenging than esophageal strictures. The stomach may be distended and filled with food, making negotiation of the stricture difficult. Although a long 5-French angiographic catheter can be tried initially, it may be necessary to use stiffer catheters such as those used for duodenal intubation.

Colorectal Strictures

The vast majority of colorectal strictures are anastomotic strictures after colorectal surgery. A limited barium enema is necessary beforehand to identify the location of the stricture. This is best done on the day before stricture dilatation. For stricture dilatation, the patient is placed in the decubitus position and a Kumpe catheter and hydrophilic guidewire used to traverse the stricture. The hydrophilic guidewire is exchanged for a 0.035-inch superstiff guidewire which is placed proximally in the sigmoid colon. Dilatation is performed with a 20- or 30-mm rigiflex balloon (Boston Scientific, Natick, MA). The balloon is inflated until the "waist" disappears and is left inflated for 2–3 minutes (Fig. 19-16). At the end of the procedure a plain film of the abdomen is obtained to rule out any free air. A limited gastrograffin enema is performed 4–6 hours after the procedure. If there is no mucosal tear or perforation, the patient can go home.

Malignant GI Strictures (Metallic Stent Placement)

Esophageal Carcinoma

Most patients with malignant esophageal strictures have locally advanced or metastatic disease that is often incurable. The object of palliation is to restore oral feeding and improve the quality of life for the patient. Rigid plastic endoprostheses have been used in the past but are difficult to insert and are associated with a high complication rate (Fig. 19-17). Complications are associated with rigid plastic endoprosthesis in 36% of patients, with esophageal perforation (5–11%), tube dislodgement (11–15%), hemorrhage (1–5%), pressure necrosis (1–3%), and aspiration pneumonia being the commonest. In published series, the procedural mortality rate is 2–4%, but in one study the rate was as high as 16%. Similarly, laser therapy has been used and offers effective palliation, but the palliation is usually short-lived and it has to be repeated every 4–6 weeks. Also, it is a high-cost procedure. Self-expanding metal stents have recently emerged as an attractive alternative for palliating patients with esophageal carcinoma.

Metal Stent Types and Design

A commonly used stent for palliation of malignant esophageal strictures is the Wallstent (formerly Schneider, Bulach, Switzerland; now Boston Scientific, Natick, MA). The author's unit predominantly uses this stent for palliation of patients with malignant esophageal strictures. There are a number of Wallstent designs currently available. The original Wallstent endoprosthesis comes in 20- and 25-mm diameters and is a straight cylindrical tube. The 20-mm stent is 110 mm long and is mounted on an 18-French delivery system, while the 25-mm version is 105 mm long and is mounted on a

Figure 19-16 cont'd The guidewire was exchanged for a 0.035-inch superstiff wire and a 30-mm rigiflex balloon placed across the stricture (arrows). **C,** The 30-mm rigiflex balloon was dilated with air (arrows) and remained inflated for 2 minutes. It is important to use air to dilate the balloon as contrast or fluid cannot be aspirated fully from the balloon so that balloon decompression is difficult. **D,** Gastrograffin enema performed the following day shows a good result at the anastomosis (arrow). The patient has been asymptomatic for 3 years since balloon dilatation.

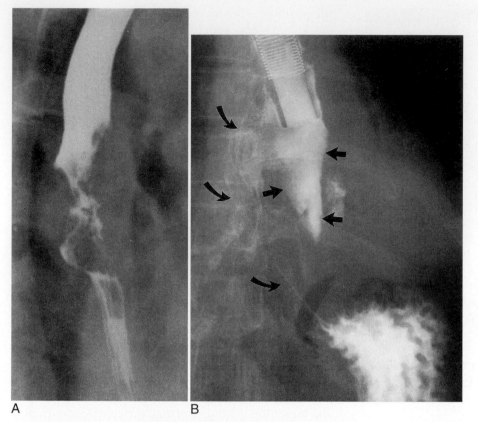

A   B

Figure 19-17   Esophageal perforation associated with insertion of a rigid plastic endoprosthesis. **A,** The 34-year-old patient with breast cancer presented with dysphagia secondary to esophageal wall metastases. Barium swallow shows an irregular stricture in the mid to lower esophagus. **B,** The patient was brought to the operating theater and under general anesthesia a rigid plastic endoprosthesis was placed. This caused a perforation (arrows) in the esophagus. Note the distal end of the endoprosthesis is actually lying outside the esophageal lumen (curved arrows). Associated collapse of the left lower lobe is seen. The tube was removed and the patient was managed conservatively for a number of weeks but eventually an esophagectomy was performed.

22-French delivery system. The stent comes in both covered and uncovered varieties. In the covered version the middle two-thirds of the stent is covered with a layer of polyurethane which is applied to the outside of the metallic mesh. The upper and lower 15 mm are uncovered. The covered and uncovered versions have different functions and are associated with different complications.

The uncovered version is prone to tumor ingrowth but is less likely to migrate as it becomes relatively fixed and endothelialized within the esophageal wall. The covered version was developed to decrease the rate of tumor ingrowth, but there is a slightly increased risk of migration. Migration is particularly a problem with the covered versions when they are placed across the GE junction. Normally, when the stent is placed in the mid-esophagus the sharp ends on either end of the stent become embedded in the esophageal wall and this helps to prevent migration. Because the stent is placed in parallel to the esophageal wall, the embedding of the sharp ends of the stent in the esophageal wall does not increase the risk of perforation. However, if an angle develops between the stent and the esophageal wall then problems may arise because esophageal peristalsis will slowly cause erosion of the sharp ends, at the lower end of the stent, through the esophageal wall which may lead to perforation. Initially, the uncovered Wallstent was

used for GE junction strictures and the covered Wallstent for strictures in other locations.

A further Wallstent design has recently been introduced. This is a conical design (Flamingo). The conical stent is wider at its upper end (30 mm) and tapers to the lower end (20 mm); a smaller version with a 24-mm upper end and a 16-mm lower end is also available (Fig. 19-18). The stent is mounted on a 15.5-French delivery catheter with a similar deployment system to the conventional Wallstent. The stent is 110 mm long with uncovered areas at its upper and lower ends – the upper 15 mm is uncovered and the lower 10 mm. There is a polyurethane covering on the remainder of the stent but, as opposed to the conventional Wallstent, the covering is on the inside of the metal mesh. Another difference between the conical stent and the conventional Wallstent is the braiding angle. The braiding angle is wider at the upper end of the stent than the lower end. This means that the metal mesh is denser at the upper end of the stent and more open at the lower end. This stent was designed particularly for use at the GE junction to reduce the rate of stent migration. Theoretical reasons for a reduction in stent migration include increased friction between the metal mesh of the stent and the esophageal wall because the polyurethane cover is on the inside of the metal mesh, the conical shape, and the

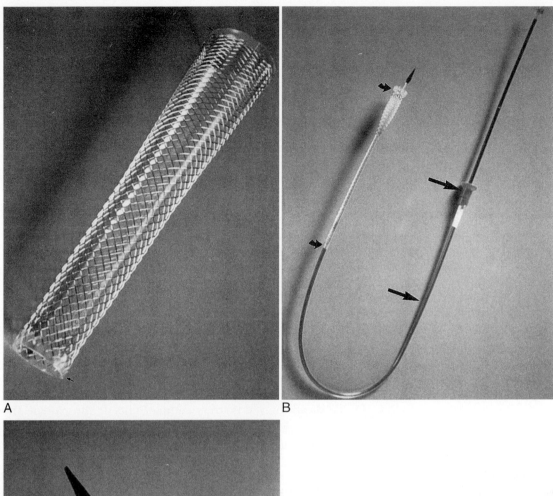

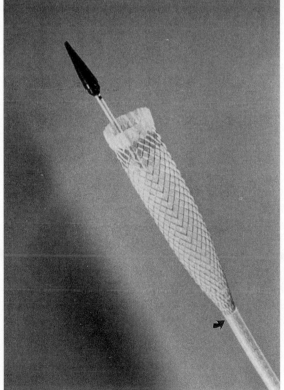

Figure 19-18   The Wallstent endoprosthesis. **A**, The conical Wallstent (Flamingo) comprises a stainless steel metallic mesh with the polyurethane covering on the inside of the metallic mesh. The upper 15 mm and the lower 10 mm are uncovered apart from at the terminal end (arrow) where there is a slim polyurethane covering. Note the more closely woven metallic mesh in the proximal end of the stent when compared with the distal end. This helps to prevent migration. **B**, The introducer catheter is 15.5-Fr in diameter and the stent (curved arrows) is enclosed by a plastic sheath at the distal end of the introducer catheter. Pulling the outer cannula (large arrow) back towards the delivery catheter hub releases the stent. **C**, Close-up of the distal end of the introducer catheter with the stent half deployed. Note the outer plastic cannula (small arrows) being withdrawn to release the stent from distal to proximal.

braiding angle. The change in braiding angle between the upper and lower ends of the stent means that the upper end of the stent is more resistant to esophageal peristalsis because it is more tightly woven. The lower end is more loosely woven and is thus easier to stretch along its length. Theoretically, peristalsic forces generated in the esophagus are accommodated by the lower end of the conical stent which stretches into the stomach, but the upper end of the stent remains fixed so that propulsion of the entire stent into the stomach is avoided.

The self-expanding nitinol Strecker stent (Ultraflex, Boston Scientific, Natick, MA) is another commonly used esophageal stent (Fig. 19-19). The stent is made of 0.15-inch nitinol wire with thermal as well as shape memory. The stent is 18 mm in diameter with a proximal end that is slightly wider, measuring 20 mm. It comes in 10 cm and 15 centimetre lengths. The stent is encased in gelatin on the delivery catheter so that as the covering sheath is withdrawn the gelatin dissolves and the stent progressively opens to its maximal diameter. Covered and uncovered varieties are available.

The Gianturco–Rosch stent (Cook, Bloomington, IL) also comes in covered and uncovered versions. It consists of a number of 2-cm long Gianturco–Rosch stents

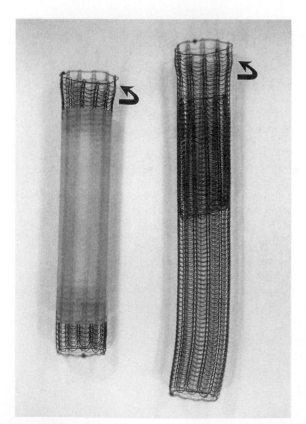

Figure 19-19   The nitinol Strecker stent. Covered (left) and uncovered (right) nitinol stents are shown. Note the slightly wider proximal end (arrows) which is 20 mm as opposed to 18 mm for the remainder of the stent.

connected together to form a longer stent. Stent lengths range from 8 cm to 14 cm with variable stent diameters.

Technique
Similar to esophageal stricture dilatation, a barium swallow should be obtained prior to the procedure to document the location and length of the stricture. The patient is sedated and placed in the decubitus position with an oral mouthpiece. The author uses a 5-French angiographic catheter and hydrophilic guidewire to access the esophagus after first anesthetizing the oropharynx with a local anesthetic spray. The catheter is manipulated into the esophagus under screening control and brought to a level just above the stricture (Fig. 19-20). A small amount of contrast is injected to outline the stricture and the guidewire and catheter are then manipulated through the stricture. The hydrophilic wire is then replaced with an exchange length 0.035- or 0.038-inch superstiff wire. The stent is then ready to be placed.

The stent is loaded on to the guidewire and inserted down through the stricture. The stent is placed so that there is sufficient overlap above and below the stricture. The delivery mechanism is simple in that the stent is covered by a sheath on the distal end of the delivery catheter. The stent can be released by pulling back the sheath on the delivery catheter outside the patient. The stent delivers from distal to proximal and the stent can be recaptured up to a point where as much as 50% of the stent has been deployed. In some cases if the esophageal stricture is very tight, it may be necessary to dilate the stricture beforehand. Once the stent is released, the delivery system is removed and the stent dilated in place with a 12-mm or 15-mm balloon. An esophagogram is performed the following day to assess stent location and the level of dilatation. The patient remains on a sloppy diet for 1–2 weeks after stent placement, after which solid food is gradually introduced.

GE Junction Strictures
Palliation of strictures at the GE junction deserve special mention. Because this proportion of the stent has to be placed in the stomach, and is therefore not in contact with the esophageal wall, there is a high propensity for stents in this region to migrate. It is therefore vitally important to choose an appropriate stent. Initially the author's unit used uncovered Wallstents in this location because the covered variety were prone to migrate. More recently, we have begun to use the conical wall stent (Flamingo) with good results (Fig. 19-21). When performing the procedure it is important to coil the superstiff guidewire in the stomach. The stomach is often collapsed, and injection of air through the initial 5-French angiographic catheter is helpful to distend the stomach so that the guidewire can be coiled into the stomach. The conical stent is placed such that the minimum amount of

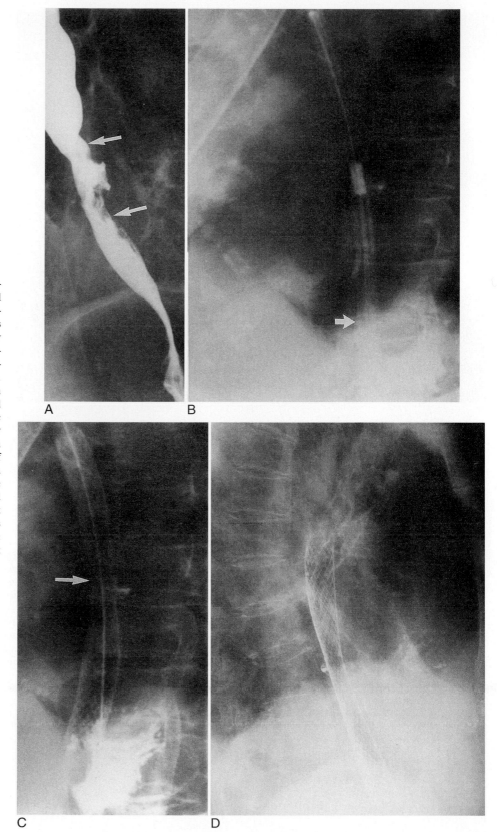

Figure 19-20 Metal stent placement in a patient with squamous cell cancer of the esophagus and considerable dysphagia. The patient was unfit for surgery. **A**, Barium swallow obtained before esophageal stent insertion shows an irregular, ulcerated stricture (arrows) in the distal esophagus. **B**, After manipulating a wire down through the stricture, a conventional covered Wallstent was placed. The distal end of the stent is partially deployed (arrow) and can be seen springing away from the distal end of the catheter. **C**, After full deployment a slight waist (arrow) is noted in the region of the stricture. This was dilated with a 15-mm balloon. **D**, Lateral chest x-ray performed 2 months later shows the stent in good position and the patient was eating a normal diet at this time.

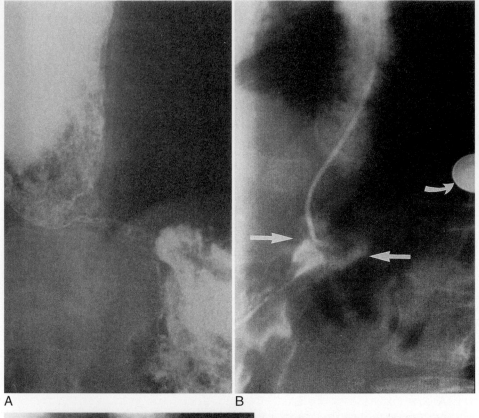

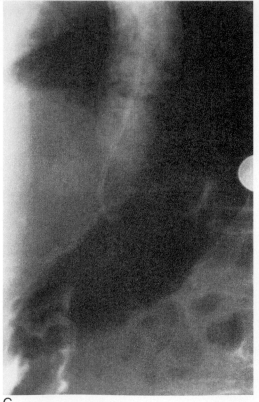

Figure 19-21   Patient with adenocarcinoma of the esophagus and marked dysphagia who required stenting before undergoing neoadjuvant radiotherapy and chemotherapy prior to esophageal resection. **A**, Barium swallow shows a tight stricture at the gastroesophageal junction with marked dilatation of the proximal esophagus. **B**, A 5-Fr angiographic catheter and 0.035-inch guidewire were used to negotiate the stricture and gain purchase in the stomach. Note that the fundus of the stomach (straight arrows) is collapsed making coiling of a guidewire in the fundus of the stomach impossible. A coin (curved arrow) taped to the patient's skin marks the position of the stricture. **C**, The stomach was inflated with air through the 5-Fr angiographic catheter to facilitate coiling of a guidewire in the stomach for better purchase. *(Continued)*

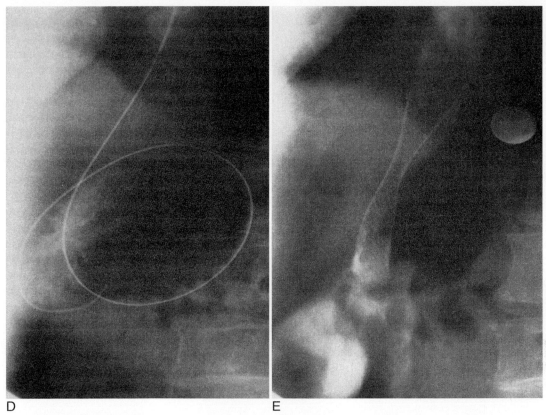

D   E

Figure 19-21 cont'd D, A 0.038-inch superstiff guidewire is inserted for stent deployment. **F**, A 24/16-mm conical Wallstent was placed across the stricture as shown. Note the waist in the region of the stricture. This was dilated using a 15-mm balloon. The patient was started on 20 mg of omeprazole daily. The patient underwent esophageal resection after neoadjuvant therapy and the stent was removed at the same time as the esophagus.

stent necessary to cover the stricture is placed in the stomach. The larger the length of stent in the fundus of the stomach, the more likely the stent is to migrate.

Malignant Tracheo-esophageal Fistulas

Malignant fistulas occurring between the esophagus and the trachea or main bronchi are a devastating complication of esophageal malignancy. Patients are often unable to swallow their own saliva without aspirating. Without treatment most patients die within a month because of malnutrition or thoracic sepsis.

Perforation of the esophagus may also occur in the treatment of patients with esophageal carcinoma. It occurs in approximately 4–6% of patients during laser treatment and in 5–8% treated with plastic endoprostheses. Again, perforation may lead to mediastinal abscess which has a high mortality and survival is short without appropriate treatment. A number of reports in the literature have indicated that placement of covered metallic endoprostheses is a highly effective means of treating these patients (Fig. 19-22). Success rates vary from 90 to 100% in excluding the fistula or perforation. It is important to

place the covered portion of the stent over the perforation or fistulous site. An esophagogram is performed the next day and, if there is any persistent evidence of perforation or fistula, a second overlapping stent is placed. In patients with high fistulas it may not be possible to place a stent in the esophagus because of the upper esophageal sphincter. It may then be necessary to place a covered metal stent in the trachea. This is usually done as a joint procedure with the respiratory physician (Box 19-10).

Box 19-10

Esophageal stent placement
Uncovered stents or conical stents with internal covering for GE junction strictures
Covered stents for non-GE junction strictures
Covered stents for tracheo-esophageal fistulas
Predilatation necessary if stricture is tight
Omeprazole 20 mg daily for GE junction stent patients

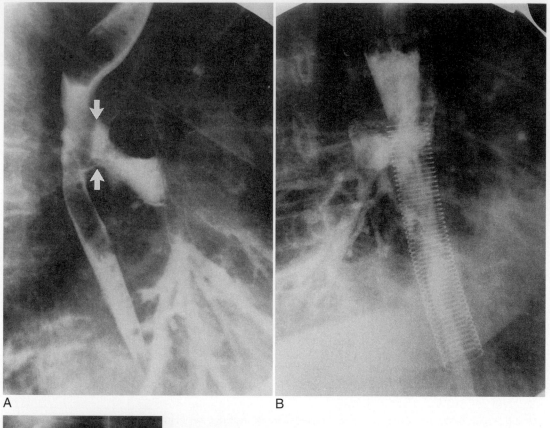

A

B

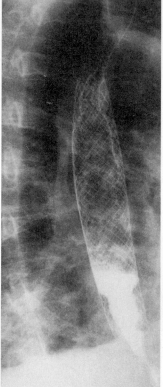

C

Figure 19-22 Esophagobronchial fistula treated with a covered Wallstent in a patient with lung cancer which had invaded the esophagus and caused the fistula. **A,** Barium swallow shows a fistula (arrows) between the esophagus and bronchial tree. **B,** The patient was brought to the operating theater and under general anesthesia a rigid plastic stent was deployed. This however did not exclude the fistula. There is contrast present within the bronchial tree on this gastrograffin swallow performed after the rigid plastic tube was inserted. **C,** The rigid plastic tube was removed and a covered Wallstent was placed. Barium swallow after Wallstent placement shows that the bronchial fistula has been excluded.

Results

The first report of successful treatment of a malignant esophageal stricture with a metal stent was made by Domschke and associates in 1990. Since then, there have been many studies in variable numbers of patients describing the placement of covered and uncovered metallic stents of different designs in various numbers of patients. Overall success rates vary from 90 to 100%, and experience at the author's institution reflects that of the literature in that it is a safe procedure that can be simply performed under fluoroscopic guidance without the need for endoscopic control. For appropriately placed stents there is almost always an improvement in the patient's dysphagia. Reported results are illustrated in Table 19-4. Comparison of metallic endoprosthesis with other therapies for palliation of malignant esophageal strictures show that metallic endoprosthesis deserve to be the first-choice treatment in palliation of patients with inoperable malignant esophageal strictures. Although similar dysphagia scores have been achieved in a comparative study between plastic and metallic stents, the use of plastic stents is associated with a much greater morbidity and mortality than that associated with metallic stents.

In yet a further study comparing palliation with metallic stents versus palliation with laser therapy, laser therapy was associated with an unsatisfactory level of dysphagia relief compared with metallic endoprostheses. In addition, laser therapy was associated with perforation rates of 6–9%.

In patients with malignant esophageal fistulas or perforations, insertion of covered metallic endoprostheses is associated with a success rate of over 95%. In the largest study reported of 39 patients with esophageal respiratory fistulas or perforations, covered Wallstents were used in 36 patients and covered Gianturco stents in three. Nineteen perforations and 18 of 20 fistulas were successfully closed, leading to a success rate of 95%. In three patients, fistulas recurred and were treated with an additional esophageal stent in one patient and tracheal stents in two patients. The other advantage of using metallic endoprostheses for treating these patients is that the dysphagia as well as the fistula is treated by the placement of the covered metallic stent. The author prefers to use covered Wallstents for the treatment of patients with esophageal respiratory fistulas but covered Gianturco stents can also be used. A synopsis of the reported literature can be seen in Table 19-5.

Metallic stents have also been placed in patients with benign esophageal strictures. However, the results have not been encouraging. In one study, 14 metallic stents were placed in 12 patients with benign esophageal strictures. Delayed complications occurred in all patients with new strictures forming in five patients either above, below or within the lumen of the stent. Stent migration occurred in six patients while formation of a new stricture occurred in one patient. These results are disappointing and caution is advised in the placement of metallic stents for patients with benign esophageal strictures.

Complications

The main complications associated with metallic endoprostheses include stent migration and tumor ingrowth. Tumor ingrowth was reported to occur in up to 20–30% of patients who had uncovered metallic

Table 19-4			**Malignant Esophageal Strictures: Metal Stent Results**					
				Mean Dysphagia Score		**Complications**		
First Author	**Year**	**Patients**	**Stent Type**	**Pre**	**Post**	**Migration**	**Tumour ingrowth or overgrowth**	**Other**
Cwikiel	1993	40	Ultraflex (u)	NP	NP		8	2
Grundy	1994	12	Ultraflex (u)	NP	NP	–	–	2
Winkelbauer	1995	26	Ultraflex (u)	3.5	0.6		2	1
Watkinson	1995	32	Wallstent (c)	3.38	0.81	8	2	3
Ellul	1995	33	Mixture	0.75	0/1	3	2	1
Grund	1995	114	Ultraflex (u)	3.5	1.5	–	76	
Saxon	1995	52	Gianturco (c)	NP	NP	5	1	9
Ell	1995	20	Gianturco (c)	NP	NP	2	1	
Acunas	1996	59	Ultraflex (u)	NP	NP		21	12
Pocek	1996	27	Ultraflex (u)	2.3	1	–	–	–
Cwikiel	1998	100	Ultraflex (u)	NP	Decrease by 1.8	4	20	17

u, uncovered; c, covered; NP, information not provided.

Table 19-5	Esophago-respiratory Fistulas or Perforation: Covered Metal Stent Results				
First Author	**Year**	**Patients**	**Stent Type**	**Success (%)**	**Complications**
Watkinson	1995	6	Wallstent-4 Gianturco-2	100	2
Saxon	1995	12	Gianturco	100	3
Weigert	1995	8	Gianturco	87.5	2
Mintlan	1996	10	Gianturco	100	4
Han	1996	10	Gianturco	100	4
Morgan	1997	39	Wallstent-36 Gianturco-3	95	8

stents in place. This problem has now largely been abolished by the use of covered metallic stents. Stent migration occurs more frequently with covered stent designs, particularly where the polyurethane cover is placed on the outside of the stent (Fig. 19-23). Conventional covered Wallstents placed at the GE junction had an overall rate of migration of 29%, but when the lower end projects into the fundus of the stomach this figure can rise to as high as 50%. A recent small study reported the use of conical stents for tumors at the GE junction. Ten conical stents were placed and there was no incidence of distal migration. Proximal migration occurred in two patients. However there was a marked reduction in the rate of distal migration from the previously reported rate of 50% to 0%.

Other complications reported with esophageal metal stent placement include food impaction which occasionally occurs. Patients should be instructed to drink carbonated beverages after eating to help clear the stent of residual debris. Transient chest pain related to stent deployment has been reported and may be severe enough to require narcotic analgesia. The reasons for this are unclear. Tumor overgrowth has been reported in some series and can occur in up to 6.2% of patients. This can be treated by placement of a further metal stent.

Hemorrhage has been reported in a total of 22 patients, proving fatal in 18. One of these patients died from stent erosion into the aorta. It is not clear in many of the others where the hemorrhage originated. At least some of these patients had either received or were receiving radiotherapy, and whether this may increase the risk of bleeding complications is unclear. The Gianturco-type esophageal stent exerts greater outward radial force than either the Wallstent or Strecker. It is not unreasonable to expect that this stent may be associated with a higher rate of hemorrhage because of the increased radial expansion and potential for erosion. However, hemorrhage has been reported with both the Wallstent and the Strecker stents, although not as frequently.

Colorectal Cancer

Recently, metallic stents have been placed in patients with colonic neoplasms who present with acute large bowel obstruction. The stents are placed as a temporizing measure to allow colonic decompression and permit elective surgery rather than emergency surgery. The mortality rate for elective surgery varies from 0.9 to 6%, compared with 22% for patients undergoing emergency surgical treatment for acute colorectal obstruction. Additionally, patients with acute large bowel obstruction are often in a poor general state of health because of the underlying disease, dehydration, and electrolyte imbalance. Placing a stent across the colonic tumor to alleviate the obstruction will also allow time for correction of any electrolyte imbalance and will allow time for the clinical condition of the patient to be optimized for elective surgery. Experience with this technique is limited but encouraging.

Figure 19-23 Esophageal Wallstent migration in a patient with recurrent gastric cancer and an esophagojejunal anastomosis. **A**, Barium swallow shows a stricture in the distal esophagus at the esophagojejunal anastomosis. **B**, A covered Wallstent was deployed across the stricture. Note that the waist (curved arrow) in the stent is present at the level of the diaphragm (straight arrow). A covered stent was placed because it was felt that the stent would not migrate because the stomach had been removed. **C**, The patient returned 6 weeks later with recurrent dysphagia. A barium swallow at this time showed that the Wallstent had migrated distally. Note the position of the proximal end of the Wallstent vis-à-vis the diaphragm. **D**, A second uncovered Wallstent was placed which provided relief of dysphagia for the patient's remaining life.

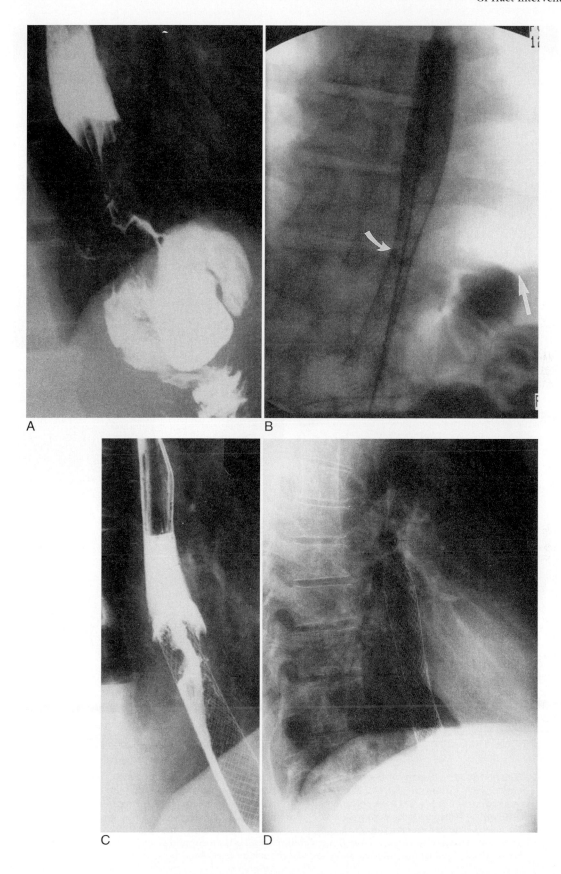

A

B

C

D

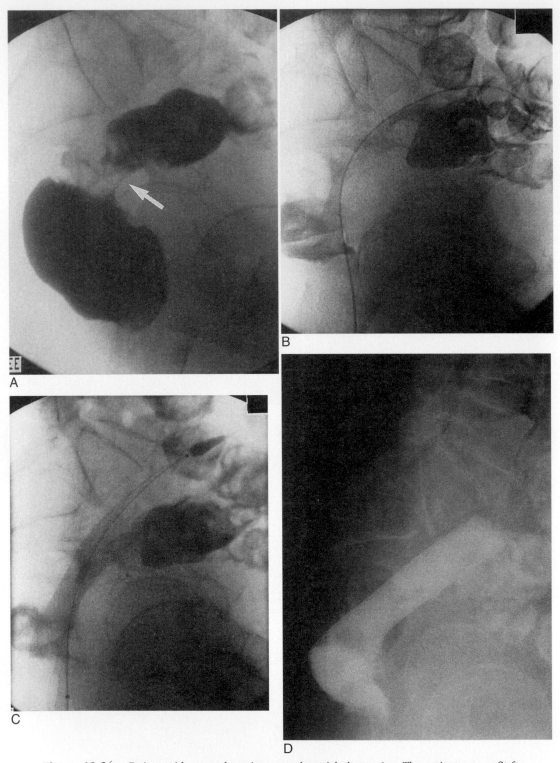

Figure 19-24 Patient with a rectal carcinoma and partial obstruction. The patient was unfit for surgery. **A**, A barium enema performed shows a stricture (arrow) in the mid rectum. **B**, The stricture was traversed using a 5-Fr Kumpe catheter and a hydrophilic guidewire. **C**, A conventional covered esophageal Wallstent was deployed across the stricture. The esophageal Wallstent was placed because the newer enteral stent was not available at this time. **D**, A limited barium enema study shows the Wallstent *in situ* with free flow of contrast both proximally and distally. The Wallstent provided effective palliation and the patient did not require a colostomy.

Technique

A preprocedure-limited barium enema is performed to delineate the site of the stricture. If there is total colonic obstruction, no attempt is made to place barium through the lesion. Endoscopic confirmation of the malignant nature of the stricture is also usually performed. Patients are sedated with midazolam and placed in a decubitus position on the fluoroscopy table. Approximately 75% of colonic neoplasms occur on the left side of the colon and it is predominantly these that are amenable to radiological techniques. In general, lesions in the radiosigmoid can usually be accessed and stented radiologically. Lesions in the descending colon or transverse colon require endoscopic guidance for stent placement.

A 5-French angiographic catheter and a hydrophilic wire are used to cross the stricture. Both ends of the stricture are delineated with contrast material and the length of the stricture is measured. A stent that will provide 2-3 cm of overlap on both sides of the stricture is chosen for placement. The author uses Wallstents (Boston Scientific, Watertown, MA), which vary in diameter from 20 mm to 25 mm and can vary in length from 40 mm to 110 mm. Once the lesion is crossed, a superstiff 0.035-inch wire is placed across the lesion and manipulated proximally into the colon. The stent is then delivered to the site of the tumor and placed so that overlap is obtained above and below the tumor. The stent is delivered and the stent delivery system removed. The stent is dilated in position with a 12- to 15-mm balloon to initiate the self-expanding process and to promote immediate colonic decompression (Fig. 19-24). A plain film of the abdomen is obtained to assess the position and degree of dilatation of the stent prior to sending the patient back to the ward. The plain radiograph is used as a marker for future comparisons. A follow-up film is obtained at 24-48 hours to assess the degree of colonic decompression and the degree of dilatation and location of the stent.

Results and Complications

Although data on this procedure are limited, preliminary results have shown metallic stents to be safe and effective in relieving acute colonic obstruction and avoiding emergency surgery. Choo and associates reported the placement of metal stents for relief of acute colorectal obstruction secondary to malignant colorectal carcinoma in 20 patients. Twelve patients underwent the placement of the metal stent for presurgical decompression of the colorectal obstruction. In 8 of these 12 patients, definitive surgery was carried out without complication within 5-7 days after stent placement. Two patients underwent tumor resection and had a colostomy fashioned. In the other eight patients the stent provided palliative decompression of the colon. Binkert and associates reported their experiences with 13 patients. Again in 10 patients the stents were placed as a preoperative decompressive procedure,

whilst in three patients the stents were placed purely for palliation. Stent placement was successful in 12 of the 13 patients, with relief of obstruction in all 12 patients. Definitive surgery was possible in eight of the nine patients treated preoperatively for decompression.

Reported complications have also been limited, with mild rectal bleeding reported in a single patient from one series. Potential complications are many, however, and include colon perforation, colorectal bleeding, prosthesis migration, and inadequate decompression of the colon. Experience with this procedure at the moment is limited and we await future developments.

SUGGESTED READING

Acunas B, Rozanes I, Akpinar S et al: palliation of malignant esophageal strictures with self-expanding nitinol stents: drawbacks and complications. *Radiology* 199:648-652, 1996.

Adam A, Ellul J, Watkinson A et al: palliation of inoperable esophageal carcinoma: a prospective randomized trial of laser therapy and stent placement. *Radiology* 202:344-348, 1997.

Adam A, Morgan R, Ellul J, Mason RC: a new design of the esophageal wallstent endoprosthesis resistant to distal migration. *Am J Roentgenol* 170:1477-1481, 1998.

Adam A, Watkinson AF, Dussek J: Boerhaave syndrome: to treat or not to treat by means of insertion of a metallic stent. *J Vasc Interv Radiol* 6:741-743, 1995; discussion 744-746.

Bell SD, Carmody EA, Yeung EY et al: Percutaneous gastrostomy and gastrojejunostomy: additional experience in 519 procedures. *Radiology* 194:817-820, 1995.

Binkert CA, Ledermann H, Jost R et al: acute colonic obstruction: clinical aspects and cost-effectiveness of preoperative and palliative treatment with self-expanding metallic stents: preliminary report. *Radiology* 206:199-204, 1998.

Canon CL, Baron TH, Morgan DE, Dean PA, Keebler RE: treatment of colonic obstruction with expandable metal stents: radiologic features. *Am J Roentgenol* 168:199-205, 1997.

Choo IW, Do YS, Suh SW et al: malignant colorectal obstruction: treatment with a flexible covered stent. *Radiology* 206:415-421, 1998.

Clark JA, Pugash RA, Pantalone RR: Radiologic peroral gastrotomy. *J Vasc Interv Radiol* 10:927-932, 1999.

Cwikiel W, Stridbeck H, Tranberg KG et al: malignant esophageal strictures: treatment with a self-expanding nitinol stent. *Radiology* 187:661-665, 1993.

Cwikiel W, Tranberg K-G, Cwikiel M, Lillo-Gil R: Malignant dysphagia: palliation with esophageal stents: long-term results in 100 patients. *Radiology* 297:513-518, 1998.

Dawson SL, Mueller PR, Ferrucci JT et al: Severe esophageal strictures indications for balloon catheter dilatation. *Radiology* 153:631-635, 1984.

Ell C, May A, Hahn EG: self-expanding metal endoprosthesis in palliation of stenosing tumours of the upper gastrointestinal tract: comparison of experience with three stent types in 82 implantations. *Dtsch Med Wochenschr* 120:1343-1348, 1995.

Ell C, May A, Hahn EG, Gianturco Z: Stents in the palliative treatment of malignant esophageal obstruction and esophagotracheal fistulas. *Endoscopy* 27:714, 1995.

Ellul JP, Watkinson A, Khan RJ, Adam A, Mason RC: Self-expanding metal stents for the palliation of dysphagia due to inoperable oesophageal carcinoma. *Br J Surg* 82:1678-81, 1995.

Grund KE, Storek D, Becker HD: Highly flexible self-expanding meshed metal stents for palliation of malignant esophago-gastric obstruction. *Endoscopy* 27:486-494, 1995.

Grundy A: The Strecker esophageal stent in the management of oesophageal strictures: technique of insertion and early clinical experience. *Clinical Radiology* 49:421-424, 1994.

Grundy A, Glees JP: Aorto-oesophageal fistula: a complication of oesophageal stenting. *Br J Radiol* 70:846-849, 1997.

Hallisey MJ, Pollard JC: Direct percutaneous jejunostomy. *J Vasc Interv Radiol* 5:625-632, 1984.

Han Y-M, Song H-Y, Lee J-M et al: Esophagorespiratory fistula due to esophageal carcinoma: palliation with a covered Gianturco stent. *Radiology* 199:65-70, 1996.

Ho CS, Yeung EY: Percutaneous gastrostomy and transgastric jejunostomy. *Am J Roentgenol* 158:251-257, 1992.

Hoffer EK, Cosgrove JM, Levin DQ, Herskowitz MM, Sclafani SJ: Radiologic gastrojejunostomy and percutaneous endoscopic gastrostomy: a prospective, randomized comparison. *J Vasc Interv Radiol* 10:413-420, 1999.

Knyrim K, Wagner HJ, Bethge N, Keymling M, Vakil N: A controlled trial of an expansile metal stent for palliation of esophageal obstruction due to inoperable cancer. *N Engl J Med* 28:329:1302-1307, 1993.

Kwak S, Leef JA, Rosenblum JD: Percutaneous balloon catheter dilatation of benign ureteral strictures: effect of multiple dilatation procedures on long-term patency. *Am J Roentgenol* 165:97-100, 1995.

Lee MJ, Kiely P: Percutaneous radiological gastrostomy and gastrojejunostomy. *J ICPS* 27:13-16, 1998.

Lopera JE, Ferral H, Wholey M et al: Treatment of colonic obstructions with metallic stents: indications, technique and complications. *Am J Roentgenol* 169:1285-1290, 1997.

Lu DS, Mueller PR, Lee MJ et al: Gastrostomy conversion to transgastric jejunostomy: technical problems, causes of failure and proposed solutions in 63 patients. *Radiology* 197:679-683, 1993.

Mainar A, Tejero E, Maynar M, Ferral H, Castaneda-Zuniga W: Colorectal obstruction: treatment with metallic stents. *Radiology* 198:761-764, 1996.

Miyayama S, Matsui O, Kadoya M et al: Malignant esophageal stricture and fistula: palliative treatment with polyurethane-covered Gianturco stent. *J Vasc Interv Radiol* 6:243-248, 1995.

Morgan RA, Ellul JPM, Denton ERE et al: Malignant esophageal fistulas and perforations: management with plastic-covered metallic endoprostheses. *Radiology* 204:527-532, 1997.

Olson DL, Krubsack AJ, Steward ET: Percutaneous enteral alimentation: gastrostomy versus gastrojejunostomy. *Radiology* 187:105-108, 1993.

Pocek M, Maspes F, Masala S et al: Palliative treatment of neoplastic strictures by self-expanding nitinol strecker stent. *Eur Radiol* 6:230-235, 1996.

Ryan JM, Hahn PF, Boland GW et al: Percutaneous gastrostomy with T-fastener gastropexy: results of 316 consecutive procedures. *Radiology* 203:496-500, 1997.

Sabharwal T, Cowling M, Dussek J, Owen W, Adam A: Balloon dilation for achalasia of the cardia: experience in 76 patients. *Radiology* 224:719-724, 2002.

Saini S, Mueller PR, Gaa J et al: Percutaneous gastrostomy with gastropexy: experience in 125 patients. *Am J Roentgenol* 154:1003-1006, 1990.

Sawada S, Tanigawa N, Okuda Y, Mishima K, Ohmura N: Clinical value of combined stents in esophageal cancer: combined use of ultraflex and self-expanding zigzag metallic stents. *Am J Roentgenol* 169:493-494, 1997.

Saxon RR, Barton RE, Katon RM et al: Treatment of malignant esophagorespiratory fistulas with silicone-covered metallic Z stents. *J Vasc Interv Radiol* 6:237-242, 1995.

Saxon RR, Barton RE, Katon RM et al: Treatment of malignant esophageal obstructions with covered metallic Z stents: long-term results in 52 Patients. *J Vasc Interv Radiol* 6:747-754, 1995.

Saxon RR, Morrison KE, Lakin PC et al: Malignant esophageal obstruction and esophagorespiratory fistula: palliation with a polyethylene-covered Z-stent. *Radiology* 202:349-254, 1997.

Song H-Y, Park S-I, Do Y-S et al: Expandable metallic stent placement in patients with benign esophageal strictures: results of long-term follow-up. *Radiology* 203:131-136, 1997.

Song H-Y, Park S-I, Jung H-Y et al: Benign and malignant esophageal strictures: treatment with a polyurethane-covered retrievable expandable metallic stent. *Radiology* 203:747-752, 1997.

Szymski GX, Albazzaz AN, Funaki B et al: Radiologically guided placement of pull-type gastrostomy tubes. *Radiology* 205:669-673, 1997.

Tan, B-S, Kennedy C, Morgan R, Owen W, Adam A: Using uncovered metallic endoprostheses to treat recurrent benign esophageal strictures. *Am J Radiol* 169:1281-1284, 1997.

Thornton FJ, Fotheringham T, Alexander M et al: Enteral nutrition provision in amyotrophic lateral sclerosis (ALS): endoscopic or radiologic gastrostomy? *Radiology* 224:713-717, 2002.

Thornton FJ, Fotheringham T, Haslam et al: Percutaneous radiological gastrostomy (PRG) with and without T-fastener gastropexy: a randomised comparison. *Cardiovasc Interv Radiol* 25:467-471, 2002.

Thornton FJ, Varghese JC, Haslam PJ et al: Percutaneous gastrostomy in patients who fail or are unsuitable for endoscopic gastrostomy. *Cardiovascc Interv Radiol* 23:279-284, 2000.

Varghese JC, Lee MJ: Percutaneous cecostomy. *Semin Interv Radiol* 13:351-354, 1996.

Watkinson AF, Ellul J, Entwisle K et al: Plastic-covered metallic endoprostheses in the management of oesophageal perforation in patients with oesophageal carcinoma. *Clin Radiol* 50:304-309, 1995.

Watkinson AF, Ellul J, Entwisle K, Mason RC, Adam A: Esophageal carcinoma: initial results of palliative treatment with covered self-expanding endoprostheses. *Radiology* 195:821–827, 1995.

Weigert N, Neuhaus H, Rosch T: Treatment of esophagorespiratory fistulas with silicone-coated self-expanding metal stents. *Gastrointest Endosc* 41:490–496, 1995.

Winkelbauer F, Schofl R, Niederle B et al: Palliative treatment of obstructing esophageal cancer with nitinol stents: value, safety, and long-term results. *Am J Roentgenol* 166:79–84, 1996.

Wollman BD, Agostino HB, Walus Wigle J, Easter DW, Beale A: Radiologic, endoscopic, and surgical gastrostomy: an institutional evaluation and meta-analysis of the literature. *Radiology* 197:699–704, 1995.

<table>
<tr><td></td></tr>
</table>

CHAPTER 20

Biliary Intervention

MICHAEL J. LEE, M.D.

Percutaneous transhepatic cholangiography (PTC) and percutaneous biliary drainage (PBD) techniques gained widespread popularity in the late 1970s and early 80s after they were first described. However, the use of both PTC and PBD has declined with the development of diagnostic and therapeutic endoscopic retrograde cholangiopancreatography (ERCP). PTC and PBD remain an important part of interventional radiology and they are performed on a regular basis at many institutions. The indications for biliary intervention are less numerous but, nonetheless widely accepted and well defined. Before embarking on any discussion of biliary intervention, it is important to understand biliary ductal anatomy within the liver.

INTRAHEPATIC DUCTAL ANATOMY

Intrahepatic ductal anatomy is modeled on the segmental anatomy of the liver as described by Couinaud. At the hilum there are two main hepatic ducts, the right and left, which join to form the common hepatic duct. The right hepatic duct drains segments 5–8 and is formed by the right posterior duct (RPD) and the right anterior duct (RAD). The RAD drains segments 5 and 8 while the RPD drains segments 6 and 7. The RPD has a more horizontal course on anteroposterior cholangiographic images of the liver while the RAD has a more vertical course. Normally, the RPD passes behind the RAD and joins the RAD on its medial side to form the right hepatic duct. The left hepatic duct is usually horizontally orientated in the left lobe of the liver and drains segments 2–4. It joins with the right hepatic duct to form the common hepatic duct and exits the liver at the biliary hilum in conjunction with the portal vein and hepatic artery. The common hepatic duct is joined by the cystic duct which drains the gallbladder, to form the common bile duct.

This standard anatomy is present in approximately 57% of patients (Fig. 20-1). There are a wide number of variations in bile duct anatomy which can have a profound effect on planning a biliary drainage. The variations that

558

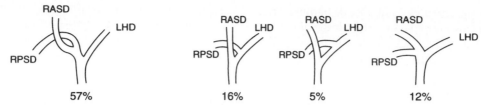

Figure 20-1   Normal bile duct anatomy and its variants. Note that in approximately 21% of patients the right posterior sectoral duct joins the left hepatic duct. In 16% the RPSD joins the left hepatic duct close to the hilum, while in the other 5% it joins the LHD at some distance from the hilum. In patients with hilar strictures and aberrant drainage of the RPSD to the LHD, left-sided drainage will drain a large amount of liver and will provide excellent liver function. (RASD = right anterior sectoral duct; RPSD = right posterior sectoral duct; LHD = left hepatic duct).

most affect biliary drainage procedures are those involving anomalous drainage of the RPD and the RAD (see Fig. 20-1). The RPD may drain into the left hepatic duct (Fig. 20-2A) or alternatively into the common hepatic duct. The RAD can also drain into the left hepatic duct but not as frequently as the RPD. In addition, occasionally the RAD, RPD, and left hepatic duct form a triple confluence so that there is no right hepatic duct (Figure 20-2B).

Knowledge of the anatomic relationships of the intrahepatic bile ducts is important before planning biliary drainage procedures particularly in patients with obstructions at the level of the biliary hilum. If a patient with a hilar obstruction has anomalous drainage of the RPD into the left hepatic duct, then a left hepatic drainage is the appropriate drainage procedure in that most of the liver will be drained by a single drainage procedure. Conversely, if a right-sided biliary drainage is performed only a small amount of liver will be drained (that drained by the RAD), which may not be enough to provide adequate hepatic function to relieve jaundice and pruritis. The RPD is said

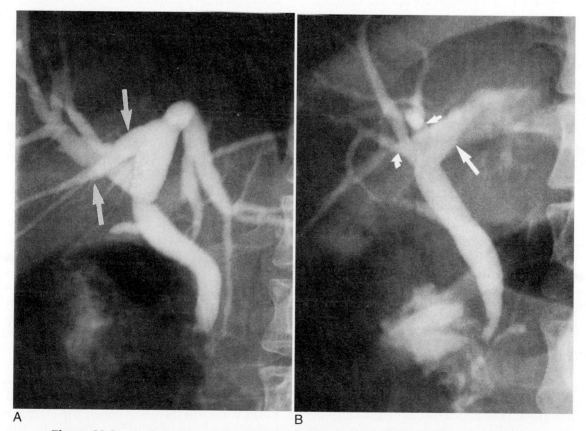

A   B

Figure 20-2   **A**, Aberrant biliary anatomy. ERCP film showing drainage of the right posterior sectoral duct (large arrows) into the left hepatic duct. **B**, Trifurcation bile duct. Note the RASD (curved arrow), RPSD (short arrow), and LHD (long arrow) forming a trifurcation at the hilar confluence.

to drain into the left hepatic duct in 23% of patients and the RAD in 5%. It is also important to be aware of anomalous drainage of right-sided ducts into the left hepatic duct when performing biliary drainages from the right side. Often, if the RPD drains anomalously into the left hepatic duct, a very acute angle may be formed by the junction of the RPD with the left hepatic duct. This may make it impossible to pass catheters or guidewires from the right side into the left hepatic duct and then down the common hepatic duct. Indeed, trying to do so may increase the risk of complications such as hemorrhage. In the author's unit we now perform magnetic resonance cholangiography on all patients prior to biliary drainage to fully assess intrahepatic bile duct anatomy and assess any variations present. In this way, an appropriate biliary drainage can be planned for the patient.

PATIENT PREPARATION

Patient preparation is similar for all transhepatic biliary interventional procedures. Antibiotic prophylaxis is mandatory before any biliary interventional procedure. Common antibiotic regimens include gentamycin 80 mg IV and ampicillin 1 g IV before the procedure. The author's unit used to use this regimen but has changed to using piperacillin/tazobactam 4.5 g IV before the procedure. Piperacillin/tazobactam consists of a penicillin (piperacillin) and a beta-lactamase inhibitor (tazobactam). Piperacillin is a broad-spectrum antibiotic with activity against Gram-positive, Gram-negative, and aerobic infections. High levels are found in bile when administered intravenously; and the addition of the beta-lactamase inhibitor protects piperacillin against beta-lactamase producing anaerobes. Piperacillin/tazobactam is an ideal monotherapy for biliary drainage procedures, but gentamycin and ampicillin can be used, where piperacillin/tazobactam is not available. For PTC a single dose is given before the procedure. For biliary drainage we now continue piperacillin/tazobactam 4.5 g IV t.i.d. for 2 days.

Coagulation parameters must be checked carefully and any bleeding tendency corrected with fresh frozen plasma and/or vitamin K. In jaundiced patients who are undergoing biliary drainage for relief of malignant biliary obstruction, we place the patients on intravenous fluids as soon as they are referred for biliary drainage. The regime we use is $2\frac{1}{2}$ liters of Hartman's solution daily for 3–4 days around the time of the drainage procedure. The reason for this is that many of these jaundiced patients have not been eating or drinking appropriately before coming into hospital, and when they do reach hospital they are fasted for different tests such as ERCP, CAT scans, ultrasound, etc. Usually by the time they are referred for biliary drainage they are quite dehydrated, which increases the risk of hepatorenal failure developing. Fluid replacement is important in these patients in the periprocedural time period to prevent hepatorenal failure. Informed consent is obtained from all patients prior to the procedure by a member of the interventional team.

PERCUTANEOUS TRANSHEPATIC CHOLANGIOGRAPHY

The indications for percutaneous transhepatic cholangiography (PTC) have fallen dramatically since the introduction of ERCP and more recently magnetic resonance cholangiography. We occasionally are asked to perform a diagnostic PTC in patients who have had a laparoscopic bile duct injury, in patients with sclerosing cholangitis, and in patients in whom ERCP is not possible because of altered upper GI anatomy. Contraindications are rare but would include an uncorrectable coagulopathy.

Technique

Percutaneous transhepatic cholangiography (PTC) is performed predominantly from the right side for diagnostic purposes. The patient is placed supine on the fluoroscopy table and the right flank is sterilely prepared. A combination of midazolam and fentanyl is used for sedoanalgesia. Under fluoroscopic control the patient is asked to take a deep breath and the position of maximal lung descent is marked. A point is chosen one or two interspaces below this point for needle access. The needle access point should also lie in the mid-axillary line. Once the point is marked on the skin, the skin is infiltrated with local anesthetic and a small incision made with a #11 scalpel blade. A 22-gauge Chiba needle (15 cm in length) is used for PTC. The needle is inserted under fluoroscopic guidance from the right flank towards the 12th vertebral body. The needle is inserted parallel to the table top in one smooth motion. The stylet is withdrawn and a syringe containing dilute contrast material is attached to the hub of the needle via an extension tube. The needle is slowly withdrawn and small aliquots of contrast material are injected every 1–2 mm until a bile duct is entered. When a bile duct is entered contrast material will flow away from the tip of the needle, slowly, akin to wax flowing down a candlestick. This is a very characteristic phenomenon and is easily differentiated from hepatic vein or portal vein branches where contrast washes quickly away either towards the heart if a hepatic vein is entered or towards the periphery of the liver if a portal vein branch is entered. If a bile duct is not entered on the first pass, successive passes are made in a fan shape down through the liver towards the biliary hilum (Fig. 20-3). It is important, however, not to withdraw the needle fully outside the liver capsule so that only one hole in the liver capsule is made. This helps to reduce bleeding complications.

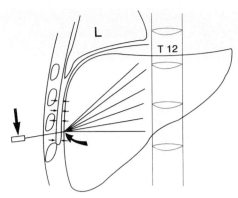

Figure 20-3   Schematic showing PTC technique. The patient is asked to take a deep inspiration and the point of maximal lung descent marked. An interspace below this is chosen for puncture. The 22-gauge needle (long arrow) is aimed towards the T12 vertebral body and withdrawn slowly while injecting dilute contrast medium until a biliary duct is entered. The procedure is repeated in a fan shape inferiorly if a bile duct is not entered. It is important not to take the needle fully out of the liver so that only one hole in the liver capsule (curved arrow) is made. Note that invariably the needle passes through the pleura (small arrows) but should not pass through the lung (L).

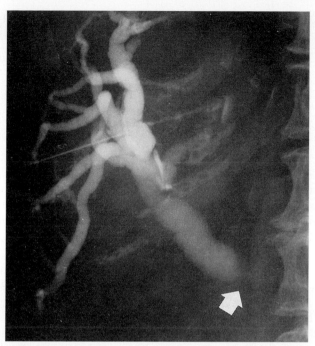

Figure 20-4   PTC in a patient with failed ERCP. A 22-gauge needle (arrow) inserted into the liver towards the T12 vertebral body was withdrawn slowly with small pulses of contrast material injected until the right anterior sectoral duct was entered. The contrast injected shows a dilated biliary system with an obstruction at the lower end of the bile duct (curved arrows). Note the left duct is often not seen with a right-sided PTC. Trendelenburg positioning may help fill the left duct.

When a bile duct is entered, contrast is injected to outline the biliary system (Fig. 20-4). With low bile duct obstructions, it is often advantageous to have a table that can tilt. In the supine position, the injected contrast material may not reach the level of the obstruction. By tilting the patient to a semi-erect position, the heavier contrast material will fall and displace the lighter bile so that the level of obstruction can be accurately depicted. Radiographs are obtained in anteroposterior (AP) and both oblique projections and the needle is withdrawn if a biliary drainage is not planned.

Results and Complications

Success rates for PTC lie between 97% and 100% in experienced hands. Technical difficulties can be experienced in patients without biliary dilatation. As many as 15–20 passes can be safely made, but after this, if a bile duct has not been entered, the procedure is best terminated. Alternatively, one can place a needle into the gallbladder and inject contrast material through the gallbladder to outline the biliary system. Of course, this is possible only if the biliary obstruction is below the junction of the cystic duct and common hepatic duct. Placing the patient in Trendelenburg will aid filling of the intrahepatic ducts if a gallbladder access is used.

Complications are minimal and occur in about 1–2% of patients. Possible complications include hemorrhage, sepsis, and bile leak leading to biliary peritonitis. The incidence of hemorrhage can be decreased by correction of any abnormal coagulation parameters beforehand and by making only one hole in the liver capsule. If the blood coagulation parameters are abnormal, the percutaneous track can be embolized with Gelfoam or autologous blood clot as the needle is withdrawn though the track. This will help to further decrease the incidence of hemorrhage and/or bile leak. Bile leakage is rare after PTC but occurs more frequently after biliary drainage. Appropriate antibiotic coverage can help minimize the significance of bacteremia and prevent sepsis developing.

BILIARY DRAINAGE

Percutaneous biliary drainage was first described by Molnar and Stockhaum in the late 1970s and enjoyed a pre-eminent position in biliary intervention until the advent of therapeutic ERCP. Nowadays, management of patients with biliary obstruction will depend to a large extent on the expertise available in any given institution. However, most patients are managed by endoscopic techniques such as stone extraction or stent placement for common bile duct (CBD) stones and stent placement for malignant biliary obstruction. At the author's institution the indications for biliary drainage are limited but

---

Box 20-1 Indications for Biliary Intervention

Failed endoscopic drainage
Hilar obstruction
Biliary problems after biliary enteric anastamoses
Injury after laparoscopic cholecystectomy

Box 20-2 Patient Preparation for Biliary Drainage Procedure

Appropriate antibiotic prophylaxis
$2\frac{1}{2}$ liters of IV fluids daily
Sonography and MRCP beforehand
Define level of obstruction
Define any aberrant biliary anatomy

---

remain important; they are shown in Box 20-1. The main indication for percutaneous biliary drainage (PBD) is when ERCP fails or is not possible due to altered upper GI anatomy.

Preprocedure Imaging

It is important before embarking upon a biliary drainage that all relevant information as to the probable cause of the biliary obstruction, the level of obstruction, and details of relevant biliary anatomy are obtained. If the ERCP has failed the endoscopists may not have injected contrast material into the biliary system. Often, even if contrast material is injected into the biliary system, it may not have outlined the whole biliary system so that bile duct anatomy cannot be ascertained. An ultrasound of the liver is important to confirm intrahepatic biliary duct dilatation, to eliminate metastatic disease, to determine the level of obstruction, and to rule out the presence of ascites. Usually an ultrasound has been performed before the ERCP; if not, it should be performed. A CT can also be helpful to check for evidence of a pancreatic tumor and again to look for liver metastases. More recently, in the author's unit we have tended to perform MR cholangiography in conjunction with ultrasound in all patients referred for biliary drainage (Fig. 20-5). We perform MRC using a torso coil and heavily T2-weighted fast spin echo pulse sequences. Coronal and axial acquisitions are obtained using breath-hold techniques if possible. MRC is particularly useful for evaluating biliary anatomy and planning the appropriate biliary drainage procedure in patients with hilar obstruction (Box 20-2).

Right-sided Biliary Drainage

This is the most common approach for biliary drainage. We use a one-stick needle system (Cook, Bloomington, IN) for biliary access (Fig. 20-6). A right-sided PTC is performed as described previously. When a bile duct is entered, contrast material is injected to opacify the biliary system. If the patient is septic, the minimum amount of contrast material is injected to allow safe performance of the biliary drainage, without overdistending the biliary system. If a favorable duct is entered by the initial needle

puncture, a 0.018-inch guidewire is placed through the needle and manipulated towards the hepatic hilum and common bile duct (Fig. 20-7). If a favorable duct has not been entered by the initial needle, a second 22-gauge Chiba needle is used to puncture a duct with a more favorable orientation to bring the guidewire to the biliary hilum. It is important, when draining patients with hilar obstruction, to gain entry into a peripheral duct, particularly if the patient is going to have a stent placed. Occasionally the 0.018-inch guidewire will not run appropriately down the duct towards the hepatic hilum. This can be remedied by turning the bevel of the needle in 90-degree aliquots and probing with the wire (Fig. 20-8). Alternatively, the needle may have to be pulled back slightly if the needle is up against the medial wall of the bile duct entered. Once the 0.018-inch guidewire has gained reasonable purchase within the bile duct and is at the level of the common hepatic duct or more distally, the needle is withdrawn and the 5-French sheath assembly placed over the 0.018-inch guidewire into the bile duct.

Problems can be encountered when a vertical bile duct has been entered in that the 5-French sheath assembly may not follow the guidewire down toward the biliary hilum. It is important to withdraw the metal stiffening cannula when the 5-French sheath assembly reaches the bile duct. The metal trocar is too stiff to follow the 0.018-inch guidewire around a 90-degree degree curve down into the bile duct. By withdrawing the metal trocar the more flexible 4-French plastic cannula and 5-French sheath should follow the guidewire down towards the hepatic hilum.

Occasionally, despite appropriate technique the plastic 5-French sheath and 4-French cannula will not follow the 0.018-inch guidewire down to the biliary hilum. In this situation, the author places the sheath assembly into the vertically orientated duct punctured, removes the 4-French plastic cannula, and place a 0.035-inch hydrophilic guidewire or 1.5 mm "J" guidewire through the 5-French sheath and this is manipulated down the duct. The 0.018-inch guidewire can be left in place during this maneuver because there is enough room in the 5-French sheath for both guidewires. The 5-French sheath will virtually always follow the larger 0.035-inch guidewire.

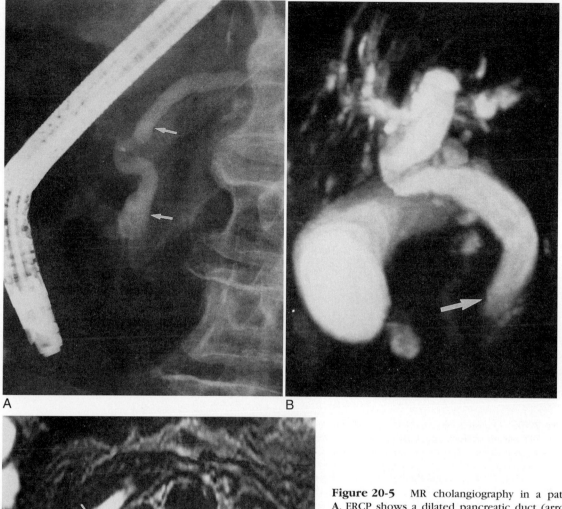

Figure 20-5   MR cholangiography in a patient with failed ERCP. **A,** ERCP shows a dilated pancreatic duct (arrows). However, the bile duct could not be cannulated at ERCP. **B,** MRCP shows a dilated bile duct (large arrow) down to the level of the ampulla. **C,** Axial images through the region of the ampulla show a small periampullary tumor (arrows) which is causing the obstruction. Note the dilated pancreatic duct proximal the periampullary tumor. This appearance was confirmed at PTC. The patient was 83 years of age and unfit for surgery. A biliary drainage was performed with metal stent placement.

Once good purchase is obtained, the 4-French inner plastic cannula and 0.018-inch guidewire are removed and a 0.035- or 0.038-inch "J" guidewire placed through the 5-French sheath into the biliary tree. At this stage, the 5-French plastic sheath is removed and a hockey-stick type catheter placed over the "J" guidewire. The "J" guidewire is then removed and exchanged for a 0.035-inch hydrophilic guidewire with a straight tip. The hockey-stick catheter and hydrophilic guidewire are manipulated down to a level just above the stricture. The guidewire is removed and contrast material is injected just above the stricture because often there is a small nipple of compressed duct above the stricture which points the way for guidewire manipulation. The hockey-stick catheter and hydrophilic guidewire are manipulated into the area where the nipple of contrast material was seen and the stricture probed with the hydrophilic guidewire until the stricture is crossed. The hockey-stick catheter is advanced through the stricture over the hydrophilic guidewire and both are manipulated into the proximal jejunum. At this point the hydrophilic guidewire is exchanged for a 0.035-inch superstiff

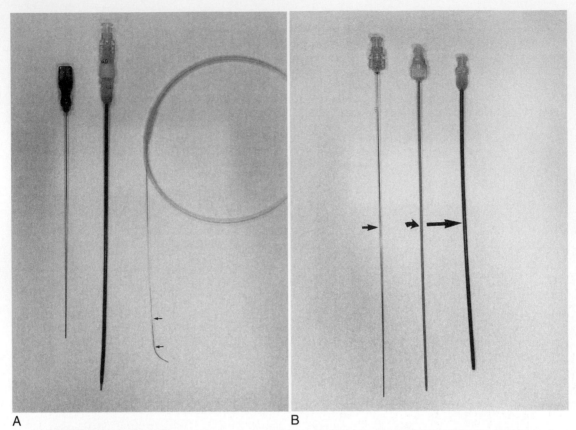

A   B

Figure 20-6 One-stick system (Neff, Cook, Bloomington, IN) used for biliary access. **A,** A 22-gauge needle, 5-Fr sheath system and 0.018-inch guidewire form the components of the system. The guidewire has a floppy, platinum curved tip (arrows). **B,** The 5-Fr sheath system consists of a metal trocar (small arrow), a plastic trocar (curved arrow), and an outer 5-Fr sheath (large arrow). When the 0.018-inch guidewire enters the bile duct, the sheath assembly is placed over the guidewire as a unit. When the sheath assembly enters the bile duct, the metal trocar is unhooked from the plastic trocar and the 5-Fr sheath fed over the guidewire into the bile duct. The metal trocar is too stiff to maneuver around acute angles in the biliary tree and should be withdrawn when the bile duct is entered or it will kink the guidewire.

guidewire and the percutaneous track is now ready for dilatation.

The percutaneous track through the liver is dilated with a 7-French dilator and a 9-French peel-away sheath placed through the percutaneous track. If the obstructing lesion is not appropriate for stenting, an internal/external biliary drainage catheter is placed to drain the

biliary system. The catheter we use is an 8.3-French Ring catheter (Cook, Bloomington, IN) with either 32 or 42 side-holes (Fig. 20-9). The 32-side-hole catheter is used for patients with low CBD obstruction while the 42-side-hole catheter is used for patients with hilar obstruction. The Ring catheter has a tapered tip which helps the catheter pass through the strictured area. The peel-away

Figure 20-7 **A,** A patient with pancreatic cancer and failed ERCP. Initial PTC shows the tip of the needle (small arrows) in the left hepatic duct. Contrast was injected to outline the biliary tree, but this bile duct was not used for access because of the steep angulation between the left hepatic duct and the common hepatic duct. **B,** The needle was withdrawn and a second puncture made into a right hepatic duct. A 0.018-inch guidewire was placed through the 22-gauge needle, and the 5-Fr sheath assembly was placed into the biliary system. A "J" wire was placed through the 5-Fr sheath and the sheath removed. **C,** A hockey-stick catheter (curved arrows) was placed over the "J" wire and manipulated down to the level of the obstruction. Note the small nipple (straight arrow) representing the proximal end of the stricture. **D,** Using a 0.035-inch Terumo guidewire, the stricture in the lower common bile duct was negotiated and a hockey-stick catheter and hydrophilic wire were used to manipulate the hockey-stick catheter into the proximal jejunum (arrows). A metal stent was then placed.

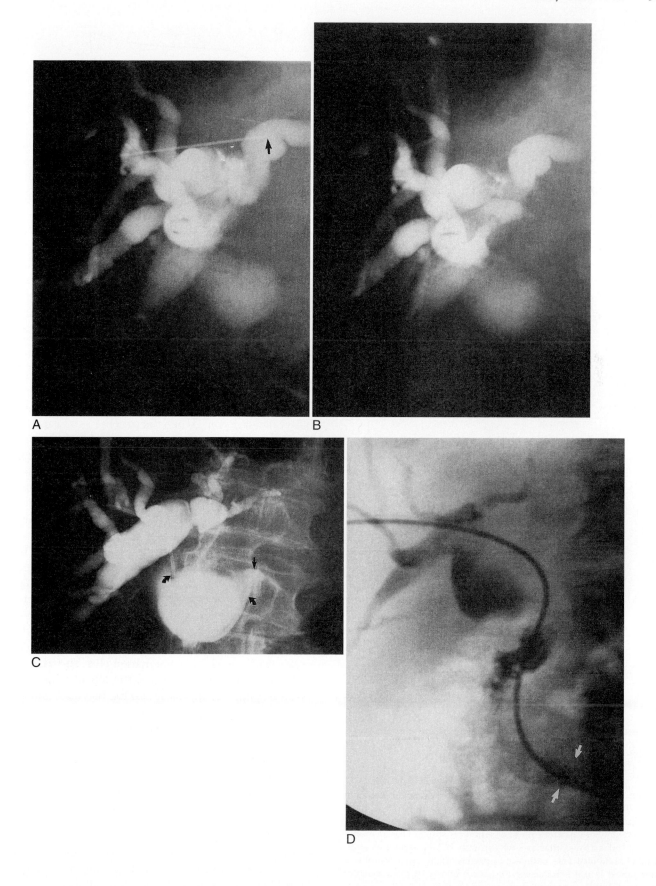

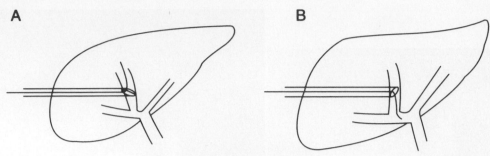

Figure 20-8   Schematic showing biliary access difficulties in vertically orientated bile ducts. **A**, Access is gained with a 22-gauge needle into a vertically orientated bile duct in the right lobe of the liver. When the bevel on the needle tip is pointing superiorly, the 0.018-inch guidewire tends to travel superiorly within the bile duct. **B**, By turning the bevel it is often possible to manipulate the guidewire in an inferior direction towards the common bile duct.

sheath protects the liver parenchyma, prevents buckling of the guidewire and catheter in the perihepatic space, and helps to direct the pushing force applied to the catheter down the bile duct. The Ring catheter is placed well into the duodenum and the guidewire removed.

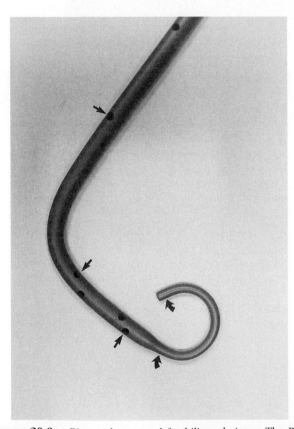

Figure 20-9   Ring catheter used for biliary drainage. The Ring biliary drainage catheter (Cook, Bloomington, IN) is 8.3-Fr, is made from polyethylene, and has 32 side-holes (straight arrows) (zoomed view of catheter tip). The catheter is stiff and has a tapered tip (curved arrows) that passes through biliary strictures with minimal difficulty. This catheter is preferentially used for biliary drainages. It is *not* suitable for long-term internal/external biliary drainage: a larger, softer catheter is used for this.

Contrast material is injected and the catheter withdrawn until contrast material is seen to opacify the biliary tree proximal to the obstruction. This implies that there are catheter side-holes above and below the level of obstruction. The catheter is placed to gravity drainage and attached to a bag.

Left-sided Biliary Drainage

In the author's unit we generally perform left-sided biliary drainages only when the patient has a hilar stricture. However, some authors prefer to use the left side for most, if not all, biliary drainages. A left-sided biliary drainage can be technically more challenging than using the right side, depending on the size of the left lobe, the anatomic configuration of the xiphisternum and costal margins, and the relationship of the left lobe to the costal margins and xiphisternum. There is a limited window of access to the left lobe through the inverted "V" formed by the xiphisternum and medial edges of the right and left costal margins. Depending on the size and position of the left lobe of the liver, the angle of entry into the left lobe may be shallow and within the inverted "V" formed by the bony landmarks of the upper abdomen; or indeed if the left lobe is small, it may be quite steep and angled up underneath the right costal margin (Fig. 20-10).

We use ultrasound to locate the left lobe of the liver, assess the angle of approach into the bile duct, and indeed guide the needle into a bile duct. In general, the segment-3 bile duct which courses inferiorally towards the inferior margin of the left lobe is chosen for entry. Depending on the size of the left lobe, a segment-2 duct which has a more horizontal course in the left lobe can be entered if the left lobe is large enough to permit access to segment 2. The advantage of using the segment-2 duct is that there is a more gentle curve with a less acute angle for manipulating guidewires and catheters down into the common bile duct. For patients with hilar obstruction it is important to gain access to the left lobe biliary system in as peripheral a location as the anatomy allows.

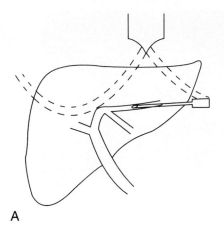

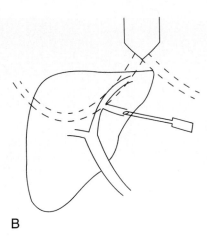

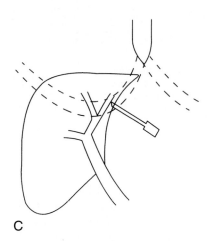

Figure 20-10   Schematic showing the various approaches to left lobe drainage which depend on the anatomy of the left lobe. **A**, In patients with a large left lobe it may be possible to enter the segment-2 bile duct which generally has a horizontal course in the left lobe and allows easy access into the common hepatic duct. **B**, In patients with smaller left lobes, the segment-3 duct is usually accessible but there is a more acute angle for entry down the bile duct. A peel-away sheath is important in this situation to ensure that the pushing force applied to catheters is directed toward the common bile duct. **C**, In patients with very small left lobes, a left-sided biliary drainage is difficult with a very acute angle of entry into the segment-3 duct making guidewire purchase and other manipulations difficult.

A 22-gauge Chiba needle is used to access the segment-2 or -3 duct and contrast material injected to outline the biliary system. A 0.018-inch guidewire is manipulated towards the biliary hilum followed by the 5-French sheath system as on the right side. The hydrophilic guidewire and Kumpe catheter are used to negotiate the stricture and are placed in the proximal jejunum. The percutaneous track is dilated over a 0.035-inch superstiff guidewire and a 9-French peel-away sheath placed. The 9-French peel-away sheath is important particularly when access is gained through a segment-3 duct as it will help to direct the pushing force applied to the catheter down the common bile duct and make placement of the catheter significantly easier. The 8.3-French Ring catheter is placed through the peel-away sheath and over the guidewire so that side-holes are left above and below the stricture (Fig. 20-11 and Box 20-3).

Palliation of Malignant Biliary Obstruction with Metal Stents

The introduction of metal stents for palliation of malignant biliary strictures has revolutionized the percutaneous treatment of these patients. The metallic biliary stents require significantly less track dilatation as opposed to plastic stents (7-French versus 10- to 12-French), can be placed at the same time as the initial biliary drainage procedure, are associated with shorter hospital stays, and are overall more cost-effective than plastic stents (Fig. 20-12). For these reasons, in the author's unit we exclusively place metallic endoprostheses for palliation of patients with malignant bile duct obstruction.

Box 20-3 Biliary Drainage: Key Points

One-stick needle system used for access
Stricture negotiated with short catheter and
    hydrophilic wire
9-Fr peel-away sheath placed
8.3-Fr Ring catheter inserted
Allow 2–3 cm of "slack" when fixing the
    catheter

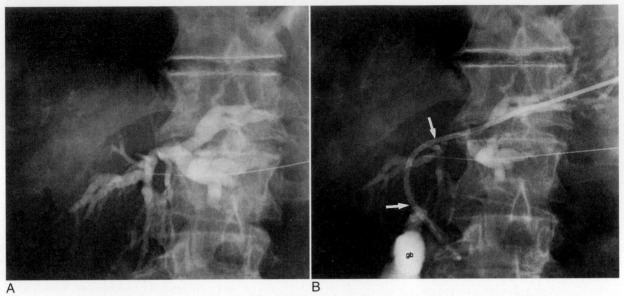

Figure 20-11 A patient with hilar cholangiocarcinoma who had a left biliary drainage performed. **A,** The initial needle puncture was too central but was used to opacify the left biliary system. **B,** A second needle was used to puncture the segment-2 duct which provided direct access down across the hilum into the common hepatic duct. A catheter (arrow) was placed across the stricture. (gb = gallbladder.)

Hilar Obstruction

Patients with hilar obstruction form a subset of patients with biliary obstruction that are technically challenging and are usually best palliated by percutaneous methods if not surgically resectable. Knowledge of liver and biliary anatomy is important before planning biliary drainage and/or stent placement. If there is anomalous drainage of the RPD into the left hepatic duct, it may be sufficient to drain the left lobe alone. If not, the author's practice is to drain both right and left lobes and stent both sides. The other significant factor that influences the approach taken is the Bismuth classification of the lesion (Fig. 20-13). If there is separate occlusion of the RAD and RPD (stage 3a), then draining the right side is of little benefit to the patient. In this situation, it is often

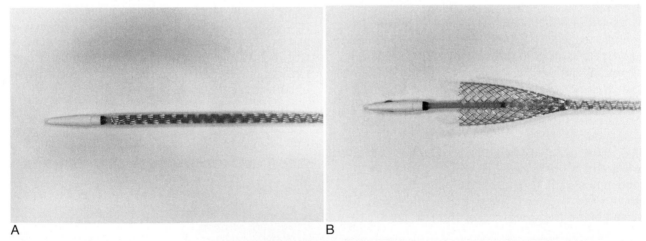

Figure 20-12 Wallstent endoprosthesis used for biliary drainage. **A,** Close-up view of the end of the 7-Fr Wallstent delivery catheter. The Wallstent is compressed on the end of the delivery catheter by a plastic sheath. **B,** The stent is deployed by pulling back the sheath on the delivery catheter. The stent deploys from distal to proximal but tends to move a little forward as it is deployed. It is important to readjust the position of the stent as it is being deployed. The author's unit generally uses a 90 × 10 mm Wallstent.

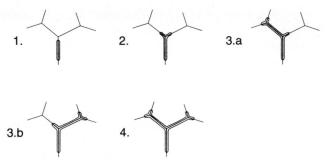

Figure 20-13 Bismuth classification. This is used to stage biliary hilar tumors. In stage 1, the tumor involves the common hepatic duct and is driven 2 cm from the biliary hilum. In stage 2, the tumor involves the biliary hilum and the right and left hepatic duct. In stage 3a, the tumor grows out along the right hepatic duct with involvement of the segmental ducts on the right. In stage 3b, the tumor encases the left hepatic duct and involves the segmental ducts on the left. In stage 4, there is segmental duct involvement in both right and left lobes of the liver.

best to drain the left side by itself provided that the left lobe is of adequate size and that there is no second-order bile duct involvement on the left side. When there is multisegmental involvement on both sides, there is very little that any drainage procedure can offer the patient.

Magnetic resonance cholangiography is a very useful preprocedure imaging test to assess both the anatomy of the biliary system and the Bismuth classification of the hilar tumor (Fig. 20-14). Most hilar malignancies are due to cholangiocarcinoma of the bile duct or the so-called Klatskin tumor. The natural history of this tumor is to grow centrally into the liver along the bile ducts. Eventually, this leads to segmental and subsegmental obstruction. With this in mind, the principle of palliation is to drain as much functioning liver as possible. Although some operators drain one side only, in the author's unit we have found over the years that optimal palliation is achieved when both sides are stented. Most of our reasons for doing this are anecdotal; but given the progressive nature of the disease, it seems appropriate to drain both sides. In addition, there is a faster resolution of jaundice and pruritis. Draining both sides also means that there are no undrained segments which may become infected at a later date and require a further drainage procedure. However, it is not always feasible to drain both lobes in every patient.

There are a number of metal stents used in the biliary tree, with the most popular being the Wallstent (Boston Scientific, Natick, MA) and the Gianturco (Cook, Bloomington, IN). We prefer the Wallstent which is a self-expanding stainless steel mesh (see Fig. 20-12). It can have many differing lengths but the preferred length for the biliary tree is 9 cm and the preferred diameter is 1 cm. The advantages of the Wallstent include the fact that it has a small delivery catheter (7-French), the

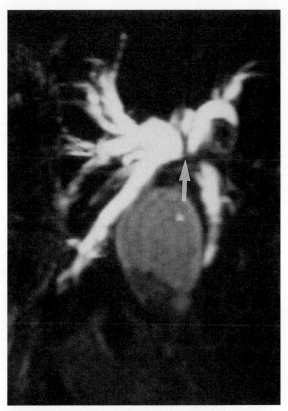

Figure 20-14 MRC in a patient with hilar cholangiocarcinoma. Coronal MIP examination from an MRCP examination shows dilated intrahepatic bile ducts with a stricture at the hepatic hilum (arrow). There is no communication between left and right ducts but intrahepatic bile ducts do not appear encased. This indicates a Bismuth type 2 stricture.

delivery system is flexible, and the stent has a large luminal diameter (1 cm).

The Wallstent consists of a 7-French delivery catheter on the end of which the Wallstent is loaded by the manufacturer. The Wallstent is compressed on the end of the delivery catheter by a sheath which is withdrawn by the operator to deliver the stent. The stent deploys from distal to proximal and tends to move a little forward as it deploys. It is important to reposition the delivery catheter during stent deployment for this reason.

There are a number of different approaches to stenting right and left lobes. In one approach, a single right- or left-sided biliary drainage is performed and two Wallstents are placed across the biliary hilum in a "T" configuration. A stent is initially placed across the biliary hilum from right to left side to form the top of the "T" (Fig. 20-15). A guidewire is placed through the metal mesh of this initial stent, down into the duodenum, and an 8-mm balloon is used to make a hole in the mesh of this stent. A second stent is placed through the hole in this initial stent to complete the "T." We have used this approach in some patients but have abandoned this approach as the junction of the right and left ducts are almost never

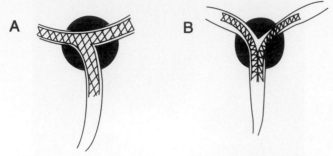

Figure 20-15 Schematic showing "T" and "Y" stenting. **A**, In patients with a horizontally orientated hilar confluence it may be possible to perform T-stenting from a single biliary drainage. The first stent is laid between the right and left hepatic ducts. A hole is made in the first stent with a balloon and the second stent is placed through the first stent into the common bile duct. However, the vast majority of patients do not have a horizontally orientated hepatic hilum, so "T" stenting is not suitable for the majority of patients. **B**, For Y-stenting bilateral biliary drainages are performed with metal stents inserted. This is the author's preferred method for stenting patients with hilar lesions.

horizontal and this procedure does not provide optimal drainage.

The approach that we currently use is based on bilateral deployment of Wallstents in a "Y" configuration (see Fig. 20-15). This means that bilateral biliary drainages are performed for stent placement.

The principles of effective palliation for hilar strictures are:

- Peripheral purchase within the biliary tree;
- Overstenting.

Over-stenting means that the proximal end of the stent is situated at least 2–3 cm above the proximal edge of the tumor. To facilitate this procedure, peripheral access into the biliary tree is mandatory when performing the initial biliary drainage.

To deploy the stents, two 0.035-inch superstiff guidewires are placed across the stricture into the duodenum. The stents are loaded on each wire in turn and placed across the stricture from right and left sides. The stents are positioned so that there is an approximate 2–3 cm of stent above the tumor. The stents are then deployed, one at a time, by simply pulling back the sheath which covers the stent on the delivery catheter (Fig. 20-16).

If the procedure has gone smoothly without evidence of hemobilia, and if the patient is not septic, we generally do not leave a safety catheter. We do decompress the biliary system if not leaving a safety catheter. We also embolize the track with either Gelfoam or a mixture of glue and lipoidol. However, if there is any doubt about the patient's condition, or if there is significant hemobilia, a safety catheter is left through both sides. An 8.3-French Ring catheter is generally used for this purpose and left for 2–3 days on gravity drainage, at which time the

Figure 20-16 A 59-year-old patient with hilar cholangiocarcinoma unsuitable for surgery (Bismuth stage 3a). **A**, Axial reformatted view from MR cholangiography shows separation of the anterior and posterior sectoral ducts on the right (arrows) with no segmental duct encasement on the left (Bismuth stage 3a). Because of the patient's young age, bilateral Y-stenting was performed. **B**, Peripheral access into the left segment-3 duct (arrow) was achieved with similar peripheral access on the right. *(Continued)*

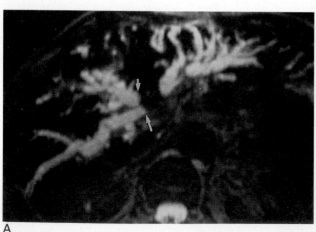

A

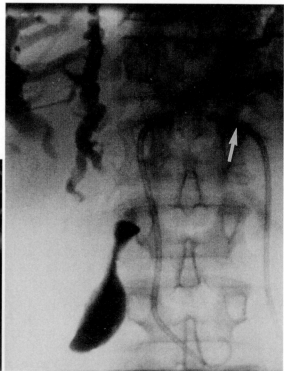

B

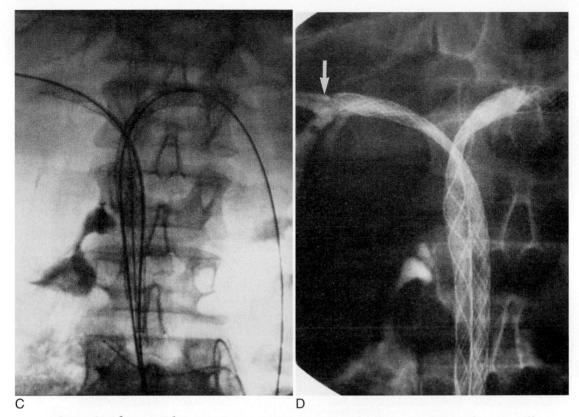

C   D

Figure 20-16   cont'd C, 90×10 mm Wallstents were deployed over 0.035-inch superstiff guidewires. Both stents were dilated with an 8-mm balloon and a safety Ring catheter was left through the right-sided stent. **D,** Two days later the safety catheter was removed over a guidewire and injection was made through a 4-Fr dilator (arrow) at the proximal end of the right-sided stent. Good flow of contrast is seen in both stents. Note the peripheral access on both right and left lobes which permits over-stenting of the tumor. The patient survived for 18 months after the procedure without further jaundice or cholangitis.

patient is brought back for a further cholangiogram. If at this time the biliary system is clear and the patient's condition has normalized, the catheter is removed.

In the author's unit we generally do not dilate the stents *in situ* unless we are not leaving a safety catheter. If we are not leaving a safety catheter then we dilate the stent in the area of the stricture with an 8-mm balloon to speed up the self-expanding process. The Wallstent is a self-expanding stent and tends to expand and shorten over time. It is an easy stent to deploy; but the shortening with time means that correct positioning is import-ant because otherwise the proximal end of the stent may shorten to lie within the tumor (Box 20-4).

Low CBD Obstruction

The majority of patients with low CBD obstruction have pancreatic carcinoma. These patients are most often palliated endoscopically, but occasionally endoscopic stent insertion fails and the patient is referred for biliary drainage and stent placement. It is important not to place

a metal stent if the patient is an operative candidate, so this information should be obtained by consultation with the referring clinician or surgeon before the biliary drainage (Fig. 20-17). If the patient is not a candidate for surgery, then a stent can be placed at the time of initial biliary drainage. For patients with low CBD obstruction, it is not as important to gain peripheral access into the biliary tree, but it is again important to overstent and to ensure that there is no duodenal encasement by the pancreatic tumor. This can be done by injecting contrast

---

Box 20-4 Hilar Strictures and Metal Stents

Double "Y" stenting best where possible
10 mm × 90 mm Wallstent used
Peripheral biliary purchase necessary
Proximal stent position 2–3 cm above tumor
"Y" stents placed simultaneously and deployed
   sequentially

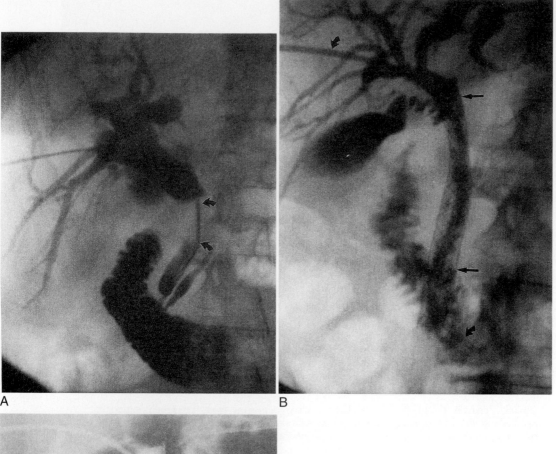

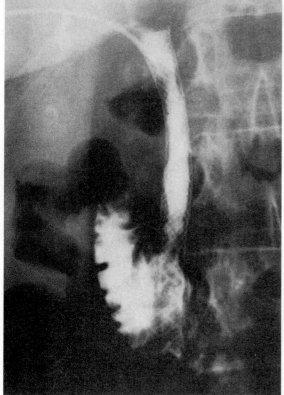

A

B

C

Figure 20-17 Metal stent placement in a patient with pancreatic cancer who had a failed ERCP. The patient had a low platelet count of 35,000 and received 6 units of platelets before the biliary drainage. **A**, Biliary drainage was performed and the stricture (curved arrows) was traversed with a hockey-stick catheter and hydrophilic guidewire. Note the normal duodenum without evidence of encasement. **B**, 70 × 10 mm Wallstent was placed across the stricture (straight arrows) and a safety catheter was left *in situ* for 3 days (curved arrows) because of some bleeding at the time of the biliary drainage. **C**, The patient returned for a tube injection 3 days later. The stent was in good position and there was good flow of contrast into the duodenum. The safety catheter was removed.

material into the duodenal loop using the hockey-stick catheter when the tumor has been crossed. It is very important to do this before stenting. Obviously, if there is duodenal encasement, the stent will not provide effective palliation and the patient may need a gastro-jejunostomy or other form of surgical decompression. Occasionally, if the patient is not fit for surgery, a duodenal stent can be placed or a long-term internal/external drainage catheter can be placed with its tip placed in the proximal jejunum (Fig. 20-18).

The stent is placed in a similar fashion as for hilar stenting. Approximately 3–4 cm of the stent is placed above the proximal edge of the tumor and the distal end of the stent is left in the duodenum. Again, a safety catheter is not left in place if the procedure has been uneventful, but the stent is balloon dilated if a safety catheter is not left *in situ* (Box 20-5).

Aftercare

Correct catheter fixation to the skin is important for biliary drainage catheters because they are subject to the effects of liver movement during breathing, movement which can be significant. This is particularly true of right-sided biliary drainage catheters. If the catheter is tied tightly at the skin entry site, the catheter will not be free to move with the liver as the patient breathes. If the catheter cannot move in and out because it is tied tightly at the skin, it will tend to back out of the liver as the patient breathes and form a loop between the liver capsule and the abdominal wall (Fig. 20-19). This can lead to drainage problems such as back-bleeding through the catheter if a side-hole migrates back into the liver and communicates with a vein (Fig. 20-20). Or indeed, a side-hole may migrate outside the liver and communicate with either the pleural space or abdominal cavity, leading to a bile leak. To avoid these problems, allow approximately 2 cm of slack in the catheter when suturing the catheter to the skin.

Daily rounds by a member of the interventional team are important to monitor these patients. The catheter is usually irrigated with 5 mL of saline every 6 hours for the first 48 hours. The patient is maintained on piperacillin/tazobactam 4.5 g t.i.d. for 2–3 days after the procedure and is also maintained on intravenous fluids (2–2$\frac{1}{2}$ liters of Hartman's solution daily for 48–72 hours). Intravenous

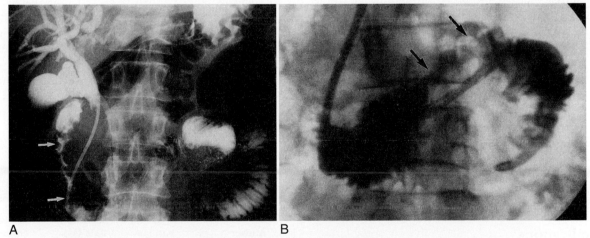

A   B

Figure 20-18   A patient with pancreatic cancer and encasement of the duodenum. **A,** During initial biliary drainage it was noted that the second part of the duodenum (arrows) and the fourth part of the duodenum (not shown) were encased. It was not practical to place a metal stent. The patient had a gastrojejunostomy to decompress the stomach. **B,** A long 14-Fr biliary Cope catheter (Cook, Bloomington, IN) was placed into the proximal jejunum and extra side-holes cut in the catheter to provide appropriate biliary drainage. The catheter was clamped at the skin and provided adequate internal drainage for 3 months until the patient died. Note the stricture (arrows) in the fourth part of the duodenum also. An alternative approach in patients with a single stricture in the duodenum would be to place a metal stent across the stricture.

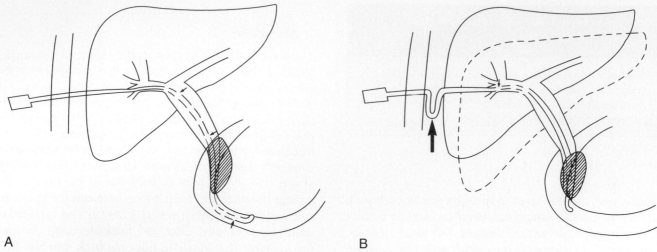

Figure 20-19 Schematic showing the catheter buckling between the skin and the liver owing to inappropriate fixation of the catheter at the skin entry site. **A,** Biliary catheter appropriately placed with side-holes (arrows) above and below the stricture in the lower bile duct. **B,** If the catheter is fixed tightly at the skin entry site, ascent and descent of the liver during respiration will cause the catheter to back slowly out of the liver and form a loop (arrow) between the abdominal wall and the liver. This may result in a catheter side-hole (small arrow) lying close to or within the hepatic parenchyma and possibly communicating with an hepatic or portal vein. If this happens, back-bleeding can occur. In addition, it can be technically difficult to straighten this loop if it is large, because any guidewire inserted may cause the loop to get bigger and the catheter may flip completely out of the liver.

fluids are important in these patients because there may often be a marked choleresis which may precipitate hepatorenal failure. The skin site should be inspected to make sure that the catheter has not backed out. The bag should also be inspected to ensure that there is no back-bleeding into the bag. If problems are encountered with the catheter, the patient should be brought down to the interventional suite for a cholangiogram and appropriate action taken for any problem that is seen.

Results

Percutaneous biliary drainage should be technically successful achieving either internal drainage, external drainage, or stent placement in 95–100% of patients with malignant bile duct obstruction. Similarly, effective palliation by catheter or stent placement should be possible in approximately 90% of patients. The success rates for metal stent placement are shown in Table 20-1.

Complications

Major complications related to percutaneous biliary drainage include hemorrhage, bile leak with potential biliary peritonitis, and sepsis. Major complications have been reported in approximately 5–10% of patients (see Table 20-1). Death has also been reported with percutaneous biliary drainage in 1–2.5% of patients. Most of these series describing percutaneous biliary drainage

were from the early 1980s; with newer techniques the mortality rate should be less than 1%.

Hemobilia frequently occurs after biliary drainage but is almost always transient. Transgression of vascular structures with guidewires and catheters is to be expected during a biliary drainage, but bleeding from this usually settles down over 2–3 days. Back-bleeding through the catheter can occur if a catheter side hole is left in the hepatic parenchyma where it may communicate with a hepatic vein (Fig. 20-21). This can be remedied by repositioning the catheter during catheter cholangiography so that there is no venous communication. Serious hemorrhage is usually evidenced by a fall in the hematocrit, abdominal pain, and obvious hemobilia.

Table 20-1 Metal Stent Results			
Author	**Patients**	**Occlusion Rate (%)**	**Survival (mths)**
Gillams (1990)	45	42	5
Lammer (1990)	61	12.7	?
Adam (1991)	41	7	3.5
Lameris (1991)	69	14	3.2–4.3
Lee (1992)	34	12	3.7
Lee (1993)	69	17	7.2
Rossi (1994)	240	17.7	5.9

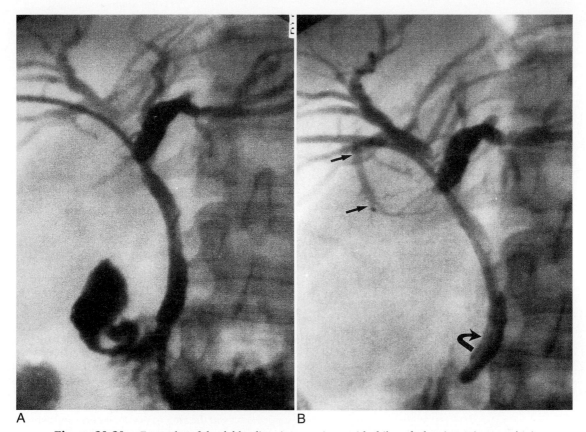

A   B

Figure 20-20   Example of back-bleeding in a patient with hilar cholangiocarcinoma. **A**, A catheter inserted from the right at the time of initial biliary drainage shows good flow of contrast both proximally in the bile duct and distally in the duodenum at the end of the procedure. **B**, The next day the patient had dark blood appearing through the catheter in the drainage bag. The patient was bought back to the radiology department for catheter injection. Catheter injection shows communication with a hepatic vein branch (straight arrows). Note also the catheter has migrated proximally (curved arrow) with the tip of the catheter now lying in the distal bile duct as opposed to the duodenum. This was rectified by inserting the catheter more distally into the duodenum using a guidewire.

Although hemobilia is frequent, severe or prolonged hemobilia occurs in fewer than 4% of patients. It is important before embarking on a percutaneous biliary drainage to correct any coagulation abnormality with fresh frozen plasma. It is also best to give the fresh frozen plasma before the procedure, during the procedure, and after the procedure as the half-life of fresh frozen plasma is short. In the author's unit we generally would administer two units of fresh frozen plasma before the procedure, two units during the procedure, and two units immediately after the procedure.

Hemobilia which presents after several days of drainage is usually more serious and requires immediate intervention. It may be due to either pseudoaneurysm formation or tumor bleeding. Replacing the catheter with a larger catheter often tamponades bleeding from a pseudoaneurysm. If this does not work and bleeding continues, embolization will be required and should resolve the problem.

Tumor bleeding occurs in patients with hilar tumors that are managed by long-term internal/external drainage catheters. We generally do not see this problem in the present day because most patients with hilar cholangiocarcinomas are managed by indwelling metal stents. Tumor bleeding, if it does occur, is difficult to deal with and may not respond to embolization or to placement of a larger catheter.

Patients undergoing percutaneous biliary interventional procedures are prone to develop septicemia as the obstructed biliary system may be infected in as many as 25–50% of patients with malignant obstruction. Bacteremia almost invariably occurs in these patients with infected and obstructed biliary systems. For these reasons, appropriate antibiotic coverage is mandatory before undertaking biliary interventional procedures. Despite appropriate antibiotic coverage, septicemia may occur in these patients. A number of patients have developed septicemic shock after biliary drainage despite adequate

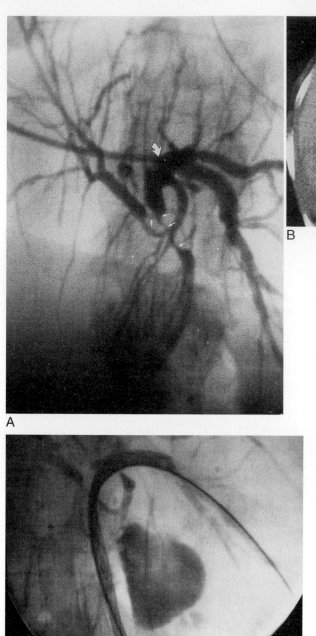

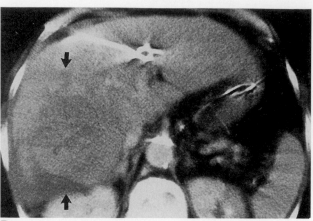

Figure 20-21 Intrahepatic hemorrhage after biliary drainage in a patient referred from another hospital. **A**, Right-sided access shows the catheter tip in the left hepatic duct (curved arrow). A cholangiocarcinoma with stricture (small arrows) is noted in the common hepatic duct, and involving the origin of the right and left hepatic ducts. Attempts to manipulate guidewires from the left hepatic duct into the common hepatic duct were unsuccessful and the patient developed pain and subsequently had a fall in hematocrit. An external catheter was left *in situ* and the patient returned to the ward. Attempts to manipulate catheters and guidewires from the left hepatic duct into the common hepatic duct from a right-sided access is not advised because of the acute angulation involved. **B**, A CT performed shortly afterwards revealed a large right intrahepatic hemorrhage (arrows). **C**, After a 7-day interval during which the patient's symptoms subsided, a left-sided biliary drainage was performed and a 90 × 10 mm Wallstent was placed from the left side across the stricture. The intrahepatic hematoma spontaneously resolved over the ensuing months.

coverage with ampicillin and gentamicin. In the author's unit we have therefore changed our antibiotic regimen to piperacillin/tazobactam 4.5 g t.i.d. The antibiotic is started either on the morning of the percutaneous biliary drainage, or the day before, if the procedure is anticipated. We also continue the antibiotic regimen for 2 days after the biliary drainage as we have had one or two patients develop septic shock 24 hours after biliary drainage.

In patients, who are septicemic before the procedure with high fever and white cell count, it is best to perform the minimum intervention necessary to drain the patient. The biliary tree should not be overdistended with contrast material, and it may be appropriate to simply place an external biliary drainage catheter rather than trying to place an internal/external catheter. After appropriate antibiotic therapy and drainage, the patient can be brought back to the interventional suite in 2–3 days and further definitive drainage performed.

Bile leak and biliary peritonitis can cause severe abdominal pain and tenderness. The presence of even small amounts of bile in the peritoneal cavity can cause a severe chemical peritonitis in some patients, while the presence of large amounts of bile in the peritoneal cavity in other patients does not appear to cause any symptoms. The reasons for this are unclear. Bile leaks can be avoided with careful technique and experience. It is important when performing a biliary drainage that dilators and catheters are not removed from the liver until the next dilator or catheter is ready to be placed. This minimizes the amount of time that the guidewire is present in the percutaneous track by itself. Obviously, if the track has been dilated, and only the guidewire is present in the track, then bile can flow out along the guidewire into the peritoneal cavity. Similarly, the use of a 9-French peel-away sheath helps to protect the peritoneal cavity from biliary leaks as the bile leaks externally through the 9-French peel-away sheath during catheter manipulations. In addition, proper fixation of the catheter and proper siting of the catheter within the biliary tree is important to prevent the catheter backing out of the biliary tree and possibly having a side-hole communicating with the peritoneal cavity. Lastly, embolizing the percutaneous track with Gelfoam or glue when removing catheters helps prevent bile leakage or bleeding through the track.

Other complications that have been reported with percutaneous biliary drainage – such as pneumothorax, empyema, or bilious pleural effusion – may occur owing to the use of a transpleural approach. Often this is necessary because of the location of the liver. It is important that the catheter is sited properly so that a side-hole does not communicate with the pleural space (Box 20-6).

Immediate complications related to metal stent insertion are usually similar to those for percutaneous biliary drainage techniques. Careful positioning of the metal stent is important to allow for stent shortening so that adequate coverage of the stricture is obtained. Migration is rare with metallic stents. Late complications of metallic stent insertion include occlusion and tumor ingrowth. The relative frequency of these is shown in Table 20-2. The incidence of occlusion and/or cholangitis requiring intervention varies between 7% and 20% in reported series.

Box 20-6 Preventing Complications

Appropriate antibiotic prophylaxis for biliary sepsis
Intravenous fluids to prevent hepatorenal failure
Back-bleeding prevented by appropriate catheter positioning
Fresh frozen plasma to correct coagulopathy
If cholangitis present, minimum intervention to drain the biliary tree
9-Fr peel-away minimizes bile leak and protects liver parenchyma
Catheter fixation allowing "slack" in the catheter

SPECIAL CONSIDERATIONS

External Biliary Drainage

External biliary drainage is rarely performed. It involves leaving a catheter in the biliary tree above the level of obstruction. In general, with hydrophilic guidewires it is usually straightforward to cross most biliary obstructions at the first sitting. However, before the advent of hydrophilic guidewires it was not unusual to perform an external biliary drainage and bring the patient back for conversion of an external drainage into an internal/external biliary drainage in 1–2 days. The indications for performing external biliary drainage now would include a patient with septicemic shock due to cholangitis in whom the minimum intervention necessary to drain the patient is appropriate (Fig. 20-22). Other indications would include a patient with a bile duct stricture or transection at laparoscopic cholecystectomy. Drainage of the intrahepatic biliary tree by an external biliary drainage catheter will help temporize the patient before definitive surgery.

When performing an external biliary drainage, the catheter used is important. The catheter needs to have a relatively small pigtail with relatively large side-holes to promote biliary drainage. A 5- or 7-French angiographic pigtail catheter is not appropriate as it does not drain well and it tends to fall out. The catheter the author uses is an 8-French locking pigtail catheter designed for percutaneous cholecystostomy (Cook, Bloomington, IN). This catheter has a small pigtail with relatively large side-holes and is easy to place and provides good drainage.

Long-term Internal/External Biliary Drainage

As with external biliary drainage, the long-term use of internal/external biliary drainage catheters is no longer common. The advent of metallic stents has proved a much more effective and more comfortable method for palliating malignant biliary obstruction. Long-term internal/external biliary drainage catheters may be used after balloon dilatation of anastomotic strictures, and in patients with duodenal encasement from pancreatic carcinoma where a metal stent cannot be placed.

The catheter used for long-term internal/external biliary drainage is usually a 10- or 12-French catheter as opposed to the 8.3-French Ring catheter placed at initial biliary drainage. The larger bore catheters are more difficult to place initially and an 8.3-French catheter is appropriate at the time of initial biliary drainage. The track can then be dilated over the ensuing week to 12-French and a 12-French Cope (Cook, Bloomington, IN) or Flexima (Boston Scientific, Natick, MA) catheter placed. When the

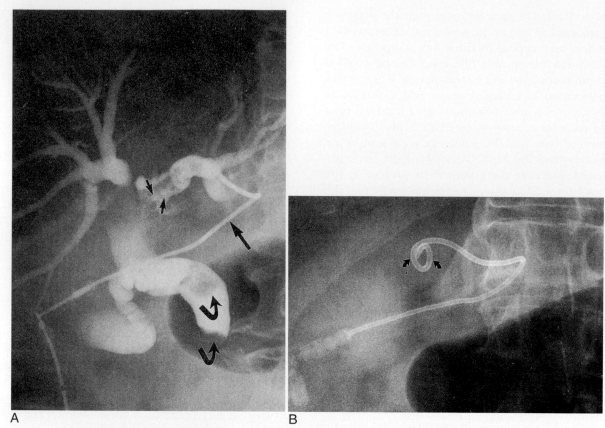

Figure 20-22   External biliary drainage performed in a 75-year-old patient with ascending cholangitis secondary to choledocholithiasis. The patient was profoundly hypotensive, in respiratory distress, and with a platelet count of 43,000. The patient was given 8 units of platelets and an external biliary drainage was performed. **A**, A left-sided external biliary drainage was performed instead of a right-sided biliary drainage so that splinting of the diaphragm and further respiratory distress would not occur. A cholangiogram performed 3 days after the procedure shows a catheter (large arrow) sited in the left hepatic duct with stones (curved arrows) in the lower bile duct causing the obstruction. Some blood (small arrows) is presented within the bile duct resulting from the biliary drainage procedure. The patient settled with external biliary drainage, and because of the patient's age a double pigtail stent was placed percutaneously after 5 days. **B**, Note the small size of the pigtail (arrows) on this catheter (Cook, Bloomington, IN). The catheter is 8.5-Fr and is ideally suited to external biliary drainage.

12-French catheter is placed, it is left to free drainage for 1-2 days and then clamped, provided the patient has no fever. If the patient tolerates catheter clamping, the patient can be discharged. The idea is that bile will drain through the side-holes above the obstruction, through the catheter, and out the side-holes below the obstruction into the duodenum. The patient is given a bag to take home and if the patient develops a fever, they are instructed to attach the bag to the catheter for free drainage and to come back to the interventional radiology department for further management. These catheters will need replacement every 2-3 months, or sooner if catheter occlusion or fever occurs.

Tissue Diagnosis of Malignant Biliary Obstruction

Obtaining a tissue diagnosis for patients with biliary obstruction is important, particularly if radiotherapy or other forms of nonsurgical therapy are being considered. The simplest way of obtaining cells for cytologic evaluation is by sending a sample of bile obtained during the initial biliary drainage, to the histopathology laboratory. The bile is best collected after the stricture has been traversed and before the final internal/external biliary drainage catheter is placed. Collecting the bile sample at this time helps increase the diagnostic yield from bile cytology in that malignant cells may be shed into the biliary tree after manipulation of guidewires, etc., through the malignant stricture. Just before placing the internal/external biliary drainage catheter, the hockey-stick catheter is placed through the 9-French peel-away sheath to a level just above the stricture and a sample of bile obtained for bile cytology. Bile cytology has an approximate 40–60% success rate in obtaining a diagnosis.

If bile cytology is negative or inconclusive, biliary brushing can be performed. For this procedure a small brush, similar to that used for bronchoscopic brushing of strictured bronchi, is placed through a 9-French peel-away sheath and vigorous brushing of the internal lumen of the stricture is performed. The brush is then removed through the 9-French sheath and a sample spread on a glass slide. This can be repeated a number of times until sufficient samples are obtained. Some operators have also used atherectomy catheters to obtain cells for diagnosis. The author has not done this as biliary brushing usually suffices.

Obviously, brushing is only appropriate for malignant strictures primarily originating in the bile duct. For patients with pancreatic carcinoma, the mass can be biopsied percutaneously.

Percutaneous Biliary Drainage after Failed ERCP

The author's unit is often asked to perform a percutaneous biliary drainage after a failed ERCP in patients with malignant biliary obstruction. Some interventional radiologists like to perform the percutaneous biliary drainage immediately after the failed ERCP, but we prefer to wait for a number of hours unless the patient is febrile or requires immediate drainage. The reasons for this approach are that patients are usually given a significant amount of sedoanalgesia for the endoscopic procedure, and indeed may even be given reversal agents at the end of the procedure. This makes it difficult to re-sedate the patient for the percutaneous biliary drainage. We have found that patients are often very uncomfortable during the percutaneous biliary drainage and this makes percutaneous biliary drainage technically difficult and perhaps more prone to complications.

The other determining factor with regard to how soon the percutaneous biliary drainage should be performed after the ERCP is whether the endoscopists have managed to inject contrast material above the level of obstruction. If they have not, the percutaneous biliary drainage can be postponed for a number of days provided the patient does not have signs of sepsis. If, however, the endoscopists have injected contrast material above the level of obstruction, the biliary drainage should be performed relatively soon after the ERCP. If the ERCP has been performed in the morning with contrast material injected

---

Box 20-7 Biliary Drainage after Failed ERCP

If no contrast material injected and patient not septic, PBD within 2 days

If septic, drain immediately

If contrast material injected above obstruction, start IV fluids and antibiotics and do PBD within 8–12 hours

---

above the obstruction, the biliary drainage is performed in the afternoon. If the ERCP is performed in the evening and contrast material has not been injected above the level of obstruction, then the biliary drainage is performed the following day. If the ERCP is performed in the afternoon or the evening and contrast material has been injected above the level of obstruction, we generally place the patient on intravenous fluids and antibiotics and perform the biliary drainage early the next morning (Box 20-7).

Interventional Management of Laparoscopic Cholecystectomy Complications

The advent of laparoscopic cholecystectomy has dramatically changed the treatment of gallstone disease. Most patients prefer a laparoscopic cholecystectomy rather than an open cholecystectomy because of shorter hospital stay, less pain, and a quicker return to work. Bile duct injuries with laparoscopic cholecystectomy have been reported to occur up to ten times more frequently than with open cholecystectomy. However, with experience, the complication rate declines and in most large series the complication rate is under 1%.

The most frequent complication is bile leakage. This usually occurs when surgical clips slip from the cystic duct, or occasionally small ducts that drain the gallbladder directly into the liver may leak after the gallbladder is laparoscopically removed. Bile tends to collect in the gallbladder fossa, subhepatic space, subphrenic space, or paracolic gutter. Bile accumulation can be managed by one or more percutaneous drains placed under ultrasound or CT guidance. If there is a leak from the cystic duct stump, then endoscopic stenting of the bile duct will help decrease the amount of leakage. The more serious complications include bile duct injury and ligation. Bile duct injury or ligation may result from aberrant biliary anatomy such as a left-sided entry of the cystic duct into the common bile duct, or indeed mistaking the common bile duct for the cystic duct.

The key points in the management of these patients include delineation of the anatomy, defining the site and nature of the bile duct injury, and diverting bile away from

Box 20-8 Laparoscopic Cholecystectomy and Bile Duct Injury

Delineate anatomy by PTC
Define site and nature of bile duct injury – PTC/ERCP
Divert bile from site of biliary leakage – external biliary drainage and/or endoscopic stent placement
Drain intraabdominal collections – percutaneous abscess drainage

the site of biliary leakage. If the bile duct is intact, and there is leakage only from the cystic duct stump, then retrograde stenting by ERCP is appropriate. However, if the bile duct has been injured with associated leakage, then drainage and stenting is best performed percutaneously. With ligation, the intrahepatic bile ducts can be drained percutaneously by leaving an external biliary drainage catheter above the level of the ligation. Any associated bile leakage can be drained percutaneously. After a number of weeks of drainage the patient returns to theater for a definitive reconstructive procedure. By allowing time for the inflammation and effects of the first surgery to settle down, the reconstructive surgery is made easier (Box 20-8).

Reintervention for Metal Stent Occlusion

The average patency rate for metallic stents in the biliary tree is approximately 6 months. Metallic stents do occlude and may require further reintervention. Occlusion is usually manifested by recurrent jaundice or cholangitis. These patients can be managed by percutaneous reintervention or endoscopic intervention. The causes of occlusion are either tumor overgrowth at the upper or lower end of the stent, tumor ingrowth through the wire mesh of the stent, or occlusive debris clogging the stent. Tumor overgrowth can be prevented by overstenting of the stricture. Tumor ingrowth cannot be prevented but occurs less commonly. For patients with tumor overgrowth above the stent, a percutaneous biliary drainage can be performed and a guidewire manipulated down through the stent into the duodenum. The tumor above the stent can then be dilated and a second Wallstent inserted in a sleeved fashion through the first Wallstent (Fig. 20-23). Similarly, patients with tumor ingrowth can be managed by balloon dilatation of the first stent in the region of the tumor ingrowth and by the placement of a second stent. Lastly, patients with stent occlusion by inspissated debris or sludge can be managed by manipulating a guidewire down through the lumen of the occluded stent and using a balloon catheter to sweep the occluded metal stent clear of debris. As with patients

for primary biliary drainage, these patients all need intravenous antibiotic coverage and also need to be placed on intravenous fluids.

Another approach to metal stent occlusion is the endoscopic or retrograde approach. Depending on the level of expertise at your institution, the referral pattern, and the clinical state of the patient, it may be appropriate to place a plastic stent through the existing metal stent to reinstate drainage.

PERCUTANEOUS MANAGEMENT OF BENIGN BILIARY STRICTURE

Percutaneous balloon dilatation of benign biliary stricture has been in use since early reports first described the technique in the 1970s. It is a procedure associated with low morbidity and may avoid the necessity of complex hepatobiliary operations.

Indications

Percutaneous balloon dilatation of biliary strictures is most often performed in patients with anastamotic strictures such as choledochojejunal or hepaticojejunal anastamoses. Patients with iatrogenic strictures of the bile duct are also suitable for percutaneous biliary dilatation. Patients with sclerosing cholangitis may benefit from balloon dilatation provided there is a dominant stricture. Biliary strictures due to pancreatitis or biliary calculi can be balloon dilated, but these are usually dilated at ERCP rather than by the percutaneous route.

Preprocedure Evaluation

In patients with anastamotic strictures, imaging findings may be misleading. CT and ultrasound may show no dilated intrahepatic bile ducts. However, patients with anastamotic strictures often have episodes of cholangitis with rigors requiring oral and/or intravenous antibiotics. The patient is usually asymptomatic between attacks, and often may not present for evaluation until a number of attacks have occurred. The most sensitive indicator of anastamotic stricture formation is the serum alkaline phosphatase level, which is almost invariably elevated. The role of magnetic resonance cholangiography in imaging these patients is unclear. It is, however, an attractive noninvasive method of obtaining cholangiogram-like images to look at the hepatico-jejunal anastamosis and intrahepatic biliary tree.

Patients with iatrogenic strictures usually present either immediately or soon after the initial surgical procedure. Usually, ERCP will first be performed in these patients and MRCP or PTC may be necessary to give full anatomic delineation of the abnormality.

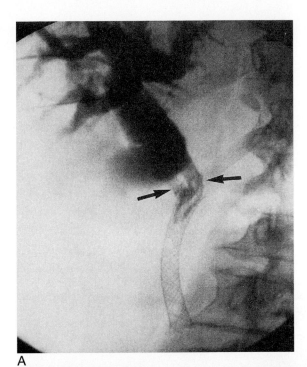

A

Figure 20-23   Reintervention for metal stent occlusion. A patient with pancreatic cancer who had a metal stent placed 5 months earlier returned to the hospital with recurrent jaundice and cholangitis. **A,** A PTC performed showed tumor overgrowth above the stent (arrows). **B,** A guidewire was manipulated down through the stent and a Ring catheter (arrows) placed into the duodenum. **C,** A second metal stent was placed through the first with an appropriate overlap above the tumor (arrows).

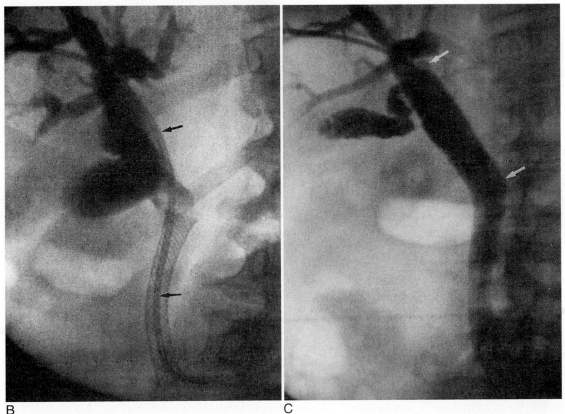

B   C

Technique

Patient Preparation

As with other biliary procedures, broad-spectrum antibiotic coverage is mandatory for biliary dilatation.

Sedoanalgesia is even more important as many patients experience considerable pain during the balloon inflation process. Indeed, in the author's unit we performed this procedure under general anesthesia in earlier years, but now with appropriate use of sedoanalgesia this is not

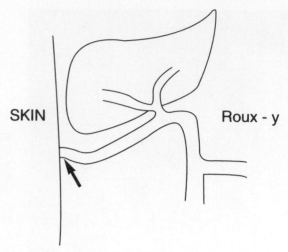

SKIN   Roux - y

Figure 20-24   Schematic showing a long Roux loop brought out to the skin after creation of a biliary enteric anastomosis. A long limb on the Roux loop (arrow) can be brought out to the skin and sutured underneath the skin. The position of the loop can be marked with metal clips or a metal ring. This provides access for any future percutaneous biliary intervention.

necessary. The combination of midazolam and fentanyl works extremely well to control patient pain. A loading dose followed by regular aliquots of both drugs should be administered throughout the procedure. If we are planning a retrograde access through a jejunal Roux loop, then a CT of the abdomen is useful before embarking upon the procedure to confirm the location of the Roux loop and also to ascertain the position of the colon *vis-à-vis* the loop (Box 20-9).

Biliary Access

The traditional method of access is transhepatic with dilatation of a track through the liver parenchyma and placement of a balloon catheter across the stricture site. A less traumatic access is the use of a retrograde access through the Roux loop. Some surgeons when fashioning the Roux loop for the hepaticojejunostomy or choledo-chojejunostomy will fix a portion of the Roux loop anteriorly underneath the abdominal wall (Fig. 20-24). The loop is then marked with either a metallic suture or a circular metallic ring. By marking the Roux loop and fixing the loop underneath the anterior abdominal wall, the loop can be accessed under fluoroscopic guidance and guidewires and catheters placed retrogradely through the loop up into the intrahepatic biliary tree. This avoids the necessity for transhepatic access. Even if the surgeon has not fixed the Roux loop underneath the anterior abdominal wall, the loop can still be used for retrograde access (Fig. 20-25). A transhepatic cholangiogram is first performed and contrast is injected into the intrahepatic biliary tree. When contrast enters the Roux loop, the loop can be punctured under fluoroscopic guidance and used for biliary access. When performing this procedure it is important to first perform a CT to ascertain where the colon is in relation to the Roux loop. Lateral screening also helps to identify the most anterior portion of the Roux loop for puncture.

Performing the Dilatation

It can occasionally be difficult to determine whether there is some evidence of narrowing at the anastamotic site. Some operators have used biliary manometry to help decide whether there is a real obstruction present or not. However, in the author's unit we have found this cumbersome and difficult to interpret. Instead, we place a 10-mm balloon across the anastamosis and inflate the balloon. Presence of a stricture is determined by the presence of a waist in the balloon. The balloon is inflated until the waist disappears (see Fig. 20-25). The number of balloon dilatations per session, the length of time the balloon remains inflated, and the number of sessions vary widely between different operators. Some authors inflate the balloon for variable periods from 30 seconds to 15–20 minutes and repeat until the waist on the balloon disappears. Others leave the balloon inflated for up to 2 hours. We inflate the balloon for 2–3 minutes and repeat the procedure until the waist disappears. In many instances the waist on the 10-mm balloon is minimal, so a 12-mm balloon is used.

The role of long-term stenting of the stricture which has been dilated is also controversial. Some authors advocate leaving a long-term stent across the anastamosis for 6–12 months. We have not tended to do this and prefer to leave the catheter across the stricture for 3–4 weeks. Normally a 10- to 12-French soft catheter (Cope Loop, Cook, Bloomington, IN) is left across the anastamosis. The catheter can be clamped and the patient discharged with the catheter *in situ*. The patient is brought back as an outpatient for a cholangiogram after 3–4 weeks. If the anastamosis looks widely patent then the catheter is removed. If the anastamosis is not patent the balloon dilatation is repeated and the catheter left for a further 3–4 weeks (Box 20-10).

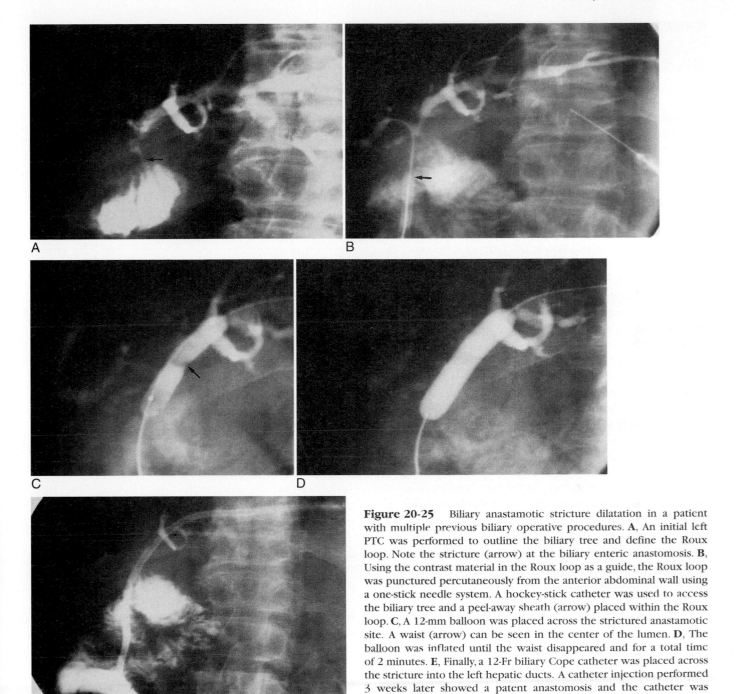

Figure 20-25   Biliary anastamotic stricture dilatation in a patient with multiple previous biliary operative procedures. **A,** An initial left PTC was performed to outline the biliary tree and define the Roux loop. Note the stricture (arrow) at the biliary enteric anastomosis. **B,** Using the contrast material in the Roux loop as a guide, the Roux loop was punctured percutaneously from the anterior abdominal wall using a one-stick needle system. A hockey-stick catheter was used to access the biliary tree and a peel-away sheath (arrow) placed within the Roux loop. **C,** A 12-mm balloon was placed across the strictured anastomotic site. A waist (arrow) can be seen in the center of the lumen. **D,** The balloon was inflated until the waist disappeared and for a total time of 2 minutes. **E,** Finally, a 12-Fr biliary Cope catheter was placed across the stricture into the left hepatic ducts. A catheter injection performed 3 weeks later showed a patent anastomosis and the catheter was removed.

Metallic Stents for Benign Biliary Stricture

The use of metallic stents for benign biliary strictures has been reported in the literature. In general, it is used as a last resort when benign biliary strictures fail to respond to balloon dilatation. In the author's unit our practice is to perform at least three separate balloon dilatations before resorting to metallic stenting. Additionally, the age and condition of the patient is important. If the patient is young, surgical revision may be the best option if balloon dilatation fails. If the patient is older, then perhaps metallic stenting is appropriate. The procedure should first be discussed with the referring surgeon or clinician. If it is decided to place the metallic stent, then a Gianturco–Rosch stent should be placed rather than a Wallstent. The Gianturco–Rosch stent exerts a stronger radial force and presents a lesser surface area for the development of intimal hyperplasia. It is therefore the preferred stent for dealing with recalcitrant biliary strictures.

Box 20-10 Biliary Stricture Dilatation: Key Points

PTC to delineate anatomy and identify Roux loop
Puncture Roux loop and negotiate anastomosis
10-mm balloon followed by 12-mm balloon
14-Fr biliary catheter inserted through Roux loop
Catheter removed after 3 weeks if open anastomosis

Results

The success rate of balloon dilatation for benign biliary strictures is shown in Table 20-2. In earlier reports the success rate varied from 50 to 90%. One of the criticisms of earlier reports was the fact that follow-up tended to be short, with a maximum follow-up of approximately 3 years. Two newer studies report longer-term follow-up with patency rates of 80–90% over 9 years. This compares very favorably with reports from surgical series.

Surgical repair of benign biliary strictures has a long-term (5-year follow-up) success rate which varies between 70 and 80% at the first attempt, but decreases exponentially after each unsuccessful attempt at surgical repair. The success rate of a third operation is approximately 60%. It would seem that surgery is the best initial option for patients with iatrogenic strictures, but percutaneous balloon dilatation should be used for the management of patients who present with anastamotic strictures. Approximately 15–25% of patients who undergo surgical repair of iatrogenic strictures will develop anastamotic strictures. A surgical policy of fixing the Roux loop underneath the anterior abdominal wall would facilitate the further management of patients who develop anastamotic strictures.

Balloon dilatation of strictures in patients with sclerosing cholangitis has a lower success rate varying between 42 and 59%. However, for patients with sclerosing cholangitis, balloon dilatation may represent the only form of treatment available, particularly for intrahepatic ductal strictures. It is always worthwhile dilating dominant strictures in patients with sclerosing cholangitis as significant improvement of patient wellbeing may occur. Indeed, the last resort for these patients is liver transplantation if multiple complex strictures are present.

Complications associated with this procedure are those associated with biliary drainage (discussed previously).

PERCUTANEOUS MANAGEMENT OF COMMON BILE DUCT STONES

Most common bile duct stones are removed endoscopically – which is the best option for most patients. In some situations, endoscopic removal is not possible. ERCP may be unsuccessful because of previous gastric surgery, because of a large diverticulum at the Ampulla of Vater, or because of other technical problems.

If ERCP is unsuccessful, a number of methods can be used to remove or manage common bile duct stones. The preferred method in the author's unit is the rendezvous procedure (Fig. 20-26). Standard biliary drainage is performed and an internal/external biliary drainage catheter left in the duodenum. After 1–2 days an ERCP is performed. An exchange length guidewire is passed through the internal/external biliary drainage catheter and used by the endoscopist to facilitate bile duct cannulation. In this way the stones can be removed endoscopically.

If the rendezvous procedure is not possible because of altered upper GI anatomy, alternatives include open surgical removal of the common bile duct stones, or transhepatic stone removal. Depending on the size of the stone(s) present, the transhepatic approach can be used to perform a sphincteroplasty by inflating a 10-mm balloon across the sphincter oddi and pushing any small stones into the duodenum with a semi-inflated balloon. Transhepatic stone removal is rarely performed, but if it is to be performed, a mature tract through the liver is required. This involves initial percutaneous biliary drainage and sequential tract dilatation up to 14- to 16-French size, followed by basket extraction of the stone(s). If the stones are larger, mechanical lithotripsy can be performed to crush the stones before removal.

Table 20-2 Benign Biliary Strictures

Author	Patients	Success (%)	Follow-up (mths)
Mueller	73	67	24
Williams	74	78	30
Russell	23	100	?
Citron	17	70.5	32
Gallacher	13	77	8-30
Lee	14	93	38
Pitt[a]	25	88	60
Davids[a]	35	83	50
Bezzi	180	82	68

[a]Surgical series.

PERCUTANEOUS EXTRACTION OF CBD STONES THROUGH T-TUBE TRACT

If the patient has a post-operative T-tube in place, then ERCP is inappropriate as any retained stones can be removed easily through the percutaneous tract (Fig. 20-27).

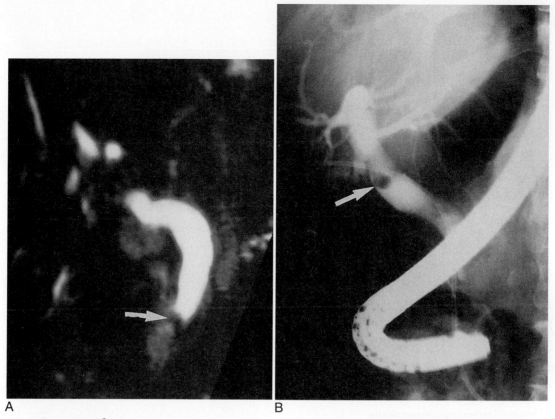

A   B

Figure 20-26   Rendezvous procedure in a patient with failed ERCP. **A**, Coronal image from an MRCP examination shows a stone (arrow) at the lower end of the bile duct in this patient who failed ERCP. **B**, A transhepatic biliary drainage was performed and a Ring catheter manipulated across the bile duct into the duodenum. Note the stone (arrow) in the common bile duct. At ERCP the next day, a guidewire passed through the percutaneous catheter was snared by the endoscopist and pulled out through the mouth. Access to the bile duct was then assured for further biliary manipulation. In this case a sphincterotomy was performed and the stone removed.

If stone removal through the T-tube tract is planned, the T-tube is left *in situ* for 4–6 weeks until a mature tract develops. Patients are brought back to the hospital for stone removal and given standard antibiotic prophylaxis. A T-tube cholangiogram is performed to confirm that the stones are still present. In many instances the stone(s) may have passed in the interval. If a stone is not present the T-tube can be removed.

If a stone is still present, extraction will be required. The T-tube is removed over a guidewire and access to the duodenum is achieved using a combination of a hydrophilic wire and Kumpe catheter. A superstiff wire is placed in the duodenum and left as a safety wire. A steerable catheter (Burhenne) is placed in the bile duct through the percutaneous T-tube tract. The handle of the Burhenne is used to deflect the tip of the catheter so that the catheter can be manipulated either up or down the bile duct, depending upon where the stone is located.

The Burhenne catheter is placed a little distal to the stone and a basket placed through the Burhenne catheter. The basket is opened distal to the stone and the Burhenne catheter and basket are slowly withdrawn until the stone is reached. The Burhenne catheter and basket are then jiggled so that the stone falls within the basket. The basket is then pulled back against the end of the Burhenne catheter to grip the stone, and the Burhenne catheter and basket are removed as a unit from the bile duct through the percutaneous tract. If the stone is too large to be removed through the percutaneous tract, the stone can be fragmented by electrohydraulic, laser, or mechanical lithotripsy. (See the section on percutaneous cholecystolithotomy in Chapter 21.) After the procedure, a 12-French catheter is left in the duodenum for 2–3 days if significant edema is present at the ampulla. If the procedure has been atraumatic then no catheter need be left.

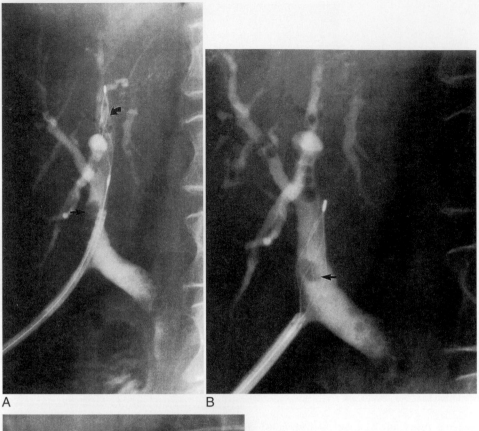

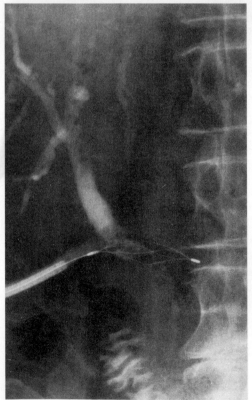

Figure 20-27   Percutaneous extraction of a retained common bile duct stone through a T-tube track. **A**, The T-tube has been removed and a steerable Burhenne catheter placed through the percutaneous track into the bile duct to the level of the stone (small arrow). A basket (curved arrow) has been placed distal to the stone. **B**, The basket is pulled back and manipulated so that the stone (small arrow) is engaged within the basket and the basket is then pulled back against the end of the Burhenne catheter. Basket, stone, and Burhenne catheter are then removed through the percutaneous track. **C**, There is some air present in the lower bile duct. The basket was traversed through the lower bile duct but no further stones were present. Contrast injection at the end of the procedure showed a clear bile duct.

SUGGESTED READING

Bezzi M, Bonomo G, Salvatori FM et al: Ten years follow-up percutaneous management if benign biliary strictures: how successful are we? RSNA 1995. *Radiol Suppl* 197:241, 1995.

Diamond T, Parks RW: Perioperative management of obstructive jaundice. *Br J Surg* 84:147–149, 1997.

Gazelle GS, Lee MJ, Mueller PR: Cholangiographic segmental anatomy of the liver: implications for interventional radiology. *Semin Interv Radiol* 12(2):119–125, 1995.

Hausegger KA, Kugler C, Uggowitzer M et al: Benign biliary obstruction: is treatment with the Wallstent advisable? *Radiology* 200:437–441, 1996.

Lammer J, Hausegger KA, Fluckiger F et al: Common bile duct obstruction due to malignancy: treatment with plastic versus metal stents. *Radiology* 201:167–172, 1996.

Lee MJ, Mueller PR, Saini S, Hahn PF, Dawson SL: Percutaneous dilatation of benign biliary strictures: single-session therapy with general anesthesia. *Am J Roentgenol* 157:1263–1266, 1991.

Lee MJ, Dawson SL, Mueller PR et al: Palliation of malignant bile duct obstruction with metallic biliary endoprostheses: technique, results, and complications. *J Vasc Interv Radiol* 3:665–671, 1992.

Lee MJ, Dawson SL, Mueller PR et al: Percutaneous management of hilar biliary malignancies with metallic endoprostheses: results, technical problems, and causes of failure. *Radiographics* 13: 1249–1263, 1993.

Lee MJ, Dawson SL, Mueller PR et al: Failed metallic biliary stents: causes and management of delayed complications. *Clin Radiol* 49:857–862, 1994.

Mathisen O, Bergan A, Flatmark A: Iatrogenic bile duct injuries. *World J Surg* 11:392–397, 1987.

McNicholas MMJ, Lee MJ, Dawson SL, Mueller PR: Complications of percutaneous biliary drainage and stricture dilatation. *Semin Interv Radiol* 11(3):242–253, 1994.

Morrison MC, Lee MJ, Saini A, Brink JA, Meuller PR: Percutaneous balloon dilatation of benign biliary strictures. *Radiol Clin N Am* 28:1191–1201, 1990.

Mueller PR, vanSonnenberg E, Ferrucci JT et al: Biliary stricture dilatation: multicenter review of clinical management in 73 patients. *Radiology* 160:17–22, 1986.

Rossi P, Bezzi M, Salvatori FM, Maccioni F, Porcaro M: Recurrent benign biliary strictures: management with self-expanding metallic stents. *Radiology* 175:661–665, 1990.

Russell E, Yrizarry JM, Huber JS et al: Percutaneous transjejunal biliary dilatation: alternate management for benign strictures. *Radiology* 159:209–214, 1986.

Schima W, Prokesch R, Österreicher C et al: Biliary Wallstent endoprosthesis in malignant hilar obstruction: long-term results with regard to the type of obstruction. *Clin Radiol* 52:213–219, 1997.

Warren KW, Jefferson MF: Prevention of repair of strictures of the extrahepatic bile ducts. *Surg Clin N Am* 53:1169–1190, 1973.

Yee ACN, Ho C-S: Complications of percutaneous biliary drainage: benign vs malignant diseases. *Am J Roentgenol* 148:1207–1209, 1997.

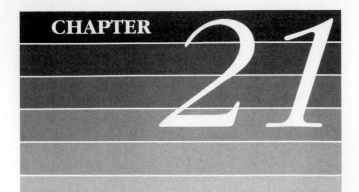

CHAPTER 21

Gallbladder Intervention

MICHAEL J. LEE, M.D.

Gallbladder intervention in the form of gallbladder decompression was first proposed as a definite technique in the second half of the last century. However, percutaneous gallbladder intervention did not gain widespread acceptance because of the fear of bile leakage and life-threatening vagal reactions. It was not until the 1980s that percutaneous drainage of the gallbladder and other percutaneous therapies for gallstones became popular.

Percutaneous gallbladder intervention can be divided into diagnostic and therapeutic techniques. Diagnostic techniques include gallbladder aspiration, biopsy, and diagnostic cholecystocholangiography. Therapeutic techniques include percutaneous cholecystostomy, biliary drainage and stent placement via the gallbladder, MTBE dissolution therapy, percutaneous cholecystolithotomy, and gallbladder ablation. Apart from percutaneous cholecystostomy, many of these techniques are infrequently performed. The advent of laparoscopic cholecystectomy, to a large extent, has meant the demise of percutaneous techniques to treat gallstones such as percutaneous cholecystolithotomy and MTBE dissolution therapy.

DIAGNOSTIC GALLBLADDER INTERVENTION

Gallbladder Aspiration

Aspiration of bile for Gram stain gained some popularity in the 1980s in intensive care units or in critically ill patients with suspected acute calculous or acalculous cholecystitis. The lack of an accurate noninvasive test to diagnose cholecystitis in this particular patient population led to the practice of gallbladder aspiration for Gram stain and culture of bile. Using ultrasound guidance, a 20- to 22-gauge needle was placed in the gallbladder and bile aspirated for microbiologic analysis. However, the accuracy of gallbladder aspiration in this clinical situation is approximately 50%, which is equivalent to tossing a coin. Additionally, one has to wait several days for culture results. One of the major reasons for the lack of sensitivity is the fact that patients are often on broad-spectrum antibiotics prior to gallbladder aspiration so that Gram stains may be negative despite the presence of acute cholecystitis. This procedure has largely been abandoned because of the low sensitivity.

Diagnostic Cholecystocholangiography

In limited clinical situations, diagnostic cholecysto-cholangiography may be performed instead of percutaneous transhepatic cholangiography. In patients with minimally sized intrahepatic bile ducts, who only require a diagnostic study, a gallbladder puncture can be used. In the author's unit we usually try to perform transhepatic cholangiography first, and only if this fails do we resort to a gallbladder puncture. A 22-gauge needle is placed in the gallbladder under ultrasound guidance and contrast material injected under fluoroscopy. Provided the cystic duct is open, contrast material will flow into the common bile duct and common hepatic duct. It may be necessary to place the patient in Trendelenburg for contrast medium to fill the intrahepatic ducts fully. If the patient requires therapeutic procedures with biliary drainage or stent placement, it is best to use a transhepatic route as it can be difficult to manipulate stents and catheters through the cystic duct into the common bile duct (Box 21-1).

Gallbladder Biopsy

The gallbladder wall can be biopsied successfully using small (20- or 22-gauge) needles, if there is a gallbladder mass (Fig. 21-1). Gallbladder masses are usually due to either primary gallbladder adenocarcinoma or metastatic disease. The procedure is usually performed under ultrasound guidance and has a success rate of over 90% in obtaining a diagnosis. It is best to use small needles to prevent bile leakage. However, if the mass is large and the gallbladder lumen is totally replaced, then cutting needles such as trucut needles can be used.

THERAPEUTIC GALLBLADDER INTERVENTION: PERCUTANEOUS CHOLECYSTOSTOMY

Percutaneous cholecystostomy is a valuable technique for the management of patients with either calculous or

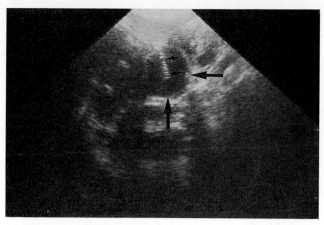

Figure 21-1   Gallbladder biopsy. Transverse image from an ultrasound of the right upper quadrant showing the gallbladder (large arrows) containing predominantly solid material. The patient was suspected to have a gallbladder cancer. A fine-needle biopsy was performed under ultrasound guidance and the needle (small arrows) can be seen within the mass. Pathology's examination of the biopsy specimen confirmed a gallbladder cancer.

acalculous cholecystitis who are critically ill and unfit for surgery. In these patients, percutaneous cholecystostomy is performed as a temporizing measure, with definitive surgery carried out at a later date when the patient has recovered from the acute illness. In acalculous cholecystitis, percutaneous cholecystostomy may be curative in that once the inflammation resolves the patient may not need a cholecystectomy. Percutaneous cholecystostomy is also useful in the management of empyema and hydrops of the gallbladder.

Percutaneous cholecystostomy has also been used for drainage of the biliary tree in patients whose cystic duct is patent and the biliary obstruction lies below the insertion of the cystic duct into the common bile duct. Transhepatic biliary drainage is usually a better alternative for long-term drainage of the biliary tree, but in selected cases percutaneous cholecystostomy may be of benefit. Selected clinical situations include patients with pancreatitis where short-term decompression of an obstructive biliary tree may be necessary, and patients with biliary cholangitis and distal obstruction of the common bile duct where ERCP has failed to provide drainage. For long-term palliation of patients with obstructive jaundice, the transhepatic route is preferred because stenting can be performed easily through the transhepatic tract. It can be difficult to manipulate a wire through the cystic duct and into the common bile duct using a gallbladder approach. Additionally, long-term catheter drainage of the biliary tree via the gallbladder in patients with distal malignant obstruction is not optimal because both pancreatic cancer and cholangiocarcinoma will eventually grow to obstruct the origin of the cystic duct. For these reasons, percutaneous cholecystostomy for decompression of the biliary

---

Box 21-1   Diagnostic Cholecystocholangiography

Use only if intrahepatic ducts minimally dilated and if transhepatic approach fails

Biliary obstruction must be at a level below junction of cystic duct and common hepatic duct

Ultrasound guidance and a 22-gauge needle are used

Trendelenburg positioning may be necessary to fill intrahepatic ducts

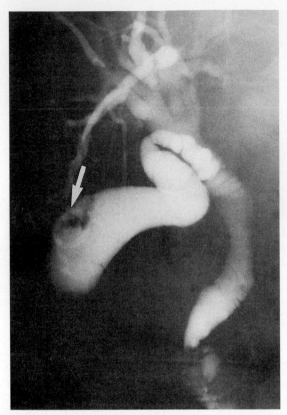

Figure 21-2   Percutaneous cholecystostomy for drainage of the biliary tree in a patient with severe cholangitis and hypotension. A percutaneous cholecystostomy catheter (arrow) was placed in the gallbladder using the Seldinger technique. A stricture can be seen in the lower bile duct, caused by a small pancreatic tumor. The catheter remained *in situ* until the patient went to surgery for a Whipple procedure.

tree is only performed for temporary decompression, and in selected patients (Fig. 21-2).

Technique

There are a number of technique variations to consider before performing a percutaneous cholecystostomy. The access route used can be either transhepatic or transperitoneal, while the catheter can be placed using either a Seldinger or trocar technique. The access route and method of catheter insertion chosen is a matter of personal preference. The author's unit has tended to place cholecystostomy catheters using ultrasound guidance and trocar technique in ICU patients, while patients who can travel to the department may have the procedure performed using a Seldinger or trocar technique.

Transperitoneal versus Transhepatic Access

Use of a transhepatic or transperitoneal approach is largely a matter of personal preference. Many authors prefer the transperitoneal approach because it is more direct and avoids the necessity of going through the liver.

Additionally, if percutaneous cholecystectolithotomy (PCCL) is being considered, a track can safely be dilated if a transperitoneal approach has been used. One of the main problems with the transperitoneal approach is that catheters and guidewires often buckle outside of the gallbladder, particularly, when using the Seldinger technique. This is due to gallbladder mobility. The closer the entry site to the fundus of the gallbladder, the more mobile the gallbladder is and the more likely this is to happen (Fig. 21-3). The Seldinger technique also increases the likelihood of this happening. Additionally, the transverse colon may occasionally overlie the fundus of the gallbladder and may result in perforation of the transverse colon if the transperitoneal approach is used (Fig. 21-4).

The author prefers the transhepatic approach because entry of the catheter into the gallbladder is closer to the attachment of the gallbladder to the liver (the bare area) where the gallbladder is relatively fixed in position compared to the fundus. The bare area represents the attachment of the gallbladder to the liver and also represents the extraperitoneal surface of the gallbladder. The bare area is situated superolaterally in the gallbladder fossa and, in an ideal world, it would be best to place catheters through the bare area into the gallbladder. Thus, any bile leakage would be extraperitoneal and tamponaded by the liver. However, in practice it is very difficult to traverse the bare area as its precise location cannot be determined by any imaging method. In the author's unit we therefore insert the catheter vertically into the gallbladder, making sure that the catheter passes through a portion of the liver en route to the gallbladder (Fig. 21-5). One of the potential disadvantages of using the transhepatic approach is that if a PCCL is required at a later stage, a large track through the liver will have to be created. Some operators are reluctant to dilate a 1-cm tract through the liver into the gallbladder. We have done this on a considerable number of patients without mishap (Boxes 21-2 and 21-3).

Trocar versus Seldinger Technique

The Seldinger technique requires fluoroscopic and sonographic guidance and is unsuitable for placement of

---

Box 21-2   Advantages and Disadvantages of the Transhepatic Approach for Percutaneous Cholecystostomy

Catheter entry site closer to the bare area of the gallbladder
Bile leaks potentially tamponaded by liver
Gallbladder less mobile closer to bare area
If large tracks required for PCCL, risk of hemorrhage increased

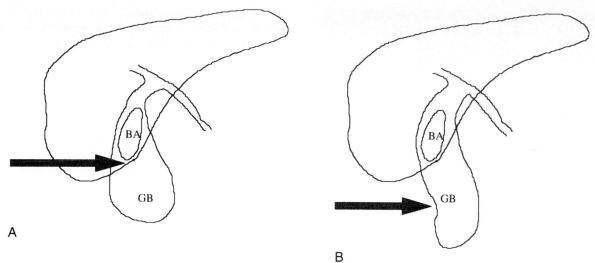

A

B

Figure 21-3   Transhepatic versus transperitoneal insertion of gallbladder catheters. **A,** Schematic diagram showing the gallbladder (GB) with bare area (BA) shown near the neck of the gallbladder. The bare area represents the extraperitoneal surface of the gallbladder or the attachment of the gallbladder to the liver. A transhepatic insertion (large arrow) will be nearer the bare area and thus the gallbladder will be less mobile in this location than if a transperitoneal access route is chosen. **B,** A transperitoneal insertion is nearer the fundus of the gallbladder, which is also the most mobile portion of the gallbladder. The gallbladder wall may indent and move away from the needle or catheter using a transperitoneal approach. In addition, dilators or even the catheter may catch in the wall of the gallbladder and cause the guidewire to buckle outside the lumen of the gallbladder. (Reproduced with permission from Stafford-Johnson D, Mueller PR, Varghese J, Lee MJ: Percutaneous cholecystostomy: a review. *J Interv Radiol* 11:1–8, 1996.)

cholecystestomy catheters in the intensive care unit or at the bedside. For the Seldinger technique the gallbladder is first located with ultrasound and a 22-gauge needle from a one-stick needle system (Cook, Bloomington, IN) is inserted into the gallbladder under ultrasound guidance.

The gallbladder is opacified with dilute contrast material and a 0.018-inch guidewire inserted through the 22-gauge needle into the gallbladder using fluoroscopic guidance. The 5-French sheath system is placed over the 0.018-inch guidewire into the gallbladder. A 0.035-inch

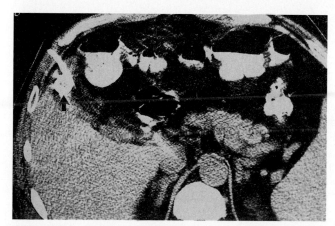

Figure 21-4   Clinical example showing a transperitoneal insertion of a percutaneous cholecystostomy catheter. The catheter can be seen (arrow) entering the gallbladder through the peritoneum. Note the position of the colon more anterior, indicating that an anterior approach was not possible in this patient.

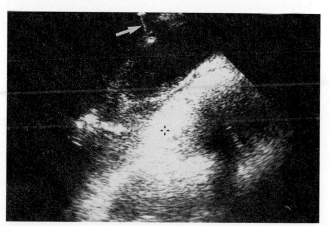

Figure 21-5   Example of a transhepatic catheter insertion into the gallbladder in a patient with acalculous cholecystitis. The catheter (arrow) is inserted through the liver into the gallbladder. Although the catheter almost certainly does not traverse the bare area, the gallbladder is less mobile with a transhepatic route.

J-shaped guidewire is then placed through the 5-French sheath into the gallbladder. As much as possible of the 0.035-inch "J" guidewire should be coiled into the gallbladder to achieve adequate purchase. Once this is done the percutaneous track is ready for dilatation.

The track is dilated using 7- and 9-French dilators and finally an 8-French pigtail with a small pigtail is placed (Cook, Bloomington, IN). Care must be taken during track dilatation that the guidewire does not kink at the gallbladder entry site. If this happens and is not recognized, further dilatation or catheter placement may cause the guidewire to buckle at this site resulting in the guidewire flipping into the peritoneal cavity. This is more likely to happen with a transperitoneal approach (Fig. 21-6). If the guidewire kinks during track dilatation the guidewire should be replaced by removing the kinked wire using the 5-French sheath and inserting a new 0.038-inch "J" guidewire or indeed a stiffer guidewire such as a 0.038-inch Ring guidewire (Cook, Bloomington, IN).

The trocar technique is the author's preferred method of accessing the gallbladder (Table 21-1). The trocar technique is particularly suited to those patients who cannot travel to the radiology department. Ultrasound is used to

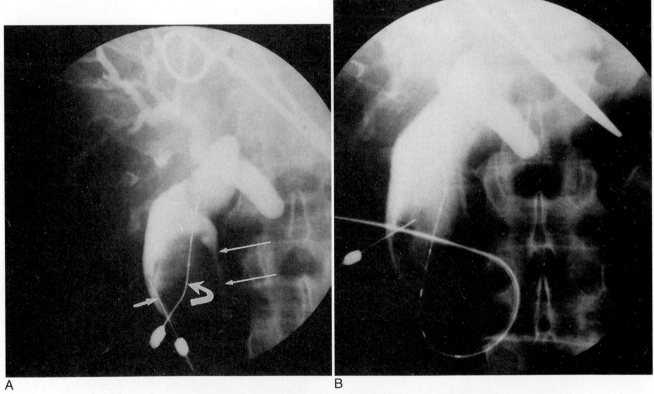

A   B

Figure 21-6   Example of the Seldinger technique and the transperitoneal approach causing buckling of the guidewire and catheter out of the gallbladder. **A,** Patient with a pancreatic carcinoma who was scheduled for a Whipple procedure had markedly elevated liver function tests. The surgeon requested a biliary decompression prior to surgery. Attempts at percutaneous biliary drainage were unsuccessful and the gallbladder was accessed with a 22-gauge spinal needle with a view to doing a cholangiogram. Note the spinal needle (small arrow) for injecting contrast material into the gallbladder. A second 18-gauge needle (curved arrow) was used to place a 0.038-inch Ring guidewire into the gallbladder. Contrast material can be seen in the pelviocalyceal system (long arrows) from the repeated attempts at percutaneous transhepatic cholangiography. **B,** During dilatation of the percutaneous track a large guidewire loop formed outside the gallbladder because of buckling of the guidewire.   *(Continued)*

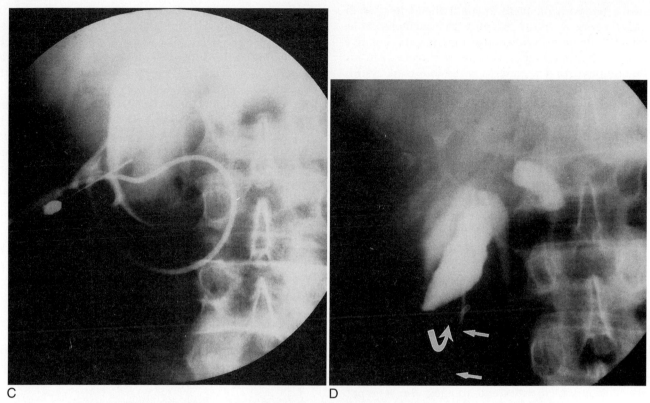

C   D

Figure 21-6   cont'd C, The catheter was placed but proved to be outside the gallbladder. **D**, Using ultrasound guidance, a second 8-Fr catheter (straight arrows) was trocarred into the gallbladder to provide decompression. The first catheter (curved arrow) was left *in situ* to drain the contrast and bile from around the gallbladder. The patient did not experience any pain or evidence of biliary peritonitis and proceeded to surgery for a Whipple resection one week later. (Reproduced with permission from Stafford-Johnson D, Mueller PR, Varghese J, Lee MJ: Percutaneous cholecystostomy: a review. *J Interv Radiol* 11:1–8, 1996.)

locate the gallbladder and an access route is chosen that passes through the liver. Local anesthetic is administered to the skin at the puncture site and an incision made with a #11 scalpel and the superficial tissues dissected with a surgical forceps. Under US guidance, insert a 22-gauge spinal needle into the gallbladder as a reference needle. Bile aspiration confirms the needle to lie within the gallbladder cavity. An 8-French pigtail catheter

(Cook, Bloomington, IN) is inserted into the gallbladder in tandem to the reference needle. Importantly, a quick thrust is required when inserting the catheter into the gallbladder rather than a gradual approach. With a gradual or incremental advance the gallbladder may move ahead of the catheter and make entry of the catheter into the gallbladder difficult or impossible. With a quick thrust, the catheter usually pierces the anterior wall of the gallbladder. This can be confirmed with ultrasound and/or by aspirating bile from the catheter. When the catheter is in the gallbladder the catheter is advanced off the cannula which is withdrawn and the catheter tip is coiled in the gallbladder. A locking pigtail catheter is necessary to prevent dislodgement.

Results

Technically, the success rate for percutaneous cholecystectomy should be 100% in experienced hands. In patients with calculous cholecystitis who are too ill to undergo formal surgery, percutaneous cholecystostomy

Table 21-1   Trocar versus Seldinger Technique

	Trocar	Seldinger
Ultrasound guidance	Yes	No
Portable	Yes	No
Fluoroscopic guidance	No	Yes
Speed of performance	Fast	Slower
Guidewire and catheter buckling into peritoneal cavity	No	Yes

acts as a temporizing measure until the patient is fit enough for surgery. In the patient with acalculous cholecystitis, percutaneous cholecystostomy may be curative and no further intervention such as cholecystectomy may be required. In ICU patients, acalculous cholecystitis is a frequent and often underdiagnosed cause of sepsis. The author's unit has used percutaneous cholecystostomy as a therapeutic trial in ICU patients with persisting sepsis of unknown origin. A percutaneous cholecystostomy is performed only if other causes of sepsis have been excluded. In a series of 82 such patients, Boland and associates showed a dramatic response in 48 patients (59%). The response usually occurs within 24–48 hours and is evidenced by a decrease in white cell count, normalization of body temperature, and reduced dependence on vasopressor support (Box 21-4).

Catheter Care

When a percutaneous cholecystectomy catheter is inserted, daily rounds by the interventional team are important to ensure that catheter kinking or dislodgement does not occur. Catheters also need to be irrigated 2–3 times per day as many of these patients will have biliary sludge which will tend to clog the 8-French catheters that are placed.

Percutaneous cholecystostomy catheters must be left in place for a minimum of 2 weeks before removal. This is to ensure that a mature track develops between the gallbladder and skin surface. If the catheter is removed before a mature tract develops, bile contamination of the peritoneal cavity may result. Before removing the cholecystostomy catheter, the author's unit performs a cholecystocholangiogram to ensure patency of the cystic duct and to exclude the presence of gallstones in the cystic duct, gallbladder, or bile duct. Obviously, if stones are present in the gallbladder the patient may require cholecystectomy, or percutaneous cholecystolithotomy if the patient is unfit for surgery. If an occluding gallstone is present in the cystic duct, the catheter should not be removed until the stone is dealt with either surgically or percutaneously. Lastly, if there is a stone in the common bile duct the patient will require ERCP and stone removal, or the stone can be removed percutaneously.

If the catheter is to be removed it is withdrawn over a guidewire and a Kumpe catheter or a 5-French dilator placed over the guidewire into the opening of the percutaneous track. Using a Tuohy–Borst adapter, contrast material is injected into the percutaneous track. If the track is mature, contrast material will outline the track all the way to the gallbladder (Fig. 21-7). If the track is immature, contrast material will spill into the peritoneal cavity (Fig. 21-8). If this happens, the catheter is reinserted over the guidewire into the gallbladder. The procedure is repeated at weekly intervals until the track is mature (Box 21-5).

Complications

The complication rate for percutaneous cholecystostomy is low compared to surgical cholecystostomy. The rate of complications for surgical cholecystostomy is approximately 24% compared to rates of 0–8% reported

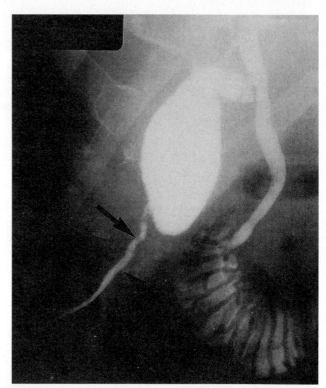

Figure 21-7 Mature track in a patient who completed MTBE dissolution therapy for gallstones. Contrast injected while the catheter was in the gallbladder shows a patent cystic duct and clear common bile duct. The catheter was then removed and a small dilator placed in the percutaneous track. Contrast injected in the track shows a mature track (arrows) with no evidence of any peritoneal extravasation of contrast material. The gallbladder catheter is safe to take out at this stage. It usually takes a track 2–3 weeks to develop around the catheter. (Reproduced with permission from Mueller PR, Lee MJ, Saini S et al: Percutaneous contrast dissolution of gallstones; complexity of radiological care. *Radiographics* 11: 759–764, 1991.)

Box 21-4   Acalculous Cholecystitis

Frequently occurs in ICU patients
No accurate noninvasive diagnostic test
Gallbladder aspiration has a 50% accuracy
Percutaneous cholecystostomy can be used as a
    therapeutic trial if other causes of sepsis excluded

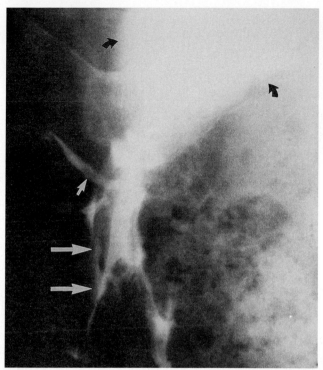

Figure 21-8   Patient with an immature track after percutaneous cholecystostomy catheter removal. The patient developed pain after removal of the gallbladder catheter. The percutaneous track was not documented to be mature before catheter removal. An injection of contrast material through the track (small arrow) after percutaneous cholecystostomy catheter removal shows wide extravasation of contrast material (large arrows) into the peritoneal cavity because of an immature track. The gallbladder itself (curved arrows) can be seen at the top of the image (Reproduced with permission from Stafford-Johnson D, Mueller PR, Varghese J, Lee MJ: Percutaneous cholecystostomy: a review. *J Interv Radiol* 11:1–8, 1996.)

for percutaneous cholecystostomy. The major complications reported include bleeding, bradycardia and hypotension which is vagally mediated, and biliary peritonitis. Locking catheters reduce the risk of catheter dislodgement and subsequent biliary peritonitis. If bile leakage is suspected, antibiotic administration is started

Box 21-5   Catheter Care
PC catheters should be left in place for 2–3 weeks before removal A catheter cholecystogram is performed to ensure no stones in the CBD A mature track must be demonstrated before catheter removal If acalculous cholecystitis, the catheter can be removed and cholecystectomy is not required

and close supervision of the patient is mandatory. Laparoscopy or laparotomy may be required if the patient does not settle. Some authors advocate the use of atropine prior to percutaneous cholecystostomy because of the risk of vagally mediated bradycardia and hypotension. However, the author's unit has not encountered a single episode of hypotension or bradycardia in over 150 percutaneous cholecystostomies. Therefore, we do not give prophylactic atropine but we do make sure that it is at hand, if required.

Patient Outcomes

In patients who recover from a bout of acute acalculous cholecystitis, percutaneous cholecystostomy usually allows the cystic duct obstruction to resolve so that the likelihood of a repeat attack occurring is low and the catheter can be removed at the appropriate time. There is usually no need for surgical cholecystectomy in these patients. In patients with calculous cholecystitis the situation is different as the gallstones remain in the gallbladder and future bouts of acute cholecystitis are probable. In elderly patients with severe intercurrent illnesses, the situation is compounded in that further bouts of acute cholecystitis may be the terminal event for some of these patients. Nonsurgical gallstone therapy has a role in treating gallstones in this subgroup of patients. In a recent study, Boland and associates reported the clinical outcome in 26 elderly patients with severe intercurrent illness who underwent percutaneous cholecystostomy for acute calculous cholecystitis. Of the 26 patients, 7 died, 7 recovered from the acute illness and underwent surgical cholecystectomy at a later date, and 12 underwent nonsurgical gallstone therapies. Nonsurgical therapies included MTBE (methyl-tert-butyl ether) dissolution therapy in 3 patients, percutaneous cholecystolithotomy in 2 patients, ERCP removal of a stone which passed from the gallbladder into the CBD in 1 patient, and long-term catheter drainage of the gallbladder in 6 patients who were terminally ill. These results emphasize the need for nonsurgical gallstone therapy options as many of these patients with severe medical illnesses are unfit for surgery.

Treatment of Gallbladder Perforation and Bile Leakage

In older patients with complicated medical illnesses, acute cholecystitis, when it occurs, can result in perforation which occasionally can be life-threatening. The author's unit has treated a number of patients with gallbladder perforation by performing percutaneous cholecystostomy and draining any localized abscesses in the abdominal cavity using percutaneous abscess drainage (Fig. 21-9). In this high-risk patient group the patient

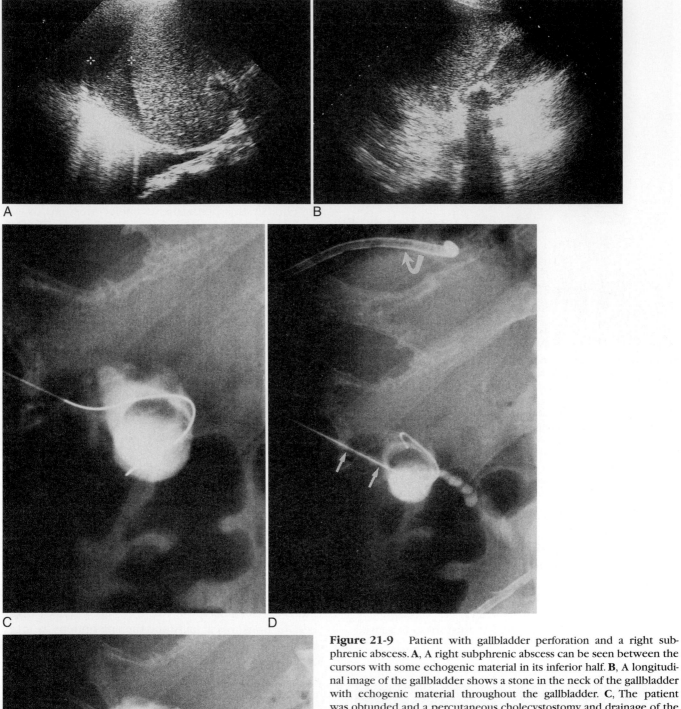

Figure 21-9   Patient with gallbladder perforation and a right sub-phrenic abscess. **A**, A right subphrenic abscess can be seen between the cursors with some echogenic material in its inferior half. **B**, A longitudinal image of the gallbladder shows a stone in the neck of the gallbladder with echogenic material throughout the gallbladder. **C**, The patient was obtunded and a percutaneous cholecystostomy and drainage of the subphrenic abscess was performed. A one-stick needle system (Cook, Bloomington, IN) was used to access the gallbladder, and the platinum tipped 0.018-inch guidewire can be seen coiled in the gallbladder. **D**, A larger 0.035-inch "J" guidewire was coiled in the gallbladder and track dilatation was performed. A dilator can be seen (straight arrows) over the guidewire dilating the track. Note the sump catheter in the right subphrenic abscess (curved arrows). **E**, An 8-Fr catheter was placed in the gallbladder for decompression. The patient recovered sufficiently in 10–14 days to have a cholecystectomy. At cholecystectomy the gallbladder was gangrenous with a perforation which had been spontaneously sealed by some omentum.

can be temporized for future surgery. Perforation of the gallbladder usually implies gangrenous change with necrosis, and surgical principles suggest that emergent removal of the gallbladder should be performed. However, this is not always possible in elderly patients with severe intercurrent illnesses. In this situation, percutaneous cholecystostomy can decompress a gallbladder and prevent the escape of more infected bile and also allow the gallbladder perforation to seal over. Imaging of the peritoneal cavity by CT or ultrasound can then help to identify any loculated pockets of puss which can be drained separately. This combination of percutaneous cholecystostomy and percutaneous drainage is potentially life-saving in these special circumstances.

NON-SURGICAL GALLSTONE THERAPIES

MTBE Dissolution Therapy

Cholesterol gallstones are the most suitable stones for MTBE dissolution therapy. MTBE (methyl tert-butyl ether) is an alcohol ether which dissolves cholesterol. Calcium bilirubinate stones or stones with a thick calcium rim on CT are usually not suitable for MTBE dissolution therapy. Additionally, gallstones with a central midus of calcium on CT are also usually not suitable for MTBE dissolution therapy.

Technique

A percutaneous cholecystostomy is performed as described previously. A 7- or 8-French pigtail catheter is coiled in the gallbladder and MTBE infused either by means of repeated hand injection or by using a computer-based pump. In the author's unit we have tended to use repeated hand injection. The procedure can be very time-consuming and can take an average of between 2 and 14–15 hours (Fig. 21-10). Frequent cholecystograms and sonograms are performed throughout the procedure to monitor the progress of the stone treatment. The MTBE therapy is stopped when cholecystograms and sonograms reveal that the stones have been dissolved. As you can see from the lengthy procedural times, MTBE dissolution therapy has fallen into disfavor more particularly since the arrival of laparoscopic cholecystectomy.

Results

In a large study by Thisle and associates, 75 patients with cholesterol gallstones were treated with MTBE. Ninety-five percent or more of the stone mass dissolved in 72 of 75 patients, 21 patients had no residual stones, but in 4 of these 21 patients stones recurred in 6–16 months. In 51 patients, residual debris less than 5 mm in diameter was present. Fifteen of these 51 patients cleared the residual debris spontaneously. Of the 36 patients with

persistent debris, no patient developed cholangitis, biliary obstruction, or pancreatitis. Five patients in total required cholecystectomy for persistent symptoms, 4 from the 51 patients who had residual fragments, and 1 from the 21 patients who originally had no debris.

In a further study by van Sonnenberg and associates involving 18 patients with gallstones, a combination of techniques was used including dissolution alone and dissolution in combination with PCCL. Dissolution alone was successful in eliminating stones in 8 of 10 patients, including 6 of 7 with gallbladder stones and 2 of 3 with common bile duct stones. Dissolution when combined with basket extraction was effective in 5 of 6 patients.

Complications

Complications associated with MTBE dissolution therapy include those associated with percutaneous cholecystostomy (as described previously) and those associated with MTBE. Side-effects of MTBE include sedation, pain, duodenal ulceration, intravascular hemolysis, renal failure, transient nausea, and emesis. The side-effects can be reduced if small amounts of MTBE are used and excess leakage into the duodenum is prevented (Box 21-6).

Percutaneous Cholecystolithotomy (PCCL)

In a patient with acute cholecystitis and severe intercurrent illness, the mortality rate for cholecystectomy ranges from 10 to 30%. In fact, the patient may never be fit for surgery. In this high-risk group, percutaneous cholecystolithotomy (PCCL) can be used to remove gallstones from the gallbladder to prevent further attacks of acute cholecystitis. PCCL can be performed irrespective of the number, size, and composition of stones.

Technique

Using the existing percutaneous cholecystostomy track, a larger track is dilated into the gallbladder. The track needs to be dilated to between 26- and 30-French. Track dilatation can be achieved by using either an 8- to 10-mm balloon or using fascial dilators. The author prefers to use a balloon for track dilatation. When the track has been dilated, a large 26- to 30-cm sheath is placed into the gallbladder (Cook, Bloomington, IN).

Box 21-6   MTBE Dissolution Therapy

Cholesterol gallstones are the most suitable
Percutaneous cholecystostomy performed
MTBE infused over an average of 2–15 hours
Time-consuming and rarely performed since
    laparoscopic cholecystectomy

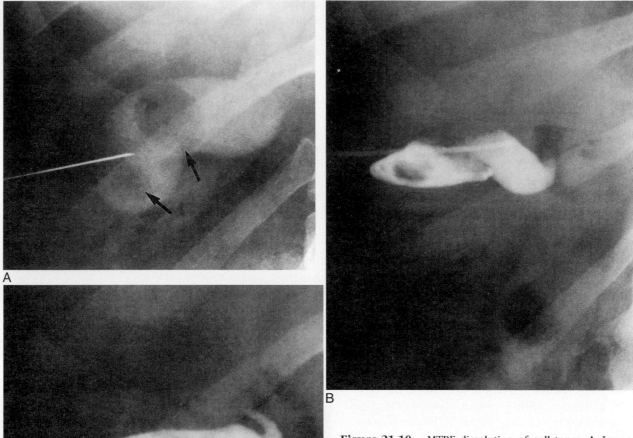

Figure 21-10 MTBE dissolution of gallstones. **A,** Image obtained after initial puncture with an 18-gauge needle shows two large gallstones (arrows) in the gallbladder. **B,** A pigtail catheter was placed and MTBE dissolution therapy commenced. Dissolution therapy was performed over three separate sessions and took approximately 15.5 hours to complete. This fluoroscopic spot image shows residual fragments after 10 hours of MTBE therapy. **C,** Fluoroscopic spot image with contrast material injected into the gallbladder at 15.5 hours shows that the gallstones have been dissolved. (Reproduced with permission from Mueller PR, Lee MJ, Saini S et al: Percutaneous contrast dissolution of gallstones; complexity of radiological care. *Radiographics* 11:759-764, 1991.)

The transperitoneal approach is preferable when large tracks are to be dilated. However, the transhepatic approach has been used in many patients without complication. In general, wait for the symptoms of acute cholecystitis to subside before performing track dilatation and stone removal. The time interval between percutaneous cholecytostomy and PCCL is usually 4-6 weeks in most patients.

If stones are small they can be removed from the gallbladder using standard basket techniques (Fig. 21-11) or using graspers or alligator forceps. Larger stones usually require some form of lithotripsy to make them small enough to remove through the percutaneous track. There are a number of ways of breaking up larger stones. These include electrohydraulic, laser, ultrasonic, and mechanical lithotripsy. The first three all require the insertion of an endoscope into the gallbladder. Mechanical lithotripsy involves using a basket to capture the stone and then the wires on the basket are tightened to actually crush the stone. This does not require direct vision and it can be performed under fluoroscopy. In the author's unit we usually perform mechanical lithotripsy first, and if this fails then ultrasonic lithotripsy is performed. Ultrasonic lithotripsy is performed in the operating room using a rigid nephroscope and the same equipment that is used for ultrasonic lithotripsy of renal stones. No matter which technique is used there are usually small stone fragments remaining at the end of the procedure which can be removed under fluoroscopy using a basket. At the end of the procedure, a large catheter is inserted into the gallbladder; we usually place a 26- to 28-French Malecot catheter to maintain the track and prevent bile leakage. The catheter remains in place for a further 2–3 days and then the patient returns for a final check cholecystogram. If this is clear and there is good flow contrast material into the bile duct and duodenum, the catheter is removed.

Results

There are a number of papers in the radiology literature describing the results from PCCL. Gilliams and associates achieved complete stone clearance in 100 of 113 patients with 73.4% of patients requiring a single-stage procedure in a mean time of 64 minutes. Picus and associates were successful in removing all of the stones in 56 of 58 patients. These stones ranged from 3 mm to 40 mm in diameter. Intracorporeal electrohydraulic lithotripsy was used to fragment large stones in 31 patients, with one stone removal session required in 32 patients, two sessions in 15 patients, three sessions in 8 patients, and four sessions in 2 patients. Cope and associates were successful in removing all gallstones from 17 of 20 patients using PCCL. Stone sizes varied from 2 mm to 22 mm and were removed in one session in 11 of 17 patients, and in two consecutive sessions in 6 patients.

Complications

Complications are mainly those reported for percutaneous cholecystostomy. Picus and associates reported major complications in 5 of 58 patients (9%). Four of these major complications were related to bile leakage after the cholecystostomy tube was removed. One patient died from extensive bowel infarction secondary to hypotension. These complications emphasize the

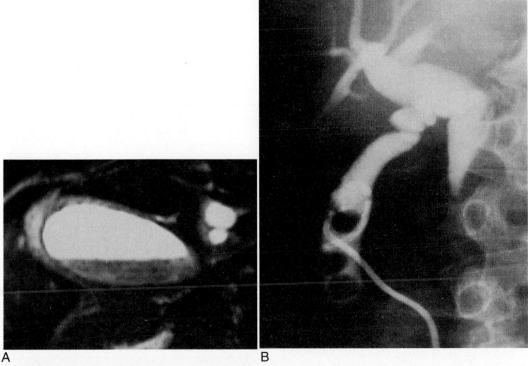

A   B

Figure 21-11   Elderly patient with acute calculous cholecystitis who was unfit for surgical cholecystectomy. The patient did not settle on conservative management with IV antibiotics and a percutaneous cholecystostomy was performed. **A,** Axial MRCP image through the gallbladder shows a rim of hyperintense signal around the gallbladder and a fluid-sludge level within the gallbladder consistent with acute cholecystitis. **B,** An 8-Fr pigtail catheter was placed into the gallbladder using a trocar technique. A catheter cholecystogram was performed when the patient's symptoms had settled. This showed three stones within the gallbladder. Note the common bile duct is moderately dilated, but this was presumed to be secondary to loss of elasticity through the normal aging process. The liver function tests were normal.   *(Continued)*

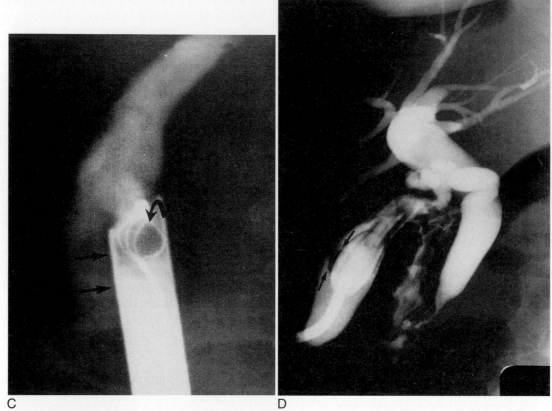

C

D

Figure 21-11   cont'd C, Six weeks after the initial percutaneous drainage, track dilatation was performed using a 1-cm diameter balloon and a 30-Fr sheath (arrow) was placed into the gallbladder. A Wittich basket (Cook, Bloomington, IN) can be seen extracting one of the stones (curved arrows) through the sheath. **D,** A 24-Fr Foley catheter was placed in the gallbladder after the procedure and 2 days later the patient returned for a catheter cholecystogram. This shows the gallbladder to be clear. There is some residual clot (arrows) present in the gallbladder. The catheter, however, was removed. The patient has had no further symptoms.

need for careful tube handling and delayed tube removal in this patient group (Box 21-7).

Gallbladder Ablation

It is well known that the risk of symptomatic gallstones recurring in patients after surgical cholecystolithotomy is high. Unfortunately, all forms of nonsurgical gallstone therapies leave a diseased gallbladder in place which has the potential for stone recurrence. In fact, symptoms of biliary tract disease reoccur in 20–50% of patients 2–5 years after the initial nonsurgical gallstone therapy. Obviously, in the patient population for which nonsurgical gallstone therapies are performed the high recurrence rate of systematic gallstones is problematic. Therefore, the idea of ablating the gallbladder so that stones cannot recur was proposed.

Technique

Gallbladder ablation was popularized in the late 1980s and early 90s with experimental animal studies and one human study. However, again with the advent of laparoscopic cholecystectomy the need for gallbladder ablation has decreased enormously and it is now rarely performed.

Complete gallbladder ablation to prevent stone recurrence can be achieved only by ablating both the gallbladder and cystic duct mucosa. The cystic duct is usually first ablated using either a laser fiber or radio-frequency ablation. In general, access will already have been gained and some form of nonsurgical therapy will have been

---

Box 21-7   PCCL

Can be performed irrespective of stone composition
26- to 30-French track required
Stones removed by basket or, if large, lithotripsy
  performed
Performed only in those patients with symptomatic
  gallstones who are unfit for surgery

used to remove the gallstones. A laser fiber or a radio-frequency catheter is then negotiated into the cystic duct and energy is delivered to the gallbladder mucosa while the laser fiber or radio-frequency catheter is slowly pulled backward into the gallbladder. This serves to destroy the mucosa of the cystic duct, with eventual scar formation.

The second step is to ablate the gallbladder. This is usually achieved by chemical sclerotherapy using sodium tetradecyl sulfate (STS) and 95% ethanol. The volume of the gallbladder is first determined and an equal volume of each sclerosant is then given. Ethanol is instilled first and left in place for 30 minutes followed by STS which is left in place for 30 minutes. The cholecystostomy tube is removed after sclerotherapy when the drainage from the gallbladder is less than 20 mL per day. Repeat sclerotherapy may be necessary if the gallbladder fails to obliterate and a persistent mucus discharge occurs through the cholecystostomy tube track.

Results

Animal results reported by Girard and Becker and associates have demonstrated successful obliteration of the cystic duct and gallbladder. Girard's team used laser ablation of the cystic duct, whilst Becker's used radio-frequency ablation. Although animal studies were successful in ablating gallbladder mucosa and cystic duct mucosa, human studies have not been as successful. Becker's team reported successful gallbladder ablation in five of eight patients. However, in three patients mucus discharge persisted, and forceps biopsy of the gallbladder in these three patients showed evidence of gallbladder mucosa regeneration.

It is likely that the extensive regenerative capability of the gallbladder mucosa makes complete ablation of the human gallbladder less likely to succeed than in the animal model. The author's unit rarely performs gallbladder ablation, anticipating that the short life expectancy of many of the elderly patients who are unfit for surgery or cholecystectomy will usually not be sufficient to make recurrent stone formation a major concern.

SUGGESTED READING

Becker CD, Quenville NF, Burhenne HJ: Gallbladder ablation through radiologic intervention: an experimental alternative to cholecystectomy. *Radiology* 171:235-240, 1989.

Becker CD, Fache JS, Malone DE, Stoller JL, Burhenne HJ: Ablation of the cystic duct and gallbladder: clinical observations. *Radiology* 176:687-690, 1990.

Boland GW, Lee MJ, Mueller PR et al: Gallstones in critically ill patients with acute calculous cholecystitis treated by percutaneous cholecystostomy: nonsurgical therapeutic options. *Am J Roentgenol* 162:1101-1103, 1994.

Boland GW, Lee MJ, Leung J, Mueller PR: Percutaneous cholecystostomy in critically ill patients: early response and final outcome in 82 patients. *Am J Roentgenol* 163:339-342, 1994.

Cope C, Burke DR, Meranze SG: Precutaneous extraction of gallstones in 20 patients. *Radiology* 176:19-24, 1990.

Gillams A, Curtis S, Donald J et al: Technical considerations in 113 percutaneous cholecystolithotomies. *Radiology* 183:163-166, 1992.

Girard MJ, Saini S, Mueller PR et al: Percutaneous chemical gallbladder sclerosis after laser-induced cystic duct oblivation: results in an experimental model. *Am J Roentgenol* 159:997-1000, 1992.

Lee MJ, Saini S, Brink J et al: Treatment of critically ill patients with sepsis of unknown cause: value of percutaneous cholecystostomy. *Am J Roentgenol* 156:1163-1166, 1991.

McGahan JP, Lindfors KK: Percutaneous cholecystostomy: an alternative to surgical cholecystostomy for acute cholecystitis. *Radiology* 173:481-485, 1989.

Mirvis SE, Wainright JR, Nelson AW: The diagnosis of acute acalculous cholecystitis: a comparison of sonography, scintigraphy and CT. *Am J Roentgenol* 147:1171-1175, 1986.

Mueller PR, Lee MJ, Saini S et al: Percutaneous contrast dissolution of gallstones; complexity of radiological care. *Radiographics* 11:759-764, 1991.

Nemcek AA, Bernstein JE, Vogelzang RL: Percutaneous cholecystostomy: does transhepatic puncture preclude a transperitoneal catheter route? *J Vasc Interv Radiol* 2:543-547, 1991.

Picus D: Percutaneous gallbladder intervention. *Radiology* 176:5-6, 1990.

Picus D, Hicks MR, Darcy MD et al: Percutaneous cholecystolithotomy: analysis of results and complications in 58 consecutive patients. *Radiology* 183:779-784, 1992.

Picus D, Marx MV, Hicks ME, Larg EV, Edmundowiez SA: Percutaneous cholecystolithotomy: preliminary experience and technical considerations. *Radiology* 173:487-491, 1989.

Stafford-Johnson D, Mueller PR, Varghese J, Lee MJ: Percutaneous cholecystostomy: a review. *J Interv Radiol* 11:1-8, 1996.

Thistle JL, May GR, Bender CE et al: Dissolution of cholesterol gallbladder stones by MTBE administered by percutaneous transhepatic catheter. *N Engl J Med* 320:663-639, 1989.

Valff V, Froelich JW, Lloyd R et al: Predictive value of an abnormal hepatobiliary scan in patients with severe intercurrent illness. *Radiology* 146:191-194, 1983.

vanSonnenberg E, Casola G, Zakko SF et al: Gallbladder and bile duct stones: percutaneous therapy with primary MTBE dissolution and mechanical methods. *Radiology* 169:505-509, 1988.

vanSonnenberg E, D'agostino HB, Casola G et al: Benefits of percutaneous cholecystostomy for decompression of selected cases of obstructive jaundice. *Radiology* 176:15-17, 1990.

vanSonnenberg E, D'Agostino HB, Casola G et al: Gallbladder perforation and bile leakage: percutaneous treatment. *Radiology* 178:687-689, 1991.

vanSonnenberg E, D'Agostino HB, Casola G, Varney RR, Ainge GD: Interventional radiology in the gallbladder: diagnosis, drainage, dissolution and management of stones. *Radiology* 174:1-6, 1990.

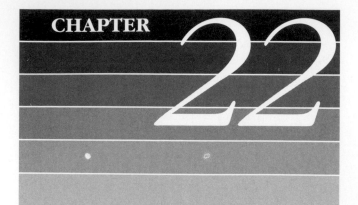

Percutaneous Genitourinary Intervention

MICHAEL J. LEE, M.D.

Although the first percutaneous genitourinary procedure was a renal cyst puncture reported in 1867, it wasn't until approximately 100 years later that the first percutaneous nephrostomy using the Seldinger technique was described. Since then, percutaneous access to the kidney has been employed for a wide variety of renal and ureteric pathology. Relief of acute urinary obstruction remains the commonest procedure performed by interventional radiologists in the genitourinary tract. However, percutaneous access to the kidney has also been used to remove ureteric or renal calculi, dissolve certain types of renal calculi, place ureteric stents, biopsy pelvicalyceal lesions, perform endopyelotomy for ureteropelvic junction obstruction, and remove foreign bodies from the collecting system.

Many of these procedures gained widespread popularity during the 1980s, but the development of extracorporeal lithotripsy and ureteroscopy has limited the number and variety of percutaneous procedures performed in the genitourinary tract at the present time. However, depending on the clinical circumstances, interventional radiologists may be called upon to perform many or all of these techniques. Obviously, an intimate knowledge of the relevant anatomy of the genitourinary system is important for the performance of these procedures.

ANATOMY RELEVANT TO PERCUTANEOUS GENITOURINARY INTERVENTION

Kidney

The kidneys are paired organs located in the retroperitoneum surrounded by fat. They are usually located between the level of the 11th or 12th thoracic to the 2nd or 3rd lumbar vertebral bodies. The left kidney usually lies 1-2 cm higher than the right. The pleura is attached to the 10th rib laterally and the 12th rib posteriorly. Normally the 12th rib crosses over the upper pole of the right kidney, whereas on the left side the upper renal pole is often covered by the 11th and 12th ribs. Because of this anatomy, percutaneous intervention through the upper pole will almost certainly be transpleural, so the risk of pneumothorax or hydropneumothorax is increased. The lower poles of both kidneys are located more anteriorly than the upper poles and this means that when performing percutaneous nephrostomy it is important to remember that the lower poles are further away from the skin than the mid and upper poles when the patient is in the prone position.

At the renal hilum the renal vein is situated anteriorly. The renal artery lies posterior to the renal vein and the renal pelvis lies posterior to both. Therefore, in the prone position the renal pelvis is the most posterior structure of the renal pedicle and nearest the skin. The renal artery divides into an anterior and posterior division as it approaches the renal hilum, with the anterior division dividing into three or four segmental branches and the posterior division giving rise to one segmental branch. The segmental renal arteries become interlobar arteries in the renal sinus and cross through the Septum of Bertin and course along the medullary pyramid and arch around the distal end of the pyramids to divide into arcuate arteries. The arcuate arteries are located at the base of the pyramids and give rise to interlobular arteries which supply the peripheral renal cortex.

Broedel's line is a relatively avascular plane in the posterolateral aspect of the kidney between the posterior and anterior intrapolar vascular territories. Because of the absence of large arterial branches this avascular plane is theoretically safer for placing catheters into the renal pelvicalyceal system. However, in practice this plane cannot be routinely identified and placement of a catheter into a calyceal fornix is usually adequate and safe for percutaneous nephrostomy (Fig. 22-1).

Percutaneous puncture and placement of a catheter directly into the renal pelvis is not recommended because of the proximity of the renal vascular pedicle and the propensity to cause arterial damage and major hemorrhage. Placement of a catheter through the peripheral cortex of the kidney is the recommended route for percutaneous access because of the proximity to the avascular Plane of Broedel and the presence of smaller blood vessels in this region (see Fig. 22-1).

Renal calyceal anatomy is also important for planning percutaneous nephrostomy. Because percutaneous nephrostomy is performed in the prone position, gaining access to a posterior calyx is the preferred entry point into the renal pelvicalyceal system. Because the posterior calyces are closer to the skin surface in the prone position, the angle of entry from a posterior calyx into the renal pelvis will be more direct and less acute than that

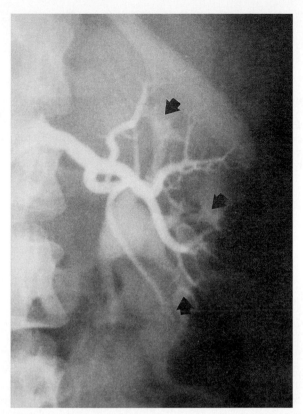

Figure 22-1   Arterial anatomy of the kidney. Selective angiographic image of the left kidney shows the arterial anatomy overlying the pelvicalyceal system. Arrows denote the calyces. Nephrostomy access is best gained through peripheral calyces where adjacent arteries tend to be smaller, rather than more centrally where the arteries are larger.

associated with an anterior calyx (Fig. 22-2). The location of anterior and posterior calyces in relation to the lateral contour of the kidney is not constant. Broedel proposed that anterior calyces are located medially and posterior calyces laterally, while Hodson proposed the opposite; i.e., anterior calyces are located laterally and posterior calyces medially. However, more recently Kaye and Reinke studied calyceal location using CT imaging. They found that the Broedel description is far more common in the right whereas the Hodson calyceal description is more often present on the left (Fig. 22-3).

Because of the variation in the anterior and posterior calyces, in the author's unit we tend to use either carbon dioxide or air to outline the posterior calyces (Fig. 22-4). In circumstances where there is marked hydronephrosis, differentiation of anterior from posterior calyces is usually not of any technical advantage. However, in renal collecting systems that are moderately or minimally dilated, delineation of the posterior calyces with air or CO_2 may make placement of the percutaneous nephrostomy catheter technically easier.

The colon is occasionally positioned laterally or even posterior to the kidney. Posterior colonic location is

Figure 22-2   Schematic showing the difference between a posterior calyceal puncture and an anterior calyceal puncture. **A**, Puncture of an anterior calyx may pose problems for guidewire access into the renal pelvis because of the more acute angle between the calyx and the renal pelvis. **B**, Puncture of a posterior calyx allows easy access of guidewires and catheters into the pelvis.

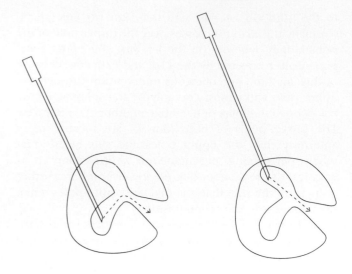

rare and if present may well result in colonic transgression (Fig. 22-5). However, it is so rare that routine prenephrostomy imaging with CT or barium studies is not warranted. Lateral colonic location is more frequent and mitigates against using a lateral access route for percutaneous nephrostomy. Therefore, in practice, a posterolateral route is chosen for gaining access to the kidney so that if the colon is located laterally it will be avoided (Box 22-1).

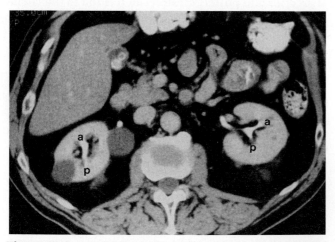

Figure 22-3   Contrast-enhanced CT scan showing the relationship of the anterior (a) and posterior (p) calyces. In the majority of patients the anterior calyces in the right kidney are situated medially and the posterior calyces are situated laterally. The opposite is true in the left kidney. In this example the anterior and posterior calyces are in the same plane on the right, while on the left the anterior calyces are situated laterally and the posterior calyces are situated medially.

Ureter

The ureter descends from the renal hilum on the anteromedial surfaces of the psoas muscle. As it passes over the common iliac artery a slightly more medial course is assumed followed by a posterolateral course in the pelvis. Finally, as the ureter approaches the bladder the ureter turns medially and enters the bladder at the ureterovesical junction. There are three areas of physiologic narrowing in the ureter. These are located at the ureteropelvic junction, the common iliac artery, and the ureterovesical junction.

Bladder

The urinary bladder is located behind the symphysis pubis. The superior wall or dome of the bladder is the only portion of the bladder covered by peritoneum. The neck is fixed in position and as the bladder fills and distends it becomes elevated well above the symphysis pubis. As the bladder fills all bowel loops are pushed superiorly out of the pelvis, allowing for safe percutaneous access.

Box 22-1   Renal Anatomy

Renal vein, artery and ureter run anterior to posterior in this order
Broedel's plane is theoretical, not practical
Anterior and posterior calyces may have different mediolateral orientations in right and left kidneys
The colon is rarely found posterior to the kidney

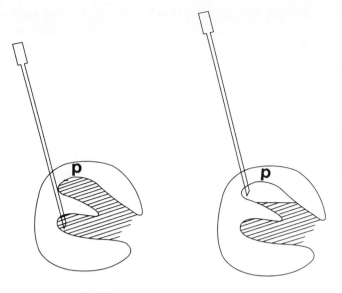

Figure 22-4   Schematic showing how the use of air can help identify posterior calyces during percutaneous nephrostomy. The air rises into posterior (p) calyces making them easier to identify.

The vascular supply of the bladder enters through the posterior and lateral aspects of the bladder wall which also makes for safe percutaneous access through the anterior wall. When planning a percutaneous suprapubic cystostomy it is important to remember that the inferior epigastric vessels run down the anterior abdominal wall on each side of the rectus muscles and are avoided by selecting an entry site close to the midline.

PATIENT PREPARATION

As for other interventional procedures, a coagulation profile and informed consent are obtained before

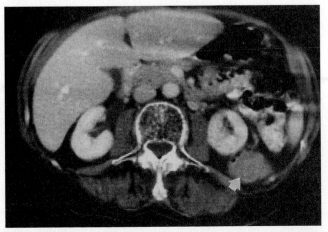

Figure 22-5   CT scan showing the colon (arrow) situated posterior to the left kidney. This is an unusual occurrence but ultrasound is recommended prior to percutaneous nephrostomy to ensure that there is no colon posterior to the kidney.

the procedure. Coagulation abnormalities are corrected if necessary. Intravenous sedoanalgesia with fentanyl and midazolam is given before and during the procedure for adequate pain relief. The patient is placed prone on the fluoroscopy table. Patients with a recent anterior abdominal wall surgical scar may need sedation and analgesia before being turned prone.

Preprocedure antibiotics are given if there is a suspicion of pyonephrosis or an infected collecting system. The antibiotic regimen chosen depends on operator preference. The author uses gentamycin 80 mg IV and ampicillin 1 g IV.

RENAL INTERVENTION

Antegrade Pyelography

Antegrade pyelography refers to the insertion of a needle into the pelvicalyceal system and the injection of contrast material to delineate the anatomy of the pelvicalyceal system and ureter (Fig. 22-6). It currently forms a starting point for many percutaneous genitourinary interventions. It was widely used in the 1980s as a diagnostic technique when intravenous urography failed to adequately opacify the pelvicalyceal system or ureter. However, with the advent of cystoscopy and retrograde injection of contrast medium into the ureter, its popularity has declined. Moreover, with the more extensive use of imaging such as ultrasound, CT, and MR, many renal and ureteric abnormalities can be fully evaluated without recourse to either antegrade pyelography or retrograde pyelography. However, it still remains the mainstay for performance of the Whittaker test and also for delineating

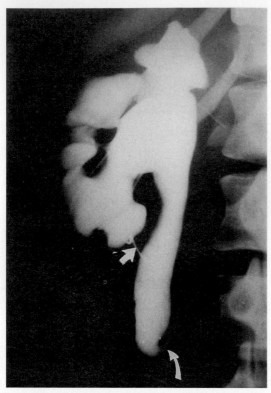

Figure 22-6   Antegrade pyelogram in a patient with right-sided hydronephrosis and pain. The needle (straight arrow) was inserted into the lower pole calyx. Contrast material injected showed a dilated collecting system with clubbed calyces and characteristic medial deviation of the upper ureter (curved arrow), indicating a retrocaval ureter.

the anatomy and cause of obstruction prior to percutaneous nephrostomy.

Technique

The patient is positioned prone on the fluoroscopy table and the kidney is located with ultrasound. Because only a single needle is being placed, the renal pelvis or a calyx can be chosen as a target. It is easier to access the renal pelvis in most instances and in the author's unit we generally choose the renal pelvis as a target. The needle can be directed into the renal pelvis using fluoroscopy alone. The commonly chosen landmark is approximately 2–3 cm lateral to the transverse process of L2. Alternatively, some authors prefer to use ultrasound alone to direct the needle into the renal pelvis or renal calyx using a freehand technique. We prefer to use ultrasound to mark the location and if there is marked dilatation of the pelvicalyceal system the needle is inserted into the renal pelvis without ultrasound guidance. If there is mild or moderate hydronephrosis ultrasound guidance is used. A 20- or 22-gauge needle can be used, but a 20-gauge needle is preferred as it is a little stiffer and can be directed through the muscles and perinephric tissues

without the tip becoming deflected as can happen with 22-gauge needles. Once urine is aspirated from the needle, the needle hub is connected to extension tubing and contrast material injected. If there is high grade obstruction, it is important to remove adequate amounts of urine before injecting contrast material to avoid over distension of the collecting system. A tilting table may help to delineate the lower level of the obstruction, particularly in the severely hydronephrotic collecting system. By placing the patient semi-erect, the heavier contrast material will gravitate towards the lower end of the ureter and delineate the level of the obstruction.

Complications

Complications encountered with antegrade pyelography are rare. Bacteremia can be induced by injecting contrast material into a high-pressure collecting system particularly if the urine is infected. If the urine is cloudy on visual inspection, it is important to decompress and remove an adequate amount of urine before contrast material is injected.

The Whittaker Test

The Whittaker or ureteral perfusion test is used to determine whether a dilated urinary system is obstructed or not. It has been regarded as the gold standard for this determination but is performed rarely. Lasix renography can often determine the presence or absence of an obstruction but does have a 10–15% false positive rate, particularly, in patients with dilated collecting systems. The Whittaker perfusion test was devised to evaluate the presence or absence of obstruction to flow in the presence of a dilated but non-refluxing upper urinary tract. It is more commonly used in pediatric patients where dilated non-refluxing ureters can pose a diagnostic dilemma. Its most common use in adults is to determine whether pelvicalyceal dilatation due to pelviureteric junction (PUJ) dysfunction is causing obstruction or not. Similarly, it can be used in adults to evaluate the adequacy of pyeloplasty for the treatment of PUJ obstruction.

The Whittaker test is basically a ureteral stress test. The ureter is perfused with known volumes of fluid at known flow rates. An antegrade needle is placed in the pelvicalyceal system and a Foley catheter placed in the bladder. Manometers are attached to both the antegrade needle and the bladder catheter and contrast material is infused through the antegrade needle using a pump at known flow rates.

On placement of the antegrade needle a sample of urine is aspirated for bacteriologic assessment. If the urine appears cloudy, it is best to delay the procedure until the Gram stain can be obtained. An opening pressure is recorded by connecting a water manometer to the antegrade needle. A water manometer is also connected to

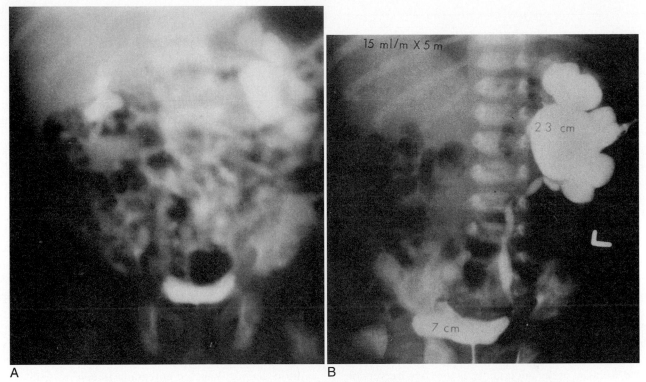

Figure 22-7   Whittaker ureteral perfusion test in a 2-month-old baby with left-sided hydronephrosis. The hydronephrosis was noted on an antenatal ultrasound scan and thought to represent a ureteropelvic junction obstruction. **A,** An IVP performed at 2 months shows a dilated collecting system on the left with no visualized ureter. **B,** A ureteral perfusion test was performed under general anesthesia by inserting an antegrade needle into the left collecting system and a small catheter was inserted into the bladder. Pressure differential after perfusion of the collecting system with 15 mL/min of contrast material for 5 minutes was 16 cmH$_2$O. This is equivalent to a mild obstruction. Because of the minimal nature of the obstruction it was decided not to perform surgery at this time but to adopt a conservative approach with regular follow-up.

the bladder catheter (Fig. 22-7). An opening pressure from the bladder is recorded. It is important to have the base of the manometers at the same level as the tip of the antegrade needle. Water manometers are usually strapped to drip infusion stands and can be set to a similar level as the tip of the antegrade needle by calculating the amount of needle length within the patient. The ureter is then perfused with contrast material diluted to a 20% concentration at a flow rate of 10 mL/min for 5 minutes. Then the perfusion is halted and pressures are again taken from the kidney and bladder. If no evidence of obstruction is present the ureter can be further stressed at a higher flow rate of 15–20 mL/min for another 5 minutes. The subtraction of the recorded bladder pressure from the renal pressure provides the differential pressure. Normal and abnormal pressure differentials are shown in Table 22-1.

Lastly, the ureteral perfusion test is repeated with the bladder full to evaluate the effect of increased bladder pressure on the urinary tract. This is important in situations where the bladder pressure is high owing to either

outlet obstruction or neurogenic disease. Intermittent or continuous high bladder pressures above 20 cmH$_2$O places the kidney at risk even in the absence of ureteral obstruction.

The ureteral perfusion test is abandoned if the opening pressure in the kidney is above 35 cmH$_2$O or if the patient develops pain during the procedure.

Table 22-1   Normal and Abnormal Pressure Differentials Associated with the Whittaker Test

Flow rate (mL/min)	Pressure Differential (cmH$_2$O)	Grade of Obstruction
10	<13	Normal
10	14–22	Mild or equivocal
10	23–35	Moderate
10	>35	Severe

Percutaneous Nephrostomy

Percutaneous nephrostomy remains the most common procedure performed on the kidney by the interventional radiologist. The most common indications for percutaneous nephrostomy include obstruction from ureteric stones and malignant obstruction from carcinomas of the bladder and prostate. The ureters may also be involved by secondary malignant deposits from cancers of the uterus, colon, breast, and abdominal lymphoma. Other indications for percutaneous nephrostomy include postsurgical damage to the ureter, ureteral fistulas, and idiopathic retroperitoneal fibrosis.

It is important to remember that nephron damage and parenchymal atrophy can begin as early as a few days to a week following the onset of obstruction. Undoubtedly, nephron damage occurs much earlier if the urine is infected. Information on how long the kidney can tolerate high grade obstruction is incomplete, but nephron damage is influenced by whether the obstruction is unilateral or bilateral, whether there is superimposed infection, and whether there is pre-existing renal or vascular disease. Because of the uncertainty as to when irreversible nephron damage begins, an obstructed urinary system should be drained as soon as possible after diagnosis.

Technique
Pelvicalyceal Access

The patient is placed prone on the fluoroscopy table and the obstructed kidney is imaged with ultrasound to determine its location and the degree of hydronephrosis. An antegrade pyelogram is performed as previously described and contrast material injected to outline the pelvicalyceal system. During antegrade pyelography the level and cause of obstruction is determined, if not known already. The only exception to this is when a pyonephrosis is encountered. If a pyonephrosis is encountered, the minimum amount of contrast material is injected and minimal manipulation of the pelvicalyceal system is carried out. Once the pelvicalyceal system is outlined by contrast material, a calyx is chosen for puncture. The calyx chosen will depend on the anatomy of the kidney and on the likelihood of any future procedures such as antegrade ureteral stent insertion. If antegrade stent insertion is likely, then a mid-pole calyx is preferable; if not, a lower-pole calyx can be chosen.

Having decided on the calyx of choice, the next step is to decide whether the calyx seen is an anterior or posterior calyx. The best way to do this is to inject either carbon dioxide or air via the antegrade needle into the pelvicalyceal system (Fig. 22-8). If CO_2 is not available, 10–15 mL of air can be injected through the antegrade needle. It is important to ensure that the antegrade needle is not in communication with a vein, so that air

embolus is avoided. The air or CO_2 will rise into the posterior calyces which can then be readily identified. At this stage, some operators like to turn the patient into the prone oblique position which, theoretically makes the angle from the calyx into the infundibulum and renal pelvis more shallow and easier to negotiate. In the author's unit we prefer to leave the patient in the prone position as usually there is little or no difficulty in negotiating a wire from a posterior calyx into the pelvis.

A single-stick needle access system (Neff Set, Cook, Bloomington, IN; Acustick, Meditech, Watertown, MA) is used to gain access into the calyx. These needle access sets are composed of a 22-gauge, 15-cm needle, a 0.018-inch guidewire, a metal cannula, a 4-French plastic cannula, and a 5-French sheath. A skin position is marked using fluoroscopy 1.5-2.0 cm lateral to the calyx chosen. The skin is infiltrated with local anesthetic, an incision is made with a #11 scalpel, and the needle is inserted under fluoroscopic guidance into the calyx. The depth of insertion can usually be gauged by, the depth of the antegrade needle inserted, to gain access to the renal pelvis; remembering that the lower pole of the kidney is more anterior, the second needle will have to be inserted a little deeper than the antegrade needle to gain access to the collecting system. A 10-mL syringe with 2 mL of saline is placed on the hub of the needle. The stylet is removed and the needle is slowly withdrawn until urine or air bubbles appear in the syringe. The 0.018-inch guidewire is then manipulated down through the needle into the calyx and into the renal pelvis. Occasionally, difficulty will be encountered in advancing the guidewire from the tip of the needle even though urine has been aspirated through the needle. Often this is because the needle tip is up against the wall of the calyx. Withdrawing the needle slightly and turning the needle so that the bevel points in different directions may aid in negotiating the guidewire into the renal pelvis. When the 0.018-inch guidewire is in the renal pelvis, the needle is removed over the guidewire and the 5-French sheath assembly is placed over the wire into the pelvicalyceal system. It is important to detach the metal stiffening cannula when the sheath system has entered the calyx. The metal cannula is too stiff to traverse the angle between the calyx and renal pelvis. Once the metal cannula is withdrawn, the 5-French sheath and inner plastic cannula are flexible enough to follow the guidewire into the renal pelvis. If the metal cannula is left in place, attempts to force the sheath system into the renal pelvis will result in guidewire kinking in the calyx and further pushing may cause the guidewire to slip out of the kidney altogether. Once the 5-French sheath is in the renal pelvis, a 0.035-inch "J"-guidewire is inserted through the 5-French sheath and either coiled in the renal pelvis, placed in the upper pole calyx, or manipulated down the ureter (Fig. 22-9).

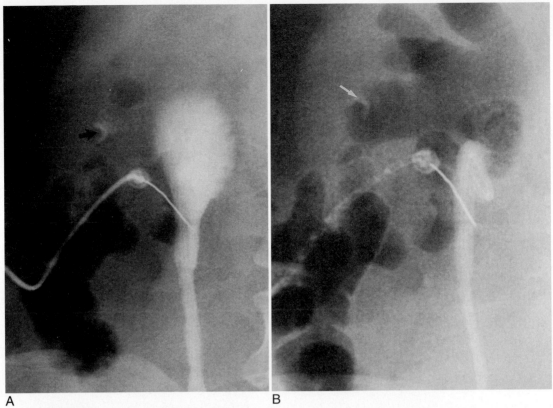

Figure 22-8   A patient with a ureteral stent which, was calcified and was not possible to remove cystoscopically. **A,** An antegrade needle was placed near the apex of the proximal end of the stent and contrast material injected. Unfortunately, owing to the low access, contrast material did not opacify the calyceal system apart from one anterior calyx (arrow). **B,** Air was injected which helped to outline the posterior calyces for puncture. Note the small amount of contrast material remaining in the anterior calyx (arrow) in the lower pole of the kidney.

Placing the Nephrostomy Catheter

When the 0.035-inch "J" guidewire is present in the renal pelvis, the tract is dilated. Some others prefer using a stiffer guidewire such as a 0.035-inch Ring–Lunderquist (Cook, Bloomington, IN) guidewire, but with experience the "J" guidewire is usually adequate. If an 8-French catheter is being placed, the tract is dilated with 8- and 10-French dilators. If a 10-French catheter is being placed the percutaneous tract is dilated with 8-, 10-, and 12-French dilators and so on. An 8-French nephrostomy catheter is placed for the vast majority of percutaneous nephrostomies. Only if one encounters a pyonephrosis should a 10- or 12-French catheter be placed. It is important to fluoroscopically monitor the guidewire while dilating the tract to ensure that kinking of the guidewire does not take place. When the track is dilated the nephrostomy catheter (Cook, Bloomington, IN; Meditech, Watertown, MA) is passed over the guidewire into the renal pelvis. The nephrostomy catheters usually come with a metal stiffening cannula which is used to provide stability for the catheter as it passes through the subcutaneous tissues, muscles, and retroperitoneal tissues on the way to the kidney. Once the catheter has entered the kidney, it is important again to detach the metal stiffening cannula and withdraw it slightly while sliding the catheter forward over the guidewire. Failure to do this will result in kinking of the wire and/or loss of purchase within the kidney.

Depending on where the guidewire is coiled, the catheter is either placed in the upper-pole calyx, coiled

---

Box 22-2   Percutaneous Nephrostomy

20-gauge antegrade needle first placed in renal pelvis
CO_2 or air injected to identify posterior calyces
Single-stick needle system used to access chosen calyx
Nephrostomy catheter metal stiffener withdrawn at calyceal level
Minimal contrast injection and manipulation in infected system

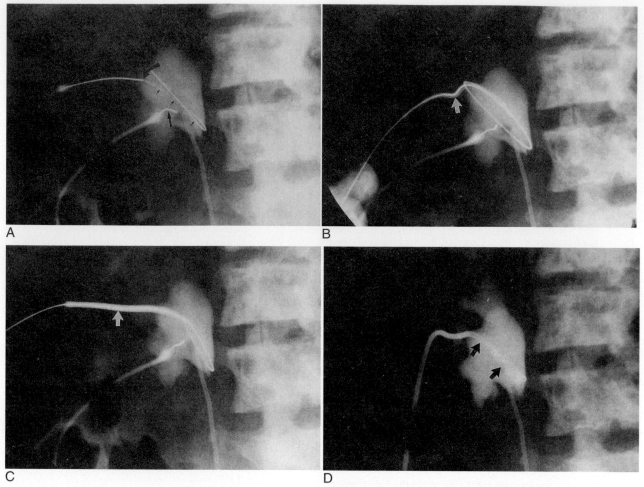

Figure 22-9 Percutaneous nephrostomy in a patient with a blocked ureteral stent and fever. **A,** An antegrade needle (straight arrow) was inserted to outline the pelvicalyceal system. A second 22-gauge needle (curved arrow) was used to puncture a mid-pole calyx and a 0.018-inch guidewire (small arrows) coiled in the renal pelvis. **B,** The sheath system (arrow) can be seen inserted over the 0.018-inch wire into the renal pelvis. The guidewire was removed and a 0.35-inch "J" guidewire inserted. **C,** Track dilatation was performed with 8- and 10-Fr dilators. The 10-Fr dilator (arrow) can be seen dilating the percutaneous track. **D,** Finally, an 8-Fr nephrostomy catheter (arrows) was inserted and coiled in the renal pelvis.

in the pelvis, or placed down the ureter over the wire. The string on the end of the catheter is then pulled to form the pigtail loop. If the catheter is down the ureter, pulling the catheter back until the tip is approximately 4–5 cm from the PUJ will ensure that, when the string is pulled, the catheter will flip back into the renal pelvis forming a nice pigtail (Fig. 22-10 and Box 22-2).

Aftercare

Catheter fixation to the skin is important and can be accomplished in a number of different ways. The author uses a Hollister ostomy disc which is placed on the patient's skin with the catheter threaded through the opening in the center of the Hollister disc. Adhesive tape is placed around the catheter and the adhesive tape is then sutured to the ostomy disc.

Alternatively, the adhesive tape which is first placed around the catheter can be sutured directly to the patient's skin. Unless there has been a lot of bleeding and clot formation, it is usually not necessary to irrigate a nephrostomy catheter. Urine contains proteolytic enzymes which will tend to break down any clot forming in the catheter and will keep the catheter patent. The author's unit tends to use irrigation only if there is thick pus in the collecting system or if there is significant clot formation after the procedure.

Results

The success rate for percutaneous nephrostomy approaches 100% in experienced hands. Difficulties may be encountered with the nondilated collecting system,

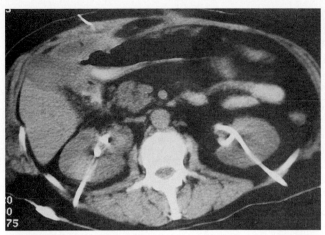

Figure 22-10 CT scan showing appropriately placed nephrostomy catheters. The catheters are placed from a posterolateral approach through the renal cortex into both collecting systems. The idea of placing catheters through the renal cortex is so that any potential bleeding will be tamponaded.

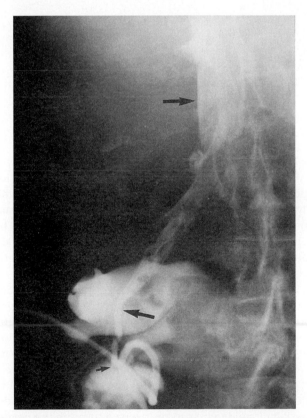

Figure 22-11 Back bleeding through a percutaneous nephrostomy catheter placed in a ptotic and obstructed right kidney. A nephrostogram performed through the nephrostomy catheter shows communication with the renal vein and inferior vena cava (straight arrows). This was due to the fact that the catheter had got pulled back into the percutaneous track such that one of the side-holes was communicating with a renal vein branch (small arrow). This was corrected by inserting the catheter more medially into the renal pelvis over a guidewire.

but these are surmountable by appropriate placement of an antegrade needle and adequate distension.

Complications

Complications resulting from percutaneous nephrostomy are infrequent and have been estimated to be around 4%. Hemorrhage (Figs. 22-11 and 22-12) and infection are the two most frequent complications requiring therapy. Some bleeding is not infrequent after most percutaneous nephrostomies. However, severe bleeding may indicate arterial damage such as a pseudoaneurysm or arteriovenous fistula. If there is significant back bleeding through the catheter with an associated hematocrit drop, then an arteriogram may be indicated with embolization of any bleeding site. However, this is a rare occurrence, and in fact in the author's unit we have only had one major bleeding complication in the last 10 years. Bleeding can be prevented to a large extent by correcting any coagulopathy beforehand and placing the catheter peripherally through the cortex into a calyx rather than placing the catheter directly into the renal pelvis (Fig. 22-13).

Sepsis is the other major complication that can complicate percutaneous nephrostomy. This almost invariably occurs in patients with either a pyonephrosis, infected stone, or infected urine. During the percutaneous nephrostomy, bacteria and endotoxins from the collecting system invariably enter the blood stream. This may cause a septicemia in some patients, often despite appropriate antibiotic cover. It is important not to overdistend

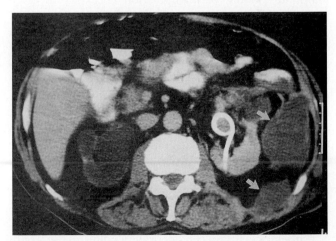

Figure 22-12 CT scan performed after a percutaneous nephrostomy in a patient who became hypotensive. Note the nonfunctioning kidney on the right side. The nephrostomy catheter is in good position but there is extensive retroperitoneal hemorrhage (arrows) around the kidney. The kidney is also displaced forward by the hemorrhage. The patient settled with conservative management and no operative or other percutaneous intervention was required. The reason for the bleeding was unclear as the percutaneous nephrostomy was uncomplicated and the patient did not have a coagulation disorder.

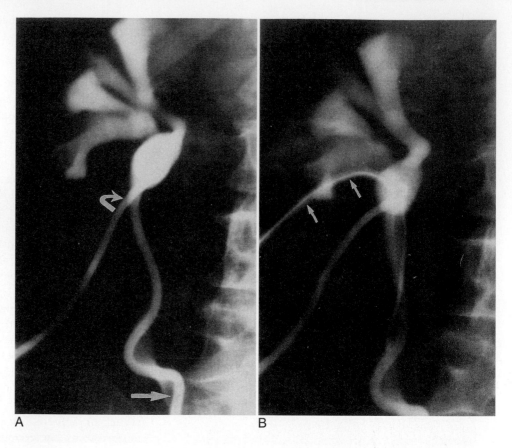

Figure 22-13 Example of a percutaneous nephrostomy catheter inserted directly into the renal pelvis. **A,** Nephrostomy catheter (curved arrow) insertion performed at an outside hospital shows that the nephrostomy catheter was inserted directly into the renal pelvis. The tip of the nephrostomy catheter (straight arrow) is in the proximal ureter and not coiled in the renal pelvis. **B,** The patient was referred for antegrade stenting and a new access into a lower-pole calyx was obtained (arrows) for the purpose. Direct manipulation of the renal pelvis is not advised because of the potential for damage to arterial or venous structures.

A

B

the collecting system in these patients and to use the minimum amount of manipulation necessary to place the catheter.

Catheter-related problems such as dislodgement and occlusion do occur. With modern pigtail catheters it is rare for catheters to become dislodged. However, if this does occur, it is important to bring the patient to the interventional suite as soon as possible. Depending on the maturity of the tract, it may be possible to probe the track and reinsert a nephrostomy catheter. Generally, in the author's unit we use an angled hydrophilic guidewire and Kumpe catheter to probe the track. If access to the pelvicalyceal system is gained, it is usually a straightforward task to place a new nephrostomy catheter. If access cannot be gained, a new percutaneous nephrostomy procedure is performed.

Catheter occlusion can occur depending on the length of time the catheter is *in situ*. It may be possible to open the existing catheter by using a guidewire. If this is not possible, the catheter can be exchanged by using a 9-French peel-away sheath. The hub of the catheter is cut and the peel-away sheath inserted over the catheter into the collecting system. The catheter is then removed and a new catheter inserted into the pelvicalyceal system. A guidewire is not used for this procedure.

Special Circumstances
Transplant Kidney

Occasionally, an interventional radiologist may be called upon to place a nephrostomy catheter in a patient with a transplant kidney (Fig. 22-14). Often, the cause of obstruction may be edema at the ureterovesical junction. The nephrostomy drainage may therefore be of a temporary nature. Rarely, the obstruction may be due to ureteric torsion or ureteric ischemia leading to a stricture.

Because the transplant kidney is superficially placed in the right or left flank, the procedure is more easily performed than in a native kidney. For percutaneous nephrostomy in the transplant kidney, a single needle puncture suffices for both antegrade pyelography and access to the pelvicalyceal system. Ultrasound is used to place a 22-gauge needle in a calyx. This needle is then used to inject contrast material for antegrade pyelography and a 0.018-inch guidewire can be inserted through the needle for access into the pelvicalyceal system. Any calyx can be chosen for access. However, if a ureteric stent is to be placed, a mid-pole calyx or upper-pole calyx is preferable. Tract dilatation is usually easier than in the native kidney because of the decreased amount of tissue between the skin and the transplant kidney. The exception to the latter statement occurs in patients who have had

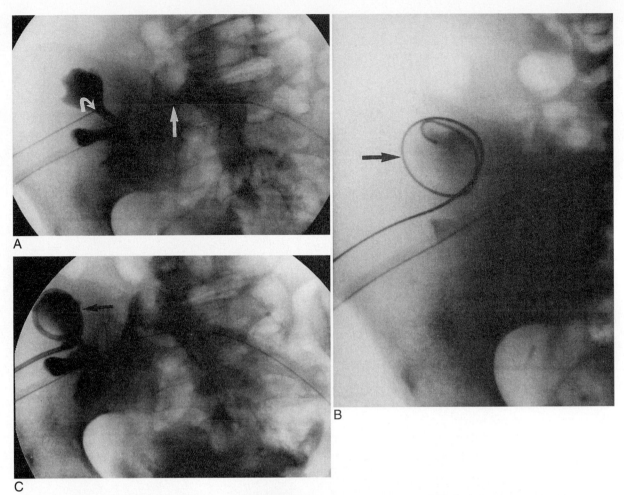

Figure 22-14 Percutaneous nephrostomy in a patient with a transplant kidney. The patient was noted to have a raised serum creatinine with hydronephrosis detected on ultrasound. **A,** A Tenchkoff catheter (straight arrow) can be seen *in situ.* Ultrasound determined that the upper-pole calyx was the largest calyx and ultrasound guidance was used to place a 22-gauge needle (curved arrow) into the upper-pole calyx. **B,** After placing the 5-Fr sheath over the 0.018-inch guidewire, a 0.35-inch "J" wire (arrow) was coiled in the upper-pole calyx. **C,** After track dilatation, an 8-Fr nephrostomy catheter (arrow) was placed in the upper-pole calyx. The hydronephrosis was due to ureteric ischemia.

more than one transplant kidney placed in the same area. Then there may be quite extensive fibrotic tissue which makes dilatation very difficult. In some cases, it may not be possible to pass the sheath system over the 0.018-inch guidance. In these situations the author has used a 19-gauge long-dwell needle to make the initial puncture and inserted a superstiff guidewire to aid track dilatation. An 8-French nephrostomy tube is placed in a similar fashion to that described for percutaneous nephrostomy in a native kidney.

Retrograde Nephrostomy Drainage via an Ileal Loop

In the patient with an ileal loop who presents with obstructive uropathy, a retrograde approach to the ileal loop is worth considering for nephrostomy drainage (Fig. 22-15). The obstruction is usually due to recurrent tumor or stricture at the anastomotic site between the ureter and ileal loop. It is prudent to perform a loopogram first to document that there is no reflux of contrast medium from the ileal loop into the ureter. This helps to confirm the presence of obstruction. Additionally, if there is bulky tumor in the ileal loop it is best to perform the nephrostomy drainage from an antegrade approach.

The ostomy site is cannulated with a Kumpe catheter and straight or angled 0.035-inch hydrophilic guidewire. The Kumpe catheter and hydrophilic guidewire are manipulated to the end of the ileal loop. When the Kumpe catheter has reached the end of the ileal loop, the guidewire is removed and exchanged for a 0.035-inch superstiff or extra-stiff wire. A 9-French peel-away sheath is placed over the superstiff wire. The peel-away sheath will usually

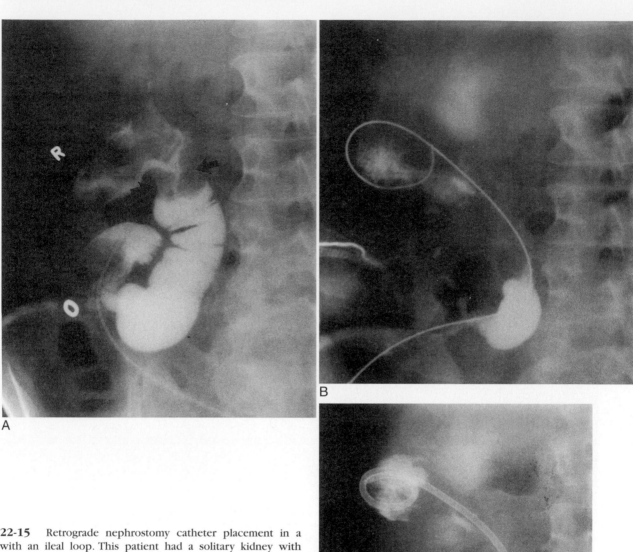

Figure 22-15   Retrograde nephrostomy catheter placement in a patient with an ileal loop. This patient had a solitary kidney with recurrent transitional cell cancer. **A**, A loopogram shows recurrent TCC at the anastomosis between the ileal conduit and the upper ureter (arrows). **B**, After manipulating a Kumpe catheter and a hydrophilic guidewire down the ileal loop towards the kidney, a superstiff guidewire was placed into the kidney which helped straighten out the ileal conduit for future catheter placement. A 9-Fr peel-away sheath was placed into the loop for added rigidity. **C**, An 8-Fr nephrostomy catheter was placed retrogradely into the kidney through the peel-away sheath and the end left in the ostomy bag for drainage. The patient survived for almost a year with this catheter in place.

reach the end of the ileal loop. This is the key step in the retrograde procedure. The 9-French peel-away sheath straightens out any tortuosity of the ileal loop and protects the guidewire and Kumpe catheter from peristalsis which, may cause the guidewire and Kumpe catheter to be extruded from the ileal loop. The Kumpe catheter is again placed over the superstiff wire and the latter is exchanged for a hydrophilic guidewire. The ureteric orifice is then sought using the Kumpe catheter and hydrophilic guidewire. It is helpful to inject contrast material because often a small nipple can be seen where the ureteric orifice arises. It is also helpful to review previous IVPs or loopograms which may guide you to the appropriate place to search for the ureteric orifice. Once the ureteric orifice is negotiated, the hydrophilic guidewire and Kumpe catheter, are manipulated up the ureter into the kidney. The hydrophilic guidewire is removed and the superstiff or extra-stiff guidewire placed up into the kidney.

Depending on the distance from the ostomy site to the renal pelvis, a nephrostomy catheter, an internal/external ureteral stent, or an internal ureteral stent can be placed. A rough estimate of the distance to be traversed can be gained by using the Kumpe catheter as a marker. An 8-French nephrostomy catheter can be placed, or, if the distance is longer, either internal or internal/external ureteral stents can be placed. Whichever catheter is placed, it is important to leave the end of the catheter in the patient's ostomy bag and not in the ileal loop. If the distal end of the catheter is left in the ileal loop, it will tend to clog rapidly. This is because the ileal loop sheds mucosal cells on a regular basis and the catheter side-holes will tend to become clogged with silt.

If it is not possible to negotiate the ureteric orifice, the patient can be turned prone and an antegrade nephrostomy performed (Box 22-3).

The Non-dilated Collecting System

Percutaneous nephrostomy in the non-dilated collecting system is technically difficult. This situation is most commonly encountered in patients with ureteric leaks after surgery. Percutaneous nephrostomy and/or stent placement is the preferred treatment but the collecting system will be decompressed because of the ureteric leak. On ultrasound the collecting system is usually decompressed and ultrasound guidance is not usually helpful. In this situation in the author's unit we give 50–75 mL of a 300% contrast material to opacify the pelvicalyceal system. When the pelvicalyceal system is opacified, an antegrade needle is inserted into the renal pelvis under fluoroscopic guidance. This needle is then used to distend the pelvicalyceal system and a calyx is chosen for

nephrostomy access. Because many of these patients will be having antegrade stents placed, a mid-pole calyx is preferable. A 22-gauge needle is placed into the mid-pole calyx and a 0.018-inch guidewire manipulated into the renal pelvis. It is important to keep the pelvicalyceal system distended by asking an assistant to maintain a steady injection of dilute contrast material into the pelvicalyceal system using the antegrade needle. This will often aid the passage of the 0.018-inch guidewire into the renal pelvis. Remember that the pelvicalyceal system is collapsed in these patients and optimal distension is important to facilitate the passage of a guidewire from the calyx to the renal pelvis. Once access is gained, the procedure can be performed in the traditional fashion.

CT-guided Nephrostomy Drainage

Rarely, CT guidance is necessary to gain access to the kidney. This almost exclusively occurs in patients with severe scoliosis who require a nephrostomy drainage (Fig. 22-16). It can be very difficult to assess the relationship of the kidney to adjacent organs in the severely scoliotic patient. Particularly, it is important to assess the relationship of the colon with the obstructed kidney in these patients. In addition, obstructed kidneys in the severely scoliotic patients can be difficult to identify with ultrasound and it can be extremely difficult to work out the relationships of the kidney with adjacent organs on ultrasound.

The patient is placed supine or prone on the CT table and a non-contrast CT through the kidneys is performed. The patient is then placed in the position which best facilitates access to the kidney. Under CT guidance, either a 22-gauge needle can be placed into the renal pelvis as an antegrade needle for opacifying the pelvicalyceal system, or a 22-gauge needle can be placed directly into a calyx and the patient transferred to fluoroscopy for the completion of the procedure. Either way, the anatomic relationship of the kidney with adjacent organs can be ascertained and a safe access route to the pelvicalyceal system planned.

Percutaneous Lithotripsy and Nephrolithotomy

Traditionally, staghorn calculi were removed surgically. However, from about 1980 onwards percutaneous nephrolithotomy became the procedure of first choice for the removal of large staghorn calculi and indeed for the removal of upper urinary tract calculi in many institutions. The subsequent introduction of extracorporeal shockwave lithotripsy (ESWL) reduced the number of indications for percutaneous nephrolithotomy but these are now well defined and commonly accepted. These include complete staghorn calculi and partial staghorn calculi or smaller renal calculi refractory to extracorporeal shockwave lithotripsy. In some institutions, renal

---

Box 22-3   Retrograde Ileal Loop Nephrostomy

Loopogram first to confirm obstruction
9-Fr peel-away sheath important to straighten out loop
Kumpe catheter and hydrophilic guidewire used to negotiate ureteric orifice
Leave distal end of catheter or stent in ostomy bag and not in ileal loop

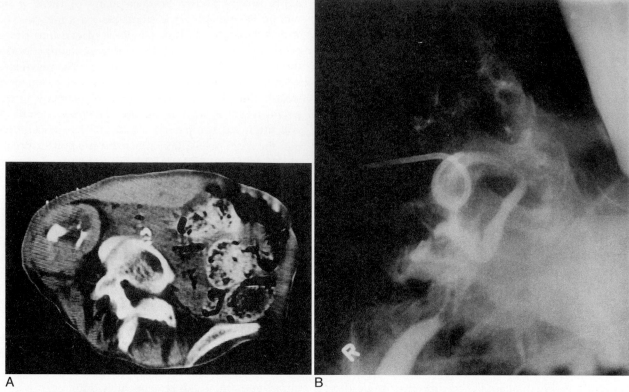

A   B

Figure 22-16 CT-guided nephrostomy drainage in a patient with severe scoliosis, renal stones and fever. **A**, CT guidance was used because of the severe scoliosis. A noncontrast CT was performed and a 22-gauge needle placed into the mid-pole calyx at CT. Note the radiopaque stones in the kidney. **B**, The patient was then moved to a fluoroscopic suite and an 8-Fr nephrostomy catheter was placed. The CT was useful to guide the initial needle puncture and to ensure that there were no intervening organs between the skin and the kidney.

stones in calyceal diverticula may also be managed by percutaneous nepthrolithotomy. In many instances, both techniques are used together for the larger staghorn calculi; if clearance is incomplete after percutaneous nephrolithotomy, ESWL is performed.

Technique

Percutaneous nephrolithotomy consists of placing a large-bore track or tracks (up to 30-French) into the kidney for stone fragmentation (Fig. 22-17). Stone fragmentation is usually achieved with a rigid 24- to 26-French nephroscope. Because of the inflexibility of the nephroscope, it is vitally important to access the kidney proximal to the stone to be fragmented. In other words, peripheral access into a calyx is vital. The nephroscope looks straight ahead and can only fragment stones in front of it. Although smaller flexible scopes can be used to enter individual calyces, this is a more tedious procedure. Close cooperation between the urologist and interventional radiologist is mandatory for appropriate track placement. In patients with large staghorn calculi, it may be necessary to place as many as two to three large-bore

tracks into the kidney. In some centers the track is created and a 24-French catheter left *in situ* for 1–2 days after which the patient is brought to the operating room for stone removal. The advantage of using this technique is that any bleeding that occurs during track preparation has usually cleared after 1–2 days and a clear view of the stone will be available at the time of stone fragmentation. Others prefer to perform the whole procedure in one sitting in which track preparation is performed and a large 30-French sheath inserted into the kidney. The patient is then transferred to the operating room where a nephroscope is inserted and the stone fragmented. Although we initially used the two-stage procedure, we now prefer a one-stage procedure. The disadvantage of the two-stage procedure is that the large 24-French catheter in the kidney is quite painful over the intervening days until surgical removal of the stone.

In general, the procedure can be performed almost entirely under fluoroscopic guidance. A 22-gauge antegrade needle is placed directly down on top of the stone in the renal pelvis. After the antegrade needle is placed urine is aspirated. If the urine appears cloudy or infected, then a simple nephrostomy tube is placed to allow drainage and appropriate antibiotic therapy started. It is imperative not to proceed with large track formation into the kidney in the presence of infection. This can lead to profound septic shock and occasionally disseminated intravascular coagulation. If the urine is clear, track preparation is performed. An appropriate calyx is chosen that will yield the maximum stone clearance from the pelvicalyceal system. In some instances, two or even three tracks may be required for this purpose.

A one-stick system (Neff Set, Cook, Bloomington, IN; Acustick, Meditech, Watertown, MA) is inserted into the peripheral portion of the calyx chosen. The 0.018-inch wire is then manipulated into the renal pelvis. To aid passage of the 0.018-inch wire into the renal pelvis, it is invaluable to have an assistant inject dilute contrast material through the antegrade needle to distend the collecting system and allow some space to develop between the stone and the surrounding uroepithelium. This will facilitate passage of the guidewire into the renal pelvis. If the 0.018-inch guidewire cannot be manipulated into the renal pelvis, access to the calyx is maintained

and a Kumpe catheter and hydrophilic guidewire used to gain access to the renal pelvis. Once access to the renal pelvis is gained, the Kumpe catheter and hydrophilic guidewire are used to access the ureter. The Kumpe catheter is placed down the ureter as far as the UV junction or into the bladder. The hydrophilic guidewire is then exchanged for a 0.035-inch superstiff guidewire (Meditech, Watertown, MA). The percutaneous track is then ready to be dilated.

The track can be dilated in two ways. The track can be dilated with serial fascial dilators from 8- to 30-French or by using a balloon catheter (10 mm × 10 cm). The author prefers to use the stated balloon catheter for track dilatation as it is much faster and you are less liable to kink the guidewire. Usually a waist will be seen in the balloon at the renal capsule and it is important to inflate the balloon until this waist disappears. During balloon dilatation any persistent waist that is seen that does not disappear despite increased inflation pressure implies that the percutaneous track will have to be dilated with larger fascial dilators such as 26- and 28-French for complete track dilatation. After balloon dilatation, a 30-French Amplatz

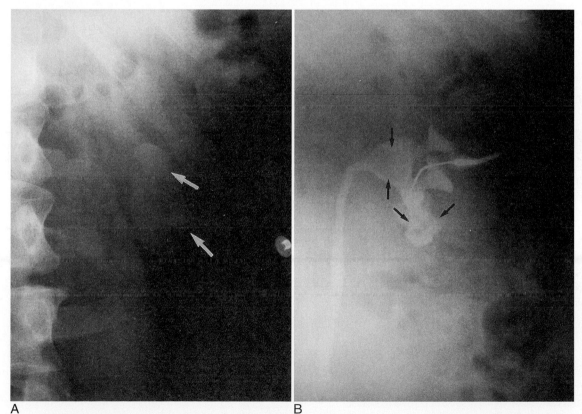

A   B

Figure 22-17 Percutaneous nephrolithotomy in a patient with uric acid stones in the left kidney. **A,** The plain film shows two stones (arrows) in the left kidney, one in the renal pelvis and one in a lower-pole calyx. **B,** An antegrade nephrostogram was performed where stones can be seen (arrows) as filling defects in the contrast medium column.   (*Continued*)

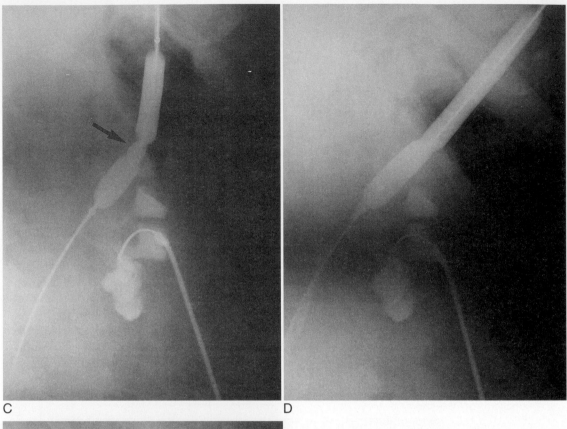

C

D

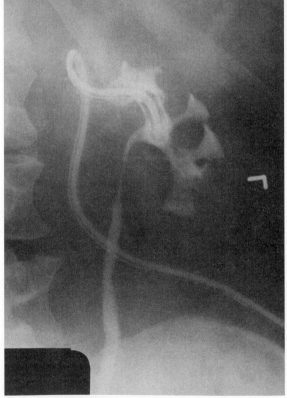

E

Figure 22-17   cont'd C, An upper-pole access was chosen to ensure complete removal of both stones. After access was gained down the ureter, a 1-cm balloon was used to dilate the percutaneous track. Note the waist in the balloon at the level of the renal cortex (arrow). **D,** The balloon was further inflated and the waist disappeared. After the balloon was removed, a 30-Fr Amplatz sheath and dilator was inserted over the superstiff wire. We usually place a second safety guidewire down the ureter and place a small balloon catheter in the upper ureter to prevent stone fragments from going down the ureter. **E,** Nephrostogram performed 24 hours after nephrolithotomy in the operating room shows that the stones have been completely removed. There is a little narrowing of the upper ureter due to edema. This settled spontaneously and the catheter was removed after 2 weeks.

sheath (Cook, Bloomington, IN) is placed over the guidewire into the renal pelvis. A second safety wire is placed down the ureter and a small balloon catheter (4–6 mm in diameter) inflated in the upper ureter to prevent stone migration. Alternatively, the balloon catheter can be inserted retrogradely at cystoscopy into the upper ureter. The patient is transferred to the operating room and the stones fragmented using either, ultrasonic lithotripsy, electrohydraulic lithotripsy, or laser lithotripsy.

In the author's unit we use ultrasonic lithotripsy under direct endoscopic visualization. Stone fragments are washed back out through the sheath using a high-flow irrigation system that is connected to the nephroscope. At the end of the procedure, a 26-French Foley balloon catheter or Malecot catheter is placed in the renal pelvis for a period of 2–3 weeks after the procedure. If there are remaining stone fragments, ESWL can be performed during this period. Two to three days after the procedure a nephrostogram is performed which helps to identify any remaining stone fragments and assess if there is any pelvicalyceal or ureteral damage. Stone fragments identified in the ureter may require further retrograde intervention. Remaining stones in the kidney can be shattered by ESWL. Renal pelvis perforation usually heals rapidly with a nephrostomy tube in place (Box 22-4).

Results

Percutaneous nephrolithotomy has proven very effective in the management of renal stones with low complication rates and results approaching those of open lithotomy. For large staghorn calculi, success rates for complete stone removal vary from 70% to approximately 90% in experienced hands. Success rates for complete removal of smaller pelvicalyceal stones are as high as 98%. Obviously, the size of the stone, location, the sitting of the percutaneous track, and the experience of the operators influence results. The main advantage of this technique over open lithotomy is that patients can return to their normal lifestyle and activities within a few days after the procedure.

Box 22-4   Percutaneous Nephrolithotomy

Access to the peripheral part of the calyx is vital
Many large tracks may be necessary depending on
  stone size
Do not proceed if infected urine is found
A 10 mm × 10 cm balloon is used for track dilatation
The entire procedure is performed in one sitting

Complications

The published complication rates for percutaneous nephrolithotomy approach 4%. The main complications are bleeding and sepsis. Bleeding may occur due to injury or laceration of a small segmental artery during track dilatation. This can be remedied by tamponading the track with a large nephrostomy catheter, or it may require angiographic embolization. Additionally, arteriovenous fistulas or arterial pseudoaneurysms may rarely occur and may require angiographic embolization.

Postprocedure sepsis occurs in up to 1% of patients. Patients with infected stones are obviously more prone to develop sepsis and it is important to look for indications of infection before the procedure. This includes ensuring that the patient does not have a fever before the procedure and that the white cell count and ESR are normal. Sepsis can occur even in patients who are adequately covered by antibiotics. In the author's experience, the subset of patients that can often have undetected infection are those with spina bifida. It is vitally important to aspirate and inspect the urine after antegrade needle placement. If there is any doubt as to whether the urine is infected or not, an immediate Gram stain should be performed before proceeding to track dilatation. If the urine is infected, then an 8-French nephrostomy catheter is placed and the patient placed on appropriate antibiotic therapy. When the urine is clear, track dilatation can commence.

Pneumothorax or hemothorax may rarely occur after percutaneous nephrolithotomy (Fig. 22-18). This complication is predisposed to by an upper-pole renal access. If an upper-pole renal access is performed, this complication should be anticipated and the appropriate catheters should be readily available for treatment.

Rarely, strictures of the ureteropelvic junction occur from injury at the time of ultrasonic, laser, or electrohydraulic lithotripsy. If this is recognised on the nephrostogram immediately after stone fragmentation, early antegrade stent placement will help to prevent the formation of a stricture.

Occasionally, foreign bodies may remain in the collecting system after percutaneous nephrolithotomy. They may include pieces of guidewires, baskets, or graspers. These are best removed endoscopically through the percutaneous track.

Percutaneous Stent Extraction

Rarely, ureteric stents cannot be removed at cystoscopy, owing either to marked encrustation or migration of the distal pigtail of the stent proximally up into the ureter. Access to the pelvicalyceal system is gained in the manner previously described for percutaneous nephrostomy and, depending on the size of the stent retained in the

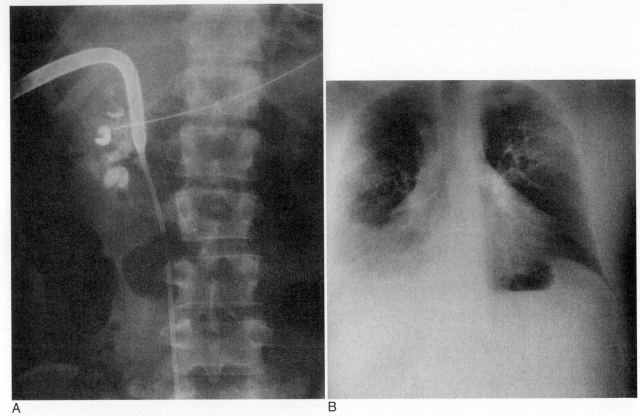

Figure 22-18   Hemothorax which occurred after placement of a percutaneous nephrolithotomy track. **A,** A two-stage procedure was performed on this patient with the placement of a large pyeloureteral stent using an upper-pole access. The patient was brought to the operating room the next day. **B,** In the recovery room after nephrolithotomy the patient became hypotensive and a chest x-ray performed showed a pleural effusion which was not there preoperatively. This was tapped and proved to be a hemothorax which is a known complication of upper-pole track formation. This was drained and the patient settled with conservative management.

ureter, an appropriate peel-away sheath is placed into the pelvicalyceal system (Fig. 22-19). If the ureteric stent is 6-French, then a 12- to 14-French peel-away sheath is placed; if the ureteric stent is 8-French, then a 14- to 16-French peel-away sheath is placed. It is useful to cut a 45-degree bevel in the end of the peel-away sheath as this will greatly aid stent engagement within the peel-away sheath. The peel-away sheath is placed into the renal pelvis as close as possible to the stent. Either a three-pronged grasper or a long alligator forceps are used to grasp the stent. The stent is then pulled through the peel-away sheath and delivered externally. It is not always possible to grasp the end of the stent and often the proximal portion of the stent is grasped. The stent then folds on itself while being pulled through the peel-away sheath. If insertion of another stent is required this can be performed through the peel-away sheath by placing a guidewire down into the bladder and placing an antegrade stent.

In a similar fashion, biopsy of suspected pelvicalyceal tumors can be performed through a peel-away sheath. A biopsy forceps can be placed through the peel-away sheath to biopsy pelvicalyceal lesions. This is rarely necessary as most patients with suspected urothelial tumors undergo retrograde biopsy or cell sampling of urine from the affected side.

URETERIC INTERVENTION

Antegrade Stent Placement

Antegrade stent placement is a well established percutaneous technique which evolved from the placement of percutaneous nephrostomy tubes. In the present day, an interventional radiologist may be called on to place an antegrade ureteric stent when retrograde stenting by the urologist fails. The usual indications are for malignant obstruction or occasionally benign disease such as strictures, stones, and ureteric leaks or fistulas.

Technique

The two key points in the procedure are:

- Getting appropriate access to the pelvicalyceal system;
- The use of a peel-away sheath.

A mid-pole access is the preferred access point for antegrade stent placement as there is a more direct route to the ureter. The peel-away sheath helps to direct the pushing force applied to the stent down the ureter rather than towards the medial wall of the renal pelvis (Fig. 22-20).

Access is gained to the kidney in the manner described for percutaneous nephrostomy. An antegrade needle is first placed and access to a mid-pole calyx is preferably achieved. Once the 5-French sheath from the one-stick system is in the renal pelvis, a "J" guidewire is placed in the renal pelvis and a Kumpe catheter placed over the guidewire. A straight or angled hydrophilic guidewire is then placed through the Kumpe catheter and directed down the ureter into the bladder. Once the Kumpe catheter is in the bladder, the hydrophilic guidewire is exchanged for a 0.035 inch Amplatz superstiff guidewire which is coiled in the bladder. The percutaneous track is dilated with 6- and 8-French dilators and the 9-French peel-away sheath is placed into the pelvicalyceal system with the tip of the peel-away sheath placed at the UPJ or just into the upper ureter. In the author's unit we use an 8-French stent (Meditech, Watertown, MA), which comes in 22-, 24-, 26-, and 28-cm lengths for patients with malignant ureteric obstruction. We tend to place a 6-French stent in patients with benign ureteric obstruction; a 22- or 24-cm length is suitable for the vast majority of average sized people. In general we place 22-cm stents in females and 24-cm stents in males of average height. Table 22-2 correlates stent length with patient height.

The stent system consists of an inner plastic cannula, a pusher catheter, and the stent (Fig. 22-21). A Nylon suture is attached to the proximal end of the stent. The stent is loaded over the inner plastic cannula so that the proximal end of the stent lies alongside the distal end

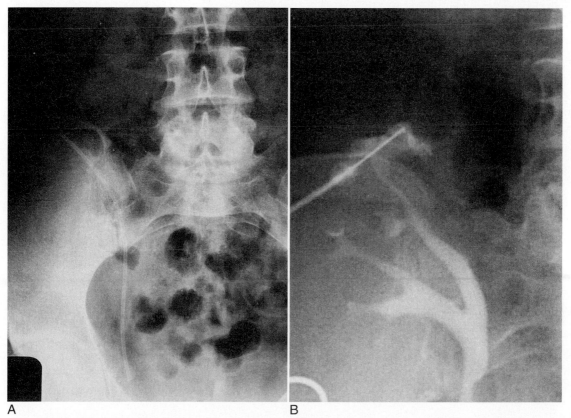

A   B

Figure 22-19 Percutaneous stent extraction in a patient with a transplant kidney in whom a ureteric stent was placed. The distal end of the stent was cut before placement because the stent was too long. The stent migrated proximally in the ureter and could not be retrieved retrogradely. **A**, Plain radiograph showing the stent *in situ*. Note the distal pigtail has been cut. **B**, Antegrade needle placed in upper-pole calyx under ultrasound guidance. *(Continued)*

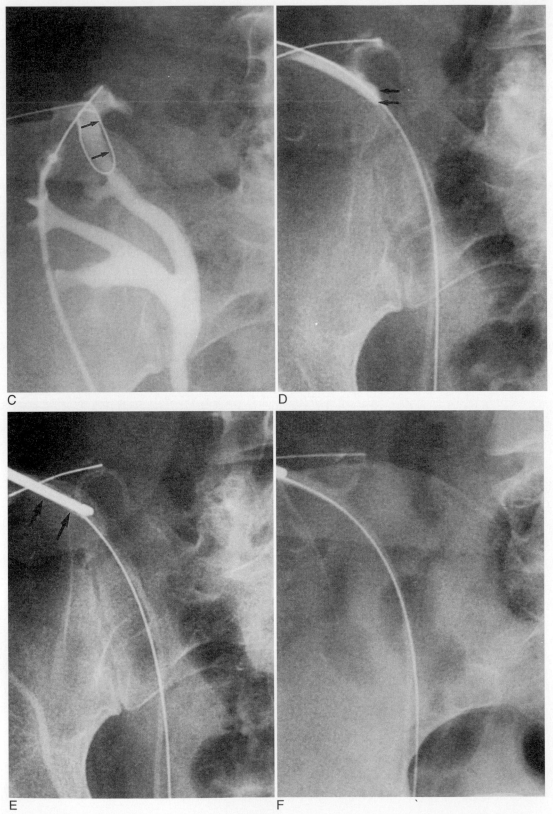

C

D

E

F

Figure 22-19   cont'd C, Upper-pole access gained using a 22-gauge needle and 0.018-inch guidewire (arrows). Note the antegrade needle is used to distend this unobstructed collecting system for guidewire manipulations. **D**, A track was dilated and a 12-Fr peel-away sheath inserted with a 45-degree bevel cut at its distal end (arrows). A small alligator forceps (arrows) was used to grasp the 6-Fr stent near its proximal end. **F**, The stent was doubled over on itself and removed. A nephrostomy catheter was left *in situ* for 2 days.

Table 22-2	Length of Ureteric Stent Required for Various Patient Heights

Height (cm)	Stent Length (cm)
<178	22
178—193	24
>193	26

Modified from Seymour H, Patel U: Ureteric stenting: current status. *Semin Interv Radiol* 17(4):361, 2000.

Box 22-5   Antegrade Stent Insertion

Access via a mid-pole calyx is best

A 9-Fr peel-away sheath helps direct the stent down the ureter

Tight obstructions are crossed with a Kumpe catheter and hydrophilic guidewire

A Van Andel catheter can be used to dilate tight obstructions before stent placement

A nephrostomy is left *in situ* for 48 hours *only* if the procedure is traumatic

---

of the pusher catheter. The pusher catheter is usually loaded onto the inner plastic cannula by the manufacturer. The distal end of the pusher catheter has a metallic marker which marks the proximal end of the stent for stent placement. The whole assembly is placed over the superstiff guidewire and inserted down the ureter into the bladder. The stent is placed in the bladder until the marker on the distal end of the pusher catheter is in the renal pelvis. The guidewire and plastic inner cannula are removed, leaving the pusher catheter and the stent through the peel-away sheath. The Nylon suture in the proximal stent is pulled to form the proximal loop. The distal loop forms automatically once the guidewire and plastic inner cannula are removed. With a little to-and-fro motion and gentle tugging on the Nylon suture, the proximal pigtail loop forms in the renal pelvis (Figs 22-22 and 22-23).

If there has been bleeding and there is clot in the collecting system, leave a nephrostomy catheter *in situ*. This is simply placed through the peel-away sheath into the renal pelvis without using a guidewire. The nephrostomy catheter can be removed after 24–48 hours when the clot has cleared from the pelvicalyceal system. If, on the other hand, the procedure has been relatively atraumatic, the peel-away sheath can simply be removed without placing a nephrostomy catheter. If the stents are for long-term drainage they are usually changed cystoscopically at 3–6 monthly intervals depending on the referring urologist (Box 22-5).

Commonly Encountered Problems

Inappropriate Pelvicalyceal Access

Occasionally a nephrostomy catheter will already be *in situ* when you are asked to place an antegrade stent. The nephrostomy catheter may have been placed at another institution and is often placed through a lower-pole calyx. Lower-pole calyceal access usually results in a more difficult angle of entry towards the upper ureter. It also means that any pushing force applied to the stent will tend to be directed towards the roof of the renal pelvis rather than down the ureter (see Fig. 22-20).

An extra-stiff or superstiff guidewire and a 9-French peel-away sheath placed into the upper ureter will make stent insertion much easier. However, the problem can be avoided altogether by using a mid-pole access where possible.

Tortuous Ureter

Many pelviureteric systems that are obstructed have kinks or tortuosities in the mid or upper ureter. These can be difficult to negotiate, but the use of a Kumpe catheter and guidewire greatly facilitates negotiation of these kinks (Fig. 22-24). If it is not possible to negotiate ureteric kinks using a Kumpe catheter and hydrophilic guidewire, then draining the system for 2–3 days reduces the amount of dilatation and often helps in the successful negotiation of these ureteric kinks.

Stent Assembly Malfunction

Initially the author's unit had problems with the proximal end of the stent becoming engaged in the distal end of the pusher catheter. This happens particularly with stent systems that do not have a metallic marker on the end of the pusher catheter. Particularly, in patients with tight obstructions, considerable force may be necessary to pass the stent through the obstruction. This sometimes results in the pusher catheter becoming engaged in the proximal end of the stent. Using a peel-away sheath helps to avoid this problem, and passing a Van Andel catheter through the stricture beforehand will also facilitate passage of the stent. Also, using stent systems with a metallic marker on the distal end of the pusher system is important, because not only does it facilitate ready identification of the proximal end of the stent, but it also helps to prevent engagement of the pusher catheter with the proximal end of the stent.

Difficulty Forming the Proximal Pigtail Loop

Occasionally, the proximal pigtail may be released from the inner plastic cannula and pusher catheter in the proximal ureter rather than in the renal pelvis. If this happens the proximal pigtail will not form as it has insufficient space in the ureter. The stent can be pulled back into the renal pelvis by using the Nylon suture

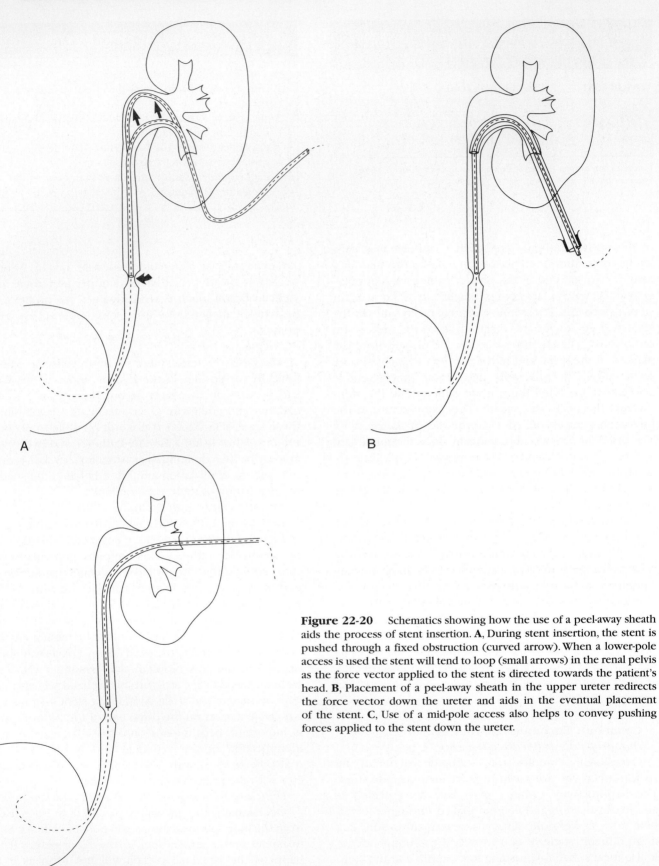

Figure 22-20 Schematics showing how the use of a peel-away sheath aids the process of stent insertion. **A,** During stent insertion, the stent is pushed through a fixed obstruction (curved arrow). When a lower-pole access is used the stent will tend to loop (small arrows) in the renal pelvis as the force vector applied to the stent is directed towards the patient's head. **B,** Placement of a peel-away sheath in the upper ureter redirects the force vector down the ureter and aids in the eventual placement of the stent. **C,** Use of a mid-pole access also helps to convey pushing forces applied to the stent down the ureter.

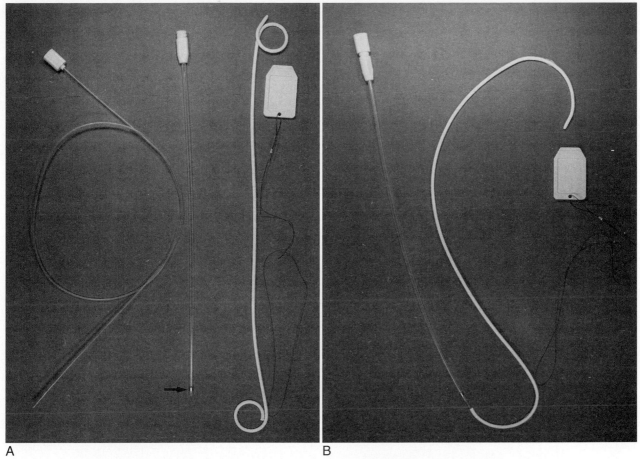

A B

Figure 22-21 An 8-Fr ureteral stent. **A**, The stent assembly comprises a stent (*right*), a pusher catheter (*middle*), and a plastic stiffening cannula (*left*). The inner plastic stiffening cannula and pusher catheter are inserted through the proximal end of the stent. Note the metallic marker (arrow) on the end of the pusher catheter which marks the proximal end of the stent. The strings on the proximal end of the stent are used to form the proximal pigtail and/or reposition the proximal end of the stent if needed. (Note the 6-Fr stent does not have a plastic stiffening cannula). In general we place the 8-Fr stent for malignant ureteric obstructions and the 6-Fr stent for patients with stone disease. **B**, The 8-Fr stent assembly is fitted together by placing the plastic stiffening cannula through the pusher catheter and stent.

which is attached to the proximal end of the stent. Sometimes when the Nylon sutures are used to do this, the proximal end of the stent may flip into a mid- or lower-pole calyx. This can be avoided by using the peel-away sheath as an anchor to fix the proximal end of the stent while traction is applied to the Nylon suture.

Tight Ureteric Obstruction

If the ureteric obstruction is felt to be tight, difficulty may be encountered in negotiating the ureteric obstruction with a hydrophilic guidewire or Kumpe catheter. The author's unit has found that the vast majority of obstructions can be bypassed by using a Kumpe catheter and hydrophilic guidewire in the first sitting. Rarely, we may leave the patient to decompress for 1–2 days and reattempt negotiation of the ureteric obstruction.

A more significant problem is the passage of the 8-French stent through the tight ureteric obstruction. This can be facilitated by passing a Van Andel catheter to predilate a track through the ureteric obstruction. The Van Andel catheter has a long tapered distal end which facilitates this process. Use of the peel-away sheath also helps to direct the force applied to the pusher catheter and stent down the ureter so that more leverage is obtained. Rarely is predilatation of the stricture with a balloon catheter necessary. If the stricture is very tight, a 6-French stent can be used.

An Empty Bladder

Many patients referred for antegrade stent insertion will have bladder catheters *in situ*. Manipulation of guidewires and catheters in the empty bladder is painful

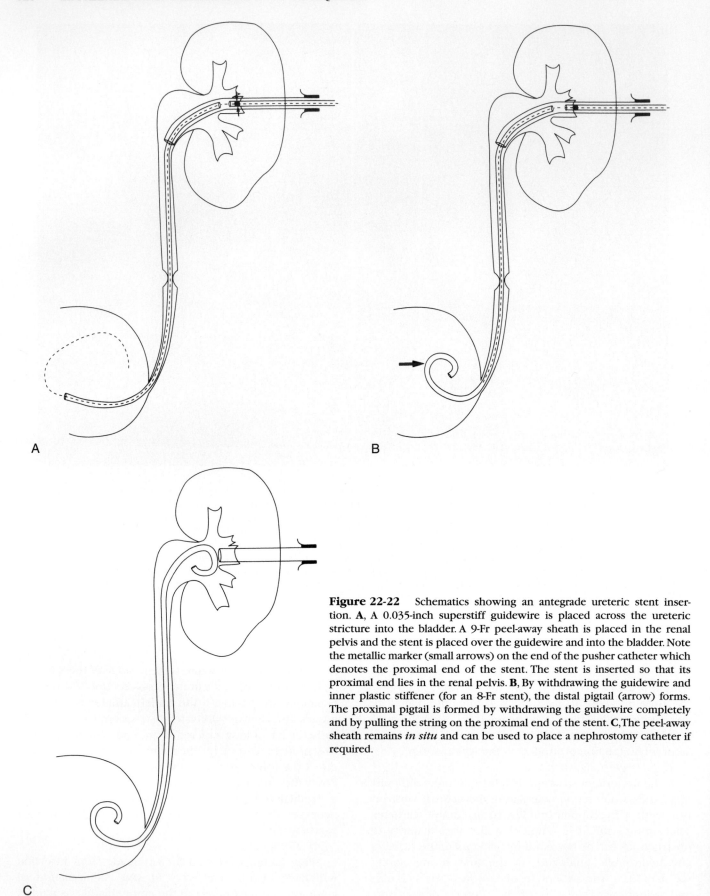

A

B

C

Figure 22-22 Schematics showing an antegrade ureteric stent insertion. **A,** A 0.035-inch superstiff guidewire is placed across the ureteric stricture into the bladder. A 9-Fr peel-away sheath is placed in the renal pelvis and the stent is placed over the guidewire and into the bladder. Note the metallic marker (small arrows) on the end of the pusher catheter which denotes the proximal end of the stent. The stent is inserted so that its proximal end lies in the renal pelvis. **B,** By withdrawing the guidewire and inner plastic stiffener (for an 8-Fr stent), the distal pigtail (arrow) forms. The proximal pigtail is formed by withdrawing the guidewire completely and by pulling the string on the proximal end of the stent. **C,** The peel-away sheath remains *in situ* and can be used to place a nephrostomy catheter if required.

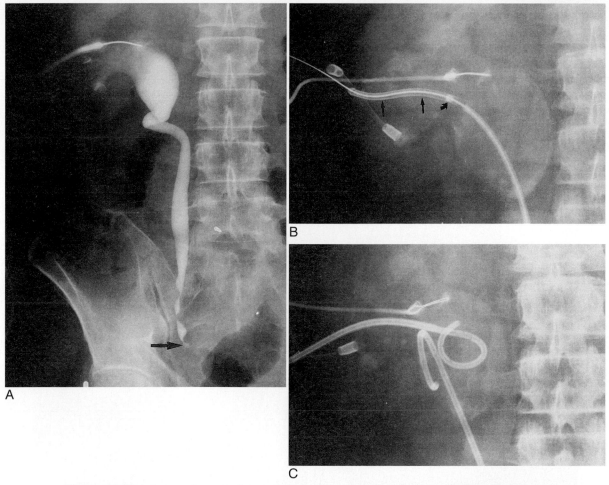

Figure 22-23 Antegrade ureteral stent insertion in a patient with an obstructing stone in the lower ureter and a failed attempt at retrograde stent insertion because the ureter had been reimplanted some years earlier. **A,** Antegrade pyelography shows a tortuous ureter with a dilated collecting system down to the level of the stone (arrow) in the lower ureter. **B,** Using mid-pole calyceal access, an antegrade stent was inserted through a peel-away sheath (straight arrows). The metallic marker (curved arrow) on the pusher catheter denotes the proximal end of the stent. **C,** By withdrawing the guidewire the distal pigtail forms in the bladder. Withdrawing the guidewire further and pulling on the string attached to the stent forms the proximal pigtail. Because of the hemorrhage in the collecting system a pigtail nephrostomy catheter was left *in situ* for 2 days. The pigtail catheter was simply inserted through the peel-away sheath without using a guidewire.

and also difficult. Clamping the bladder catheter before the procedure, or putting 100 mL of dilute contrast into the bladder via the Kumpe catheter is useful to circumvent this problem (Fig. 22-25).

Results

Use of an appropriate mid-pole access and a peel-away sheath, results in a success rate approaching 100% for antegrade stent placement. In a study by Lu and associates, use of the peel-away sheath resulted in a 96% success rate compared to 81% when a peel-away sheath was not used. The 3-month and 6-month patency rates in this study were 95% and 54%, respectively. Newer stents are now available with hydrophilic coating which should make negotiation of tighter strictures easier and should increase the technical success rate. The author's experience with these newer stents is as yet limited.

Complications

Complications are similar to those seen with percutaneous nephrostomy. The author's unit has encountered a number of cases of renal pelvic perforation particularly without the use of the peel-away sheath when the force applied to the stent may be directed towards the medial

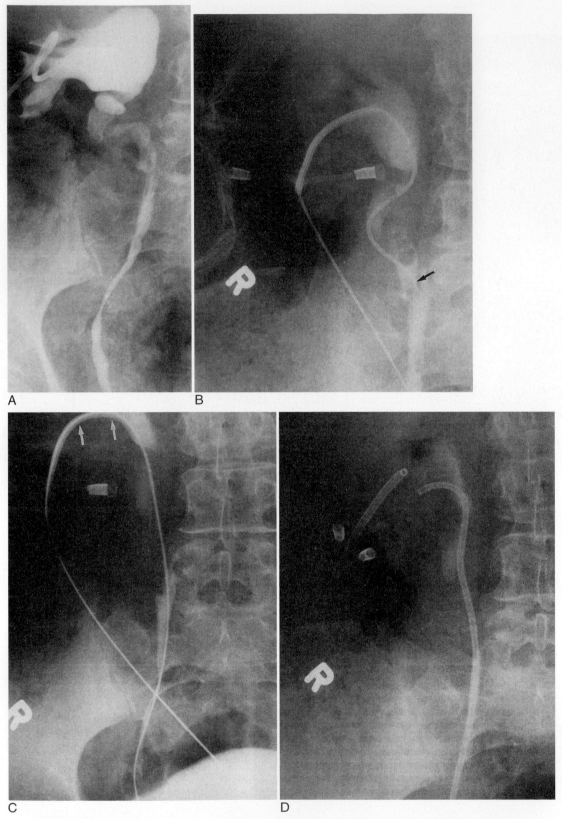

Figure 22-24   Tortuous ureter. **A**, A tortuous upper ureter was noted in this patient who required an antegrade stent because of pelvic malignancy. **B**, Using a Kumpe catheter (arrow) and hydrophilic guidewire, the upper ureter was negotiated without difficulty. **C**, Placement of a superstiff guidewire into the bladder straightened the tortuosity for eventual stent placement. Note the peel-away sheath bridging the percutaneous track into the upper ureter (arrows). **D**, An 8-Fr antegrade stent was inserted without difficulty. A nephrostomy catheter was not left *in situ* because of the relatively atraumatic nature of the stent placement.

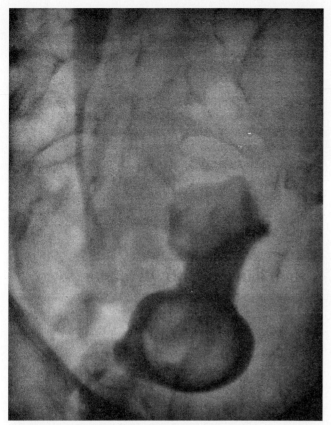

Figure 22-25 The empty bladder. Many patients referred for antegrade ureteric stent placement will have bladder catheters *in situ* as in this patient. It is important to clamp the Foley catheter and fill the bladder either antegradely or retrogradely with some dilute contrast material to allow room for guidewires, etc., to coil within the bladder.

wall of the renal pelvis and not down the ureter. This usually resolves with percutaneous drainage and has not posed a significant problem.

Balloon Dilatation of Ureteric Strictures

Usually benign ureteric strictures occur after instrumentation for stone disease. Ureteric strictures can be dilated antegradely or retrogradely. If the retrograde route is not possible or has failed, you may be asked to dilate the ureteric stricture from an antegrade approach. First, a percutaneous nephrostomy is performed as described previously. Using a Kumpe catheter and hydrophilic guidewire, access through the stricture is gained and the catheter manipulated into the bladder. The hydrophilic guidewire is exchanged for a 0.035-inch superstiff guidewire and a 6- or 8-mm balloon manipulated over the guidewire and across the stricture (Fig. 22-26). The balloon is inflated until the waist disappears on the balloon, and is left inflated for approximately 2 minutes. It is then deflated and removed. A 9-French peel-away

sheath is placed down as far as the ureteropelvic junction and an 8-French stent placed antegradely across the stricture into the bladder, as described previously.

Results of balloon dilatation of ureteric strictures have shown a limited success rate. Quoted long-term success rates vary from approximately 50 to 70%. It is undoubtedly worth a trial in the first instance as the alternative may involve ureteric reimplantation or some other urologic operation.

Ureteral Occlusion

Ureteral occlusion is occasionally performed in patients with malignant strictures of the ureter associated with severe ureteric bleeding episodes, or occlusion may be indicated in patients with underlying malignancy and ureteral or vesical fistulas. Percutaneous nephrostomy is performed in the usual fashion and a Kumpe catheter and hydrophilic guidewire manipulated down the ureter. The catheter is positioned just above the malignant stricture. Many different agents have been used for ureteral occlusion, including coils, Gelfoam and glue. In the author's unit we use a combination of coils and glue. The ureter can be packed with coils and glue through the Kumpe catheter which is an end-hole type (Fig. 22-27). In this manner the ureter can be completely occluded. Obviously, the patients will have an indwelling nephrostomy catheter for the remainder of their lives.

Endopyelotomy

Traditionally, the gold standard for treatment of ureteropelvic junction (UPJ) obstruction has been open pyeloplasty. Quoted success rates for this procedure are in the region of 90%. More recently, with the more widespread use and interest in minimally invasive techniques, antegrade and retrograde methods have been described for treating UPJ obstruction without the need for open surgery (Fig. 22-28). These techniques consist of either antegrade or retrograde balloon dilatation, or more recently, antegrade or retrograde techniques that produce a longitudinal full-thickness cut in the ureter. It is well known that such a cut in the ureter will cause regeneration of normal uroepithelium to bridge the defect, while minimizing damage to the ureteral blood supply.

If antegrade balloon dilatation is performed, a percutaneous nephrostomy is undertaken, as described previously. Access is gained to the renal pelvis and a short Cobra catheter is used to cross the UPJ with the help of a hydrophilic guidewire. The Kumpe catheter does not have enough rigidity for use in the capacious renal pelvis. An oversized balloon catheter is then placed across the UPJ and inflated until extravasation of contrast material occurs. The idea behind balloon dilatation is that disruption of the ureter and extravasation of contrast material

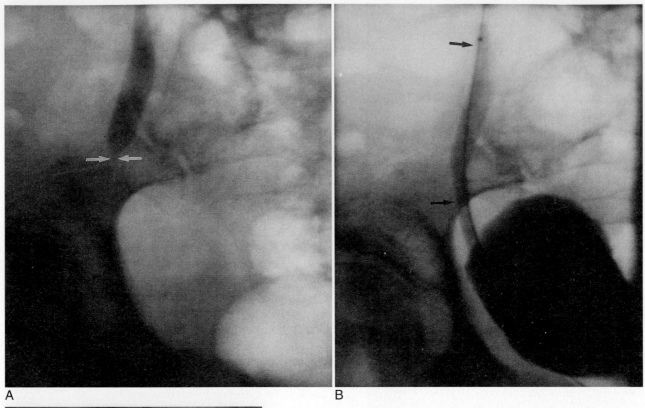

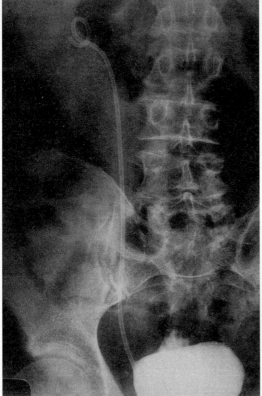

Figure 22-26   Ureteric stricture dilatation. **A**, This patient had ureteric instrumentation for removal of a ureteric stone and developed a stricture (arrows) in the lower ureter. This was approximately 8 cm in length. **B**, A percutaneous nephrostomy was performed and a 6 mm × 8 cm balloon (arrows) was used to dilate the stricture in the lower ureter. **C**, An 8-Fr stent was placed at the end of the procedure and left *in situ* for 3 months. The patient made an uneventful recovery and did not require surgery.

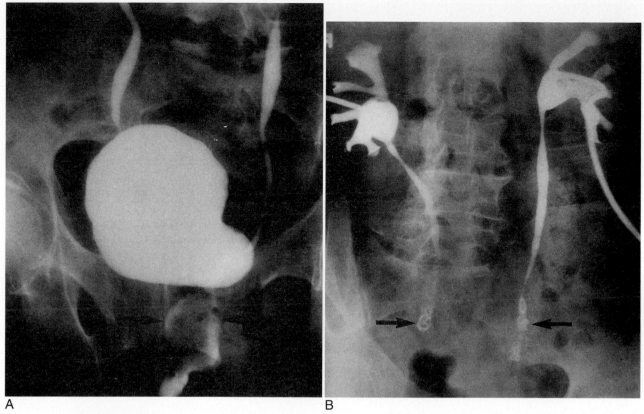

A   B

Figure 22-27   Ureteral occlusion in a patient with an inoperable pelvic malignancy and a vesi-covaginal fistula. The patient was uncomfortable because of a constant urine leak. **A,** IVP shows the leak (arrows) from the bladder into the vagina. **B,** Bilateral nephrostomy catheters were placed and both ureters occluded with a mixture of coils and glue (arrows). This completely dried up the vesicovaginal fistula and the patient had bilateral nephrostomy catheters for her remaining days. The patient succumbed 2 months after the procedure.

must be seen before the procedure is terminated. An antegrade stent is then placed in the bladder. The particular stent placed has a 14-French proximal end which lies across the UPJ and an 8-French terminal portion which resides in the bladder. The stent is left *in situ* for 3 months, after which it is removed.

More recently ureteral cutting balloons have been developed which result in simultaneous balloon dilatation and incision of the ureteropelvic junction. Again, this technique can be performed either retrogradely or antegradely. It is important before using a cutting balloon to ensure that there are no crossing blood vessels adjacent to the UPJ. This is usually accomplished by performing a preprocedure CT scan. After access to the ureter is gained in either retrograde or antegrade fashion, the cutting balloon catheter is placed across the UPJ, the cutting wire is placed in a posterolateral position, and an endopyelotomy is performed by simultaneously inflating the balloon and activating the cutting wire. The current is continuously applied to the cutting wire until the

waist on the balloon disappears. The balloon is then left inflated for 1–2 minutes before removal. Again, it is important to leave a 14-French/8-French internal stent across the ureteropelvic junction.

Overall results using cutting balloon catheters approach those of open pyeloplasty. While this technique is still in its infancy, it shows great promise for the treatment of this condition.

BLADDER INTERVENTION

Suprapubic Cystostomy

Suprapubic cystostomy is often used for providing bladder decompression in patients with acute urinary retention. Small-bore 10-French catheters are usually placed by trocar technique and are very effective for the relief of urinary retention where transurethral catherization has failed or is contraindicated. Long-term bladder

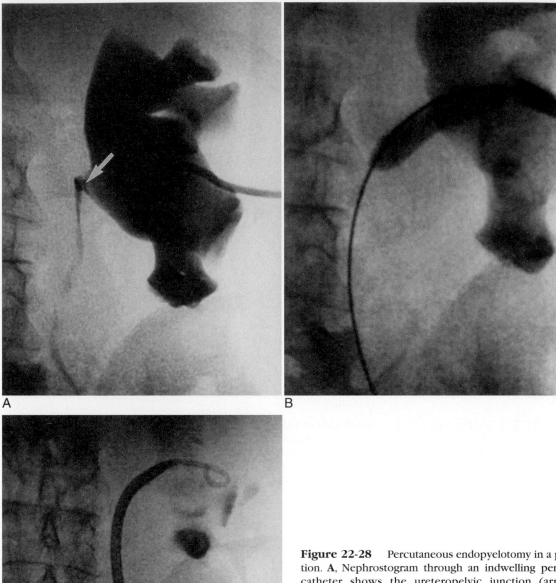

A

B

C

Figure 22-28   Percutaneous endopyelotomy in a patient with UPJ obstruction. **A**, Nephrostogram through an indwelling percutaneous nephrostomy catheter shows the ureteropelvic junction (arrow) obstruction. **B**, A 10 mm × 4 cm balloon was placed across the UPJ and inflated until the waist disappeared. **C**, A stent was inserted across the UPJ, after dilatation. The stent used tapered from 14-Fr in its upper end to 8-Fr in its lower end. The stent was removed after 3 months. Follow-up at 1 year shows no evidence of recurrence.

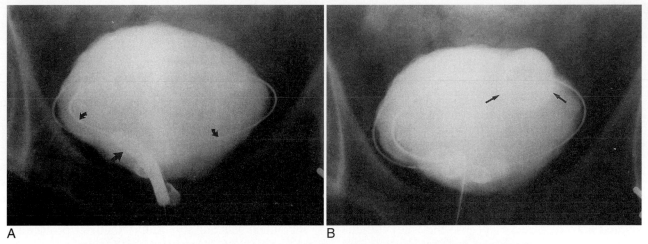

Figure 22-29 Suprapubic cystostomy in a patient who required a long-term bladder catheter. **A,** After gaining access to the bladder using a right paramedian needle puncture, a 0.038-inch super-stiff wire (curved arrows) was inserted into the bladder and coiled. Tract dilatation was performed with a 7-mm balloon catheter after which a 22-Fr peel-away sheath (straight arrow) was placed into the bladder. **B,** A 24-Fr Foley catheter was inserted over the guidewire through the peel-away sheath and into the bladder. Contrast material (arrows) can be seen in the Foley balloon. This is only for the purpose of documenting that the catheter is in the bladder. The balloon is emptied of contrast material and refilled with saline.

drainage can also be achieved by the use of suprapubic catheters. Large-bore catheters (16-French or greater) are necessary for long-term drainage as the small-bore catheters tend to block easily. Traditionally, suprapubic bladder catheters for long-term drainage have been placed in the operating room under general or regional anesthesia. More recently, radiologic suprapubic placement of bladder catheters has been described as an effective alternative to the operative procedure (Fig. 22-29).

Indication

The most common patients referred for long-term suprapubic cystostomy include those with bladder neck outflow obstruction from prostatic hypertrophy or prostatic cancer, where surgery is either not possible or contraindicated. Patients with neurogenic bladders form the second largest patient referral group. Rarely, in the author's unit we have performed percutaneous suprapubic cystostomy for patients with urethral trauma, radiation cystitis, vesicocolonic or vesicovaginal fistula, urinary incontinence, and pyocystis.

Technique

The procedure is performed in the radiology department on a standard fluoroscopy table. Local anesthesia and intravenous sedoanalgesia (mizadolam and fentanyl) are used. The patient is placed supine on the fluoroscopy table and the bladder filled with dilute contrast medium. Bladder filling can be achieved either by a transurethral Foley if present, or by placing a 20-gauge spinal needle into

the bladder under ultrasound guidance if a transurethral Foley catheter cannot be placed. The bladder needs to be filled almost to capacity to displace loops of small bowel out of the pelvis.

An 18-gauge sheath needle or a one-stick needle is placed into the bladder in a vertical, paramedian position, approximately 2–3 cm above the pubic symphysis. It is important to use ultrasound to guide the needle into the bladder to make sure that no small bowel loops lie between the bladder and the needle puncture site on the anterior abdominal wall. This is particularly important for patients with small-capacity bladders which may not distend very well. A 0.035-inch superstiff guidewire is then coiled in the bladder and the percutaneous track is dilated. The percutaneous track can be dilated with sequential fascial dilators, but the author prefers to use a balloon catheter for dilatation. The advantage of using the balloon catheter is that it is a single-stage dilatation and is less painful than using the sequential dilators. Additionally, the guidewire is less likely to kink during dilatation. The balloon catheter used is $7\,cm \times 7\,mm$ (Meditech, Watertown, MA). The balloon is inflated until the waist disappears and is left inflated for 3 minutes. The balloon catheter is then removed and a peel-away sheath placed over the superstiff guidewire into the bladder. The peel-away sheath should be two French sizes larger than the proposed Foley catheter to be placed (Box 22-6). Foley catheters between 16- and 20-French are appropriate for long-term bladder drainage and these are placed over the guidewire, through the peel-away

Box 22-6   Suprapubic Cystostomy

Distend the bladder well and use ultrasound to make sure no bowel loops are adjacent to puncture site

A balloon catheter (7 mm × 70 mm) is used for track dilatation

The peel-away sheath used should be two French sizes larger than the chosen Foley catheter

Patients are placed on long-term trimethoprim and sulphamethoxazole

sheath and into the bladder. Because the Foley catheter has no end-hole either, the tip of the Foley catheter can be cut or a 15-gauge needle can be inserted through one of the distal side-holes and out through the tip of the Foley catheter, through which the guidewire can be loaded retrogradely through the Foley catheter. The Foley balloon is inflated with 5 mL of saline and the peel-away sheath finally removed. The catheter is pulled snugly against the anterior abdominal wall for catheter fixation. There is no need for skin fixation devices or sutures.

Results

In the author's unit we have found that a single-stage suprapubic catheter insertion is not possible in two groups of patients. In obese patients or patients with extensive midline scarring, it is difficult to dilate an appropriate track in a one-stage procedure. In these patients, we place a 10- or 12-French nephrostomy catheter into the bladder after initially dilating the track with fascial dilators. Two or three weeks later when the existing track is mature, we bring the patient back for track dilatation with a 7-mm diameter balloon. At this stage the track is usually easily dilated and an 18- or 20-French Foley catheter can be placed.

The success rate for percutaneous suprapubic cystostomy approaches 100%, comparing very favorably with surgical cystostomy. Two-stage procedures may be required for some patients as described above. Long-term efficacy is also excellent with appropriate catheter care. Percutaneous suprapubic cystostomy can be performed on an outpatient basis, but follow-up care is important. Long-term bladder catheters are associated with an increased risk of infection and stone formation. Patients should therefore remain on low-dose trimethoprim/sulfamethoxazole to prevent bladder infection. Catheter exchange is performed every 2–3 months. This can be performed at the bedside or in the doctor's office once the percutaneous track is mature. The existing Foley balloon is deflated, the catheter removed, and a new catheter inserted through the existing track. This can be performed without the use of a guidewire.

Complications

Complications associated with percutaneous suprapubic cystostomy are minimal. Minor complications such as hematuria are extremely common but this is usually not significant and resolves spontaneously. Localized cellulitis at the skin site may occur but again is rare with good hygiene. Occasionally, treatment with systemic antibiotics may be required. One of the most feared complications is traversal of a small bowel loop by the catheter en route to the bladder. Attention to technique is important to prevent this complication. Adequate distension of the bladder and ultrasound evaluation of the proposed needle puncture site will ensure that small bowel loops are not present between the anterior abdominal wall and the bladder. Catheter problems such as occlusion do occur but can be rectified by simple catheter exchange.

SUGGESTED READING

Banner MP, Amendola MA, Pollack HM: Anastomosed ureters: fluoroscopically guided transconduit retrograde catheterization. *Radiology* 170:45–49, 1989.

Bing KT, Hicks ME, Picus D, Darcy MD: Percutenous ureteral occlusion with use of Gianturco coils and gelatin sponge: II. Clinical experience. *Semin Vasc Interv Radiol* 3:319–321, 1992.

De la Toille A et al: Treatment of ureteral stenosis using high pressure dilation catheters. *Prog Virol* 7:408–14, 1997.

Faerber GJ, Richardson TD, Farah N, Ohl DA: Retrograde treatment of ureteropelvic junction obstruction using the ureteral cutting balloon catheter. *J Urol* 157:454–458, 1997.

Krebs TL, Papanicolaou N, Yoder IC, Tung GA, Pfister RC: Antegrade pyelography and ureteral perfusion in children with urinary tract dilatation. *Semin Interv Radiol* 8(3):161–169, 1991.

Lee MJ, Papanicolaou N: Extracorporeal lithotripsy and percutaneous interventions in symptomatic urinary tract lithiasis. *Postgrad Radiol* 11:27–44 (see also Editors' comments, 25–26).

Lee WJ, Smith AD, Cubelli V, Vernace FM: Percutaneous nepthrolithotomy: analysis of 500 consecutive cases. *Urol Radiol* 8:61–66, 1986.

Lee WJ, Smith AD, Cubelli V et al: Complications of percutaneous nephrolithotomy. *Am J Roentgenol* 148:177–180, 1987.

Lee MJ, Papanicolaou N, Nocks BN, Valdez JA, Yoder IC: Fluoroscopically guided percutaneous suprapubic cystostomy for long-term bladder drainage: an alternative to surgical cystostomy. *Radiology* 188:787–789, 1993.

LeRoy AJ, May GR, Bender CE et al: Percutaneous nephrostomy for stone removal. *Radiology* 151:607–612, 1984.

Lu DSK, Papanicolaou N, Girard M, Lee MJ, Yoder IC: Percutaneous internal ureteral stent placement: review of technical issues and solutions in 50 consecutive cases. *Clin Radiol* 49:256–261, 1994.

Maher MM, Fotheringham T, Lee MJ: Percutaneous nephrostomy. *Semin Interv Radiol* 17:329-339, 2000.

Pender SM, Lee MJ: Percutaenous suprapubic cystostomy for long-term bladder drainage. *Semin Interv Radiol* 13(2):93–99, 1996.

Pfister RC, Newhouse JH, Hendren WH: Percutaneous pyeloureteral urodynamics. *Urol Clin N Am* 9:41–49, 1982.

Reznek RH, Talner LB: Percutaneous nephrostomy. *Radiol Clin N Am* 22:393–406, 1984.

Segura JW, Patterson DE, LeRoy A et al: Percutaneous removal of kidney stones: review of 1000 cases. *J Urol* 134:1077–1081, 1985.

Seymour H, Patel U: Ureteric stenting: current status. *Semin Interv Radiol* 17(4):351–365, 2000.

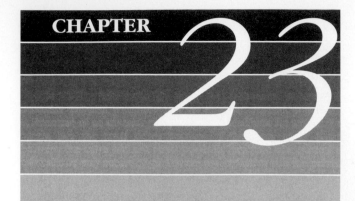

CHAPTER 23

Image-guided Breast Biopsy

SUSAN PENDER, M.B.

The sensitivity of mammography for detection of abnormalities in the breast is proven, but its specificity for breast cancer is suboptimal. Therefore any woman with a clinical or screening-detected abnormality which is either suspicious for cancer, or indeterminate, requires further assessment.

Following a thorough work-up, including additional imaging and, in the case of screening-detected abnormalities, clinical examination, tissue sampling may be necessary to obtain a histologic diagnosis.

In the past, a patient with an impalpable mammographic lesion, which was suspicious for malignancy, required surgical excision to confirm the diagnosis, prior to definitive surgery. This resulted in a large number of unnecessary open biopsies for benign disease. Seventy to eighty percent of lesions referred for surgical biopsy are benign. This has significant implications in terms of morbidity, cost, and bed occupancy. Stereotactic automated large-core biopsy has been shown to obviate the need for surgery in 76–85% of cases and to reduce the cost of diagnosis by up to 58%. The costs can be further reduced if ultrasound guidance is used.

It is suggested that 90% of patients with symptomatic or screening-detected breast cancer should have a preoperative diagnosis made before surgery. This significantly decreases the number of surgical procedures performed in women with breast cancer and increases the likelihood of achieving clear resection margins at the first operation in those undergoing breast conserving surgery. When performing a surgical biopsy, the aim is to resect the smallest volume of tissue necessary to establish a diagnosis, as most lesions will prove benign. With this approach, scarring and deformity are minimized. The aim of therapeutic surgery for carcinoma is to excise the tumor completely and achieve clear margins. The benefits of preoperative diagnosis by percutaneous biopsy include the chance to counsel patients about therapeutic options if a diagnosis of breast cancer is established, and optimal utilization of operating time and hospital beds. The surgeon can plan a single-stage therapeutic procedure based on whether the cancer is an *in situ* type or invasive, and on its extent. Preoperative diagnosis also obviates the need for frozen sections.

PATIENT SELECTION AND PREPARATION

A patient may present for image-guided breast biopsy either as a result of an abnormality detected on a screening mammogram or because she has a palpable breast lump. Following appropriate assessment – which may include additional mammographic views, ultrasound, and clinical examination by a breast surgeon – the imaging and clinical data are assigned a level of suspicion using the Breast Imaging Reporting and Data (BIRAD) system recommended by the American College of Radiology:

1 – Normal
2 – Benign

3 – Indeterminate
4 – Probably malignant
5 – Malignant.

All significant radiologic or clinical abnormalities (those with a code of 3 or higher) require needle biopsy. If a biopsy is performed then the pathologist similarly codes the result according to the same categories. There must be concordance between clinical, radiologic, and pathologic findings to decide that an abnormality is benign (requiring no further intervention) or malignant (requiring therapeutic surgery). Concordance is best established at a multidisciplinary meeting, attended by radiologist, surgeon, pathologist, and preferably an oncologist and breast care nurse. If the results are discordant then repeat percutaneous biopsy, or a diagnostic surgical biopsy in certain cases, should be considered.

Fine-needle aspiration, core biopsy, and mammotomy are all performed on an outpatient basis. The procedure and potential complications are explained to the patient and informed consent is obtained. If the patient is undergoing ultrasound-guided biopsy, the possibility of a pneumothorax is explained, although this is extremely rare.

Patients undergoing breast biopsy are typically a very anxious population. Even so, the procedure is invariably performed using local anesthetic only and sedoanalgesia is not necessary. A coagulation screen is performed only if the patient has a known coagulopathy or is on anticoagulant therapy, as direct pressure is applied to achieve hemostasis (Box 23-1).

CONTRAINDICATIONS

It has been argued that if there is a high probability that a lesion is benign, but the patient wishes the entire lesion to be removed regardless of whether the histology proves to be benign or malignant, that she should proceed to wire localization and excision.

There are occasions where the pathologist requires the entire lesion to make the correct diagnosis. Papillomas and radial scars fall into this category. In the case of papilloma, the entire lesion must be examined to exclude papillary carcinoma. Radial scars are associated with tubular carcinoma (30% of cases) and less commonly other carcinomas, which occur between the spicules and may be missed on core biopsy owing to sampling error. Again such patients should proceed to wire localization and excisional biopsy.

NEEDLE SELECTION

Fine-needle Aspiration (FNA)

FNA can be used to aspirate cystic lesions or obtain a cytologic specimen from a solid lesion. The technique is performed with a 21- to 25-gauge needle; the 23-gauge is preferable, and needles with a sharp beveled tip and clear hub are most commonly used. In experienced hands accurate results can be achieved with FNA, with sensitivities of 73–96% and specificities of 76–100% reported in the literature. However, these results can be difficult to reproduce in practice and in most centers core biopsy has replaced FNA as the main method of tissue diagnosis for breast disease. The accuracy of FNA is very dependent on the experience of both the operator and the cytopathologist. Sample inadequacy is a problem for lesions under 2 cm and occurs more commonly with benign than malignant lesions (Box 23-2).

Core Biopsy

Core biopsy was introduced in the 1980s and initially manual needles such as the trucut were used. Core biopsy gained widespread acceptance following the

---

Box 23-1 Patient Preparation for Biopsy

Complete clinical and radiological information should be available
BIRAD category 3 or greater require biopsy
Biopsy can be performed in an outpatient setting
Coagulation screen rarely necessary
Local anesthesia is usually sufficient for pain control

Box 23-2 Advantages and Disadvantages of FNA

Advantages

Relatively simple
Quick, less traumatic than core biopsy
High success rate in small or hard lesions
Potential for immediate, same-day reporting
Cheap
In theory, more of a lesion can be sampled than with core biopsy

Disadvantages

Expertise required to both obtain and interpret specimens
Cannot distinguish between *in situ* and invasive disease
Cannot determine estrogen receptor status
Microcalcifications usually not apparent
Risk of false positive diagnosis with some lesions

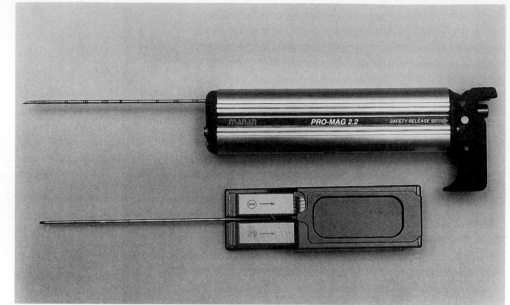

Figure 23-1 Automated biopsy guns used for core biopsy. Both have a 10-cm 14-gauge needle inserted.

introduction of the automated, spring-loaded biopsy devices. These include the Biopsy gun (Bard, Murray Hill, NJ) and the Manan gun (Manan Medical Products, Wheeling, IL) (Fig. 23-1).

These devices are used with a large-gauge cutting needle, a minimum diameter of 14-gauge being necessary to obtain results comparable to excisional biopsy. These needles have a notch just proximal to the tip and an outer cutting trocar (Fig. 23-2). They ideally produce a core of tissue 1–2 cm in length and 1–2 mm in width. When deployed, the needle moves forward at high velocity, the tissue falls into the notch, and the cutting trocar then moves forward to cover the notch (Fig. 23-3). The needle can then be withdrawn. While the larger gauge needle may theoretically cause an increased complication rate, this remains very low. In practice, disposable biopsy guns are not favored for core biopsy of the breast as they are often not sturdy enough to deploy into relatively hard tumors.

Core biopsy allows the pathologist to differentiate invasive from noninvasive tumors and to determine estrogen receptor status (Box 23-3).

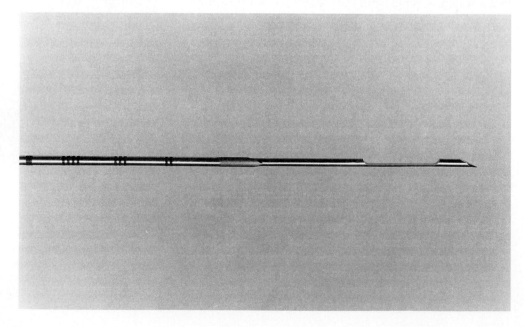

Figure 23-2 Fourteen-gauge core biopsy needle. The outer needle is pulled back to show the inner needle with tissue notch at the distal end.

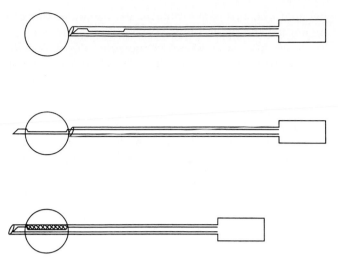

Figure 23-3   Core biopsy. The diagram at the top shows the needle position pre-fire. The center diagram demonstrates the position of the inner needle when it has been fired. The lower diagram shows the final position as the outer needle moves forward to cover the notch containing the tissue sample.

Vacuum-assisted Core Biopsy (Mammotomy)

The vacuum-assisted biopsy device (Mammotome, Ethicon-Endosurgery, Cincinatti, OH) is a recent development which is designed to improve the results of core biopsy and decrease the risk of sampling error. The Mammotome uses a 14- or 11-gauge probe which has an aperture at the distal end and a rotating cutter. A single insertion is made with the probe.

Box 23-3   Advantages and Disadvantages of Core Biopsy

Advantages

Decreases the number of inadequate samples, compared to FNA
Diagnosis of invasive carcinoma may be confirmed
Microcalcifications frequently identified
Specific benign lesions may be diagnosed
Estrogen receptor status may be established
Less expertise required for interpretation of specimens than for FNA

Disadvantages

Small increased risk of sampling error, compared to surgical biopsy, especially for calcifications
Reporting takes 3–48 hours
Sampling small or hard lesions may be difficult
More traumatic than FNA
More expensive than FNA
Potential for tumor seeding along needle track?

The lesion is localized as for core biopsy using stereotactic guidance. The probe is positioned so that the aperture is at the level of the center of the lesion. The vacuum is applied and tissue is aspirated into the aperture. The rotating cutter is advanced forward and the sample captured. After the cutter has advanced fully forward, rotation and suction cease. The cutter is withdrawn, transporting the sample to the collection chamber, while the outer probe remains in the breast. Using this method several samples or contiguous samples can be obtained in a relatively short time. Retrieval rates of 99–100% have been documented for calcifications, compared with 86–94% with 14-gauge automated core biopsy. However, most or all of the abnormality being sampled – for example a cluster of microcalcifications – may inadvertently be removed at mammotomy, especially if the abnormality is small. In these cases a MicroMark clip can be introduced via the Mammotome probe, to facilitate localization for subsequent surgery, if necessary (Box 23-4).

In 95% of cases it should be possible to make a preoperative diagnosis using core biopsy, which is quicker and less expensive than vacuum-assisted biopsy. The cost of a Mammotome probe is approximately 10 times that of a core needle for an automated biopsy device.

Advanced Breast Biopsy Instrumentation (ABBI)

The ABBI system is a sampling device which is used with a dedicated prone stereotactic unit. It is an expensive procedure, the cost of a cannula being approximately 25 times that of a 14-gauge automated needle and $2\frac{1}{2}$ times that of a vacuum-assisted biopsy probe.

The center of the lesion is located stereotactically as for automated core biopsy and mammotomy. The ABBI system uses a cannula which ranges in diameter from 5 mm to 20 mm. It contains a snare wire which traps the

---

Box 23-4   Advantages and Disadvantages of Vacuum-assisted Biopsy

Advantages

Stereotactic or ultrasound guidance
Single insertion of the probe
Device does not have to be "fired"
Sample flexibility
Vacuum ensures a good sample and minimizes complications

Disadvantages

Expensive
Takes longer to set up and perform than core biopsy

sample by electrocautery. The smallest cannula possible should be chosen. The core of tissue removed is up to 20 mm in diameter, but includes the lesion and the breast tissue between it and the skin. This procedure does scar the breast and initial reports suggest that it has a higher complication rate (1.1%) than automated core biopsy (0.2%) or mammotomy (0.1%). In some cases the procedure has to be converted to open surgery.

While the ABBI system has the potential to remove an entire lesion, the size of the sample obtained means that for the vast majority of malignant lesions an adequate margin would not be achieved. In studies to date, malignant lesions diagnosed using the ABBI system have had positive margins in 64–100% of cases. It remains to be proven whether or not the ABBI system has a role to play in the diagnosis or treatment of breast disease (Box 23-5).

IMAGE GUIDANCE

Stereotactic mammography and ultrasound are the modalities routinely used to guide percutaneous breast biopsy procedures. Both modalities can be used for guidance of fine-needle aspiration, core biopsy, and vacuum-assisted biopsy. In general, if a lesion is visible on ultrasound, then this is the modality of choice for biopsy guidance. Stereotactic guidance is usually best for calcifications. Other systems have been developed for image guidance, such as magnetic resonance imaging and scintimammography, but these are not yet in general use.

Ultrasound Guidance

Both clinically palpable and mammographically detected impalpable breast lesions can be biopsied under ultrasound guidance. High-frequency ultrasound with a 10- to 15-MHz linear array transducer is now routinely used for breast imaging. A minimum of 7.5 MHz is required. Color and power Doppler are also widely available. These developments mean that most mammographically detected abnormalities, including some calcifications, can be imaged and biopsied under US guidance. In some patients with a palpable abnormality, mammography can be normal and the lesion is visible on ultrasound alone. There are also cases where stereotactic biopsy fails for anatomic reasons – for example in a small breast, or where a lesion is very close to the chest wall. In these cases US-guided biopsy is often successful. While the learning curve is longer for ultrasound than for stereotactic biopsy, US guidance allows real-time visualization of the needle passing through the lesion and should be more accurate in expert hands. It is also quicker to perform and less uncomfortable for the patient. There is no ionizing radiation involved and it does not require dedicated equipment.

Stereotactic Guidance

There are two types of stereotactic unit, the dedicated prone biopsy table and the add-on unit, which is fitted to an existing erect mammography unit (Box 23-6). The latter allows the unit to be used for both routine mammography and stereotactic procedures. The dedicated prone biopsy tables use digital imaging. The older add-on stereotactic units did not have digital imaging but newer units do. Digital imaging has the advantage that the images are immediately available and multiple check images can be obtained, improving the accuracy of sampling while minimizing procedure time. There are postprocessing facilities, such as selective magnification, black/white inversion, and contrast alteration which improve accuracy when sampling calcifications (Boxes 23-7 and 23-8).

Box 23-5 Needle Selection

Trucut core biopsy favored

Mammotomy probe 10 times more expensive than trucut needle

ABBI sampling cannula 25 times more expensive than trucut needle

Vacuum-assisted core biopsy and ABBI technique may remove all microcalcification being sampled

---

Box 23-6 Comparison of Prone Table and Add-on Unit

Prone Table

Patient prone, vasovagal reactions reduced
Localization images in digital format
Likelihood of movement minimized
Expensive
Large floor space required
Can be used for a single procedure only
Some posterior and axillary lesions cannot be biopsied

Add-on Unit

Patient erect and seated
Localization images in digital format or on film
Potential for movement, but decreased if using digital format
Less expensive
Can be located in a smaller room
Can be used for mammography as well as biopsy and localization procedures

Box 23-7 Comparison of Ultrasound and Stereotactic Guidance

Ultrasound Guidance

Patient supine, more comfortable

Continuous needle visualization, more accurate sampling

No ionizing radiation

Low cost

Long learning curve

Quick to perform

Access to all areas of the breast

Stereotactic Guidance

Patient prone or seated

Needle not continuously visualized

Uses ionizing radiation

More expensive, especially if dedicated prone table used

Short learning curve

Slower to perform, although digital imaging decreases procedure time

Access to axillary and posterior lesions may be limited

PERFORMING A CORE BIOPSY

Core biopsy is performed using an automated spring-loaded biopsy device, preferably with a 23-mm throw and a 14-gauge needle with a 19-mm notch. When the needle tip is positioned for the biopsy, either with ultrasound or stereotactic guidance, it must be considered that the needle tip will move forward another 23 mm when the gun is fired. In the pre-fire position the needle tip should lie at the near edge of the lesion. When the gun is fired, the center of the lesion will then lie within the needle notch (see Fig. 23-3). It is essential to ensure that the needle tip will not end up in an unsafe position when the gun is fired – for example in the chest wall with US guidance, or in the detector when using stereotactic guidance.

Box 23-8 Image Guidance

Ultrasound guidance preferred if lesion visible

Minimum of 7.5-MHz ultrasound probe required

Stereotactic biopsy preferred with digital units

Lesions in the axilla or close to the chest wall not suitable for stereotactic biopsy

Ultrasound-guided Core Biopsy

Ultrasound-guided core biopsy is performed with the patient in the supine position with the arm raised and the hand placed behind the patient's head. She is turned obliquely in the direction which allows the minimum distance between the skin and the chest wall at the portion of the breast containing the abnormality. A foam pad or a small rolled blanket will help the patient to maintain the optimal position. This positioning decreases the amount of tissue that the needle has to traverse and keeps the lesion relatively stable in position.

In the author's unit, while we use sterile drapes to minimize contamination of the biopsy site, we do not sheath the ultrasound transducer, preferring instead to clean the probe and distal portion of the cable with an agent such as chlorhexidine. We use sterile gel as a coupling agent to maximize visualization of small or subtle lesions, which may become difficult to define as the procedure progresses and there is some hematoma formation at the biopsy site. When an optimal transducer position has been selected, the skin is marked along the edge of the footplate with a skin marker. It is then easy to return to the same position for each biopsy.

The skin entry site of the biopsy needle is usually made 4–6 cm from the site of the lesion as seen on ultrasound. This allows the needle to be kept parallel to the chest wall at all times as it is guided to the edge of the lesion, which is necessary to avoid a pneumothorax. The needle tip should always be visible (Figs 23-4 and 23-5). If these principles are applied, even posterior lesions lying on the chest wall can be biopsied safely. It has been shown that it is technically easier and causes less discomfort to the patient if a radial approach is used, where the long axis of the needle is parallel to the radial anatomy of the breast lobule.

Stereotactic Core Biopsy

Stereotactic guidance uses the principle of parallax, to locate a lesion in three dimensions within the breast. The patient is positioned in the mammography unit and compression applied using a compression plate with a rectangular aperture. The approach is determined from the original mammogram: either craniocaudal, lateral, or oblique. The shortest route possible should be chosen. However, when using an add-on unit, where the patient is sitting upright, many operators prefer the craniocaudal approach, as the likelihood of movement during the procedure is minimized.

The detector may be either film or digital. A zero-degree or straight scout view is obtained and the lesion positioned as centrally as possible in the aperture. When a good position has been achieved, the corners of the

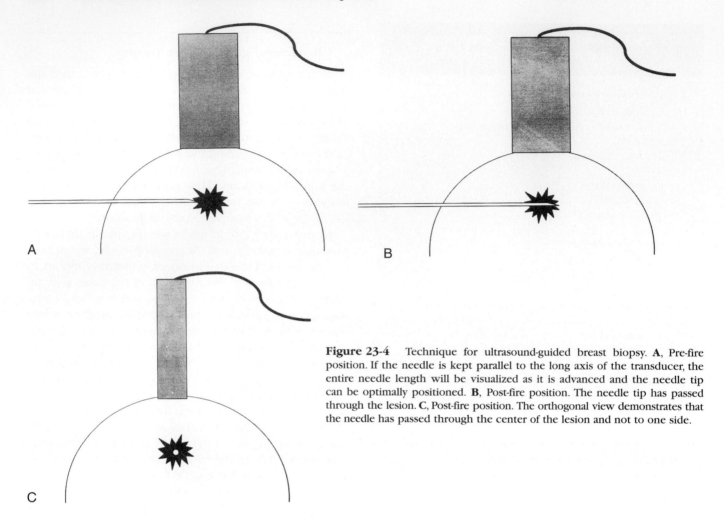

Figure 23-4   Technique for ultrasound-guided breast biopsy. **A**, Pre-fire position. If the needle is kept parallel to the long axis of the transducer, the entire needle length will be visualized as it is advanced and the needle tip can be optimally positioned. **B**, Post-fire position. The needle tip has passed through the lesion. **C**, Post-fire position. The orthogonal view demonstrates that the needle has passed through the center of the lesion and not to one side.

aperture are outlined on the skin, which makes it easy to detect any movement as the procedure progresses and minimizes sampling error due to movement. Two stereotactic views are performed by angling the tube 15 degrees to both the right and left of the perpendicular, a difference of 30 degrees in total between the two images. The x and y coordinates of the lesion's position in the aperture are readily seen. The apparent movement of the lesion between one stereotactic image and the other is used to calculate its depth within the breast – this is the z coordinate. Both the reference marks and the center of the lesion are targeted on both views (Fig. 23-6).

The computer software then calculates the depth of the lesion by measuring the apparent movement of the lesion relative to the fixed reference marks. The needle guide is moved either manually or automatically to the correct position. For targeting to be accurate the length of the biopsy needle being used must be entered into the unit software. The stereotactic device will also calculate the stroke margin available to allow a safe biopsy and prevent the needle from hitting the detector on the other side of the lesion when the biopsy gun is fired. A long-throw biopsy gun (23 mm) should be used for sampling breast tissue.

The lesion's coordinates are either manually or automatically entered into the unit and the needle guide is aligned on the correct trajectory. The skin is cleaned and local anesthetic is injected. Skin and subcutaneous infiltration with local anesthetic is usually sufficient, while deep infiltration may obscure the lesion on subsequent films. A 3- to 5-mm nick is made in the skin with a #11 scalpel and the tip "wiggled" gently to loosen the subcutaneous tissues. Care is taken not to move the breast. The biopsy gun needle is advanced through the bushings in the needle guide to the hub. The housing is removed and the stereotactic views repeated.

It is important to be familiar with how the particular unit is calibrated. Some units are calibrated so that the needle tip lies at the center of the lesion on the pre-fire films, and with these units the needle should be withdrawn approximately 5 mm before firing. Other units position the needle tip at the proximal edge of the lesion.

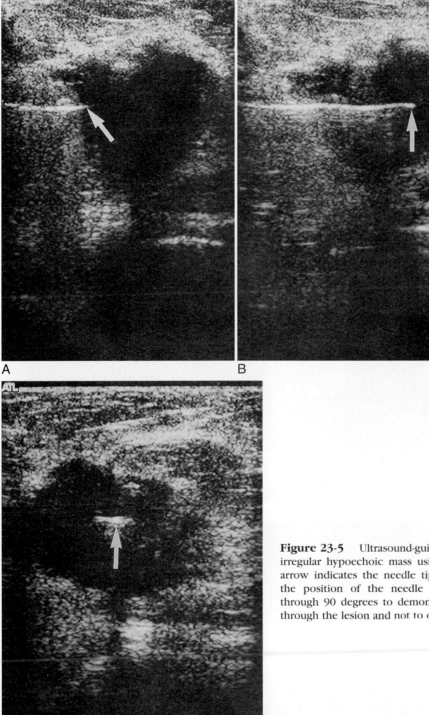

Figure 23-5   Ultrasound-guided core breast biopsy in a patient with a 15-mm irregular hypoechoic mass using a 10-MHz transducer. **A**, Pre-fire position. The arrow indicates the needle tip. **B**, Post-fire position. Again the arrow indicates the position of the needle tip. **C**, Post-fire position. The probe is rotated through 90 degrees to demonstrate that the needle (arrow) has in fact passed through the lesion and not to one side of it.

When the needle tip is optimally positioned the gun is fired. Post-fire stereotactic views should be performed to confirm that the tip of the needle has passed through the lesion.

The needle is withdrawn and the sample carefully removed from the notch. This can be done gently with a needle or by floating the sample off the notch in saline. The sample is placed in formalin or initially on a glass slide with a drop of sterile saline, if specimen radiography is required to prove the presence of calcifications. At least five samples should be obtained. Usually the center of the lesion is targeted in addition to positions at 12, 3, 6 and 9 o'clock between the center and periphery of the lesion. Intermediate positions may be targeted and often more than five samples are required when sampling calcifications. At the end of the procedure a repeat view (0 degrees) is performed which may show air in needle tracks through the lesion or small foci of hemorrhage, again confirming that the correct area has been sampled (Box 23-9).

Specimen Radiography

If the purpose of the biopsy is to sample calcifications, then it is essential to perform a radiograph of the specimens obtained, to confirm that there are calcifications present. The presence of calcifications within the specimens significantly increases the chance of making the correct histologic diagnosis.

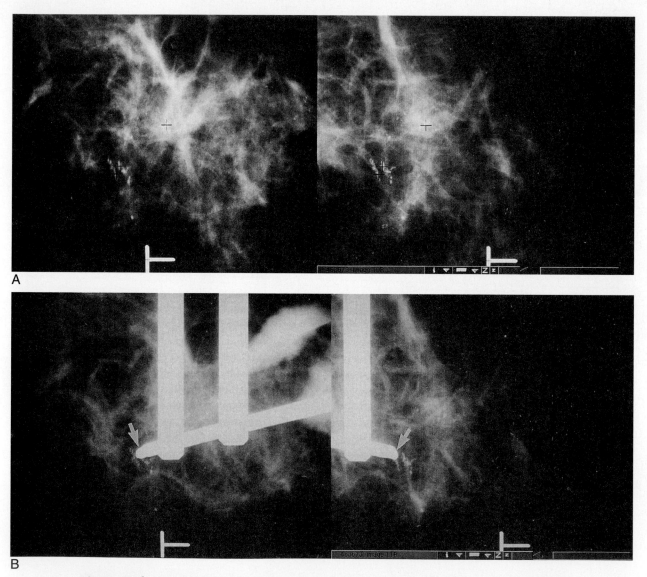

Figure 23-6 Stereotactic core biopsy of a cluster of microcalcifications. Histopathology confirmed high nuclear grade ductal carcinoma-in-situ. **A,** Digital stereotactic pair. The cross-hairs indicate selected targets. **B,** Pre-fire stereotactic pair. The arrows indicate the position of the needle tip.

(Continued)

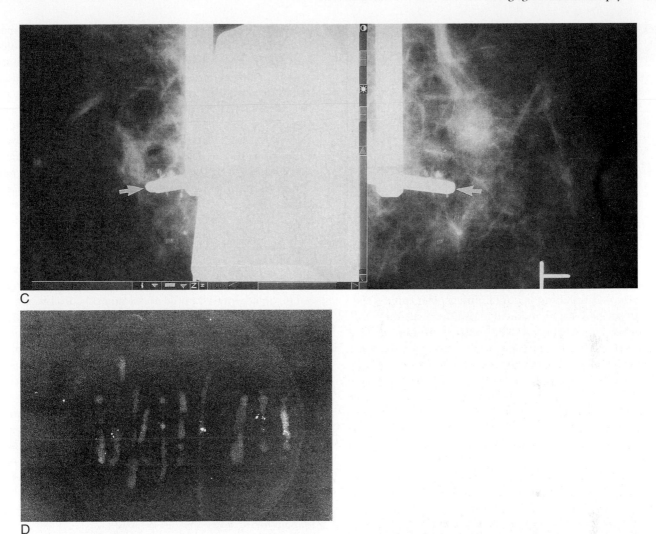

C

D

Figure 23-6   cont'd C, Post-fire stereotactic pair. Again the arrows indicate the needle tip which has passed through the lesion. The artefact on the left image is caused by the housing of the biopsy device. Some devices do not allow removal of the housing once the device has been fired. **D,** Specimen radiograph, demonstrating calcifications in several of the cores.

Each specimen is removed from the needle and placed on a glass slide. It is useful to place them in a row, side by side, so that those containing calcifications can be easily identified on the radiograph. Each sample should be gently arranged in a linear fashion rather than coiled. The samples should be moistened with a little saline. The glass slide is placed on a 4 × 4 pad. It may be helpful to place these in a Petri dish for ease of handling. Excess saline is removed by tilting the slide and allowing the 4 × 4 pad to absorb the saline. Magnification radiography is performed using a standard mammography unit or a dedicated specimen x-ray device (Faxitron, Buffalo Grove, IL) (see Fig. 23-6). If digital imaging is being used, the postprocessing facilities can be used to optimize the visualization of calcifications. Some pathologists prefer that those samples containing calcifications are identified and placed in a separate container of formalin.

AFTERCARE

When a stereotactic biopsy procedure has been performed, the patient is disengaged from the mammography unit and an icepack applied to the biopsy site. (icecubes in a "ziplock" plastic bag will suffice). The patient holds this in place herself, applying pressure, for 15 minutes. A more vigorous pressure dressing has been suggested by some investigators, if an 11-gauge vacuum device has been used. After 15 minutes, the site is examined to ensure that there is no active bleeding. A simple adhesive dressing is applied to the needle insertion site and the patient is allowed to get dressed.

The patient is warned that she may experience some discomfort and bruising once the local anesthetic wears off, and that this can be minimized by applying an

---

Box 23-9   Stereotactic Core Biopsy

Shortest route possible to the lesion should be chosen
15-degree views to right and left performed to calculate
  lesion depth
Post-fire stereotactic views performed to confirm needle
  position
At least five samples should be obtained
Specimen radiography is performed if microcalcifications
  were sampled

---

icepack at home at regular intervals during the evening. She is advised to have some painkillers available to take, but to avoid preparations containing aspirin (unless they are prescribed for a medical condition) as they may exacerbate the bruising. The patient should rest as much as possible for 24 hours and avoid excessive exertion as this may make the wound bleed. If bleeding does occur, she should apply pressure for 15–20 minutes. If bleeding continues, she should telephone a designated contact number or attend the emergency department.

The dressing can be removed after 24 hours. The patient may replace it with a simple adhesive dressing if she wishes, but it is unlikely that a dressing will be needed for more than 2 days. The patient can resume her normal activities the following day.

RESULTS

A large number of studies have shown sensitivities ranging from 85 to 100% and specificities of 98–100% for core biopsy. In addition, concordance rates of 87–96% have been demonstrated between 14-gauge automated core biopsy and surgical biopsy.

False negative rates are reported to be very low (0–4%). Results compare favorably with data published in the literature for surgical "miss" rates following wire localization for surgical biopsy. The recent development of the vacuum-assisted biopsy device (Mammotome) has further reduced the risk of sampling error and can significantly decrease the rebiopsy rate for calcifications.

One recent study has shown calcification retrieval rates of 85% using a digital add-on device, with preoperative absolute sensitivity for ductal carcinoma-in-situ (DCIS) of 69%. These results are similar to those previously reported with dedicated prone units. Most of the studies in the literature use prone tables and report high success rates for sampling both masses and calcifications. Similar results can be achieved using add-on units, especially if these are digital.

When interpreting the results of image-guided breast biopsy, correlation must be made with both the clinical and the imaging findings. Cases where results do not correlate should be considered for further image-guided biopsy or surgical excisional biopsy. For example, a histologic result of normal breast tissue is not acceptable where the mammogram or ultrasound demonstrates a discrete mass, because this indicates that there has been a sampling error. Discordance between the imaging and pathologic findings is one of the occasions where rebiopsy may be recommended. The most common cause of a recommendation for rebiopsy is a diagnosis of atypical ductal hyperplasia (16–56%); others include inadequate tissue or possible phyllodes tumor. One recent study has shown a significantly lower rate of rebiopsy for 11-gauge vacuum-assisted biopsy (9%) than for 14-gauge automated core biopsy (15%). The likelihood of failing to obtain an adequate sample at automated core biopsy, and therefore failing to avoid rebiopsy or a surgical procedure, is higher for calcifications than for mass lesions. Studies to date show that surgery is avoided in 84–87% of masses and 66–72% of calcifications. The use of vacuum-assisted biopsy appears to further reduce the need for rebiopsy or surgery particularly for calcifications.

There is debate regarding the necessity for excisional biopsy of specific lesions diagnosed on automated core or vacuum-assisted biopsy. These include radial scar, papillary lesions, and lobular carcinoma-in-situ. It is now widely accepted that multidisciplinary correlation of biopsy results is best achieved at regular meetings where the radiologist, pathologist, and surgeon are present and management decisions can be made.

With experience it should be possible to provide a preoperative diagnosis in more than 90% of women with breast cancer. Adequate training and audit of individual performance and results is essential if this goal is to be achieved (Box 23-10).

COMPLICATIONS

It is reasonable to define clinically significant complications following breast biopsy as those that require

---

Box 23-10   Core Biopsy Results

Sensitivities of 85–100% and specificities of 98–100%
  reported
Concordance rates of 87–96% with surgical biopsy
Discordance between histology and clinicoradiologic
  findings should prompt repeat biopsy
Commonest cause of rebiopsy is atypical ductal hyperplasia on histology

surgical or medical intervention. Significant complications following core or vacuum-assisted breast biopsy are rare. They include hematoma formation, infection, and pneumothorax. If every attempt is made to control hematoma formation at the time of the procedure, and the needle is kept parallel to the chest wall at all times, then the complication rate should be negligible. In the largest series of percutaneous large-gauge core breast biopsies (3765 cases), performed under stereotactic guidance, significant complications occurred in only 0.2%. In this series the authors reported three hematomas requiring surgical drainage and three infections requiring drainage, antibiotic therapy, or both. In one series of 345 vacuum-assisted biopsies, significant complications occurred in only two cases.

Needle track seeding has been reported in patients who have undergone core biopsy of malignant lesions, but this is exceedingly rare.

SUGGESTED READINGS

Berg WA, Krebs TL, Campassi C et al: Evaluation of 14- and 11-gauge directional, vacuum-assisted biopsy probes and 14-gauge biopsy guns in a breast parenchymal model. *Radiology* 205:203–208, 1997.

Brenner RJ, Fajardo L, Fisher PR et al: Percutaneous core biopsy of the breast: effect of operator experience and number of samples obtained on diagnostic accuracy. *Am J Roentgenol* 166:341–346, 1996.

Burbank F: Stereotactic breast biopsy of atypical ductal hyperplasia and ductal carcinoma-in-situ lesions: improved accuracy with directional, vacuum-assisted biopsy. *Radiology* 202:843–847, 1997.

Burbank F, Parker SH, Fogarty TJ: Stereotactic breast biopsy: improved tissue harvesting with the Mammotome. *American Surg* 62:738–744, 1996.

Dershaw DD, Morris EA, Liberman L et al: Nondiagnostic stereotaxic core breast biopsy: results of rebiopsy. *Radiology* 198:323–325, 1996.

Dershaw DD, Liberman L: Stereotactic breast biopsy: indications and results. *Oncology* 12:907–916, 1998.

Diaz LK, Wiley EL, Venta LA: Are malignant cells displaced by large-gauge needle biopsy of the breast? *Am J Roentgenol* 173:1303–1313, 1999.

Dowlatshahi K, Yaremko ML, Kluskens LF, Jokich PM: Nonpalpable breast lesions: findings of stereotactic needle-core biopsy and fine-needle aspiration cytology. *Radiology* 181:745–750, 1991.

Elvecrog EL, Lechner MC, Nelson MT: Nonpalpable breast lesions: correlation of stereotactic large-core needle biopsy and surgical biopsy results. *Radiology* 188:453–455, 1993.

Farjedo LL: Cost-effectiveness of stereotactic breast core biopsy. *Acad Radiol* 3:521–523, 1996.

Helbich TH, Rudas M, Haitel A et al: Evaluation of needle size for breast biopsy: comparison of 14-, 16-, and 18-gauge biopsy needles. *Am J Roentgenol* 171:59–63, 1998.

Hendrick RE, Parker SH: Principles of stereotactic mammography and quality assurance. In Parker SH, Jobe WE eds: *Percutaneous Breast Biopsy*, Raven, New York, 49–59, 1993.

Homer MJ, Smith TJ, Safaii H: Prebiopsy needle localization: methods, problems, and expected results. *Radiol Clin N Am* 30:139–153, 1992.

Jackman RJ, Nowels KW, Shepard MJ, Finkelstein SI, Marzoni FA: Stereotactic large-core needle biopsy of 450 nonpalpable breast lesions with surgical correlation in lesions with cancer or atypical hyperplasia. *Radiology* 193:91–95, 1994.

Jackman RJ, Marzoni FA, Nowels KW: Percutaneous removal of benign mammographic lesions: comparison of automated large-core and directional vacuum-assisted stereotactic biopsy techniques. *Am J Roentgenol* 171:1325–1330, 1998.

Kopans DB: *Breast Imaging*, Lippincott–Raven, Philadelphia, 1998.

Liberman L: Advanced Breast Biopsy Instrumentation (ABBI): analysis of published experience. *Am J Roentgenol* 172:1413–1416, 1999.

Liberman L: Percutaneous imaging-guided core breast biopsy. *Am J Roentgenol* 174:1191–1199, 2000.

Liberman L, Dershaw DD, Rosen PP et al: Stereotactic 14-gauge breast biopsy: how many core biopsy specimens are needed? *Radiology* 192:793–795, 1994.

Liberman L, Dershaw DD, Glassman JR et al: Analysis of cancers not diagnosed at stereotactic core breast biopsy. *Radiology* 203:151–157, 1997.

Liberman L, Feng TL, Dershaw DD, Morris EA, Abramson AF: Ultrasound-guided core breast biopsy: utility and cost-effectiveness. *Radiology* 208:717–723, 1998.

Parker SH, Burbank F: A practical approach to minimally invasive breast biopsy. *Radiology* 200:11–20, 1996.

Parker SH, Jobe WE, Dennis MA et al: US-guided automated large-core breast biopsy. *Radiology* 187:507–511, 1993.

Parker SH, Burbank F, Jackman RJ et al: Percutaneous large-core breast biopsy: a multi-institutional study. *Radiology* 193:359–364, 1994.

Philpotts LE, Shaheen NA, Carter D, Lange RC, Lee CH: Comparison of rebiopsy rates after stereotactic core needle biopsy of the breast with 11-gauge vacuum suction probe versus 14-gauge needle and automatic gun. *Am J Roentgenol* 172:683–687, 1999.

CHAPTER 24

Musculoskeletal Intervention

A. GANGI, M.D., S. GUTH, M.D., J. L. DIETEMANN, M.D.,
AND C. ROY, M.D.

Interventional musculoskeletal procedures are performed to an increasing degree by radiologists. The techniques described in this chapter are the standard commonly used techniques or the newer techniques that offer the most promise. Percutaneous musculoskeletal procedures, like other interventional procedures, are usually performed using ultrasound (US), fluoroscopy, computed tomography (CT), or magnetic resonance (MR) guidance.

Fluoroscopy and CT are the most frequently used guidance techniques. Fluoroscopy offers direct imaging in multiple planes but has the disadvantage of poor soft-tissue contrast. CT is well suited for precise interventional needle guidance because it provides excellent visualization of bone and surrounding soft tissues. Damage to adjacent vascular, neurological, and visceral structures can also be avoided with CT guidance. Fluoroscopic CT guidance is rarely necessary.

A combination of CT and standard fluoroscopy for interventional procedures has been recommended for complex procedures (Fig. 24-1). For fluoroscopy, a mobile C-arm is positioned in front of the CT gantry. With the use of CT and fluoroscopic imaging the structure to be punctured can be visualized 3-dimensionally and anatomic structures can be precisely located, which in many cases is not possible with standard fluoroscopy alone. Two mobile monitors are placed in front of the interventional radiologist, displaying the last stored image and the fluoroscopic image. The operator can switch from CT to fluoroscopy and vice versa at any time.

MUSCULOSKELETAL BIOPSY

Histopathologic and bacteriologic studies are often required in musculoskeletal lesions to establish a definitive diagnosis. In such cases, percutaneous musculoskeletal biopsy (PMSB) has become a routine procedure that is safe and cost-effective.

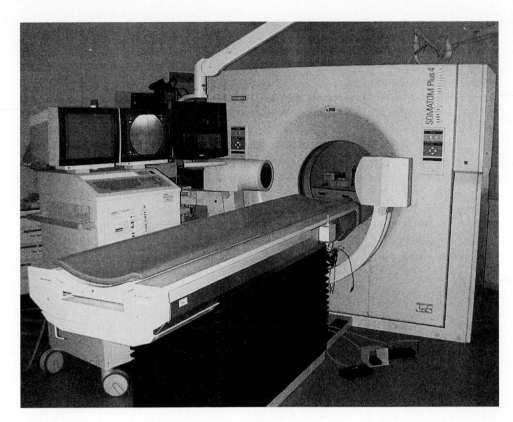

Figure 24-1 Interventional room with combination of CT and fluoroscopy.

Indications

Percutaneous bone biopsy is performed whenever pathologic, bacteriologic, or biologic examination is required for definitive diagnosis or treatment (Box 24-1). Major indications include primary or secondary bone tumors, or less frequently soft tissue masses. Bone metastases are the most common indication for biopsy. Biopsy is performed to prove that the visualized lesion is indeed a metastasis before treatment and/or to identify the primary tumor if possible. In certain tumors, such as breast tumors, the biopsy may provide information with regard to the hormone sensitivity of the lesion which has direct therapeutic implications. In patients with suspected primary bone tumors, biopsy is not routine and is performed only if doubt persists as to the nature of the lesion or if histology will influence the therapy chosen. Suspected infected lesions are another indication for

PMSB where identification of the responsible organism is required to institute appropriate therapy (e.g., septic arthritis, discitis, osteomyelitis).

Contraindications

The expected results of biopsy should outweigh the risks of the procedure. Careful review of imaging findings and of previous studies should assist the radiologist in avoiding unnecessary biopsies (benign bone islands, subchondral sclerosis, etc.). The risk of tumor seeding should be considered with primary bone tumors and sarcomas. If the biopsy is to be performed before surgical resection, the needle pathway should be chosen in consultation with the surgeon. In this way, the needle pathway can be chosen so that it will lie in the area of surgical resection. Well-known contraindications include bleeding diatheses, biopsy of inaccessible sites (odontoid process, anterior arch of C1), and soft tissue infection with high risk of bone contamination (Box 24-2).

Technique

A CT scan is performed to localize the lesion. The entry point and the pathway are determined by CT; avoiding nervous, vascular, and visceral structures.
- For peripheral long-bone biopsy, the approach used should be orthogonal to the bone cortex.

Box 24-1 Musculoskeletal Biopsy: Indications

Bone metastases
Primary bone tumor if diagnosis is in doubt
Soft tissue masses
Suspected infectious lesions

Box 24-2 Musculoskeletal Biopsy: Techniques

Needle pathway should lie in surgical resection area for primary bone tumor biopsy

Odontoid process and anterior arch of CI are not suitable for PMSB

Review of previous studies and all imaging findings helps avoid unnecessary biopsy

CT guidance or dual CT and fluoroscopic guidance preferred

Box 24-3 Musculoskeletal Biopsy: Preferred Routes

Anterior access in the cervical spine

Transpedicular or intercostovertebral route in the thoracic spine

Posterolateral or transpedicular route in the lumbar spine

Needle approach orthogenal to bone cortex for long bones

Needle approach tangential to bone cortex for flat bones

This approach angle avoids the tip of the needle becoming deflected by the bone cortex. In addition, the shortest approach to the lesion should be chosen that avoids tendons as well as nervous, vascular, visceral, and articular structures (Fig. 24-2).

- For flat bones such as scapula, ribs, sternum, and skull, the authors use an oblique approach angle of 30–60 degrees. This is a compromise. This tangential approach is preferred to avoid damage to underlying structures because these bones are relatively thin. The tangential approach also provides more bone bulk to biopsy in these flat bones (Fig. 24-3).
- For the pelvic girdle, a posterior or lateral approach is used to avoid the sacral canal and sacral and femoral nerve plexuses (Figs 24-4 and 24-5).

- For vertebral body biopsy, different approach routes are selected depending on the vertebral level: the anterior route is used at the cervical level; the transpedicular and intercostovertebral routes at the thoracic level; and the posterolateral and the transpedicular route at the lumbar level. For the neural posterior arch a tangential approach is used to avoid damage to underlying neural structures (Figs 24-6 through 24-8; Box 24-3).

Bone biopsy is usually performed under local anesthesia. Sedoanalgesia may be necessary for painful lesions or if the patient is very anxious. General anesthesia is required for pediatric bone biopsy. The procedure is carried out under strict sterility. The skin, subcutaneous tissue, muscle, and the bony periosteum are infiltrated by

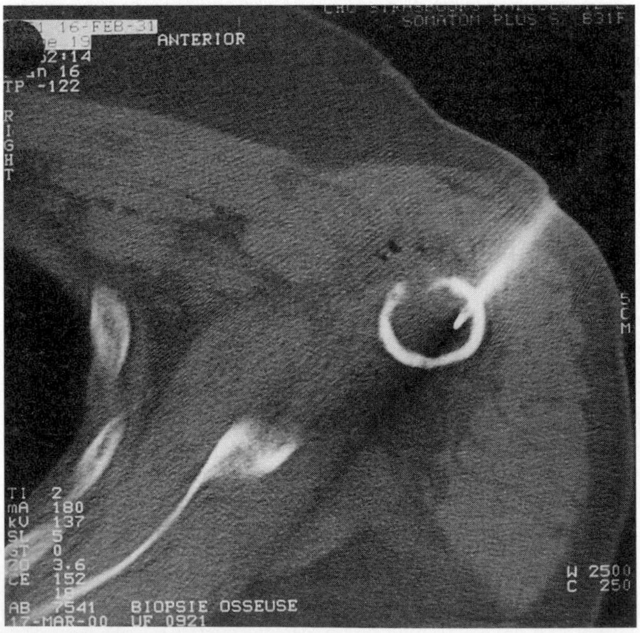

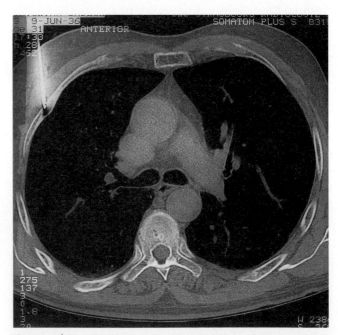

Figure 24-2 Percutaneous biopsy of a humeral lytic lesion with a 14-gauge needle. To avoid damage to the long head of the biceps tendon, a lateral approach is used.

Figure 24-3 Percutaneous biopsy of a rib. An oblique approach to the flat bone is used to avoid slippage and damage to the pleura and lung. During needle positioning, the rib is locked between two fingers.

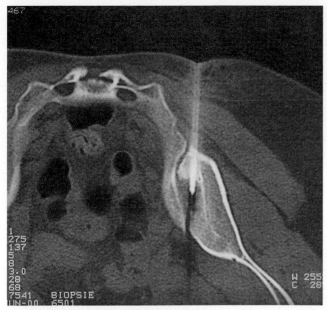

Figure 24-4   Sacroiliac biopsy. Posterior approach with a 14-gauge needle. The trocar needle is inserted with the help of a surgical hammer under local anesthesia.

local anesthetic (1% lidocaine) with a 22-gauge needle. For bone biopsy, CT guidance is routinely used. CT images are repeated to confirm the correct placement of the needle tip before sampling. For pathologic examination, the specimen is fixed in 10% formalin. If bacteriologic analysis is necessary the specimens are not fixed and are sent for Gram stain and culture. Soft tissue and

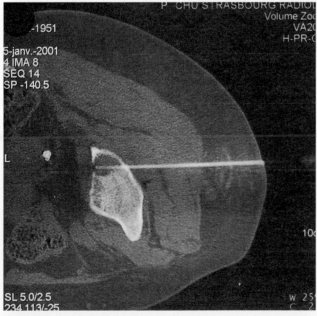

Figure 24-5   Acetabular biopsy performed using a lateral approach to avoid damage to the sciatic nerve.

subperiosteal lesions without ossification are directly punctured with a 14- to 16-gauge trucut biopsy needle.

For bony lesions with mild ossification or a small amount of bone cortex surrounding the lesion, and for most vertebral body lesions, the authors use a 14-gauge Ostycut bone biopsy needle with a surgical hammer used for bony penetration (Ostycut, Angiomed/Bard, Karlsruhe, Germany). For bony lesions with mild bony sclerosis, and for primary tumors or lymphomas, we use an 8-gauge trephine needle (Laredo type). For bony lesions with dense ossification, or with dense cortical bone surrounding the lesion, drilling is necessary. In the latter instance, we use a 2-mm diameter hand drill or a 14-gauge Bonopty Penetration set (Radi Medical Systems Uppsala, Sweden) (Box 24-4).

Results

In the authors' unit, 440 percutaneous musculoskeletal biopsies were performed on an outpatient basis. Sixty-three percent of patients were female and 37% were male ranging in age from 4 to 87 years (mean 58 years). Fifty-five percent of patients had lytic lesions, 24% had sclerosing or mixed lesions, and 18% had vertebral compression fractures. The anatomic area biopsied was the vertebral column in 68%, pelvic girdle in 14%, and peripheral long bones in 14%. Vertebral lesions were at the cervical level in 3% of patients, at the thoracic level in 15%, at the lumbar level in 45%, and at the sacral level in 7%. Specificity for diagnosis was 100%, sensitivity was 93.9%, positive predictive value was 100%, and negative predictive value was 87.5%. These results concur with other results in the literature.

Complications associated with PMSB are rare. Bone infection (osteomyelitis) is the most feared complication, but with strict adherence to sterile precautions this is rare. Soft tissue hematomas can occur but are rarely significant. Pneumothorax has been described in particular with biopsies of the bony skeleton encasing the thorax. Neural and vascular injuries have also been described, but

---

Box 24-4 Musculoskeletal Biopsy: Needles

Soft tissue or subperiosteal lesions without ossification are biopsied with 14- to 16-gauge trucut needles

In vertebral body biopsy or lesions with thin cortex, an Ostycut needle is used

For lesions with mid bony sclerosis or primary bone tumors, an 8-gauge trephine needle is used

For lesions with dense sclerosis or thickened cortex, a hand-drill is used

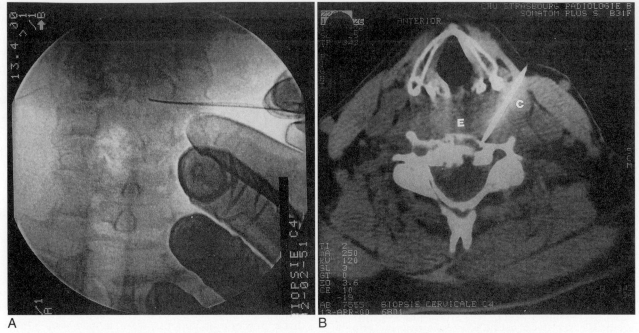

Figure 24-6   Discovertebral biopsy of C4. **A,** The vascular structures are pushed by hand out of the needle path. **B,** The needle is inserted between the carotid sheath (C), esophagus (E), and trachea using CT and fluoroscopic guidance.

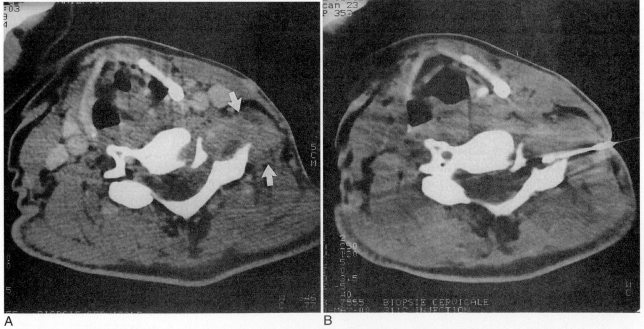

Figure 24-7   Cervical biopsy. **A,** CT with injection of contrast medium shows a tumor (arrows) affecting the neural foramen and lateral portion of the vertebral body. **B,** Biopsy performed with an 18-gauge needle. This lateral approach avoids neurologic and vascular damage.

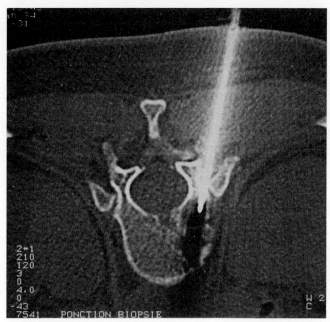

Figure 24-8   Transpedicular biopsy of T12. The biopsy is performed with a 14-gauge trocar needle. Cortical perforation is performed with the help of a surgical hammer.

with CT guidance and appropriate planning of access routes the rate of these injuries should be very low.

Murphy and associates, in a large review of 9500 percutaneous skeletal biopsies, identified 22 complications (0.2%). They reported nine pneumothoraces, three cases of meningitis, and five spinal cord injuries. Serious neurological injury occurred in 0.08% of procedures and death in 0.02%.

Only three complications were observed in the authors' series of 440 patients. These consisted of paravertebral hematomas in two patients which resolved spontaneously and a needle tip which broke off in cortical bone in one patient. This low complication rate seems to be related to the consistent use of CT or dual guidance which provides optimal needle access planning and monitoring during the biopsy procedure.

INTRAARTICULAR INJECTION OF CORTICOSTEROIDS IN FACET SYNDROME

The term "facet syndrome" was introduced by Ghormley. Facet pain is attributed to segmental instability, synovitis, and degenerative arthritis. The signs of facet syndrome are local paralumbar tenderness, pain on hyperextension, absence of neurologic deficit, absence of root tension signs, and hip, buttock, or back pain during straight leg raising. In the absence of precise diagnostic clinical features or criteria, the diagnosis of facet syndrome relies exclusively on the result of a diagnostic block. This entails the injection of local anesthetic (and corticosteroid if positive) into the facet joint.

Injection of local anesthetic agents acts on the nociceptive fibers within the synovium, whereas intracapsular corticosteroids reduce inflammation of the synovium. The choice of injection level(s) is based on the location of focal tenderness over the joint(s) or the presence of osteoarthritis involving the joints. The block test with intraarticular injection of local anesthetic into the facet joint must produce complete pain relief to support the presumptive diagnosis.

Indications

Intraarticular injection of steroids is performed on patients in whom diagnostic facet joint blocks prove that the facet joints are the source of back pain.

Technique

Facet-joint injection in the lumbar spine is a simple and safe procedure that can be performed under CT or fluoroscopic guidance. Facet joint degenerative disease usually affects multiple levels and both sides, so multilevel facet joint injections (L3–L4, L4–L5, and L5–S1) could be necessary.

The patient is placed in a prone position on the CT or fluoroscopy table. A CT scan of the affected level is performed to determine the needle pathway and skin entry point. A 22-gauge needle is advanced vertically into each joint (Fig. 24-9). Once the needle is in the joint, a solution of cortivazol and bupivacaine 0.25% is injected into the joint. Cortivazol is provided in a 1.5-mL solution (3.75 mg of long-acting steroid) and with the addition of 1.5 mL of bupivacaine 0.25% a 3-mL solution is obtained. Usually the injection is performed bilaterally and 1.5 mL of this solution is injected into each side. A global dose of 3.75 mg of cortivazol per session should not be exceeded.

Results

The value of corticosteroid injection into facet joints remains controversial. In the literature, immediate relief varies between 59 and 94%, and long-term relief varies from 27 to 54%. In the authors' experience with 166 facet blocks, immediate pain relief was obtained in 62% of patients but long-term relief was observed in only 31% (with long-term relief defined as absence of pain for at least 6 months).

The complications of lumbar facet joint injection are rare with either fluoroscopic or CT guidance. Severe allergic reactions to local anesthetic are uncommon. Steroid injections can produce local reactions, which occur most

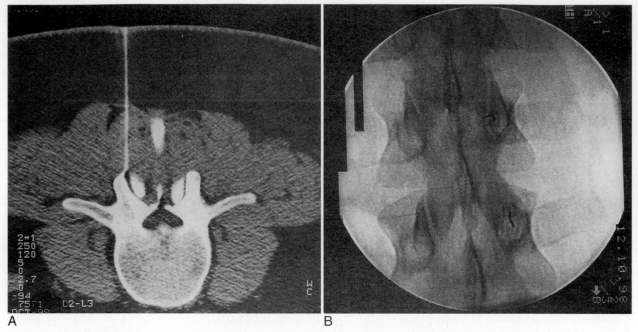

Figure 24-9 Facet-joint injection in an outpatient. A 22-gauge spinal needle is inserted inside each affected facet joint. Arthrography is not performed systematically. The procedure can be performed under (**A**) CT guidance or (**B**) fluoroscopic guidance.

often immediately after the injection. These reactions last 24–48 hours, and they can be relieved by application of ice. The greatest complication is septic arthritis and this can be avoided by appropriate aseptic technique. The only serious complication the authors have observed was due to the injected corticosteroid, with a temporary episode of agitation occurring in one patient. This settled with conservative management (Box 24-5).

PERCUTANEOUS EPIDURAL AND NERVE ROOT BLOCK

The lumbar spine causes pain, suffering, and disability more frequently than any other part of the body.

Box 24-5 Facet Joint Injection

Corticosteroid injection is performed only if local anesthetic injection provides complete pain relief
Fluoroscopic or CT guidance and 22-gauge needles are used
Multiple joint injections may be necessary
Procedure efficacy remains controversial
Immediate pain relief varies from 59 to 94%
Long-term pain relief poor, varying from 27 to 54%

In the past 20 years, the growing crisis of disability resulting from low back pain has led to the recognition that the problem cannot be solved by better or more frequent surgery. Some minimally invasive interventional procedures are available to relieve pain and to minimize the risk of disability. These procedures offer new hope for lumbosacral pain control either with or without conventional pain therapy. Nerve root inflammation is responsible for much low back pain and sciatica. Percutaneous periradicular infiltration (PPRI) consists of an injection of corticosteroid and local anesthetic into the epidural space at the level of the offending disc.

There is no clear, single explanation as to why a disc herniation causes back pain and/or sciatica. Physical pressure on a peripheral nerve alone does not produce pain; it produces paresthesia. It is likely that there are neuromechanical factors involved in explaining the mechanism of symptom production in a herniated disc. Periradicular injection of longacting steroids is effective in relieving pain, probably because it decreases inflammation of the epidural space.

Indications

The major indications for PPRI are treatment of acute back pain and/or neuralgia of discogenic origin (without nerve paralysis) resistant to conventional medical therapy, or postdiscectomy syndrome.

Technique

The procedure is performed on an outpatient basis. In the authors' unit, all epidural injections are performed under CT guidance, although MRI can be used for epidural and foraminal injection if appropriate needles are available.

If a lumbar level is to be injected, the patient is placed in the prone position on the CT table. CT determines the needle entry point and access route. The skin is infiltrated with local anesthesia and a 22-gauge spinal needle is placed near the painful nerve root under CT guidance. When injecting longacting corticosteroid (cortivozol 3.75 mg) into the epidural space, it is essential to ensure that the needle tip is not in the dural space, by aspirating through the needle; the absence of returned cerebro-spinal fluid (CSF) through the needle confirms an extradural location (Fig. 24-10). Sterile air contained in a 15-cm plastic tube is injected to further confirm the extradural position of the needle tip (Figs 24-10, 24-11, and 24-12). After this, 2–3 mL of longacting corticosteroid (cortivazol) solution is injected, mixed with a solution of 1% lidocaine (2 mL). If the dura is traversed by the needle tip because of an adhesion of the dural sac to the ligamentum flavum or because of a procedural mishap, the needle must be pulled back slightly and attempts made to aspirate CSF. If there is no CSF aspirated, the corticosteroid solution is injected without local anesthetic and in these cases only hydrocortisone should be used. During injection, the patient may experience a spontaneous recurrence of pain lasting a few seconds, brought on by stretching of the dura.

At the cervical level, the patient is placed in the supine position with the head slightly turned and hyperextended. The skin is infiltrated with local anesthestic and a 22-gauge spinal needle is placed from a lateral approach near the painful nerve root using CT guidance. When aspiration through the needle confirms the absence of CSF or blood, 1.5 mL of contrast material is injected (Fig. 24-13). This outlines the epidural space and confirms the needle tip position. When happy with the position of the needle tip, inject 2–3 mL of hydrocortisone. The use of CT guidance avoids the risk of vertebral artery injury or intradural injection.

Results

A review of 470 periradicular injections performed using CT guidance demonstrated that the short-term benefit of PPRI is quite high, with good pain relief in 78% of patients with extraforaminal herniations and in 65% of patients with disc herniations at another localization. Long-term pain relief (persistence of relief for at least

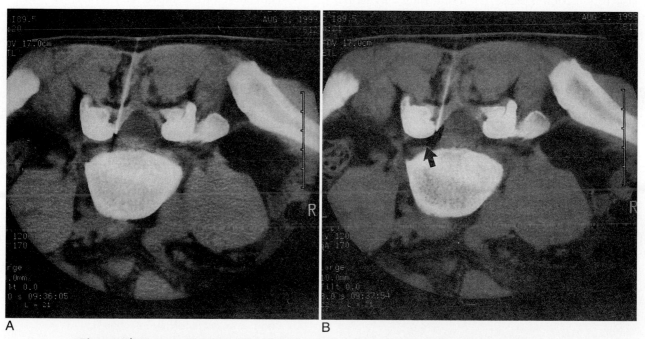

A   B

Figure 24-10   L5–S1 periradicular injection of steroid in an outpatient with recalcitrant back pain. **A**, A 22-gauge spinal needle is positioned in the epidural space. **B**, Before injection of the corticosteroid the epidural position of the needle tip is confirmed by the lack of aspiration of CSF. One milliliter of sterile air (arrow) is then injected to outline the epidural space and to again confirm needle tip position.

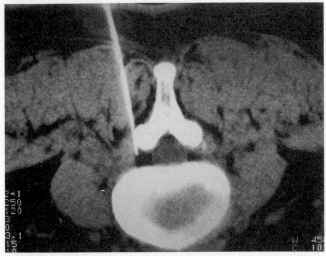

Figure 24-11   Foraminal PPRI. This approach is used in foraminal and extraforaminal disc herniations. The 22-gauge spinal needle is inserted into the affected foramen and longacting corticosteroid mixed with lidocaine is injected.

6 months) was satisfactory only in patients who had PPRI for extraforaminal disc herniations. Sixty-eight percent had good pain relief 2 years at PPRI (an average of three sessions of PPRI).

Meningitis with neurologic damage (quadriplegia, multiple cranial nerve palsies, nystagmus) is described after epidural or intrathecal injection of steroids if strict sterility is not respected. A sterile technique will limit the risk of infection. Precise CT monitoring also helps avoid accidental intrathecal injection of corticosteroid or lidocaine. In 2% of patients, pain was accentuated during

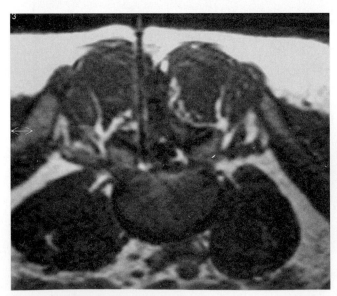

Figure 24-12   Periradicular infiltration under MR guidance. The procedure is performed with a specially adapted 22-gauge spinal needle (MR Eye, Cook, Bloomington, IN).

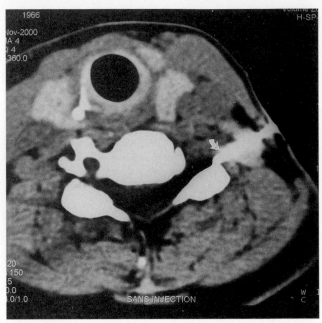

Figure 24-13   Cervical PPRI. A 22-gauge spinal needle (arrow) is inserted near the foramen from a lateral approach. Before injection of corticosteroid, 1.5 mL of contrast medium is injected to confirm the position of the needle tip.

the first 24 hours after the procedure. Other possible complications of PPRI include the risk of calcification if triamcinolone hexacetonide is used as the long-acting corticosteroid. The use of this product is not recommended for the above reason.

At the cervical level, vertebral artery injury or intra-arterial injections have been described. Precise CT control and the use of contrast media before injection to confirm an extradural location can avoid this (Box 24-6).

PERCUTANEOUS NUCLEOTOMY

The long-term outcome, complications, and occasionally suboptimal results which accompany open disc surgery have led to the development of other treatment

---

Box 24-6   Percutaneous Periradicular Infiltration of Corticosteroid

A 22-gauge spinal needle and CT guidance is used
Epidural space location is confirmed by lack of CSF aspiration and sterile air injection
Short-term pain relief best in patients with extraforaminal disc herniations
Long-term pain relief only in patients with extraforaminal disc herniations

techniques that avoid a surgical approach through the spinal canal with an extensive disc ablation. Percutaneous removal of the nucleus pulposus has been performed using a variety of chemical and mechanical techniques for the past several years. These techniques consist of removing all or part of the nucleus pulposus to induce more rapid healing of the abnormal lumbar disc. Percutaneous nucleotomy is now widely used, as it is much less invasive than surgical discectomy. To date, the most promising of these minimally invasive therapies used for treatment of disc herniations is percutaneous laser disc decompression (PLDD).

The advantage of this percutaneous technique is that disc decompression can be achieved without damage to other spinal structures. All minimally invasive techniques like PLDD are based on achieving a reduction in volume in the offending disc. In this procedure the laser energy is transmitted through a thin optical fiber into the intervertebral disc. The aim of PLDD is to vaporize a small portion of the nucleus pulposus. The ablation of a relatively small volume of the nucleus pulposus results in an important reduction of intradiscal pressure which reduces the effect of the disc herniation on adjacent nerve roots.

Indications

Patient selection is crucial for treatment effectiveness. Eligible patients must have positive and consistent neurologic findings (leg pain of greater intensity than back pain, positive straight-leg-raising test, decreased sensation, normal motor response and tendon reflexes). Patients must also have failed 6 weeks of conservative therapy and/or epidural injections. Other eligible patients are those with contained disc herniations determined by CT or MR imaging.

Contraindications

The contraindications are nerve paralysis, hemorrhagic diathesis, spondylolisthesis, spinal stenosis, previous surgery at the same level, significant psychologic disorder, significant narrowing of the disc space, workplace injuries where monetary gain is an issue, and local infection of cutaneous/subcutaneous or muscular layers.

Technique

In the authors' unit, PLDD is performed under dual guidance with a combination of CT and fluoroscopy. Some authors perform this procedure under fluoroscopy guidance alone. However, vaporization of the nucleus pulposus can be visualized only with CT.

The patient is placed in the prone position on the CT table. Two mobile fluoroscopy monitors are placed in front of the physician along with a CT monitor.

At any time the operator can switch from CT to fluoroscopy and vice versa. Needle positioning is performed under fluoroscopic guidance and vaporization of the disk is monitored by CT. Rolls are positioned under the abdomen to open up the disc spaces so that the lumbar spine is in a semiflexed position; this is particularly helpful for the L5–S1 level. Needle access is from a posterior approach, avoiding the nerve root and visceral structures. At the L5–S1 level, curved needles are usually necessary. The procedure is performed under local anesthesia with strict sterile precautions. Through a skin incision an 18-gauge needle is inserted into the disc. The tip of the 18-gauge needle must reach the posterior part of the nucleus pulposus (Fig. 24-14). The patient is monitored for pain during the whole procedure and the needle has to be repositioned if radicular pain occurs. To confirm contained disc herniation, or if any doubt persists, a discography can be performed just before PLDD. After removal of the stylet of the 18-gauge needle, the optical fiber is inserted into the disc. The distal part of the optical fiber should extend 5 mm beyond the needle tip.

The laser (diode laser 805-nm, or Nd:YAG laser 1064-nm wavelength) is turned on to produce 15–20 watts in 0.5- to 1-second pulses at 4- to 10-second intervals depending on patient comfort. Recommended laser doses for PLDD range from 1200 to 1500 joules for L1–L2, L2–L3, L3–L4, and L5–S1 levels, and from 1500 to 2000 joules for L4–L5. These short exposure times mean that there is no heating of the adjacent bone structures. A CT scan is performed after every 200 joules at the disc level to visualize the vaporized area (see Fig. 24-14). The patient must be able to communicate and respond to pain during the entire procedure, so that general anesthesia is absolutely contraindicated. If pain occurs, the intervals between laser pulses are increased and aspiration is applied to reduce pressure within the disc. If vaporization has not occurred after 500 joules, the fiber should be removed and its tip put into 1 mL of iodinate, which is used as a colorant to increase the absorption of the beam. The patient's blood can also be used as a colorant. The laser fiber is reinserted and the procedure is continued.

For 2 weeks after the intervention, positions that induce hyperkyphosis as well as athletic activities should be restricted. Resolution of leg pain usually occurs within 1–8 weeks.

Results

Two hundred and forty-eight patients with herniated lumbar discs and radicular pain were treated by PLDD on an outpatient basis. There were 138 male and 110 female patients. The oldest was 71 years and the youngest was 12 years (mean 40 years). The longest follow-up was

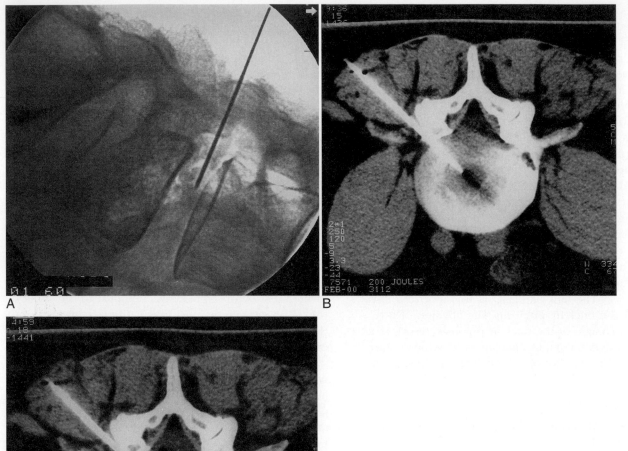

Figure 24-14   Percutaneous laser disc decompression (PLDD) at L4–L5. **A**, An 18-gauge spinal needle is inserted into the nucleus pulposus under fluoroscopy. **B**, A CT scan confirms optimal needle positioning. **C**, Vaporization (black areas) can be visualized only with CT.

8 years; the average follow-up was 28 months. The Macnab criteria were used to grade the response to treatment. The overall success rate was 76% according to MacNab's criteria with 55% having a "good" response and 21% having a "fair" response. In four cases, the PLDD was performed at two levels. After 6–12 months, a reduction in disc herniation was observed with CT or MR imaging. Thirty-two patients with poor results or recurrence were later treated surgically with a satisfying success rate (66%).

Complications of PLDD under CT and fluoroscopic guidance are rare. The major complication of percutaneous

nucleotomy is septic discitis. One patient suffered from a spondylodiscitis. Another suffered for 6 weeks from severe backache due to an aseptic thermal discitis (3 years' follow-up). One patient was readmitted 24 hours after PLDD with severe recurrence of leg pain because of free fragment extravasation of disc material with upward migration.

These results provide encouraging information that substantiate the validity of percutaneous laser nucleotomy for contained lumbar disc herniation. The most critical elements to successful PLDD are proper

patient selection, correct needle placement, and optimal
disc vaporization. Further randomized comparative
studies with surgery are necessary to confirm these data
(Box 24-7).

ALCOHOL ABLATION OF BONE METASTASES

Injection of alcohol is widely used for pain treatment
(neurolysis) in tumor management. Tumor invasion of
bone, from either a primary or a metastatic lesion, is the
most common cause of pain in cancer patients. Alcohol
ablation of bone metastases is aimed at treating the
excruciating pain that cancer patients often develop.

Indications

Percutaneous alcohol ablation of bone metastasis
(PABM) can be performed:

• In patients with painful severe osteolytic bone
  metastases
• If conventional anticancer therapy is ineffective and
  high doses of opiates are necessary to control pain
• When rapid pain relief is necessary (radiation or
  chemotherapy usually requires a 2- to 4-week delay).

Technique

The procedure is performed under sedoanalgesia or
general anesthesia to control pain associated with alcohol injection. After defining tumor location and size on
contiguous pre- and post-contrast CT scans, the optimal
puncture site and angle are defined. Contrast-enhanced
CT is performed to determine the necrotic part of the
tumor. Following local anesthetic (lidocaine 1%) administration in the skin and subcutaneous tissues, a 22-gauge
needle is placed in the tumor. Initially, contrast medium
(iohexol) 25% diluted with lidocaine is injected into the
lesion (Fig. 24-15). Intratumoral instillation of lidocaine is

performed to reduce the pain provoked by the injection
of alcohol. The distribution of contrast media within the
tumor is imaged by CT and predicts the diffusion of
ethanol in the lesion (see Fig. 24-15). If diffusion of the
contrast medium extends beyond the tumor boundaries,
and particularly if it reaches contiguous neurologic
structures, the procedure is discontinued.

Depending on tumor size, 3–30 mL of 96% ethanol are
instilled into the tumor. In large tumors, alcohol is selectively instilled into regions considered to be responsible
for pain, usually the periphery of metastases and osteolytic areas. After injection of 2–3 mL of alcohol, the distribution in the tumor is again evaluated by CT. The
ethanol is visualized by the dilution of contrast media
and by hypodense areas (injected alcohol has a low CT
attenuation value of −200 HU). If the alcohol is acciden-
tally injected and comes to lie in contact with neural
structures or other vital structures, the alcohol must be
immediately diluted with the injection of an isotonic
solution. If the distribution of alcohol is uneven within
the tumor (particularly in large metastases), the needle is
repositioned in regions of poor diffusion and the injection is repeated.

Results

Ninety-one patients with 124 bone metastases in various locations underwent bone alcohol ablation. In the
authors' small series, satisfactory results were obtained in
71% of the patients based on the reduction of opiate
doses. One of the major advantages of the injection of
alcohol into bone metastases is the rapid relief of pain
occurring within 24–48 hours. Duration of pain relief
ranged from 2 to 9 months (none of the patients survived beyond 9 months). In five patients, the alcohol
ablation was not performed because of a rich vascular
blood supply seen after contrast medium injection.

Possible complications are neurolysis and massive
tumor necrosis with fever and hyperuricemia. In the
authors' series, fever was observed in 15 patients in the
first 72 hours. In one patient with extension of a vertebral metastasis into the brachial plexus and severe neuralgia of C5, C6, and C7, a paraparesis was observed after
instillation of alcohol into the corresponding territory

RADIO-FREQUENCY ABLATION OF BONE METASTASES

Percutaneous ablation of bone metastases with radio-
frequency (RF) energy can be used in a similar manner
to alcohol ablation. Radio-frequency energy is able to
produce a much more predictable necrotic lesion than
alcohol, although alcohol is cheaper to use.

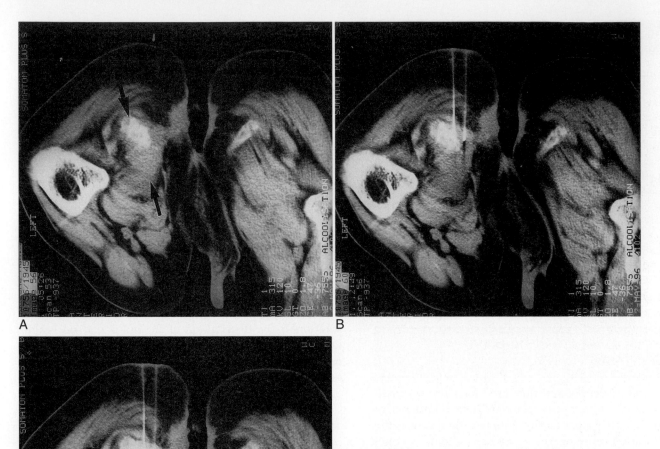

Figure 24-15   Alochol ablation of painful metastasis in ischium. **A,** Axial CT shows metastasis (arrows) with a soft tissue component in the left ischium. **B,** Two 22-gauge spinal needles are inserted into the tumor. **C,** After injection of 3 mL of contrast medium diluted with lidocaine, 6 mL of 96% ethanol was injected into the lesion.

Indications

In the authors' unit, RF ablation is reserved for tumor ablation and pain management if alcohol ablation is contraindicated. RF ablation is more suited to the treatment of lesions in sensitive regions because of the predictable size and shape of the lesion produced by this technique. Thermocoagulation is contraindicated if the lesion is close to neurologic structures and in bone tumors that are sclerotic.

Technique

Radio-frequency ablation is widely used for treating liver tumors. In the authors' unit we use an electrode with continuous saline infusion to increase the induced lesion size (Berchtold, Germany). The infusion electrode (16- to 18-gauge) is inserted into the tumor and a power of 40 watts is used for 10 minutes with continuous infusion of saline (82 mL/h) (Fig. 24-16). For large lesions (≥4 cm), the procedure should be repeated

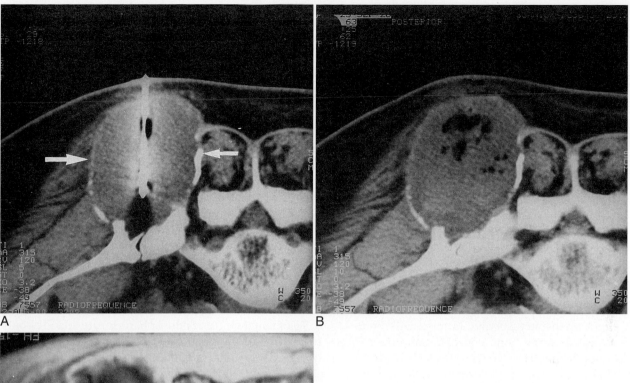

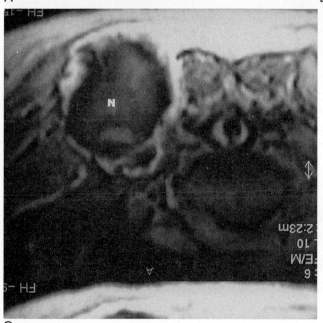

Figure 24-16   Alcohol ablation of large sacroiliac metastasis from thyroid cancer. **A**, Four injections of alcohol were performed in different parts of the metastasis (arrows). **B**, CT scan after the procedure shows some low-density alcohol inside the lesion. **C**, Two weeks after the procedure, MRI with injection of gadolinium shows a large amount of necrosis (N) within the tumor. Only a peripheral ring of contrast enhancement is visualized. The patient's pain resolved.

after modification of the position of the needle electrode. CT is used to guide the needle position within the lesion.

Results

The induced coagulation inside bone with a single energy delivery is about 35 mm in diameter. The ablation is monitored 1 week later with MRI using a dynamic injection of gadolinium. If the ablation is not complete it is repeated. Large bone metastases require multiple sessions. For lesions larger than 4 cm, two to three sessions, at weekly intervals, are usually necessary. As with alcohol ablation, fever is usual after the ablation. Local sepsis and neurologic complications can be avoided by strict sterility and a thorough knowledge of anatomy, respectively (Box 24-8).

PERCUTANEOUS CEMENTOPLASTY

Percutaneous cementoplasty (PC, or vertebroplasty) with acrylic glue (polymethylmethacrylate, PMMA) is a procedure aimed at preventing vertebral body collapse

and pain in patients with pathologic vertebral bodies.
Percutaneous cementoplasty seems to be a promising
technique for relieving pain in patients with bone
failure. The pain-reducing effect of cement cannot be
explained by the consolidation of the pathologic bone
alone. In fact, good pain relief is obtained after injection
of only 2 mL of methylmethacrylate in metastatic bone
lesions. In these cases the bone consolidation effect is
minimal. The methylmethacrylate is cytotoxic owing to
its chemical and thermal effect during polymerization.
The temperature during polymerization is high enough
to produce coagulation of tumoral cells. Therefore, good
pain relief can be obtained with a low volume of glue in
patients with metastatic bone lesions.

Lesions with epidural extension require careful injection to prevent epidural overflow and spinal cord compression by the cement, particularly in tumoral lesions.
The procedure is contraindicated in patients with hemorrhagic diathesis and in the presence of infection.

Indications

Percutaneous injection of acrylic glue is indicated in:
- Painful vertebral body tumors (particularly metastasis
  and myeloma), especially when there is a risk of
  compression fracture
- Patients with symptomatic vertebral hemangiomas
- Severe painful osteoporosis with loss of height and/or
  with compression fractures of the vertebral body
- Painful metastases to the acetabulum.

Technique

The procedure can be performed under fluoroscopy
alone in the lumbar and lower thoracic spine, but a combination of CT and fluoroscopy is safer. Fluoroscopy is
mandatory during injection of the glue. CT is particularly
useful in the thoracic spine and in other difficult areas to
reduce complications.

The procedure is performed under local anesthesia
usually combined with sedoanalgesia. The patient is

placed in the prone position for lumbar treatments and
in a supine position for cervical treatments. A 15-gauge
needle is used in the cervical spine, a 10-gauge needle in
the thoracic and lumbar spine. The needle entry point
and the access route are determined by CT, avoiding
nerve roots and visceral structures (Figs 24-17 and 24-18).

An anterior approach is used in the cervical area, a
transpedicular or intercostovertebral route in the thoracic area, and a posterolateral or transpedicular route in
the lumbar area.

Cortical perforation requires the aid of a surgical
hammer. When the needle is in the optimal position
(needle tip in the anterior third of the vertebral body),
the imaging mode is switched to fluoroscopy. A package
of methylmethacrylate (Simplex/Howmedica, Palacos
low-viscosity/Schering Plough) contains a 40-g packet of
powder and a 20-mL tube of fluid monomer. The acrylic
glue or cement is prepared by mixing the powder and
the fluid monomer together.

Because the cement is not sufficiently radiopaque,
2–3 g of tantalum (tungsten, or barium) are added to only
10–15 mL of the mixture and aspirated in a screw
syringe. During the first 30–50 seconds after mixing, the
glue is thin but then becomes pasty. The acrylic cement
has to be injected during its pasty polymerization phase
to prevent distal venous migration. Two to eight milliliters of acrylic glue are injected using a screw syringe
(Cemento, Optimed, Germany). At this stage, the intervention has to be performed quickly because the glue
begins to thicken after 3–5 minutes (depending on the
temperature of the operating room) and any further
injections become impossible.

The injection of the glue is monitored under strict lateral fluoroscopy (Box 24-9). The injection of acrylic glue

is stopped immediately whenever epidural or paravertebral opacification is observed to prevent spinal cord compression. When vertebral filling is insufficient, a contralateral injection is performed to complete the treatment. After vertebral body opacification, the stylet of the needle is replaced and the needle is removed before the cement begins to set. Six to seven minutes after mixing; the methylmethacrylate begins to harden. During this hardening time, the methylmethacrylate becomes hot (90°C). The patient should be sedated and given analgesic medication to control pain. Monitoring of the arterial pressure is necessary during the procedure

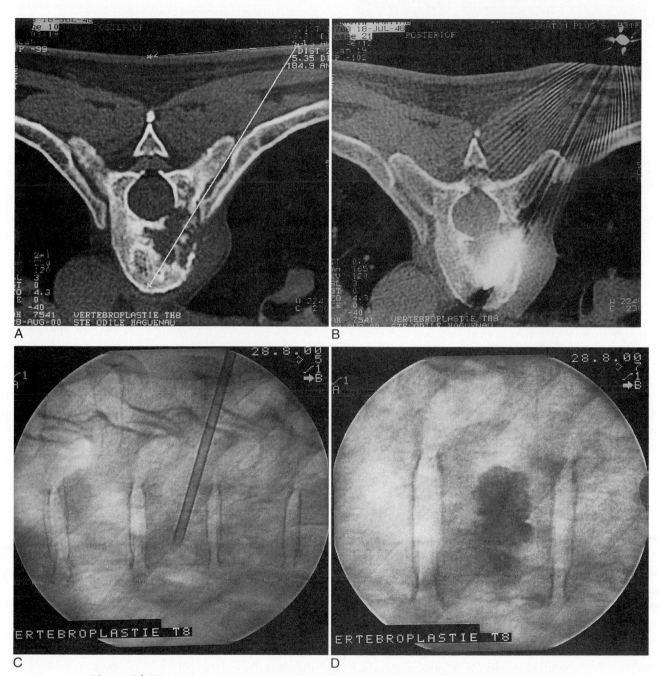

Figure 24-17   Percutaneous vertebroplasty of a painful lytic metastasis in the T8 vertebral body. **A,** An intercostovertebral access route is chosen on this CT image. Note the partial rupture of the lateral wall of the vertebral body. **B/C,** A 10-gauge vertebroplasty needle is positioned in the anterior part of the metastasis under (B) CT and (C) fluoroscopic guidance. **D,** Injection of polymethyl methacrylate (PMMA) is performed under strict lateral fluoroscopy monitoring.

(Continued)

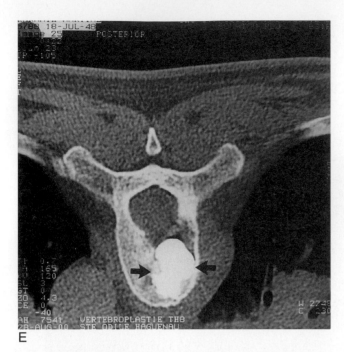

Figure 24-17   cont'd E, CT postprocedure shows the cement (arrows) in position in the metastasis.

because methylmethacrylate injections can induce brief drops in arterial pressure. Total procedure time ranges from 20 to 60 minutes. In patients with osteoporosis and symptomatic hemangiomas, optimal filling (2.5–7 mL) of the vertebral body is required to obtain both effects of percutaneous vertebroplasty: bone consolidation and pain relief (Fig. 24-19).

In patients with tumoral pathologies, percutaneous cementoplasty is usually performed for excruciating pain. In these cases, a low volume (1.5–3 mL) of acrylic glue affords good pain relief (see Box 24-9).

Results

Percutaneous cementoplasty was performed in 310 patients; indications included severe painful osteoporosis (173 patients), vertebral myeloma and metastases (123 patients), and symptomatic hemangiomas (14 patients). A total of 407 vertebral bodies were injected. The average volume of cement injected was 2.8 mL (ranging from 1.8 to 6.5 mL). The analgesic effect appeared within 6–48 hours after the procedure. Results were evaluated according to the reduction of opiate analgesic doses and using a visual analog scale.

Percutaneous cementoplasty is a successful technique for pain management and consolidation of pathologic vertebral bodies. The most critical elements for successful vertebroplasty are proper patient selection, correct needle placement; good timing of cement injection, strict fluoroscopy control of the injection, and the

operator's experience. The pain relief obtained with this technique does not correlate with the volume of glue injected, especially in metastases where 1.5 mL of glue is usually enough to reduce the patient's pain considerably.

In osteoporosis, satisfactory results were obtained in 78% of patients. In vertebral tumors, satisfactory results were obtained in 85%. In patients with hemangiomas, satisfactory results were obtained in 78%.

Complications

Complications related to vertebroplasty include cement leaks into the epidural space, epidural veins, neural foramen, disc space, intercostal artery, paravertebral veins, and paravertebral soft tissues.

Epidural leak of methylmethacrylate may cause spinal cord compression. This risk is minimized by monitoring the injection of cement into the vertebral body using high-quality fluoroscopy and by adding tantalum to the acrylic glue to provide adequate radiopacity. Radiculopathy is the major risk with neural foramen cement leaks. In the authors' series, three complications occurred immediately after vertebroplasty with the filling of either an epidural vein or neural foramen causing intercostal neuralgia. Obviously, orthopedic or neurosurgical support should be available when performing these procedures. Venous leaks into paravertebral veins can lead to pulmonary cement embolism. In the authors' series, an asymptomatic pulmonary embolism was detected in two patients; in both, paravertebral venous opacification was observed. To avoid major pulmonary infarction, the glue should be injected slowly during its pasty polymerization phase under fluoroscopic guidance, and the injection should be stopped immediately if a venous leak is observed.

Cement leaks into paravertebral soft tissues have no clinical significance, while cement leaks into the disc space are usually also without clinical consequence. However, the latter may increase the risk of adjacent vertebral body collapse in osteoporotic patients.

In the authors' series one patient had a leak of acrylic cement into an intercostal artery. This was asymptomatic.

In cementoplasty of the hip, the risk of intraarticular injection is the main problem. This complication can be reduced with continuous monitoring of the injected glue under fluoroscopy.

Other general complications related to vertebroplasty and hip cementoplasty include infection, temporary pain, and allergic incidents. Infection can be avoided by using a strict sterile technique while performing the intervention.

Temporary pain can be observed after the procedure. Patients are usually free of symptoms after 24 hours. The postprocedural pain is usually proportional to the volume of glue injected. In the authors' series the

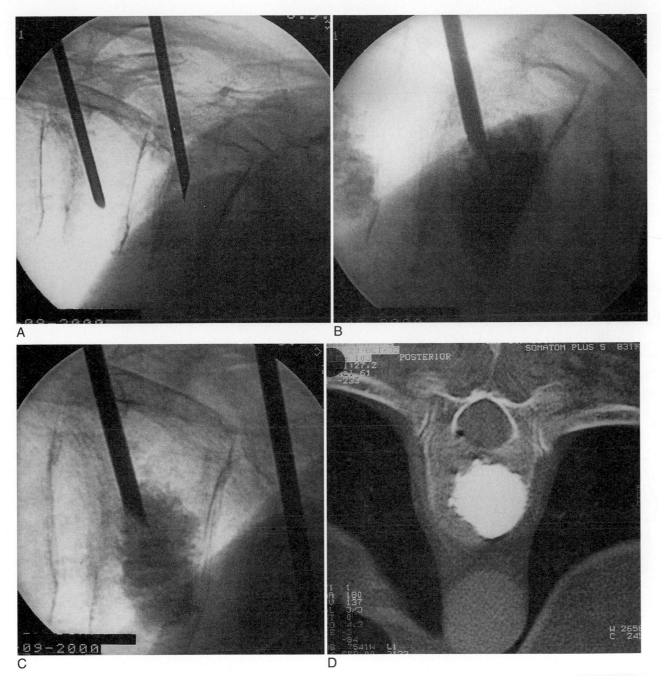

Figure 24-18   Percutaneous vertebroplasty of T12 and L1 in osteoporotic collapse fractures. **A**, Transpedicular insertion of two 10-gauge needles under fluoroscopic guidance. The bevel of the needle is used to direct the needle. **B/C**, When the needles are in the anterior part of the vertebral bodies, the PMMA is prepared separately for each level and injected under fluoroscopic guidance. If necessary, the needle position is modified during the injection for optimal vertebral body filling. **D**, DCT scan at one level after the procedure shows the cement in good position.

majority of patients had good packing of the vertebral body with more than 5 mL of acrylic glue injected.

The risk of allergic incidents and hypotension is limited in these procedures, because the quantities of acrylic glue injected in percutaneous cementoplasty are far less than those used in orthopedic surgery (Box 24-10).

PERCUTANEOUS MANAGEMENT OF OSTEOID OSTEOMA

Osteoid osteoma is a benign neoplasm of bone which occurs most often in men. The age range is from 2 to

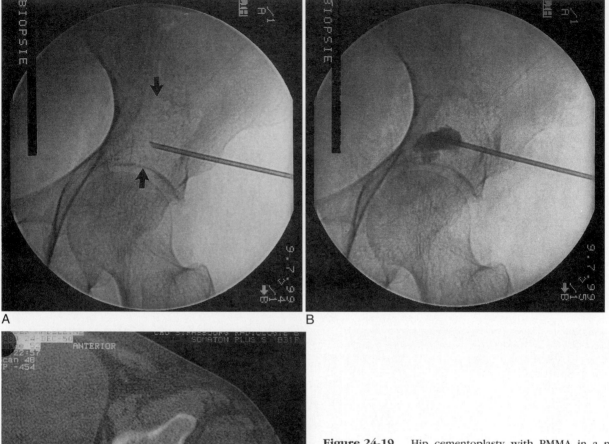

Figure 24-19 Hip cementoplasty with PMMA in a patient with a painful metastasis. **A,** A 14-gauge needle is inserted into the metastasis (arrows) under fluoroscopic guidance. **B,** PMMA is injected under fluoroscopic guidance to avoid intraarticular leak. **C,** CT image after procedure showing the cement in good position in the roof of the acetabulum.

Box 24-10 Vertebroplasty: Complications

Spinal cord decompression from epidural cement leak
Radiculopathy from neural foramen or epidural vein leaks
Pulmonary embolism from paravertebral vein leaks
Osteomyelitis
Allergic or anaphylactic responses

---

50 years, but 90% occur before the age of 25. Osteoid osteoma produces local pain that is worse at night and improves dramatically with aspirin. The characteristic signs of this tumor in clinical and radiologic examinations can lead to a high level of diagnostic confidence for this condition. Effective treatment of this tumor depends on complete removal of the tumor nidus. The conventional treatment is surgical or percutaneous excision. The ability to precisely control the treated area, a high degree of precision, applicability in joints, and an excellent dose–response characteristic makes interstitial laser photocoagulation (ILP) a valuable treatment method for osteoid osteomas.

Contraindications to the procedure are hemorrhagic diathesis, and lesions closer than 5 mm to vital neurologic structures.

Indications

Patient selection is crucial for treatment effectiveness. The indications are osteoid osteomas visible by CT, MR imaging, or scintigraphy, with positive and consistent clinical findings.

Technique

ILP consists of percutaneous insertion of optical fibers into the tumor. The tumor is coagulated and destroyed by direct heating. With a low-power laser technique, a well-defined coagulation necrosis of predictable size and shape can be obtained in bone tissue. Experimental work has shown that a reproducible area of coagulative necrosis is obtained around the fiber, with good correlation between energy delivered and the lesion size, and with conservation of the biomechanical properties of the bone tissue in the treated area. The size of most osteoid osteomas falls within the range that can be coagulated effectively by one or two fibers (Figs 24-20 and 24-21).

The procedure is performed under CT-guidance. CT is used to measure the diameter of the nidus. The largest diameter of the nidus determines the energy that will be necessary to coagulate the tumor. For diameters larger than 10 mm, the authors usually use two fibers to ensure tumor destruction. The needle entry point and access route are determined by CT, avoiding neural, vascular, and visceral structures. Penetration of the needle into the nidus is always extremely painful; therefore ILP is performed under general anesthesia or local anesthetic limb blocks.

Subperiostal nidi or cortical nidi without major ossification are directly punctured with an 18-gauge spinal needle (Becton Dickinson, Rutherford, NJ). In cases with mild ossification or a small amount of cortex surrounding the lesion, a 14-gauge bone biopsy needle is more appropriate (Ostycut, Angiomed/Bard, Karlsruhe, Germany). In tumors with dense ossification, or if dense cortical bone surrounds the lesion, drilling is necessary. In these cases we use a 2-mm diameter hand drill or a 14-gauge Bonopty Penetration set (Radi Medical Systems, Uppsala, Sweden) to allow insertion of the 18-gauge needle.

The 18-gauge needle tip is inserted into the center of the nidus. Before the optical fiber is placed, it is inserted in an 18-gauge needle mounted in a side-arm fitting to measure the appropriate length of the fiber. The 400-μm fiber is then inserted through the needle; the needle is withdrawn about 5 mm so that the tip of the bare fiber lies within the center of the tumor.

The diode laser (Diomed 805-nm) is turned on in continuous wave mode, at a power of 2 watts for 200–600 seconds depending on the nidus size (energy delivered 400–1200 joules). CT imaging is performed during the procedure to detect vaporization.

After a period of 6–12 months, sclerosis of the nidus is observed on follow-up CT examination.

Results

From 1993 to 2000, 79 patients with osteoid osteomas were treated by ILP on an outpatient basis or with an overnight stay. Patients ranged in age from 4 to 48 years. ILP was successful in 78 patients. Pain relief occurred rapidly: 88% of patients were completely pain-free within 24 hours of the procedure, and 6% within 48–72 hours. One patient was pain-free only after 2 months because of a reflex sympathetic dystrophy syndrome. Immediately after the procedure the majority of patients had substantial local pain and were hospitalized overnight for treatment with narcotics and discharged within 24 hours of the procedure. Return to normal activities was prompt: most patients were able to return to work or school within a week.

Treatment was unsuccessful in one patient. In five patients pain recurred after variable pain-free periods ranging from 6 weeks to a year, and in these patients follow-up CT examinations revealed a residual nidus. These were treated successfully with a second ILP procedure.

Complications of ILP are very rare. Only one complication was observed among the authors' 79 patients. This consisted of a mild reflex sympathetic dystrophy of the wrist. One week after the procedure, this patient reported burning pain, which was different from the previous pain. The patient described a new symptomatology consisting of burning pain, hyperalgesia, hyperesthesia, and vasomotor disturbances. Symptoms were entirely relieved after 2 months of treatment. Possible complications of ILP are infection, hematoma, and reflex sympathetic dystrophy (Box 24-11).

Box 24-11   ILP of Osteoid Osteomas

Precise image localization of the nidus and appropriate clinical symptomatology are required

ILP is performed under general anesthetic using CT guidance

One needle and one laser fiber are sufficient for nidus diameters up to 10 mm

Nidus vaporization is seen as ILP progresses

Success rates of 80–90% reported.

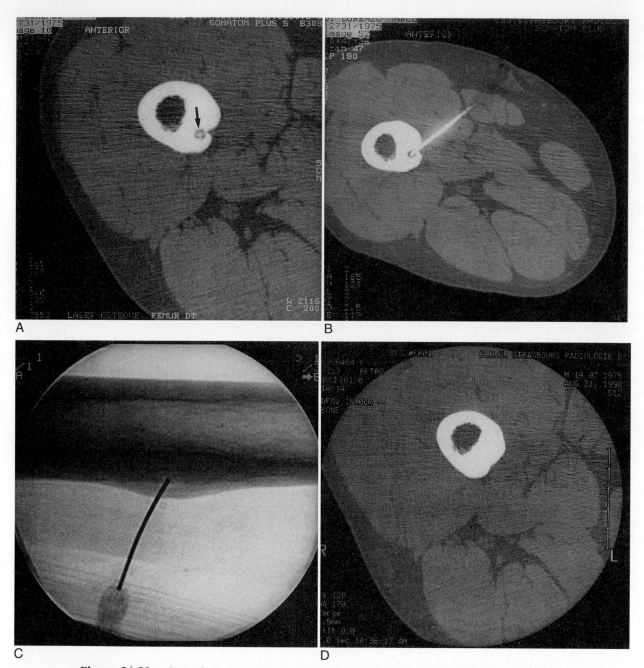

Figure 24-20   Osteoid osteoma of femoral diaphysis treated with interstitial laser photocoagulation (ILP). **A**, Axial CT image showing the tumor nidus (arrow) in the femoral cortex. **B**, An 18-gauge needle was inserted into the nidus under CT guidance and 1000 joules of energy delivered to the tumor nidus. **C**, Fluoroscopic image showing the needle tip within the tumor nidus. **D**, CT scan 18 months after photocoagulation shows ossification of the nidus. The patient's pain resolved after ILP.

SUGGESTED READINGS

Bush K, Hillier S: A controlled study of caudal epidural injections of triamcinolone plus procaine for the management of intractable sciatica. *Spine* 16:572–575, 1991.

Choy DS, Ascher PW, Saddekni S et al: Percutaneous laser disk decompression: a new therapeutic modality. *Spine* 17:949–956, 1992.

Cotten A, Boutry N, Cortet B et al: Percutaneous vertebroplasty: state of the art. *Radiographics* 18:311–323, 1998.

Deramond H, Depriester C, Galibert P, Le Gars D: Percutaneous vertebroplasty with polymethylmethacrylate: technique, indications, and results. *Radiol Clin N Am* 36:533–546, 1998.

El-Khoury GY, Renfrew DL: Percutaneous procedures for the diagnosis and treatment of lower back pain: diskography,

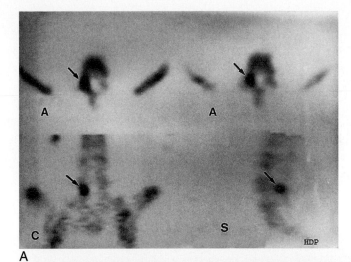

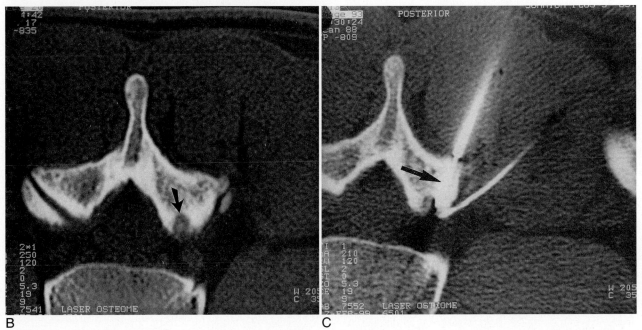

Figure 24-21   ILP of an osteoid osteoma in the articular process of L4. **A,** Bone scan confirming markedly increased uptake (arrows) of the radiopharmaceutical in the right articular process of L4 on these axial (A), coronal (C), and sagittal (S) images. **B,** Axial CT image confirming the location of the tumor nidus (arrow). **C,** A 14-gauge needle (straight arrow) was inserted into the nidus. The adjacent exiting nerve root was too close to the lesion, so to avoid neurologic damage, a 22-gauge curve spinal needle (curved arrow) was positioned between the nidus and the nerve root. The curved 22-gauge needle was continuously perfused with saline (80 mL/h) to protect the nerve root during ILP. The nidus was then ablated by ILP.

facet-joint injection, and epidural injection. *Am J Roentgenol* 157:685-691, 1991.

Gangi A, Dietemann JL, Schultz A et al: Interventional radiologic procedures with CT guidance in cancer pain management. *Radiographics* 16:1289-1306, 1996.

Gangi A, Dietemann JL, Gasser B et al: Interstitial laser photocoagulation of osteoid osteomas with use of CT guidance. *Radiology* 203:843-848, 1997.

Gangi A, Dietemann JL, Gasser B et al: Interventional radiology with laser in bone and joint. *Radiol Clin N Am* 36:547-557, 1998.

Gangi A, Dietemann JL, Mortazavi R et al: CT-guided interventional procedures for pain management in the lumbosacral spine. *Radiographics* 18:621-633, 1998.

Ghormley RK: Low back pain with special reference to the articular facets with presentation of an operative procedure. *JAMA* 101:1773, 1933.

Jensen ME, Evans AJ, Mathis JM et al: Percutaneous polymethylmethacrylate vertebroplasty in the treatment of osteoporotic vertebral body compression fractures: technical aspects. *Am J Neuroradiol* 18:1897-1904, 1997.

Laredo JD, Bellaiche L, Hamze B et al: Current status of musculoskeletal interventional radiology. *Radiol Clin N Am* 32: 377-398, 1994.

Maldjian C, Mesgarzadeh M, Tehranzadeh J: Diagnostic and therapeutic features of facet and sacroiliac joint injection: anatomy, pathophysiology, and technique. *Radiol Clin N Am* 36: 497-508, 1998.

McCulloch JA, Transfeldt EE: *MacNab's Backache*, 3rd edn, Williams & Wilkins, Baltimore, 1997.

Murphy WA, Destoutet JM, Gilula LA: Percutaneous skeletal biopsy: a procedure for radiologists . *Radiology* 139:545-549, 1981.

Panjabi MM, Hopper W, White AA, Keggi KI: Posterior spine stabilization with methyl methacrylate biomechanical testing of a surgical specimen. *Spine* 2:241-247, 1977.

Rosenthal DI, Hornicek FJ, Wolfe MW et al: Percutaneous radiofrequency coagulation of osteoid osteoma compared with operative treatment. *J Bone Joint Surg Am* 80:815-821, 1998.

Tohmeh AG, Mathis JM, Fenton DC, Levine AM, Belkoff SM: Biomechanical efficacy of unipedicular versus bipedicular vertebroplasty for the management of osteoporotic compression fractures. *Spine* 24:1772-1776, 1999.

CHAPTER 5

Tumor Ablation

GREGORY M. SOARES, M.D., AND
WILLIAM W. MAYO-SMITH, M.D.

Many solid tissue malignancies are poorly responsive to systemic chemotherapy, surgical resection, or local radiation therapy. Patients presenting with these tumors often have poor life expectancy and multiple co-morbid diseases. Though surgical resection remains the only potentially curative treatment, the small number of patients who are suitable surgical candidates limits its usefulness. Even in appropriate candidates, surgical morbidity is not trivial. *In situ* image-guided tumor destruction or ablation has become an attractive option. It offers the possibility of an effective, minimally invasive and less costly approach, often achievable in an outpatient setting. Available ablation techniques can be broadly classified as chemical, embolic, or thermal (Box 25-1). Embolic therapy such as transarterial chemoembolization (TACE) is discussed elsewhere.

CHEMICAL ABLATION

Chemical ablation is achieved with image-guided instillation of a chemical agent. The most common chemical agent used for tumor ablation is ethanol. Percutaneous ethanol injection (PEI) has been shown to be a safe, inexpensive, and effective treatment for small (3–5 cm) hepatocellular carcinomas (HCC). Ethanol works by protein denaturation leading to coagulative necrosis, thrombosis of small vessels, and formation of fibrotic and granulomatous tissue. It is effective for an encapsulated tumor, like HCC, which is surrounded by liver tissue made firm by underlying disease (cirrhotic liver). The alcohol diffuses throughout the tumor but is prevented from diffusing into the normal liver parenchyma by the tumor capsule and surrounding cirrhotic parenchyma. Unfortunately, PEI is less effective for treating metastases since they are often firm tumors surrounded by normal liver tissue (Box 25-2).

PEI is performed by placing a small (19-gauge) needle into the center of the tumor. Absolute ethanol (96%) is injected during continuous sonographic monitoring. Alcohol droplets appear as a hyperechoic cloud. The volume injected is based on the tumor size, considered as a sphere, using the equation

$$\text{Injected volume } (V) = 4\pi(r + 0.5)^3/3$$

Box 25-1 Solid-tumor Ablation Techniques

Chemical

Percutaneous ethanol injection
Transarterial chemoembolization

Thermal

Cryoablation
High-intensity focused ultrasound
Microwave ablation
Interstitial laser photocoagulation
Radio-frequency ablation

Box 25-2 PEI for Liver Tumors

Ethanol ablation, effective for hepatocellular
  carcinoma (HCC)
Less effective for liver metastases
10–20 mL ethanol injected per treatment session
Multiple treatment sessions often required
Multiple needle tracts in the liver should be avoided

In the authors' unit we generally use 10–20 mL of ethanol per treatment session. Injections are repeated as needed on a weekly basis until the calculated volume is achieved. Multiple needle tracts are avoided to decrease the risk of alcohol leaking into the peritoneal cavity, which can be very painful.

Though CT can be used for image guidance, ultrasound is the preferred modality for performing PEI. CT imaging is usually employed for treatment follow-up (Fig. 25-1).

Ethanol injection for HCC results in complete tumor necrosis in 70–80% of cases (see Fig. 25-1). Cure rates equal those of surgery in selected patients. Results for metastases are less favorable with complete necrosis rates closer to 50%. PEI has not gained widespread popularity in the United States probably due to the need for multiple treatments and its decreased efficacy in treating colorectal metastases.

THERMAL ABLATION

Tissue functions normally in a narrow range of temperatures. If the local temperature is made sufficiently abnormal, the cells within the environment are permanently

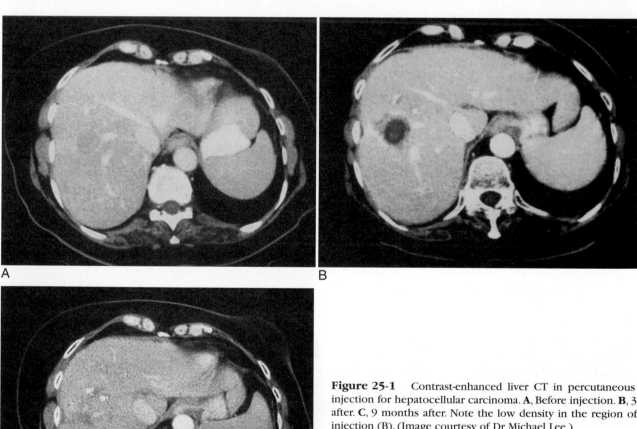

Figure 25-1   Contrast-enhanced liver CT in percutaneous ethanol injection for hepatocellular carcinoma. **A**, Before injection. **B**, 3 months after. **C**, 9 months after. Note the low density in the region of alcohol injection (B). (Image courtesy of Dr Michael Lee.)

damaged. If extremes of temperature are applied, the cells are destroyed, and coagulative necrosis ensues. Thermal energy can be effectively used to destroy tumors through either freezing or burning.

Cryoablation

In situ tumor destruction by freezing is called cryoablation. Cryoablation has been used to treat neoplasms of skin, rectum, bone, and larynx as well as solid organ tumors. Cryoablation has been widely studied as a treatment for nonresectable liver cancers. Tumors must be cooled to at least −35°C to achieve complete necrosis. At this temperature, ice crystals, formed during rapid freezing, result in mechanical destruction of normal cell structures, cell death, and coagulative necrosis. Cryoablation often requires the use of large cryoprobes, generally 3- to 8-mm outer diameter. The probes use circulating liquid nitrogen to cause freezing and tumor necrosis. The ablation is performed during laparotomy or laparoscopy, with intraoperative ultrasound for probe placement and iceball monitoring (Box 25-3).

As freezing occurs the iceball appears sonographically as an echodense hemisphere with posterior acoustic shadowing (Fig. 25-2). Tumor beyond the leading echogenic edge is therefore difficult to evaluate once the iceball forms. Magnetic resonance imaging has been studied experimentally as an image guidance modality during cryotherapy to circumvent this problem. This requires open magnet platforms, nonferromagnetic anesthesic and surgical equipment, and MR-compatible cryoprobes. In clinical practice, effective tissue necrosis occurs by repetition of the freeze/thaw cycle two to three times per treatment. The low temperature required for effective tumor cell necrosis is difficult to maintain at the periphery of tumors because, blood vessels act as a heat sink. Effective freezing near peripheral vessels is therefore hampered.

Complication rates with hepatic cryoablation range between 15% and 50%. Complications include pleural effusions, hemorrhage, biliary fistulas, abscesses, cold injury to adjacent organs, and a 4% mortality rate. Blood loss up to 750 mL has been reported which may be

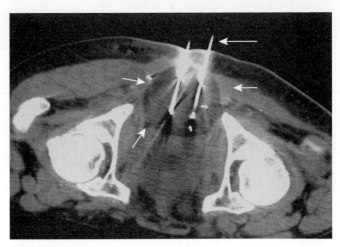

Figure 25-2   A 56-year-old man with nonresectable, painful rectal carcinoma recurrence treated with percutaneous cryoablation. CT image of the pelvis with the patient in the prone position demonstrates two cryoablation probes (long arrow) in the tumor. Note the low-density "freeze ball" around the probes (short arrows). (Image courtesy of Dr David Iannitti.)

related to the large probe size or liver surface cracking during thawing. Suturing or packing of the liver is often required after cryoablation. For these reasons, and because the cryotherapy equipment is expensive, less invasive technologies with similar or better efficacies have gained popularity.

Heat–Tissue Interaction

Percutaneous, image-guided therapics using heat have utilized diverse thermal energy sources. All thermal ablation techniques are loosely based on the Pennes' "bioheat equation," which can be approximated as

Coagulation necrosis (tumor kill) = Energy deposited × (Local tissue interaction − Heat lost)

From this equation (regardless of the energy source), the determinants of effective ablation are governed by the tissue being ablated and its surroundings. The intent of each of these treatment modalities is destruction of malignant cells and an acceptable tumor-free margin. When cellular temperatures are elevated above approximately 50°C, cytotoxicity results through denaturation of intracellular proteins and cell membrane destruction. If the temperature is raised to between 60°C and 100°C, near instantaneous protein coagulation and cell death occurs.

All thermal ablative methods are hindered by the inverse relationship between heat deposition as a function of increasing distance from the energy source. This results in less uniform attainment of cytotoxic temperatures distal to the epicenter. All thermal ablative

---

Box 25-3   Cryoablation

Tumors cooled to −35°C for complete necrosis
3- to 8-mm diameter cryoprobes used
Laparotomy or laparoscopy required to place probes
Complication rates vary from 15 to 50%
Mortality 4%

Table 25-1   Comparison of Thermal Modalities

Modality	Availability	Number of Sessions	Complication Rate	Cost
Cryoablation	↑↑	↓	↑↑↑	↑
Microwave	↓↓↓	↑	↑↑	↑↑↑
Laser	↓↓	↑↑	↓	↑↑↑
High-intesity US	↓↓	–	–	↑↑↑
Radio-frequency	↑↑↑	↓	↓	↓

methods are also limited in the maximum quantity and rate of heat energy that can be delivered, since exposure of tissue to extreme temperatures causes vaporization and gas formation that insulates distal tissue from further heating.

Strategies have been applied to each thermal energy modality to improve tumor kill. Generally, these approaches include increasing the amount or rate of energy delivered, improving the tissue conduction of the heat released by the energy delivered, or potentiating the deleterious effect of heat on the tumor. Thermal energy sources have included sound (high-intensity focused ultrasound), light (lasers to induce photocoagulation), and other electromagnetic energy sources (microwaves and radio-frequency energy).

HIGH-INTENSITY ULTRASOUND, MICROWAVE, AND LASER ABLATION

High-intensity ultrasound utilizes multiple small piezoelectric crystals to deposit sound energy in tissues, which induces heat destruction of cells. However, foci of energy deposition and tumor destruction remain small and require excessive and complex imaging guidance to be widely applied. Microwave coagulation has been studied most extensively in Japan with only minimal experience in the United States. Most reports describe multiple treatment sessions even for lesions as small as 1.5–2.0 cm. Complications of microwave therapy include burning in the electrode entrance tract and on the skin. Image guidance generally consists of continuous ultrasound monitoring.

Interstitial laser photocoagulation (ILP) uses intense pulses of light created by a laser to generate heat. The laser light is conveyed to the tissue by optical fibers passed through 19-gauge needles. The needles are arranged in arrays within the tumor using ultrasound guidance for placement and monitoring of therapy. CT or CT fluoroscopy may aid with difficult tumor localization. Generally, between four and eight needles are placed for each 3- to 4-cm lesion; 12 needles may be required for large or multiple lesions. Complete tumor

necrosis in lesions less than 4 cm has been reported in 40–60% of lesions. A comparison of thermal ablation techniques can be seen in Table 25-1.

RADIO-FREQUENCY ABLATION

Mechanism of Action

Radio-frequency (RF) energy has been used for surgical electrocautery since the early 1900s. Cushing and Bovie described the use of electrosurgery to aid the removal of intracranial neoplasms in 1928. In the late 1970s, Organ showed that alternating electrical current in the RF range in living tissue resulted in agitation of ions and frictional heat. As with all thermal energy sources, sufficient heating causes coagulation necrosis. Early experiments investigating the use of RF to create deep thermal injury in solid organs used equipment similar to that of the Bovie knife. Lesions were limited in size, but enthusiasm for the modality grew. Radio-frequency ablation (RFA) has been applied in the treatment of cardiac conduction anomalies, trigeminal neuralgia, osteoid osteomas, and neoplasms of liver, kidney, adrenal, spleen, bone and soft tissue, breast, lung, and prostate. RF techniques have been refined and continue to be modified. RFA has now emerged as the most predictable and safe means to treat solid neoplasms percutaneously.

RFA can be achieved with monopolar or bipolar electrode systems. Most work on RFA has focused on monopolar systems. Monopolar electrode RFA creates an electrical circuit within the patient between an active probe within the tumor and large dispersive grounding pads on the patient's back or thighs. The active electrode consists of a metal needle(s) with an insulated shaft(s). The electrode is placed in the tumor using image guidance. Percutaneous access to the lesion is similar to needle placement for a biopsy. Ultrasound, computed tomography, and magnetic resonance have been used as guidance modalities.

RF electrodes consist of an insulated shaft and an active tip from which current emanates, causing heat and tumor necrosis. As noted previously, tissue temperature declines rapidly at increasing distances from the energy source. Heat conduction in tissue is limited and adjacent flowing blood acts as a heat sink (dissipating heat). Several engineering strategies have been developed to induce maximal tumor necrosis from a single RF treatment. One strategy employs a single electrode with multiple tines emanating from its tip, much like the struts of an umbrella. A second design employs a cluster of three electrodes placed a fixed distance apart to ensure complete tumor necrosis distal to and between the electrodes (Fig. 25-3).

Several manufacturers have placed temperature-measuring devices at the tips of the electrodes to measure temperature locally during treatment sessions and ensure complete necrosis. A sustained temperature greater than 50°C at 1 minute after treatment indicates satisfactory ablation. One manufacturer produces a water-cooled electrode to prevent the active tip from getting too hot. This limits tissue vaporization at the tip, which would otherwise insulate distal tumor and limit effective heating. Another strategy to augment energy deposition uses rapid alternation of high- and low-energy application, or energy pulsing. Pulsing algorithms increase the mean thermal energy deposited and widen the effective zone of coagulation. Preferential cooling is achieved adjacent to the electrode during the low-energy periods without significantly decreasing tissue heating deeper in the tumor.

A final approach to increasing relevant necrosis volumes addresses the heat sink effect of flowing blood. Perfusion-mediated tissue cooling greatly determines the extent and effectiveness of thermal energy deposition. Studies have shown that the Pringle maneuver of temporary cross-clamping the portal vein and hepatic artery in the porta hepatis during RF treatment results in larger volume coagulation. The obvious drawback to this approach is the inherently greater invasiveness. Alternative techniques using catheter-delivered temporary (occlusion balloons) or permanent embolic material (Gelfoam, PVA, or Lipiodol) before RFA may achieve similar results. Using some or all of these approaches, contemporary RFA equipment is capable of producing single sphere burns of 3.5–5 cm (Box 25-4).

The benefits of image-guided, percutaneous RFA over open or laparoscopic RFA include its less invasive nature, the use of intravenous conscious sedation versus general anesthesia, the repeatability of the treatment, and its lower cost. Most RFA can be performed on an outpatient basis. Open or laparoscopic RFA can provide better access to tumors not detected by imaging with the ability to move or resect structures that may hinder the RF treatment. Additionally, open or laparoscopic RFA provides the option to decrease perfusion-mediated cooling with a Pringle-type maneuver.

Patient Preparation

Since the RFA technique is similar to image-guided needle biopsy, patient preparation is also similar. Obviously, special attention must be paid to the patient's coagulation profile and platelet function since RF probes are between 14- and 17-gauge outer diameter. Anticoagulants (warfarin, low-molecular-weight heparin) and antiplatelet agents (clopidogrel, NSAIDs) should be stopped with sufficient time for coagulation status to normalize (or be appropriately substituted with short-acting clotting factors if anticoagulation can be ceased for only a brief window).

As with percutaneous biopsies, preparation begins with patient selection. In most cases this entails pre-procedural CT, US, or MR examination of the tumor to be treated. In addition to determining the surgical resectability of lesions, imaging allows evaluation of adjacent structures. Tumors that can be safely and effectively resected for cure dictate surgical evaluation. Therefore, a close relationship with oncologists and oncologic surgeons is imperative. If the lesion is amenable to RFA, histologic sampling to confirm malignancy should be considered. If lesion pathology is unavailable prior

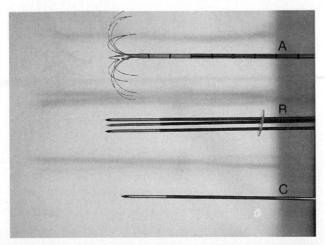

Figure 25-3 Three radio-frequency electrodes. **A**, Retractable "umbrella" electrode. **B**, Cluster water-cooled electrode. **C**, Single water-cooled electrode.

Box 25-4 **Strategies to Increase Tumor Kill**
Coaxial multiple probe or cluster array electrodes
Cooled-tip RFA electrodes
Radio-frequency energy pulsing
Inflow occlusion to eliminate perfusion-mediated cooling

to RFA, but imaging is sufficiently characteristic, then percutaneous biopsy can be performed at the time of RF treatment. The biopsy needle may even be employed as a tandem needle guide. Obviously, if histopathologic diagnosis will dictate RF treatment, this approach mandates on-site cytopathology personnel for the biopsy procedure.

Relative contraindications to performing RFA may include excessive tumor burden, untreatable diffuse or distant disease, active signs of infection, uncorrectable coagulopathy, and inability to obtain informed consent. Prior to treatment the patient must receive a directed history and physical examination. Preprocedural laboratory studies should include complete blood count, coagulation profile, blood chemistries (tailored to the organ system being treated), electrocardiogram, baseline appropriate tumor markers, and blood type and match. Often a brief sonographic evaluation of the lesion in question is performed at the time of initial consultation to aid in choosing and scheduling the most efficient imaging modality for guidance (Box 25-5).

Image Guidance

All percutaneous ablation techniques require diagnostic imaging. Though RFA can be performed with open or laparoscopic approaches, even these techniques require image guidance to treat deep lesions. Imaging must guide placement of ablation devices into tumor, provide some information regarding the course of treatment, and provide a method for postprocedure follow-up. The best lesion conspicuity is provided by MRI, which also allows multiplanar imaging for lesions that require complex access. However, procedure time and magnet availability limits the applicability of MRI to RFA at most centers. Additionally, special MR-compatible equipment is necessary. One major advantage of MRI is its ability to detect signal intensity changes relating to tissue temperature and thus guide treatment.

CT and CT fluoroscopy are excellent for guiding probe placement especially in circumstances where ultrasound may be limited. This includes tumors adjacent to, or hidden by, gas-filled bowel, tumors in very obese patients, and some thoracic lesions. CT fluoroscopy provides near real-time guidance with an acceptable level of radiation dose to patients and personnel. Contrast enhancement before treatment or during the procedure can additionally increase lesion conspicuity.

Most reported RFA has relied on ultrasound (US) guidance. Ultrasound is cheap, available, and portable. Although it is limited relative to MRI and CT regarding tissue contrast, US is adequate for most situations (Fig. 25-4). Tumor–tissue contrast may in the future be improved with the advent of sonographic contrast agents. Since all cross-sectional modalities are useful for image guidance, combinations are often employed. Experience and comfort with each approach may be the best guide to the ideal targeting method (Box 25-6).

Performing the Ablation

After all preprocedural imaging tests have been reviewed, the patient examined, and laboratory studies evaluated, the procedure is performed. Signed, informed consent is obtained and IV access procured. Vital signs, heart rhythm, and oxygen saturation monitoring are continuously performed. In the authors' unit we use a combination of fentanyl and midazolam for conscious sedation. Intravenous fluids and oxygen by nasal cannula are administered as necessary. Prophylactic antibiotic coverage varies from institution to institution and has not been definitively proven to be of benefit.

Box 25-5   Patient Preparation

Preprocedure ultrasound, CT, and/or MRI of target organ
Imaging also to exclude significant extrahepatic disease
Histologic diagnosis required beforehand
Coagulation screen, tumor marker profile, and blood chemistries obtained
Directed history and physical examination

Box 25-6   Image Guidance for RFA

MRI

High tumor conspicuity
Multiplanar imaging
Temperature-sensitive sequences
Specialized equipment necessary
Availability limited

CT/CTF

Conspicuity between MRI and US
Ideal when US limited (obese, thorax, gas)
Wide availability
Less operator dependence
Near real-time with CTF

US

Least tumor–tissue contrast (usually adequate conspicuity)
Portable/cheap
Most available
Operator/location dependent
Contrast agents required

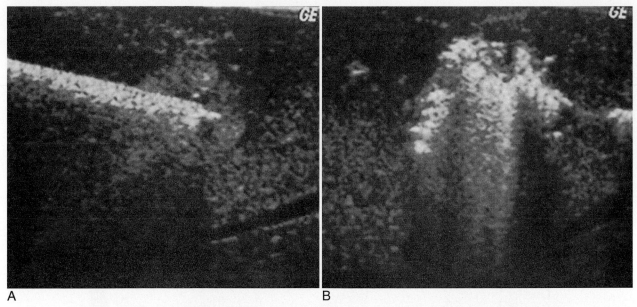

Figure 25-4 Ultrasound-guided targeting of HCC. **A**, Echodense shaft of multiprobe array within hyperechoic tumor. **B**, Hyperechoic "cloud" due to vaporization at site of ablation. (Image courtesy of Dr Damian Dupuy.)

The appropriate grounding pads are placed on the patient's back or thighs. The site of planned percutaneous access is prepared in sterile fashion and the superficial tissues and organ capsule are infiltrated with local anesthetic. Placement of the active probe is performed utilizing the chosen image guidance modality analogous to placement of a percutaneous biopsy needle (Fig 25-5). If large volumes are to be ablated, overlapping spheres should be planned to ensure complete treatment. If US is the guidance modality used, intended spheres of ablation must be chosen in the deep part of the lesion first, later withdrawing into superficial parts of the lesion, to avoid obscuration of treatment areas by acoustic shadowing. Once the electrodes are confirmed to be in the correct location, the RF energy is applied. The time varies depending on the tissue being treated. Treatment times of 12 minutes are recommended for liver tumors. Bone and kidney lesions may require less treatment time (Box 25-7).

Monitoring the effectiveness of tumor necrosis at the time of treatment is done by measuring the temperature

of the treated site at the conclusion of treatment. If MR is used for guidance, repeat MR imaging using temperature-sensitive sequences are useful. If using CT for image guidance, a post-treatment contrast-enhanced CT can be used to document the extent of tumor necrosis (Fig. 25-6). Color-flow and power Doppler have not been found sufficiently accurate to immediately predict areas of necrosis. Sonographic contrast agents are being studied for this application and show some promise for the future. Since the ability to predict coagulation

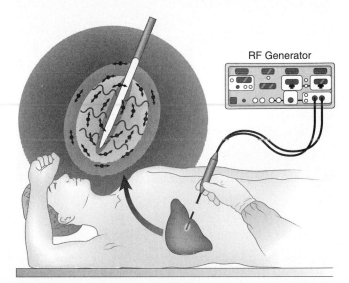

Figure 25-5 Schematic of radio-frequency ablation procedure. (Image courtesy of Dr Damian Dupuy.)

Box 25-7 RF Ablation Techniques

RF probe placed analogous to biopsy needle
Overlapping spheres planned if tumor is large
Treatment times of 12 minutes recommended for liver
tumors
Measure temperature of treated site at end of treatment

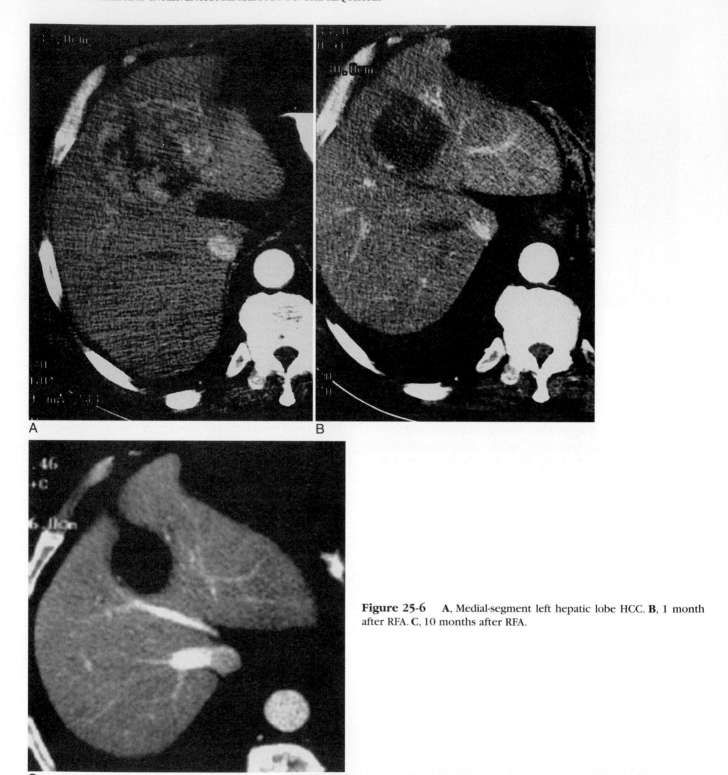

Figure 25-6 **A**, Medial-segment left hepatic lobe HCC. **B**, 1 month after RFA. **C**, 10 months after RFA.

necrosis volumes accurately is difficult, close post-procedural follow-up and imaging should be part of every ablation treatment plan. Patients need to be aware of the importance of multiple postprocedural imaging studies.

Postprocedural Follow-up and Imaging

Appropriate imaging follow-up depends on the type of tumor being treated, the organ in which the tumor is located, the confidence of the radiologist that an effective treatment has been performed, and local preferences. Contrast-enhanced CT is probably the most common imaging modality used to assess treatment response. Areas that enhance generally imply untreated or recurrent tumor. The CT examination protocol is tailored to the type of tumor and its location. MR is useful in patients with renal failure or in patients who have allergies to iodinated contrast agents.

Usually a follow-up phone call is made 24 hours after the treatment and a clinic visit scheduled around the time of the 1-month imaging follow-up. Appropriate tumor markers are obtained at this time. If residual or recurrent tumor is suspected at any time during follow-up, repeat ablation treatments are performed or alternative treatments suggested.

RFA for Hepatic Malignancy

RFA has been most extensively evaluated in the treatment of hepatic malignancies. Factors predicting success of therapy include tumor size, tumor type, and local anatomic structures. Approximately 90% of lesions smaller than 2.5 cm can be ablated completely. The corresponding ablation rates for larger lesions are: 70–90% of lesions 2.5–3.5 cm, 50–70% those 3.5–5.0 cm, and ≤50% of those above 5 cm. Small hepatocellular carcinomas can be treated as effectively with RFA as with PEI. RFA usually requires fewer treatment sessions than PEI. For HCC most operators consider RFA when there are four or fewer lesions smaller than 3.0 cm. If there is a greater number of lesions, or the size is >5 cm, RFA is used along with chemoembolization, chemoinfusion, or systemic chemotherapy.

RFA for liver metastases is less efficacious. Early results suggest that the overall 5-year survival rate for colorectal metastases might approach that of surgical series (25–40%) with fewer complications. However, no randomized controlled trials have been performed.

There are no absolute contraindications to liver RFA. Relative contraindications include low platelets and coagulopathy. Extrahepatic disease may not preclude RFA if it is felt that hepatic disease will more significantly affect the patient's morbidity or life expectancy. RFA for hepatic tumors is associated with very low complication rates, generally below 2%. Complications include pain, pleural effusion, hematoma, and abscess formation (Box 25-8).

RF Ablation of Renal Tumors

The conventional treatment for patients with renal tumors has been nephrectomy or partial nephrectomy in suitable candidates. However, there are many elderly patients with small renal tumors that are unsuitable for total or partial nephrectomy. Indeed, many of these elderly patients often have coexisting morbidity, which

---

Box 25-8 RF Ablation of Liver Tumors

Complete ablation in 90% of lesions <2.5 cm
70–90% ablation in lesions 2.5–3.5 cm
50–70% ablation in lesions 3.5–5.0 cm
Less than 50% ablation in lesions >5 cm
Complication rates <2%

---

makes surgery undesirable. There has been recent interest in the use of RF ablation to treat such patients. Early work in animals, and with renal tumors in humans that were treated with RF ablation intraoperatively and then resected after ablation, indicate promising results. There have also been some recent preliminary results in patients treated with RF ablation as the sole treatment technique.

Reports suggest that lesions up to 3 cm and exophytic lesions have the best results when treated with RF ablation (Fig. 25-7). Larger lesions and central lesions are more challenging. Renal parenchyma is highly vascular and central tumors are surrounded by a heat sink effect. Ablation of central tumors may also be associated with slightly more risk of ureteric damage. In contrast, exophytic lesions are surrounded by fat, which is a poor heat conductor and thus provides an insulating effect, which accentuates tumor necrosis by RF. Follow-up thus far is short, and long-term results will be needed to fully assess the efficacy of RF ablation for small renal tumors.

RF Ablation of Bone Metastases

RF ablation has been used to treat patients with bone metastases causing intractable pain. Pain control can be very difficult in these patients, and RF ablation can offer help in patients where conventional options have failed, or are not possible. In a recent study, Callstrom and associates treated 12 patients having a single painful osteolytic metastasis in whom radiation therapy or chemotherapy had failed. They found that at 4 weeks after treatment the mean worst pain had decreased by 3.1 points on a scale of 0 to 10. The mean pain score before treatment was 6.5, and this decreased to 1.8 four weeks after treatment. Eight out of ten patients who were using analgesics also reported reduced use at some time after RF ablation. Importantly, pain interference in general activity decreased from 6.6 to 2.7 points. This indicates an improved quality of life.

Results thus far are preliminary, and larger studies with longer follow-up will be required to fully document the use of RF ablation in this patient group.

RF Ablation of Lung Tumors

Primary non-small-cell lung cancer is usually discovered at an advanced stage (stage T3). These patients often

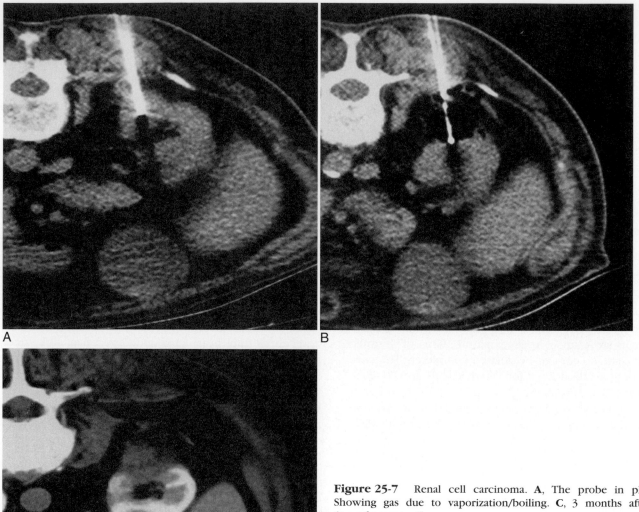

Figure 25-7   Renal cell carcinoma. **A**, The probe in place. **B**, Showing gas due to vaporization/boiling. **C**, 3 months after RFA (no enhancement).

have coexisting emphysema with low forced expiratory volumes, making them unsuitable for surgery. Some preliminary work exists to suggest that RF ablation may have a role to play in providing local tumor control in some of these patients.

Compared to solid organs such as the liver and kidney, the air present in normal lung tissue limits the penetration of RF energy. There is no definite information available with regard to the ablation size that can be achieved in patients with lung tumors. However, because of the insulating effect of the surrounding aerated lung, comparable liver ablation sizes can be achieved in significantly less time.

Experience with lung tumor ablation is still preliminary and many issues need to be addressed. The outcome of ongoing studies is eagerly awaited.

FUTURE DIRECTIONS

RFA and other thermal ablation techniques require well-designed, large (multicenter) clinical trials to confirm their utility and better define suitable patient populations. Research will continue into methods of increasing coagulation or "kill" zones. Given the likelihood of suboptimal treatment with thermal ablation alone, research into combined therapies employing transarterial chemoembolization, temporary blood flow occlusion, and infusion chemotherapy is continuing.

SUGGESTED READINGS

Amin Z, Donald JJ, Masters A et al: Hepatic metatases: interstitial laser photocoagulation with real-time US monitoring and dynamic CT evaluation of treatment. *Radiology* 187:339-347, 1993.

Bilchik AJ, Wood TF, Allegra D et al: Cryosurgical ablation and radiofrequency ablation for unresectable hepatic malignant neoplasms. *Arch Surg* 135:657-664, 2000.

Callstrom MR, Charboneau JW, Goetz MP et al: Painful metastases involving bone: feasability of percutaneous CT- and US-guided radiofrequency ablation. Radiology 224:87-97, 2002.

Charnley RM, Doran J, Morris DL: Cryotherapy for liver metastases: a new approach. *Br J Surg* 76:1041-1041, 1989.

Dupuy DE: Radiofrequency ablation: an outpatient percutaneous treatment. *Med Health RI* 82:213-216, 1999.

Dupuy DE, Goldberg SN: Image-guided radiofrequency tumor ablation: challenges and opportunities: II. *J Vasc Interv Radiol* 12:1135-1148, 2001.

Dupuy DE, Mayo-Smith WW, Abbott GF, DiPetrillo T: Clinical applications of radiofrequency tumor ablation in the thorax. *Radiographics* 22:259-269, 2002.

Dupuy DE, Zagoria RJ, Akerley W: Percutaneous radiofrequency ablation of malignancies in the lung. *Am J Roentgenol* 174:57-59, 2000.

Gazelle GS, Goldberg SN, Solbiati L, Livraghi T: Tumor ablation with radio-frequency energy. *Radiology* 217:633-646, 2000.

Gervais DA, McGovern FJ, Wood BJ et al: Radiofrequency ablation of renal cell carcinoma: early clinical experience. *Radiology* 217:665-672, 2000.

Gervais DA, McGovern FJ, Arellano RS, McDougal WS, Mueller PR: Renal cell carcinoma: clinical experience and technical success with radiofrequency ablation of 42 tumors. *Radiology* 226:417-424, 2003.

Giovannini M: Percutaneous alcohol ablation for liver metastasis. *Semin Oncol* 29:192-195, 2002.

Goldberg SN, Dupuy DE: Image-guided radiofrequency tumor ablation: challenges and opportunities: I. *J Vasc Interv Radiol* 12:1021-1032, 2001.

Goldberg SN, Gazelle GS, Mueller PR: Thermal ablation for focal malignancy: a unified approach to underlying principles, techniques and diagnostic imaging guidance. 174:323-331, 2000.

Livraghi T, Goldberg SN, Lazzaroni S et al: Small hepatocellular carcinoma: treatment with radio-frequency ablation versus ethanol injection. *Radiology* 210:655-661, 1999.

Mayo-Smith WW, Dupuy DE, Parikh PM, Pezzullo JA, Cronan JJ: Image guided percutaneous radiofrequency ablation of solid renal masses: techniques and outcomes of 38 treatments in 32 consecutive patients. *Am J Roentgenol* in press.

McGahan JP, Dodd GD: Radiofrequency ablation of the liver: current status. *Am J Roentgenol* 176:3-16, 2001.

Pavlovich CP, Walther MM, Choyke PL et al: Percutaneous radio frequency ablation of small renal tumors: initial results. *J Urol* 167:10-15, 2002.

Pearson AS, Izzo F, Fleming D et al: Intraoperative radiofrequency ablation or cryoablation for hepatic malignancies. *Am J Surg* 178:592-599, 1999.

Ravikumar TS, Kane R, Cady B et al: Hepatic cryosurgery with intraoperative ultrasound monitoring for metastatic colon carcinoma. *Arch Surg* 122:403-409, 1987.

Sek I T, Wakabayashi M, Nakagawa T et al: Ultrasonically guided percutaneous microwave coagulation therapy for small hepatocellular carcinoma. *Cancer* 74:817-824, 1994.

Wood BJ, Ramkaransingh JR, Fojo T, Walther MM, Libutti SK: Percutaneous tumor ablation with radiofrequency. *Cancer* 94:443-451, 2002.

Index